D0205596

# Ericksonian Approaches to Hypnosis and Psychotherapy

# Ericksonian Approaches to Hypnosis and Psychotherapy

*edited by*

*Jeffrey K. Zeig, Ph.D.*

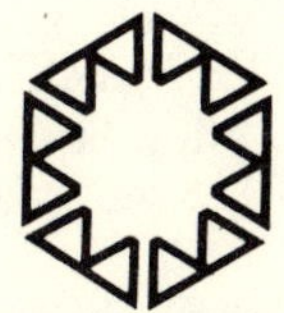

BRUNNER/MAZEL, Publishers • New York

All royalties from this book are the property of The Milton H. Erickson Foundation, Inc., 1935 East Aurelius Avenue, Phoenix, Arizona 85020. Royalties will be used to foster educational and scientific efforts that pertain to Ericksonian psychotherapy and hypnosis. Directors of The Milton H. Erickson Foundation, Inc. are: Jeffrey K. Zeig, Ph.D., Sherron S. Peters, Elizabeth M. Erickson, and Kristina K. Erickson, M.D.

**Library of Congress Cataloging in Publication Data**
Main entry under title:

Ericksonian approaches to hypnosis and psychotherapy.

Proceedings of the International Congress on Ericksonian Approaches to Hypnosis and Psychotherapy, held Dec. 3-8, 1980, in Phoenix, Ariz.
Includes bibliographies and index.
1. Erickson, Milton H.—Congresses.
2. Hypnotism—Therapeutic use—Congresses.
3. Psychotherapy—Congresses. I. Zeig, Jeffrey K., 1947- . II. International Congress on Ericksonian Approaches to Hypnosis and Psychotherapy (1980 : Phoenix, Ariz.)
[DNLM: 1. Hypnosis—Congresses. 2. Psychotherapy—Congresses. WM 415 E685 1980]
RC490.5.E75E75 616.89'14 81-18115
ISBN 0-87630-276-2 AACR2



*Published by*
BRUNNER/MAZEL, INC.
19 Union Square
New York, New York 10003

To
ELIZABETH M. ERICKSON

## ABOUT MILTON ERICKSON, M.D.

Milton H. Erickson, M.D., was generally acknowledged as the world's foremost authority on hypnotherapy and brief strategic psychotherapy, and was one of the most creative, perceptive and ingenious psychotherapeutic masters of all time.

Among Dr. Erickson's professional accomplishments, he received his degrees from the University of Wisconsin, and he was founding president of the American Society of Clinical Hypnosis; founding editor of the American Journal of Clinical Hypnosis; and founding director of the Education and Research Foundation of the American Society of Clinical Hypnosis. He was associate professor of psychiatry at the Wayne State University College of Medicine. Dr. Erickson was a Life Fellow of the American Psychological Association and a Life Fellow of the American Psychiatric Association.

He authored more than 140 scholarly articles on the subject of hypnosis and co-authored five books: *Experiencing Hypnosis: Therapeutic Approaches to Altered States; Hypnotherapy: An Exploratory Casebook; Hypnotic Realities: The Induction of Clinical Hypnosis and Forms of Indirect Suggestion* (all co-authored with Ernest Rossi, Ph.D.); *Practical Applications of Medical and Dental Hypnosis* (co-authored with Seymour Hershman and Irving Secter, D.D.S.); *Time Distortion in Hypnosis* (co-authored with Leslie Cooper, M.D.). The collected papers of Milton H. Erickson, M.D., appear in a four-volume set edited by Ernest L. Rossi. There are a number of other volumes on Ericksonian psychotherapy and hypnosis both in print and in progress.

Dr. Erickson surmounted a considerable number of health problems throughout his adult life. He was confined to a wheelchair from 1967 on and stated that anterior poliomyelitis was the best teacher he ever had about human behavior and its potentials. Dr. Erickson had a color-vision deficiency, and he saw clearly, and attired himself in, the color purple. Although born in 1901, Dr. Erickson was a young man with a deep appreciation of the moment-to-moment creativity involved in daily living. He died after a brief illness on March 25, 1980.

“Each person is a unique individual. Hence, psychotherapy should be formulated to meet the uniqueness of the individual's needs, rather than tailoring the person to fit the Procrustean bed of a hypothetical theory of human behavior.”

Milton H. Erickson, M.D.

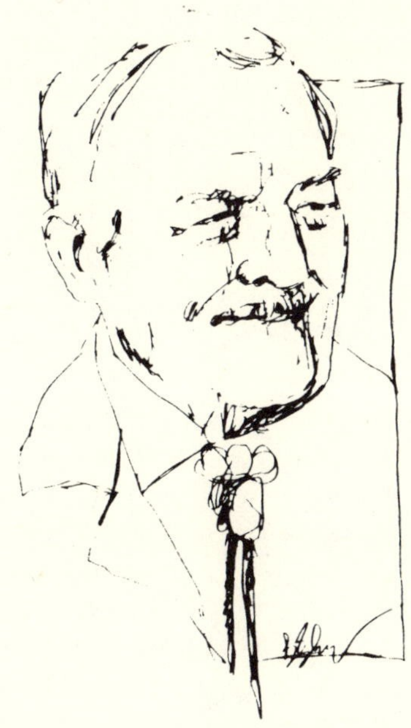

# Contents

# Acknowledgments

The Erickson Congress and this volume of its proceedings were made possible by virtue of the fact that many people volunteered many hours of their time.

The editorial board for the proceedings consisted of Mariam Cohen, M.D., Pat Johnson, Ph.D., Jill Littrell, Ph.D., Art Schimelfenig, Ph.D., George Davies, M.S.W., Miriam Gottlieb, Ph.D., Philip H. McAvoy, M.S., Chris Monaco, M.C., and Mark Woods.

Without the volunteer help of the organizing committee and supporting staff, there would not have been an Erickson Congress. The organizing committee consisted of Sherron S. Peters, Administrative Director; Joyce Vesper, Ph.D., Travel and Public Relations Coordinator; Caryl Ainley, Ph.D., Publicity Coordinator; H. James Schulte, M.D., Continuing Education Coordinator; Roy Cohen, Ph.D., Exhibits Coordinator; and Marilyn Green, On-site Coordinator.

Approximately 100 volunteers accomplished such tasks as bulk mailings, making posters, working the registration tables, checking badges, etc. These people are too numerous to name individually. Certain members of the coordinating staff should be singled out because of their exceptional contributions: Art Schimelfenig, Ph.D., Candy Schimelfenig, David Wenner, M.S.W., Kim Price, Ph.D., Edward R. Hancock, M.C., Chris Monaco, M.A., Bonnie Shcolnik, M.C., Donna Mosher-Todd, M.C., Lee Boeke, M.C., Ann Wright-Edwards, M.S., Dennis Elias, M.C., Jim Showalter, M.S., Susan Maxwell, Ph.D., Mary Menacker, M.Ed., Veronica Navlet, M.S.W., Renee Sheahan, M.S.W., and Patricia Mills.

The contributions of some of the faculty and moderators of the Erickson Congress unfortunately could not be recorded in this volume. However, their participation added immensely to the high quality and overall educational excellence of the Conference. On behalf of the Board of Directors of The Milton H. Erickson Foundation, I take this additional opportunity to thank Leonard Ravitz, M.D., David Akstein, M.D., Charles Stern, Ph.D., Lars-Eric Unestahl, Ph.D., Lindsay Wilkie, L.R.C.P., T.E.A. von Dedenroth, M.D., Dan Golman, Ph.D., Jean Lassner, M.D., Marc Lehrer, Ph.D., Hilton Lopez, M.D., Walt Mac Donald, M.S.W., Robert B. McNeilly, M.D., Eric Steese, Ph.D., Paul Lounsbury, M.A., Charles Mutter, M.D., Audry Ruben, R.N., David Ruben, M.D., and Nancy Winston, M.S.W.

I am grateful to Susan Barrows, Editorial Vice President of Brunner/Mazel, for her efficiency and gentle prodding.

Two people were instrumental in promoting the International Congress on Ericksonian Approaches to Hypnosis and Psychotherapy. Barbara Bellamy worked long, hard hours as my personal secretary. Sherron S. Peters, Administrative Director of the Congress, shared in all major decisions. She did a remarkably efficient job conducting registrations and handling the numerous administrative tasks.

JEFFREY K. ZEIG, PH.D.

# History of The International Congress on Ericksonian Approaches to Hypnosis and Psychotherapy

*Sherron S. Peters*

The International Congress on Ericksonian Approaches to Hypnosis and Psychotherapy began as the vision of a student who traveled great distances many times to study with Milton H. Erickson, M.D. With each visit, the student left hungry to learn more and anxious to visit again. Erickson was generous with knowledge and time. Realizing the student had little money for training, Erickson made no demand for payment, and even opened his guest house so the student could avoid lodging expenses.

For six and one-half years the door remained open. It became clear to the student that in this too brief period Erickson had sown the seeds that would grow to yield a lifetime of knowledge. Grateful, and knowing he could never repay Erickson, the student committed himself to pass on knowledge in the same spirit as it had been given to him.

The student, Jeffrey K. Zeig, Ph.D., began fulfilling his promise by organizing the International Congress on Ericksonian Approaches to Hypnosis and Psychotherapy. Intended to be a tribute to and celebration for Erickson, the Congress was conceived with several goals in mind.

First, through the Congress interested professionals would be provided with an exceptional opportunity to learn about Ericksonian techniques, not only from international experts, but from Erickson himself.

Second, the Congress was scheduled to coincide with Erickson's 79th birthday, and was intended to be a birthday celebration, with the invited speakers being his long-time friends and colleagues.

Third, through those attending the Congress, Erickson would be offered the tribute of witnessing the dramatic impact of his life's work.

In March 1979 Jeff requested permission from Erickson to hold the Congress. While Erickson didn't reject the idea, he certainly didn't approve it readily. Following the March proposal, Jeff approached Erickson many times to see if he had reached a decision, and it began to appear that Erickson didn't want the Congress to take place. In retrospect, it seems more likely that Erickson wanted to insure sufficient initiative and motivation in Jeff to complete such an enormous task, because not until June 1979 did Erickson give his permission.

Dr. and Mrs. Erickson were part of the organizing committee and, with Jeff, selected the speakers to be invited. As Jeff's fiancée, and because of my background in business, I joined the group as Administrative Director.

Initially, the selected faculty consisted of about 30 people. However, as the Ericksons became more interested and excited about the project, the number of invited presenters quickly grew from 30 to 63 people. As well as having recognized expertise in Ericksonian hypnosis and psychotherapy, each invited speaker was a friend, colleague and student of Erickson. Together they were to comprise the most gifted faculty ever to speak on the topic of hypnosis.

It was a humbling experience inviting people like Gregory Bateson, Jay Haley, and the 60 other renowned experts. We were asking a lot of them. Each speaker was to compose a formal paper on Ericksonian hypnosis and psychotherapy suitable for publication. Each was also expected to take part in at least two major events, and to leave his private practice for one week. For what we were requesting we had little to offer in return. We could not pay an honorarium, and only offered to pay partial expenses with the possibility of more being paid if sufficient revenues were generated.

With few exceptions, all who received invitations accepted. Bateson and Haley agreed to present keynote addresses. Other speakers offered to do workshops and take part in conversation hours. Two special interaction hours were planned—one consisting of Erickson, Bateson, Haley and Rossi, and the other to include Watzlawick, Weakland and Fisch. Of the 63 Congress faculty, 40 members were from the United States and 23 were from 18 other countries.

Having secured the faculty, we established the Milton H. Erickson Foundation to handle all financial arrangements. The Foundation eventually acquired State and Federal nonprofit status. The original Board of Directors of the Foundation were: Dr. and Mrs. Milton H. Erickson, Jeffrey K. Zeig, Ph.D., and myself, Sherron S. Peters.

Financing the project was the next issue to be resolved. We estimated that we would need as much as $10,000 seed money to print and mail preliminary brochures, buy a typewriter and file cabinet and pay legal fees.

Because of Erickson's growing popularity, Jeff speculated that publishers would be willing to provide a substantial advance against the royalties for the published proceedings of the Erickson Congress. As it turned out, publishers were interested in Erickson books, but were not willing to provide a very substantial advance for proceedings from a Congress that had not been held yet.

Therefore, we had to come up with other ideas for procuring seed money. Jeff had been videotaping Erickson's seminar classes. Since one of these week-long seminars was of exceptional quality, we decided to transcribe the videotapes of that week into book form, and the idea for the *Teaching Seminar* book was born. A contract for the two books was finally signed with Brunner/Mazel Publishers, who provided us with an advance sufficient enough to begin the project.

Although the advance from Brunner/Mazel against the royalties of the two books provided us with part of the seed money necessary to initiate the project, it fell short of our financial needs. To generate additional capital, we offered a substantially reduced registration fee for registrations made prior to March 15, 1980. Brochures advertising the Congress and the early registration offer were printed and mailed in November 1979.

Budgetary limitations precluded our renting or leasing office space. Instead, our home became the headquarters for The Milton H. Erickson Foundation. Two rooms were converted to office space with the intention that they would accommodate both Jeff's private practice and Foundation work. However, as word about the Erickson Congress spread and response grew, our entire home yielded itself to workspace. The diningroom table became the bookkeeping and advance registration area, while the breakfast nook was used for overflow secretarial work and editing space. The guest room stored files and video equipment. Work lists were taped to the kitchen cabinets and refrigerator. For lack of space, work stacks and filing were placed on the floor around the livingroom until they could be handled.

Bulk mailings were the most time-consuming and frustrating jobs in the entire Congress preparation. Over 70,000 brochures were mailed. To maintain low overhead expense, all mailings were done from our livingroom, with the help of a handful of dedicated volunteers who had joined the organizing committee. Each mailing required 15 to 20 hours of boring, hard work.

The reward for the work came in the tremendous response received from interested professionals. Registrations began flooding in from all parts of the country and from around the world. From February to July 1980, it was not unusual to receive 50 to 100 pieces of mail per day.

We had no idea how much interest would be stimulated by the proposed Erickson Congress. In fact, during the initial planning stages of the Congress, two of our major speakers were consulted on the number of attendees we could expect. One suggested that we would be lucky to get 200 people. Another speaker was willing to wager two steak dinners to one that we would receive no more than 750 registrations. By March 1980, we had already received well over 750 registrations and it appeared to Jeff and me that we could look forward to collecting those two steak dinners.

On March 25, 1980, Dr. Erickson passed away. An awesome sense of loss was felt by everyone who had known, loved and respected him. For those of us who had worked on organizing the Congress, it was devastating to realize that he would not be at the Congress, that the banquet held on the evening of December 5th would not be a birthday celebration, and that Dr. Erickson would not be with his friends and colleagues gathering nine months later to honor him and his work. Our consolation was that Erickson died with the knowledge that over 750 people had already registered for the Congress. He had at least a glimpse of the profound impact and interest his work had stimulated around the world.

The death of Erickson raised the question of whether or not the Congress should be postponed or even cancelled. It was felt this decision should be made by the Erickson family, and the organizing committee was prepared to respect and follow through with their wishes. The unanimous decision of the Ericksons was that the December Congress should take place on schedule. Since it was Erickson's wish not to have a funeral, the family thought it appropriate that the Congress be held as a memorial tribute.

After Erickson's death, the Erickson family members united to provide their total support of the Congress. They worked many hours notifying each speaker and registrant of Erickson's death. They assumed total responsibility for sending thank you letters, often handwritten, for the numerous donations made to the Foundation in memory of Dr. Erickson. It was the courage and strength of the Erickson family, together with their help and support, that renewed energies and transformed disappointment into excitement.

Then, in July 1980, another devastating blow came with the death of

Gregory Bateson. Bateson, who was a close friend and colleague of Dr. Erickson, was scheduled to present a keynote address entitled "Science or Power." Bateson was irreplaceable. Once again we were faced with notifying our registrants and faculty of a tremendous loss.

The consensus of several major Congress faculty members was that a replacement speaker had to be found as soon as possible. This was a very difficult task for many reasons. Our faculty already included virtually every available authority on Ericksonian hypnosis and psychotherapy. In addition, the Congress was five short months away, and we feared it might be impossible to find a keynote speaker on such short notice. Consequently, we moved outside the field of hypnosis and Ericksonian technique, searching for a person with a complementary expertise who would provide a unique vantage point from which to comment on Erickson's work. In late July 1980, an invitation to present a keynote address was extended to and accepted by Carl A. Whitaker, M.D. As one of the preeminent practitioners of family therapy in the world and as one who shared many philosophies that are hallmarks of Erickson's work, Whitaker proved to be an excellent choice.

In October 1980 the workload became overwhelming and volunteers came to our home daily to help complete the endless tasks. Three sources of volunteers filled the ranks. Initially, interested friends in the field of psychotherapy helped with the mailings, served as organizing committee members, and joined the editorial staff for the *Teaching Seminar* book. The second source was from Jeff's patients, who became very involved and worked hard on the preparation of the Congress. Those who could not afford to pay for therapy instead donated their time to the Foundation. Some of these people ran errands while others answered phones. One young man spent days folding and stapling hundreds of brochures. Another young woman worked for weeks to complete a 6′ × 6′ latchook rug of the Foundation's expanding heads logo. The rug was used as a backdrop on the stage of Symphony Hall during the Congress. The third source of volunteers was students. Most were enrolled in counseling and psychology programs at Arizona State University. This group volunteered hours of work in return for free registration at the Congress. These people served as monitors at the Congress, and with the exception of one paid professional the entire video portion of the Congress was organized and run by volunteers. In total, 100 people volunteered. It is a tribute to our volunteer staff that the Congress ran smoothly and on schedule.

The Congress began on Thursday, December 4, 1980 with 14 half-day precongress workshops. On Friday morning, December 5th, seven half-day workshops were held. Some of the workshops were large in size, totaling as many as 500 attendees. The Convocation to the Congress was held Friday afternoon.

Almost half of the registrants attended the Congress banquet and dinner dance held the evening of December 5th. Carlos Sluzki, Director of Mental Research Institute, presented a special toast. Faculty members, representing several international hypnosis societies, made special presentations of tribute to Erickson.

The faculty presented their papers at the General Sessions, which began on Friday, December 5th, and continued through to the afternoon of December 8th. Two General Sessions ran simultaneously. Concurrent with the General Sessions, two conversation hours and two media events were held. The media events included film presentations of Bateson, Whitaker, and Erickson. A biographical slide presentation on Erickson's life was shown continuously throughout the Congress.

The tone of the Congress was one of cooperative learning. The faculty did an outstanding job in offering attendees a unique and varied learning experience. Through workshops, papers and conversation hours, the faculty presented Erickson's influence in the fields of medicine, dentistry, psychiatry, psychology, anthropology, and forensics.

Some speakers were still feeling the loss of Bateson and Erickson, and a certain tone of eulogy emerged. Stories of special personal experiences with Erickson were shared by some faculty members. The Congress, being unexpectedly presented within the framework of a memorial meeting, provided attendees with an extraordinarily rare blend of insights into the work, the person, and the genius of Milton H. Erickson, M.D.

The full Congress schedule didn't provide attendees with much time to see the Phoenix area. However, many who had read Erickson's work and were familiar with the special meaning Squaw Peak had in Erickson's life and therapy took time to climb the mountain.

On the afternoon of December 8th, the Closing Remarks brought the Congress and a year and a half of work to a close. For Jeff and me that day will always have a very special place in our hearts because, not only did it mark a successful ending, but it also marked a happy beginning—we were married that evening.

# Convocation

The International Congress on Ericksonian Approaches to Hypnosis and Psychotherapy was conceived as a training event that would recognize and extend the contributions that Milton H. Erickson, M.D., made to the health sciences. Dr. Erickson was scheduled to be the featured speaker.

The Congress was both academic and clinical. The meeting centered on the presentation of 50 academic papers, and 21 four-hour clinical workshops were presented in three time blocks on Thursday morning, Thursday afternoon, and Friday morning. The Convocation on Friday afternoon opened the academic assembly.

In an attempt to present some of the emotional flavor of the Congress, the Convocation is presented here as it was recorded.

*Jeffrey K. Zeig:*

My name is Jeff Zeig and I would like to welcome you here, and now I can remind you of certain things so that you can really understand that learning about Ericksonian approaches is not the kind of task you won't find easy and so that you can comfortably lay to rest the idea that you don't know more than you know you know. But is there really any reason to understand until you take an easy breath and remind yourself that what your conscious mind does now is awfully unimportant?

The Erickson Congress is distinguished on a number of accords. We have an outstanding faculty here. It consists of more than 60 people from 12 nations, and they are all locomotives and there are no cabooses. A friend of mine looked over the program, and she said that it was an embarrassment of riches. I think that is an excellent description.

We are also distinguished on a number of other accords. This Erickson meeting is the largest meeting that has ever been held in the name of hypnosis. I think that it is also the largest meeting that has ever been convened that will honor a person who was strictly a clinician rather than a theorist in the field of psychotherapy. Traditionally, psychology has provided more recognition for theorists than it has for therapists. But we are congregated here to pay tribute to Erickson, and Erickson was interested in how to therapeutically influence individuals—not in how to correctly describe personality.

Our debt to Milton Erickson is enormous. Erickson was a man whose genius at doing psychotherpay was legendary, and his impact on the field of psychotherapy will be tremendous. Currently, many people consider Erickson's methods to be state of the art in the field of psychotherapy. Erickson was known by many as the world's greatest communicator.

I think Erickson's genius at living was even more extraordinary than his genius at doing psychotherapy. He was a wonderful model of living "the good life." He could create a tremendous aura of electricity, vibrancy, excitement, and aliveness around him. And it was that aura of being glad-to-be-alive that was really so much part and parcel of the man who was Milton Erickson.

This Congress was conceived for a number of reasons. I had originally thought of it as a 79th birthday gift for Dr. Erickson. For six-and-a-half years, while I was his student, he provided training for me at no fee. I didn't have any money, and he didn't choose to charge me.

Early in March 1980, I told Dr. Erickson that 750 people were registered for the Congress. I reminded him that the Congress was my way of saying "thank you" for all of the things that he had done for me—and that it wasn't enough. There are many people here in this room today who could have told Erickson something similar—that whatever "thank you" they could say simply wouldn't be enough.

This Congress was also convened as an opportunity for Dr. Erickson to see the impact of his work. It was also to be an opportunity for Erickson and his friends to visit once more.

A little bit over two years ago I had the vision of this meeting room, Symphony Hall, filled. I had the vision of being able to introduce Dr. Erickson to you and have him present himself and his ideas to you personally. That vision was almost a reality.

A little over a year ago, I visited Dr. Erickson and spontaneously asked him, "What's your goal?" He replied immediately, "To see Roxanna's baby." His goal was to see the birth of his 26th grandchild. Now, I knew that Dr. Erickson's mind worked like that. I knew that he would have a goal to which he was directed. It would not be an obsession; rather it would be a light that would draw him into the future. Another purpose of this Congress was that it was to be one more goal for Dr. Erickson—a light after which he could strive—and it was that kind of light because he really did want to be here with you.

Erickson was a member of the organizing committee of this Congress. He personally approved and was involved in the selection of all the faculty.

So we meet here to honor a legend. Our purpose is not to mourn Erickson. He was a firm believer that life is for the living and he wouldn't have wished to be mourned in any way. Our purpose here is to celebrate Erickson, to teach something about Erickson's methods and perhaps even to institutionalize the contribution of someone who, I think, will stand out as being the Einstein of psychotherapy.

On the stage here we have an ironwood tree. It's my honor to introduce you to this ironwood tree and to welcome you to what I hope will be be an uncommon conference for a very uncommon person.

* * * *

I next would like to introduce Sherron Peters. Sherron is the Administrative Director of the Congress. Without the tremendous amount of work that Sherron put in, this meeting would not be convened here today.

*Sherron S. Peters:*

On behalf of the Board of Directors of The Milton H. Erickson Foundation, I warmly welcome you to the International Congress on Ericksonian Approaches to Hypnosis and Psychotherapy.

In attendance, we have physicians, dentists, psychologists, psychiatrists and counselors from every state in the United States and from more than 20 countries. We have a delegation from Holland alone of over 60 people; from Canada we have over a hundred. The total registration of the Congress is about 2000.

We are very proud of our distinguished faculty. More than a dozen of the Congress faculty have been presidents of their own national hypnosis societies and numerous others have served as officers to their national hypnosis societies. Besides having an internationally renowned faculty, we also have internationally known therapists who are in attendance to the Congress, including Carlos Sluzki and Bob Goulding. . . .

I would also like to tell you that The Milton Erickson Foundation is now establishing the Erickson Archives. The Foundation is collecting audiotapes and videotapes of Dr. Erickson as well as letters, autographs and interesting anecdotes about him. The purpose of this project is to have one central location as a repository for historical materials about Erickson. Erickson's lectures were often taped and these audiotapes and videotapes are currently in the possession of many different individuals. One purpose of the Erickson Foundation is to establish an archive so that these historical tapes can be made available to students here in Phoenix. It was Dr. Erickson's policy to freely transmit his knowledge and this policy will be continued through the Erickson Archives. The Foundation will pay for duplicating expenses. If you have any tapes that you can contribute or you know of people who do have tapes, please have them contact Jeff Zeig or myself at the Erickson Foundation.

And now, ladies and gentlemen, it is my pleasure to introduce Elizabeth Erickson and Kristina Erickson.

*Elizabeth M. Erickson:*

I am extremely gratified beyond words at this wonderful Congress. I would like to express my heartfelt thanks to all of the local people who have worked so hard in the preparation and to all of the speakers and attendees who have come so far to join in this assembly.

I also want to say that I know that my husband would have been extremely gratified, as he already was with his knowledge of the advance preparation and planning which was being made. I want to say that I know, definitely, one thing he would have said, because there were a few previous occasions on which he was given some special tribute and he said this every time. He would take me to one side and lean back, look around with a smile on his face and say, "If only Mom and Dad could have seen this." *(Laughter and applause.)*

*Kristina K. Erickson:*

I feel that I am speaking as several persons here. I am speaking as a member of The Milton H. Erickson Foundation. I am speaking also as a physician who has had the opportunity to know and study both my father's work and that of many others. I also speak as a member of the Erickson family and, finally, I speak as myself, the youngest daughter of Milton Erickson.

As his daughter, I find that this Congress is awesome. I see his picture everywhere. I see his name; I see purple everywhere. I find it overwhelming because to me my father was—and he found humor in this, because it was one of his favorite stories—he was just my daddy. My father had his picture and a writeup in, I believe, *Life Magazine* or some other such magazine. I looked at the story; my brother and sisters showed it to me. I leafed through it and said, "Well, what's so great about daddy?" And my father loved it. He repeated that to me many times. We'd sit in our house which, as most of you know, is fairly modest. He would get a big award and he'd say, "Okay, so what's so great about daddy?"

But he was, as I say, my dad, as well as the person who those of you in attendance at this Congress see him to be. Despite his many contributions, and the enormous amount of hours that he spent in his work—writing, teaching and giving individual attention to people who contacted him—he also maintained a homey simplicity. And he enjoyed the aspect of life of being just daddy or grandpa or Kristie's dad or Roxanna's dad.

But I think that the most valuable thing that I learned from my father is something that Jeffrey mentioned that my father did every day of his life—he enjoyed living. He believed in the value of each human as an individual and he believed that each person had worth, dignity and an intrinsic privilege to enjoy life.

My father, despite increasing disability and illness as the years went on, took pleasure in each and every day. Every time I visited him he was taking pleasure in the plants growing around the house, what one of the grandchildren had done, what one of the students or persons who had visited had said. Each little item, he enjoyed. He liked life.

He derived immense satisfaction from knowing that this Congress was to take place and, in that sense, I feel that he did not miss this Congress, that he did participate in it in advance.

I wish on behalf of my entire family, on behalf of myself, to thank everyone who has helped to create and organize this conference, as well as each and every one of you who has come from so far or who has come from near to be a part of it. Again, thank you very much.

*Jay Haley:*

I am honored to be invited to address this meeting and to welcome you. I will speak quite briefly because I will be addressing you at much greater length later today. Let me just begin by expressing the appreciation of all of us for the extraordinary efforts of Jeff Zeig and Sherron Peters and the others who organized this meeting. It's really extraordinary.

I think that we can regret only that Milton Erickson couldn't have lived just awhile longer so he could be here. We really should have thought to arrange this meeting years ago; then we could have had him present as well as Gregory Bateson. But now these men won't join us at a meeting again.

I think that all of us owe a great debt to Milton. To some of us, the debt is really a personal one because he contributed to our lives. I think that we also owed him a debt as a model for professional therapists everywhere. I think that he really had class. His originality and ideas, his ethical conduct, and his generosity set an example for all of us. I think that he also set an example for all of us in how to deal with personal handicaps. He not only surmounted but he turned to advantage his physical handicaps in ways that I don't think anyone has done before. He had the courage to rise above his pain and difficulties and to make use of them to live an active and long life of hard work.

Whether one thinks about his personal struggles or his professional contribution, we can only really be in awe of this great and good man.

I think that the size of this gathering is a tribute to the magnitude of the man we came to honor. The miscellaneous collection of people here is an example of the diverse kinds of people involved in his life. There are really some remarkably mixed backgrounds at this meeting, as I understand it. I think, too, that everyone here had different purposes in coming. People are here to honor Erickson, to have an experience, to learn something, to meet other people of similar interests, and so on.

I hope that you find what you seek here. I think that one of the things that all of us found in our personal contact with Erickson is that, if we met with him for professional reasons, we also always found ourselves influenced by him personally. And I hope that each of you find yourself touched at this meeting, both professionally and personally. Thank you.

# Ericksonian Approaches to Hypnosis and Psychotherapy

PART I

# *Keynote Address*

*I think that attending the Congress was very moving for Jay Haley. Both of his important teachers, Bateson and Erickson, had died within four months of each other. Haley was touched personally as well as intellectually by his contact with these two great men.*

*Haley does not lack any of the intellectual or personal power of his mentors. His keynote address was rich with perceptive insights and warm wit. It received the highest ratings of any of the presentations at the Congress. Moreover, it was delivered by a man with class.*

Chapter 1

# The Contribution to Therapy of Milton H. Erickson, M.D.

*Jay Haley*

I will present some personal experience with Milton Erickson and try to communicate some of my understanding of this extraordinary man and his work. I have published my views of Erickson's therapy extensively, but to me he remains a mysterious person. Although I met with him for many years, I never fully understood him. In hundreds of hours talking together, I explored his life and work; yet I know him less well than other men I have associated with more briefly. I studied a number of therapists over the years, and Erickson more extensively than anyone. Having learned many of his therapy techniques, I applied them in my practice and teaching. Not a day passes that I do not use something that I learned from Erickson in my work. Yet his basic ideas I only partially grasp. I feel that if I understood more fully what Erickson was trying to explain about changing people, new innovations in therapy would open up before me.

Erickson was by no means secretive about his work. Quite possibly he was the most visible therapist the world has ever known. For many years he gave seminars and workshops to large audiences in this country and abroad. He wrote over one hundred publications. Thousands of visitors came to talk with him, individually and in groups. His lectures, demonstrations, and conversations have been recorded more than those of any other clinician. He gave generously of himself and his knowledge to anyone who was interested. Although Erickson liked to show you that you still had much to learn, he did not attempt to be mysterious or obscure. He really tried to simplify and explain his ideas so everyone could understand them. Often he was frustrated when his ideas were only partially understood by many of us. I don't know how many times over the years I asked him why he did something in therapy and he answered, "That's obvious." I would say, "Milton, it's not obvious," and I pursued him only to find a new and unexpected complexity in his thinking.

It was not only the unusual nature of his ideas that made Erickson difficult to fully understand. One problem was the way he talked with people. Erickson tended to join the person he was talking with in that person's language. His style of therapy and teaching was to converse in the language of the other person; within that framework he suggested new ideas. This style of "accepting" the person's language as a way of joining gave professionals with quite incompatible theories the idea that Erickson operated within their ways of thinking. He could talk in many ideological languages, so that colleagues and patients often had the illusion they shared and understood his theories and were later surprised by an unexpected idea. Erickson's own beliefs and premises about therapy were not self-evident. When one asked him about a theory, the response was often a case example which was a metaphor with many referents.

Erickson's use of stories in his conversations gave people of diverse views metaphors where they discovered their own ideas. Each anecdote was put in such a way that quite different people thought it was designed precisely for them. When some of my trainees visited Phoenix and met with Erickson in a group, they returned and reported on the experience. One of them mentioned a story that Erickson had told about him. One of the others said no, that story was actually about *her*. Yet another said the other two did not understand that the story applied to his particular experience. It turned out that all of the group thought they had each received a personal metaphor from Erickson designed just for them. Each felt that he or she had been understood by Erickson and really understood him. Yet they were people of quite diverse backgrounds and perspectives, and the metaphors were stories and cases that Erickson had told many times before (although his way of telling the story would vary). Some of the stories were ones I had heard many years before and I knew they applied personally to me.

The fact that Erickson talked on many different levels of meaning at the same time also complicated the problem of getting a flat statement of his views. When asked what to do with a therapeutic problem, Erickson would offer advice and usually a case illustration to show how he dealt with a similar problem. Yet that case example was not merely a description of a case. It might also be a metaphor designed to change or resolve some personal problem of the person he was talking with. That is, Erickson could talk about a case in a way that educated one about the general nature of that problem, taught how to use a particular therapy technique and encouraged or imposed a change in one's personal life or ideas.

One of Erickson's greatest skills was his ability to influence people indirectly. This is one of the reasons so many people were uneasy in his presence. Anyone talking with Erickson could never be quite sure whether he was only offering professional advice or subtly suggesting a change in an unstated personal problem. A story or a case example is an analogy drawing a parallel between one situation and another. While the case example would pair a therapy technique and a problem, it could also be an analogy in relation to the person being talked with and the person in the case example. Erickson liked to change people outside their awareness. If they were on guard against his influence and resisted the idea Erickson was offering, it was usually some other idea that Erickson was actually interested in imposing. He liked to offer an idea to resist and one to influence, at least.

Erickson would tell the same case example in different ways to different people. While the essentials of the case remained the same, what he emphasized in the complex story would vary with the analogy he was communicating to that particular listener. This complex process of metaphoric influence could occur routinely while Erickson was in conversation with people or while he was doing a case consultation. It was as if doing one thing at a time bored him, and he needed to communicate in more complex ways.

What Erickson said and did had multiple purposes and he taught in complex analogies. Therefore, it is difficult to say flatly that a particular idea or technique was his view. His theory was offered to us in metaphors with many referents, told with different analogies, emphasized in different ways for different people, and varying with the social context.

A major difficulty in grasping what was new in Erickson's theories is the problem of language. He was talking about new premises about human beings and ways to change them in a language constructed to express past views. (One is reminded of Harry Stack Sullivan, who struggled to describe interpersonal relations in a language constructed for describing individuals.) I think Erickson was offering something new in the world—a presentation of the intricacies of interpersonal influence (at least that was the set of ideas he talked to me about). Yet he had available only a language developed for a quite different conception of people. The language for describing an individual is simply not adequate to describe Erickson's therapy.

I think the language of hypnosis and hypnotherapy is too primitive and limited to encompass the complexities of many of Erickson's trance inductions and his use of hypnotic influence in therapy. How can one talk about a hypnotic induction in the language of "sleep" when the subject is hypnotized while walking up and down the room? Or how can one talk about the complex interpersonal influence of a conversational trance induction in the language of the "unconscious"? As an example, Erickson attempted to explain the fact that if a subject followed the directive to have a negative hallucination, he must see the object in order to avoid seeing it. Erickson sometimes used the term "unconscious awareness" to describe this phenomenon. Yet the term "unconscious" is by definition something outside of consciousness, or awareness.

Clearly such terminology is too cumbersome to explain the subtle processes which interested Erickson. He was elaborating a new way of thinking about people, about hypnosis, and about therapy without a descriptive language that could express that new view. It was like trying to talk about quantum theory in a language of levers and weights. I believe that is why he turned more and more to metaphor, which is not a way to describe an idea rigorously but it can cover the complexity he was trying to communicate.

Many people here today never met Erickson. Others are so young they saw him only in his old age. Granting that he was a formidable man even when old and frail and in a wheelchair, I would like to communicate something of what he was like in his middle years when he was vigorous.* I think his success as a therapist was partly the result of the personal power that exuded from him. Not only did his personality have an impact, but his power was increased by his reputation as a hypnotist who influenced people outside their awareness. Quite a number of people were simply afraid of him.

I discovered Erickson's power when I first heard of him in 1953. While on Gregory Bateson's research project on communication, I told Bateson that I would like to take a workshop being offered by a hypnotist coming to San Francisco. I wanted to study the communicative aspects of hypnosis. Bateson asked me who was giving the workshop, and I told him

---

*Many people think of Erickson as an old man who was frail and spoke with extreme difficulty. I think that is unfortunate. In his prime he had more control of his vocal inflections and his body movement than anyone I knew. That was part of his mastery of skills in influencing people. He had extraordinary ability to communicate with others. There is too little visual record of that skill remaining. Some years ago I asked him about videotaping his work, and he said he would rather not allow it. He did not want to be remembered as a helpless old man who communicated with difficulty. Finally, he allowed that videotaping, and so, many people only know him in his frail period and do not have any idea what he was like at the height of his power.

it was Milton H. Erickson. "I'll call him," said Bateson, "and ask if you can attend." In that way I found out that Bateson knew Erickson, just as he seemed to know anyone of importance in the social science field. It turned out that Bateson and Margaret Mead had consulted with Erickson and Mrs. Erickson about the films of trance dances they had made in Bali. They were consulting to determine when the dancers in masks went into trance. (In fact, it was Bateson and Mead who encouraged Erickson to publish that extraordinary description of communication he wrote up in "A Study of an Experimental Neurosis Hypnotically Induced in a Case of Ejaculatio Praecox.")

Bateson called Erickson at his hotel in San Francisco (we were in Menlo Park) and asked if I could attend the workshop. Erickson said I was welcome. They chatted awhile, and Bateson hung up the telephone and said, "That man is going to manipulate me to come to San Francisco and have dinner with him." Interested in manipulation, I asked, "What did he say to you?" Bateson replied, "He said to me, 'Why don't you come to San Francisco and have dinner with me?'" Even straightforward statements by Erickson were suspect with Gregory Bateson and with other people who feared his power.

Erickson clearly enjoyed his reputation as a powerful person who influenced people both in and outside their awareness. I recall that once our project was having an evening seminar with Erickson and Don D. Jackson was present. As we were discussing hypnosis, Jackson was holding a pencil in one hand and turning it round and round. Jackson said, "I can't stop turning this pencil, and Milton, I think you have something to do with it." "Well," replied Erickson, "you can continue to turn the pencil." He proceeded to give Jackson a few suggestions and then he had him stop the turning. Later I asked Erickson privately just what he said to Jackson that made him turn the pencil that way. I wanted more information about his ways of inducing special behavior in someone while ostensibly merely having a conversation. "I didn't have anything to do with it," said Erickson. "But Jackson seemed to think I was doing something, so I took advantage of that."

To illustrate another aspect of Erickson's formidability as a hypnotist and a person, let me describe an incident which truly impressed me and John Weakland. One evening we took the Ericksons out to dinner to a Mexican restaurant on one of our visits here. It was an authentic type of Mexican restaurant, as I learned when I put some of their standard hot sauce on my food. I gasped and my eyes watered uncontrollably. Erickson kidded me about that. Somehow out of the conversation came Erickson's claim that he could survive any hot sauce that could be served to him. To demonstrate, he called the waitress and sent her for the chef. He asked the Mexican chef to put together the hottest sauce he could make in the kitchen and deliver it to the table. The chef seemed pleased with the challenge. He came back in a little while with something in a small dish and he placed it before Erickson. He stayed to watch him eat it, with some anticipation. Erickson took a spoon, dipped it into the hot sauce, and then put it in his mouth and rolled it around his tongue. His face did not change expression, nor did his eyes show the slightest sign of watering. "Delicious," he said. I was impressed—and even more impressed when I watched the astonishment of that Mexican chef.

Besides his skill in influencing people, there was simply something about Erickson that made him difficult to oppose. I recall a psychiatrist telling me about an experience with Erickson here in Phoenix. The psychiatrist was a mature, responsible man with an important position in the field. He told me that Erickson spent an eight-hour day with him, and the psychiatrist said he never had lunch, because Erickson did not. He told me that he got so hungry. I asked him why he did not tell Erickson he was hungry and wanted some lunch. He said that somehow he felt he could not say that to Erickson while he was busy instructing him about therapy. Months later he was still angry at having gone hungry like that. I told him that Erickson must have thought he was important. He didn't often spend eight hours with a visitor, so it was quite a compliment. That pleased the psychiatrist and seemed to help make up for the lost lunch.

Erickson was always quite comfortable with power. He did not mind taking it or using it. I recall his saying that he was on a panel and "there was no power there, so I took over the panel." With his willingness to take and use power, I think it is fortunate that he was a benevolent man. If the kind of influence he had was turned to destructive purposes, it would have been most unfortunate. Erickson was not only benevolent, but he was consistently helpful to people, both in and out of his office.

I spend my time restraining therapists from being helpful. I don't believe benevolent helpfulness should be imposed on people and therapy should not be done unless people have clearly requested it. Yet somehow I was never concerned with that issue with Erickson. He would set out to change whomever he thought ought to be changed whether they had requested that in any direct way or not. I never had a doubt about his ethics or benevolent intentions, nor was I concerned about his exploiting anyone for any personal advantage.

A similar issue arises about using individuals or families for demonstration purposes before audiences. I have been opposed to using people for teaching purposes because I think it exploits them. Yet I was never concerned about that issue with Erickson. He not only used people to demonstrate for large crowds at his workshops, but he also did helpful therapy with them before that audience while he was demonstrating hypnosis. He always managed it so that the subject got a fair exchange of benefits for being used in the demonstration. He also protected the person so that changes he was inducing were not even known to the audience. He had the ability, through his extraordinary use of language, to have a private exchange with a subject while doing a public demonstration.

Although Erickson condemned stage hypnosis, he was really a great performer himself at hypnotic demonstrations. He could simultaneously teach a hypnotic technique, give therapy to a subject, illustrate a point at issue with a colleague, and entertain the audience. The speed with which he worked could be the envy of any stage practitioner.

As an example, I recall a demonstration Erickson once did before a large audience. He asked for a volunteer and a young man came up and sat down with him. Erickson's only trance induction was to ask the young man to put his hands on his knees. Then he said, "Would you be willing to continue to see your hands on your knees?" The young man said he would. While talking with him, Erickson gestured to a colleague on the other side of the young man, and the colleague lifted up the young man's arm and it remained in the air. Erickson said to the young man, "How many hands do you have?" "Two, of course," said the young man. "I'd like you to count them as I point to them," said Erickson. "All right," said the young man, in a rather patronizing way. Erickson pointed to the hand on one knee, and the young man said, "One." Erickson pointed to the vacant other knee, where the young man had agreed to continue to see his hand, and the young man said, "Two." Then Erickson pointed to the hand up in the air. The young man stared at it, puzzled. "How do you explain that other hand?" asked Erickson. "I don't know," said the young man. "I guess I should be in a circus." That hypnotic induction took about as long as it took me to describe it here.

It was always a pleasure to watch Erickson do one of his stage demonstrations. Some of his most interesting ones were his demonstrations of dealing with resistance to hypnosis. He would begin by asking for a volunteer to come up from the audience and be resistant. As always with Erickson, he was managing it so that if the person was resistant he was cooperating.

Erickson enjoyed showing that inducing a trance could not be described simply. He illustrated the many ways it could be done. I recall one demonstration where he showed that one could induce a trance without saying a word. He asked a resistant subject to come up on stage and a young man came up. Erickson just stood there saying and doing nothing. I could see the young man going into a trance. Later I asked Erickson what subtle thing he did to bring that about. He said he induced a trance by *not* doing anything. The young man came up in front of all those people to be hypnotized and Erickson did not do anything. "Somebody had to do something," said Erickson, "so the young man went into a trance."

I am reminded of my neophyte days when I was learning to use hypnosis in therapy. I would have a patient sit down and I would go through an induction procedure. I began to notice that a number of patients went into a trance when they first sat down in the chair in my office. What I was doing was waking them up so I could hypnotize them. I began to realize, and I think it was after that demonstration by Erickson, that when people came to be hypnotized it was not necessary to do more than get out of their way. Erickson used the social context when doing hypnosis and always thought in a larger unit than just himself and the subject. Hypnotic subjects are often better subjects on stage when in a triangle with the audience than when in a dyad alone with the hypnotist.

Besides his power to influence people outside awareness, Erickson had another ability which made some people uneasy in his company. He was an extraordinary observer and could just about read a person's mind from his or her posture and body movement. He put great emphasis on the therapist being an acute observer, treating posture and responsive movement as a language in itself.

Erickson liked to improve a trainee's ability to observe. Once when John Weakland and I visited he called us into his office briefly to look at a patient. It was a woman sitting in a chair with her eyes closed. Later, when the woman had left, Erickson asked us what we had observed. The question was so general that we found it difficult to answer. We made wise comments, such as the fact that we noticed it was a woman and even that she was in a trance. Erickson dismissed our observations and pointed out that one half of the woman's face was slightly larger than the other half and her right hand was slightly larger than her left. He said that was obviously important for diagnosis and we had to agree.

Generally people do not choose to be closely observed; trainees of Erickson were uneasy with his skill in observation. I once spent some time talking with a psychiatrist who had been a psychiatric resident in training with Erickson in Michigan many years before. He told me about the residents' respect, if not fear, of Erickson. He said that Erickson had high expectations of a student—he would pose a question and then stare at the resident with what they called his "ocular fix." His powers of observation, which he insisted the residents develop, were becoming legendary. For example, this psychiatrist told me that one day his wife was walking across the hospital grounds and Erickson stopped her. "You're pregnant, aren't you?" he said. "Yes," she said, surprised because she had just learned the fact herself. "How did you know?" she asked. Erickson said, "Your forehead has changed color."

Erickson had high expectations of himself as a clinician and held the same expectations of trainees. He expected a therapist to be an acute observer, but more than that he expected a wide range of skills. He would emphasize how a therapist should use his own movement and posture to influence a patient. Often he would illustrate with a head movement or another body movement how one should offer an idea with special emphasis. He also expected a therapist to control his voice so that words could be given special emphasis when an idea was being communicated. He liked to say a sentence and put emphasis on certain words so that he was communicating a different sentence by that emphasis. When discussing how he phrased something to a patient, Erickson would duplicate the vocal emphasis he had used. Sometimes the differences he was emphasizing were so subtle they were difficult to grasp.

Erickson expected a clinician to have a thorough knowledge of types of psychopathology, a broad understanding of human beings and their normal social situations, common sense, keen observation, and an ability to use the self in a wide range of ways from being authoritative to being helpless. He also expected a therapist to have an actor's control of his use of body movement and vocal intonation. After observing Erickson, I began to realize what abilities were necessary to become a master therapist. At that time I began to think about turning to a less exacting profession, like being a supervisor or teacher.

One of the most important aspects of Erickson that permeated his work was his sense of humor. He found humor everywhere and enjoyed practical jokes and puzzles as well as puns and turns of phrase. It was his humor that saved him, I think, from being overwhelming in his power. Something about the absurd nature of human beings and their problems was taken for granted by him. Let me give an example. I once consulted him about a case of a young couple. The wife was exasperated by her husband following her around wherever she went, particularly when she did housework on the weekends. If she went into the kitchen, he went into the kitchen, and if she went outside, he went outside. Her main objection was his following her from room to room and watching her when she vacuumed the house. She had protested to him, and he said he tried to stop, but somehow he could not. He found himself following her around and watching her vacuum.

I asked Erickson what I might do to solve the problem with this couple. He said the solution was obvious. I should talk privately with the wife and get her to agree to follow my instructions. The next Saturday she should vacuum as usual, and when her husband followed her from room to room she should make no comment. After she finished vacuuming, she should take the bag full of dirt and go back to each room where she had vacuumed and make a pile of dirt on the floor. She should say, "Well, that's that," and not touch that dirt until she vacuumed the following Saturday so that it remained there all week. I instructed the wife as Erickson suggested. Her husband stopped following her around the house.

The therapy of Erickson, more than that of any other therapist, seems to force us to consider whether the map of logic is the appropriate one to explain the behavior and dilemmas of human beings. He lived quite comfortably with paradox, while most people try to avoid that. When he could, he framed his actions in paradoxical ways. Let me cite an example from one of Erickson's social experiments.

A unique aspect of Erickson was his interest in experimenting with people and situations. Not only did he do experiments in the laboratory, but, concerned with laboratory bias, he liked to do them in the field in natural situations. Typically, with whatever group he was with, Erickson might be doing an experiment to see how someone would respond to this or that. He once told me that at a party he might choose someone and apply his "ocular fix" just to see how the person would respond. Or he would set himself the task of having someone move from one chair to another without ever directly asking for that move. Sometimes it seemed to be a way he kept from being bored in situations where his active mind found what was happening to be too routine. At other times he would do more formal experiments in social situations.

I recall an experiment where Erickson said he wished to demonstrate that one could make a person forget something by constantly reminding him of it. Erickson was a master in the control of amnesia and he worked with it in hypnosis as well as in ordinary social relations. The experiment he described was the following. He was teaching a seminar with a group of students at a table. He arranged that a young man who was a chain smoker sit on his right without any cigarettes. While they were discussing the important academic subject of the seminar, Erickson turned to the young man and offered him a cigarette. As the young man reached for the cigarette, Erickson was asked a question by someone on his left. Turning to answer the question, Erickson inadvertently pulled the cigarettes away from the young man before he could take one. The group went on with the discussion and then Erickson seemed to recall that he had been offering a cigarette. He turned, offered one to the young smoker again, and again someone on his left asked him a question, so that he inadvertently pulled the cigarettes away from the young man when he turned to answer it. Of course the interruptions had been prearranged. All the students except the smoker were aware of the nature of the experiment. After repeating this procedure several times, the young man lost interest in the cigarettes and did not reach out for one when it was offered. At the end of the seminar, the students asked the young man, if he had obtained a cigarette. He did not remember having been offered any, having amnesia for what happened. Erickson argued that what was important was the offer and the inadvertent turning away and deprivation. The young man could not blame Erickson for depriving him, because it was clearly not Erickson's fault; yet he was being deprived. This rather classic double bind was responded to by simply forgetting the sequence.

It was constant experimentation of this kind which, I think, gave Erickson not only his wisdom about human behavior but led him to new therapy techniques. For example, Erickson had a procedure for helping a person addicted to medication, such as a tranquilizer. If he refused to give the medication, the person would simply go to another doctor who would provide it. Therefore, Erickson would agree to write a prescription when it was requested, and he would begin to look for a prescription blank among the items on his desk. As he was looking, he would start a conversation with the patient which became increasingly interesting. The conversation would continue until the interview ended. Only after the interview was over would the person realize the prescription had been forgotten. The person would not go to another doctor, because the business with Erickson had not been completed. The person could not blame Erickson for the deprivation, because he was obviously willing to provide but he had *inadvertently* not provided. Just as with the cigarettes, he had benevolently offered it and been distracted. He said the person would begin to lose interest in the medication and forget about it.

Many of us have difficulty adopting Erickson's techniques because of the skill required in carrying them out. The teaching of interpersonal skills has not been part of academic training for a therapist. One of the values of hypnosis is that it teaches one how to give directives. With hypnotic training one learns how to motivate people, how to direct them to behave, how to follow up the response, and so on. This learning is necessary if one does a therapy based upon skill. What set Erickson apart as a hypnotist was his interest and concern with the interpersonal processes of trance induction, not simply the ritual procedure. He argued that a hypnotic induction needed to vary with the type of person the hypnotist was, the nature of the subject, and the particular situation they were in. He liked to see each hypnotic relationship as unique, just as he did with therapy.

The young people here today might find it difficult to realize what it was like to hear Erickson when the ideology of the field was so different. As an example, in the 1950s I was on Gregory Bateson's research project in a Veterans Administration Hospital. I was studying the communication of, and doing therapy with, a 40-year-old man defined as psychotic. He talked, among other things, about how he had cement in his stomach, seeming at times to literally believe that. Constantly he complained about his digestion and this awful feeling in his stomach. At that time the more avant garde of the psychiatric field had made a step forward, or deeper, into the unconscious. From being concerned with the genital stage and the oedipal conflict, the shift in the study of the psychosis had been made to the oral stage. It was a time when the breast was said to be the dream screen and the underlying cause was related to mother's stony breast, which John Rosen talked about, as well as the poison of mother's milk. Being in the avant garde, I was of course interpreting to this poor fellow ideas about his mother and his oral fixation and so on, which I assumed to be the basis of his delusion about having cement in his stomach. The logic of the symbolism was irrefutable.

At about this time I began to talk with Erickson and I asked him what he would do with these delusionary comments of the patient about the cement in his stomach. Erickson said, "I would go with the patient to the hospital dining hall and try out the food." I was astonished at such a shallow approach to this problem. Erickson went on to say that he would teach the patient about digestion, what foods digest easily and quickly, and which digest with difficulty. I felt that Erickson simply did not understand how to approach a psychotic delusion of this kind. It was only some time later that I inadvertently went to the hospital dinning hall and discovered the quality of the food. By then I was taking a more practical approach with the patient and even thinking that therapy might do better if he were out of the hospital in the real world rather than sitting on a ward complaining about his stomach.

Several years later, when our project had made great advances, Erickson was still ahead of us. I recall in about 1958 I had been working for some time with psychotics out in the real world in a practical way and we were even doing therapy with the whole family. We had discovered the communication approach and we were clarifying the communication of offspring and parents and bringing out their feelings and ideas about each other. Our goal was to bring about more harmony and closer relationship among the family members. I talked with Erickson at this time about our approach and he said that he thought the attempt to bring about closeness between young adult psychotics and their parents was an error. "This is not a time for closeness," he said, "it is a time when the young person should be disengaging from the family." I felt, of course, that Erickson did not understand the importance of communication theory and was not familiar with the new emphasis on the family that we were developing. It was a few years later that I realized that the problem with a young adult psychotic is not bringing about togetherness with his family but helping parents and offspring disengage and the family survive that change.

I do not wish to imply that Erickson was always ahead of us, or that he always knew and did not himself learn. We too had our influence on him, as I discovered to my surprise one day. In those days Erickson had his own way of doing therapy with a person diagnosed schizophrenic. As an example, he was seeing a woman who was a school teacher and at times she was quite crazy. He persuaded her to keep her delusions locked in the closet of his office where they would be secure and not interfere with her teaching. She did that and saw Erickson irregularly. Then she was going to move to another city and she was worried because she might go mad in that other city and Erickson would not be available. She said she didn't know what to do. Erickson said to her, "If you have a psychotic episode, why not put it in a Manila envelope and mail it to me." The woman agreed to do that and in the other city she continued to function well. Occasionally, she sent Erickson a psychotic episode in a Manila envelope. What impressed me with that case was not only that he would think of having the woman put her psychotic episodes in envelopes, but that he saved all those envelopes. He knew that one day she would return and would want to see them. She did just that.

If you examine this therapy, it appears that Erickson was assuming the woman could not be changed but only stabilized. Later, when I was visiting Erickson, he introduced me to a young woman who was showing him her wedding pictures. After she left, he told me that she had been schizophrenic and had made a good recovery. I pointed out that previously he seemed to assume one could only stabilize a schizophrenic, not cure one. I asked him if this was not a change from his past, more traditional view of schizophrenia. He said it was and added, "After all, I've learned something from you people too."

It was Erickson's willingness to change his ways and experiment with new techniques that was his greatest asset. He was a pragmatist. Looking at Erickson and his therapy from the broadest view, it seems apparent in his pragmatism and in other ways that he was very American in his views. The stories and examples he presented were out of life on a farm and the values of small towns. Whether he was talking of stealing apples from an orchard, going swimming, or expressing enthusiasm about college life, his expression seemed to be middle America. He had a basic understanding of growing up in the United States that clarified for him the stages of family life and the processes of normal living. He knew the different regions of the country and their particular ideas, style and prejudices. He understood other cultures because he knew this one so well and could contrast it.

Erickson expressed a different psychiatric tradition from the one with its roots in Europe, where there was a focus on classification and diagnosis. Although Erickson was interested in diagnosis, his main interest was in producing change. He sharply focused on the subject of therapy as an art in itself and he emphasized the practical skills needed to carry it out. He was pragmatic and would shift what he did if it was not working, quickly adopting some other procedure rather than continue with a failing method because it was traditional. Not concerned with schools of philosophy, Erickson focused quite specifically upon the real world and real problems. He recommended that a therapist use techniques which worked and discard those which did not, independent of tradition. He did not suggest you look to a prominent person to lend support to your practices, but rather that you defend your work by its results. These ideas are considered characteristic of American pragmatism, just as is Erickson's emphasis upon taking action rather than being an observer and waiting for change.

In the 1950s there was an explosion of innovative therapies in the United States. The subject of how to change people came into vogue rather than a concern with how to study and classify them. The behavioral therapies developed and so did the family therapies. Everyone became less philosophical, more pragmatic, and more concerned with social change. Erickson was premature in the field in that when these changes in therapy came about he had already changed. One way to describe his contribution to the present revolution in the field of therapy is to point out that his position about what to do in therapy was exactly the opposite of what was done by traditional therapists. It is difficult to believe that he went to such an opposite extreme from the mainstream of therapy. It is also difficult to believe that the mainstream of therapy could have been so wrong that doing the opposite was appropriate. Let me summarize some aspects of his contribution by contrasting it with the prevailing views of a few years ago.

## HYPNOSIS

In the 1940s and 1950s the field of therapy was largely prevented from using hypnosis. Psychiatrists did not learn hypnosis, and social workers would probably have had their casework buttons torn off if they wanted to hypnotize a client. It was so little taught in clinical training that traveling workshops had to be done to teach it at all. While this condemnation of hypnosis was happening, Erickson was using hypnosis in therapy, developing a wide range of techniques and advocating that it be a basic skill taught to clinicians.

## SYMPTOMS

At that time the field of therapy was not symptom-focused. It was argued that symptoms were unimportant and the real problem was the roots in character structure and personality. As a result, clinicians not only did not know how to change symptoms but argued that one should not. Some vague disaster would occur. Erickson took the opposite position and based his therapy specifically on symptoms. He argued that you change character structure by centering therapy on the specific problem. As he said, the symptom is like the handle of a pot; if you have a good grip on that handle, you can do a lot with the pot. He taught that one should not ignore a symptom but learn all the details about it. As one examined the frequency, intensity, and so on, a proper symptom became something to admire in the way it was involved in all aspects of a person's life. The therapists who ignored symptoms and said one should not deal with them never learned to appreciate the complexity of symptomatic behavior. They also never learned to change what the patient wanted changed.

## INSIGHT AND THE UNCONSCIOUS

Erickson deviated most from his colleagues on the issue of insight and the nature of the unconscious. In the 1940s and the 1950s the proponents of insight therapy gained their greatest power. At that time therapists made only interpretations. It was generally assumed that a person's problem was a product of repression and the ideation must be made conscious. Erickson, who had experimented extensively with unconscious repression, slips of the tongue, memories and dreams, had by the 1940s apparently abandoned that notion as relevant to therapy. It was thought that if a therapist did not bring about insight, he was doing shallow therapy. Erickson took the position that insight therapy did not produce change and even implied that interpretations about internal dynamics could prevent real change.

Erickson's view of the "unconscious" was the opposite of the psychodynamic view of that time. Insight therapy was based upon the idea that the unconscious was a place full of negative forces and ideas which were so unacceptable that they had to be repressed. According to that view, a person needed to watch out for his or her unconscious ideas, and to distrust the hostile and aggressive impulses striving for expression. Erickson took the opposite view and accepted the idea that the unconscious was a positive force which held more wisdom than the "conscious." If a person just let his unconscious operate, it would take care of everything in a positive way. Erickson emphasized trusting one's unconscious and expecting it to fullfill the greatest good. As an example, he said that if he misplaced something and forgot where it was, he did not agitatedly try to find it. He assumed his unconscious had set it aside and would bring it forth at the proper moment.

As a result, you never find in Erickson's therapy statements such as, "Have you noticed that when you mention your husband it is after you mention your father?" or "Have you wondered if you have an unconscious desire to resist this therapy?" He did not assume that insight into unconscious ideas that were repressed was relevant to change. This is why his therapy seemed so strange to an insight therapist. For example, how could such a therapist understand arranging that a depressed woman schedule a certain period of time each week to be depressed? Or how could an insight therapist understand paradoxically encouraging a symptom?

As always, Erickson offered the opposite of insight by encouraging amnesia and changing people outside their awareness. Rather than help patients understand the hidden meaning in dreams or fantasies, he would change them so they dreamed and fantasized differently. He considered an "interpretation" to be an absurd reduction of a complex communication. Similarly, he did therapy with analogies and metaphors differently from the therapists of his time. Erickson was introducing a new theory of change in the ways he used analogical communication. In the past, clinicians worked with the analogies of patients to gain information, as in asking the patient about fantasies and dreams. Or they thought that making the patient aware of the metaphorical meanings in his analogies would cause change, as in discussing the parallels between the content of a fantasy and a real life situation.

Erickson took quite the opposite view; making people aware of the parallels in their analogical presentations would not cause change and would even prevent change. The awareness would reduce the complexity of the issues being changed. If, for example, he was talking about food and eating as a way of influencing a person to have more enjoyment in sex and to be less inhibited, he would be careful not to let the person become conscious of the parallel between eating and sex. As he put it, if they begin to be aware, one should "drift rapidly away from the subject." What he seemed to be suggesting was that therapy done in this way had two requirements: First, one must talk about something that is analogical with something about the patient one wishes to change. That is, one talked about A in order to change B when they had similarities. Once the analogy was being drawn, the therapist also needed to take a position on how A should be in order to change B. Merely talking about A and drawing the analogy was not sufficient, and making the analogy conscious would destroy the change. For example, to talk about eating food as analogic to sex is not sufficient in itself. The therapist must also take a position that food should be enjoyed. For example, he might say there should be pleasure in the appetizers to wake up the gastric juices before the main course. It is saying how something should be when talking about the analogical area that is the cause of change. I think that is what gave Erickson so often the quality of being an ethical lecturer; he emphasized how things should be in one area to change another area.

Consider another example of how Erickson worked outside awareness. If one sees a person caught up in a repeating cycle of behavior with other people, the traditional approach is to make the person aware of the cycle on the assumption that if he becomes aware of it he can stop repeating his behavior. Erickson did not bring about awareness of the cycle but simply set out to change it. He might even induce amnesia for behavior in the cycle so the person would do something and forget he did it. Therefore he would do it again. This repetition would force the other people in the cycle to respond differently and so the repeating pattern would change.

Although Erickson did not offer the usual insight, he was an educator. He would teach patients that life is more complex than they thought by using riddles and puzzles. Often he did explicit teaching about medical and other issues. He was teaching people about their sexual organs and instructing them in specific sexual practices long before "sex therapy" became permissible and fashionable. That too added to the controversy about him.

## POSTURE OF THERAPIST

Traditionally, the therapist was an objective consultant to a patient. He or she was an observer who reflected back what was produced and helped the person understand his or her problems and motivation. Rather than intervene into a person's life, the therapist took a position on the outside as a non-participant observer. If asked if his job was to change someone, the therapist would say it was not, it was to help people understand themselves so they could choose to change if they wished. The therapist was not really responsible for change, so if therapy failed it was the patient's fault. Therapists took money from patients to change them, while declining to take responsibility for changing them. A curious paradox of the field.

If we ask what the opposite of the traditional therapeutic posture would be, there we find Erickson. He assumed it was his responsibility to change a patient. If change did not occur, he had failed. I can recall him saying, often in a grim tone, "That case is still defeating me." He was not an objective observer or a consultant; he was an active intervenor into the person's life. He assumed that what he did and said was the cause of change, not some objective awareness that the patient achieved. He would visit the home or office of a patient and escort them to places they feared.

Even psychoanalysts who were thought to be closely involved with their patients thought that Erickson entered too much into a patient's life. I recall Frieda Fromm-Reichmann's comment. She had the reputation of being a therapist most intimate with her patients in intensive therapy. When we said we were studying Erickson, she said, "Couldn't you have chosen a therapist to study who is less involved with his patients?"

Even though Erickson was personal with patients, he was not a pal as many humanistic therapists are. He kept his professional distance while being a friend and confidant. As with many aspects of Erickson, his closeness and distance were paradoxical.

As an example, he was once defining the nature of hypnotic trance as a focusing of attention, and he said amnesia was a product of that attention. He said that he could be talking with a patient about something emotionally moving, and at that point he would kick off his shoes. He would put the shoes on again and later ask the patient about that action. The patient would not remember it happening. Although Erickson was talking about concentration and amnesia, I was thinking about *him*. He could be closely involved enough with the patient to bring out something emotionally moving and simultaneously he would be distant enough to experiment with kicking off his shoes.

## BRIEF THERAPY

At that time it was assumed that long-term therapy was necessary to bring about change. Brief therapy was just a matter of doing less than you did in long-term therapy; you just gave less insight. Erickson worked in quite an opposite way by doing therapy as briefly as possible. When he did long-term therapy, it was when he could not solve the problem more briefly. Instead of seeing someone methodically several times a week, he worked intermittently and for different lengths of time.

Even the way he talked about brief therapy was paradoxical. He said the way to get a quick change was to proceed slowly. He would say, for example, if you get a one-second change in a symptom that exists 24 hours a day, you have made a major change. Often with hypnosis he would increase a one-second change by geometrical progression—from one to two to four and so on. The small change inevitably led to the larger one. As Erickson put it, if you want a large change you should ask for a small one.

Erickson's brief therapy also occurred in the real world. He practiced a therapy of common sense in that he had resources in the community to help his clients, whether it was a hairdresser, a clothing salesman, a waiter in a restaurant, or whatever might be needed. He was familiar with the day-to-day operations of normal living, knew what average families were like and understood what children did at different stages of development. He was familiar with the problems of growing old and knew intimately the difficulties of dealing with pain and physical illness.

## DIRECTIVE THERAPY

Traditionally a therapist was non-directive. It was considered wrong to tell someone what to do, whether in large issues or in what to talk about in the room. There was a naive assumption that one could talk with a patient for months, even years, without directing him in what should be said or done.

Erickson took the opposite position. He argued that change came about by the therapist being directive. He also assumed that whatever one said or did in the presence of a client was directive; the problem was how to do that skillfully rather than assuming it was not happening.

## INVOLVING FAMILY MEMBERS

Traditionally, it was not proper to see the relative of a patient; many therapists would not even talk to one on the telephone for fear some terrible damage would be done to the therapy. As always, Erickson, quite the opposite, was willing to see relatives and was one of the earliest therapists to bring family members together in an interview. Sometimes he would see parents and child together, sometimes separately, just as he would see couples both together and individually. He was one of the first to have worked out specific procedures for persuading reluctant relatives to come in when they declined. As an example, when a husband would not come to therapy with his wife, despite an invitation, Erickson would begin to arrange that he come in. Talking to the wife, Erickson would say, "Your husband would probably understand the matter this way," and at another point he would say, "I'm sure your husband would have this view." Each time he would suggest a view or an understanding that was incorrect and not the husband's view. When the wife went home, the husband would interrogate her about the therapy session. She would reveal the misunderstandings of his views that Erickson expressed. Soon the husband would say that he wanted an appointment to "straighten that psychiatrist out" and he would come in.

Erickson was quite comfortable with families. While Freud said he did not know what to do with relatives of patients, Erickson said he did. More than any other therapist of his time, Erickson defined symptoms as contracts between relatives—not merely the expression of an individual. He was also willing to do therapy with friends and colleagues. Not concerned with maintaining a mystical relationship with a patient, he could see a person both professionally and socially.

In summary, traditional therapists were non-directive, consultants to the individual patient. At their most active they encouraged patients to talk and express themselves. They did not use hypnosis, did not give directives, avoided relatives and did not interview families and did not deal with symptoms. They relied almost entirely on interpretations to cause change in both individual and group therapy.

Erickson developed an opposite approach on each of these variables. He was an active participant in the lives of patients, used hypnosis, gave both paradoxical and straightforward directives, included relatives in therapy, did not make insightful interpretations or do group therapy, encouraged amnesia, and focused specifically on symptoms.

If we look at the multitudinous schools of therapy today and the general trajectory of the field, it would seem that the mainstream has largely swung toward Erickson's position. His approach in therapy is now acceptable and taught, while the position of his opponents is becoming an historical curiosity. If Erickson were 50 years old at this time and at the height of his strength, I think he would dominate the field of therapy. One might think it is sad that he was 20 years ahead of his time and so not fully appreciated when he was in his younger years. However, I think it is better to think about how he helped to create our time. If Erickson had not done his work and taught so widely, we would not have the therapeutic ideas and opportunites we have today.

Choosing any aspect of Erickson and his work to talk about means neglecting some other aspect. The complexity he appreciated in human beings was well expressed in himself. If one emphasized Erickson's concern with people in the real world, one must also recall that he quite fully developed the world of fantasy. To Erickson the human mind was a many chambered room with entrances and exits which often operated independently of each other. One can have secrets from other people, as well as secrets from oneself. Erickson was as comfortable with the interior of people and their dream states as he was with a child's difficulties with arithmetic in school.

In this presentation I have tried to cover some general and specific issues about Erickson. Doing so, I face Erickson's view that making explicit and conscious any idea about human life reduces a complex subject to an oversimplification. That problem applies to what I have said here about this extraordinary man and his work. In time I think other people will understand him more fully than we do now. Therefore, in closing, let me paraphrase a comment once made by A. N. Whitehead about a speaker. I hope that in this presentation I have left unobscured the vast darkness of the subject of Milton Erickson.

PART II

# *Ericksonian Psychotherapy: An Overview*

*F. William Hanley, M.D., is a longtime friend of the Erickson family. Dr. Hanley is a psychiatrist in private practice in Vancouver, British Columbia, where he conducts seminars on hypnosis for professionals. He is commonly referred to as "Mr. Hypnosis" in Western Canada.*

*In his chapter, Hanley develops and illustrates some of the major principles that Erickson espoused. Hanley is not a passive interpreter of Ericksonian techniques; his case examples illustrate his own development and interpretation of Ericksonian principles.*

*Richard Van Dyck, M.D., is president of the Netherland Society of Clinical Hypnosis. Dr. Van Dyck and his colleagues in Holland have established a school of directive psychotherapy and published two volumes in Dutch that are highly esteemed in the Netherlands. The Dutch group is now attracting international attention. They soon will be acknowledged generally as leaders in the field of strategic approaches to psychotherapy.*

*Van Dyck describes a famous case in which Erickson used a symbolic approach in couples therapy. Van Dyck clarifies the mechanisms of Erickson's multi-level tactics so that one can more easily understand their dynamic effect. However, he does not stop at that point but presents some important guidelines so that clinicians can incorporate Ericksonian approaches in their own practice.*

*Paul Carter, Ph.D., is a remarkably effective communicator who relies on unconscious learning in teaching Ericksonian approaches. He has conducted workshops on Ericksonian techniques throughout the United States and Europe. His half-day workshop at the Erickson Congress, co-led with Stephen Gilligan, was one of the most highly rated of all the preconference workshops.*

*Carter uses a systems approach to explicate three principles of Erickson's methodology. He uses some of his own cases, as well as some of Erickson's, to illustrate the importance of the systems approach.*

*John Beahrs, M.D., a psychiatrist in private practice in Portland, Oregon, has authored major articles on Erickson's method, including "The Hypnotic Psychotherapy of Milton H. Erickson," published in the* American Journal of Clinical Hypnosis *(Vol. 14, 1971). In his presentation at the Congress, Dr. Beahrs developed important philosophical underpinnings to Erickson's work. Beahrs is no stranger to philosophical investigation. He has written two volumes integrating philosophical and clinical approaches:* That Which Is: An Inquiry Into the Nature of Energy, Ethics and Mental Health and Unity *and* Unity and Multiplicity: Multilevel Consciousness of Self in Hypnosis, Psychiatric Disorder and Mental Health.

Chapter 2

# Erickson's Contribution to Change in Psychotherapy

*F. William Hanley*

## INTRODUCTION

In 1974, in his Foreword to the book *Change,* Erickson stated, "Psychotherapy is sought not primarily for enlightenment about the unchangeable past but because of dissatisfaction with the present and a desire to better the future. In what direction and how much change is needed neither the patient nor the psychotherapist can know. . . . I have viewed much of what I have done as expediting the currents of change already seething within the person and the family." He then spoke of the actual nature and kinds of change so long overlooked by the formulation of theories about how to change people and referred to the opening of new pathways to expedite the resolution of human impasses.

What can we learn of Erickson's contribution to understanding the actual nature and kinds of change that are possible in psychotherapy and the new pathways he trod?

In this chapter, Erickson's own words will be used frequently when referring to his ideas and unique methods. There is considerable evidence from Erickson's writings and teachings that Erickson was one of the world's foremost authorities on Ericksonian psychotherapy. As I discuss what Erickson's contribution to change in psychotherapy means to me, I will illustrate this with cases from my own practice.

How does a person learn to ride a bicycle? How does a person change from a pedestrian to one with the skill to maintain his balance upright on two wheels and to propel himself forward? How does one teach a person to ride a bicycle? One might assure the person that riding a bicycle is possible, that he/she has the ability to ride the bicycle even without knowing that he/she has that ability; one might confirm that assurance by showing other people riding bicycles or by demonstrating oneself. One might point out the existence of the seat, explain the functions of the pedals and how to rotate them and the functions of the handlebars in steering. One can remind the person that, as a child, he/she balanced himself as he/she walked along the top of a wall. One can ask the person to get on the bicycle, to hold the handlebars and begin to rotate the pedals. But just how and when the person learns and what kind of bicycle riding he/she does, neither the teacher nor the learner can know. All the teacher can do is believe with complete confidence that the person can ride the bicycle, i.e., that the person can look forward to being able to ride the bicycle sooner or later and to get on the bicycle when he/she is ready to ride it. The teacher, from his/her experience, will know how to guide the individual in his/her learning.

## OBSERVATION

Erickson's first step in the change process of psychotherapy was to make careful, detailed observations of the patient. *"Really look at your patient and really listen to your patient."* Erickson noted the walk, the posture, the minute movements of the head saying yes and no, the pupillary reflexes, the pauses and hesitations in movement and speech, the voice intonations and the omissions. He observed that therapists pay too little attention to nonverbal communication; by noticing nonverbal messages he obtained a tremendous amount and variety of useful information not usually gathered in psychotherapy. He was thus able to make a more accurate and meaningful evaluation of the symptoms and thereby provide himself with much wider scope in intervention. He also emphasized the importance of being aware of context. *"Always pay attention to the situation in which the symptom occurs."* Erickson began with a comprehensive and often amazingly precise and full gathering of data.

### *Case Example One*

Recently I saw a new patient while a student was also present. The patient came into the room, sat down in the chair indicated by a gesture of the hand and, on request, readily began to talk about her fatigue, her anxiety, her nervousness, her recurring feelings of depression, her wondering about a physical origin for her symptoms. "I don't know why I'm this way. I have no worries—I have a good home; I have no problems with my three children; my husband and I get along quite well; he is very good to me; he's a good provider and I have everything I need; we have a good social life. I have a part-time job that I like. I think I must have hypoglycemia."

"Tell me about your marriage and your dissatisfaction with some things." She quickly responded with her inner thoughts and feelings. The student asked how I knew to ask about her marriage. He had not noticed that as she was mentioning her husband, she crossed her legs and turned slightly away. Even before that movement, there was a slight shaking of the head.

Erickson was always noting the multiple-level communications he was receiving. He showed how to read the signs that said, "This way to the problem" or "Look the other way," when there were no words on the signs. He showed that, by really looking, one could see the signs that said, "Caution, bump ahead" and "Turn here." Much of his inventiveness grew out of his observational skill. Alexander Graham Bell, when asked about inventing, replied, "Look at what everybody else has looked at and see what no one else has seen."

## ORIENTATION TOWARD THERAPEUTIC CHANGE

Erickson saw therapy as a cooperative enterprise and himself an agent of change. *"The personality of the patient is of primary importance."* What the hypnotist or the therapist can do to enable the patient to accomplish certain things is important. Everything he said and did with a patient was oriented toward therapeutic goals. He let the patient hear the word "change" in many ways: "You can look forward to learning all about your problem. You can do many things and you don't know how you do them. You can do things that you don't know you can do. You can make certain changes that are satisfying to you. You won't find out how to talk to that person until after you've found it out and be willing to be surprised to find out that you speak to that person in a really confident manner."

## UTILIZATION

Erickson was prepared to use any behavior that the patient offered in working toward the therapeutic goal for that patient. *"In rendering aid, there should be full respect for, and utilization of, whatever the patient presents.*" Every manifest behavior, every psychological state, understanding, attitude, and resistance that the patient brings into the situation has a positive potential and can be used, wholly or modified, to lead to new, more adequate behavior. This is done by introducing new ideas (changing perception and meaning). For example, a cut on the lip of a child can become a source of satisfaction and even of prestige because of the number of stitches it requires.

He often used the unexpected, the sudden, the illogical or shock to expedite the currents of change. He showed that by identifying the patient's current reality, often suddenly and unexpectedly, that reality could be brought into the therapy room and utilized for change.

*Case Example Two*

Ellen came for help to break away from the brutal, alcoholic man with whom she was living. She was the daughter of a brutal, alcoholic father and had divorced a brutal, alcoholic husband. The present man was pressing her to move with him to another city where he had obtained a job. "I don't want to go with him. I know it's going to be a continuation of the same thing but he is so possessive and demanding and so persistent that I can't get away from him. He keeps at me until I break down in tears and then I agree to do what he wants. This is the one chance for me to get away. I want to live my own life." When she was sounded out on ways she might do this, she began to find excuses.

A suggestion that she might simply disappear from the apartment was met with the assertion that she had nowhere to go, that she had no money to support herself, that she would be cut off welfare, and that George would probably find her and beat her up. She continued to complain about his brutal behavior and said, "He's a sadist." "Did you hear what you just said?" "Yes, he's a sadist". "Do you know what you are saying?" She stared wonderingly, open to new ideas, her attention fixed and her pattern interrupted. (If you meet the patient at the patient's level and really enter his/her system, he/she will automatically go into a trance.) "Every sadist needs a masochist and you are the greatest masochist I have seen for a long time." Her masochism was described to her in detail. She began to cry. After a time she fell silent, staring ahead. In a few minutes she said quietly and firmly, "I have a girlfriend I can stay with. I have a little money put away and they won't cut me off welfare. He'll never find me; I'll just leave a note on the kitchen table saying that I'm leaving." Rousing herself, she got up and, without making another appointment, decisively walked out.

That night, when I arrived home from a meeting, I learned that a man had telephoned trying to find the whereabouts of his girlfriend. He told my answering service, "She saw Dr. Hanley this afternoon and when I got home tonight there was a note on the kitchen table saying she was leaving."

A few months later the patient returned to continue therapy, stating, "I've come to you because you understand me."

Erickson utilized the often unrecognized potential in a situation. He exemplified this in his own life. In the Foreword to *Change,* he said, "I would have preferred to say much more about this book than I do here. Unfortunately, ill health prevents me from doing that, but thereby leads me to come to the point at once." There is a Japanese proverb that says, "My granary has burned down, now I can see the sun."

## INDIRECT FORMS OF SUGGESTION

There are more than 20 ways to say "sit down," half a dozen of which are nonverbal.

All indirect suggestions are multi-level ways of communicating with the patient's unconscious. Orienting the patient toward change is itself an indirect suggestion to get well, i.e., to change for the better. Erickson devised many ways of giving suggestions indirectly. He used stories and anecdotes, analogies, metaphors, puns, jokes, binds and double binds. He himself considered that the interspersal approach was one of his two important contributions to the use of suggestion.

### *Case Example Three*

John was a 43-year-old man whose chief complaint was discomfort in the stomach. He had this pain for years and had much medical and surgical treatment. His childhood was severely emotionally deprived. He was a hardworking, driving, impatient person who was living a very restricted life. Fishing was his only recreation. His stomach symptoms began when he married and began to raise a family. He complained that he had gone over his background many times with his psychiatrist but it didn't do any good and he didn't want to spend any more time on that.

Hypnosis was induced by using the imagery of a boat. As he rocked gently in the boat he was offered a full, varied and satisfying lunch, which he was allowed to eat slowly and with complete enjoyment. Fishing was then begun, and it was suggested that he fish deep below the surface and near the surface, on the right side of the boat and on the left side, at the front of the boat and at the back, that he fish everywhere and catch any interesting and useful fish in that water. Then he was encouraged to row to another location, and to row hard and enjoy the rowing and then to fish again as thoroughly as before. It was suggested that he eat the fish he caught and really enjoy the eating of his own fish.

After a few sessions John's symptoms had subsided. He reported that they didn't bother him as much, and he was thinking he should do something for recreation during the week. He soon began swimming lessons.

In hypnosis it was subsequently suggested to John that he row his boat to an island, that he land on the island and explore the territory and describe the interesting things he found. He began to take more walks and to enjoy things in a leisurely way.

## HANDLING OF RESISTANCE

Resistance to change is always present and Erickson devised ingenious ways of both displacing and utilizing resistance. One such way is to provide the patient with choices that he/she can reject.

### *Case Example Four*

A patient complained of severe headache every evening, beginning about suppertime and lasting all night. She was childless and she and her husband had a happy marriage. "We've never had a cross word in the ten years since we married." In hypnosis, she was given the suggestion to be free of headache one evening during the week, to unload that headache for just one evening. She was told that this might be Monday evening or Wednesday evening and that she could let me know what happened when she returned on Friday. (She could resist by rejecting one of these evenings.) On Friday she reported, "Well, it didn't work the way you said. I had a headache again every night this week—except last night (pause). Last night my husband and I had the first fight we've had for years. It cleared the air of a lot of things and I felt much better afterwards." She resisted by rejecting both nights and choosing her own night to "unload."

Instructing a patient to continue the symptom is another effective method that Erickson used.

*Case Example Five*

A patient telephoned to ask for an appointment to have hypnosis for his headache of about ten years' duration. He had been to a number of doctors, including a psychiatrist, but the headache, which occurred at work, had not changed. He hoped I could help him to get rid of it. He was assured that hypnosis might help, given an appointment and told, "I want to see you with that headache. Do you think you can hang on to it until you see me on Tuesday?" He came to the appointment and apologized. "I don't have a headache today. Some time after I spoke to you it improved." He demonstrated that he wasn't going to be told what to do.

## THEORY

It is said that Erickson developed no explicit personality theory. He spoke of the importance of the actual nature and kinds of change so long overlooked by the formulation of theories to change people. With Erickson, practice was primary and unfettered by broad generalizations. The French author Vauvenargues (1715-1747) said, "Reason defeats us more often than nature." Other notables in the field of psychology formed schools by taking certain data, mostly verbal communications from patients, and constructing thories, i.e., putting their own meanings onto the data. Therefore, we have schools founded upon intrapsychic events, upon behavioral items, upon feeling states, etc. Erickson saw and heard the whole person and responded meaningfully and therapeutically to the whole person.

The lack of comprehensive generalizations explaining phenomena can be disturbing. Without them, we tend to deny the phenomena or to view them as magic. We are like the Irishman when he first saw the steam engine. He remarked, "I can see it works in practice all right but does it work in theory?"

I believe that Erickson had an *implicit* model. Instead of the automobile model, i.e., the repair and replacement model which focuses on pathology, his work indicated that he was using a growth and adaptation model. The individual is continuously trying to grow and adapt like a plant, sending its roots wherever it will get most nourishment, moving towards the light, strengthening its stem, healing its wounds and growing new leaves to replace those lost by accident or disease. Where some would see certain behavior as a repetition compulsion, Erickson would see it as the attempt to adapt, to change by using patterns available from the past. He would help the patient to find more satisfactory or adaptable behavior, sometimes from the past, sometimes by modification of present behavior, sometimes by complete reversal of perception and meaning, so that the patient would learn how to use this behavior until the adaptation was accomplished and growth resumed. Recognizing that each patient was different, he would give each patient a new experience, an opportunity to use his/her creative potential in living. Every case is an individual problem requiring its own unique approach. In this service he improved the quality of the available psychotherapeutic tools and invented, from his observation of how change occurs in everyday life, a wide variety of new tools, some designed to be used for specific parts of the change process, others for the process as a whole.

## CODA

Erickson showed people how the parts of the bicycle function; he introduced them to their own abilities to sit appropriately and to move their legs and arms appropriately, to balance comfortably; he enhanced these learnings and understandings and repeatedly oriented people toward the goal of learning to ride that bicycle. He helped them become aware that they could learn quickly or suddenly or even slowly. When they fell off he would point out how nice that was, that one really learned how to balance by falling off, and now could they fall to the right side. And now, would they mind trying to decide which side to fall to while they concentrated on turning those pedals.

Many people who thought they could never learn to ride a bicycle and who seemed to others as though they would never ride a bicycle discovered with Erickson that they could ride a two-wheeled vehicle.

Erickson also contributed the knowledge that it is possible to ride a unicycle.

## REFERENCES

Erickson, M.H. Foreword. In: *Change: Principles of Problem Formation and Problem Resolution.* P. Watzlawick, J. Weakland, & R. Fisch. New York: Norton, 1974.

Chapter 3

# How to Use Ericksonian Approaches When You Are Not Milton H. Erickson

*Richard Van Dyck*

In his commentary on the writings of Milton Erickson, in the last chapter of *Advanced Techniques of Hypnosis and Therapy,* Haley (1967) relates an incident that made a deep impression on him:

> Once many years ago, a research investigator was engaging in long conversations with Erickson to obtain generalizations about his therapeutic procedures. The young man wanted clear statements about his "method" and Erickson was doing his best to educate him. At a certain point, Erickson interrupted the discussion and took the young man outside the house to the front lawn. He pointed up the street and asked what he saw. Puzzled, the young man replied that he saw a street. Erickson asked if he saw anything else. When he continued to be puzzled, Erickson pointed to the trees which lined the street. "Do you notice anything about those trees?" he asked. After a period of study, the young man said they were all leaning in an easterly direction. "That's right," said Erickson, pleased. "All except one. That second one from the end is leaning in a westerly direction. There is always an exception."

Of course, Haley himself was the research investigator. His account of this event stayed with me. The incident appears to hold a basic formula for understanding aspects of Erickson's work in therapy as well as in teaching. Noticing individual exceptions and basing his approach upon

---

I wish to thank Kees van der Velden and Jeffrey Zeig for helpful suggestions and comments in preparing this paper.

them are indeed cornerstones of his work. Pointing things out with a parable or providing a somewhat confusing experience rather than endlessly arguing is another backbone of Erickson's approach.

I mention the above incident because it also is representative of the way I learned about Erickson. In 1968 I accidentally came across Haley's *Strategies of Psychotherapy* (1963) and read about Erickson for the first time. Subsequently, I read everything I could find, both about him and by him. Consequently, until rather recently when I met Erickson briefly and also came into contact with Kay Thompson and Jeffrey Zeig, both of whom worked with Erickson and knew him well, reading was the main source of my information about him.

Impressed with Erickson's therapy, I tried to understand and apply what I picked up from the sources that were available. As I am involved in training, I have tried to transmit this understanding to beginning therapists. These attempts are the background of my paper. It is addressed to those who recognize that trying to learn from an exceptionally gifted individual may be a difficult problem for those of us who have more limitations to our talents. It is also addressed to those who are not sure that they would have noticed that not *all* the trees were leaning to the east before it was pointed out to them.

In this paper I will mention some of the difficulties that are inherent in analyzing Erickson's work. After discussing a case history, I will identify particular elements in his style which may not be fit for large-scale application. I will then attempt to point out conditions which seem favorable to the process of trying to incorporate Ericksonian elements.

It has been argued many times that Erickson's willingness to adapt to unique circumstances makes it difficult to adequately discuss his work. One is faced with the choice between making limited observations which are correct for a single individual case or formulating more general statements which frequently turn out to be inapplicable to other therapy cases.

The only way to respect both accuracy and variety lies in moving into higher levels of abstraction. However, statements such as, "Ericksonian psychotherapy is based on extreme flexibility," while indisputable, do not provide leads for finding an Ericksonian solution to a particular problem. To be sure, this kind of difficulty arises during the description and transmission of any psychotherapeutic system. But most other founders of a school make a virtue out of remaining predictable to some degree and they generally attempt to stay within the confines of the theories that they have developed. Conversely, Erickson did not develop any limiting theories to begin with and he seemed to make it a virtue never to use the same solution twice if he could think of a new one. Since it is therefore up to others to find some limits, I will make an attempt by discussing a case history which can be found in *A Teaching Seminar With Milton Erickson* (Zeig, 1980).

In the seminar, Erickson tells about a couple from Pennsylvania who consulted him. The husband was a psychiatrist who, after 13 years, had not yet organized a successful practice. Both he and his wife were in individual therapy with the same analyst for several years. They traveled to Phoenix seeking marital therapy from Erickson. Erickson mentioned that he took no systematic history and, following a brief conversation, he sent them to complete separate tasks without explaining whether or how the task related to therapy. The husband was to climb Squaw Peak, investing three hours in the project. Similarly, the wife was to spend three hours at the desert botanical gardens.

The next day they reported their experiences to Erickson. For the husband it had been "the most wonderful thing he had done all his life"; climbing Squaw Peak changed his perspective. The wife, on the other hand, reported that she spent the "most boring three hours" of her life at the gardens; all she saw was "more and more of the same old thing."

Without further comment, Erickson sent the couple to complete new tasks. Now the wife was to climb Squaw Peak and the husband to visit the botanical gardens. Their report the next day showed the same discrepant pattern. The husband found it wonderful and awe-inspiring to see all the different desert plants. His wife, who climbed that "goddamned" Squaw Peak, cursing Erickson and herself for doing so, still cursed when she reported about it. Only briefly did she feel some satisfaction upon reaching the top. Erickson then asked them each to choose a task for the next afternoon, admonishing them to do it *separately*, and then he told them to come back the following day and report to him. When they came in the next morning, the husband said that he returned to the botanical gardens and again had enjoyed every minute of it, regretting having to leave. To her puzzlement, the wife decided to climb Squaw Peak again. She did so, cursing even more fluently than she had before, both on the way up and on the way down. Again, she felt only a momentary satisfaction upon reaching the top. After they had given these comments, Erickson said: "All right, glad to hear your reports. Now I can tell you your marital therapy is complete. Go down to the airport and return to Pennsylvania." This they did.

A few days later, Erickson received a telephone call from the couple, detailing the following: Upon returning home, they had each separately gone for a ride "to get the cobwebs out of their minds." Next, they had each separately fired their analyst. In addition, the wife had reached the decision to file for a divorce which was eventually the outcome of this marital therapy.

When this couple was seen by Erickson, he had accumulated over 40 years of experience in psychotherapy. To fully appreciate the subtlety of his approach I think one must already be somewhat of an Ericksonian. I would like to use this case to try to explain why his interventions had the effect they did and to explore whether they would work the same way if any of us were to use a similar approach.

First, this story is typical of Erickson's later work in several respects. Although no formal hypnotic induction techniques were used, the therapy contained moments of tension and confusion which forced the patients to make an inner search for solutions. The case history also typifies what Erickson did *not* do. He avoided raising issues for conscious discussion with the couple. Jeffrey Zeig (Note 1) presents a metaphor for Erickson's style: Erickson was much like a watchmaker, who, without ever opening the case to check out the parts, could somehow reach around it, subtly do something out of eyesight and make the clock run again. This image is certainly descriptive of the way Erickson brought change into the life of this couple with only a limited amount of verbal information. Erickson stated that the few facts which were known to him were all he needed. His interventions showed the same sort of parsimony. Having listened briefly to the couple's history, he gave simple assignments. His prescriptions overtly reflected only on the way they spent their afternoons but turned out to have a decisive influence on their married life.

Erickson presented this story as an example of his "symbolic therapy." Everything that goes on has meaning on more than one level. With this in mind, we can suspect that the last assignment, to think of a task for themselves and to carry it out *separately,* related not only to that afternoon, but also covertly pertained to the rest of their lives. We can also suspect that groundwork for this had been laid by Erickson's instruction that earlier assignments also had to be completed separately. We know that Erickson worked with implications. What are the implications of the statement: "Your marital therapy is complete"? It means: "No improvement is to be expected. More therapy will not be useful. Now is the time to make decisions. Do not wait for further results."

I have indicated some of the stylistic and technical qualities of this therapy. They are:

- confusion which necessitates an internal search,
- interventions based upon very limited background information,
- parsimony of therapeutic interventions,
- specified tasks which activate decision making on the part of the patient,
- multi-level communication,
- use of implications rather than direct discussion about important issues.

More elements could be found in this therapy; others, no less important than those listed, could be found in other case reports. But that is not the purpose of this paper. Rather, let us now ask in what way this therapy could have had the effect it did. The question is worth asking because there is uncertainty in the whole procedure. Given this uncertainty, one must wonder how the couple acted upon it so quickly and firmly. Assuming that the answer is not to be found in any information which is omitted from the case report, an important part of the answer surely lies in various unique aspects of the situation. For one thing, at the time of this treatment, Erickson was an internationally reputed therapist with an aura of being incredibly successful. A psychiatrist himself, the husband must have been aware of this. Consequently, for this couple to obtain therapy from Milton Erickson was the virtual equivalent to finding a foolproof solution. This is underlined by the fact that they came all the way from Pennsylvania, further structuring the situation strongly toward a conclusion within a limited period of time. We do not know exactly how the couple perceived their difficulties, but after several years of individual psychotherapy this shift to marital therapy may indicate a major move toward a new perception of their problems. So, the stage was set for further swift and dramatic developments.

The fact that they meticulously executed the assignments they were given, even though they must have been puzzled as to how these related to their difficulties, further illustrates their investment in the therapeutic effort. Apparently, Erickson had quickly reached the conclusion that they were, as persons, too different to remain together. It is not clear which element or elements led him to conclude that this difference was not merely a difference in appreciation of outdoor activities, but was far more fundamental. Rather than telling them so or hinting at it, he provided them with experiences which they could interpret themselves in this way at the appropriate time. It is the nature of metaphors that two people who receive the same symbolic assignment may very well have different experiences with it. Certainly, this couple did. The wife's execution of the last task was especially interesting. Given the freedom to choose her own project, she resumed the activity she had detested, once again climbing "the mountain of her marital distress." Erickson's message that the therapy was completed must have been the final puzzle for the couple.

In ancient times, the wealthy went to the oracle of Delphi to seek advice from the Gods about important decisions. The answer received was usually vague and unspecific, requiring considerable further interpretation by the receiver before it could be acted upon. Of course, in this process of interpretation, the receiver had to confront his beliefs, hopes, fears and expectations in order to be able to reach any conclusion at all.

In essence, this couple was given a verdict much like a Delphian oracle. Only through their own interpreting activity could they decode the message. This assured that they would become aware of thoughts of divorce only when they were ready to deal with them and this occurred earlier for the wife than the husband. The metaphorical strategy, in providing a certain protection to the patients, made it feasible for Erickson to raise the possibility of divorce.

Now, what about all of us doing symbolic therapy from now on, sending couples to the botanical gardens and up and down Squaw Peak, or to comparable local sights? I think that the gravest peril for Erickson's contributions to psychotherapy lies precisely in such attempts at mimicry of the great master. Let me point out some of the dangers invoked should we follow this example on a large scale. To begin with, not many of us are likely to be consulted by couples from a distance of over 2000 miles, which itself represents a difference in what people expect and are ready to do. Furthermore, although you may be provoking an inner search by using a metaphor, people will more quickly abandon that search if it seems fruitless. Some may think you just have a strange habit of expressing yourself in an unnatural and vague way. And most important, you are likely to have insufficient knowledge about your patients for formulating interventions if you limit yourself to the amount of information gathering that Erickson did overtly. That is, unless you yourself have several decades of therapeutic practice behind you and have developed your own ways to make accurate assessments without asking many questions, you are less likely to succeed with such parsimony.

So, the first guideline for trying to use Ericksonian elements in therapy would be: *It is better not to use some Ericksonian approaches*, particularly those elements that are connected with his being as famous and as experienced as he was. (And in case you are almost as famous and experienced as Erickson was, you may be *able* but *unwilling* to use Ericksonian elements because you are likely to be trying to accomplish something of your own.)

Care should also be taken with many of the elements that contributed to the *stylistic* and *aesthetic* qualities in Erickson's work. These are the aspects of his work which elicit much of the fascination and admiration that one feels when reading his cases. While they make his therapies into an art, they are not indispensable to a satisfactory outcome for a treatment. In this category one finds the *parsimony* of his interventions, especially the way he achieved this later in his life. Related to this are remarkable feats such as treating two problems at the same time, one overtly and at a request of the patient, the other covertly, without even checking that the patient is aware of the existence of this problem. Erickson and Rossi (1979) analyze a therapy where Erickson not only directs his treatment at the chief complaint of hyperhydrosis, but at the same time, without the patient's awareness, he directs his efforts towards her sexual functioning, which he suspects to be a problem too.

This also ties in with another fascinating stylistic element: gathering information and gaining impressions without overt questioning. Of course, this provided Erickson with various opportunities to use surprise and confusion on his patients when accurate revelation appeared to have no overt basis in information given. But, until we can achieve the same degree of accuracy with our observations, we should employ overt and, if necessary, elaborate questioning.

We should also be aware of the fact that most of us will not ever achieve the same extremes of flexibility and creativity. I must admit that, besides admiration, I also experienced some feelings of slight depression at the time when I read Haley's *Uncommon Therapy* (1973). However, such feelings can be outgrown. Upon finding that a certain approach worked well, we may want to use it again, rather than trying to invent a new solution to a similar problem.

I now turn to the question of which Ericksonian principles are suitable for larger scale application in psychotherapy and how this could be promoted. To be sure, much has already been done in this respect. Largely as a result of the contributions of Milton Erickson and those that came after him, goal-directed approaches to psychotherapy have gained status in the field. Brief therapy is no longer looked upon as a poor substitute to long-term treatment and symptom relief is no longer considered a waste of time. In hypnosis, there is already a clear departure from earlier unsophisticated methods, which sought to eliminate symptoms by direct and repetitious suggestion.

Still, this process of assimilation has not been exhausted. We now have at our disposal a treasury of examples through case studies and commentaries, which is continually augmented by new books and articles as numerous specific interventions are inventorized. Erickson's joint publications with Rossi (Erickson & Rossi, 1974, 1975, 1979; Erickson, Rossi, & Rossi, 1976) are undoubtedly the most comprehensive works in that respect.

While these efforts toward detailed analysis should continue, we should not ignore the plight of the beginning therapist. Is he equipped to use Ericksonian techniques? Can he apply varieties of double bind or amnesia, be indirect and permissive, use metaphors, pace before leading, employ the utilization approach? How well does he manage the buckshot approach and how often does he succeed in providing a useful positive framework? I name only a small selection of the elements that come jumping at us from the literature. I think each of these items is worth incorporating into the therapeutic armamentarium, but, to date, we lack all but intuitive knowledge to do so.

Nathan Epstein (1980) argues that in therapy we should distinguish macro stages and micro moves. The first are the major blocks of any therapy and include assessment, contract setting, treatment, and closure. The micro moves are the interventions used in the therapy procedure to carry out these macro stages. Epstein states:

> When therapists discuss techniques of therapy, they invariably talk about "Micro Moves." This area is what makes therapy so challenging, rich, and exciting, and such an opportunity for creativity on the part of the therapist as well as the patient. It comprises much of the "art" of therapy. However, our group has come to feel that it is a mistake to present too much material on the "Micro Moves" to beginning therapists. In our opinion, it only serves to confuse and frighten them, and in many instances, to encourage them to perform as "wild therapists" in a highly undisciplined manner in the course of their attempts to model themselves on the "master therapists" they have either observed in action or whose papers they have read.

This commentary deserves attention when thinking about presenting Ericksonian elements to beginning therapists. It is clear that Erickson's own writings are overwhelmingly on the level of what Epstein calls micro moves, and I think Epstein makes a strong point by stressing the need for a larger framework for organizing these micro moves. To be sure, Erickson was not a strong advocate of rational, logical and systematic learning techniques. Rather, he liked to rely upon "unconscious learning" in his patients as well as in his students. He worked with models, examples, stories, analogies, metaphors, and other methods that foster intuitive, global learning.

In my opinion, Epstein's reasoning is sound when it concerns beginning therapists. The analogical modeling approach may be preferable to transmit *skills,* but analytic knowledge and critical thinking must be incorporated to maintain the quality of therapy. So, my second proposition for using Ericksonian approaches would be in accord with Epstein: *For the benefit of beginning therapists, emphasis should be placed on the study of macro stages rather than micro moves in learning about Ericksonian therapy.*

Although the bulk of the effort and attention has so far gone to Erickson's micro moves, I actually think that some of Erickson's major contributions may turn out to be in the area of macro stages. Epstein's proposal seems to fit well into the usual, rational therapeutic approach: assessment, contract setting, therapy, and closure. It is most appropriate as long as "all the trees are indeed leaning in an easterly direction." Erickson's contribution to macro stages was in providing uncommon therapy that departed from the basic scheme when needed. However, we know little about the assessment that Erickson did. We know he had an eye for discovering unusual idiosyncrasies in his patients. We do not know how he did it and we should welcome clarification on this issue. It is clear that by initiating a positive framework he could thereby influence the assessment in a constructive direction. Contract setting is often absent in his work. Instead of making overt agreements, Erickson maneuvered the patient into a position where he was under pressure to generate his own alternative behavior. Therapy usually consisted of fostering change through providing active experiences. Neither was closure a definite stage in his work. He sometimes maintained an active correspondence with former patients for years.

My last topic is how to learn and use the micro moves or specific techniques and approaches. I previously pointed out that Erickson's own teaching is mainly by example; he has given us detailed descriptions of how he proceeded in a great many cases. I think most of us have tried the following: After reading about a case that strikes us as being similar in some regard to a patient we are currently treating, we decide to try a particular approach that Erickson has developed. This may or may not be successful and, gradually, by trial and error, we build up some experience that allows us to be more accurate. Unfortunately, trial-and-error learning must be repeated over and over again if we limit our teaching procedures to the communication of examples. The clinical experience that has been collected by several people now needs recording and analysis. Although Erickson gave many good descriptions of numerous procedures, he did not dictate when to use and when *not* to use a specific approach, and why this should be so.

Picking up the work at that stage, to develop more formalized ways of evaluating procedures, we must clarify various issues. For example, when might a positive framework not apply? And when is it better to be direct and concrete? I realize this detours somewhat from the spirit of Erickson's magic, since, despite his accurate choice of interventions, he does not seem to have had any passion for the formalization of procedures. He probably would not have covered as much new ground in therapy as he actually did, had he tried to map and chart as well as to explore. No doubt his passion for discovery was greater than his interest for systematic charting, but if we want to make use of these discoveries, the more tedious work of analyzing the inner consistency of each type of intervention and especially the demarcation of the field of application will be essential.

After incorporating macro stages and micro moves, I think we, as students, can turn to the last stage in the project of learning from Erickson—one which is truly in his spirit. One of the things he was a master at was turning personal idiosyncrasies into important assets for his patients, as well as for himself. He has demonstrated in an impressive way how to use aspects of his own person to a constructive purpose, including those that would be classified disadvantageous by any standard. Such an undertaking is something that each therapist will have to achieve for himself. It is important that we realize that, to accomplish this properly, we will have to learn to apply our *own* talents and characteristics, rather than to imitate those aspects of Erickson's personality that are not natural to us.

## REFERENCE NOTE

Zeig, J.K. Personal communication, 1980.

## REFERENCES

Epstein, N. Discussion: Engagement techniques in family therapy. *International Journal of Family Therapy*, 1980, 2(2), 97-98.

Erickson, M.H. & Rossi, E.L. Varieties of hypnotic amnesia. *American Journal of Clinical Hypnosis*, 1974, *16*, 225-239.

Erickson, M.H., Rossi, E.L., & Rossi, S.I. *Hypnotic Realities*. New York: Irvington, 1976.

Erickson, M.H. & Rossi, E.L. *Hypnotherapy: An Exploratory Casebook*. New York: Irvington, 1979.

Haley, J. *Strategies of Psychotherapy*. New York: Grune & Stratton, 1963.

Haley, J. *Advanced Techniques of Hypnosis and Therapy: Selected Papers of Milton H. Erickson*. New York: Grune & Stratton, 1967.

Haley, J. *Uncommon Therapy: The Psychiatric Techniques of Milton H. Erickson*. New York: Norton, 1973.

Zeig, J.K. *A Teaching Seminar with Milton H. Erickson*. New York: Brunner/Mazel, 1980.

Chapter 4

# Rapport and Integrity for Ericksonian Practitioners

*Paul Carter*

*In the universe, when a star dies,*
*We continue to see its light*
*For thousands of years to come.*
*Milton, I see you and I am in love.*

You may notice that there are many techniques and analyses of cases that I do not mention in this paper. I intend to focus only on a few principles for the sake of simplicity. Please feel free to enjoy the case examples in all the greater complexity that you know.

## PREFACE

When you learn to ski, you learn individual techniques, the sum of which will allow you to move skillfully and freely down the slope; with continual adjustments to changes in the terrain and snow, you hope to have some choice as to the final place at which you arrive. In order to enjoy skiing and truly master the art, however, you must learn to integrate your movements with your changing perceptions at speeds too fast for the conscious mind. You are forced either to stop yourself or to become a master by relaxing your conscious control and trusting your unconscious intelligence and ability for high-speed integration. At this point, you discover that you are not learning just a sport or a way to move from here to there. You are learning a new concept of "I," a new relationship between "I" and "you," between skier and mountain. You are not separate; you are part of a completely connected and simultaneous system. You are learning about your capacity to create, move, communicate, and love beyond what you consciously know to be possible. You are moving beyond yourself.

Some of you may have had this kind of experience in your profession, in another sport, in music, in dance, in marriage, or in some other context. Perhaps you have not known this experience fully yet. For many people, Dr. Erickson was the context for this kind of experience. Although they may have learned what they came to Erickson for, they inevitably learned much more. An important part of that "much more" was an experience and conception of integrity.

## INTEGRITY—WHOLENESS

"Integrity" is defined by *Webster's* as the state of being complete or whole, the unimpaired or unbroken state of anything. Dr. Erickson often said that what a therapist needs to do is *not* get in the way of the client's progress. Thus, to respect a client's integrity means to treat him or her as a complete human being and *not* get in the way of his/her progress.

Each one of Milton's therapies, each of his "double binds," "confusion techniques," "paradoxical directives," and each of his communications was shaped by and had the shape of integrity. I want to propose in this paper that by practicing some of the principles of "integrity in systems," you will naturally begin developing Ericksonian therapies, communications, and ideas. I will relate three of these principles to some specific techniques and examples of Erickson's work. The first idea is that systems, and in particular people, have integrity. The second is the idea that every part of a system is valuable and important to the balanced functioning of the whole. The third idea is that no part of a system can have unilateral control over the whole.

## SYSTEMS HAVE INTEGRITY

Dr. Erickson was fond of asking his trainees for their definitions of psychotherapy. After listening patiently, he would often offer his answer by telling a story about "Joe."* As a child, Milton was walking into town when he heard everyone saying, "Joe is back. Joe is back!" Joe had spent most of his teenage years and his twenties in and out of numerous county and state penal institutions. Though he had been out of state for several years, everyone remembered Joe. The morning after Joe's return, almost every store had been broken into, and someone's boat and trailer were missing. Nobody was surprised. That afternoon Sally rode into town for supplies; Joe stopped her carriage and asked her if she would

*For the complete case report. see *A Teaching Seminar with Milton H. Erickson*, edited with commentary by Jeffrey K. Zeig, New York: Brunner/Mazel, 1980, p. 211.

accompany him to the Saturday night dance. Sally looked at Joe and said, "If you're a gentleman, you can." The next morning, all the stolen merchandise had been returned, along with the boat and trailer. Saturday evening Joe showed up at the farmhouse where Sally lived with her father. Eventually Joe and Sally were married, and Joe became one of the most respected farmers in the area. Years later, Joe's comment to Milton was, "It took a long time to grow up." Milton would smile at his trainees and say, "And that's all the therapy Joe needed: 'If you're a gentleman you can.' Years of criminal behavior and institutions, diagnostic tests and rehabilitation, and all she said was, 'If you're a gentleman, you can.' That's psychotherapy."

Systems have integrity. People are already whole. Joe was already a whole human being. A basic premise at the heart of Erickson's work was that people don't need to have something new added to them or, conversely, something wrong removed from them. When teaching hypnosis, he would remind a trainee, "I am not asking you to use a new skill that you don't have. I'm only asking you to be willing to use a skill you have but don't *know* you have." Joe always had the ability to be a gentleman. Sally helped Joe discover the ability he had but didn't know he had.

Erickson told me about a couple who came to see him a year after they had been married. They wanted Milton's advice on how to consummate their marriage. The woman came from a very proper and religious family, and the husband complained that she would not even kiss him. She said she thought kissing was vulgar, and she was afraid of what she had never done. Milton looked directly into her eyes and said, "Mrs. C., I'll bet you that you can stand with your toes touching one end of this sheet of typing paper, and your husband will face you with his toes touching the other end of this same paper, and no matter how hard you may try, you won't be able to kiss him." With a look of bewilderment, she agreed to Milton's wager. Milton took a piece of paper and asked a student in the room to very carefully place it right in the doorway. He asked her husband to stand on the other side of the doorway with his toes at one end of the paper. Then, Milton had a student close the door and asked the woman to put her toes on the other end of the piece of paper. They were standing facing each other with their feet on each end of the paper, and she couldn't kiss him. After a moment Milton asked them both to sit down again, and he looked at her and said, "Never limit yourself when there are no limits given." Since she lost the bet, he told her to ride all the way home with her husband, and she was not allowed to kiss him until after they had finished dinner and had retired to the bedroom. She was further not allowed to kiss her husband during the day for the first week after therapy. That was all the therapy he gave to that couple. Nothing new was added; limits were only confused to allow a couple to discover what they already could do.

The technique that perhaps best demonstrates Dr. Erickson's trust in the integrity of his clients is the technique referred to as "Pseudo-orientation in time into the future." The client imagines some future date by which time his problem has been solved. From the perspective of this future date, the client reviews the series of experiences, particularly interactions with his therapist, that led to his change and solution to his problem. In other words, the client designs the progression of the therapy. Implicit, of course, is the assumption that the client's unconscious has the knowledge of precisely what he needs and how to go about solving his own problems. This assumption is a powerful statement about the completeness of an individual person.

Erickson applied a slightly different technique, but with the same basic assumption, with clients who had had repeatedly failed with other therapists. He would have the client describe in detail all the failures, and even as they described these, they could go into a trance state. Once they were in a trance state, he would have them repeat a detailed description of their failures and then describe exactly what it was that they needed to do in order to solve their problems. Then Milton would ask them to come out of trance and suggest that they do exactly what they had told him while in a trance state, i.e., what they needed to do. Therapy was very successful.

The implicit assumption in all of these examples is that you have what you need. Therapy is a process of delimiting in order to realize your real possibilities.

## EVERY PART OF A SYSTEM IS VALUABLE

When you combine the idea that people are already whole with the idea that every part of the system is important to the balanced functioning of the whole, many of the paradoxical techniques that Dr. Erickson used make very natural, logical sense. If someone comes into your office and tells you that he wants to go into hypnosis but knows that it is impossible for him, naturally, knowing the wholeness of the person, you know he can go into trance. Moreover, knowing the value of every part of the system, you know that you should find a way to support the part that has expressed itself in the impossibility of going into trance. Thus, it would be only natural to communicate something like the following: "You do believe it is impossible to go into trance, even though you can, but perhaps it is impossible for your head to go into trance, even though your arm can," or "It is impossible for you to go into trance even though you can sit comfortably. So don't go into trance as you relax deeper and deeper. You know it is impossible for you to *go into a trance state,* and I know it is impossibly easy to go into a trance."

As a therapist you can make an exercise for yourself: Take one statement of desired outcome, and then think of any different possible statements that would be opposed to that desired outcome. Then simply know deep inside yourself, with confidence, that since the person is whole, he can achieve the desired outcome. Be aware also that in some way the opposing parts are important to the person. Next, begin constructing statements that support both the desired outcome and the oppositional statements to the desired outcome.

The correlate to the importance of every part of the system is the idea that, rather than attempting to get rid of any part of the system, you need to find a way to make use of every part of the system. By extending the part, developing it, and developing possible ways to express that part, you find a way to achieve and meet the total needs of the personality. Numerous examples are mentioned in Erickson's articles on utilization. In those examples, the basis of the trance induction is the utilization of some part that previously prevented the client from experiencing suitable trance or a successful therapeutic relationship. Erickson recorded one case which exemplifies a common problem (Erickson, 1959). A woman came who was compulsively distracted by different details—the room, the desk, floor, the external environment in general. Erickson, in talking with her, simply utilized that pattern and extended her awareness of the minutia in the room—the paperweight, the clock, the way the second hand moves. In the process of detailing all the minutiae, he gave her suggestions to relax by slowing down the pace in which he described the details of the room.

This idea itself can be a very fruitful kind of exercise for therapists interested in developing an Ericksonian approach. Pick some rigid pattern that you have found in a client of yours and simply require that you make use of that pattern as the method of inducing the trance state or, in other words, a state of openness and responsiveness to therapy. For example, with the couple that I described earlier the pattern stated by the woman, "I can't kiss," was used as part of Erickson's prescription; he told her "You can't kiss, until after you've gotten home, and you've finished a good meal, and you've retired to the bedroom." Thus the actual change is based on the previous pattern that was a limit to change. This kind of patterning not only builds tremendous success into therapeutic directives; at the same time, it insures the integrity of the system, by demonstrating support for all parts of the system.

On the other side of the coin, many clinicians have experienced the results of operating without this integrity model. I'll mention a few cases here; I'm sure most readers can supply their own. A man once came to me and asked me to help him to quit smoking. After several months, he was successfully breathing and enjoying his life without the aid of cigarettes. However, six months later, he came back with his wife and complained that ever since he had stopped smoking, their relationship seemed to have become more and more difficult. As we explored their communication, a package of cigarettes was brought into the room, and I asked the man to make use of them however he wanted. We very quickly discovered that in their communicational system cigarettes had been the cue to let each other know when something was wrong and it was time to talk. It was their way of facilitating a family discussion, and apparently since he quit smoking, they had not developed any other way of comfortably sitting down and discussing some of their difficulties. I have simplified the description of this case just to emphasize the point that every part has some important value to the total system. Often you never know exactly what it is. Erickson, after giving a client a specific and explicit directive, would often follow it with the suggestion to carry out that directive "in a way that meets the total needs of your personality." In this statement Milton would support this principle of integrity in his client.

A woman came to me who had one breast removed in an attempt to treat a malignancy. Her physicians gave her no certain prognosis but felt the operation had been very successful. Several months after the operation, she developed terrifying hallucinations that a vulture was flying over her house. The hallucination thoroughly disrupted her life. Every 20 minutes she felt forced to run outside and look for that vulture. She said she wanted very much to get rid of the vulture, and so I told her to go ahead and try that. We discussed various ways in which she could get rid of the vulture, and she decided to poison it. She came back a week later and reported that she had poisoned it. The vulture died, but two vultures had come back in its place, and they were even more terrifying. Fortunately, systems do have some kind of self-protective integrity. She had tried to get rid of the part represented as a vulture, and she'd successfully killed off one. But two came back. I suggested to her that rather than kill them, she ought to try to trap them. She set up a trap. Knowing that the best bait was herself, since the vultures were just waiting to come down, rip open her flesh, and, in her words, "ravage her," she went home and lay out in the sun, pretending to be dying. When the vultures swooped down on her, she threw her arms around them and held onto them until they both agreed to come together to my office, as I had told her to do. In my office the next day, she said that she felt a lot stronger and couldn't understand why. So I asked her to keep those vultures inside her, and I asked her unconscious mind to help her integrate those vultures into her life in a way that would be suitable to the total needs of her personality. Rather than throwing away a part of herself, she was integrating a part that was to give her the strength to continue to have a more and more successful therapy.

The nice thing about trying to find a way to integrate all parts of the system into your work rather than throw some away is that the parts will not come back later to interrupt your therapy. If you have tried to remove some part from the therapy, it will usually come back later to interrupt the successful therapy that you've been doing. Integrity seems to act with its own checks and balances.

Examples of this can be found in all different kinds of systems, certainly not just human systems. I'd like to describe briefly a couple of interesting ones. One example can be seen in the result of fire prevention programs in California and several other states. They were so successful at preventing fires that they disrupted much of the ecology that was supported by the fires. Deer starved that had fed on the manzanita that grew only after a fire had cleared away the taller trees. Now the program has been shifted to intentionally setting controlled fires—an Ericksonian technique if there ever was one. Fires are an important part of the integrity of the eco-system.

An experiment was done in which two kittens were raised in small cardboard boxes from the time of their birth. One of the kittens was not allowed to walk for the first several months of its life. The other kitten had holes poked through the bottom of its box so that its legs stuck through. The kitten's box was coupled to the first kitten's box; both boxes had wheels on them so that they moved easily. Thus, one kitten could move around with its feet moving through its environment, and the other kitten simply moved around in the same space without any movement of its legs through its environment. For the first several months of their life both kittens had the same visual experiences. One kitten experienced the kinesthetic integration, and the other kitten did not have any kinesthetic integration. After several months, both kittens were removed from the boxes and set free in the room. The kitten that had the benefit of the kinesthetic integration walked around the room exploring normally. The other kitten walked around the room as if completely blind, walking confidently into walls, bumping into chair legs. In a sense, we can use this as an analogy for integrity at the psychological level as well. The implication is that if you fail to integrate all the different psychological needs and parts of the person, even though you may very well develop one part, the person will still behave as if psychologically crippled. It is the integration of the perceptual systems and the integration of the parts of the person that lead to a successful life within its environment. Integration of all parts is a key to integrity.

## NO PART CAN HAVE UNILATERAL CONTROL OVER THE WHOLE

If there is one principle of integrity that distinguishes Milton's work from most others, it is in his ability to support the notion that no part can have unilateral control over the system. Milton emphasized letting go of partial control in lieu of using what Gregory Bateson referred to as wisdom, defined as "the intelligence of the system as a whole" (Note 1). Milton's favorite way of stating this idea was, "Your conscious mind is very intelligent, and your unconscious mind is a hell of a lot smarter than you are." The prerequisite of all his hypnotic techniques and particularly his dissociation techniques was his trust that the unconscious knows what is best for a person, the unconscious being understood as the intelligence of the system as a whole. When you accept that a person's conscious mind-sets are a limited and partial perspective, then it is only logical to utilize a person's unconscious mind to make decisions of integrity. Thus, the general form of directives can be built as follows: First, identify what you want; second, ask your unconscious to help you do what you want "in a way that is fitting for all parts of your person"; and third, let yourself trust your unconscious, with its fuller perspective, to discover the solution with greatest integrity.

A woman came to me with tremendous fears of abandonment, depression, and a general feeling of not deserving to live. As part of her therapy, while in a trance state, I asked her to choose some way to learn to breathe more fully that would fit with all her needs. She told me she would like to play saxophone. Out of the trance state, she informed me that she hated the saxophone, but that she would find one and bring it to our next session, "if that was what I wanted." I assured her it was. All week I was uncertain about having asked her to do something she hated. Maybe I should have asked her to bring a flute. When she came in, she insisted that I immediately give her a lesson with the saxophone.

So I began to show her how to "*handle* the instrument with *care,* and place your *lips* on the mouthpiece and *blow,* and at first you'll only be *able to play* for one minute before your lips start *hurting* so bad that you will have to *stop.* But after *stopping* and *starting* 10 or 20 times a day for several weeks, you will *get used to it,* and your *lips* will actually begin to *enjoy* the sensations." To make a long story short, six weeks later she came to my office to thank me for the hypnosis: "Two weeks after you showed me how to learn saxophone, my husband began liking me. I asked him why, and he told me that I was appreciating him more and that's all he would say. Then I noticed he was right. For the first time in my life I was enjoying sex, and I *really* did enjoy my husband. I want to thank you for that and your hypnosis, but I've decided to quit the saxophone. I like the flute much better. I know you want me to play saxophone, but it's just too big for me." Her unconscious mind had picked the perfect way for her to learn what she wanted, and neither of us would have thought of that consciously. In retrospect, I can appreciate her perfect choice. The saxophone was something she hated, which satisfied her self-hatred. It also could teach her how to go slowly through a painful experience and learn to *enjoy* feeling and caring. All I had told her was to choose a way to learn to breathe that would suit *all* of her needs.

## CONCLUSION

I want to suggest that we live in an age of more and more potent technology. The work of Milton Erickson demonstrates some of the most powerful technology known in the area of human communication and change.

Learn to work with some of the principles of integrity. Assume and support the completeness of all individuals. Practice integrating all parts into your work. That is the challenge: How do you integrate your needs with others' needs, your quiet with your boisterous, your soft with your hard, your spiritual with your physical, your body with your mind?

As a therapist, you can begin by accepting and utilizing every part of a person. Remember, you are a person, too, and remember, your conscious mind is very intelligent, and your unconscious mind is a hell of a lot smarter than you are.

## REFERENCE NOTE

1. Bateson, G. Personal communication, 1974.

## REFERENCE

Erickson, M.H. Further techniques of hypnosis—Utilization techniques. *American Journal of Clinical Hypnosis, 2*, 3-21, 1959.

Chapter 5

# Understanding Erickson's Approach

*John O. Beahrs*

## INTRODUCTION

To help understand Erickson's approach, I will discuss his work from two perspectives. A clarification of his basically conservative life position, his "theology," loosely speaking, is the first perspective. Erickson's theology is rarely if ever stated explicitly and therefore is sometimes assumed to be lacking. Without this grounding in basic values, however, Ericksonian psychotherapy in its most positive form is meaningless. Because of his theology, Erickson's psychotherapy avoids becoming manipulation without respect or technique without integrity, and supports society with values and direction.

The foremost tenet of his theology that is essential to understanding Erickson's approach is his basic integrity. Faith, commitment, solid values, discipline, and a sense of direction are vital aspects of this tenet. Another tenet is his awareness that life and consciousness are experienced simultaneously at many levels; because he spoke "simple commonsense psychology" to levels not conscious or directly observable to most people, much of his communication seemed "bizarre" but at the same time absorbing and effective. Another aspect of his theology is a belief that everything is basically OK, including all human beings and all of their aspects and parts. This position must be reconciled with the problem of evil in individuals and societies. Struggling with this problem has led many of its proponents into major difficulties. That Erickson avoided these pitfalls and instead rose to greater heights, I see as a major reason for examining his work closely at all levels. The "OKness principle" is based on an awareness of polarity and paradox in everything. This view gives us the option of looking on any aspect of reality in either a positive or a negative manner; and generally, the former feels and works better. We must keep our logical categories clear, especially in distinguishing when value judgments are appropriate. Reframing and paradox are the natural therapeutic offshoots of this awareness of polar opposites in reality. Effective reframing and paradoxical interventions should be literally true at a content level and striking only because they are unconventional.

Autohypnosis is the second perspective from which I want to look at Erickson's work. Autohypnosis is an unique mode of experiencing and behaving that was perfected by Erickson and which may help bridge the gap between psychoanalytic theory and the practice of hypnotherapy. Erickson's earliest clinical experience involved hypnosis, which he explored in as many of its ramifications as he could. Indirect hypnosis permeates nearly all his work. Speculating on personal aspects of Erickson's methods, I suggest the possibility that the flexibility of perception and cognition characterizing the hypnotic state may provide cues to how he operated. He probably functioned in a nearly continuous autohypnotic mode while working with patients, so that what in other contexts would be a symptom could appear as a skill of the highest order. He emphasized the necessity of keeping reality-testing accessed and in charge, so that potentially psychotic primary process thinking was instead tertiary process, approaching unusual creativity. The paradox of flexibility in outlook based on the safety of a strong value structure is a consistent reflection of Erickson's greatness.

One view of narcissistic and borderline personality disorders shows these to be similar phenomenologically to normal expressions of hypnosis. (This view will be explained and developed later in this chapter.) Although recent advances in psychoanalytic theory provide better understanding of narcissistic and borderline personalities, the implicit value judgment of "defect" or "psychopathology" carried by this framework does not appeal to most patients. It is often more effective to help the patient take charge of his own autohypnotic behavior from a position of feeling good about himself. Symptoms then become skills. The power of positive reframing can be seen in these cases even at the level of formal psychiatric theory. New data from hypnosis research support this approach and suggest major revisions of the psychoanalytic method without any violation of basic theory. The result ultimately may approach Ericksonian psychotherapy, and the convergence of psychoanalytic theory and hypnosis research in the study of multi-level consciousness may provide a link between Ericksonian psychotherapy and the psychiatric and research communities at large.

## A "THEOLOGY" WITHOUT A THEOLOGY

"There is no place for theology in mental health." I have heard Erickson (Note 1) say this himself; this position has been restated by most of his interpreters, myself included, while describing his work. Erickson (Note 2) makes a similar point in the Congress brochure: "Each person is a unique individual. Hence, psychotherapy should be formulated to meet the uniqueness of the individual's needs, rather than tailoring the person to fit the Procrustean bed of a hypothetical theory of human behavior." A responsible therapist should try to meet the patient at the patient's level, with respect for the *patient's* "theology" and willingness to speak the patient's own language. Any theology of the therapist's is seen as a disrespectful imposition of a limited belief system on another person for whom that system probably has only limited relevance. The result is often the patient's "resistance" to any threat against the basis of his own self-esteem and sense of identity; the flexibility and malleability that epitomize Erickson's methods are sacrificed.

I am concerned, however, that summarily denouncing theology as valueless in psychotherapy not only smacks of "flow with it" pop psychologies, such as that popularized by Perls (1969), but also misses what is most critical to understanding Erickson's approach. I am convinced that Erickson's work cannot be characterized by an amoeba-like lack of structure that adapts to and "flows with" whatever happens; nor is it a consummate skill in opportunistic "manipulation." Rather, a conservative element, best summarized by the word "integrity," pervades his basic personality and life but is rarely discussed in analyses of his work. In my opinion, a lack of appreciation of this conservatism prevents a full understanding of Erickson and his work. I will attempt to supply that missing element in this chapter. Commitment, faith, respect, direction, discipline, values and responsibility all come to mind as I reflect on this basic quality. I find evidence of it in his personal life and family commitments, as well as in all of his work with patients. Where any of these qualities was missing, he quickly took measures to restore the patient's centeredness into a congruent value system and sense of direction. What has often been mislabeled as "manipulation" could also be considered skillful validation of the patient's own values so that the patient, feeling better about his own basic being, could be more true to himself. That this method works so often can be seen as ratification of a basic faith that values necessary for healthy living are inherent in all of us and only need skillful permission in order to flower and bear fruit. A high-order "theology" is suggested. I will try to define and clarify

Erickson's own "theology" and show how it contributed to his success at all levels of living.

The uniqueness of Erickson's theology lies in its being a "theology" without theology, so to speak, that reached a level of faith and commitment rarely surpassed. That *lack* of theology at one level could lead to the highest levels of theology at another is a fundamental paradox in the character of a man often looked on as the master of paradox. His awesome flexibility and adaptability to difficult psychiatric situations are based on a rather fixed life position, but that relationship is not often appreciated, even by mental health professionals.

Returning to Erickson's home from a jaunt up what is now one of my favorite spots, I found Milton in a serious and reflective turn of mind. "You know, John, that you have *never really seen* Squaw Peak. You *do not know* Squaw Peak, even in the slightest." I replied, "That is absolutely true, Milton. At no time have I had the experience of actually *being* Squaw Peak, that which would be necessary to truly 'see' or 'know' that favorite spot of mine in the truest sense. Yet every time I see, hear, feel, and climb it from any new perspective, however slight the difference, I know *more* of it than I had before, and I find that to be entirely satisfactory." His relaxed nodding and deliberate "That's right" indicated that this awareness was also satisfactory to him. I felt a profound sense of communion in faith, belief and shared mutual respect. We both implied that there *is* a Squaw Peak that is really "out there," but all we can know of it is our sense impressions and beliefs, which we form by integrating the sense impressions into *our* Squaw Peak; each individual's own Squaw Peak is a unique composite of perceptions and beliefs differing from everyone else's. Watzlawick (1976) calls the former, that which "really exists—out there," a "first order reality." Any belief system, from perception of the most simple objects all the way to the most lofty philosophical and scientific theories, can only be like *my* Squaw Peak, unique to me and differing significantly from anyone else's comparable belief system. These belief systems are "*second*-order realities." The first, Reality with a capital R, can be assumed basically only on *faith*, and it is faith in something beyond ourselves that can be depended upon from which we take roots, making orderly living possible (Beahrs, 1977a). The second, the realm of *beliefs*, is the "reality" of our own theorizing. Clear awareness of the distinction between first- and second-order reality, with behavior appropriate toward each, can be seen as a major tenet of Erickson's theology.

I want to emphasize that Erickson's adaptability was not based on relativism but on a faith in a greater Reality without making this faith dependent upon any one fixed belief system. Many others who appreciate the subjectivity of most belief systems have unfortunately been led to a skeptical rejection of anything really real. It is as if there is no tree "really" falling in a forest unless there is someone to observe it, and even if there were, it would not be an individual tree unique from the observer's perceptions. No first-order Reality exists, just an infinite number of second-order realities with no criteria for judging them except, perhaps, utility. Although Watzlawick challenges the subjectivity of our "realities," his work carries an implicit assumption of the greater Reality beneath these; so did the entire body of Erickson's life and work—a point that is too often missed and should not be.

I have dealt with the philosophical aspects of Reality more fully elsewhere (Beahrs, 1977a), reaching the conclusion that forming any functional belief system or "reality" *must depend* on a primary Reality independent of the observer, ultimately taken on faith. I refer to this as "That Which Is" and use it synonymously with a concept of God. Lack of faith in this basic leads to a state that Lowen (1972) and I describe as identical to clinical depression. I cannot comprehend how one can jump to *no* Reality from awareness of the uniqueness of our beliefs about it. In rejecting theology as having "no place in mental health," Erickson must be referring to the impossibility of any second-order belief system *about* Reality being *the* "truth" and to his aversion to imposing his own truth on another person. Everyone has his own perceptions that are, in their own way, as good as those of anyone else, and it is simply decent living to treat others with the respect that they deserve. Working with *their* realities is more respectful, assures their understanding and cooperation, enhances their pride and self-esteem instead of "resistance," and *works better*.

I often compare belief systems to two-dimensional photographs of a three-dimensional object. To warrant the attention of many photographers, the subject must be worth photographing; many photographs are taken of Mt. Rainier, portraying its grandeur from various perspectives. In all the photographs the unifying stability and dependability of "The Mountain" shine through. If basically adequate, any photograph from any perspective is no more "true" or "false" than another; it is a valid portrayal of one aspect of the Reality, but different from equally valid photographs taken from different perspectives. None of them approaches really seeing or knowing the Reality as it is, but we know *more* of it when we view it from more perspectives. Barber (Note 3) says of the different theories about hypnosis: "They're all true but only part of the story." Erickson often said similar things about interpretations of his own work. In his foreword to a Bandler and Grinder work (Erickson, 1975), he prefaces an endorsement with "Although this book . . . is far from being a complete description of my methodologies, as they so clearly state. . . ." In other words, it is a good photograph, but no more.

Erickson is unique among theorists in having preferred to keep his "system" at the level of first-order Reality. With no "official photograph" or orthodoxy, his work can be viewed and organized into psychological systems from many different perspectives. Each is only a perspective; none portray Erickson in his entirety. But viewing his work from many perspectives will help us understand his approach better and help us avoid dangerous misunderstandings. Thus, his theology finds more potent expression precisely because of the deliberate *lack* of a theology, another paradox from the master of paradox. How well this strategy is progressing can be assessed by taking a close look at this volume.

Keeping one's system at a first-order level is not something everyone can get away with, of course, and Erickson seems to be alone in this regard. Most pioneers in psychotherapy provide their own self-portraits, unaware of the fact that even their own beliefs about their work might limit awareness of ramifications of their own work. That Freud and Berne, for example, were often more expansive than most of their followers may partly reflect the irony of their having not limited themselves to the narrow theology about their work that they provided. Under no circumstances would Erickson provide a theology! He insisted that any system was limited and limiting and that his followers must develop their own systems fully. Thus, evolution continues and Erickson's work itself gains increasingly broader appreciation as more and more aspects become evident.

I feel honored to join the ranks of photographers portraying Erickson's work. Like Erickson, I appreciate good photography and have developed modest skill in it. Unlike Erickson, I take delight in developing bigger and better second-order realities to structure my own life and work. While I enjoy living life as fully as possible at many levels, including expanding my ability as a psychotherapist, I am a philosopher at heart—*explicitly* so, in this regard the opposite of Erickson. Recognizing and defining the limitations of my own beliefs enhances rather than detracts from my joy in theorizing. By keeping in mind that the Reality behind my beliefs is infinitely more expansive and that my beliefs can be only different perspectives, I hope to minimize the danger of being limited by the "Procrustean bed of a hypothetical theory" and be able to enjoy the best of both worlds. I am delighted to accept Ericksonian psychotherapy as a quality photographic subject and hope to provide a photograph from a different enough perspective that we can understand Erickson's approach more than we would without it.

I emphasize the underlying conservatism of his basic values for two reasons: 1) This perspective of Ericksonian psychotherapy is rarely portrayed, and 2) it may help make Ericksonian psychotherapy easier for many to understand, for each in his own unique way. The psychotherapy may then no longer be Ericksonian, but the individual therapist's *own* system, developed to its fullest extent—Erickson's explicitly stated goal. What, then, *is* Erickson's "theology," which he has worked so hard to keep *im*plicit and which I wish to *ex*plicate?

Shortly after my initial study with him, Erickson (Note 4) told me, "You know, my work isn't really all that complicated, elaborate or unfathomable. There's nothing mystical. It's really quite simple: all of what I do boils down to *simple commonsense psychology*." That was a concise statement of Erickson's own self-portrait and I believe it is not only subjectively honest but may also reflect more about his methods than many elaborate interpretations. A Mozart sonata may carry as much information in its simplicity as a Wagnerian opera, each having its own beauty.

What is "simple commonsense psychology"? As best as I can see, it is simply what has been known and accepted about human behavior by most people at all times. People do what makes them feel good and what makes those they care about feel good and reflects on themselves. People do what they feel will fulfill their goals or, if they lack goals, they do their best to define some goals or sense of direction in life. People do what they think agrees with or furthers their basic values and beliefs about what is important in life. People like to have fun. They also like to discipline themselves when they feel that this will be to some later advantage. People do what enhances their pride in themselves and their sense of having some place in the order of Reality. While people like to feel safe, they also seek a certain amount of adventure and like to rise to challenges in life. People enjoy loving and being loved. People enjoy a certain amount of competitive aggression. People feel better when they can identify with and have faith in something beyond themselves.

These statements are indeed simple. Why do so many people, especially those called "psychiatric patients," seem to violate this common sense and appear to strive toward negative outcomes, all the while stating that they are unhappy and would like things different? And why did a psychiatrist who emphasized that all he did was "simple commonsense psychology" appear bizarre, unorthodox, and even frightening? To deal with these questions I will discuss another tenet of

Erickson's theology: that consciousness and behavior within a human being may occur simultaneously at more than one level.

If we assume that in some sense there is more than "just one of us" in all people, the apparent contradictions resolve. What most of us term healthy living requires that the "commonsense psychologies" of *all* the different levels, parts, or aspects of the personality must *coordinate* in a collaborative endeavor that is advantageous not only to the overall self but to all its aspects. If any *part* follows commonsense psychology but two or more parts are out of synchrony or at open odds, both of the questions just raised become simple. A negative outcome might be likely by default if an individual's parts are sufficiently discordant and equally matched so that the overall self's power for action is paralyzed. Likewise, one part might get its way, but the result is not what the consciously experienced "self" wants. When we think in this manner, the possibilities are virtually limitless. Erickson's treatments for these individuals appear bizarre because his commonsense methods were directed to one aspect of consciousness that was important but not experienced as "conscious" by the overall self and not visible to most observers. Most of our responses to others are determined by what we see and hear at the overt level of words and behavior, and these responses are considered "appropriate." If we responded to what seems hidden, what otherwise might be commonsense might appear bizarre.

My favorite model for understanding and working with human behavior is to liken the human mind to a symphony orchestra. Like the overall self, it is a complex whole with a personality of its own, but it is composed of many component parts. Each orchestra member has its own sense of identity and unique personality, but they all function together in a coordinated collaborative endeavor to the advantage of the whole and of each one. The music is made by the composite of parts but transcends being a mere algebraic sum; it is held together and organized by the leadership of an *executive,* the conductor. The conductor makes none of the actual music but is in charge—at one level a paradox, at another level simple commonsense psychology.

The concept of the "unconscious" is as critical to understanding Erickson's work as it is to Freud's (1916), though their conceptions of it differ considerably. Erickson did not see the unconscious as a teeming cauldron of untamed fury crying for suppression for society's sake, to be dealt with by a complicated hierarchy of "defense" mechanisms. The unconscious, rather, was seen as the source of all life and growth. Being a repository of all our learning and experiences, it clearly contains information that exceeds what is usually available to awareness. In Erickson's view, the unconscious is actually more likely than the conscious to be cooperative, realistic, dependable, and workable. Erickson tried to access this unconscious consciousness in every way, while dealing with the conscious respectfully to preserve its pride and avoid resistance. The result is often his legendary *indirectness*, which develops from his respect for the conductor's right to feel in control rather than manipulated.

I shared my symphony orchestra analogy with Milton, since I had a hunch that the conductor—like Gallwey's (1974) "Self 1" and Lowen's (1975) "Ego"—might parallel Erickson's concept of a properly functioning "conscious." The "unconscious" would then correspond to the overall orchestra itself, like Gallwey's "Self 2" and Lowen's "Body." Erickson replied that the analogy was "exact," and he was not prone to making absolute statements. *Ideally* the analogy is exact, but only when things are going "as they should" (Erickson, Note 1). He elaborated, emphasizing two points in addition to the necessity of mutual cooperation. Each part must "know his own *role*" and do his best to fulfill it without attempting to usurp a role that belongs to another part. Furthermore, all parts "must treat each other with *respect*." He emphasized that the triad of coordinated cooperative function between levels of consciousness, adherence of each to its appropriate role, and mutual respect is necessary not only for healthy living but also for effective psychotherapy. He had earlier called effective psychotherapy "commonsense psychology." Are these formulations then the same?

A model of "unity in multiplicity" that attends to these many levels of experience and behavior without set expectations may provide a vehicle for understanding how the simple can be made complex or what appears complicated made simple and easy. Erickson clearly preferred as much simplicity as possible and was not disturbed by criticism of his views as simplistic or credulous. I increasingly prefer simpler working models, especially when they fit the data as well as or better than the more complicated. Simplicity feels better and seems to work better. My conductor-orchestra analogy does not require any specific model for the psychodynamics of mental disorder; the ways in which a complex cooperative whole can "go wrong" are manifold. The therapist must know the two requirements of Ericksonian psychotherapy I have cited elsewhere (Beahrs, 1977b): *Observe* at as many levels and with as many senses as possible, and be *flexible*, behaving in a way "formulated to meet the uniqueness of the individual's needs." I have elaborated on the implications of simultaneous multi-level consciousness elsewhere (Beahrs, 1982); Watkins (1978) has similarly explored what makes up a "therapeutic self," also applicable to Erickson's work.

Not only are Erickson's methods basically simple, but he has also been thought to hold simplistic or "credulous" theories about hypnosis, since he stated that what a subject reports about his hypnotic experience or observably does while hypnotized is all that is really going on. This criticism is accurate at the level of Erickson's stated belief. Less credulous views, which are increasingly supported by laboratory data and are actually more congruent with his methods, were often heatedly and emotionally rejected by Erickson. He was hostile to Hilgard's (1977) concept of the "hidden observer" in hypnotized subjects, despite increasing acceptance of this concept by clinicians and researchers. Erickson was emphatic that, "if a hypnotized subject is hallucinating a chair, he *really sees* that chair. Why do we need to waste our time with some hypothetical construct like an 'observer' if that's not needed to explain the data?" (Note 1). He rejected the "new Ego sub-systems" of Gill and Brenman (1959) with even greater fervor. The scientist's reply, of course, is that the construct *is* useful if it is needed to explain data that would otherwise remain anomalous. An example is Orne's (1959) demonstration that simulators of a subject negatively hallucinating a person bump into that person as they believe they "should," while hypnotized subjects who *really* "don't see" the person respectfully and unobtrusively walk around the person while giving all other appearances of not seeing him. I can hardly imagine a better demonstration of consciousness simultaneously occurring at more than one level. Who sees and who doesn't see whom and what?

I have trouble understanding Erickson's motives for summarily rejecting scientific data that could go far toward explaining how he works! What makes his commonsense psychology *seem* bizarre is precisely that he would talk to an observer (anything that can respond must be "observing") that is hidden (unconscious). He defined hypnosis as "communication with the unconscious" (Beahrs, 1971). Multi-level consciousness is likely to occur throughout life, as well as during hypnosis. With most "observers" remaining "hidden," I can see this construct as a valuable extension of Hilgard's research that could guide further research in useful directions. Why would a man of Erickson's stature condemn work that could bridge the immense gulf between scientific research and clinical experience, a gulf that deprives everyone concerned of valuable information?

Since Erickson did not live long enough to answer this question, I can only speculate. At an emotional level, he may have felt that remaining at the level of primary or first-order reality was so important that he discouraged anything that might threaten this status. The original hidden observer theory is somewhat limited, but Watkins and Watkins (1979) have already presented convincing data that, depending on the setting, there may be many "hidden observers," each with a unique personality. The implication is that we may all be covert multiple personalities, with potentially infinite levels. I am not certain whether Erickson would have found the expanded versions of Watkins and myself more congenial. In any case, since the original "hidden observer" concept has proven rapidly amenable to modification, it is hardly "limiting" in the negative sense that he avoided.

Perhaps the message in this is simple. We are all human, Erickson no less so than any of us. We all have our second-order realities, whether or not we actively propound them. These all have their limits, and we all resist challenges to these limits if we consider our constructs sufficiently important to our basic values. I doubt that Erickson would have any problem with this way of looking at the issue. He always encouraged his students to extend their limits beyond his own. Another aspect of commonsense psychology is that it feels good to grow, evolve, push our limits and extend our capabilities. This growth can only come from within the capabilities and implied limitations that constitute our uniqueness.

That important mental processes are experienced and may direct our actions at a hidden level is hardly new to Erickson, Hilgard, Watkins or myself. Credit for the concept of the unconscious is generally given to Freud (1916), but it was implicit centuries earlier in the work of such philosophers as Spinoza (1677): "Experience teaches us no less clearly than reason that men perceive themselves to be free because they are aware of their actions but not aware of the causes from which these arise." While psychoanalytic concepts of the unconscious differ from those of hypnotherapists, they are not incompatible. Hypnotherapists do not deny that unconscious motivations are at times frightening and may lead to defensive processes. Nor do psychoanalysists deny that the unconscious must be given its proper place as the basic life mover. Defining what is unique to the hypnotic view as exemplified by Erickson requires stepping to another level, another tenet of Erickson's theology, which I refer to as the *OKness principle*: Everything that exists, including all human beings and all their aspects or parts, is OK in its basic being. "OK" literally means "approved" or "endorsed." As a principle, it refers to a life position of approval or endorsement of our basic being—whatever judgments are made about the goodness or badness of certain of our behaviors.

The OKness principle can be seen as another way of stating the position of *faith*. What is, is. It feels best and works best to define this inscrutable and unchangeable basic being as positive and to make the most of what *is*, as opposed to what "should be" according to some "Procrustean theory." It does not get tricky until we read the fine print: "and all their aspects or parts. . . ." Most of us would be strained to find anything OK in our aspects that resemble a "little Hitler." Pascall (Note 5) raises this challenge to the OKness principle most explicitly: "If you attempt to reconcile Adolf Hitler to the idea that any person or part of a person is OK, doesn't the very problem of Evil evaporate?" The implication is that if we were to define an evildoer as basically OK we would then lose any rationale for fighting evil and it would fester and grow to levels first abhorrent and then intolerable, as during the 1930s.

We have trouble finding anything OK about a part of a person that sabotages all his attempts to better his life or to achieve healthier relationships, and which reduces that person to a chronic mental patient or criminal. Yet, *looking for and finding* this OKness in even the most negative aspects of life and validating it in a way that furthers more positive outcomes *is precisely what we must do* if we hope to achieve anything near to Ericksonian psychotherapy. This is both the challenge and the key to the door: We have to learn to positively reframe events, experiences and behaviors that seem to threaten our basic values, only to find that these values are strengthened as a result. We must not forget two basic points. In order to do this reframing comfortably, we must be rooted strongly enough in our own basic values that we can encounter and embrace other value systems with a sense of OKness without any threat to our own. Whether or not there is any place for theology in mental health, practitioners will not be able to do what is necessary for Ericksonian psychotherapy without first facing and resolving this central issue for themselves. With deeper and more solid roots, we can send out more branches without fear of being uprooted.

Too quick or glib an acceptance of the OKness principle has led to its abuse by today's pop therapy cults. These have become like religions in their own right, often without a God and with less than desirable results. The pop therapy premise, an outgrowth of nineteenth-century romanticism, seems to be that the OKness of "human potential" can fully surface and flower only when free of restrictive sociopolitical or theological limitations. If we experience ourselves fully, "flow with it," "let it happen," "express our feelings fully," then all will be well. Current statistics for crime and terrorism, alienation in human relationships, escapism such as drug abuse and suicide, as well as our politico-economic quagmire, hardly bear out this claim, yet a large segment of society finds it difficult to reject these premises.

The pop psychology "ethic" described above bears such striking superficial resemblance to much of Erickson's approach that most people can be forgiven if they draw an unfortunate erroneous parallel between the two. A theology without theology, striving to avoid the straitjacket of Procrustean theories, respecting and developing all aspects of a person's being—all these formulations seem to be shared by both. Pop psychology's advocates may even cite Erickson's stature to support their own antitheologies, and conservative individuals who seek more structure and direction in society might easily perceive Erickson as a threat and reject him outright, if they do not take the time and trouble to gain a full understanding. While understandable, these misunderstandings are unfortunate and possibly tragic. To avoid these misunderstandings is another reason why I emphasize Erickson's integrity, commitment, responsibility, discipline and basic values.

The pop therapy ethic misses Erickson's point. We do *not* need to be free of sociopolitical or theological restrictions in order to live fully; it is quite the reverse. He refers to the structure we need with terms similar to what I have emphasized: "discipline," "sense of direction," "basic values," and the like. All these imply the integrity from which his flexibility and adaptability flowed, like branches from a solidly rooted tree. Technicians who "start at the top," so to speak, with the branches instead of the roots may lack this integrity.

Erickson's overall conservatism extended also to a skeptical attitude toward today's many activistic "liberation" movements. In the sense of maximizing our potential as human beings, liberation was certainly one of his primary goals, but he felt that liberation is achieved more by an individual's accepting and dealing with himself as he really *is,* not as he believes he "should be." That which is includes one's biological and early social parenting, sex and innate abilities. Erickson's approach emphasizes the uniqueness of every person. Full respect for and use of our unique differences lead to fulfillment of the potential we have in common. Hence, our equality emerges at another level, a sharing of our basic humanness. At one level each of us is unique; at another we all follow the rules of simple commonsense psychology. For myself, the most liberating change in my life to date could be formulated as *liberation from the need to be liberated.* My own perceived need to rebel had been more the ball and chain. Accepting the basic "givens" of my life enhanced my sense of freedom and enabled me to expand my power for action beyond what it had been. This liberation reveals again the ever-present face of paradox, and I believe it is the essence of Erickson's approach.

In order to "derive" the OKness principle, I start with a variant of the idea of multi-level consciousness, one well known to the ancient Greeks and described by such diverse contemporary sources as Jung (1961), particle physicists and Eastern mystics. It is possible to look on all that exists as *polarity* and *paradox.* For a proton there is an anti-proton, for a male a female, for consciousness the unconscious, for good evil. More importantly, *even the same* event, experience, or behavior can be considered in different ways that would lead to opposing positions or value judgments toward it and each can be equally "true" factually. Elaborating on commonsense definitions of good and evil within a quasi-mechanistic framework has already led to the conclusion (Beahrs, 1977a) that they are inseparable and interdependent, and that few if any events can be seen from only a single perspective of good *or* bad. This observation permits us considerable leeway in how we wish to look upon any situation. We can *choose* to view the situation from perspectives that would emphasize either its OKness or the converse. We can dwell on the restrictiveness of our upbringing, biological sex, limits in innate abilities or whatever and cry for "liberation," or we can choose to focus on the same innate *assets* and develop these to the fullest. This interdependence of good and evil, the ability to see polar opposites in any event or process, is the philosophical underpinning of *reframing* (redefinition) and therapeutic paradox.

Milton Erickson as a person exemplified the advantages of choosing to emphasize the more positive. Few would want to suffer two attacks of anterior poliomyelitis. Few would even survive and many only as physical and emotional cripples. That Erickson capitalized fully on the positive aspects of his handicap is legendary; he developed his powers of intellect and observation to the point that his life work was the topic of an international congress, and his personal and family life reflected far above average fulfillment. Few would see any advantage in dyslexia, least of all intellectually inclined persons. Yet we know how Erickson's assiduous study of the dictionary in his effort to overcome his learning disability led to a unique appreciation of the structure of language and thought that became second nature to him and permeated all of his work.

It is much easier to change our *attitude* toward an aspect of reality than the reality itself. We cannot change our early parenting, biological sex or the structure of our basic being. A few handicaps can be cured, a few more given some palliative relief and many more are to be endured. *All* can be *reframed.* Since positive change is the goal of most therapists, it follows that what can *most easily* be changed should be the focus of attention—*attitudes* and the beliefs that underlie them. Negative reframing is commonplace in long-term psychotherapy, often euphemistically labeled "confrontation" or "awareness." If a patient is considered complacent (feels OK about some aspect of himself that we feel he shouldn't), we may confront him with all of its negative aspects so that he will become more aware and motivated to change. This process sometimes works or long-term therapy would have long ago sunk into oblivion. That this therapy is *long*-term may be partly a consequence of this approach, however. The explicit *or implicit* not-OKness simply does not feel good to a patient. Commonsense psychology tells us that feeling good about ourselves enhances our motivation, and that we usually fight off anything that detracts from our self-respect even when we can see its rationale. I wonder how much "resistance" arises simply by this means; I wonder how much is necessary.

While negative reframing is by no means illogical, the content of confrontation often being quite accurate, it just doesn't feel good and is likely to lead to avoidance behaviors. The essence of *brief* therapy, as described by Watzlawick et al. (1974), is the "gentle art of reframing" —*positive* reframing. The classic case is Tom Sawyer, forced to spend a tedious day whitewashing the fence and fearing an even worse calamity, ridicule by the other boys. The perfect redefining question of "How often does a boy get the opportunity to whitewash a fence?" turns the ridicule of others to envy and soon he is being *paid* by the other children for the "opportunity" to do his work for him. A comparable classic from psychotherapy is the stutterer who had to be a salesman. Rather than treating the stuttering, known to be a resistant behavior pattern, attention was directed to the patient's attitude toward it. He was asked to think about how someone listening to a stutterer will "hang on his every word" and to consider other ways in which his "defect" was really an asset. This reframing was underscored by a paradoxical directive: "Even if for some reason you don't fully comprehend you might feel like relaxing some, I advise you to purposely maintain an optimal amount of stuttering so that you preserve that advantage which is uniquely yours." It was paradoxical, to be sure, but *also literal truth.* I increasingly believe that therapeutic reframing and paradox should be *literally true* at a content level. It *seems* so counter-sensical, absurd, or amusing simply because it runs counter to our normally rigid, structured way of viewing things. The relaxed smile of partly conscious awareness that often accompanies a patient's acceptance of a paradox or reframing betrays recognition of that fact. Since that rigidity in belief structure is often what we most want to loosen in treatment, a positive reframing that leads to a shift in attitude while preserving and enhancing the patient's self-esteem will necessarily change behavior and increase motivation instead of resistance.

Seeing all that exists as polarity and paradox provides us with a basis for either negative or positive reframing. We can define things as not-OK or as OK without in either case violating logic or the data. The OKness principle emerges, then, as not any more "true" than a "not-OKness principle," for which many arguments are hard to refute. The OKness principle as a life position is just *equally* true and it *feels* better and *works* better. Whether or not these factors may even be criteria for "truth" at a higher level is a question beyond the scope of this discussion.

One of the difficulties for most of us in implementing the OKness principle is our appropriate fear of aspects of ourselves that are like a "little Hitler," thoughts and impulses including destructive aggression and denigration of values that are necessary for cooperative personal and social living. Just as we saw earlier that one of Erickson's hallmarks was *keeping his categories clear,* so we need to be clear in this regard, especially in defining the categories in which negative value judgment are and are not appropriate. If we consider a continuum made up of our basic being, feelings, thoughts and impulses, and observable *behavior,* it is easy to see that value judgments are appropriate to behavior and not to our basic being. This awareness allows us to preserve the OKness principle where it is most applicable, without letting the problem of evil "evaporate" into Hitlerism and without abrogating the discipline required for a healthy society. Treatment of an offending person or part-person with *respect* for his *basic being,* with clear confrontation of the negativity of his behavior, rarely runs counter to that person's or part's own assessment. When the confrontation is done with respect for his basic pride, the negative behavior often ceases to be relevant. What was once a "little Hitler" might even become a center of positive creativity, ratifying not only the OKness principle but Fromm's (1973) contention that the worst of destructiveness often follows from frustrated creativity. It also suggests that "simple commonsense psychology" may include some commonsense ethical values that are to everyone's advantage, not unlike the Golden Rule. Here is the theology of Milton Erickson, a "theology" without a theology in the sense of rigid doctrines, yet one whose values and faith in a greater Reality are solidly grounded.

Much severe mental disorder is associated with confusion of the categories of basic being, feelings, thoughts and behavior. Many patients torture themselves with guilt and elaborate defensive structures around *feelings* that they believe are not what they "should" be feeling, while they *actually do* some really bad-news deeds and feel like victims helpless to control themselves. This is only a reversal of logical categories. The therapist has to accept the person and his feelings as OK at the same time as he confronts the patient with both the negativity and the controllability of the behavior and shows respect to the person's dignity. The "flow with it" and "let happen whatever is happening" dictums abused by pop psychology are fully appropriate in the category of feelings (Beahrs and Humiston, 1974). Feeling fully and flowing with even an unpleasant feeling, as opposed to doing what one feels like doing, may carry the implicit assumption of basic OKness with the same force as an overt positive reframing, but at a deeper level than is usually conveyed by words alone. Words were more Erickson's style, however. He was much more likely to ask questions carefully worded to stimulate the patient to do his own reframing than he was to supervise a patient through an awareness continuum.

Even in regard to behavior, while Erickson was not someone to run away from a strong confrontation when indicated, he preferred whenever possible to reframe the behavior itself. If anything positive could be found in it he was likely to emphasize and elaborate upon this and to suggest ways of doing it even more effectively within a positive framework. Since most people strongly resist changing bad habit patterns, this method is more likely to secure cooperation instead of resistance, with the paradoxical effect that the undesirable behavior itself might change more quickly with less subjective effort. Behavioral reframing works, again, only when the content of the reframing is literally true. I find it liberating and refreshing to find out how often this fact actually proves true. The awareness helps me to let go of unnecessarily rigid beliefs and behavior patterns while strengthening rather than loosening my values and integrity. It also helps me to deal with negative behavior in others more effectively, with respect for their values but in no way threatening to abrogate my own.

In these ways one can understand the elegant paradox of how the flexibility and adaptability of Erickson's creative methods flowed outwards like branches from the roots of his basic faith and values. At one level these were rigid and immovable, but his flexibility depended upon them. An unswerving faith in the OKness of the commonsense psychology by which all people operate led him to *look for the OKness where this seemed to be missing*. When this search involved reframing on levels far from our usual structures of thinking, Erickson seemed to be operating far beyond most "ordinary" people. The fact that reframing was usually therapeutically effective is the primary ratification of the underlying faith itself.

Erickson was not the only psychiatric innovator to propound the OKness principle. It had been well stated by Perls (1969) and Berne (1966), each the founder of a major school of psychotherapy. In what way, then, does Erickson differ from these others? The amorality of Perls' own personal life and its extension to the pop therapy "ethic" in general can probably be traced to a failure to distinguish categories sufficiently to deal with the problem of evil. To "flow with it" is appropriate for feelings, but limits must be placed upon behaviors. Transactional analysis often falls victim to the problems of any systematic theory, no matter how workable it may be at some levels. Describing nearly universal behaviors as "games" and "rackets"—implicitly not-OK terms—violates the basic principle of Berne's psychotherapeutic system. Even implicit negative reframing in clinical practice has the same consequences as any negative redefinition, not least the arousal of unnecessary resistance.

Erickson avoided these problems by keeping clear his logical categories, maintaining a strong sense of his own values and not allowing himself to be limited by ascribing to any theoretical or methodological orthodoxy. Fully implementing the OKness principle requires the solid faith that it is there when it appears most lacking, the willingness and flexibility to look for it and often find it where least expected and the ability to utilize it so that it is enhanced at all levels. I know of no psychotherapist who has carried this method to anywhere near the level achieved by Milton Erickson.

## AUTOHYPNOTIC BEHAVIOR AS SYMPTOM, SKILL, AND CREATIVE PSYCHOTHERAPY

Understanding how Erickson *did* his work, at a level beyond pure technique, might be facilitated by taking a close look at the psychological state of mind from which he operated. Many ramifications of Ericksonian psychotherapy have evolved from a thorough grounding in the use of hypnosis. Erickson and Rossi (1977) clarify how many of the former's most profound insights had "come" to him in the form of autohypnotic experiences even early in his life. Knowing this, it would seem difficult to fully understand Erickson's approach without some understanding of spontaneous autohypnosis.

Early in my psychiatric practice, a 33-year-old woman was brought into the emergency room agitated and disoriented, talking and responding to something neither seen nor heard by objective observers. She appeared to be oblivious to all other attempts at communication. Though quite young, she had been diagnosed as schizophrenic for ten years and had been treated with heavy doses of Thorazine for similar episodes with minimal effect. Because of my clinical experience with both hypnosis and schizophrenia, I perceived her quite differently. "This lady is not schizophrenic. She does not have any loosening in her thought processes. She is simply in a hypnotic age regression, although I don't know why. If I talk to her as I would any regressed hypnotic subject, I wonder if she will hear me and shift more into a 'normal' state of hypnosis?" Following Erickson's method of joining the patient's system, I talked with her as I would any subject who had entered a similar state in a controlled hypnotic setting. Within 20 minutes she was indistinguishable from any deeply hypnotized subject, having good rapport with me and accepting suggestions that her hypnotic ability was an important skill that she could use under her full direction and control. Except for a fleeting one-minute episode a week later, her psychosis did not recur. Instead, she was a virtuoso hypnotic subject. *What was once a symptom had become a skill.* She was by no means "cured" in a characterological sense; she was still an immature person whose subsequent development in psychotherapy could be looked upon as a delayed maturation. She *was* cured, however, of the floridly psychotic behavior that had led to her having been treated as schizophrenic, and she was cured of this in only 20 minutes.

What happens once can happen again. I became increasingly attentive to other disturbed behavior that might be looked upon as spontaneous hypnosis and also subjected to a similar, rapidly effective treatment paradigm. In quick succession I dealt with a couple of intractable patients who proved to be classic multiple personalities, and one episodically psychotic woman whose communications were rich, expansive, pregnant with information, "bizarre" in an almost Ericksonian sense, and yet clearly psychotic. In each case clarification of what was going on, validation of its positive aspects and instruction to do them even more positively led to improvement. When the psychotic symptoms had become a normal hypnotic skill, what was usually left was an immature or overly rigid character structure whose spontaneous hypnotic behavior could be considered an attempt to cope with a difficult situation otherwise beyond the person's perceived abilities. Frankel (1976) subsequently suggested that taking charge of spontaneous hypnotic ability may be a desirable shortcut to long-term therapy.

In each of these cases there was a disorder of *self-identity*. Some patients split into sub-parts that don't coordinate well; multiple personality is at the extreme end of this continuum. For others the boundary between their self and their environment is diffuse; total symbiosis is at the extreme end of another continuum. Both processes usually occur simultaneously, though the expression of one may predominate. Kernberg (1975) and Kohut (1971) have defined these processes as the essence of "narcissistic" and "borderline" personality disorders, generally considered as among the most difficult challenges facing modern clinical psychiatry. Kohut (1966) discovered that these patients often form a unique type of intense transference and therefore might be "analyzable"; this discovery led him into a study of narcissism comparable to Freud's early work with neurosis. Narcissism is no longer seen as a primitive precursor to object relations; instead, it is the essence of such essential qualities as intuition, empathy, humor, creativity, and wisdom. I am not sure whether the psychoanalytic community has fully awakened to the significance of this immense positive reframing that has occurred within their own system—what was once seen as a severe developmental defect is now seen as essential to the highest levels of living. Kohut explicitly redefines the goal of psychoanalytic treatment from "curing" the patient of narcissism to helping him transform it from "pathological" into "healthy" narcissism, being quite clear about what distinguishes one from the other. This redefinition may provide a bridge between the psychiatric community at large and Ericksonian psychotherapy, as well as shedding some light on how Erickson might have operated.

When I began to see many narcissistic and borderline patients in more "simple commonsense" terms as using autohypnosis to their disadvantage, I had to face the task of looking in depth at what is meant by "hypnosis." Freud (1920) compared hypnosis to love; each involves some dissolution of ego boundaries between self and object so that, although at one level the patient lost some identity, at another it was actually enhanced. Hilgard's (1977) recent demonstration that dissociative behavior is manifest in normal hypnosis (one or more "hidden observers" perceive and experience simultaneously with but differently from the conscious hypnotized subject) suggests that both splitting and merging contribute to hypnosis. Both of these "mechanisms" are involved in severe narcissistic personality disorders, and I have already shown that many of these patients were using autohypnosis in a maladaptive manner.

Another philosophical and treatment issue followed: To what extent is it useful to perceive ourselves as a whole or "cohesive self," defined by Kohut (1971) as that which experiences itself as having extension in space and continuity in time? When is it more useful to see ourselves as being divided into many parts, with each having some sense of self-hood of its own? When is it more useful to see ourselves as a part of a greater whole? Since we truly exist at all these levels at the same time, I use the term "useful" instead of "true." All levels of organization from elementary particles through cells to societies must be experiencing their identities simultaneously, each in its own way. When does emphasizing one of these perspectives *work,* when not, and how can we change the latter to the former? I have worked out some of the ramifications of such an approach in my second book (Beahrs, 1982). I hope that these new ways of looking at personality may help bridge the gap between the seemingly inscrutable work of Milton Erickson and the psychiatric community at large.

While *ex*plicit formulation of the issues of unity and multiplicity is still in progress, I suspect that *im*plicit awareness of their relationship led to much of Erickson's success. He was acutely aware of multi-level consciousness and used his keen powers of observation to notice when some hidden aspect of a person needed to be contacted and dealt with. The same skill in observation helped him know enough about that part in advance to contact it in a way that would both validate its intrinsic OKness and make it want to change whatever attitudes and behaviors might need changing. Looking at Erickson's work in this light has treatment implications for us therapists who prefer to work within some theoretical structure while yet maximizing our flexibility. Seeing any of us as a covert multiple personality, being aware of the hidden observers or orchestra members who may perceive us more accurately than a patient's overt overall self, we may want to assume an attitude somewhat like that of a CIA agent in the field, saying and doing only what we would feel comfortable being observed by everyone present. This attitude would influence us toward a more overall OK position because we would want the patient and all his parts to view *us* as OK.

Watkins (Note 6) states, "With any patient I assume that there are at least two 'personalities.' One wants to get well, or he would not be coming to my office. The other does not want to get well, or he already would be well. Too much, or the wrong kind of reassurance to the first might make an implacable enemy of the second, sabotaging treatment." "Resistance" or resistant parts is another issue in Ericksonian treatment. Many therapists who talk about bypassing, neutralizing, or turning around a patient's resistance to achieve a desired end convey an implicit negative judgment against the part that is doing the resisting. They miss

Erickson's and Watkins' point—that the resistant part is probably resisting for a valid reason and possibly expressing very potently the life survival instinct that so often appears to be missing in psychiatric patients. The goal should be instead to contact that aspect, looking for its positive force, and make it an ally instead of conceiving it as resistance.

Freud's early work (1916) provides an interesting historical twist on spontaneous hypnosis. He developed much of his original psychoanalytic theory from studying patients much like those I am talking about now, those whose symptoms resemble hypnotic behaviors. He was a competent hypnotist, and one can wonder why, if the disorders he saw were expressions of hypnotic behavior easily managed as such, he did not do so. I believe that ultimately Freud gave understanding a greater priority than treatment. If phenomena A (hysterical and narcissistic disorders) are really the same as phenomena B (hypnosis), which we understand no better than the former, then to "explain" A as "really" B only shifts the burden of what *needs* to be explained. Freud's dissatisfaction with pseudo-explanations has led to the accumulation of much scientific data we might otherwise be lacking, but adequacy of theory and what works in practice do not always correlate as well as theorists would like. More pragmatically, if phenomena A are essentially the same as B, and we know what to *do* with B, we can apply methods effective with B to dealing with A whether or not we fully understand the dynamics of either. Despite theoretical controversy about the nature of hypnosis, there is remarkable consensus on certain basics of how to *use* it, and that knowledge can logically be extended to any phenomenologically identical psychopathology. A further advantage of the hypnotic approach is that most therapists make implicit positive value judgments about hypnotic behavior. It feels better to take charge of a misused ability, so that *what was once a symptom becomes a skill.* I do my best to follow this maxim as much as feasible in my own clinical work.

Given this phenomenological identity, any insights into spontaneous hypnosis gleaned from the research lab should also carry over to clinical work with these "psychopathologies." The implication that, even in borderline patients, intact hidden observers may be present and may perceive the therapist accurately, no matter how intense the transference may be overtly, suggests a possibly major revision in psychoanalytic method without significantly violating its theory. Talking directly to the hidden aspects or "communicating with the unconscious," as Erickson defined the hypnotic modality (Beahrs, 1971), might serve the same function as working through the transference but more expeditiously. Psychoanalytic therapy would become archaic while remaining valid in principle. Going from Kohut's psychoanalytic theory to Hilgard's "hidden observer" requires that we recognize that the "vertically split-off sectors" of the patient's personality are always there, with a *simultaneous consciousness of their own*. This conclusion, nearly unavoidable from hypnosis research, can bridge the gap. I feel also that this position can be framed in terms that enhance a patient's self-respect. Kohut's formulation of narcissism as the essence of creativity is certainly an auspicious start.

Few of us can function like Erickson, rising to the highest level of competence while rejecting theory as "Procrustean" and limiting. Most of us need some theoretical structure as a base of operation, to strengthen our roots in a theology we have seen as essential for Erickson himself as for the rest of us. As long as we see theory as having that purpose alone, plus whatever joy we may get in working with ideas apart from their practical application, I can find little problem in theories. Recognizing that any theory is only an approximate model and that its limits will be transcended by most difficult patients in clinical practice, we are not prevented from also seeing each patient as a unique individual. For those of us who both need and like theoretical structure, it may help to become proficient within several seemingly different frameworks. For each individual, one framework will work better than another, and which works for whom will not always fit our preconceived ideas. Although some theory can strengthen our rootedness, responding to the uniqueness of each patient inevitably forces us to keep updating our theories so that they become our tools instead of our master. Gedo and Goldberg (1973) show how different models work better for several specific cases, but all their models are psychoanalytic. That psychoanalysis is itself only one of many models is an extension of their views, which extrapolated to its logical conclusion merges inextricably into Ericksonianism.

In an earlier paper (Beahrs, 1977b) I reported that I had functioned in an autohypnotic manner for a considerable period of time in coping with a major life challenge. Most striking was that when working with patients I seemed to be functioning almost like Erickson, being unusually attentive to subtle communication by "hidden" parts of the patient that seemed then as clear and obvious as the overt words and behavior, and responding to these as naturally as I would to "normal" communication. "Bizarre" to be sure, but logically appropriate, strikingly effective—and, even more interesting, it seemed almost as if it "just happened." For years I had despaired of achieving anything like that mode of functioning so that I did not consider it to be a significant life priority. Yet here it was, "just happening" without any effort, when I was in a somewhat altered state of consciousness to boot. I hypothesized that much of the therapeutic effectiveness of my unusual interventions was precisely due to the *unconventionality*, which itself creates a climate for change, and the *logical appropriateness*, which made the resulting change more likely to occur in an appropriate direction.

Even though Erickson rejected it, Gill and Brenman's (1959) formulation of hypnosis as an adaptive "regression in the service of the ego" fits my experience quite well, and I suggest it may be important in "how to do" Ericksonian psychotherapy at a level beyond pure technique. This is the psychological state of mind from which the work is done. Elsewhere (Beahrs, 1982) I have distinguished hypnotic from nonhypnotic behavior as relatively toward the righthand end of three continua of human experience: 1) voluntary vs. involuntary, "hypnotic" behavior seeming to flow effortlessly and even "just happen"; 2) usual structured perception vs. fluidity of perception, with an almost infinite capacity for modification and extension of our "perceptions" in the state we call hypnotic; and 3) "reality" thinking vs. "regressed" or "creative" thinking. The hypnotic end of these continua certainly fits Erickson's style. Erickson had a well-known personal preference for a relative preponderance in executive control by what we usually call the "unconscious." The unconscious functions more economically, with less sense of effort, is able to accurately process information at many more levels simultaneously, and is able to utilize all the modes of thinking and problem-solving acquired during the individual's life. Applying these assets to the issue at hand characterizes autohypnotic behavior when it is being employed adaptively. Considered this way, the Ericksonian therapist is as much a hypnotic *subject* as he is a hypnotist, with his patient being as much a hypnotist as a subject.

Some words of caution are in order. Autohypnotic behavior is hardly to be recommended for everyone and certainly not for anyone all of the time. There is often a fine line between the highest levels of creativity, approached by Erickson, and frank psychosis. Although patients with narcissistic disorders may be in an autohypnotic state, as discussed, they *are* disturbed. They do not get along very well with themselves or their environment. What distinguishes this state from adaptive hypnosis or "healthy" narcissism? I believe the answer lies in the third of the three continua within which I have defined hypnosis, the level of cognition. "Regression" per se usually implies primary process, primitive or magical thinking based more on symbolism and wish fulfillment than on assessment of data and probabilities. Although it is more flexible and has its role in dreams and the creative process, primary process without that assessment of data and probabilities, which we call secondary process or reality-testing, generally amounts to psychosis. Normal hypnosis is not just regression, but regression "in the service of the ego." This wording implies that it is functional and serves the interests not only of the ego but the overall self. Therefore, the primary process must be available, with its flexibility and malleability, but also full reality-testing must be *simultaneously* present. Without close supervision from the latter, there is too much tendency to over-read or misread the subtle cues that are perceived so clearly, especially when they do not fit our usual beliefs about life and reality too closely. This tendency may lead either to obsessing with the "occult" or even to frankly delusional thinking.

A theoretical *belief* is only a problem when confused with *observation* or experience. Keeping our categories clear, *any* observation or experience is nothing more or less than an observation or experience and could not amount to a psychosis. Only when a *belief* is attached can it qualify for that judgment. When not shared by other people but still not refutable, it is likely to be called "occult." When it flagrantly violates what can be measured and tested, it becomes delusional. Because most belief systems are not flexible enough to deal with the almost infinite potential for what can be observed and experienced within our unconscious or inner self, they may present a twofold liability: 1) They may rigidly influence us to exclude awareness of important perceptions that do not fit the system but considered in themselves are valid. 2) There is a tendency to interpret striking experiences erroneously in terms of preexisting beliefs, which can merge unavoidably into psychosis. Possibly these are two *behavioral* reasons for Erickson's theology of avoiding theologies.

Kohut differentiated pathological from healthy narcissism by the presence of a schism or horizontal split between the intuitive-empathic-creative aspects of life and the reality-testing functions. When the patient was functioning at one level, the other was likely to be excluded. When the levels are integrated, we have an expanded type of thinking, which Arieti (1976) terms *tertiary* process and which constitutes the essence of creativity. When spontaneous hypnosis is a problem, it may simply be that it is not yet sufficiently integrated with reality testing and behavior control and not yet "in the service of the ego"—primary instead of tertiary process. When what was once a symptom has become a skill, all levels function together as a harmonious whole. Reality-testing is not abdicated but may "drop back" to the level of an observer that remains operational and in charge, like the conductor sufficiently strong to let the orchestra "play itself" most of the time. The strength of this observer may be what distinguishes it from the hidden observers present in disturbed patients, who helplessly watch the drama play itself before their eyes until they find out how to take charge and help out. When the conductor is permitting the orchestra to play itself, there is no doubt to anyone concerned as to who the executive actually is.

In summary, I want to emphasize several basic precautions that a student of psychotherapy must learn. Without this, attempting to understand and practice Ericksonian psychotherapy could be ludicrously ineffective at best and dangerous at worst. First is a need to examine and be fully aware of one's own theology and value system and to be able to keep this clear and distinct from that of one's patients or clients. Such a student must have sufficient experience in dealing with human behavior to provide a structure protective to both himself and his patients. As even Erickson maintained, this experience can best be gained by thorough grounding in "basics" in an accredited professional training program. He must be able to keep his categories clear. He must not confuse second-order belief systems with the first-order Reality beyond them that can only be fully appreciated on faith; when dealing with different levels of consciousness he must keep clear about what is appropriate to each level and not confuse one with the other. The student must clearly differentiate between thoughts, feelings, behaviors, and a part-self's basic being, and he must be able to distinguish observations and experiences from the beliefs that are often attached to them, being able to discern when and at what levels a person's beliefs are appropriate. This is all no mean feat, but I do not know of any shortcuts. First and foremost is to become deeply rooted in one's own basic integrity, without which a person has no business practicing psychotherapy in the first place. The rest is a lifelong process of growth and discovery, which can keep even the oldest of men young—and Milton Erickson always remained young.

## REFERENCE NOTES

1. Erickson, M.H. Personal communication, 1976.
2. Erickson, M.H. International Congress on Ericksonian Approaches to Hypnosis and Psychotherapy brochure, 1979.
3. Barber, T.X. Personal communication, 1977.
4. Erickson, M.H. Personal communication, 1972.
5. Pascall, G. Personal communication, 1979.
6. Watkins, J.G. Personal communication, 1979.

## REFERENCES

Arieti, S. *Creativity, the Magic Synthesis.* New York: Basic Books, Inc., 1976.

Beahrs, J.O. The hypnotic psychotherapy of Milton H. Erickson. *American Journal of Clinical Hypnosis.* 1971, *14*, 73-90.

Beahrs, J.O. *That Which Is, An Inquiry Into The Nature of Energy, Ethics, and Mental Health.* Portland, Oregon: Integrated Arts, Inc., 1977 (a).

Beahrs, J.O. Integrating Erickson's approach. *American Journal of Clinical Hypnosis.* 1977, *20*, 55-68 (b).

Beahrs, J.O. *Unity and Multiplicity: Multi-Level Consciousness of Self in Hypnosis, Psychiatric Disorder and Mental Health.* New York: Brunner/Mazel, 1982.

Beahrs, J.O., and Humiston, K.E. Dynamics of experiential therapy. *American Journal of Clinical Hypnosis.* 1974, *17*, 1-14.

Berne, E. *Principles of Group Treatment.* New York: Grove Press. 1966.

Erickson, M.H. Preface to Bandler, R., and Grinder, J. *Patterns of the Hypnotic Techniques of Milton H. Erickson, M.D.*, Cupertino, California: Meta Publications, Inc. 1975.

Erickson, M.H., and Rossi, E.L. Autohypnotic experiences of Milton H. Erickson. *American Journal of Clinical Hypnosis.* 1977, *20*, 36-54.

Frankel, F.H. *Hypnosis: Trance as a Coping Mechanism.* New York: Plenum Medical Book Co., 1976.

Freud, S. *Introductory Lectures on Psychoanalysis* (1916). New York: Doubleday, 1943.

Freud, S. *Group Psychology and Analysis of the Ego* (1920). New York: Norton, 1975.

Fromm, E. *The Anatomy of Human Destructiveness.* New York: Holt, Rinehart & Winston, 1973.

Gallwey, W.T. *The Inner Game of Tennis.* New York: Random House, 1974.

Gedo, J.E., and Goldberg, A. *Models of the Mind: A Psychoanalytic Theory.* Chicago: The University of Chicago Press, 1973.

Gill, M.M., and Brenman, M. *Hypnosis and Related States: Psychoanalytic Studies in Regression.* New York: International Universities Press, 1959.

Haley, J. *Strategies of Psychotherapy.* New York: Grune and Stratton, 1963.

Hilgard, E.R. *Divided Consciousness: Multiple Controls in Human Thought and Action.* New York: John Wiley & Sons, 1977.

Jung, C.G. *Memories, Dreams, and Reflections.* New York: Random House, 1961.

Kernberg, O. *Borderline Conditions and Pathological Narcissism.* New York: Jason Aronson, 1975.

Kohut, H. *The Analysis of the Self.* New York: International Universities Press, 1971.

Kohut, H. Forms and transformations of narcissism. *Journal of the American Psychoanalytic Association*, 1966, *14*, 243-272.

Lowen, A. *Depression and the Body.* New York: Coward, McCann & Geoghegan, 1972.

Lowen, A. *Bioenergetics.* New York: Coward, McCann & Geoghegan, 1975.

Orne, M.T. The Nature of hypnosis: Artifact and essence. *Journal of Abnormal and Social Psychology*, 1959, *58*, 277-299.

Perls, F.S. *Gestalt Therapy Verbatim.* Lafayette, California: Real People Press, 1969.

Spinoza, B. *Ethics*, 1677.

Watkins, J.G. *The Therapeutic Self.* New York: Human Sciences Press, 1978.

Watkins J.G. and Watkins, H.H. Ego states and hidden observers. *Journal of Altered States of Consciousness.* 1979, *5*, 3-18.

Watzlawick, P. *How Real is Real?* New York: Random House, 1976.

Watzlawick, P., Weakland, J., and Fisch, R. *Change: Principles of Problem Formation and Problem Resolution.* New York: Norton, 1974.

PART III

# *Hypnotic Induction*

*Stephen Gilligan, currently a Ph.D. candidate in psychology at Stanford University, is destined to become a major figure in the field of clinical and theoretical approaches to hypnosis. His article on induction techniques is one of the best papers written on the subject; it is concise and well thought-out and deserves careful study. His chapter includes important material on principles of Ericksonian communication. He also reminds us of the importance of integrity on the part of the practitioner.*

*Marion Moore, M.D., is a psychiatrist in private practice in Memphis, Tennessee, and a former vice-president of the American Society of Clinical Hypnosis. He spent almost 30 years studying with Erickson. Moore was not only one of Erickson's closest colleagues, but also Erickson's personal physician and one of Erickson's closest friends. In his chapter on principles of induction, Moore develops the important point that Ericksonian techniques must be geared to the individual and necessarily reflect the individual style of the clinician.*

Chapter 6

# Ericksonian Approaches to Clinical Hypnosis

*Stephen G. Gilligan*

I would like to discuss in this paper what I consider to be some essential aspects of an Ericksonian approach to hypnosis and hypnotherapy. I want to first contrast briefly the Ericksonian view of the hypnotic relationship to other more traditional views, and then to identify what I consider to be the general principles of communication in the Ericksonian approach and their application to the specific situation of hypnotic inductions. Finally, I want to comment about the need for integrity in applying these principles and techniques. Each of these topics is a major one, and in a short discussion I can convey only a general sense of their significance. Therefore, my remarks will be highly selective and necessarily incomplete. A more comprehensive treatment of these issues will be found in my forthcoming book, *Hypnotherapeutic Changes: An Ericksonian Approach.*

## THE HYPNOTIC RELATIONSHIP

The first issue is the nature of the hypnotic relationship. Below I list the three main views of the hypnotic relationship: 1) the authoritarian approach; 2) the standardized approach; and 3) the utilization approach.

The *authoritarian approach* emphasizes the power of the hypnotist. This approach, spawned by Mesmer and others, is still explicitly exploited by stage hypnotists and is consequently often the conceptualization held by the uninformed layperson. Even many trained clinicians implicitly adhere to this view, which in its extreme form involves some powerful and charismatic operator (usually a male) exercising some strange power over some hapless and weak-willed subject (often a female). In essence, the operator gets the subject to do something he or she wouldn't ordinarily do (e.g., bark like a dog or stop smoking). This approach generally assumes that the unconscious is some passive receptacle into which suggestions are "placed" or some fertile ground which the hypnotist "digs into" so that he can "plant" suggestions. Frankly, I don't think the unconscious should be treated like a piece of dirt. For this and other reasons—such as the fact that direct suggestions generally don't work very well, and people often don't like to be told authoritatively what to do—this approach has rather limited value.

Many people have realized these limitations and subsequently developed what might be called the *standardized approach.* This conceptualization, adhered to by many experimentalists, is in part a reaction to the misplaced emphasis of the authoritarian approach on the power of the hypnotist. The standardized approach generally assumes that hypnotic responsiveness is determined by some inherent trait or ability of the subject. The hypnotist really isn't important—the subject is either hypnotizable or he isn't. This view further assumes that you can assess a person's "susceptibility" to trance by presenting 10 or 20 minutes of standardized and repetitive suggestions and then administering some quick behavioral tests such as hand immobility or heaviness. If the subject passes most of these tests, he is considered a good hypnotic subject; otherwise, too bad. I might note that the hypnotist is considered so unimportant in this approach that suggestions are sometimes put on tape. So, if you're a busy person, you can put the tape on, go out and drink coffee for 10 or 20 minutes, and then come back and administer the tests.

There is nothing inherently wrong with this approach, especially in a research setting, where sometimes it is necessary. However, it doesn't work very well for a lot of subjects, especially those in clinical situations. The standardization approach interprets the large percentage of unresponsive subjects as evidence that some people are just not susceptible to the phenomenon of trance. I think their unresponsiveness is more a reflection of the limitations of the approach. The standardized inductions are usually poor in quality and essentially tell the subject to relax about 40 or 50 times. The standardized form demands that the subject attempt to fit his experience into some predetermined structure; it cannot handle or utilize any difficulties a subject might be having, such as a nagging internal dialogue.

Another problem in the standardized approach is that trance is defined in terms of the number of behavioral items passed on a test. I think this is like defining love in terms of the number of kisses emitted by a person or saying that I can't dance because I don't know the fox trot. I think this approach misses a major point about trance: *It is a subjective internal experience whose behavioral manifestations will vary across individuals.*

This point is central to the Ericksonian approach, which I put under the heading of being the *utilization approach*. In contrast to the authoritarian and standardized approaches, it stresses the *interactional* nature of the hypnotic relationship. Neither hypnotist nor subject is of prime importance; what is of major importance is the *interaction* between the two. The hypnotic endeavor is a *cooperative* effort in which responsibility is mutually assumed. The hypnotist's task is to guide and supervise the subject; the subject's task is to decide if, how, and when to respond to the hypnotist's communications.

The utilization approach also assumes that each person is unique in terms of the strategies used to create his or her own experience and that, consequently, the hypnotist's effectiveness depends upon how well he is able to adapt his strategies to those of a given subject. Thus, standardized communications are not used. The approach further assumes that unconscious processes can operate in an intelligent, autonomous, and creative fashion and that people have stored in their unconscious all the resources necessary to transform their experience. This is what trance is all about: It is an opportunity for the subject to set aside his identification with any limiting conscious processes and shift into a context (i.e., trance) where he/she can access and utilize unconscious resources for therapeutic gain.

## PRINCIPLES OF ERICKSONIAN COMMUNICATION

The question thus becomes: How does the hypnotist facilitate hypnotic processes in the subject? Instead of standardized techniques, he has to use general principles to guide his efforts. I consider the most important of these principles to be 1) accept and utilize the client's reality, 2) pace and lead the subject's behavior and 3) interpret "resistance" as lack of pacing.

The first principle—accept and utilize—was stressed again and again by Erickson and is the essential theme of Erickson and Rossi's *Hypnotherapy* (1979). Briefly stated, *accepting* means assuming and communicating to the subject that "What you're doing at this point in time is exactly what I'd like you to be doing. It's fine; it's perfect." *Utilizing* means assuming and communicating the attitude that "What you're doing right now is exactly that which will allow you to do X." The process of accepting and utilizing is one of communicating that what the subject is doing is fine *and* it will allow him/her to do something else (e.g., experience trance).

Bandler and Grinder (1975) discussed these principles in the more process-oriented terms of *pacing and leading the subject's behavior. Pacing* communications essentially feed back the subject's experience; they add nothing new. Their major intent is to enhance the rapport between hypnotist and subject. This enables the subject to be more trustful and cooperative and the hypnotist to be more understanding. Once rapport has been developed, the hypnotist can *lead* by introducing behaviors that are different from, but consistent with, the subject's present state and slightly closer to the desired state (e.g., trance).

According to these principles of Ericksonian communication, the effective hypnotic communicator assumes all experience is valid and utilizable and then behaviorally paces and leads toward the desired state. He freely admits that he does not know exactly which path will lead to the desired state and really does not know which techniques will work best. But he does know that he can "get in tune with" the subject, thereby establishing a rhythmic, continuous feedback loop in which one closely observes, accepts, and utilizes the subject's ongoing response. In this sort of interaction, the trek toward the desired state unfolds in a nonlinear, spiral-like fashion.

Within this feedback loop of interaction, the principles of pacing and leading can be applied in many different ways and at many different levels. One of the simplest forms of pacing and leading involves direct verbal description of the subject's ongoing behavior. This is often a good way to start a hypnotic induction. For example, you, as hypnotist, might note to a subject:

1) You're sitting there, *(pacing statement)*
2) You're looking at me, *(pacing statement)*
3) You're breathing in and out, *(pacing statement)*
4) eyes blinking up and then down, *(pacing statement)*
5) and as you shift in your chair *(pacing statement)*
6) you can also begin to shift into a state of comfortable relaxation. *(leading statement)*

The first five clauses are all pacing statements; they simply describe the undeniable reality of the subject's observable behaviors. The final clause, however, uses pacing to introduce a leading statement (develop relaxation).

Of course, just any leading statement will not do. Sometimes you will lead too quickly or inappropriately. But that's fine; you simply observe how the subject responds and pace and utilize that. If he/she follows, fine, that becomes your new state to pace; if not, fine, simply pace what he/she is doing. This whole interaction is one of pacing and leading, pacing and leading, again and again and again and again.

Pacing and leading can be done nonverbally, too. For instance, if you wanted to calm down an excited client, you could begin to mirror or reflect back his nonverbal excitedness by speaking in the same breathless, high-pitched and frantic way. After a while you could begin to lead by slowing down just a bit and relaxing just a bit more. If you lead too quickly and the subject continues in his frenetic rhythm, that's fine; you can shift back into the quick pace once again, talking about how fast things can really get and then again begin to gradually slow down. You can continue this process until the subject reaches the desired state.

Another way to nonverbally pace and lead is to synchronize one of your behavioral parameters—such as the tonal inflections in your voice—to a different behavioral parameter of the subject—say his breathing rate—so that every time he breathes out, your tonal inflection goes down. You might nod your head subtly every time the subject blinks his eyes and then begin to nod occasionally when the subject is *not* blinking. This leading can be gradually increased to the point that you can elicit eyelid flutters from the subject, a response that can easily be utilized to develop a trance. This technique, which I call *cross-behavioral pacing and leading,* is usually quite effective. It is indirect and thus bypasses the subject's conscious processes.

Pacing and leading can be more complex and sophisticated. For example, a co-therapist and I worked with a psychotic who terrorized the psychiatrists on his ward with gross hallucinations of dead babies, hot dogs coming out of his ears, and other bizarre images. When we first interviewed him, he looked wildly about and asked us if we saw the hallucinations. We agreed with him in a matter-of-fact fashion and then looked crazily into space before asking him if he saw *our* hallucinations. Of course, this was all done quite elaborately and dramatically. He was understandably stunned by our response. He tried to counter with more hallucinations, which we again accepted and then led by introducing more of our own. After a while we disappointedly confessed that we had asked to see him because we were interested in becoming better hallucinators and had been told that he was an expert. However, we pointed out, there had obviously been a mistake; after all, we had 10 good hallucinations, while he only had three mediocre ones. Besides, we continued, the guy on the next ward had half a dozen hallucinations of a much better variety.

Needless to say, this produced a state of confusion in the patient, which we used by offering to teach him to be a better hallucinator. He agreed, so over the next several months we showed him how to generate other hallucinations, how to hallucinate in a relaxed fashion, and how to have comforting hallucinations. We gradually led from scary and uncontrolled hallucinative processes, to more relaxed and valuable sorts of hallucinations, and then to dropping hallucinations altogether.

Another client of mine was a successful corporate president who suffered from intense internal conflicts. As part of the therapeutic strategy, I hypnotized him and had him visualize himself at a "board meeting" where all of the different "parts" of himself were present. He was directed to use his position as "chairman" to solve the various disagreements between the "board members." This was done over several sessions and produced favorable results.

The point to be drawn from these examples is that you take what the person gives you and use it. That becomes your strategy. One of the profound consequences of this way of thinking and acting is that there really is no such thing as "resistance" in a utilization approach. *Everything the person is doing is exactly what you would like him to be doing.* Your task is to generate communications that use ongoing experiences. When you are not fully using them, the subject will tell you, usually indirectly and nonverbally. You will find yourself accusing the person of being "resistant" or branding him/her as "nonsusceptible." You are reacting to communications from the subject that are saying, "What you're doing is not pacing me at this time. You're not using some behavior or experience of mine." Neither the hypnotist nor the subject is a "bad person" or "wrong" or "sick" or "crazy." "Resistance" is just a message that you need to synchronize yourself with the subject again. I think this is a radical concept that is incredibly useful to the clinician.

## THE PROCESS OF INDUCTION

How do these utilization principles apply to the specific situation of inductions? The main strategies or principles that the Ericksonian hypnotist uses to induce trance are: 1) Secure and maintain the subject's attentional absorption; 2) access and develop unconscious processes (associational strategies); and 3) pace and distract conscious processes (dissociational strategies).

The first thing you want to do in an induction is to secure the subject's attention and then maintain that absorption. To do this, you use nonverbal processes in certain ways: 1) Stay externally oriented; 2) remain flexible; 3) communicate meaningfully; and 4) be confident.

The first—staying externally oriented—is critical, because your major task as a hypnotist is to use the subject's ongoing processes. It is therefore rather important that you remain aware of what the subject is doing all the time. To best do this, you might develop what Bandler and Grinder call an *up-time state,* which I call an *externally-oriented trance.* In this state the hypnotist breathes comfortably and focuses fully and continually on the subject. He gets into a rhythmic feedback loop where he feels strong contact with the subject. In this state the hypnotist's behavior is not mediated by conscious processes; rather, he allows himself to drop into trance and let his unconscious respond. Stated another way, the sole contents of the hypnotist's consciousness are the subject's behavior, rather than the internal imagery that normally pervades thinking processes. It is as if the notion of mind extends beyond the normal boundaries of the body to include the subject. This is not a state of total empathy; it is a paradoxical state in which the hypnotist simultaneously experiences complete rapport with the subject *and* an observational detachment from the interaction. This process enhances both the hypnotist's and subject's feelings of rapport. It also helps both participants to develop focused but effortless styles of processing. Furthermore, it helps the hypnotist to detect subtle aspects of the subject's experience.

Now all of this may sound a bit strange, but I train my students to develop and use this style of processing while operating as hypnotists. Most of them find it easy to develop and almost all of them claim that it markedly enhances their effectiveness as hypnotists. It is a process not unlike those used by great entertainers and athletes. These master practitioners spend endless hours using conscious, analytical processes to develop and refine their skills, but they "stop thinking" and let their unconscious do it for them when it comes time for the actual performance. An effective Ericksonian hypnotherapist thinks long and hard before and after a clinical session, but while actually interacting with a client, he lets his unconscious use the products of those contemplations.

I learned of this process from Erickson, who used it rather often. For example, during the early part of my training with him I watched him do a marvelous piece of work with a patient. Assuming that his sophisticated strategies had to be generated from complex conscious cognitions, I was determined to identify the exact thought processes he used. After the patient left, I poised pencil on paper and resolutely began to interrogate him.

"Milton, do you make a lot of pictures?"

"No," he slowly but firmly stated.

"No pictures," I muttered, crossing that category out on my sheet. "OK. Do you have a lot of internal dialogue in that situation?"

"No," he again convincingly replied.

"OK. No internal dialogue. Let me write that down here. OK. Well, do you have kinesthetic sensations? You know, feelings in the body, that sort of thing."

"No."

I was beginning to grow both suspicious and confused. "Let's see. No pictures, no internal dialogue, no kinesthetic sensation. Well, Milton, I don't understand. How do you know what to do?"

"I don't know. I don't know what I'm going to do, I don't know what I'm going to say. All I know is that I trust my unconscious to shelve into my conscious that which is appropriate. And I don't know how they're going to respond. All I know is that *they will respond.* I don't know why. I don't know when. All I know is that they'll respond in an appropriate fashion, in a way which best suits them as an individual. And so I become intrigued with wondering exactly *how* their unconscious will choose to respond. And so I comfortably await their response, knowing that when it occurs, I can accept and utilize it."

He paused, his eyes twinkling. "Now I know that sounds ridiculous. *But it works*!!"

And after my initial confusion, I checked it out and found that indeed it did work.

The second process involves *remaining flexible* when you're in this externally-oriented trance state. If a technique doesn't work, fine, use another one. If a communication does not seem appropriate, fine, shift to a different one. *There are really no mistakes you can make in well-intentioned hypnotic communication.* There are only outcomes, and every outcome is useful. You offer behavioral communications and then observe and use the responses. To do this, you must really stay in tune with the subject, not trying to fit him/her into any rigid, preformed category.

Another interaction I had with Erickson illustrates the importance of this point. It was one of the most important learning experiences in my life. After years of diligently studying his approach, I felt I had a fairly good grasp of his sophisticated strategies, yet clearly sensed that I was lacking something. My work was not as effective as I knew it could be, but I was unclear about how I was limiting myself. Finally, on the last day of a week-long visit with Erickson, I respectfully requested some guidance in the matter. Instead of launching one of his lengthy and indirect answers, he stated in a simple but intensely meaningful fashion, "You've got a tendency to overcompartmentalize your experience, and it gets in the way of your unconscious." He then immediately ended the session.

As I walked out with a colleague, I confessed my disappointment about not being given any useful feedback, but sympathetically suggested that it was because Erickson was getting old, and besides, he never did have a good conscious understanding of what he did. In other words, I "compartmentalized" his response! Several months later, at the end of a similar training session, I again advanced the question, to which he replied a bit more sternly, "You've got a tendency to overcompartmentalize your experience, and it gets in the way of your unconscious!" My disappointment was even more marked this time, for Erickson was clearly getting a bit senile; he didn't even remember what he had told me before.

Four months later, my despair deepened when a third phrasing of the question was met with the same response. Why was Milton being so uninformative? Why couldn't he remember what he had told me before? Did he give such unhelpful advice on such matters to all his students? If so, what happened to his emphasis on unique solutions for each person? I gave the question one more try several months later, to which he replied: "You've got a tendency to overcompartmentalize your experience, and it gets in the way of your unconscious!" FLASH!! Four times and eight months later, I was startled with the blinding (or rather unblinding) insight: *I had a tendency to overcompartmentalize my experience, and did it ever get in the way of my unconscious*!! When I finally looked at Erickson, his eyes were twinkling. "That's right," he said softly.

My realization really unfolded and developed over the next months. It became all too clear that most of my time as a hypnotist was spent in internal dialogue, trying to classify the subject's behavior and then come up with some sophisticated response. The more I indulged in these conceptual evaluations, the less I attended to what the subject was actually experiencing and doing. In addition, I was forced to "objectify" the subject into this or that class, thereby limiting the degree of possible rapport. As I relinquished the need for such "compartmentalizations," my appreciation of the uniqueness of each individual grew. Most importantly, my communications became more fitting and my work more effective.

Of course, I sometimes find myself mired again in this evaluative mode. But when I do, I think back to Erickson's simple but persistent suggestion. It is difficult to resist such a suggestion.

The final two points are that you must communicate in a meaningful and confident fashion to the subject. This process was a major part of what Erickson emphasized in his writings. Your nonverbal delivery must unequivocally communicate to the subject that what you're saying is important and that he/she can respond to it. In many respects your nonverbal communication is more important than your verbalizations. If what you're saying *seems* meaningful and important, the person will feel compelled to respond.

Once the subject is attentive, you use rapport to develop unconscious processes; that is, you want to develop hypnotic experiences in the subject. You can accomplish this in a number of ways. A nice technique to begin an induction is with questions that access trance-relevant experiences from the person's memory. For instance, you might ask general questions:

- Do you remember what you felt like during your last trance?
- What did it feel like when you were in the deepest trance you've ever been in?

Or, if the subject has no previous trance experience:

- Can you imagine and begin to describe to me what it would be like for you to begin to develop a trance?
- Do you remember a time when you felt very relaxed?

Or, if you wish to develop a particular trance phenomenon, such as age regression, you might ask more specific questions:

- Did you have a nickname as a child?
- Did you have a favorite game as a youngster?
- Did you have an imaginary playmate as a child?

There are countless numbers of these questions, which essentially ask the subject to revivify some naturalistic experience relevant to trance processes. It is important to realize that the subject's response to such inquiries will depend in large part on *how* they are delivered. Generally speaking, the subject will access and become absorbed in the revivified experiences to the extent that the hypnotist asks the question(s) in a meaningful, compelling, and expectant fashion.

The subject's responses can then be developed, either through further questions or through other, more elaborate techniques. Many of these techniques are well known already, so I will not say much about them except that most traditional techniques are suitable, as long as you adapt them to the particular subject. For example, you might use progressive relaxation techniques with kinesthetically-oriented subjects, or guided imagery methods with visually-oriented persons. With a person whose conscious processes (e.g., internal dialogue) interfere with the development of trance, you might tell metaphorical stories. Such stories, which were a trademark of Erickson's work, have content that is dissimilar to the subject's experience or problems, but specify processes or themes that are quite similar to those salient in the subject's experience. So you talk about other people going into a trance, or interactions with other clients, or even personal experiences. The subject is consciously distracted because he/she thinks, "Gee, that's not about me," and yet unconsciously identifies with the story and thus gains access to the experiences suggested by it.

This last point leads to the third induction principle, that of pacing and distracting the conscious processes. Distraction or confusion techniques are useful because accessing techniques alone will generally be effective only to the extent that the subject allows them to be. That is, the subject not only must be willing to participate, but must also be *able* to let unconscious experiences develop. Many subjects have difficulty doing this. Specifically, their conscious processes interfere by continually questioning, analyzing, or trying to help with the development of the hypnotic experience. To the extent that such conscious participation occurs, the hypnotist needs to employ techniques and strategies that depotentiate such interference.

There are many ways in which this can be done. For example, the hypnotist can use techniques that totally occupy the subject's internal processes with tasks irrelevant to the trance development. One such technique involves instructing the subject to count backwards (silently) from a thousand to one by three's. While the subject does this, the hypnotist goes on with his induction patter. If the subject seems to be able to do this without any problem, you can use an overloading technique such as having him verbalize the letters of the alphabet in a forward fashion while visualizing them backward. The subject begins by verbalizing an "a" to himself, at the same visualizing the letter "z"; the letter "b" is then verbalized while "y" is visualized; and so on. If you try this yourself, you quickly will realize how overloading and disorienting it can be. Meanwhile back at the unconscious, the hypnotist is using accessing techniques for the development of trance.

In addition to distraction techniques, Erickson developed a large body of confusion techniques. Briefly stated, underlying the use of confusion techniques are the following assumptions: 1) There are many automatic and predictable patterns in a person's behavioral processes; 2) the unexpected discontinuation of any of these patterns will create an uncertainty state dominated by undifferentiated arousal (e.g., confusion); 3) the arousal will increase unless the person can cognitively attribute it to something; 4) most people strongly dislike uncertainty states and are motivated to avoid them; 5) consequently, most people will grab onto the first thing that enters their consciousness that reduces the uncertainty.

Based on these assumptions, most confusion techniques involve the following five steps.

1) *Identify* a dominant pattern in the subject's behavior.
2) *Pace* the pattern for awhile.
3) *Interrupt* or *overload* the pattern in a way which confuses the subject.
4) *Amplify* the confusion a bit.
5) *Use* the confusion by introducing a simple leading statement (e.g., "drop into trance").

These principles can be understood through a few examples. My first experience of involuntarily dropping into trance illustrates how relatively simple interruption techniques are easily effected. I was sitting in Erickson's office. As I intently listened to him tell a number of metaphorical stories, I was strongly dominated by the cognitive pattern of analyzing and then "compartmentalizing" every statement he made in terms of what it "really" meant. I was therefore startled when all of a sudden he intently looked at my hand, pointed to it, and said in the most surprised and incredulous fashion, "Isn't that your left hand *not* lifting? . . . Yet? . . . Now?" My recollection of the experience is still rather hazy. All I remember is seeing the room swimming about and feeling my hand beginning to involuntarily float upwards. I found myself looking right into Erickson's eyes as he said, "That's right, close your eyes and drop into trance *nowww*!!!" Believe me, I did so at once. He then added, "And let your unconscious do the work for you." I did that also. The most effective confusion techniques are those that use the very pattern that is keeping the person out of trance—in this case, my "compartmentalization" processes—as the basis for the induction. Again, whatever the person is doing is exactly that which will allow him to experience trance.

Other confusion techniques involve *overloading* the subject's conscious processes. For example, a double induction is a process in which two hypnotists perform simultaneous inductions on one subject. The hypnotists play off each other, both verbally and nonverbally. After a while, most subjects find it nearly impossible to continue to pay full attention to all they are experiencing. Some simply give up and retreat into trance; others become so disoriented that simply instructing them to "let go fully and simply drop all the way into trance" is usually quite effective.

Many clinicians tell me that they like this double induction technique, but they can't use it because they work alone. There is no need for despair. A modified procedure is to instruct the subject to pay close attention to a taped induction. While the tape is playing, you do a "live" induction in the other ear.

Confusional overload can also be accomplished by telling stories involving spatial and/or temporal disorientation. One story I have found to be particularly effective involves an automobile trip in which the driver is unclear about the exact sequence of directional turns. An abbreviated example of this technique, which I call the *autohypnosis directional maneuver*, is as follows:

> (After about 15 minutes of general inductional communications) And there are so many directions you can follow when you allow your unconscious to do it for you . . . just as there are many different directions you can follow physically. . . . I'll give you an example. . . . Some summers ago, I was traveling all alone on the highway in my car, just paying close attention to the sound of the engine, and knowing that slowly but surely I was heading into another state. And in that state there was a particular destination I was headed for, a particular person I wished to see, a particular experience I was looking forward to in that other state. . . . However, while I knew the general set of directions regarding how to get to where I wanted to go, I could not for the life of me remember the proper order in which those turns occurred. I did know that from where I was *there then*, I thought to myself, I don't want to be *here now*; I want to be *there now*, and all I can remember is that to get *there now*, or at least soon from *now* from *here*, I take a combination of three *right* turns and *three left* turns . . . but I don't know quite which is the *right* series of *rights* and *lefts* . . . but I do want to get *there* and I am *here now*, and so I said, all *right*, *pay attention very closely* (embedded suggestion to subject), because we've got to make it *right* or we'll be *left* behind. . . . And *then* I said, all *right*, let's begin. . . . I'll take a *right here* (I think that's *right*), and *then* a *left* and *now* I'm *left* with two *lefts* and two *rights*. So all *right*, I'll take another *left*, which means I'm now *left* with a *left* and a *right* and a *right*. If I take a *right*, I'll be *left* with a *right* and a *left*, but if I take a *left*, I'll be *left* with a *right* and another

> *right*. . . . But I don't think that is *right*, so I'll take a *right* first, and *then* a *left*, and *now* I'm *left* with a *right*, and so I take the *right*, and . . . dead end. It's the *wrong* way. And so now I've got to go back to the starting point, so as not to get completely *left* behind . . . so I begin to back track and *now* take three *rights* and three *lefts* again, except that each turn is *now* the opposite from the other direction. . . . *Everything is reversed*. . . . *Now* which was *then* a *right* is *now* a *left* . . . and that which was *left then* is *now* a *right*. . . . so for every *right then* it is *right now* to take a *left* . . . and for every *left then* it is *right now* to take a *right*, and *now* I'm back at the beginning, ready to begin again . . . and so I begin. . . .

You can then repeat the story with a different sequence of directions and continue until the subject looks completely confused, at which point you can offer trance suggestions within the story. For example, to continue from above:

> . . . And after a while I became so tired, so confused, that I didn't know and didn't care where to turn next. . . . I couldn't tell a *right* from a *left*, nor a *left* from a *left*. . . . I couldn't figure out whether taking a *left* was *right*, or whether taking a *right* was *right*. So I pulled off to the side of the road, turned off the engine, and sat there with my eyes closed, and said to myself, *"To hell with trying to figure it out. Stop all this activity and just relax into a trance!!"* (This statement is uttered in a slower, softer, but more intense and emphatic fashion.) and I did. (The hypnotist now shifts to a more relaxed, almost relieved tone.) . . . And I was able to *just allow that trance to develop*. . . . There was the recognition that there is no need to pay attention to anything except the need to attend to one's own internal needs . . . and what a nice thing to know that you can simply let *your unconscious do the work for you*.

All of these statements are valid and consistent with each other. Also, the effectiveness of the story depends in large part on the hypnotist's nonverbal communications. As with any Ericksonian technique, the hypnotist needs to capture and maintain the subject's conscious attention and must therefore speak meaningfully, impressively, and congruently. In addition, because the intent is to create and then use informational overload, the hypnotist begins with a relatively quick tempo, increases and intensifies it even more when the subject starts to get confused, but then dramatically reduces it (to a slower, softer voice) right at the point of utilization. Finally, it is quite useful to employ special tonal markings to subtly emphasize both (a) the directional and ambiguous terms (e.g., right/left) and (b) the several embedded suggestions regarding paying attention and dropping into trance. When these and other nonverbal techniques are judiciously applied, the story will usually work quite well as an induction device.

One final technique for depotentiating conscious processes is boredom. As Erickson used to say, "I've got an unconscious mind, and they've got an unconscious mind. Therefore, as long as we're in the room together, sooner or later they'll go into trance. And if nothing else works, I'll bore them into trance. It might take them five minutes, 10 minutes, 30 minutes, one hour, several hours, or many hours. That's fine; I can wait." And, boy, could he ever wait. You might tell two or three hours of metaphorical stories, gradually wearing down the person to the point that he/she is unable or unwilling to offer any conscious resistances to shifting into trance. In fact, many people retreat into trance to get away from all those boring stories.

To summarize, induction is a process in which the hypnotist uses his body as a musical instrument, tuning it to get into rhythm with the "behavioral dance" of the subject. The hypnotist works to secure and hold the subject's attentional processes, thereby making it possible to access unconscious processes to develop hypnotic experiences. To the extent that the subject's conscious processes interefere with this development, the hypnotist uses distraction, confusion, and boredom techniques. In short, the most effective induction strategy is one that maximally uses the subject's ongoing experience as the basis for trance development.

## THE INTEGRITY OF THE HYPNOTIST

Before closing, I'd like to comment briefly on the issue of integrity. Simply put, the principles, strategies, and techniques of the Ericksonian approach are incredibly powerful tools. And while tools are value-free, *their capacity to enhance or create is equivalent to their potential to oppress or destroy.* I think that one need only look at similarities in the communication patterns of great humanitarians like Christ and great oppressors like Hitler to realize this. The important point here is that the effect of a tool on the quality of human experience depends on its user. Consequently, the integrity of the hypnotist is a major issue.

Incidentally, I don't think you can ignore this issue, even if you try. As Bateson, Haley, and others have pointed out, you cannot *not* affect another person's behavior. In this sense, all behavior is manipulation. What the Ericksonian approach does is make explicit a lot of the ways in which we are constantly influencing each other. By becoming aware of such patterns, you can use them systematically; that is, you can align your behavior with your intent, thereby making you a powerful communicator. What becomes critical, then, is getting clear about your intent.

*This is not a trivial matter to be sidestepped or disregarded.* In training mental health professionals, I have noticed that failing to come to grips with it creates many problems. Some trainees have difficulty acknowledging that they can and do powerfully influence human behavior and thus find themselves unable to use Ericksonian techniques in any powerfully effective fashion. Other trainees are initially overpowered by an insecure need to prove themselves and consequently wield techniques in a domineering and insensitive fashion. Both types of student are controlled by their ability to manipulate, the former by attempting to dissociate from it, the latter by using it irresponsibly. In both cases, the true power to enhance experience is stifled.

Once a person becomes aware of the intent and effect of his behavior, he can use communication in powerful manner. Here the issue of integrity becomes particularly important. By integrity I mean the degree to which the hypnotist is able to *refrain* from imposing his own solutions and beliefs on the subject, to *refrain* from having to prove his own worth at the subject's expense, and instead fully to *support* the person in his/her quest for change.

The hypnotist's integrity has many practical consequences. Lacking integrity, even the highly skilled hypnotherapist will find that his clients can develop hypnotic phenomena but *not* hypnotherapeutic changes; or they will become impressed with his abilities but *not* their own; or they will try to take on his beliefs and life-style rather than developing their own. In short, the hypnotist lacking integrity will be in no position to really help the client.

Conversely, the hypnotist operating with integrity can easily secure rapport with the client. By trusting the hypnotist, the client begins to trust himself more. He consequently becomes more willing to examine his shortcomings and more able to develop new ways of being. He also becomes more willing, both in trance and waking states, to comply with directives, no matter how strange or bizarre they may seem. This is important to the Ericksonian practitioner, who uses many unorthodox strategies.

In fact, I firmly believe that the most powerful aspect of Erickson's communication was his integrity. Before training with him, I would read about all these wild things he did with his patients and I could never quite figure out how he could get these people to cooperate with him. After watching him in action, it became crystal clear that he had an unwavering intention to fully respect and support his patients and students. He wasn't out to manipulate or control for his own personal gains. Consequently, people would really let go and fully cooperate with him.

In conclusion, this whole issue of integrity needs to be thought about long, hard, and often. You must clearly decide whether you wish to support or oppress others. Of course, the second choice cannot always be implemented. Most hypnotic subjects will quickly learn to distrust and hence not cooperate with a nonsupportive hypnotist. Choosing to *support* the subject is a lot easier, since there really can be no "resistance" when one is totally aligned with another individual. Besides, it's a far more personally satisfying and professionally effective position. Simply stated, the more integrity you develop, the more fun and success you are likely to experience, and I think that's what "it" is all about.

## REFERENCES

Bandler, R. & Grinder, J. *Patterns of the Hypnotic Techniques of Milton H. Erickson, M.D.* Vol. 1, Cupertino: Meta Publications, 1975.

Erickson, M.H. & Rossi, E. *Hypnotherapy: An Exploratory Casebook.* New York: Irvington Publishers, Inc., 1979.

## Chapter 7

# Principles of Ericksonian Induction of Hypnosis

*Marion R. Moore*

When I was first asked to present at this meeting, I was rather overwhelmed with numerous thoughts and feelings. The amount of time that I spent with Dr. Erickson over the years taught me many, many things about his methods of doing inductions or having patients experience and respond to inductions. To put these learnings into written form is a very difficult task.

Erickson's induction procedures were so extremely variable that to pinpoint the basic principles one would have to review the context from which they emerged. For example, consider the history of his fight with poliomyelitis at the age of 17, when he overheard the doctors tell his mother that he was not going to be alive the next morning. His mother then moved the bed and the mirror around to where, if that was going to be his last day, at least he would see the sunset, because he always loved to see sunsets and sunrises. He survived that night, of course, and during his fight to recuperate in the next months and even years he observed in great detail the people around him: their body movements, facial expressions, movements of hands, head, face muscles, feet, their walking, their stance, the broadness of their gait, the quickness or conversely the slowness of their step, their tension or calmness, their pulse rate and its change, their blood pressure and its change, as well as their respiration changes. All these had different meanings in different situations at different times for each individual. Erickson constantly watched everything that took place about him, learning what habit patterns humans have, recognizing that each was uniquely distinct and different, although some principles could be generalized and have similiar meaning to a number of people.

He continued his observations of people and their reactions, both pitiful and grandiose, happy and depressed, and accepting and rejecting of self and/or others. He observed his patients' responses in overcoming personal losses or gains, and their emulations, frustrations and empathic feelings. This knowledge became very much a part of his life and later became incorporated into his hypnotic inductors.

In an early psychology class, Professor Clark Hull gave a demonstration of hypnosis. Erickson searched out Hull's subject and took him to his room. There Erickson began his first night of work in learning about hypnosis: how the conscious and the unconscious begin to differ and yet are the same in many ways. These differences and similarities cause an astonishing number of patterns of human response. This knowledge stimulated Milton Erickson to go further into his study of humans and their behavior, their uniqueness and their common foibles as they go through their lives from birth to death.

He studied individuals with respect to each period of the family life cycle. He observed how individuals are affected by the families they are born into, the families they grow into, the person they marry and the children they raise, who eventually start their own families, leaving behind their parents with the remaining periods of their lives to complete. Through all of these events, Erickson observed how each individual was markedly affected or unaffected, stimulated or understimulated or overstimulated. These observations became the mental notes that Erickson used consciously and unconsciously with the hundreds of patients that he saw in the course of his career.

It was not until many years later that Erickson realized other people had not made similar observations. He first assumed that every doctor had made these observations and that there was much common knowledge shared by himself and his fellow colleagues. When he found out that most therapists had not made many of these observations, it was quite a shock to him. His assumptions then had to be changed and his focus broadened. He began to test the principles suggested by his observations and when he was satisfied with them, he began discussing his observations with colleagues.

Along with Erickson's observation of the impact of the family life cycle on the individual, he noted that all experience has an impact on the individual so that language becomes infused with meaning unique to that individual. It became apparent that an observer could discern the unique meaning of a word by observing the impact of the word on the individual. The process by which language can elicit unique responses in the conscious and unconscious behavior of the individual had profound implications. Intuitively Erickson knew that by relying upon this information effective inductions could be tailored for each individual.

The preceding point can be clarified by example. The word "sky" means different things to different human beings. Many imagine the blue sky only; others see the blue sky with pretty clouds; others see a cloudy sky. Some envision a more articulated sky, perhaps a deeper gray sky with rain, or one might see a dark, dark sky with very little light peeping through overhead. The same word "sky" elicits a unique image and concomitant behavior for each individual. This was most fascinating to Erickson. Not only this word, but many words, thoughts and ideas were presented to people to elicit responses so that he could then observe their unique reactions.

He also discovered that an air of mystery would frequently help a person go into a trance. This air of mystery could sometimes be created by limiting conversations with patients to a few words. Each word was selected to allow the patient to explore and discover new feelings within him/herself that would benefit his/her health. Each word was selected to stimulate the person to expand his limiting frame of reference.

All of these principles emerge again and again as we review Erickson's work. They constitute the basic truths that Erickson taught and utilized, day by day, year by year, in his therapy and in his teaching.

I first knew Dr. Erickson when he was walking most of the time with the aid of a cane. He moved about quite well for a person who had as much anterior horn cell damage as he had incurred during his bout with polio. The pure determination in overcoming handicaps was fueled by a tremendous and constant drive within him. On numerous occasions he experienced various degrees of discomfort within his own previously diseased body. Perhaps this battle with polio and its attendant pain allowed Erickson greater awareness of people whose bodies were "normal." His struggle was also an inspiration to patients and students.

Erickson's constant concern was with the patient and his or her problems. Erickson's own problems were totally secondary and forgotten during his teaching and working with patients. He sought to help individuals adjust and find new ways of thinking and being and to help individuals overcome the barriers which stymied their own efforts toward change.

Erickson explored every level of a person's being: inner experiences, reactions to inner experience, feelings regarding external events and concerns. Additionally, he explored individuals' desires to stay within their own limited area of understanding. Erickson recognized that patients, sometimes being frightened of the new, would not dream of venturing forth into other areas. Such people wanted only to make a particular or "specific" change in their lives. Erickson utilized his unique ability then to foresee that they needed more if they were to accomplish their specific goal. He proceeded unafraid and undaunted in working with them, telling stories, teaching them unconsciously and broadening both their concepts of life and their own inner being.

His strategy was designed to help effect a workable, beneficial change that would come from within each patient. Although the process of change was not consciously understood by the patient, the change, having been negotiated with the patient's unconscious, was sanctioned by the patient. The result of change was the patient's altered manner of viewing and understanding his world. Such a change would have salubrious consequences throughout life.

There are many examples in which a former patient, after many years away from Erickson, would ask, "Well, how did you achieve a particular change with a particular person?" Actually, of course, the former patient was asking about his own past symptom and prior treatment. When Erickson delineated the process through which change had been achieved, the former patient, not recognizing the process he had undergone, would then say, "Oh, my goodness! You do it exactly the way I've been doing it!" The awareness that he had learned through his own individual work with Erickson many years before would never be realized. Dr. Erickson would never tell the former patient that he taught them that way. His usual and only comment would be "That's nice" or "That is good." The credit always goes to the patient, not to the therapist.

Erickson's therapeutic techniques and numerous hypnotic inductions were so diverse and so unique that it took many students numerous years to analyze and delineate his strategies. Inductions, each tailored according to a patient's unique requirements as manifested during the assessment phase of therapy, differed across individuals. For one particular person, he would select among a variety of methods, e.g., looking toward a spot, or feeling a sensation of lightness in the hand, in the arm, or whatever part of the anatomy was available to his vision at that particular moment. A flushing at the throat or a blushing in the face would immediately be noticed by Erickson and he would make a general comment about it. That comment could deepen the trance and function as a suggestion for the patient to go further into exploring inner feelings.

In later years one of his favorite ways to induce a trance state was to utilize a lead glass crystal on which was etched a reindeer. This was situated on his desk, and he often had patients look *toward* "the reindeer in the ice." While talking to them, he interspersed suggestions. Each suggestion was easily understandable but global enough in its denotation to allow each patient to find a trance state via his own unique process. Erickson often used the term "monoideaism" to refer to the presentation of a suggestion which was broad enough in its meaning to allow the patient to find his own uniquely focused fashion of entering trance.

Milton Erickson used many types of inductions, such as eye fixation, hand levitation and visual imagery. He often used interesting stories and even questions that the patient could not answer consciously. He would suggest vague feelings left unspecified at the conscious level which would stimulate the patient to wonder. For example, he might say, "You are experiencing a different feeling and you don't yet know what it is" (one of his particularly nice induction sentences). He was a master at distracting people from focusing on their surroundings and thoughts. He occasionally aroused in them unconscious curiosities which would stimulate a shift in present awareness.

Some people were more likely to enter a trance state with arm levitation than other methods. If that was the best way for them, he used it. For others he had merely to have them close their eyes, take a deep breath, and "really wonder how comfortable it is in a very deep sleep." A simple suggestion could easily lead to a trance, particularly in a person who was well prepared prior to seeing Erickson and who felt the mystique surrounding him. In fact, some patients while moving to their chair have dropped into a trance at the first glance of Erickson. He had merely to raise his hand in a gesture of welcome and say, "Hello, it's nice to see you today," and they would immediately go into a trance.

Erickson used the visualization technique, having patients imagine, for example, a house-tree-man or a blackboard and circle. If he knew that a patient appreciated the mountains, he might have him/her see the mountains in all their glorious splendor in the springtime, the summer, the fall, or the winter. Then, as the patient became comfortable, he would have him/her continue visualizing that scene while he merely talked, allowing him/her to being unconsciously understanding his/her own feelings. He might at times present other scenes, scenes which could induce beneficial change. By proceeding in such an indirect manner, Erickson stimulated changes which were more likely to be accepted by the patient.

Erickson's ability in teaching patients to break away from previous learnings, ideas and habits was unique. From every patient he learned something he could use in the future. Again, the goal of his induction procedures was to turn the person's mind inward and thus limit his attention to external stimuli. This protraction of attention would quickly stimulate a deep trance. During the trance, changes could be induced which would generalize to the rest of the patient's life.

Erickson was also a master at instilling feelings of confidence and hope. Additionally, he spurred patients to elevate the level of their goals, i.e., to heighten their expectations. He let each and every patient know that he or she had a unique mind and body, capable of responding in many different ways, both consciously and unconsciously. This instillation of hope and conviction helped to make the end result of any psychotherapeutic response more easily attainable. Erickson wanted his patients to attain a degree of wellness in their own way, not in the way that he might have desired. He merely sought the way that would be best for the patients, the way that patients could continue to meaningfully utilize throughout the rest of their lives, a way that would enhance and continually perpetuate the changes that they came for and the changes that they needed so badly to have well adjusted lives in their own homes, communities or jobs.

In his inductions, he would often pace his breathing with that of the patients, speak in rhythm with their breathing, or respond in synchrony with their other body movements. He would even pause, sometimes for a minute or two, to allow the patient to seek understanding from various areas of the unconscious, without the conscious mind being aware of the inner search. This important pause thus became a deepening process for the induction of trance.

Perhaps the major principle of the inductions that Dr. Erickson utilized over his lifetime was to allow the patient to begin to independently change feelings and ideas from his past and to respond in new ways. His unique inductions often were a major part of the day's therapy. One cannot forget that inductions are the beginning of change, and the operator merely facilitates this movement for the patient.

Erickson wanted those concerned to remember that the operator works to help the patient use his own hidden abilities, but the patient does the hardest work and deserves the credit for the changes that are made.

PART IV

# *Ericksonian Language*

*David Gordon, M.A., is a marriage, family and child counselor in Santa Cruz, California. He is one of the principal proponents and teachers of neurolinguistic programming. Gordon, an acknowledged expert on anecdotal communication, has authored an important volume entitled* Therapeutic Metaphors.

*Anecdotal communication was one of the hallmarks of Erickson's method. Through anecdotes, Erickson ingeniously demonstrated how much power effective therapeutic communication could have.*

*Gordon presents a model for describing Ericksonian anecdotal methods. Additionally, he reminds us that noting what is evoked by the communication is more important than focusing on possible meanings in the delivered message.*

*Donna Slosar, M.S.W., is a talented psychotherapist on the faculty of the School of Social Work at St. Louis University. Her chapter addresses Erickson's style of gearing communication to have maximal impact on the listener's unconscious. Presenting a transcript from one of Erickson's teaching seminars, Slosar presents a unique and interesting conception of unconscious processing of communication.*

*Stephen Lankton, M.S.W., is in private practice and consultation in Gulf Breeze, Florida. He has done brilliant work advancing Ericksonian and Ericksonian-based approaches; he outlined some of his clinical applications of neurolinguistic programming in his recent book,* Practical Magic.

*Lankton, a remarkably effective communicator, presents workshops throughout North America and Europe. His pre-congress workshop was one of the most well attended, and participants rated his effectiveness as the best of any of the 21 pre-conference presenters.*

*Lankton's chapter underscores the similarity of patient responses to both hypnotic and "nonhypnotic" psychotherapies. To facilitate description, Lankton presents 12 discrete communication operations most commonly used in promoting hypnotic responsiveness. Understanding this framework will help practitioners to structure more potent communications.*

Chapter 8

# Ericksonian Anecdotal Therapy

*David Gordon*

I was returning from high school one day and a runaway horse, with a bridle on, sped past a group of us into a farmer's yard . . . looking for a drink of water. The horse was perspiring heavily. And the farmer didn't recognize it, so we cornered it. I hopped on the horse's back . . . since it had a bridle on, I took hold of the rein and said, "Giddy up" . . . headed for the highway. I knew the horse would turn in the right direction . . . I didn't know what the right direction was. And the horse trotted and galloped along. Now and then he would forget he was on the highway and start into a field. So I would pull on him a bit and call his attention to the fact the highway was where he was supposed to be. And finally about four miles from where I had boarded him he turned into a farm yard and the farmer said, "So that's how that critter came back. Where did you find him?" I said, "About four miles from here." "How did you know he should come here?" I said, "I didn't know . . . the horse knew. All I did was keep his attention on the road."

. . . I think that's the way you do psychotherapy.

*M.H. Erickson, reported in Gordon, 1978*

A metaphor is a story or anecdote that is capable of accessing in its listener an intended content area without the content being explicitly identified. Thereby, the listener is offered a new and more useful perspective. This change of perspective is generally attributed to the inherent virtues of the analogies and/or resolutions employed in the metaphor. Given this orientation, metaphors can be considered special opportunities to learn within the particular analogical environment created by the storyteller. Since virtually all of Milton Erickson's therapeutic interventions entailed the creation of learning environments that had inherent within them the opportunity for developing a new perspective, most of his work can be accurately and usefully characterized as metaphorical. Anyone who has explored Erickson's ideas and case histories about the induction of hypnotic states knows that the hallmark of his approach is the creation of experiential environments that lead naturally to altered states and hypnotic phenomena. Also characteristic of Erickson's therapeutic work was his passion for getting his patients to do things in the world that would give them the opportunity to acquire the learnings they needed.

The specific purview of this paper is Erickson's use of the anecdotal form of metaphorical intervention (e.g., the story which opened this paper). The above anecdote is obviously instructional, and its lesson seems clear. Why not, then, simply make the intended statement directly? And if the creation of metaphorical environments is justified, how did Erickson go about creating them?

There are several answers to the first question regarding the usefulness of metaphoric communication. Metaphor can, if properly structured, avoid the necessity for explicit identification of the content area to which it is to be applied. Some clients may find open discussion of their problems incapacitating or even impossible if the relevant information is out of their conscious awareness. In working with a particularly prudish woman, for example, Erickson was able to discuss her sexuality by talking with her about her hair and the need to "part her hair with a one-toothed comb." In such situations, the ability to communicate in a meaningful way about a specific context, without having to explicitly identify that context, is of manifest advantage.

Coincident with this advantage is the undeniable (although often overly depended upon) experience that a metaphor can provide the substance from which its listener is free to carve whatever understandings he or she finds consciously or unconsciously appropriate. Such a metaphor, then, acts as the proverbial elephant that stands ready to satisfy the wide-ranging interpretations of any number of blind men. This particular quality of metaphorical communication has led to a genre of therapeutic storytelling characterized by awful or surprising situations that are somehow pleasurably resolved (often as a result of a *deus ex machina* of some kind). Even though it is usually unspecified in this type of metaphor just how the client is to accomplish change, these stories many times do effect changes in their listeners. Erickson made the point repeatedly that any time you make a communication, those listening will necessarily understand it in their own language, that is, make sense out of it in terms of their personal model of the world. Whether they will relate the metaphor to their personal experience in a way that is impactful or trivial, useful or destructive, is a measure of the skill of the teller.

One source of the power of a metaphor lies within the illuminative information contained in the analogies that are used. To draw an analogy between a person and a flower is automatically to imbue that individual with characteristics such as "growing," "beautiful," "delicate," "pollinatable," and so on. If instead the analogous character is drawn as a leopard, that same person becomes "stealthy," "strong," "independent," and so on. The analogies contained within the content of the metaphor itself, then, will convey to the listeners a new and hopefully more useful perspective as a result of the novel information and associations inherent in the analogy. If you tell your client that he or she lives life like a caged bird, for example, that client will probably consider in what ways he/she may be "locked in," what is in the "cage," what would happen if they "got out," and so on. That the client can take advantage of this opportunity for "gilt by association" depends upon that person's ability to extract the appropriate analogical associations and then to utilize them to generate a new perspective. Erickson's own use of metaphor, however, involved much more extensive internal structure than simple analogy.

Consider, as an example, a case reported in *Uncommon Therapy* (Haley, 1973) in which Erickson cured a boy of enuresis by talking to him about how one's iris constricts when taking aim with a bow and arrow. To talk to the boy about his "problem" with enuresis would inevitably access the memory of past failures, guilt or shame, fear of parental displeasure and so on. Once accessed, these attitudes about the problem will, of course, affect (and have been affecting) the boy's thinking with respect to his situation. One does a different kind of thinking when considering becoming competent at archery. What made it possible for Erickson to have the intentional and directed impact he had on the boy's thinking?

In order for a metaphorical communication to exert directional and intentional impact it must do two things: (a) It must access the relevant context to which the learnings are to be applied, and (b) it must then alter that individual's responses within that context in a way that leads to more appropriate and useful behaviors and experiences. In using metaphors, the accessing of the appropriate context is accomplished by creating an anecdote that is "isomorphic" with the identified target context. Isomorphism refers to the sharing of similar form or structure of two otherwise unrelated things. With respect to shape, for instance, a basketball and the earth are isomorphic—they are both spheres. An example within the context of metaphors is the isomorphism that can be created between a car running out of gas and a starving person. That is, gasoline serves the same function in an automobile as does food for a person—both provide energy.

In Erickson's anecdote at the beginning of this paper, the isomorphism between "lost horse being led home" and "confused client being led to appropriate experience" is fairly overt. When, however, the nature of the isomorphism is not so readily available to conscious awareness (either through the client's inattentiveness to the fact that a metaphor is being used or because the isomorphism being used is sufficiently subtle), there arises the possibility of having a therapeutic impact without the client's conscious understanding of the process. For instance, the isomorphism between gasoline/food and automobile/person makes it possible to access and talk about the functional relationship between food and a person without explicitly identifying "person" as the target of application.

The isomorphism can be even less obvious and still be effective in terms of creating the necessary associations. The mastery of archery seems to be a million miles away from enuresis. Yet Erickson was able to utilize elements inherent in archery to establish isomorphisms with respect to the experience of bladder control in a way that compelled the application of the one to the other. Isomorphism makes it possible to access implicitly those interrelationships and functional distinctions that are relevant to the target change. (For a thorough presentation of the generation of isomorphic environments see Gordon, 1978.)

In general, the creation of an isomorphism between a client's problem situation and the content of the metaphor is not in and of itself sufficient to effect a change. Once the isomorphism between the problem context and the content of the metaphor has been created, there are several possibilities for its utilization. One is to rely upon the ability of the listener to consciously or unconsciously detect, understand and appropriately utilize lessons contained in the metaphor's resolution and/or the information implied by the analogy. Erickson's anecdote about the lost horse is an example of such a utilization. The perspective we are to glean from that story is contained in its resolution and, perhaps, in the analogical considerations of being a horse with a "bridle," the "highway" and so on.

Another level of possible utilization is to use the context of the metaphor as an opportunity to convey to the listener specific ideas and suggestions through the use of such hypnotic patterns as presuppositions, analogue marking and embedded commands. Probably the best known example of this utilization is Erickson's (1966) work with Joe, a terminally ill cancer patient in great pain. In order to assist Joe in creating anesthesia for his pain, Erickson told Joe an extended metaphor about the growing of tomato plants, embedding in it many post-hypnotic suggestions with respect to the kinds of responses Erickson wanted Joe to have. Here is an excerpt:

> . . . One puts a tomato seed in the ground. One can *feel hope* that it will grow into a tomato plant that *will bring satisfaction* by the fruit it has. The seed soaks up water, *not very much difficulty in* doing that because of the rains that *bring peace and comfort* and the joy of growing to flowers and tomatoes. . . ."

In this brief excerpt from Erickson's work with Joe you will find several examples of Erickson's using the topic's analogical possibilities to mark out for Joe's unconscious mind certain experiences ("peace and comfort"), to embed appropriate commands ("feel hope") and to presuppose for Joe a more useful orientation ("will bring satisfaction" presupposes that satisfaction can be had). Erickson's use of these patterns of communication makes it possible for him to access in his client those experiences and ways of thinking about those experiences that Erickson considers appropriate and useful to achieve the client's desired state. (For a detailed presentation of Erickson's hypnotic patterns see Bandler and Grinder, 1975.)

A third pattern in Erickson's utilization of metaphorical environments is based on the observation that, to a great extent, the nature of an individual's behavior and experience is a function of the kinds of responses that person has with respect to a specific context. Take, for instance, the context of "things not turning out the way one wanted them to." For some individuals their response to unwanted results is "despair." For others an unwanted result triggers the response of being "challenged to try again." Obviously, behavior that is based on a response of despair will be very different from behavior generated from a response of being challenged. The response of despair may lead to behavior such as self-pity, blaming others or inaction, while responding to an unwanted result as a challenge could generate renewed attempts at getting what was originally desired.

Accordingly, Erickson frequently structured his anecdotes to elicit and instill in his clients what he considered to be more appropriate responses within the contexts either he or his client had identified. In other words, Erickson would create a metaphor that was isomorphic with the context within which he wanted a different response, then take his listener through it, eliciting the new responses when and where appropriate. His work with the enuretic boy is an example of this pattern. Erickson creates the isomorphism between archery and body control, then elicits in the boy the response of "closing down."

In this next anecdote, Erickson accesses in his listeners the context of "being ridiculed," then elicits "humor" as a response.

> In the sixties my son was in Phoenix College and the professor announced to the class for no good reason at all, "Anybody who dares wear bermuda shorts in this class will be thrown out immediately." Naturally, my son heard that and thought, "You can learn something!" So he was the last one to arrive in the classroom . . . wearing bermuda shorts. And the professor said, "Mr. Erickson you've heard what I said about bermuda shorts, now leave this room AT ONCE!" Well, gladly he walked out . . . he didn't quite close the door behind him. Outside the door his buddy was waiting for him with a pair of jeans. Robert stepped into the jeans, zipped them up, re-opened the door, walked in . . . everybody knew he was wearing bermuda shorts. And when my son Robert took his seat that unfortunate teacher said, "That is about the most stupid thing I've ever seen in my life." And Robert said with a tone of wonderment, "I wasn't even half trying!" And that's the way it should be (Gordon & Anderson, 1981).

Another very fine example of Erickson's use of this pattern is his work with a suicidal woman while using her as a demonstration subject in a hypnosis lecture (see Gordon & Anderson, 1981, and Zeig, 1980, p. 148). Erickson put the woman in a trance, then accompanied her on a metaphorical trip to the arboretum, zoo and seashore. In the course of visiting these places, Erickson elicited in her responses of curiosity, wonderment, appreciation, maternal desires and so on. Erickson later found out that that woman immediately joined the Navy, traveled the world, married happily and was raising several children. One of the things that made it possible for Erickson to have this impact was his ability to access the contexts within which change was needed and then reorient responses with respect to those contexts.

It should be noted that Erickson's use of metaphor extended beyond telling stories and anecdotes to include creating for his clients real-world experiences that were actually metaphors (and therefore isomorphic). A famous example of Erickson's use of this pattern is his work with the Pennsylvania couple that, after many years of analysis, came to Erickson for marriage therapy (for the complete case, see Gordon & Anderson, 1981, and Zeig, 1980, p. 145). Erickson sent them individually to climb Squaw Peak and visit the Desert Botanical Gardens, in order to get a different perspective on life. Much to their shock, Erickson then informed them therapy was completed and sent them home . . . where they promptly discharged their psychiatrists, cleaned their offices, got a divorce and eventually found mates with whom they could be happy.

A full appreciation of Erickson's exquisite use of anecdotal communication must include not only the apparent lesson of the story, but also the universally evocative aspects of the chosen analogy, the intricate and often subtle isomorphisms he used to evoke the appropriate associations, the ubiquitous and person-specific interweaving of hypnotic patterns and Erickson's ability to access in his listeners new and more useful responses within the identified context. I hope that this chapter has served to stir, rather than satisfy, your curiosity about what is possible. Certainly, these skills are deserving of our attention, for when Milton Erickson taught, people learned.

## REFERENCES

Bandler, R. & Grinder, J. *Patterns of the Hypnotic Techniques of Milton H. Erickson, M.D., Vol. 1.* Cupertino, CA: Meta Publications, 1975.

Erickson, M.H. The interspersal hypnotic technique for symptom correction and pain control. *American Journal of Clinical Hypnosis*, 1966, *3*, 198-209.

Gordon, D. *Therapeutic Metaphors.* Cupertino, CA: Meta Publications, 1978.

Gordon, D. & Anderson, M. *Phoenix: The Therapeutic Patterns of Milton Erickson.* Cupertino, CA: Meta Publications, 1981.

Haley, J. *Uncommon Therapy.* New York: W.W. Norton, 1973.

Zeig, J.K. *A Teaching Seminar with Milton H. Erickson, M.D.* New York: Brunner/Mazel, 1980.

Chapter 9

# Utilizing the Language of the Unconscious

*Donna M. Slosar*

If asked to describe myself professionally, my best and most telling response would be that I am a third generation Ericksonian. I first met Milton H. Erickson in May 1978 at his office in Phoenix for what I thought would be a once in a lifetime meeting. I resisted him for the first three hours. Subsequently, I have been laughing and crying as I discover all I knew that he knew I didn't know yet.

Erickson, for some unknown reason, delighted in my approach to learning. When I'm being humble, I think his interest was simply that I was young, and as an old man, he liked to have youth around; in my delusions of grandeur I like to think that he recognized some creativity that I've yet to discover. It will always remain a mystery to me whether he felt obligated to treat a first class nut in order to keep her off the street or whether in fact he was asking that in some small way I attempt to carry on his tradition for ingenious adaptation to life. I only know that we spent hour upon hour together personally and professionally. When he'd ask, "Will you come back soon?" I would reply, "Can birds fly?" And this bird flew often and at many levels. I am grateful and honored to be able to add to this tribute to Milton H. Erickson, who was not only a great therapist, but an even greater friend, and an enduring inspiration to those whose lives he touched.

One of the distinguishing features of Erickson's therapy was his ability to function at many different levels simultaneously and never to be satisfied in doing two things at once if he could be doing four. While most therapists use one or another technique to achieve a specific purpose, Erickson often combined techniques and many times utilized several at once.

Coming from a farm background, he planted choice words as seeds for change in the fertile field of the client's unconscious. He fully appreciated the importance of knowing the land, of assessing its fertility, of preparing the soil, of planting the seed at precisely the right time, of nurturing the fragile seedling, and finally, of rejoicing in the harvest which his partnership with nature had produced. Among the tools he used to bring about the harvest were clinical techniques such as pacing and leading (Gordon, 1979); reframing (Watzlawick, Weakland, and Fisch, 1974); paradox (Watzlawick, Beavin, and Jackson, 1967); and hypnotic trance induction (Erickson, Rossi, and Rossi, 1976).

In the introduction to *Change* (Watzlawick, Weakland and Fisch, 1974) Erickson stated:

> I have viewed much of what I have done as expediting the currents of change already seething within the person and the family—but currents that need the "unexpected," the "illogical," and the "sudden" move to lead them into tangible fruition.

This statement is the essence of what I think Erickson meant by "utilization."

The purpose of this paper is to examine the process of utilization as it is specifically related to Erickson's use of the language of the unconscious. It seems that it was precisely Erickson's unique facility with words—with language—that enabled him not only to recognize but also to respond so elegantly to the currents seething within the client.

I use the word "elegantly" deliberately. Many of us perform more "elephantly." Elegance demands that one use the most efficient means to reach the desired end. Erickson never wasted words—neither his nor the client's. Words were precious seeds to be planted for thought and change. When people around him would needlessly intellectualize the obvious, he became impatient. He often explained his verbal shorthand with comments such as "Basically, I'm lazy—why do or say more than I have to?" Paradoxically, he often communicated many things by saying nothing.

However, anyone who knows of Milton H. Erickson knows that he was anything but lazy. How many people teach themselves to walk again after two attacks of polio? Or single-handedly paddle a canoe from Wisconsin to St. Louis with two paralyzed legs, a bandanna and a can of beans?

Lest we become discouraged with our lack of elegance in using language, let us recall that Milton used his paralyzed body as a laboratory to study not only his own physical self, but also the complexity of human communication. Few of us have had a similar opportunity to stop, look and listen to life as Erickson did.

## ERICKSON'S USE OF WORDS IN THE THERAPIST-CLIENT INTERACTION

In order to understand Erickson's utilization of the language of the unconscious, it is necessary to examine his use of words within the larger context of the therapist-client interaction. For purposes of analysis, I would like to divide the interactional process into four phases:

1) observation of behavioral cues;
2) listening for client's unconscious language cues;
3) responding with language cues outside of conscious awareness of the client, yet matching cues given unconsciously by the client;
4) noting the client's conscious and unconscious behavioral response to Erickson's use of language.

Keep in mind, however, that it is the limitations of our conceptual tools which necessitate our consideration of these processes in a sequential fashion when, in actuality, they may occur in a different order, for example, as a cyclical chain, or even simultaneously.

### *1) Observation of Behavioral Cues*

Erickson stated that he never personally experienced a situation where events could not be explained by examining minimal sensory cues which people were unaware they were using. Erickson was always a keen observer, seeing the subtlest signs of change in bodily movement. In his later years he complained that he had been too directive with clients when he was young, and that he had learned to simply let things develop in a session and make use of things as they developed, responding to cues from the client. He often admonished students watching him work, "Don't watch me, watch the client!"

### *2) Listening for Client's Unconscious Language Cues*

Erickson seemed to hear more than most of us. He was well aware that trance alone would not and could not ensure change. He listened to what the client said while in trance. Erickson characterized the patient in trance as childlike. He stated that in a trance the client thinks like a child. Depending on one's theoretical metaphor, one could speculate that this childlike use of language is specific to the logic and syntax of the nondominant hemisphere, or, since some speculate that most repression occurs early in life, its expression is appropriately stated in a child's language form.

### *3) Responding with Language Cues that are Outside the Conscious Awareness of the Client, Yet Matching the Precise Language Cues Unconsciously Being Sent from the Client*

Erickson suggested that what he said was not important. It was the client's interpretation of what he said that was important. Therefore he used words with multiple meanings, puns, incomplete sentences, and dangling participles so that each client could "fill in the blank" with what was important for the individual client. (His "misuse" of grammar drove some people crazy!) Erickson directly told clients that their unconscious could hear and process what he said to them without their conscious mind understanding. He pointed out in his detailed work with Rossi (1976) that people's conscious minds were always correcting what did not seem logical, yet the unconscious mind received the uncorrected version, translated it, and made the appropriate association.

An interesting phenomenon began to occur as Milton grew older and his health failed. People would empathize with his difficulty in breathing, moving, and even using his voice inflection. Attributions ran rampant and group members were sure Milton had made a mistake in pronunciation, or become forgetful of names or dates due to his age or physical handicaps. Erickson, as ever, took advantage of the conscious bias and deliberately used the handicaps as ways of disguising hidden meanings to his very benevolent listeners.

Along the same line, as students (inundated with books and workshops on metaphor) became more and more conscious of the symbolism and utility for which Milton would use his storytelling, slight changes appeared in the words used in his old familiar stories. Erickson again baffled the listener who was sure he understood the fuller meaning of the metaphor—only to discover later that Milton's precise choice of words communicated another awareness outside of conscious understanding. It is fascinating to speculate what technique Milton would have devised next, now that we are analyzing his precision in the use of these words too!

### *4) Client's Conscious and Unconscious Behavioral Response to Erickson's Use of Language*

Erickson described trance as an active process of unconscious learning. He preferred that therapy occur without the client being consciously aware of what was happening. Many people left his sessions feeling confident that nothing personal had transpired between Erickson and themselves, only to report some weeks later, by phone or letter, that they were experiencing certain spontaneous changes in their behavior. Erickson thoroughly delighted in witnessing the client's bafflement at how or when the messages had been communicated at an unconscious level. He believed that the unconscious was quicker and more perceptive than the conscious mind and encouraged people to trust the functioning of their unconscious without constantly filtering information through the programmed biases of conscious thinking.

## AN ILLUSTRATION

I would now like to examine one of Erickson's sessions, slowing it down in order that we may savor the elegance of his marvelous use of language.

This was a three-day workshop in 1978 conducted by Erickson for a group of professionals. As usual, Erickson first got the lay of the land and began exploring the openness of the individual group members to trance work. One person, who had been with Erickson at a previous workshop, easily slipped into a deep trance. Erickson complimented him on the depth of the trance and asked: "Do you know where you are?" The client elaborated a number of specific visual experiences which he and Erickson enjoyed together in the trance.

The other group members, many of whom had never experienced hypnosis, were utterly amazed that this person was in such a deep trance and communicating with Erickson. Dr. Erickson then pointedly asked:

*E:* Where are you?
*Cl:* Nowhere . . . um . . . and it's nice. I'd rather be there with you than any place else.
*E:* How do you feel about nowhereness? (No awareness)
*Cl:* Just really good. It's OK.
*E:* Why do you say nowhereness is OK?
*Cl:* I like being here. It's comfortable.

Erickson said nothing, and the client continued in trance. As Erickson moved his body a microphone dropped and made quite a clatter. Erickson laughingly commented, looking at no one in particular: "Somebody dropped something?" Only one person (Client 2) replied with words, and enthusiastically said: "But what?!" This person was seated next to Erickson, a seat chosen on coming into the room. Erickson recognized her willingness and immediately guided her through her first traditional trance experience.

Both of these clients readily experienced trance phenomena, yet each gave a different unconscious language cue as to whether the trance would be utilized for change at this point in time.

Erickson then conducted his usual training session by responding to different members, answering questions, guiding trance inductions, and telling stories. As stated so clearly in Jay Haley's keynote address at this Congress (see Chapter 1), there would be as many different interpretations of what Erickson did in these sessions as there were people present. Again, we become overwhelmed by this man's ability to communicate in such diverse ways at so many different levels to so many different people. For our purposes here, I will trace only the language cues transmitted between Client 2 and Dr. Erickson. This person was unaware of most of this communication as it occurred during the sessions, but later shared with Dr. Erickson and me her astonishment in experiencing new behaviors and awareness when she returned to her family. As will be seen, the new behaviors correlate well with exact words she and Erickson were transmitting outside of her conscious awareness.

As Erickson described the details of this case to me, Client 2 was experiencing ambivalent feelings regarding her sexuality. These stemmed from sexual repression which was rooted in an all-enveloping traditional Catholic upbringing, which included an extensive period of training as a nun and was complicated by a premarital affair with a prominent and notable man. Among the themes identified by Erickson and addressed through the language of the unconscious were:

1) inhibited sexual response
2) value conflict
3) expression of self in role of mother

What follows is a brief outline of the patterns of cues and responses addressing these themes in the sessions.

*1) Inhibited Sexual Response.*

*A) Client's use of words*

The client consistently used the word "but" (perhaps a homonym for "butt") during the first part of the interview:

But, what?!
Yes, but . . .

No, but . . .
I agree, but . . .

Coming out of a trance, she related:

I didn't see any people—their bodies weren't noticeable. I only saw faces. Now, I also remember smelling *strawberries*—That's funny, I was in a boat with my cousins on a lake and there were no strawberries—but I can still smell them, now.

These words seem to indicate that unconsciously she avoided sexual awareness of bodies, hers and others, and that there was something good about her sexuality (strawberry) in the air, yet she could not recognize it yet.

Speaking of her deep experience of trance on the second day and comparing it to her first trance, she said: "If I had gone all the way yesterday, it wouldn't be so beautiful today." Unconsciously, this can be a reference to her sexual deprivation and the fulfillment she is anticipating.

On discussing her decision to leave the convent, she stated jokingly, "I guess my unconscious was kicking me in the butt." Consciously she made an intellectual decision to leave the religious life because of changes within the structure. She consciously had no thought of marriage or children. Unconsciously, she seemed to be stating where the problem was located!

Speaking to Erickson, off the cuff, later in the session as he was talking about discipline, she said, "You'd let a kid play in the dirt, wouldn't you?" It appears she was unconsciously recognizing Erickson's permissiveness and his desire to free her from sexual hangups.

*B) Erickson's choice of words*

It should be stated here that Erickson used many of his favorite stories in these sessions. We might say that in his usual fashion Erickson made sure that only the names and words were changed to instruct the innocent! He told the story of a young girl brought by parents to see him for a problem of enuresis. In this metaphor Erickson used the following words, which, because of his intonation and pronunciation, could be translated by the client to match her frame regarding sexuality.

The young girl's problem was bed wetting *(bad wedding)*

As the years went on she developed a bladder infection *(badder infection as the years go by.)*
When she laughed in the waking state she'd wet her pants.
(Erickson could be impliying that when the client tried to appear jovial, she messed herself up and found problems. Another possible meaning could be that in a state of awakening she would not only be happy but sexually responsive, i.e., lubricated.)
Her (the little girl's) sisters called her bad names—They knew she was a bed wetter *(bad wedder)*
(Religious associates looked down on her because of her sexual activity and for marrying outside the church.)

As the client was reluctant to come out of a trance Erickson commented:

It's hard to *awaken*—but you'll *make it.* (Erickson seems to be implying that awareness will be hard work but will result in good lovemaking.)

Erickson then told the story of a fellow who was in the State hospital and refused to believe that he had a stomach. This time around with the story, Erickson identified the fellow by the name of Herbert. He used these sentences.:

*Herb became my patient.* (Obviously an invitation for the client to really work with Erickson on this problem.)
I listened to Herbert (her butt). (I, Erickson, have heard your words, your need, your problem, i.e., the butt of it!)
Herbert knew he had been given rotten fish. (Her butt, her sexuality, had been misled—not misfed—by others.)

Milton told another of his favorite case histories regarding a person deep in depression whom he treated by having her plant African violets.

He repeated again and again that at the end of his treatment with her there were:

. . . African violet(s) (I can violate) in the kitchen
. . . African violet(s) in the dining room
. . . African violet(s) in the bedroom, etc. . . .

Listing all the rooms of the house, he finally said there were so many violets in her house, there was no room for depression.

The client saw this later as a critical communication—in that she shed her guilt and was comfortable with sex. There was no room for despair.

*2) Value Conflict*

*A) Client's words*

> I knew I should leave the convent—it just wasn't right for me. (She seems to be saying that the decision was not right for her to do.)

Talking about her jealousy of a younger sibling, the client confessed that she was selfish. Erickson asked her what she thought would happen if siblings were not jealous. The client replied:

> They just—they just disappear. (Again a childlike phrasing of *they adjust* and by doing so lose their identity.)

*B) Erickson's response*

Erickson related a familiar and tedious story of Pete who Erickson followed from a juvenile correctional institution to his death as an old man. Interspersed in this telling were these phrases:

> I knew what convict (convent) loyality was all about. (Erickson is stating that he can understand the value frame of loyalty and tradition within the client's religious background.)

He then related the story about the doctor telling his mother that he (Erickson) would not live till morning. He used these words:

> The doctor said *I'd be dead by morning* (mourning) and I did not want to die. (Erickson may have been referring to the religious concept "dead to the world" or to the useless mourning of the client's loss of grace. In any case, he is challenging a set value pattern that seems dysfunctional.)

The final set of word cues and reponses that we will examine have to do with the theme of motherhood.

*3) Expression of Self in Role of Mother*

*A) Client word cues*

The client related dreams in which her mother was present. The dreams were serious, but the client added these words to her ruminating about the dreams.

You know, *I really need a good belly* laugh.

This could be interpreted to mean that she had a wish to become pregnant. She further stated, patting her tummy while continuing to talk consciously about her relationship with her mother:

My mother feels good. (The part of me that is a mother is good.)

And again,

My *mother's life is full of* belly laughs.

This appeared to be another affirmation of her joy in being a mother. It should be noted that consciously she and her husband had decided to have no more children.

*B) Erickson's response in words*

As Erickson recounted the story of his doctor's conversation with his mother, these words were used:

*Move the dresser up* against the bed. *I was going to see one more sun (son) set* (yet) (Here Erickson, the good M.D., appears to be linking sexual activity with propagation.)

When the client was referring to her need for a good belly laugh, Erickson responded:

Would you like to *wake up with a good belly* laugh—go on. Enjoy it!

Intriguing as these communications are, I would be reluctant to attribute meaning to them without concrete evidence that changed behaviors were manifested in the client's functioning. Erickson cared little what a client understood about change; he measured growth by action. Through follow-up contact, Erickson verified that certain behaviors of the client had in fact changed.

*1) Sexually*

A. Her sexual spontaneity and activity increased in frequency and quality. For the first time, she not only caught sexual jokes but really laughed with them.

B. She reported spontaneously noticing that for the first time since childhood she could leave the covers of her bed unmade. She had not realized how compulsively she always made her bed neatly no matter what other household chores were left undone. (No need to cover up one's sexuality!)

C. She reported she spontaneously *really* saw a naked woman at a local spa and realized that she had never *seen* the full body of an adult prior to that.

*2) Values Orientation*

In her dealings with religious women she found she felt comfortable working with them. She no longer avoided them and could discuss openly her negative as well as positive reactions to religious life. Prior to these sessions she spoke well of "convent days" but avoided contact and was quite condescending in dealings with religious people.

*3) Motherhood*

She began without conscious planning to spend larger quantities of time with her children and delighted more and more in their development. She related that they actually looked smaller to her and she realized she had been relating to them as young people more than as young children.

Shortly after therapy ended she became pregnant. She now lives happily nested with a brood of young children.

Like a good farmer, Erickson didn't care about curing people. He was more interested in *growing* them. His attitude toward change was positive and filled with humor, curiosity, and wild expectations. Truly, he was a man of his word. He used the illogical, the unexpected, and the sudden to bring others to tangible fruition.

## REFERENCES

Erickson, M.H. & Rossi, E.L. Two level communication and the microdynamics of trance and suggestion. *American Journal of Clinical Hypnosis,* 1976, *18,* 153-171.

Erickson, M.H., Rossi, E.L., & Rossi, S.I. *Hypnotic Realities. The Induction of Clinical Hypnosis and Forms of Indirect Suggestion.* New York: Irvington Publishing, 1976.

Gordon, D. *Therapeutic Metaphors.* Cupertino, CA: Meta Publications, 1979.

Watzlawick, P., Beavin, J.H., & Jackson, D.P. *Pragmatics of Human Communication: A Study of Interactional Patterns, Pathologies and Paradoxes.* New York: W.W. Norton, 1967.

Watzlawick, P., Weakland, J., & Fisch, R. *Change: Principles of Problem Formation and Problem Resolution.* New York: W.W. Norton, 1974.

Chapter 10

# The Occurrence and Use of Trance Phenomena in Nonhypnotic Therapies

*Stephen Ryan Lankton*

Milton Erickson bridged the gap between classically understood hypnosis and "nonhypnotic" psychotherapies. Erickson showed us there are more similarities than differences among psychotherapies. Indeed, Erickson defined hypnosis as a state in which "the client concentrates on his own thoughts, memories, values, and beliefs about life" (Note 1). Because trance phenomena like catalepsy, amnesia, age regression and hallucination are the spontaneous result of prolonged or accentuated involvement in internal processing, they occur not only in hypnosis, but in other psychotherapies as well.

Hypnosis and nonhypnotic therapy have similarities that are rooted in three principles of Erickson's work. First, communication in both therapy and hypnosis elicits an unconscious search process in the client. Second, the client may develop a sense of recognition or understanding which will activate recognizable ideomotor responses. Third, this search process facilitates common trance phenomena. Trance phenomena and the search responses which accompany them are therapeutic choice points in nonhypnotic therapies.

Diverse labels have been attached to trance phenomena, so that age regression may variously be called "unfinished business," a "Child ego state," or a "neurotic affect and transference reaction," depending on the therapist's background.

To systematically analyze how these phenomena are utilized by hypnotic and nonhypnotic therapies alike, one must examine communication processes which therapeutically stimulate a client to search for memories, values, and beliefs about life. Therefore, discrete communication operations will be discussed within four analytic schemes, namely process operations, content operations, linguistic operations and input operations. Within this framework, trance phenomena are discussed and examples of their occurrence are presented.

## PROCESS OPERATIONS

In process operations, three patterns are identified by which verbal and/or nonverbal communication is expressed. These are matching, reversal and disruption.

*Matching* involves mirroring the client's communication channel, reflecting the particular mode of the moment. To match movement, gesture, breathing, or tone to that of another requires careful attention to the rhythm of change. In hypnotic therapy, the hypnotist may match the rhythm of his speech to the rhythm of the client's respiration; Erickson used this technique to build rapport with the client. In a similar vein, Erickson might speak the same type of verbal gibberish (word-salad) as a client (Erickson, 1967, p. 500). Matching can be used simultaneously, with other patterns of both a verbal and nonverbal nature.

*Reversal* involves an opposite response, that of deliberately projecting the reverse of what the client is doing. For example, Erickson might speak slowly to a resistant client who is speaking rapidly, while making a paradoxical statement such as "You can't go into a trance."

*Disruption* is a technique for interrupting the ongoing process and related associations. It may be accomplished in a number of ways, including distraction, humor, making an irrelevant comment, and so forth. It is particularly useful when hypnotists issue a direct command which they do not want challenged. For instance, in the "Monde" film (produced by Herbert Lustig, M.D.), when Erickson tells Monde to use her learnings in a directed fashion and then immediately asks her, "You're not cold, are you?", a seemingly irrelevant comment about temperature disrupted conscious consideration of his instruction (Lustig, 1975).

Just as several channels of verbal and nonverbal communication may exist at the same time, two or more of these operations can occur simultaneously. Thus, the hypnotist might match voice tone, tempo, volume, and body posture while reversing the client's verbal content.

## CONTENT OPERATIONS

In content operations, one utilizes various patterns to influence client verbal responses: specifying response questions, detailing communications, and meta-comments.

A *specifying response question* is designed to elicit more complete background information for assessment purposes. Questions might include: "Who, where, and how specifically . . . ?" as well as "What prevents you?" and "What would happen if you did?"

A *detailing communication* specifies desired behavioral responses. For example, Erickson might instruct a client to "sit down, lean back, uncross your legs like this, and listen to my words" (Note 2). Here Erickson detailed four responses he expected from the client.

A *meta-comment* is a comment about a communication. Meta-comment refers to both the simple labeling of an event and an ongoing explanation of some experience or communication. These are abundant in all forms of psychotherapy. In hypnotherapy, meta-comments allow the hypnotist to subtly shift the meaning an experience or symptom has for the client, as when the hypnotist says, "Your unconscious mind wants one thing while your conscious mind wants something else." Jay Haley (1963) speculated that Erickson employed such content operations to achieve therapeutic control.

Both process and content channels can be used singly or in combination. For example, the hypnotist could match body posture, voice tone and breathing of the client, while meta-commenting, "I'm going to tell you the real reason why you came to see me today," then follow this with the detailing communication, ". . . so sit down in that chair, relax, close your eyes and listen to my words." The very next moment, the hypnotist might employ a process reversal like, "Not that fast, I don't want you to go into a trance this soon," thus achieving response inhibition or fractionation which would serve to deepen the trance.

## LANGUAGE OPERATIONS

The grammatical syntax of the verbal communication used by the hypnotist can also be divided into three distinctive categories. These are search language, induction language and metaphor.

*Search language* initiates an internal search process within the client. This technique utilizes unspecified, vague, and general language forms to stimulate the client to search for personal meaning. Erickson frequently used deliberately vague phrasing like "You're going to recall *some* forgotten experience," "*Everybody* has had the experience of forgetting," or "Your *unconscious* contains a vast storehouse of *learnings*."

*Induction language* employs embedded commands, indirect suggestion, and presuppositions of consciousness, time and number to suggest options to the client. Statements like "You will *begin to wonder* . . . ," "You really can, Joe, *feel relaxed* . . . ," and "Can you *uncross your legs* and just relax *once again*," illustrate this technique.

*Metaphor* refers to a noncausal linking of facts which involves matching content and processes in the client's situation, or to an illustrative anecdote or explanation used which incorporates symbolism. Metaphor develops a theme using search language and induction language. Erickson's metaphors often began with a simple lead-in line like "I had a client one time from the midwest who . . .".

Following a brief discussion of input operations, the way in which these language operations initiate unconscious search processes and the role of the search process in the development of hypnotic phenomena in nonhypnotic therapy will be presented.

## INPUT OPERATIONS

Input operations (Grinder, DeLozier, & Bandler, 1977) involve the differing effects upon client visual, kinesthetic and auditory experiences, due to the verbal and nonverbal communications of the hypnotist or therapist. These include packaging, directing, and associating input.

*Packaging* input consists of the communicator's determining a client's perception of reality, then incorporating these subjective needs into his response patterns through the verbal matching of language processing words. For example, when the client specifies that he doesn't *see* how he is going to overcome his difficulty, Erickson would "package" his verbal communication with visually oriented verbs and nouns like "clear," "picture," "focus" or "bright." If the client says there is no *harmony* in his marriage, Erickson would utilize auditory packaging phrases such as "tune-in," "hear," "listen," "two hoots and a holler," or "amplify." Kinesthetically based words include: touch, relax, comfort, sit, hold, grasp, feel, embrace, solid, and grip. Obviously, many words and phrases lend themselves to this type of feedback. Most important, then, is judicious packaging by the therapist for each client's individual framework.

*Directing* assists the client in selecting the most useful sensory processing mode. This can be done by congruent changes in gestures, directed eye movement, tone shifts, and so forth. When Erickson wanted a client to consciously think with pictures, he might point or glance upward, influencing the client to break eye contact. Moving his eyes upward, he would initiate the related visualization process. Once eye closure had been established, Erickson would systematically direct the client to the desired sensory mode via stories, illustration, and analogy.

*Associating and anchoring,* pairing a particular stimulus with a specific client experience, may be induced consciously or unconsciously, using any of the sensory input channels or verbal labeling. Cueing is used as a re-induction signal in hypnotherapy. A signal (a simple word, sound or touch) successfully associated with a trance state, when subsequently presented, will cue and initiate that same trance state again. Often, re-induction signals are learned in a single trial association. On a more subtle level, the hypnotist can be reasonably certain the client will associate to comfort when he says "comfort."

## SEARCH BEHAVIOR AND RESPONSE

The client's ability to make sense of communications received reflects the sensory channel the client uses for input, his perception and his previous learning. Perception and previous learnings are mediated by ego images which consist of auditory, visual, or kinesthetic impulses with varying degrees of cathexis (Fenichel, 1945). During the momentary search process, the person unconsciously, and at times consciously, attempts to locate previous representations which give meaning to present input. If the hypnotist says, "You have had comfort, have you not?", he has used search language consisting of the complex noun "comfort" and deletions (comfortable where, when, with whom, etc?). The "have you not" is a verbal reversal which will maximize the probability of getting a "yes" response, even from an incongruent client.

The first portion of the statement, "You have had comfort, have you not?", influences the client to sort through internal representations from his/her past and fill in the deletions in the most relevant manner. He will select his most common imagery, and then respond in the manner most typical for him, when presented with deleted complex nouns and deleted noun phrases. Following the search process, the client's ideomotor responses inform the hypnotist of the images and habit patterns developed by the client. These responses allow the hypnotist to modify communication, depending upon the desired goal in the session.

The internal search process is identifiable in any ongoing communication. The best indicators include flattened cheeks, lowered center of respiration, slowed respiration, slowed blink and swallow reflexes, decreased gross motor movement, eye scanning patterns, and increased pallor. These indicators also signify hypnogogic or light trance states. Hypnotists train themselves to notice these responses, whereas non-hypnotic therapists usually do not.

When a person is spoken to, he makes meaning of words, tone, and facial expressions through subjective associations. The client is internally assembling and examining previous pictures, words and feelings. The more ambiguous the therapist communication, the greater the likelihood a person will apply the communication personally. In everyday communication, lack of specificity can create a discrepancy between intended communication and message received. In hypnosis, however, vague phrasing can be helpful.

Classical hypnosis and the various psychotherapies appear to differ most in the way elicited responses are utilized. Typically, hypnotherapists think about eye closure and similar "classical" induction ideas. This orientation alerts the hypnotist to words which retrieve certain valuable memories from the client's history, as the following induction example will illustrate.

*Transcript 1*

*Hypnotist:* Please be seated like this and notice, really notice, how you can easily learn. (Pause)

*Client:* Sits and places hands on thighs and places feet on floor. Head tilts; left ear orients to hypnotist. Face becomes immobile and respiration slows.

*Hypnotist:* You can at least learn that you already know more than you think you know.

*Client:* Looks down and right quickly, then stares ahead and defocuses.

*Hypnotist:* And your experience becomes like that in a dream now, but you couldn't say how.

*Client:* Exhales deeply, blink slows, face and stare are immobile.

*Hypnotist:* You can remember better when you close your eyes.

*Client:* Closes eyes and swallows.

The hypnotist begins by matching the client's behavior to facilitate rapid rapport. This is accompanied by subtle meta-commenting with the word "please," setting a nonauthoritarian tone. As the client searches through memories related to nonauthoritarian relationships, he will likely find images associated with relaxed musculature. Also, search language used by the hypnotist (deletions and unspecified verbs) invites the client to recall associated experiences (such as associations to the word "easily").

Next the hypnotist uses induction language (presuppositions: "at least," "more than"), search language (deletion and unspecified verbs: "think" and "know") and continues to match posture and voice tempo to client respiration. The client continues the search response. Eye movements suggest he has begun the remembered feeling of "easily" (eyes down and right). The defocused stare suggests he is thinking in pictures (probably about previous learning experiences). Continued relaxation responses indicate that relaxation and learning memories have been successfully associated.

Then, the previous structure is emphasized and search language (complex noun "experience," and unspecified verb "becomes") introduces associations to the word "dream." Similar associations are then related to not speaking. The client's response suggests ideomotor behavior associated to dreaming with medium trance depth.

Finally, the hypnotist uses search language to build the final association needed for eye closure. The client complies easily because he is now operating from that portion of his memory where he is experiencing nonauthoritarian, relaxed and dream-like states.

The structure of the hypnotic communication process and client responses can be made explicit in several ways. Two relevant applications are: 1) comparison of nonhypnotic therapeutic communications, and 2) demystification of both hypnotic and nonhypnotic therapy (Stevens, 1975, p. 247 ff.).

Hypnotists are alert to the development of certain search phenomena in their clients. These include: relaxation, catalepsy, eye closure, and dissociation of feeling state from visual imagery. The hypnotist fosters search behavior in the client until the therapeutic associations are built and these interventions alter the customary search-response pattern.

The notion of ideomotor behavior is used to explain how musculature and reflex activity are affected by remembered or constructed images. If the client recalls images associated to pleasant experiences, a smile and increased muscle tonus will be noted. Undesirable images produce muscle distortions. Lacking a well-formed response, the client will begin search phenomena, or hypnotic response. Erickson pointed out that any change in internal imagery (auditory, visual, kinesthetic) results in a noticeable change in the client's expression or behavior (cf. Assagioli, 1965). The classical hypnotic phenomena mentioned below may spontaneously occur as the search process continues.

Nonhypnotic therapies, even family interactions, involve these patterns of communication (cf. Berne, 1972; Laing, 1967; O'Connell, 1970) and similarly elicit the hypnotic responses which will be detailed below. The pattern is as follows: unspecified speech—search—naming or otherwise referring to a desired experience—retrieving the desired experience—using the groups of retrieved experiences in therapeutic patterns.

## AN ILLUSTRATION

The following transcript is provided so that the reader can get an idea of how hypnotic responses show up in "nonhypnotic" therapies. Examples are presented of how some of the above-mentioned communication operations are utilized in practice.

*Hypermnesia* is that phenomenon which occurs in deep trance, when a person can recall events from the past in much greater detail than is possible within a "normal" waking state. The person may not remember events "accurately," but since a therapist is working to alter a "map" rather than a "territory," this distinction is largely irrelevant. The client recreates whatever was real for him or her at that time, and during hypermnesia these realities can become especially vivid and detailed, as the following Gestalt therapy transcript illustrates. The client, Violet, is very depressed, anorexic and withdrawn. She frequently sits with her feet in the chair and her arms wrapped around her legs, as if to hide. She is not actively suicidal, but did speak of taking her life just prior to the referral. This transcript is her eleventh therapy session.

*Transcript 2* (Lankton, Note 3)

1) *Lankton:* (Finishing with another client) Now, Violet, what are you experiencing (actually turning and sitting like Violet is sitting; legs crossed, palms up on lap, head erect, and lips together without a smile)?
2) *Violet:* (Jerks back as she notices him) I didn't know it was my turn to work (sarcastic tone of voice).
3) *Lankton:* (With sarcastic voice, like hers) You never know what you will experience, until you make yourself available for new experience.
4) *Violet:* (Pupils dilate, face muscles flatten, blink slows, respiration slows. She nods her head slowly, as if to show agreement.)
5) *Lankton:* (Waits, still matching her behavior).
6) *Violet:* I feel crowded!
7) *Lankton:* And how is it for you to feel crowded? Give yourself room to experience being crowded (pauses) and put words to it.
8) *Violet:* (Defocuses her eyes and stares, changes posture as she pulls her legs to her chin and entwines her arms around her legs).
9) *Lankton:* Stay there—with yourself and come to know where you are crowded. (Leans forward but does not further match her specific behavior)

*10) Violet:* (Closes her eyes) I'm crowded in, closed in.

*11) Lankton:* What do you experience enclosing you?

*12) Violet:* I'm in a box. Now I feel like I was (voice gets more faint) just too little. (Begins to cry as her face muscles lose all tonus and pallor increases)

*13) Lankton:* (Changes voice to a softer, melodic tone) Say that in the present tense—"I am just too little."

*14) Violet:* (Haltingly at first) I . . . I'm just too little . . . I can't push it . . . I can't push the . . . (changes to original voice tone) I don't know what I'm talking about.

*15) Lankton:* (Changes to original tone of voice) You have some unfinished business back there. You will know where after you experience it. Perhaps the safety in this room releases you to find out what you need to finish elsewhere. Go there and re-experience what you will find.

*16) Violet:* I don't know . . . (pauses, moves her eyes up to the left and then she begins to stare ahead) . . . I'm too big to fit in here. I can pull my legs up like this. This refrigerator is big, bigger than those boxes. It opens really hard, makes a funny noise. I like it. (It) feels smooth inside. There is not as much room in here as I thought there was. (Pauses) I could go to sleep in here. The door is closed and it's dark, really dark. I don't think I want to be in here any more. The door won't open—I can't get out, I can't get out . . .

*17) Lankton:* Make noise!

*18) Violet:* Ahh, Mommy, I can't get out, can't get out, let me . . . HELLLLLPP (cries and leaps from chair)!

*19) Lankton:* You're out! (holding her) Can you finish this situation by being here and being free?

*20) Violet:* I'm scared. I'm right here, hanging on tight (to therapist's hand).

*21) Lankton:* How are you scaring yourself? There is nothing scary here.

*22) Violet:* (Standing and speaking to the group with a growing smile) I made noise when I was scared. I got out of there. I moved. I thought. I thought about what I needed even when I was scared. That was a good decision. Guess that was what I did (sits down and begins recovering from the unexpected incident).

This transcript was chosen for analysis for three reasons: 1) because it is representative of Gestalt therapy; 2) because amnesia preceded therapy; and 3) because the client relieved an early, repressed, incident. Violet had no conscious memory of having been locked in a refrigerator.

Following this therapy session, her mother confirmed that she had, at age two, become locked in a refrigerator. She had fainted and was near death upon being discovered. The family had kept this a secret. Following this incident, Violet had become a quiet, passive youngster. Therapy was directed toward building the kinds of need identification and expressive responses Violet lacked in areas of eating, feeling, and social intercourse.

Vivid recall during regression is typical of hypermnesia. It frequently assists the therapist to clarify details or to make explicit influential dialogues from their clients' early years. Therapy goals and theoretical persuasion determine how details gathered during hypermnesia will be utilized by different therapists. Possible uses include gathering diagnostic information, creating therapeutic change (i.e. believing, thinking, or feeling differently in the face of an old memory), verifying recollections received from "normal waking state," and changing portions of problematic imagery which intrude into consciousness.

Analysis of this session reveals the same communication operations found in hypnosis. In lines one through five I incorporate search language ("experience," "make available") and behavioral matching (posture, tone, tempo). Induction language is used to suggest that she will have the experience. The client demonstrates search phenomena in line four and finally locates the original experience linked to current feelings of being crowded.

The rest of her memory consists of visual images as shown in lines eight through 16. In lines seven through 10, I continue matching, search language and induction language as Violet reconstructs this experience which was outside conscious remembrance. In line 11, I ask a specifying question about the experience to enhance her reliving the experience and to prevent dissociation. Line eight illustrates her total immersion as her internal imagery stimulates increasingly more congruent ideomotor behavior.

I continue to match changes demonstrated in lines nine, 13, and 15. In line 15, I again use search language ("business," "back there," "know," "experience") and induction language (presuppositions: "you will," "after," "you will find"; and deletions producing embedded commands: "experience it," "find out," "go there," "re-experience"). A new operation is purposefully used when I remind Violet that there is "safety" available. Following this use of association, Violet's retrieval of the experience begins.

In line 16, Violet finds her legs in the chair as she acts from visual/kinesthetic maps. As she becomes more fully engaged in the process, she displays deep trance phenomena. She positively hallucinates the old incident and this entails negative hallucination for events in the room. She age regresses to a powerful degree and experiences, hypermnesia. In lines 17, 18, and 19, I guide her with detailing responses. My directive, "make noise," leads her to access a past learning. Previously unable to formulate the age appropriate response to express her needs, she had been operating as a two-year old, until she made this new therapeutic association.

Lines 20 and 22 illustrate how a client can quickly move out of total age regression and use an age-appropriate meta-comment. This indicates how valuable this regression has been in the service of the ego, as she demonstrates synthesis and integration. She can now consciously think of the trauma without withdrawing, or being hostile or quiet, her previous reaction when these images were only preconscious and unconscious.

## SIMILARITIES BETWEEN HYPNOSIS AND WAKING STATE

Hypnotic phenomena occur as the result of communication and concentrated internal attention, not from some physical difference between the normal waking state and trance states. Biofeedback studies of EEG and oxygen consumption during meditation, sleep, hypnotic trance, and waking reveal that the hypnotic state is most similar to the waking state. "The patterns during hypnosis have no relation to those of the meditative state; in a hypnotized subject the brain wave activity takes the form characteristic of the mental state that has been suggested to the subject" (Ornstein, 1973, p. 266). In other words, the physiological phenomena produced by communication and internal search process are most like those of the normal waking state.

It follows that communication in psychotherapy and other waking states produces and uses trance phenomena under various guises. This hypothesis has encouraged me to define the structure of the language and nonverbal communication which produces or initiates these search and association processes, to demystify and improve the quality of both hypnosis and psychotherapy.

Successful communication enables another person to perceive or to conceive portions of experience common to the speaker (Laing, 1972, p. 79). Commnication commonly has properties or elements of hypnotic suggestion, frequently in the same semantic order and for the same duration as purposeful hypnotic communication. Therefore, normal communication and nonhypnotic psychotherapies comprise a series of inductions. Therapeutically, these vary in style and skill, reflecting the therapist's or communicator's past training.

Psychology and sociology have much to gain from the study of Ericksonian clinical hypnosis. Practical applications of this approach should provide refinements of communication in such areas as educational settings, clinical psychotherapy, and child rearing.

## REFERENCE NOTES

1. Erickson, M.H. Personal communication, Phoenix, Arizona, August, 1975.
2. Erickson, M.H. Personal communication, Phoenix, Arizona, November, 1977.
3. Lankton, S. *Violet.* A videotape of private group therapy practice, Ann Arbor, MI, 1979.

## REFERENCES

Assagioli, R. *Psychosynthesis.* New York: The Viking Press, 1965.

Berne, E. *What Do You Say After You Say Hello.* New York: Grove Press, Inc., 1972.

Erickson, M.H. Use of symptoms as an integral part of therapy. In J. Haley (Ed.) *Advanced Techniques of Hypnosis and Therapy.* New York: Grune & Stratton, 1967.

Erickson, M.H., & Cooper, L. *Time Distortion in Hypnosis.* Baltimore: William and Wilkins, 1959.

Erickson, M.H., Rossi, E., & Rossi, S. *Hypnotic Realities.* New York: Irvington Publishers, Inc., 1976.

Fenichel, O. *The Psychoanalytic Theory of Neurosis.* New York: W.W. Norton & Co., Inc., 1945.

Grinder, J., DeLozier, J., & Bandler, R. *Patterns of Hypnotic Techniques of Milton H. Erickson, M.D., Vol. II.* Cupertino, CA.: Meta Publications, 1977.

Haley, J. *Strategies of Psychotherapy.* New York: Grune & Straton, 1963.

Laing, R.D. *The Politics of Experience.* New York: Ballantine Books, 1967.

Laing, R.D. *The Politics of the Family.* New York: Vintage Books, 1972, p. 79.

Lankton, S. *Practical Magic: A Translation of Basic Neuro-linguistic Programming into Clinical Psychotherapy.* Cupertino, CA.: Meta Publications, 1980.

Lustig, H. (producer) *The Artistry of Milton H. Erickson, M.D.* Haverford, PA: Herbert S. Lustig, M.D., Ltd., 1975 (video).

O'Connell, V.F. Crisis psychotherapy. In J. Fagan & I. Shepherd (Eds.) *Gestalt Therapy Now.* New York: Harper and Row, 1970, p. 248.

Ornstein, R. *The Nature of Human Consciousness.* San Francisco: W.H. Freeman and Co., 1973.

Stevens, J. Hypnosis, intention, and wake-fullness. In *Gestalt Is.* Moab: Real People Press, 1975.

PART V

# *Erickson's Influence on the Work of the Mental Research Institute*

*The current Mental Research Institute group, led by Paul Watzlawick, Ph.D., John Weakland, Ch.E., and Richard Fisch, M.D., have provided seminal and enduring contributions to developing, explicating, and researching strategic therapy techniques.*

*In their chapters Watzlawick and Fisch develop some of the theory behind the interactional approach. Watzlawick eloquently argues that the solutions that people apply to problem situations perpetuate their problems. Ericksonian therapy is based on effect rather than understanding. When Erickson worked with individuals, his thinking was grounded in understanding the effect of his communication on the system in which the patient was enmeshed. Watzlawick emphasizes that "action precedes understanding."*

*Fisch points to the fact that the issue in brief psychotherapy should be effectiveness rather than length of treatment. The problems that people have "relate mainly to their failure to take action or their persistence in entrapping or stalemating actions." The effectiveness of strategic approaches should lead us to change our philosophy so that we are no longer constrained by theoretical orientations based on psychopathology. This reasoning is in line with Erickson's admonition that theory can be a Procrustean bed that limits the practitioner's flexibility.*

*Our diagnosis implies a plan of treatment. If we diagnose problems in terms of pathology, we limit the range of our interventions. Both*

*Watzlawick and Fisch would agree with Erickson's dictum that resources for change are dormant within the patient. The patient does not need to be taught anything new. With proper diagnosis and intervention, potentials for change that are inherent in the system can be made manifest.*

*Weakland's chapter speaks to the influence that Erickson's thinking may have had in developing the concept of the double bind. In the history of human thought, there are few concepts that can be seen as radical departures from the prevailing Zeitgeist. The double bind was certainly such a concept. Although Erickson was not a part of the group that formulated the double bind, Haley and Weakland had visited Erickson before the formulation of the 1956 paper by Bateson, Jackson, Haley and Weakland.*

*In his chapter, Weakland specifies the double bind and delineates its historical development. He points out some of the theoretical assumptions underlying the original article, including the fact that "all behavior is markedly dependent on and shaped by communication." Such theoretical issues certainly were emphasized recurrently in Erickson's work. Whether these concepts developed in parallel or through mutually interactive influences is unimportant. They have shaped the direction of psychotherapy and are now the basis of contemporary approaches.*

Chapter 11

# Erickson's Contribution to the Interactional View of Psychotherapy

*Paul Watzlawick*

The title of my presentation seems absurd, if by interactional psychotherapy we mean a treatment method based not on hypothesized intrapsychic processes, but on observable patterns of interaction and, therefore, communication *between* people, such as, for instance, couple or family therapy. To this the purist may object by pointing out that hypnosis is very much a form of interaction. The interactionist's answer would be that, while hypnosis is an interactive process, as are transference and countertransference phenomena in classical psychoanalysis, the interaction is strictly between the therapist and his individual patient, and, furthermore, the goal of therapy is to bring about changes inside the individual's mind.

What I have been asked to present to this Congress is the influence of Milton H. Erickson's genius on human systems and not just on individuals. As one reads his articles and books, one notices how he gradually moved from a strictly intrapsychic epistemology, based on the traditional ideas of intrapsychic dynamics—from the alleged curative value of insight and the monadic view of the skin-encapsulated human being as the ultimate unit of study—to a view that more and more took into account the social contexts in which human beings function or suffer. I, for one, would find it impossible to pinpoint this transition in time. However, I should imagine that long before family therapists became aware of the vicissitudes of change in human systems, Erickson had already discovered and utilized the almost incredible degree to which a patient's family and larger social contexts can help or hinder change.

This may not be everyone's view of Erickson's work or of hypnosis in general. We must not forget that hypnosis still plays the role of the fool or the court jester in the solemn halls of orthodoxy. The jester, as you remember, got away with his undeniable truths precisely because he was a fool who could be taken seriously only in a very selective way. Similarly, even today hypnosis is seen by many as a somewhat outlandish way to further the aims of the true doctrine, namely to lift repressed material into consciousness. Once it has achieved that, it should hop along and no longer interfere with the promotion of insight.

In order to delineate the frame of my presentation clearly, let me repeat: When I refer to interactional psychotherapy, I mean a treatment modality that is applied to disturbances which arise out of the way people relate to each other in the observable here and now, and not to inferred intrapsychic processes. When I refer to the influence of hypnotherapy on interaction, I mean that aspect of hypnosis which attempts to bring about change in the here and now by getting people to behave differently, not to its utilization for uncovering individual experiences submerged in the darkness of the past.

While there is by no means agreement among interactional therapists as to the best definition of those disturbances inherent in the network of relationships, it seems useful to think of them in terms of a "game without end." This is another way of saying that the system *qua* system is rule-governed, but that the repertory of its rules does not include the solution to the particular problem. Upon observation, systems can then be seen running again and again through the coping mechanisms contained in the body of their rules—its program, if you will—without ever arriving at an adequate solution. The game, i.e., the system's rule-governed behavior, is thus without end, except for the extreme cases where the end is literally the destruction of the system (in evolution, the extinction of an entire species; on the human level, insanity and consequent removal of the identified patient from the system, through divorce, homicide or suicide). Where the game goes on without end, we find—again by mere observation in the here and now—that what perpetuates the game, the problem, are precisely the solutions attempted and stubbornly applied again and again.

If you can accept this definition of systems pathology, there are two very different ways of dealing with it. One would be the traditional attempt to promote insight into these repetitive, self-defeating patterns of interaction. Over the decades of our work at MRI, my colleagues and I have become increasingly skeptical about the clinical usefulness and efficacy of such attempts. We all know the fallacy of believing that reason is the supreme human faculty which, once restored to its lofty throne by means of insight, will make people behave rationally and sanely. We all know the patient who after years of therapy has all the insight into his murky past he will probably ever have (to say nothing about the beautiful touch he now has with his feelings), and yet does not seem to benefit from having bathed in the crystal light of reason. Fortunately, a self-sealing explanation may be found for this phenomenon. It vindicates the true doctrine and is of great value to the therapist (and his bank account)—namely, that the lack of therapeutic results proves that the patient's past has not yet been sufficiently illuminated and that deeper therapy is still needed.

The other approach is to get people to behave differently and thereby abandon their problem-perpetuating, attempted solutions. If problems persist in the here and now as a result of wrong solutions, then the genesis of the problem is immaterial and its analysis is an exercise in futility. It then becomes imperative to change the supposed problem-solving behavior. Because systems caught in a game without end are caught precisely because they cannot generate from within themselves rules for the change of their rules—the meta-rules which would enable them to engage in different problem-solving behaviors—it stands to reason that the new behaviors must be introduced into the system from the outside. Sometimes this happens through a fortuitous outside event; if not, it becomes the task of therapy to provide this input.

This is, however, what the hypnotherapist has always been doing, even though he has traditionally limited himself to individual patients. Erickson, who was an eminent systems thinker, demonstrated that this can be done even more fruitfully within entire systems of relationships. This is the point where interactional therapy, as we are trying to research and practice it at MRI, begins to profit from his ingenious techniques.

What he taught us above all was a different use of language. Traditionally, the language of therapy is the language of interpretation, explanation, confrontation and the like. It is an explanatory language and must be so because it stands in the service of consciousness-raising. By contrast, the language of hypnosis is deontic or injunctive, because its ultimate message, no matter how carefully veiled, is: "*Do* something!". The relevance this has for our work can be shown by a quotation from a book that has nothing to do directly with our field. It is from George Spencer Brown's (1973) *Laws of Form*:

> It may be helpful to realize that the primary form of mathematical communication is not description, but injunction. In this respect

> it is comparable with practical art forms like cookery, in which the taste of a cake, although literally indescribable, can be conveyed to the reader in the form of a set of injunctions called a recipe. Music is a similar art form. The composer does not even attempt to describe the set of sounds he has in mind, much less the set of feelings occasioned through them, but writes down a set of commands which, if they are obeyed by the reader, can result in a reproduction, to the reader, of the composer's original experience (p. 77).

What is therapy, if not the attempt to convey to another person experiences as difficult or even as impossible to communicate in descriptive, explanatory language as it is to describe the taste of a cake?

Another aspect of hypnotherapy that is immediately relevant to interactional therapy follows from the one just described. It is the essence of Erickson's prescription: "Take what the patient is bringing you;" his insistence on "learning the patient's language." This is again a significant departure from traditional therapy in which we were trained to teach our patients a new "language," i.e., the conceptual system of a given school of thought regarding human behavior. Only after the patient has learned to think of himself, his world and his problems in these new terms is change attempted within this new frame. This process is time-consuming, to say the least.

Erickson taught us to do the opposite: to learn the patient's language and to use it to facilitate the task of getting people to behave differently. This is of eminent importance in couples and family therapy. Families have their own myths, outlooks, jokes, value systems and shared reality distortions and they consequently speak their own "languages," enriched with individual "dialects." If we want to change such a system, we must learn the language and its dialects. This represents a total reversal of traditional psychotherapeutic procedure. The therapist, not his patients, must learn something new, just as a good hypnotist carefully listens to his subject's language and then gives his suggestions in terms that are most congenial and therefore least resistance-provoking to his client.

As already mentioned, Erickson was an accomplished thinker in terms of systems. A splendid example is the case of the couple who ran their small restaurant together and who constantly quarreled about the best way of running it. The wife insisted that the husband should be in charge because she would rather stay home; the husband pointed out that she would never let him do that, because she thought that without her supervision he would ruin the business. After a detailed exploration of this interaction, in which cause typically produced effect which fed back on cause, Erickson gave them a behavioral prescription. Each morning the husband was to go to the restaurant half an hour before his wife. This simple change, apparently so "remote" from the "real" problem, totally threw the ingrained mechanism of their vicious-circle interaction out of kilter. When the wife now arrived at the restaurant, she was hopelessly behind in her routine and the husband had already completed part of her seemingly irreplaceable functions. Soon she realized that she could arrive an hour late or even later and also she found that she did not have to stay with him until closing time. She thus found more and more time to devote to their home and he became increasingly capable of running the restaurant alone.

I shall not waste time and try to speculate what different a course this treatment would have taken along the more orthodox lines of explanation and interpretation in the service of producing insight. Instead, let me point out several other things.

The case provides an excellent illustration of the system-theoretical maxim that a small, peripheral change in a system's functioning may produce large repercussions throughout its entire structure. Incidentally, it is the simple elegance of this kind of intervention that makes it most questionable to the more monadic-minded therapist because, as Karl Popper once remarked, nothing causes more resistance than simple solutions for longstanding problems.

Erickson's intervention also illustrates another characteristic of a successful intervention. The simplicity of the injunction makes its communication easy and diminishes the chances of misunderstanding and noncompliance. Furthermore, the demanded action was completely inexpensive, nondangerous and not degrading; it therefore evoked a minimum of resistance. Finally, the injunction called for a piece of—for lack of a better word—*physical* behavior rather than mere verbalization. By this I do not want to imply that in the interactional view a verbalization would not be considered a behavior, but only to suggest that injunctions aiming at behavior in the more immediate sense are more effective. Here, too, the parallel to hypnosis and its scant reliance on verbalizations on the part of the subject is obvious.

Erickson has taught us not only the *avoidance* of resistance through the choice of the most appropriate form of suggestion and intervention, but also the skillful *use* of resistance to promote rapid change. In traditional therapy resistance is supposed to be "interpreted" and, when the therapist eventually runs out of interpretations, it is considered a sign that the patient is not yet ready to benefit from therapy. However, already Aristotle, in his *Rethorica,* wrote about *preempting* resistance, suggesting the acceptance and use of resistance for its own resolution. This technique mirrors the philosophy behind Judo. The Judo fighter, rather than opposing the other's thrust, not only yields to but even increases it. The force therefore spends itself into a void and throws the opponent off balance.

The way this is practiced in hypnosis can be applied to psychotherapy in general through the permission and the encouragement to engage in the resisting behavior. In terms of the theory of human communication, this simple intervention changes an escalating symmetrical communication pattern into a complementary one, with the therapist in the superior, one-up position. To *permit* resistance changes its interactional effect. Just as one cannot rebel against somebody who demands rebellion, the demand to resist leaves only two choices: either to comply (which by definition is no longer resistance) or to refuse to comply (which is tantamount to giving up the particular resistance). Following John Weakland (Weakland & Jackson, 1958), we call this peculiar form of communication an "illusion of alternatives." Erickson was exposed to it early in his life when he had to help out on his father's farm. His father would offer little Milton an illusionary choice by asking: "Do you want to feed the chickens or the hogs *first*?" Erickson later refined this form of intervention into a particularly powerful tool.

The elegance of the illusion of alternatives lies in the fact that through it a deviation is put into the service *of its own correction.* Here we observe the anticipation and application by gifted therapists like Milton H. Erickson, Don D. Jackson, Victor Frankl, John Rosen, Mara Selvini Palazzoli and others of a principle that for a long time seemed limited to physics, engineering and related sciences, especially cybernetics, namely, the principle of error-control. Complex systems, whether they be natural or man-made, maintain their stability in the face of a seemingly overwhelming number of potentially destabilizing factors (from their environment and from within) by simply picking up an existing deviation from a vital norm and reversing its mathematical sign, thereby counteracting the disturbance. The capability of a house thermostat to maintain an even temperature in the face of a fantastically complex interplay of forces of random genesis—an interplay that has so far defied the meteorologists' attempts to express it in a mathematical model—is a good example. All the thermostat does is identify deviations from the desired norm (71°F), turn minus into plus or plus into minus, and thereby switch on or turn off the house heater. By the way, it is precisely the simplicity and the apparently mechanistic nature of this procedure and its underlying epistemology that makes it unappealing to those colleagues who prefer to do what John Weakland has called "romantic therapy."

Time limitations force me to pass over many other Ericksonian techniques that have direct relevance to interactional therapy, such as the confusion technique, the particular language forms of his suggestions, the principle of the unresolved remnant, symptom prescriptions and the like.

But there are two special points I want to make before concluding. One refers to the use of stories, puns, jokes, metaphors, even word-salad and occasional references to 17 similar cases already treated this year. What Erickson seems to have intuitively grasped, long before modern brain research postulated the asymmetry theory of the human brain, was that language forms loosely called right-hemispheric have a far greater therapeutic potential than the left-hemispheric brilliance of rational explanations and interpretations. Anybody who has watched Carl Whitaker do family therapy will know to what extraordinary extent right-hemisphere language can be applied to interactional therapy.

The second point I wish to make is of a more general nature and, at least to me, seems to chart the course that psychotherapy is likely to take in the not too distant future.

If we ever arrive at a unified theory of hypnosis, one of its basic characteristics will most probably be that hypnosis entails a shift in attention. New accents are set, new punctuation is introduced into the old, familiar, repetitive stream of events that so far merely led to more of the same. Let us not forget that most of the situations that we encounter in therapy (as well as in our own lives) are in and of themselves unchangeable. No amount of therapy will regrow a leg lost in an accident or resurrect a loved one who has died. What can be changed, however, are the ways in which people conceptualize and try to come to terms with immutable facts. What therapy can do is change the sense, value and significance that we ascribe to such events and to the world in general. In this sense, *any* successful suggestion puts our patients' reality into a different conceptual and emotional frame. It is this technique of *reframing* that can be most fruitfully transplanted from hypnosis to the nontrance states of interaction.

Couples, families and, of course, also individuals come to us because they suffer, and they suffer because of the way they have constructed their reality, without knowing that they themselves are the architects of that mythical reality "out there." Like everybody else—humans or animals—they can then see only *one* possible, feasible, logical, reasonable course of action. And if—as already mentioned—this attempted solution does not bring about the desired change, they try more of the same, but will not examine the frame, i.e., the premises, of their attempted solutions.

Anybody who knows the phenomenon of self-fulfilling prophecies will appreciate that successful therapy literally constructs new and less painful realities. Although to the best of my knowledge Erickson has never put it in these terms, his main contribution to interactional therapy is that he turned the established philosophies of therapy upside down, by showing that action precedes understanding, and by teaching us how to become active therapists.

## REFERENCES

Brown, George Spencer. *Laws of Form*. New York: Bantam Books, 1973.

Weakland, J.H. & Jackson D.D. Patient and therapist observations on the circumstances of a schizophrenic episode. *Arch. Neurology Psychiatry, 79*: 554-74, 1958.

Chapter 12

# Erickson's Impact on Brief Psychotherapy

*Richard Fisch*

In preparation for this First Congress on Ericksonian Approaches to Hypnosis and Psychotherapy I was originally asked to make some comments on Erickson's contribution to brief therapy. However, it did not seem accurate to describe his work as a "contribution" because what he accomplished was revolutionary in its implications. Therefore, I felt that "impact" was a more fitting term. A contribution implies adding to a body of thought and thereby extending a direction already established. Erickson's impact was to open the door to a new way of thinking about human problems, thereby changing the approach needed for the resolution of those problems.

Erickson effectively eliminated the traditional dichotomy between brief and long-term treatment. That dichotomy existed because of the continued acceptance of traditional, fundamental assumptions about the nature of human problems, primarily the assumptions regarding the notion of individual psychopathology. For the most part, contributors to brief therapy have devised different techniques for dealing with psychopathology or delimiting the area of pathology on which to work. However, few contributors have offered revised views on how to look at the problems people encounter.

There have been nonpsychoanalytic approaches, notably behavior therapy and Transactional Analysis, which can provide shorter treatment. But these approaches also are pathology-oriented and lack the time-saving maneuverability of interactional models. Thus, as with other "briefer" approaches, behavior therapy and TA are useful in some types of problems but not in all, and the dichotomy between long-term and all other methods persists.

The trouble with that dichotomy is that it confirms the notion that longer treatment is somehow fuller, more complete, more thorough, and therefore a more reliable way of handling human problems. The concomitant implication is that, while "briefer" approaches can be useful, they are resorted to as expedients. Brief approaches are something one may have to do in the face of shortages: shortages of treating personnel, shortages of time, shortages of patient resources, e.g., incapacity for insight. Short-term therapy is regarded as appropriate for the resolution of crises. However, implicitly and explicitly, the notion of pathology still defines the resolution of the crisis as a preliminary step to longer treatment to alter those "defects" presumed to leave some patients, or families, still vulnerable to subsequent crises. Freud characterized this dichotomy when talking about the utility of hypnosis and direct suggestion, in conjunction with analysis. He referred to it as alloying the pure *gold* of analysis with the *copper* of these adjuncts.

Despite years of psychotherapeutic activity and considerable effort by many thoughtful clinicians to shorten treatment, "brief psychotherapy" remains the stepchild of human problem solution. Family therapy has not made much of an impact on this dichotomy either. Many family therapists have simply substituted the idea of family pathology for individual pathology, "family dysfunctional homeostasis" for "unconscious conflict," and making family members aware of the covert rules of the family for analytic insight.

Thus, even many proponents of brief psychotherapy support the idea that it is either a shortened application of conventional long-term treatment or one that is applicable to only some patients and problems.

> The two most dependable criteria for successful prognosis using this method are the same ones noted by Malan: the ability of the therapist to grasp the patient's conflicts quickly, and the patient's willingness and ability to utilize interpretations.

and

> A method of brief psychotherapy has been described, characterized by early vigorous interpretation of negative transference and separation anxiety. Its purpose is to . . . show him how his conflicts have led to his self-destructive actions and inhibitions in the past, and to suggest other ways of handling his conflicts (Lewin, 1970).

> In contrast (to long-term therapy) brief therapy deals with a specific problem constellation. It may aim for the resolution of a present

> conflict or discomfort, and its objectives indeed may be of an emergency or stopgap nature.
>
> or
>
> Considerable discussion in the literature has been devoted to selection criteria.
>
> or
>
> From a logistical point of view, it is more advantageous to regard the brief therapies as a range of procedures, including potentially long-term brief contact therapy. . . .
>
> or
>
> Brief therapy thus helps patients look beyond the symptom to the conflict. Removing symptoms may relieve the patient of a painful or even crushing burden, and this is not to be minimized, but it is not the only option in brief therapy. When possible, we can try to help patients to become less vulnerable to subsequent stresses (Barten, 1971).

In short, "brief therapists" still view the problem as representing an exceptional state of affairs within the individual or in the family, an exceptional state in which there is some defect or deficit not encountered in "normal" people. This view has perpetuated an illusory dichotomy between brief and long-term therapy. What has been needed is a fundamental change to "therapy" period. Therapy should be measured not by its brevity or length, but whether it is efficient and effective in aiding people with their complaints or whether it wastes time.

In order to make that fundamental change, we must reformulate basic assumptions about the nature of human problems in less pessimistic terms.

In his work, Erickson opened the door for change and in that way had a major impact on brief therapy, as well as on therapy itself. There were a number of features to his work which accomplished this change. First and, I think, foremost was what he persistently did *not* do. One's premises, be they explicit or implicit, dictate what one does and also what one doesn't do. It is in this latter case that one's most fundamental assumptions are borne out. Erickson did not ask for lengthy histories before he intervened in the problem. Concomitantly, he did not attempt to elicit "interpretable" information or try to get his patients to gradually achieve insight. "Insights" or understandings encouraged were actively directed by him for the purpose of enhancing patient willingness to carry out subsequent needed tasks. Erickson did not emphasize "the session" as much as events outside his office. It was rare for him to push for more and more improvement. Rather, he would move in quickly to intervene and pull back as quickly once some small but definite improvement occurred. He might stop treatment or impose a hiatus before getting back to any further work. He did not measure the session by the clock, but rather by the task to be performed in that contact. He did not "support" in the usual sense; he did not urge; he did not "confront with reality." Medications and hospitalizations played little if any part in his work, even though he was empowered to use them. He did not place importance on getting people to "express their feelings."

In short, he did not do all of those familiar things regarded as necessary for traditional therapy. In this manner of speaking, he cut out a lot of the work of conventional treatment, long-term or "brief." If one can cut out a great deal of work and still resolve problems, the implication is that the job to be done is not as difficult as was thought, and, if not as difficult, further questions about the presumed complexity and deep-seatedness of human problems are raised.

However, in addition to not doing things, Erickson did some intriguing things. While he did not spend time getting a psychological history, he did spend considerable effort in obtaining a rather detailed picture of the symptom, problem, or complaint and how it was performed, as well as how it was performed in conjunction with others involved in the problem. He did not try to get the patient to feed back to him his own ideas about the problem (commonly called developing "insight"); rather he would readily "speak the patient's language." He would not interpret resistance to the patient, but would use it to expedite client performance of therapeutic tasks. He simply did not waste time arguing with patients, focusing instead on the task the patient was to perform to resolve his or her problem.

In the performance of these tasks, he would extend his influence on the patient while reducing the patient's dependence on him by enlisting the use of people and facilities within the community. For example, he would direct a sloppy woman to a hairdresser or to a fashion consultant. He would put a shy and fearful young man through an ordeal by enlisting the aid of an attractive and, to the patient, threatening divorcee. It was not unusual for him to impose difficult and ordeal-like assignments on patients, often patients who seemed most fragile.

In all of these above tactics, important messages are conveyed: that he and the patient are to get down to business, that change is expected, that there are some simple things to consider and understand and tasks to be undertaken, which, however arduous, can and are to be accomplished. Finally, when the task is completed and change is realized, we are to part company, at least for a significant while. Therefore, patients cannot be seen as fragile or vulnerable to mysterious forces within or around them. Rather, patients are quite ready to give up or modify their problems (there is not some deep-seated need for them), and the problems people have relate mainly to their failure to take some action or their persistence in some entrapping or stalemating action. There is little room in this conceptualization for "pathology," for viewing problems as exceptional. Erickson's own descriptions of his strategies and goals are most often put in the vocabulary of ordinary and quite normal life cycle events: of courtship and marriage, of child-bearing and child-rearing, and so on, as Jay Haley has so clearly delineated in his book on Erickson, *Uncommon Therapy.*

It is his simplicity of thrust, this aura of normality conveyed by the patient's response to his approach, that makes Erickson's work so intriguing. Another significant feature of his work is the consistency of this approach. He did not work this way with selected patients or particular types of problems; he did it with every case he saw, regardless of the bizarreness, or the catastrophic swath the symptoms imposed, or the chronicity. We all know of therapists who have used some innovations in their work but, effective as they might be, these moves were regarded as quirks, as fortuitous but unreplicable strokes of brilliance or imagination. Thus, the possibility for any change in the traditional view of problems was discounted. I recall a seminar with a psychoanalyst who, in the privacy of the small coterie, described how he departed from his usual way of working. During the course of analysis with a woman who was frigid he advised her to breathe into a paper bag prior to intercourse and she reported that this had helped her immeasurably. The important point is not his intervention but that he regarded it as an atypical fluke in treatment and so continued his analytic work with her as if nothing "really" had happened. Another colleague would, on occasion, use some rather innovative interventions, but only when time did not allow for long-term insightful work, for example, when he was covering for a colleague who was away on vacation. I know that on one occasion he got excellent results with a problem for which the "temporary patient" had been in treatment for years. Yet, he always regarded these variations as untrustworthy expedients. What makes Erickson's work so compelling is that he worked innovatively with *all* cases, regardless of the presenting problem or how the patient might be defined by usual diagnostic categories, from "adjustment reactions" to "schizophrenia."

Thus, over and over again, one is confronted by a consistent thread in his "style," in his approach. It is apparent that it is an approach indicating that usual and traditional methods of struggling with patients are simply not necessary; that despite the apparent complexity of a problem, its chronicity, bizarreness or the catastrophic effects it may have, one is dealing with a basically human state of affairs and with people who are basically resilient.

For example, Erickson had seen a young woman who was living with her family. She had multiple problems: She was depressed, terrified of riding on buses or trains, enormously shy and fearful of social involvement, and extremely prudish. She wanted to break out of those strangleholds but felt hopeless about the prospect of ever achieving independence from her parents. Most of Erickson's interventions were directed toward her presumed fragility. Specifically, he patiently but firmly badgered her into moving out of the parental home, got her to talk about and then wear sexually provocative clothing, to talk about sex and finally to rekindle a relationship with a man who had almost given up on her. With the rapid reflowering of the relationship, he ultimately got her to "set the date" and marry the young man.

In another case, one in which parents were hanging on to their married daughter, insisting that she, her husband and their new child live in a cottage in back of their own, Erickson intervened to interdict a mutually paralyzing situation. Because the daughter had been diagnosed "schizophrenic," her parents doubted her ability to adapt to marriage or raise her child; therefore they made their insistent offer. Unfortunately, this fed into the doubts their daughter had about herself. In this case, Erickson maneuvered the parents out of the "protective" posture by appearing to support it. Then he drew a picture of endless sacrifice on their part—he commiserated about the cross they had to bear. Subsequently, the parents decided not to pursue their demands.

In a case analogous to the first, Erickson treated a fearful young man by engineering a night on the town which was designed to be a horrible ordeal for the patient. He was fearful of any contact with women, worst of all an attractive divorcee, and agonized if such a contact were to occur in a restaurant. The night on the town, as you can guess, consisted of just such features, with Milton staging several scenes in the restaurant.

In brief, the treatment was worse than the young man's problem of social avoidance and, following this ordeal, he decided to go back to the same restaurant.

Now, these kinds of interventions are something a therapist simply cannot employ if he views the patient's problem as "mental illness," "a lack of coping skills," "deep-seated," "a learning deficit," or as a "needed symptom." It is this feature that makes Erickson's work so intriguing and comprises much of the impact he has had on brief therapy. His work provides a new way of looking at people and their problems, and this different view is not just simpler than traditional models but seems to make irrelevant the whole notion of pathology.

To my knowledge, Erickson never laid out an explicit formulation of his underlying assumptions about problems. He was good at describing what he did with patients and was able to give a much clearer picture of his way of working than one gets from most therapists. Still, when it came to detailing his treatment rationale, he was less precise, often utilizing entrancing parables and stories. Thus, it has fallen to others to put into some comprehensive and explicit form those assumptions on which Erickson appeared to operate. The main point I am making about his impact on brief therapy, and really on therapy as a whole, is that it wasn't his imaginative interventions, his personal "style" or strengths, but the fact that he boldly and persistently (with every kind of problem under the sun) showed others what can be accomplished, simply, quickly and consistently. Once shown that, thoughtful therapists can no longer remain within the constraints of the older framework of intermeshed pathology, of strange unconscious forces, of "sick" people or "sick" families, or of mental and emotional cripples.

The work we have been doing at the Brief Therapy Center at MRI owes its greatest debt to Milton. His work has had enormous impact on the approach to human problems we have evolved. We started 14 years ago, seeing patients in a research study of brief therapy and, for the most part, simply emulated some of the techniques and interventions Erickson had used with analogous problems. Over time, we could see some central theme in this way of working or, more accurately, see a way of framing it as a comprehensive view of human problem formation and problem resolution. The techniques of intervening are thus logical extensions of this underlying rationale and for that reason need not be viewed as mysterious flourishes of brilliance or "charisma." If therapy is to be more efficient and effective, it needs to move from an aura of artistry to craftsmanship. This, we believe, is an important step, for if Erickson's work is to have its fullest and continuing impact it must be transmissible to open-minded therapists and problem solvers and not be regarded as some awesome but idiosyncratic "style."

## REFERENCES

Barten, H.H. (Ed.) *Brief Therapies*. New York: Behavioral Publications, 1971.

Haley, J. *Uncommon Therapy: The Psychiatric Techniques of Milton H. Erickson*. New York: W.W. Norton, 1973.

Lewin, K.K. *Brief Psychotherapy*. St. Louis, MO: Warren H. Green, Inc., 1970.

Chapter 13

# Erickson's Contribution to the Double Bind

*John H. Weakland*

In order to discuss Erickson's contribution to the double bind, one first must define the territory. For the double bind, this is no simple task. During 25 years of use this term has become familiar in psychiatry and psychology, and to some extent has even passed into common speech. But, as many even more common, and apparently quite simple, terms in our field illustrate (for example, "communication," "normality," "mental illness," and "reality"), familiarity is not synonymous with clarity of reference. It may be associated more with casual and loose usage. On the other hand, it would not be useful or appropriate here to attempt some ultimate definition of the double bind because we could go on at great length and still not be final. Indeed, that is just what has happened in the past; efforts to specify the double bind conclusively have always been inconclusive.

Defining the double bind would not make the present task easier because that other key word, "contribution," is ambiguous, and because mainly, as we shall see, Erickson's contributions in this area were indirect and general rather than direct and specific. He published only one article explicitly focused on the double bind (Erickson and Rossi, 1975), which appears to contain, with some variation in details, an unpublished earlier manuscript of uncertain date on "A Therapeutic Double Bind Utilizing Resistance" (included in Rossi, 1980). Erickson's failure to publish articles on the double bind does not mean that his contribution was minimal, only that it largely occurred in other ways—and ones rather typical of him.

For the above reasons, as a workable compromise in the problem of defining our territory, I will begin with the original statement of the double bind. Subsequently, I shall supplement this definition with comments on related general themes. Finally, I will consider Erickson's relationship to these concepts.

The point of departure, then, is the paper "Toward a Theory of Schizophrenia," by Bateson, Jackson, Haley and Weakland, first published in 1956. This paper ranged rather widely in only 14 pages, but it included three things that are specifically relevant here. First, it presented the term "double bind" together with the first formal statement of its "necessary ingredients," as follows: 1) two or more persons; 2) repeated experience; 3) a primary negative injunction; 4) a secondary injunction conflicting with the first at a more abstract level, and like the first enforced by punishments or signals which threaten survival; 5) a tertiary negative injunction prohibiting the victim from escaping from the field. In the original article, each of these specifications was amplified by brief discussion or illustration.

Second, the expectable or observed effects of such a combination of messages were discussed, and the conclusion was drawn that it would lead to the kinds of communicative behavior characteristically exhibited by schizophrenic patients.

Third, it was mentioned—even if only late and briefly—that in addition to and opposite to such a pathogenic double binding, therapists might impose therapeutic double binds to "force the patient to respond differently than he has in the past."

Erickson did not make a direct contribution to this original paper. Any credit due for the views expressed therein (or blame, which has certainly also arisen), and for the term "double bind" itself, must go to the Bateson research project and especially to Gregory Bateson as project director and senior author.

Nevertheless, I believe indirectly Erickson did make a significant contribution even to the original statement. As Jay Haley (1976) described in his account of the Bateson series of research projects, he and I solicited Bateson's support and made periodic visits to Phoenix—about twice a year—to confer with Erickson, starting late in 1953. We were initially motivated by a general interest in hypnosis, which increased as we began to think of hypnosis as communication by the hypnotist that could influence a subject's behavior in extraordinary ways. Then, as our project began to focus more on schizophrenia, I became struck by the parallels between the symptomatic behavior of schizophrenics, and behaviors producible in trance as reported by many writers on hypnosis (Note 1). Also, except for John Rosen (1953), at that time Erickson was almost the only person who believed that psychotherapy with schizophrenic patients was possible.

By the time the four authors began to draft "Toward a Theory . . . ," Jay and I had been visiting Milton for about two years, and we had brought back both tapes of our meetings and verbal reports. Both he and I certainly were greatly influenced—though often also confused—by Erickson's unorthodox ideas about treatment approaches and problems. Extensive discussion in our project conferences of ideas and materials we brought back from Phoenix influenced Bateson and Jackson, though not without critical examination and at times resistance. At this late date it is impossible to recall or trace any specific ways that Erickson's ideas fed into our original paper. Such an endeavor seldom makes sense anyway; I doubt that much in that joint paper could meaningfully be apportioned even among its four authors. Nevertheless, it is plain, not only from memory but from surviving transcripts of our project conferences (and even a few bits of the original tape recordings of these meetings), that at the time the article was being roughed out in project conferences there was considerable interplay in our discussions between our own materials, concepts and ideas, and illustrative materials clearly obtained from Erickson. In this sense, he certainly contributed to the production of the original double bind statement.

Of course, this was only the beginning. Subsequently, the Bateson group maintained its contact with Erickson, while continuing to think, talk and write more on the double bind, and on related ideas about communication, family interaction, pathology and therapy. Meanwhile, the original paper seemed to stir up wide interest and further writings. Again, rather than trying to uncover specific details of interaction which are largely lost in the past, some further specification of Erickson's contribution can be approached by a brief review of developments, which will then serve as a basis for some broad comparisons between major emphases in writings on the double bind and those found in Erickson's own work.

While a considerable amount of both approving and critical writing was stimulated by "Towards a Theory . . . ," much of the work was narrowly focused, e.g., efforts at very precise specification, attempts at counting double binds in samples of communication, experimental testing of responses, and so forth. After some time, this kind of work declined in amount, while the double bind notion—at least in some form—was disseminated increasingly widely by reprintings of the original article and discussions in secondary sources.

While members of the Bateson group had written additional papers (e.g., Weakland, 1960; Bateson et al., 1963) aimed at clarification and further development of the original concept, most efforts at precise description and quantification missed the main point, which lay at a different level. Bateson tried to clarify this difference early on by pointing out that "The double bind is more like a language" than a proposition, and that "You can't count the jokes in a conversation either." The basic difference involved is between focusing on certain details to illuminate a broad perspective by illustration, and focusing on details in ways that obscure or distort a broad perspective. To do the former was characteristic of Erickson himself (though he often seemed to leave the perspective only implicit), while it seemed to us that many writers on the double bind were enmeshed in the latter kind of operation.

In any case, after the original statement, the Bateson group members soon became increasingly involved with ideas and approaches growing out of the double bind work (particularly cybernetic models of causality on the one hand and family therapy on another), rather than with the concept of the double bind itself.

After a considerable lapse, and partly on the basis of further work, in 1969 Bateson produced a restatement of views about the double bind (Bateson, 1976). Then I produced my own reconsideration, "The Double Bind Theory by Self-Reflexive Hindsight" (1974). Also, Sluzki and Ransom assembled a general reconsideration, including an extensive bibliography, in *Double Bind: The Foundation of the Communicational Approach to the Family* (1976). Finally, less closely related to the original work, and perhaps even viewable as a sort of quasi-memorial service, the "Beyond the Double Bind" conference of 1977 (Berger, 1978) may be mentioned.

In my judgment, now as in 1974, what is most basic in this long sequence of thought, observation and writing does not lie in the specifics of the original article, such as the listing of double bind conditions and the posited connection with schizophrenia. Still less does it lie in the details of subsequent refinements or critiques. Rather, what is most basic lies in certain broad ideas or orientations already presented in that first article, though mainly in implicit form. The existence and importance of these ideas and orientations have been demonstrated and clarified by the remarkable extent to which they have been taken up, utilized, and carried forward in various ways—often under labels other than double bind, and as much in application as in exposition.

Four major points now can be considered. First, the most important thing about the original double bind statement is that it proposed, in terms of the specific example of schizophrenia and a pattern of communication labeled the double bind, that communication between persons could be a central factor in determining even extreme, "aberrant" forms of behavior such as being "crazy," which formerly was not really seen even as behavior. Since it was already common knowledge—despite academic concepts of communication as just the transfer of "information"—that our ordinary everyday behavior is influenced by how people talk to us, a basic implication can be gleaned: *All behavior is markedly dependent upon and shaped by communication.* This thought was not yet spelled out, yet it was soon to become an important basis for a comprehensive family-interactional reconceptualization of problems and treatment.

Second, our attempted specification of the makeup of the double bind—whether or not it was fully accurate and adequate—indicated that communication is complex as well as powerful, and also that this complexity must and can be described and taken into account in estimating behavioral effects—that it is useless or actively misleading to look for "the real message," oversimplified and in isolation, in any communication.

Third, in referring to the possibility of therapeutic double binds, the article proposed explicitly, though not yet generally, that therapy should involve deliberate alteration of patients' behavior by communicative means. Such a view was in contrast to the prevailing concepts of treatment which centered on encouraging insight or on nondirectiveness. This point aroused opposition, but it has been basic to subsequent development of family therapy and brief therapy.

Fourth, while in the original article the double bind was presented mainly in an oversimplistic, linear way—as something a "binder" imposed on a "victim"—in subsequent writings this position was modified toward an interactional and systemic view. We began to consider both that additional parties might be involved, and that the erstwhile "victim's" communications might be such as to provoke the double bind communications addressed to him or her. We moved rapidly from a linear, cause-and-effect, view of behavior to a circular or cybernetic causal view. This had profound effects on the way we and others approached understanding behavior in families and other systems of interaction, regarding both homeostatic maintenance of behavior and the spreading effects of changes.

By this point, those familiar with Erickson's work should realize that all four major points parallel recurrent emphases in his practice and writings. Yet it may not be that obvious. In these matters as in most others, Erickson preferred the illustrative anecdote or case example to explicit statement of principle. Both have their place and use, and perhaps our efforts at explicitness, in writing and in discussions, about our own views may in turn have had some value for him; I would like to think so. In any case, let me draw the parallels—all of which are exemplified in Erickson and Rossi's (1975) double bind article:

1) Erickson did not label communication as important for behavior—he took this for granted—but most everything he said and wrote illustrated the point.
2) Erickson's concern with the subtlety and complexity of communication appears over and over, as for example in both his close attention to the planning, delivery and nuances of his own messages, and in his attention to the verbal and nonverbal messages he received.
3) The deliberate, calculated use of messages to produce desired results was perhaps the most evident feature of Erickson's work. Indeed, after some experience with him one might wonder if he ever did anything *else*, and many people—usually not those in much direct contact with him—have shown concern about, or opposition to, such "manipulation." To digress slightly, my own view is that one of his greatest achievements was to begin breaking down the false dichotomous equation in human interaction: "Spontaneity" leads to good ends, and "calculation" leads to bad ends.
4) On the question of concepts of causation Erickson was, if possible, even less explicit than he was on the preceding points. Perhaps this is because this point is more abstract than the others, and with good reason and good results he adhered to the concrete rather than the abstract. Nevertheless, it is clear enough that he did not subscribe to a linear cause and effect model, as evidenced by many cases showing that while he took past events of patients' lives seriously, he never believed their future was locked in. Alternatives were always open. In addition, he repeatedly indicated that he saw the situation of hypnotist and subject or therapist and patient as an interaction, not a one-way street.

So here are some profound parallels between Erickson and—in a general sense—the double bind and its developments. Perhaps there are others. Perhaps nothing more specific can be said with certainty about the extent of his contribution. Perhaps the question should not be put in this way, since the matter is one of human interaction and influence, and therefore more circular than linear. Also, while Bateson preceded Erickson on some of the more specific formulations, Erickson preceded Bateson on some of the general emphases. Perhaps the most that can be said with assurance is that we, along with others, were in touch with Milton Erickson, and from our interaction, new steps toward understanding and dealing with human problems developed. And as Erickson recognized about his own work, a positive outcome is more important than allocation of credit.

## REFERENCE NOTE

1. Weakland, J.H. Schizophrenia and hypnosis: Phenomenal similarities and their potential relevance. Unpublished manuscript. Circa 1974.

## REFERENCES

Bateson, G. Double bind, 1976. In: *Double Bind: The Foundation of the Communicational Approach to the Family.* C.E. Sluzki & D.C. Ransom (Eds.), New York: Grune & Stratton, 1976, pp. 237-242.

Bateson, G., Jackson, D.D., Haley, J., & Weakland, J.H. Toward a theory of schizophrenia, *Behavioral Science,* 1956, *1,* 251-264.

Bateson, G., Jackson, D.D., Haley, J., & Weakland, J.H. A note on the double bind—1962, *Family Process,* 1963, *2,* 154-161.

Berger, M.M., Ed. *Beyond the Double Bind.* New York: Brunner/Mazel, 1978.

Erickson, M.H. & Rossi, E. L. Varieties of double bind, *American Journal of Clinical Hypnosis,* 1975, *17,* 144-157.

Haley, J. Development of a theory: A history of a research project. In: *Double Bind: The Foundation of the Communicational Approach to the Family.* C.E. Sluzki and D.C. Ranson (Eds.), New York: Grune & Stratton, 1976, pp. 59-104.

Rosen, J.N. *Direct Analysis.* New York: Grune and Stratton, 1953.

Rossi, E.L., Ed. *The Collected Papers of Milton H. Erickson on Hypnosis.* 4 vols. New York: Irvington Publishers, 1980.

Sluzki, C.E., & Ransom, D. C. *Double Bind: The Foundation of the Communicational Approach to the Family.* New York: Grune and Stratton, 1976.

Weakland, J.H. The "double-bind" hypothesis of schizophrenia and three-party interaction. In: *The Etiology of Schizophrenia.* D.D. Jackson (Ed.), New York: Basic Books, 1960, pp. 373-388.

Weakland, J.H. The double-bind theory by self-reflexive hindsight. *Family Process,* 1974, *13,* 269-277.

PART VI

# *Ericksonian Approaches in Psychiatry*

*Sheldon Cohen, M.D., is a psychiatrist and psychoanalyst in clinical practice in Atlanta, Georgia, and previously served on the faculty of the Schools of Medicine at Tulane University and Emory University. He is the current editor of the* American Journal of Clinical Hypnosis; *Erickson was the founding editor.*

*Cohen's efforts are directed to comparing and contrasting Ericksonian and Freudian schools by comparing the personalities of the respective founders. Subsequently, he points out some of the basic differences between Erickson's methods and psychoanalysis. His insights are perceptive and cleverly stated.*

*M. Erik Wright, Ph.D., M.D., died suddenly in May 1981 while this book was in preparation. Dr. Wright was Professor of Clinical Psychology and Psychiatry at the University of Kansas. He was an internationally noted teacher and practitioner in the field of hypnotherapy, past president of the American Society of Clinical Hypnosis, and past coordinator of the American Board of Clinical Hypnosis.*

*Dr. Wright's chapter begins with the presentation of theoretical background. Erickson's practice was more of a "healing ministry" and as such allowed more flexibility than could be found in "scientific psychotherapy with self-imposed limitations." The "ministry of healing" format was especially applicable to understanding Erickson's hypnotic approach to sex therapy. Wright's chapter speaks to the philosophical and sociological background of Ericksonian interventions.*

Chapter 14

# Ericksonian Techniques and Psychoanalysis

*Sheldon B. Cohen*

I appreciate Dr. Zeig's invitation to relate the work of Milton Erickson to psychoanalysis. Perhaps I was given this opportunity because I am one of the few card-carrying analysts who also utilize hypnosis in their practice.

In relating the work of Milton Erickson to psychoanalysis, the dilemma that immediately presents itself is quite simple. How do we define the territory? Whose concept of psychoanalysis and whose notion of "Ericksonian" should we use? When I first received this title I was uncertain as to what was meant by "Ericksonian." Therefore, in the intervening months I sampled much of the work of Milton Erickson and carefully read selected papers. I also used the opportunity to re-immerse myself in the basic literature of psychoanalysis, something which I have previously accepted as learned and assimilated long ago. While much of this reading was familiar, it had unexpectedly novel and fascinating aspects.

In deciding what type of psychoanalysis or whose conception I would use, I decided to go back to the original source, Sigmund Freud. I trust that the presentation of psychoanalysis will not seem too dated since it appears that the basic tenets espoused by Freud hold for all who practice psychoanalysis today, although many modifications and refinements have been developed by others.

My method will be, to some extent, to compare and contrast Sigmund Freud and Milton Erickson; I will try to relate their works. Also, I will note the contributions Erickson made to psychoanalysis. After discussing the paucity of psychoanalytic practitioners using Ericksonian technique, closing remarks will be directed to contrasting Freudian and Ericksonian approaches.

In reading Freud and Erickson, switching back and forth between the two, what struck me most was the pleasurable experience of reading their productions. They both wrote well.

Many other parallels exist between Freud and Erickson. Both were physicians and progressed from an organic involvement in medicine, initially in the laboratory, to an increasing inquiry into that "far country" of the human mind. Each man was a product of his time. Freud emerged from the classical, cultured Vienna of the late Victorian period; Erickson was a representative of mid-twentieth century America, and hence was more pragmatic and action-oriented. Both were brilliant innovators and apparently neither took notes, both having photographic memories. They were outstanding teachers, lecturers and authors. Each was a founding leader-father of a society devoted to his concepts. Their life-styles were strikingly similar in many ways. Both led a modest, quiet, conventional life as the head of a large family. Their offices were in their homes. Both were collectors of art, Freud being particularly interested in Egyptian pieces; those who visited Milton Erickson will remember his collection of simple, graceful sculptures carved from ironwood by the Seri Indians.

While reading the following quotation I would like you to think about whether it was written by Freud or Erickson, or perhaps by neither:

> Stimulated by a chance observation, we have for a number of years been investigating the most varied types and symptoms of hysteria with reference to the exciting cause, the event which evoked the phenomenon in question for the first time, often many years before. In the great majority of cases it is impossible to discover this starting-point by straightforward interrogation of the patient, be it ever so thorough; partly because it is often a matter of experiences which the patient finds disagreeable to discuss, but chiefly because he really does not remember and has no idea of the causal connection between the exciting occurrence and the pathological phenomenon. As a rule it is necessary to hypnotize the patient and under hypnosis to arouse recollections relating to the time when the symptom first appeared; one can then succeed in revealing this connection in the clearest and most convincing manner.

Who wrote the foregoing? It certainly could have been Milton Erickson describing amnesias in patients and the need to approach the symptoms in an indirect manner. However, the quote is correctly identified as the opening paragraph of Freud's classical paper "On the Psychical Mechanism of Hysterical Phenomena" written in collaboration with Breuer in 1892.

The ebb and flow of the vital, mysterious juices that course through our bodies and minds, along with the opportunities and adversities that fate presents, combine to produce cycles in our lives. Just as there are cycles of living, there are similar rhythms in the professional lives and productivity which we may see, particularly in those whom we term artists. One could describe the cycles of Erickson's professional life in many ways. One could certainly begin with the student-experimental-institutional role in which Erickson initially was cast, and look at similar geographical and professional interests, terminating in his last role as teacher-friend-seer. One could look upon his professional life in terms of the language that he used at various times. Also important are those people with whom he collaborated.

Just as Picasso, the master painter-sculptor, went through his classical Blue Period, Erickson went through a classical psychoanalytic period—a time of investigation of psychoanalysis. It is perhaps a fitting coincidence that the same year that has seen mounted such a spectacular display of the work of Pablo Picasso has also seen the publication of the collected works of Milton Erickson, other books about him, and the Congress in Phoenix. Indeed, one could take the analogy even further with the "Sold Out" sign outside of the Museum of Modern Art and the oversubscription to the Erickson Congress.

In the late '30s and early '40s, Erickson published approximately 10 papers directly relating to psychoanalytic concepts, the majority appearing in the *Psychoanalytic Quarterly* (Erickson, 1937, 1939a, 1939b, 1941). Four of the clinical papers were co-authored by Lawrence S. Kubie (Erickson & Kubie, 1938, 1939, 1940, 1941) and one by Lewis Hill (Erickson & Hill, 1944).

In "The Use of Automatic Drawing in the Interpretation and Relief of a State of Acute Obsessional Depression," Erickson and Kubie described the resolution of a classical oedipal conflict by unconscious hypnotic means:

> . . . the following case is reported in detail because by means of a nonpsychoanalytic technique, it illustrates a certain type of symbolic activity which is comparable in character to that studied by psychoanalysis in dreams and in psychotic states, and because of its clear demonstration of certain of the dynamic relationships which exist between conscious and unconscious aspects of the human psyche. Finally, it is reported because of our interest in this

> general type of technique as a means of uncovering unconscious material, and because of the challenge this may offer to certain phases of psychoanalytic technique (Erickson, 1938).

The case concerned a 24-year-old woman who inexplicably became "worried, unhappy and depressed." After attending a lecture by Milton Erickson which dealt with automatic writing, she asked to have this technique utilized with her. Under hypnosis she made several drawings consisting primarily of rectangles, squares, triangles, and connecting lines. At the time they made no sense to her, but later she put them together to mean that her best friend was having an affair with her father. She had absolutely no conscious data to support her thoughts but said, "When you said symbolism, I suddenly remembered that Freud said cylinders symbolized men and triangles, women, and then I recalled that cigarettes were cylinders and that they could symbolize a penis. Then the whole meaning of the picture just burst into my mind all at once, and I guess I just couldn't take it, and that's why I acted like I did. Now I can explain the picture to you."

The patient went on to describe the symbols for father, mother, herself and her friend and how one of the drawings connected her father with the friend. She finally remarked, "I know the interpretation of this picture is true, but only because I feel it is true. I have been thinking everything over and there isn't a solitary fact that I know, on which I can rely. . . ." Acting on these feelings, she arranged a confrontation in Dr. Erickson's office in which she secured a confession from her friend. Following this her agitation and anxiety disappeared. In commenting on the case it was noted that "the skillful use of orthodox psychoanalytic technique could not possibly have uncovered the repressed awareness of the father's liaison in a mere handful of sessions. . . . For at least a few of those patients for whom analysis is not applicable, such an approach as this, only because of its speed and directness, might be useful."

Erickson acknowledged that he became a substitute father for the patient and thereby gave her permission to know the facts about her real father. These few hours of therapy, without any effort to make conscious the usual oedipal material, provided an almost immediate relief from disturbing symptoms.

This case is illustrative of the series of papers in which Erickson, using conventional psychoanalytic language, demonstrated a number of the Freudian mental mechanisms, elucidated the dynamics of symptom origin, and produced symptomatic change in patients. Essentially, he proposed a direct pipeline from the patient's unconscious to the therapist's unconscious, thereby bypassing consciousness.

In view of the foregoing, it should be expected that the analytic literature, especially that related to hypnosis, would reflect Erickson's findings. Consequently, as I thumbed through the index of *Hypnosis and Related States,* a comprehensive book whose authors had a strong psychoanalytic bias (Gill & Brenman, 1959), I noted references to Erickson. Alas, as I pursued these references in the text, this turned out to be wish fulfillment, because these were many references to Erik Erikson, but only two references to Milton Erickson!

## USE OF ERICKSONIAN TECHNIQUES BY PSYCHOANALYSTS

As I was preparing this paper, I asked a senior colleague, a man immersed in psychoanalysis since the late 1940s, what he knew about Ericksonian techniques. His response was, "Very little." I then asked if he knew any of our approximately 30 analytic colleagues in Atlanta who use hypnosis or any related techniques and he said, "Only you." Because of his extensive analytic contacts, I asked if he was familiar with any analysts in the United States who used these techniques. He said that he was not and furthermore he kept close tabs of the analytic literature. He was unaware of recent articles having to do with analysis and Ericksonian techniques.

Assuming that people who have strong interest in an area identify with appropriate professional organizations, I went through a random sampling of 200 members of the American Psychoanalytic Association and found that none of them were members of the American Society of Clinical Hypnosis. This organization was founded by Milton Erickson and is the professional organization most likely to have members utilizing his techniques. Although a similar random sampling of the American Academy of Psychoanalysis yielded similar negative findings with ASCH membership, I personally know of five Academy members who have a significant interest in hypnosis; four of them are members of the Editorial Board of *The American Journal of Clinical Hypnosis*. Undoubtedly, there are other psychoanalysts who belong to one of the two major hypnosis organizations, and a reasonable number of psychoanalysts may be familiar with at least some of the work of Milton Erickson; however, hypnosis and Ericksonian techniques lie outside of the "direct" mainstream of American psychoanalysis. It is certainly possible in Ericksonian fashion that much more "indirect" permeation has taken place.

*Setting and Style of Treatment*

In many ways, Erickson was a psychoanalyst par excellence. The essence of psychoanalysis is the ability to tune in to the undercurrents of the patient's life, make sense of them and convey this meaning to the patient through interpretations and confrontations. Erickson had an unusual capacity to grasp these undercurrents, but his technique was to present his understandings metaphorically and to direct the patient's behavior in such a way that the patient's actions would become more adaptive, frequently without any conscious realization of what the underlying conflicts had been. In contrast, Freud considered making the unconscious conscious to be of paramount therapeutic importance.

Erickson denigrated psychoanalysis at times and some of his students have done this in an exaggerated fashion. There appear to be very basic differences between Erickson's methods and psychoanalysis. People who come for psychoanalysis expect long-term therapy, desire basic characterological change, and are more or less permanently in the same geographical location as their therapist. On the other hand, those whom Erickson saw frequently were not "patients" but demonstration subjects who were students or health care personnel associated with the institutions or seminars where Erickson was teaching. Even many of his patients, who came from considerable distances or saw him when he happened to be in their home town, knew that they could spend only a limited amount of time with him. This "now or never" setting was a powerful motivator for change. Consequently, even though Erickson was strikingly successful in treating certain aspects of "analytic failures," it is highly questionable whether the patient populations treated by Erickson and by psychoanalysts were the same.

Erickson, for a variety of reasons, was able to use effectively techniques that no psychoanalyst would think of using and which should probably not even be attempted by most other therapists. Although psychological shock can be highly effective, how many therapists would (or should) direct a young woman to completely disrobe in their offices even when the therapist's wife is present (Rossi, 1973)? Erickson obviously projected a powerful, benevolent, positive transference only partially explained by the fact that he was crippled (Rossi, 1973). One of the tenets of psychoanalysis, indeed of psychiatric treatment, is "professionalism," i.e., separating the therapist's and patient's personal lives outside of the therapeutic sessions. Erickson, on the other hand, at times utilized family members in therapy and entered into social situations which, of course, were carefully and therapeutically designed. Thus, he did not hesitate to have physical contact with patients, take them to restaurants, or in his teaching seminars to relate identifying information to his students by showing them pictures and naming the cities and occupations of his patients. Certainly one can see that not only are such techniques inapplicable to psychoanalysis, but that they could easily cause analysts to totally reject everything that Erickson taught because it seems so "wild."

Perhaps the essential difference between psychoanalysis and Ericksonian technique is simply that in the Freudian gospel of psychoanalysis, there is the holy trinity of theory, research and therapy, the least of which is therapy. By contrast, Ericksonian gospel is virtually synonymous with therapeutic endeavors; research occupies a quite secondary position and theory is almost insignificant.

Although their techniques were dissimilar there was much common ground between the work of Sigmund Freud and Milton Erickson. Erickson, the master therapist of the twentieth century, can perhaps be considered as Freud's legitimate psychotherapeutic heir. Having opened with a quotation from Freud, I would like to close with another which aptly describes Milton Erickson:

> It is not a modern dictum but an old saying of physicians that these diseases are not cured by the drug but by the physician, that is by the personality of the physician, inasmuch as through it he exerts a mental influence (Freud, 1905/1953).

## REFERENCES


Erickson, M. The experimental demonstration of unconscious mentation by automatic writing. In: *The Collected Papers of Milton H. Erickson,* Vol. III, E. Rossi (Ed.), New York: Irvington Publishers, 1980.

Erickson, M. Experimental demonstrations of the psychopathology of everyday life. In: *The Collected Papers of Milton H. Erickson,* Vol. III, E. Rossi (Ed.), New York: Irvington Publishers, 1980.

Erickson, M. Demonstration of mental mechanisms by hypnosis. In: *The Collected Papers of Milton H. Erickson,* Vol. III, E. Rossi (Ed.), New York: Irvington Publishers, 1980.

Erickson, M. On the possible occurrence of a dream in an eight-month-old infant. In: *The Collected Papers of Milton H. Erickson,* Vol. III, E. Rossi (Ed.), New York: Irvington Publishers, 1980.

Erickson, M. & Hill, L. Unconscious mental activity in hypnosis—psychoanalytic implication. In: *The Collected Papers of Milton H. Erickson,* Vol. III, E. Rossi (Ed.), New York: Irvington Publishers, 1980.

Erickson M. & Kubie, L. The use of automatic drawing in the interpretation and relief of a state of acute obsessional depression. In: *The Collected Papers of Milton H. Erickson,* Vol. III, E. Rossi (Ed.), New York: Irvington Publishers, 1980.

Erickson, M. & Kubie, L. The permanent relief of an obsessional phobia by means of communications with an unsuspected dual personality. In: *The Collected Papers of Milton H. Erickson,* Vol. III, E. Rossi (Ed.), New York: Irvington Publishers, 1980.

Erickson M. & Kubie, L. The translation of the cryptic automatic writing of the hypnotic subject by another in a trancelike dissociated state. In: *The Collected Papers of Milton H. Erickson,* Vol. III, E. Rossi (Ed.), New York: Irvington Publishers, 1980.

Erickson, M. & Kubie, L. The successful treatment of a case of acute hysterical depression by a return under hypnosis to a critical phase of childhood. In: *The Collected Papers of Milton H. Erickson,* Vol. III, E. Rossi (Ed.), New York: Irvington Publishers, 1980.

Freud, S. & Breuer, J. On the psychical mechanism of hysterical phenomena. In: *Collected Papers (Volume I) Sigmund Freud,* E. Jones (Ed.), London: Hogarth Press, 1953.

Freud, S. On psychotherapy. (1905). In: *Collected Papers (Volume I) Sigmund Freud,* E. Jones (Ed.), London: Hogarth Press, 1953.

Gill, M. & Brenman, M. *Hypnosis and Related States—Psychoanalytic Studies in Regression.* New York: International Universities Press, 1959.

Rossi, E. Psychological shocks and creative moments in psychotherapy. *The American Journal of Clinical Hypnosis,* 1973, *16,* 9-22.

Chapter 15

# The Sexual Therapy of Milton H. Erickson: A Ministry of Healing

*M. Erik Wright*

Early in his professional career Milton H. Erickson came to view himself principally as a "healer," even though some of his efforts were directed towards research. This self-perception meant that both in his psychiatric practice and in his psychiatric concerns there occurred a philosophical and professional separation from the mainstream of American psychiatry. The major energies of his psychiatric contemporaries were directed towards the development and understanding of diagnostic classifications, etiological origins, and systems of psychopathology which would bring rationality and respectability to a psychiatry which had yet to establish its own Medical Specialty Board. In his institutional jobs and then in his private practice, Erickson engaged in exploring methods for the direct relief of patient distress. He experimented with direct interventions which would help change patient behavior so that the patient's life situation might become more tolerable. Further, he developed a view of the patient as part of a social system and not as an isolate within whom resided both the causes and the solutions for the ongoing distress.

An analysis of the chronology of Erickson's published writings, as well as the reports of those who have known him over long periods of his life, makes it quite reasonable to hypothesize that Erickson became aware of the serious inadequacies and limitations which the model of "scientific physician" offered as a framework for a system of treatment to relieve human distress. The existing state of scientific knowledge concerning human psychological functioning in the first seven decades of the twentieth century, the uncertain methodology of scientific investigations in this area, and the uncertain verifiability of even such findings as had been published supported Erickson's conviction that a therapeutic practice guided principally by the "knowledge" available through such a "science model" would be premature, pretentious and problematic for both the help-seeker and the help-giver.

An alternative model for seeking and giving help did exist. This model had demonstrated its social value over many millenia, if deep acceptance by large segments of humanity and continued contemporary relevance to human affairs are used as indices of social value. It had served in many parts of the world as a framework for helping humans cope with psychological distress. With varying titles and in differing systems of ideas, the shaman, the guru, the holy person, the priest, the minister, the rabbi, and the faith healer have all helped individuals to achieve inner solace, psychological comfort, and positive functioning. Individuals have been helped to cope with personal tragedy as well as with the joyous events of birth, marriage and other rituals of passage. The "healing" ministry has always been based upon a system of convictions, beliefs, and moral judgments which do not need proof. Such a system is based upon faiths which provide the "healer" with inner convictions of righteousness about both the healing procedures and the eventual outcome of that ministry. Practitioners are not working in a "profession" but are engaged in a "vocation," a "calling." They respond to something beyond the self which directs both the function and the intent of the practitioner, and provides strength when difficult situations occur.

Such "healers" have much freedom in the choice of how to give help. They can respond to intuitions and inspirations from within that can be seen as reflections of their special call. They are not obligated to have a rationale or an explanation for what they do. Furthermore, seekers of help who recognize the helper as a "minister of help" are then able to draw upon their own inner resources of social faith conditioning to find hope and support for their own salvation. A "ministry of healing" is free to draw upon the rich folklore of such healing methods as confession, penance, fasting, prayer, self-abnegation, forgiveness, taboo, metaphors, homilies, mysterious statements, and allusions, etc., free from the obligations and burdens of "scientific" proof. Finally, there is a significant difference in the social contract which the seeker of help makes between the self and the "minister of healing" from that which is made with a "scientific practitioner." Whatever happens because of the interaction between the seeker of help and the minister of healing, it is perceived as part of a broader scheme of events which both may readily acknowledge as being determined in part by forces beyond their ken. The "science"-type therapy contract offers only success, partial success, or failure, for which both the seeker of help and the giver of help have to accept responsibility.

By temperament, personal disposition, and life history, Milton H. Erickson fit more comfortably into the "healing ministry" framework than into the "science" model. For example, there was his choice of communication modes with patients and associates, modes which he used and developed extensively in his treatment practice. Most healing ministries, dating back to ancient times, had learned that simple, direct communications between the help-seeker and the help-giver were far too limiting, too easily understood, and too free from fantasies of extraordinary knowledge. Therefore, the language of healing communication took on such forms as homilies, parables, metaphors, allusions, symbolic mystery words, folk tales and the like. These obtuse, indirect forms gave listeners much greater flexibility to make their own idiosyncratic interpretations of the communications and to adapt the perceived messages to their own state of need. They permitted the help-seeker to attribute to the healer as much extra knowledge and insight into the problem as was needed, indeed to attribute to the help-giver an understanding and power to heal which was far greater than anything that the healer could possibly possess.

For the healer, this mode of communication made possible greater freedom in suggesting action options than would be feasible (or acceptable) via direct communications. Demands could be implied without confrontation, while continuously enhancing the sense of mystery which indirect messages carry. Milton Erickson adopted these modes of communication early in his therapeutic practice and showed a great fondness for using them with his patients, friends, associates and pupils. In time, not only the content, but also his quality of speech, mode of delivery, features of dress, and interpersonal relationship patterns became so integrated into this "ministerial" communication mode that the mode became Milton Erickson.

In his work with patients with sexual difficulties (with the shy, the guilt-burdened, the anxious), he developed great skill in using these modes of communication to give his patients a bridge by which they could cross over to a state of being which permitted them to comfortably discuss their sexual function problems.

A second aspect of Erickson's ministry of healing derived from his strong sense of morality, from his conviction in the correctness of his own code of sexual values, and from his assured belief in what constituted a normal pattern of sexual functioning. The faith in the rightness of his own beliefs about sexual experience and sexual expression gave Erickson, in the context of the "ministry of healing," the readiness to comfortably accept any deviant sexual practice, function, or attitude which a patient might bring to the interaction. Just as the wayward sinner may be warmly welcomed back into the spiritual fold, so could Erickson easily express compassion to the patient whose sexual practices or problems deviated from the healer's beliefs about what was normal. The inner clarity of the healer's convictions about where and how normal sexual satisfaction and expression would be found (e.g., married with at least two happy, healthy children, etc.), given the context which the healer-patient created, seemed to give those patients who accepted this context both immediate support and hope for achieving a better way of sexual living in the future.

Erickson's faith in his own convictions concerning the nature of sexual expression freed him from the need to have patients search, sometimes laboriously and often fruitlessly, within themselves for a definition of what would constitute a satisfying outcome of therapy. The goals were clear for Erickson. Therefore, the healing energies needed only to be directed towards helping the patient learn ways of acting which would actualize that goal. The strategies of problem-solving which would facilitate healing were the central concern of the relationship.

Healing ministries have a long tradition of granting the healer permission to assume varied roles and functions in the service of the ministry. For example, the roles of healing "father" may include stern father, gentle father, forgiving father, responsible father, and omniscient father, to mention a few. Erickson was well aware of the variety of roles and functions which the healing ministry made available to help guide a confused or wayward help-seeker towards a goal such as sexual maturity. He was especially creative and innovative in the utilization of these roles in specific situations. His deep faith in his own healing ministry allowed him to experiment freely with these alternatives and liberated him from the self-imposed limitations which so many of the contemporary systems of "scientific psychotherapy" impose upon their practitioners.

Erickson might use himself in one of these "father" roles to psychodramatically reactivate a father-child relationship which the patient associated with a sexual difficulty. Then, he would guide the patient through a change in perception of the father, help the patient to modify the image of self in that relationship, and then lead the patient to achieve an altered view of the sexual problem itself. From his many published case studies, it is clear that Erickson was able to manage a unique flexibility in his scheduling of patients. When there were indications during a given session that far more time than had been originally been scheduled was needed, Erickson apparently had no problem in using as much time as he felt was necessary until he had reached those therapeutic goals which he had set for the session. Thus, many significant healing encounters which might possibly have foundered within the limits of a scheduled 50-minute therapeutic hour could be securely explored and experienced by the patient and the therapist when no such fixed time constraints were present.

Many years before the "new sex therapy" interventions became widely accepted into psychotherapy, Erickson clearly recognized the importance of accurate knowledge about one's sexual anatomy and physiology as a component factor of competent sexual functioning. He did not hesitate to become the "sex educator" or the "kindly family doctor" in presenting the facts of life to the patient in distress. Furthermore, he did not limit his sexual instruction to the biological sphere. Erickson's concept of sexual education included sexual socialization and awareness of the social nature of human sexual fulfillment. He could easily become the responsible father giving the growing adolescent direct guidance in the modification of hair styling, selection of clothing, and the social behaviors appropriate to dating and intimacy. If dancing would develop sexual socialization, then Erickson would bring the patient into contact with a dance instructor.

He placed strong emphasis upon the acceptance of one's own body and the development of a positive self-image as a potential sexual partner. The self-review by the patients of their own physique while in Erickson's presence would have Erickson's supportive and evaluative commentary. This experience would frequently be used as a medium for restructuring negative perceptions of the body into neutral, and then positive, self-acceptance. Again, in the tradition of a ministry of healing rather than in the ideology of the clinical professional, Erickson was ever ready to make wide use of resources in the community, such as the cosmetologist, the dressmaker, or the dance instructor. When required, he might accompany the patient to these external community resources in order to assure adequate contact and utilization. He was not reluctant to focus upon himself as the source of approval or disapproval of a patient's actions (e.g., clothes that had been chosen). He might focus upon his own "masculinity," for example, to serve as a frame of reference by which the patient might assess her sexual attractiveness or evaluate the adequacy of some newly acquired sociosexual skill.

Erickson's artistry in communication made it possible for him to convey a suggestion to the listener and concomitantly transmit a confident expectation that this suggestion would be accepted, that it would be acted upon, and that the listener would achieve the anticipated benefits. His suggestions generally stopped short of being outright demands or orders. Instead, listeners were led to feel that the decision to act had come from within. Perhaps some of the motivational effectiveness of these suggestions, these communications, emanated from the depth of Erickson's faith in his healing mission and from his own positive conviction that only good would happen to the patient who accepted his guidance.

Another important principle of Erickson's approach to sex therapy was his belief that patients who came for help did so because they could not, on their own, bring about the changes in their own life which were needed to resolve their sexual problems. Whether it was the bride who could not permit herself the sexual consummation of her marriage, or the groom whose marriage was being threatened by his erectile insufficiency, each of these patients deeply wanted, at some level of his or her personhood, to be able to respond appropriately to sexual expectations. However, these patients were caught up with disabling convictions about their own sexual self which blocked sexual functioning. Each had sought to deal with these disabling convictions but by themselves had been unable to bring about change. Therefore, each had found the path to Erickson as a therapist, the healer. The act of coming to him was a statement of faith and hope by patients that the sexual problem could be relieved even though they concurrently brought within themselves the inner psychological stresses which maintained the sexual dysfunction.

For Erickson, a crucial key to the possibility of change for the patient rested in the patient's readiness to develop his faith in Erickson's healing power and to have hope and belief grow that Erickson's power would lead to a more satisfying mode of sexual experience. In a healing ministry, the central task is that of linking up the faith of the help-seeker with the faith of the healer so the strength and faith of the healer can flow across the bond so formed to the one seeking help, and thereby create a state of coexistence. Within this state of coexistence the patient could, without conflict or resistance, come to accept Erickson's guidance and direction. In this state, the healer could become more sensitive to the communications from the patient and respond more adequately. Erickson considered this special coexisting communication state to be the essence of the hypnotic trance. The healing ministries of many faiths have long known of this phenomenon and of the special conditions which arise between persons when faith and hope in one of the persons join with a reciprocating faith and hope in a healer. Under such conditions, communications often have very profound impact upon the psychological and physiological functions of the help-seeker.

Within the context of this relationship of faith, Erickson guided the patient to place the closely held sexually disabling convictions, the "I cannots," into a new array of sexual convictions which included many enabling sexual convictions, the "I can" kind. The tyranny of the disabling convictions thus became diminished, although they were still present and ready to be activated if needed. However, as the presence of the other possibilities made their influence felt, the disabling convictions were no longer the only choice. In addition, the positive enabling sexual assertions, the "I cans," which had been admitted into awareness, gave energy to the patient's hope and also gave testimony to the power of Dr. Erickson's faith. As soon as it seemed feasible, the disabling sexual conviction was relegated to the past, to the "what used to be." The patient's attention was focused upon the choices which were available through the enabling sexual assertions. The choice had been shifted away from the all-constricting, disabling sexual conviction to a consideration of what kind, what level of which enabling sexual function should be considered first. Which enabling sexual function would be most compatible with the newly evolving perceptions of self?

Erickson carefully nurtured the faith factor with its core of trust, of readiness to believe, and of hope. He linked it to expectations about the changes in sexual function which were soon to occur. The patient was led to design the specifics of these changes with Erickson's guidance. Small changes were positively reinforced. The pace of sexual function change was carefully monitored by Erickson so that this aspect of life did not become incoordinate with the other aspects of the patient's life.

When required, Erickson actively intervened in the social environment of his patient and would contrive social contacts between the patients under his care. Or he might arrange for social interactions between a patient and some other person when Erickson judged that the potentials of the social contact would be of benefit to both of the involved parties. His faith in his own ministry of healing gave Erickson the inner security necessary to make such arrangements without fear that a negative outcome was possible. The patient never went alone; Erickson knew that his "karma" would sustain the patient and continue the healing process.

Erickson's cosmology of the sexual function was also an important component of his approach to sexual therapy. For him, human sexuality expressed the same cosmic destinies as those found in all other mammals. Within this schema, sexual functioning in females and males was fundamentally different. Human sexual behavior was, of course, shaped into many varieties by the particular culture or society into which the individual was born and raised. At each stage of the life-cycle the manifestations might be quite different. Yet, the cosmic sexual function of each human male remained the same, namely, the delivery of mature sperm to the os of the female womb. All else was embellishment, cultural potentiation to assure the achievement of this fundamental sexual destiny. At this moment, the sexual function of the male was completed. Whatever else followed for the male was guided by other meaningful social needs.

The sexual functioning of the human female, however, was far more extensive in time (duration) and in complexity. Her sexual function embraced not only all that was necessary to make possible the reception of the male sperm at the os of her uterus, but also the sexual functions of fertilization, implantation, pregnancy, delivery of the neonate, lactation, and the nurturance of the offspring to that point of independent living which her particular society judged appropriate. This total sexual function influenced, at different levels of consciousness and social acculturation, each sub-aspect of her sexual expression and sexual experience.

The scope, character, and goals of Milton Erickson's sex therapy interventions were very strongly guided by this cosmology of sexual function for the male and the female. For most sex therapists of the past two decades, the central focus for therapeutic intervention was, and remains, the improvement of the capacity of either the woman or the man who has experienced problems in sexual intercourse to function more effectively in this activity, and also to experience satisfactions in the coital encounter. Erickson departed substantially from this narrow concept of sex therapy. The goal of his healing ministry was the restoration of the woman or the man back into the mainstream of their cosmic sexual destiny. Time and again in his published case reports Erickson made clear that a critical index of successful outcome was marriage for the patient and the birth of two or more offspring. The facilitation of adequate sexual functioning so that conception could become possible might be a necessary part of the healing ministry, but it was only a part of the sexual function which needed to be restored.

Jay Haley, in his studies of Milton Erickson's therapy, has made abundantly clear through Erickson's cases how Erickson perceived his patients and their problems within the framework of a developmental life-cycle. For Erickson there were different life obligations and different tasks to be learned at each stage. There were problems to be solved in the periods of infancy, adolescence, sexual maturity, parenthood, grandparenthood, and in the final stages of each individual's life. In this life-cycle, the most significant time for expression of the sexual function was during the sexual period of reproduction, which included parenthood. The combination of this life-cycle orientation and Erickson's sexual function cosmology may account for the relatively narrow age range of the patients in Erickson's published cases of treatment of disturbed sexual function. This approach to sexual therapy seems to contrast with the approach of most other contemporary sex therapists, as well as the "enlightened" social avant garde. For them, active sexual encounter and pleasuring are seen as appropriate behavior for the total life-cycle, and not just a hallmark of the reproductive years. However, Erickson's age-limited choice of patients for sex therapy remains fully compatible with the concept of a healing ministry which gives much greater emphasis to other kinds of human needs and functions in the later, sexually non-reproductive years of the life-cycle.

There have been many psychiatrists and psychologists who have criticized Erickson's therapy as atheoretical or even antitheoretical. He has been characterized as a pragmatic therapist who functioned idiosyncratically with each clinical case, unguided by any system of related conceptual theorems. These criticisms are completely irrelevant in the light of my preceding analysis, which provides an appreciation and understanding of Erickson's approach to sexual therapy as one part of his general treatment approach to patients. When his therapeutic interventions are understood as manifestations of this ministry of healing and when his interventions are seen as deriving their strength, versatility and direction from Erickson's deep faith, hope and conviction about human destiny, then it is clear that there is a consistent and cosmic system of guidance which directed his interventions. Furthermore, the effectiveness of so many of his interventions was a consequence of Erickson's mastery of those modes of healing communication and interpersonal communion which have been part of the ministry of healing since ancient times.

PART VII

# *Erickson and Family Therapy*

*Erickson is commonly considered an eminent systems thinker and one of the precursors of family therapy. Although Erickson often did family therapy, he did not necessarily bring all the family members together during a session. However, even when doing individual treatment, Erickson remained cognizant of the effect of his interventions within the patient's family and social context. The application of Ericksonian techniques to family systems is fertile ground for future investigation. Ericksonian methods can be powerful techniques for changing systems. Carrell Dammann, Ph.D., and Alan Leveton, M.D., are two family therapists who are developing Ericksonian approaches to family therapy.*

*Carrell Dammann, a clinical psychologist, has been a family therapist for more than 15 years. She is founder and director of the Atlanta Institute for Family Studes and a part-time instructor and supervisor of doctoral students in the family studies program at Georgia State University.*

*Dammann's chapter is an overview of Erickson's contribution to family therapy. She describes three assumptions about the nature of change and the role of the therapist which are particularly applicable to working with families. Therapy should be directive in its nature, and Dammann alludes to the idea that direct manipulations by the therapist more often are centered on the context rather than the client. Confronted by an altered context, the client then self-determines a new response pattern.*

*The use of secondary gain is addressed. The therapist assumes that, given the client's environment and perspective, the system makes sense. Therefore, the client is never asked to change directly. Rather, his world is changed by the therapist in such a way that the symptoms no longer fill the same function. When secondary gain is changed, the symptom must change.*

*Alan F. Leveton is an accomplished family therapist and teacher; he has been a supervisor of family therapists for more than 15 years. Dr. Leveton is founder and medical director of The Family Therapy Center in San Francisco.*

*One of the hallmarks of Erickson's approach was his playful and gentle style of guiding the associations of his patients and students. Erickson perceived the therapist's task as creating situations in which strong healing associations were elicited. Leveton's chapter is one of the finest explications of Erickson's technique of guiding associations.*

Chapter 16

# Family Therapy: Erickson's Contribution

*Carrell A. Dammann*

The greatest truths are often simple and obvious, so I will try to stay simple and obvious in my remarks. One of my most consistent experiences over almost two decades of studying the work of Gregory Bateson, Milton Erickson, and Jay Haley has been to catch myself wagging my head and saying, "Of course, that's obvious. Why didn't I think of that before?"

John Brockman, in his volume, *About Bateson,* related a delightful conversation with cultural anthropologist Edward T. Hall, who pointed out:

> . . . that the most significant, the most critical inventions of man were not those ever considered to be inventions, but those that appeared to be innate and natural. To illustrate the point, he told a story of a group of cavemen living in prehistoric times. One day, while sitting around the fire, one of the men said, "Guess what? We're talking." Silence. The others looked at him with suspicion. "What's talking?" one of them asked. "It's what we're all doing. Right now. We're talking!" "You're crazy," another man replied. "Who ever heard of such a thing?" "I'm not crazy," the first man said, "You're crazy. We're talking." And it became a question of "Who's crazy?" The group could not see or understand because "talking" was invented by the first man. The moment he said "We're talking" was a moment of great significance in the process of evolution (Brockman, 1977).

The ideas and innovations of Erickson and Bateson, as well as their formalization and articulation by subsequent generations of their students and chroniclers, are clearly a significant step in the evolution of the social sciences and the practice of agents of change.

While basic truths have a beguiling simplicity, the technology they spawn is usually one of great complexity. Once Edison had invented the light bulb, people had to get busy designing and building a massive array of lamps. With a full awareness of the sea of emerging technology in which we now find ourselves awash, I will try to speak as simply as I can about Erickson's contributions to the field of family therapy. I shall try to abstract from the tangled threads of Erickson's influence some assumptions that are now basic to family therapy theory and practice.

Most of the ideas Erickson contributed to family therapy are those very same things he contributed to hypnosis and individual therapy. These contributions are profound and fundamental. They are summarized in the following three assumptions about the nature of change and the role of the therapist:

1) The therapist is *responsible for creating a context* in which change can take place.
2) Change comes about as a result of the accurate assessment and management of the *resistances to change* existing in the system.
3) *Change is discontinuous* in that it occurs at various points throughout the life-cycle. Brief and problem-focused therapy is most appropriate for facilitating adaptation.

Each of these assumptions has had effects on the field of family therapy as it has evolved over the last quarter century. The effect of Erickson's work on family therapy has been most clearly transmitted through his influence on Jay Haley's work at the Philadelphia Child Guidance Center and the Family Therapy Institute of Washington, D.C., and through the continuing influence of his work on the Palo Alto Group at the Mental Research Institute.

The first assumption is that the therapist is responsible for creating a context in which change can take place. Commonly, directives are used to facilitate this process. Although the traditional psychiatric practice is to try to avoid giving direct advice or telling the patient what to do, the hallmark of Erickson's work was his development of the use of tasks and directives with patients and his use of therapeutic "double binds." This break with traditional protocol is clearly a consequence of Erickson's work in hypnosis where, to paraphrase Paul Watzlawick, "One cannot not be directive" (Watzlawick, Beavin, & Jackson, 1967). The use of a complex technology of tasks and directives in family therapy is clearly the outgrowth of Erickson's influence on Haley, Weakland, Bateson, et al. In *Strategies of Psychotherapy,* Haley (1963) cites Erickson as saying, "The patient must be told to do something, and that something should be related to his problem in some way."

> When asked what he thought crucial to inducing therapeutic change, Erickson replied that he thought it was like teaching a child in school. It is not enough to explain to the child that one plus one equals two. It is necessary to hand the child some chalk and have him write "one" and then write "one" again and make a plus sign and write "two." Similarly, it is not enough to explain a problem to a patient or even to have the patient explain a problem himself. What is important is to get the patient to do something. Erickson points out that it is insufficient to have a patient with an oedipal conflict discuss his father. Yet, one can give the patient the simple task of writing the word "father" on a piece of paper and then have him crumple it up and throw it in the wastebasket and this action can produce pronounced effects (Haley, 1963, p. 45).

It is an important distinction to note that Erickson's approach does not propose that the therapist is responsible for making things change. Rather, the therapist is responsible for creating a context in which change can take place. This context in which change can take place is the probable or inevitable result of following the therapist's directives. To quote Haley's definition of strategic therapy:

> Therapy can be called strategic if the clinician initiates what happens during therapy and designs a particular approach for each problem. When a therapist and a person with a problem encounter each other, the action that takes place is determined by both of them, but in strategic therapy the initiative is largely taken by the therapist (Haley, 1973, p. 17).

The goal of the directive therapist is to create a task or situation that forces or allows the patient or family to experience some aspect of the problem in such a way that they must question their most basic perceptions or thoughts or feelings about the problem and/or they must alter the usual sequence of behaviors about the problem. Traditional therapies have been based on the assumption that insight leads to change. Ericksonian therapies might be characterized by the obverse principle, namely, change leads to insight.

Many a strategic family therapist knows that secretly warm feeling in a final session when someone in the family makes a profoundly simple observation about the function a symptom had been serving in the family. I recall one mother in a final family session poignantly noting that, since her acting-out daughter was successfully leaving home, she guessed she would have to go back where she left off early in her marriage and learn to fight with her husband. She successfully arrived at this observation entirely on her own with no assistance or prodding from a helpful therapist.

On the other hand, insight is a possible but not necessary corollary to change. (Usually it is more necessary to the "well trained" therapist than to the client.) Clients in families often attribute change to something incidental or irrelevant to the therapy rather than to the therapy itself.

I remember one of the first "monster families" we treated at the Atlanta Institute. The 23-year-old identified patient had been in and out of every psychiatric facility in Atlanta at least twice a year for the last ten years. She had been terrorizing her family and the community and had defeated a long line of therapists. The family was seen in brief therapy and the problem reframed in a way that forced the parents to cooperate with respect to the daughter's behavior, in spite of their continuing bitterness over their ten-year divorce. The daughter's behavior changed dramatically in a matter of weeks and she moved to the country with her boyfriend and got a job. After 18 months of being problem-free, the family, in a follow-up call, attributed the change to "the fresh country air."

Let us consider the second assumption. Change comes about as a result of the accurate assessment and management of the resistances to change existing in the system. This is perhaps best illustrated in Milton's own words taken from an article written with Ernest Rossi, "Varieties of Double Bind":

> My first well-remembered intentional use of the double bind occurred in early boyhood. One winter day with the weather below zero, my father led a calf out of the barn to the water trough. After the calf had satisfied its thirst, they turned back to the barn but at the doorway the calf stubbornly braced its feet and, despite my father's desperate pulling on the halter, he could not budge the animal. I was outside playing in the snow and, observing the impasse, began laughing heartily. My father challenged me to pull the calf into the barn. Recognizing the situation as one of unreasoning stubborn resistance on the part of the calf, I decided to let the calf have full opportunity to resist since that was what it ap-

> parently wished to do. Accordingly, I presented the calf with a double bind by seizing it by the tail and pulling it away from the barn while my father continued to pull it inward. The calf promptly chose to resist the weaker of the two forces and dragged me into the barn (Erickson & Rossi, 1975).

This story is a lovely metaphor for the family therapist, who must start from outside the system. From this vantage point, there is an objective view of the interactional nature of the resistances that maintain the problem. The therapist must assess the areas of resistance which will allow the most leverage for change. She or he must then enter the system and grab the calf by the tail in order to intervene in such a way as to produce *predictable* change.

The Ericksonian approach differs greatly from the traditional approach to a symptom. The symptom, rather than being viewed as a refractory manifestation of an intrapsychic conflict, is seen as a significant communication in an interpersonal encounter. The therapist must be able to speak the patient's language if he or she is to be effective.

When a patient claimed to be Jesus Christ, Erickson might respond, "I understand you have experience as a carpenter." Erickson's use of symptoms was like the Judo master who uses the force of his counterpart's move by directing it rather than by opposing it. Haley remarked that:

> Typical of Erickson's directives to patients is his accepting the patient's behavior, but in such a way that a change is produced. At the most abstract level, his directives can be seen as encouraging symptomatic behavior by the patient, but under therapeutic direction. He never, of course, tells the patient to cease his symptomatic behavior. Rather, he directs the patient to behave in a symptomatic way, at times adding something else to this instruction. Since the behavior occurs under therapeutic direction, it becomes a different kind than when it is initiated by the patient (Haley, 1963, p. 46).

The first step in this process in family therapy is an accurate assessment of the structure and function of the symptom in the interpersonal arena. This analysis often leads the therapist into the once easily dismissed territory of secondary gain. The therapist starts asking such questions as, "What happens in the family or in a given situation because of the symptom?" "What might happen if the symptom suddenly went away?" "Whom is the symptom protecting?" The interest is in the consequences of the symptom rather than the antecedents, and the assumption is that the symptom serves some function in an ongoing relationship.

I am reminded of a patient whose symptom was trichotillomania, pulling out large quantities of her hair resulting in bald spots. She was an otherwise lovely girl, and was living with a rather unsuitable young man who refused to marry her as long as the symptom persisted. Other than her symptom, she was in all respects more competent and responsible than her boyfriend. For some time he had been out of school and out of work, and was undecided about his direction in life. The symptom both balanced the relationship and precluded any possibility of marriage. Giving up the symptom and giving up the boyfriend were both accomplished in a course of brief therapy.

The utilization techniques that characterize Ericksonian approaches to therapy have been criticized by some as manipulative gimmicks. Actually, they are a natural outgrowth of a respect for the interpersonal and contextual importance of symptomatic behavior. From this view, the concern of a therapist that someone "not get over a symptom too quickly" is quite genuine. Through our study of Erickson's work we have come to recognize that therapy often moves in stages, and that the initial change in a symptom is unstable and vulnerable to systemic resistances at other levels. Thus, the prediction or encouragement of relapse can be crucial. The proper use of double binds is seen as manipulative only by those who do not view behavior from a systemic or contextual perspective.

This leads us to the third assumption for which Erickson must be given much credit. Change occurs at discontinuous points throughout the life-cycle. Brief and problem-focused therapy is most appropriate for facilitating adaptation.

Again we are confronted with a dramatic departure from the traditional focus on the long-term pathological and intrapsychic aspects of a symptom. A symptom in family therapy or systems framework often is viewed as an indication that the family has encountered difficulty making a necessary transition to the next stage of an unfolding life-cycle. This view is implicit throughout the work of Milton Erickson.

The symptom indicates that someone has gotten stuck trying to negotiate a bend in the river and subsequently created a log jam. The role of the therapist is to break up the log jam and channel the family members back into the proper stream of movement. This assumption of an interactional dilemma rather than deep-seated individual pathology is a more hopeful perspective for a change agent and leads to a brief, problem-focused therapy. In *Uncommon Therapy,* Haley says,

> If one thinks of therapy as the introduction of variety and richness into a person's life, the goal is to free the person from the limitations and restrictions of a social network in difficulty. Symptoms usually appear when a person is in an impossible situation and is trying to break out of it. It was once thought that focusing upon symptoms was "merely" relieving the symptom as the person became adjusted. This view was held by clinicians who did not know how to cure a symptom and so did not realize that, except in rare instances, a symptom cannot be cured without producing a basic change in the person's social situation, which frees him to grow and develop. Anxiety spells, for example, cannot be relieved unless the therapist intervenes to help the patient find more alternatives in life (Haley, 1973, pp. 43-44).

One of the features that I find appealing in Ericksonian style is what I call an "anthropological" rather than a "missionary" approach to working with families. There is a healthy respect for the diversity of effective family systems within the framework of a culturally appropriate developmental process.

The influence of Erickson and Bateson in the area of brief, problem-focused therapy has culminated in the articulation by Watzlawick, Weakland, and Fisch (1974) of the concepts of first and second order change. First order change represents gradual increments or decrements in one's lifes and experience, i.e., more of, or less of, the same. First order change is an essential and fundamental process in one's life. It is also useful in therapy and teaching.

By contrast, second order change is the reorganization of interrelating parts in a system, where elements must recombine or emerge in a significantly different way. It is abrupt and discontinuous rather than gradual. It is irreversible in the sense that, "You can't step into the same river twice." Changes required of the family system at critical points in the life-cycle are second order changes and require second order approaches to therapy. It is useful for us to think in terms of first and second order interventions in therapy and to learn to match our intervention appropriately to the nature of the problem.

Clearly what we now call strategic family therapy is a useful patchwork quilt full of vibrant colors—the handiwork of many gifted artisans. The old masters, from whom they inherited their tools and learned their artistry, were Milton Erickson and Gregory Bateson. Their lives continue to flow through all of us.

Erickson and Bateson were more interested in asking questions than in giving answers. Their work focused on an understanding and respect for the vast complexities and levels of communication. The serious student of their work cannot be interested in acquiring a "technique." Rather, he or she is engaged in a never-ending search for skills and knowledge, and for understanding of how to use oneself therapeutically in a given context.

Milton Erickson always taught by telling stories and he *never* explained them. So I will close by sharing a story. Having been what I called "A Sorcerer's Apprentice," studying Erickson's work for many years, I finally made a pilgrimage to see him. As always, he was most generous with his time and precious energy. Several months after I returned home, as he promised, Milton sent me a recipe for cinnamon pie. At the bottom of the card he penned a note which read, "Of course, every good cook must adjust the seasoning to suit their own particular taste."

## REFERENCES

Brockman, J. Introduction. In: *About Bateson,* John Brockman (Ed.), New York: Dutton, 1977.

Erickson, M.H., & Rossi, E.L. Varieties of double bind. *The American Journal of Clinical Hypnosis,* 1975, *17* (3), 143-157.

Haley, J. *Strategies of Psychotherapy.* New York: Grune & Stratton, 1963.

Haley, J. *Uncommon Therapy: The Psychiatric Techniques of Milton H. Erickson, M.D.* New York: W.W. Norton, 1973.

Watzlawick, P., Beavin, J., & Jackson, D. *Pragmatics of Human Communication.* New York: W.W. Norton, 1967.

Watzlawick, P., Weakland, J., & Fisch, R. *Change: Principles of Problem Formation and Problem Resolution.* New York: W.W. Norton, 1974.

Chapter 17

# Family Therapy as Play: The Contribution of Milton H. Erickson, M.D.

*Alan F. Leveton*

Now, I would like to begin by telling you of a couple I saw after my first trip to see Milton Erickson in Phoenix.

A couple came to see me with a dramatic situation. She was a young woman in her twenties; he, an older man in his late thirties. They were "madly in love." He drank intermittently and too much. She fell down with akinetic-like seizures, as many as 15 an hour. She would fall into flaccid unconsciousness, like a puppet with its strings suddenly cut. As long as she continued to fall down, he remained sober and watched her carefully. When she gained strength, he drank and was unfaithful. As in any system, there was a strong pull to induce certain behavior in me that would preserve the status quo. This invitation was strongly put. They urged me to "be the doctor," to pursue the wraith of a possible brain injury. I was to make him noble for his sacrifice to her faints. She would faint during our session; he would rush to her, looking imploringly and accusingly at me. The fact that my office was on the second floor meant that she often had to be assisted down the stairs. I didn't want to do it, but the image of us carrying her down the stairs was less threatening than the fantasy of my being on a witness stand answering a lawyer's sarcastic question, "You let her go down the stairs knowing she might fall, doctor!?"

She had been worked up medically, neurologically. There had been an old head injury; compensation money was involved. Nothing much was helping her from the medical side. Indeed, there were doubts that she was "medically ill." It was clear that an intervention was needed that would raise the threshold of her resistance to lapses of consciousness and reduce the secondary gain.

I was just beginning to use hypnosis and thought of it as a separate kind of therapeutic activity. I felt bound to announce, "I'd like to use hypnosis to help you find some other ways of doing what you are doing that won't inconvenience you as much."

She countered with a long and detailed story that her mother had told her about gypsies—how they hypnotized young children to find out their secret thoughts and so steal them away. Her mother had warned her most strongly never to let herself be hypnotized, and she had fearfully promised her mother that would never happen. Her manner was earnest. Of course, I could understand a daughter's promise. Oh my! I'd better be cautious about enthusiastically using the word "hypnosis" with her!

But Erickson never cared a fig about what you called something, or even how you got to your destination. You could get somewhere by walking, driving a car, or imagining you had wings. I could let the word "hypnosis" go. It was more important to get a sense of her unconsciously active self and arrange for that self to get what it wanted and needed in some other way. What *my* inner-self needed was to not be discouraged, to accept what was given and work within the possibilities. What she needed was a guarantee that no one would make her disloyal to her mother, discover secrets, or kidnap her. What he needed was some other reason for staying sober.

I thought: Gypsies and swearing oaths to your mother are in fairy tales and so are things that come in "threes," like three wishes, three tasks.

I agreed that her mother was right *about secrets* (that she might be wrong about some other things was implied tonally). I suggested that she write down three secrets and find a safe place to hide them so they couldn't be stolen away. We would not "do any hypnosis," but she might remember some place where, when she was little and safe at home, she felt secure—a place to which no gypsies would dare to come.

She did. It was a pond near her house with reeds that sheltered ducks, with hidden flowers, soft sounds of wind and wavelets. She enjoyed describing her special pond . . . so bright was the sunlight reflected on the cusps of the little waves that they tired her eyes; so warm was the sun that she felt relaxed and drowsy; so pleasing was the memory that to see and to feel it more fully she might shut her eyes.

Around the pond she noted her favorite trees, where she could seek shelter from the sun. Those trees had been there a long time and she found them most attractive. They guarded her pond. Their roots penetrated deep into the nourishing soil; their leaves permitted the sun's light to pass through in a muted way; their branches reached as far upwards into the air above as their roots penetrated deeply below. Her boyfriend could stay very alert and watch her closely, and soberly note how firmly safe she was by her trees, by her pond.

And what do you imagine was the most interesting quality of those trees? That they stood securely upright. They could do this because their roots were so strongly anchored and because of the wonderful, strong flexibility of their trunks. They were neither so limp they couldn't stand, nor so rigid that they might break in a strong wind. In the expectable winds by that pond they could make slight adjustments as they stood upright. They could sway, even sway noticeably, but not fall down—just what she knew they needed to do and could do, even if someone else might be disappointed to see them standing there.

After this session, she could stand on her own feet and no longer needed to be carried out of the office. She had markedly fewer seizures at home. She began a business which involved making storage racks out of a kind of wood she particularly liked. She asked her boyfriend to do the carpentry. He balked, grew restless, began to drink again. She discovered she really wanted the business to work, grew impatient with his unreliability, and asked him for real support. She told him that if he couldn't help her in this way, she wanted him to leave.

Here is my understanding of this couple's system: I believe they were organized around her being incapacitated. This gave him an opportunity to be a noble and competent rescuer. The system was unstable and destructive to both because she had to be "sick" to keep it going, and he could never test his true strength outside the relationship. Ambivalence was high. They both appreciated and resented their mutual dependence. If the system didn't change, I would eventually become another exasperated and frustrated helper.

There was no point in telling her she was not having "medical" seizures. Other doctors had already tried that. She could always faint while being confronted and was willing to be bruised in the process. He could not be told to leave her alone. Someone had to catch her falling body and this took all his time. He could not discover if he could be self-sustaining, industrious, or freely generous. Each yearned for something better. There was simply too much pain in the status quo.

In all probability she was already in a trance situation. He watched her closely, expecting her to faint. She observed him watching her and had an ability to respond to his expectation. He was a gypsy and their secret was that her ability to stand up for herself had been "stolen away."

I remembered Erickson had reassured a frightened subject by letting her write a question on a piece of paper. She could keep it hidden in her purse, giving her a reassuring sanctuary for her secret. I did the same. I had not asked her to break a promise made to her mother about hypnosis. In asking her to close her eyes, I blocked the visual cues her boyfriend was sending in his leaning forward expectantly towards her. And in asking him to watch her closely, I satisfied his need to be a vigilant helper.

In reminding her of *her* pond, I reawakened the self that was a competent, complete child dreaming of herself away from her mother. When she was "at her pond" my words held her in an intermediate space. (Later, I want to connect this idea to Winnicott's notion of "transitional space.") She was held between the eidetically recalled objects of original perception and the abstract qualities inherent in those recalled objects. I held her between her remembered trees and the "tree-ness" they represented. I held her between nouns and adjectives. I could watch as she daydreamed away with no fear of gypsies, secrets, or hypnosis. I could use the attributes of her pond-world to remind her of her useful lessons to support her independence and yearning for personal strength. I could do this in a way Erickson taught me, that is, obliquely. There was no need for a direct confrontation in which she might have to admit that her mother had frightened her, that she was stronger than she appeared, that she could faint to keep her boyfriend from drinking, that he needed her fainting, or that I was using hypnosis.

Erickson had demonstrated that patients could be held in a state of reverie and distracted from their repetitive patterns. I used that reverie to explore new possibilities of behavior. I introduced change by analogy and metaphor without charging head-on at resistances. I learned that I could participate in the patient's reverie so that her memories could suggest to my imagination symbols that might allow her to transform her original situation.

In this case I was not able to find a single theme broad enough to encompass both the woman and man simultaneously. My most focused work was with her. She made the initial changes. They separated. I then saw them individually. Later she continued her career work. He left the area and a year later married another woman.

## THEMES

I want to focus on these "Ericksonian" themes in this chapter: 1) There is a child that is both real and dormant in ourselves and our patients. 2) There is a way in which that child can be approached. 3) There is a place in which that child can play and learn. 4) There is a way to introduce new play while holding the individual or family group in a state of trance or reverie. 5) The therapist does this from the position of being a kind, imaginative, protective parent.

That leads me to the story of one of my interactions with Erickson:

*An Ericksonian Reverie*

I came to Erickson both early and late. Early, because in my training years his were the only published transcripts of actual interviews with patients that I could find. I had never seen my teachers at their work, nor had they seen me at mine. Any verbatim transcript of therapy was intensely interesting to me. But "hypnosis" had no currency in my circles and "manipulation" was a taboo that precluded the study of something as active as trance work. Naturally, I had to reject him. In the intervening years I learned that he was a Picasso of American psychiatry. His influence was in Philadelphia and Palo Alto, on double bind theory, paradoxical intervention, and brief therapy. I came to Phoenix late in Erickson's storytelling years to discover firsthand what was not easily communicated through the written word—his kindness, his deep understanding of the life-cycle, his belief in the healing powers of a benign unconscious.

On the first day Erickson put my wife, Eva, into a trance. He caught my guarded fascination as I watched. I was determined to go into trance the second day, but was in turmoil the night before. One strong childhood memory returned and I knew somehow I had to tell it at the beginning of the second day.

I told Erickson that my father had taught me to play chess when I was ten years old and continued to play with me as long as he won. At age 12, I won my first game. He never played chess with me again. In his sly, oblique style, Erickson told someone else present in the room, "Alan's father taught him that you can lose by losing and you can lose by winning." He dropped his eyes, searching and collecting from his file of stories. He then began to tell story after story about events between his children and himself, events in which he took delight in their progressive ability to get their way with him. I learned that he had the credentials to be a good father, one who enjoys the achievements of his children.

It was clear I didn't have to nod agreement or laugh at his jokes or answer rhetorical questions. I could be another kind of "son" in relation to the other kind of "father" he was. I could be free to play in my own reverie.

Two repeated words seemed to be there as strong anchors in his long discourses: "now" and "you." "Now" always seemed to be a steadying force and bridge between stories. "Now" meant he was "holding the floor." He would take responsibility for providing continuity. He would not let me drop into a silent, unattended, frightening void.

It was his use of "you" that sent me into a trance reverie. "You" sounded like the vibrant tolling of a great bell, opening doors to the delights and astonishments of my childhood. As he talked, many images and memories came to me. I don't even know what they all were. The sound of passing trucks, the ringing telephone, the birds outside, all receded from my conscious attention. I was in the world of reverie, in the world of my childhood, exploring my block, finding the nooks and crannies of my house, climbing the backyard fence, and, most importantly, being at the tops of the trees in which I spent so many hours daydreaming.

Notice Erickson's use of the word "you" in this rather typical induction:

> Now I am going to talk to you. When you first went to kindergarten you learned to form a mental image of some kind; you didn't know it at the time, but it was a permanent mental image. In grammar school you formed other mental images. You were developing mental images and you can recall all those images. Now you can go anywhere you wish. You can feel water, you may want to swim in it. You can do anything you want. You don't even have to listen to my voice because your unconscious will hear it. Your unconscious can try anything it wishes, but your conscious mind isn't going to do anything of importance (Erickson & Rossi, 1976, pp. 7-8).

I believe that the "you" he is addressing is the child playing unselfconsciously in the charmed circle created by the watchfulness of an attentive and available parent.

Erickson always had the child self of the patient in his thoughts.

> Children are uncluttered by rigid, conscious sets and therefore children can see things that adults cannot (Erickson & Rossi, 1976, p. 259).

> Adults are only children grown tall. The unconscious is much more childlike in that it is direct and it is free. When you have a patient in a trance, the patient thinks like a child and reaches for an understanding (Erickson & Rossi, 1976, p. 255).

Erickson speaks with the loving tones of a father or a grandfather who creates a sanctuary for daydreaming and reverie by the kind constancy of his voice and the pacing of his speech. He calls to that inner child and invites it to listen and not listen, to be here and to be there, to be now and to be then. He gives you permission to enter an intermediate zone between full wakefulness and sleep. It is safe there because Erickson will be the guardian of that zone. He talks to the "you" that demonstrably has learned many skills and mastered life enough to be there with him, a surviving you, and one that knows how to play, to remember, to do new things, to ignore social conventions, to go anywhere that reverie might lead.

When I said to my woman patient, "You can notice the special qualities of your pond-trees," I was talking to that resourceful and independent child that she had truly been, and I called it forth.

Where was I in Erickson's induced trance? Where was my patient when I held her in reverie and daydream? What does Erickson mean when he says, "Now you can go anywhere you wish. You can feel water. You may want to swim in it"?

I had given these questions much thought for many years while both doing play therapy and playing with my own children. I did not know how applicable the answer might be to an understanding of an Erickson-induced trance state. I noticed that children at play became entranced with their fantasies in a way that showed their use of space was unique to that play. A room might be a cave or a whole world. A chair might be a rocket ship and the rug below, the surface of an alien planet. A tiny toy dinosaur might destroy a city. Before play began, my office was an office. After play was over, it was again an office. In the midst of play, if I was not careful and diplomatic, suddenly and with jarring impact it might become an office again.

The English pediatrician-psychoanalyst D. Winnicott (1971) wrote about this phenomenon in his studies of children and how they learned about the world. He called the child's first "magical" possessions, the blankets and teddy bears, "transitional objects" because they were somewhere between the self and the not-self. He observed trustworthy parents playing with their children and noticed a "potential space" between the mother and the baby, a third area of human living, one neither inside the individual nor outside in the world of shared reality.

This potential space has no fixed boundaries or attributes. It can be filled with play, reverie, experiences that instruct a child about his or her culture. Its center is the caring parent. You might get an idea of the dimensions of this transitional space by watching how closely a child clings to its parent and how far the child ventures forth. A child venturing forth might look back to its parent's face for reassurance, or return to its mother's lap for a moment of contact. Some parents indicate the world outside is a frightening place and bind the child to a tight circle of fear. Other parents encourage a precocious freedom that leads to recklessness. Some parents have no idea about play, and are limited in their playfulness resulting in an impoverished realm between parent and child. Others thrust ideas and play on the child and jar it out of spontaneity and unself-consciousness.

Erickson was there at the center of his work as the parent-therapist. You could venture forth in a potential space in which you could play, remember, master, and learn. He did not challenge the content of your reverie or the reality of your memory. He stocked his reverie room with images and words and let you play with them as you wished.

His real room was like that, filled with actual objects that meant something to him, but something also to me: the African idol, the framed letter, the fragment of glass, the ironwood carvings, the gifts. Outside his office there was the rose bush, Squaw Peak, the Botanical Gardens. His stories had lists of places, things, events.

His pattern of indicating these was closest to what I experience when I do play therapy, following the child's action and gently adding other toys and actions to play out possible resolutions of the child's conflicts. It is close to what happens when I use experiential tasks familiar to family therapists: family sculpture, family drawing, role-playing, movement. These are also in the realm of play. Themes are explored through action, often nonverbally and metaphorically.

Here is a portion of a trance induction balanced between the "free play" of the subject and the kind of play done in the presence of a person who offers specific possibilities.

> Now, the next thing for her to do is actually to develop the hallucination or let us say a specific landscape, one she has not seen previously but a landscape she would like. Now . . . who knows what she would put in a landscape? Birds, trees, bushes, rocks (Erickson & Rossi, 1976, pp. 285-288).

Erickson left room for her to create a private landscape. He offered, as he so often did, a list of objects she might use; it was a simple list—"birds, trees, bushes, rocks." He did not insist; he provided possibilities; he created a context for her to daydream, to be in a state of reverie. (I prefer the term "reverie" to "trance" because it suggests a broader range of activity, one closer to people's ordinary lives. Some may debate what is a hypnotic trance but everyone knows what it means to daydream in a state of reverie.)

Gaston Bachelard (1969), who was a great student of reverie, talked of a poet's ability to evoke

> . . . a state of new childhood, of a childhood which goes farther than the memories of our childhood, as if the poet were making us continue, complete a childhood which was not well finished (accomplished), and yet was ours (p. 106).

> . . . in waking life itself, when reverie works on our history, the childhood which is within us brings us its benefits (p. 20).

Erickson was the master of inducing and directing reverie in the shelter of the transitional space he created.

### *A Circus Reverie*

Now, I saw a couple whom I approached as though Erickson were my invisible consultant. I tried to imagine what they were like as children. This time I was intent upon creating a shared, simultaneous reverie for both husband and wife. I created a space in which they could play. I gave them room to daydream and provided specific objects and images with which to play. In that intermediate zone that surrounded our work we entered into a shared reverie, partially theirs and partially mine, which offered some new possibilities for relating.

Martha and Robert came to see me because their daily life was a torment of repeated, painful impasses. If Martha wanted to go out, Robert wanted to stay in. If Martha wanted a child, Robert sarcastically mentioned divorce. Both had the wide and piercing eyes of people who must defend against attack and be instantaneously ready to counterattack. They said there was much shared hatred, yet they had never parted in seven years of marriage.

Martha's family was depressed. Her father was a business failure; her mother drank. Her brother, being male, was supposed to enter a profession. Instead, he became a drug addict. She, as a female, was expected to be dutiful and marry early. She graduated from a first-rate college, entered a profession, and married late. Just before going away to school, she had made a serious suicide attempt. I asked her in trance to be a young girl coming home from school. Almost her entire perception was of the façade of her house and its window blinds. All that mattered to her was whether they were drawn or not. If drawn, she expected to find her mother drunk or dead. If opened, the house might be empty. There was no clear background—no trees, flowers, bushes, rocks. No landscape save the awful message of the windows.

Robert had been under the gaze of shaming parents. He was "too intellectual" for the family and had his "head in the clouds." He remembered a beating at the hands of a younger asthmatic brother. It was unthinkable to hit back. He could not shout either. A small movement of his father's hand towards his chest and a worried glance from his mother served to remind him that his father's heart was "bad," and anger might be the death of him.

In my mind was the fear that they had such strong dependency needs, such suspicion and such hostility that they couldn't imagine being together *or* apart. Death was also in the air. I worried that a second suicide attempt might occur. I wanted to introduce a useful distraction. Their main activity with me was to attempt to get me into a coalition against one another. Almost all of their spontaneous images were of city life—houses, schools, lectures, driving to my office in two cars, dealing with their professions, dealing with their answering services. The natural world seemed absent.

I surprised them with a constructed toy, presented without comment during their hour. I strapped two wooden clowns together, a long pole held crossways between them. At each end of the pole were heavy weights so the entire construction could balance on a tightrope strung between two chairs. They were startled and intrigued. No one had ever given them an unasked-for present. The circus clowns, balanced on their high wire, responded to air currents flowing in the room. The removal of any part of the toy meant it would fall down. Yet, as it was, all it could do was stay in trembling motion, suspended in the air.

The clowns were an excellent pendulum for trance focus. I began talking about circuses. Circus acts required exquisite cooperation and concentration from each partner. Circuses weren't always at the Civic Auditorium. They often were under canvas. In the old days, they moved from town to town by caravan, traveling over rural roads through quiet, pre-dawn woods. There were many quiet places and many trees.

Martha and Robert were in a shared reverie, eyes fixed on the balancing clowns. They were together and relating to a third region other than the supercharged interpersonal conflict. Partly, each was relating to my efforts at directed distraction; partly, each was responding to internally-stored memories that would fit the flow of my verbal landscape.

My conscious attitude was one of a parent who calms the children by an unexpected gift and launches into a story to hold their attention, watching each to make sure there would be no interruptions. I also was a parent who sought to introduce certain themes of my own choosing, to teach them some new ways they might look at their lives.

My early training would have led me to point out to this couple the obvious, that they were hyperalert and paranoid about each other's motives. With Erickson at my shoulder, I sought to reduce their vigilance by creating a context in which there was nothing to watch. In earlier days I might have explained to each that they had justifiable fears of rage—she because of her mother, he because of his brother and father. Within the stories of circus life I could describe the kind of courage that performers had to develop in order to be at ease with the high wire, how the circus tent itself had to be made taut by the tent crew that drove in the ropes and poles with strong blows of their sledgehammer, how the watchfulness of the trapeze artists was repaid by the grace of their movements and the rush of flying through the air . . . even in slow motion to be caught by the partner in great sweeping arabesques. And there was that sense of wonder, that the circus family could work so well together, that the small frictions and quarrels were forgotten in the movement of performance which could be enjoyed in reflection as they leisurely traveled through the woods to the next town.

All the talk of tents and trees eventually led to a camping trip in the real woods for them. The idea came somewhere out of the circus play and my interplay with them. It was not an assigned task; it just emerged as a good thing to do for these city people. They wanted to do it. That trip was pivotal. They found that they could cooperate. They stored up images of the pine forest they camped in. He gave some mighty shouts in those woods. She took time to have long, lazy daydreams nestled in the roots of a particular tree.

I believe the therapy gave them a bit of childhood they had never fully experienced. In my formal training years I would have labeled it a "corrective emotional experience," but that would have taken far longer than a reverie. Their original family situations provided little freedom for trusting play and imagination. I was able to create a potential space. The things I did filled that space with words and objects satisfactory to them, intriguing, playful, offering new possibilities. I had the special satisfaction and pleasure that comes when play is good and shared.

### *Trees*

I noticed that in this paper many trees appear—the trees I climbed, the trees that offered stability by a pond, the trees of a wide world traversed by circuses, and the trees sent out into the world to honor Erickson.

It is fitting to end this paper by repeating a story Erickson told in a trance session reported in *Hypnotic Realities*.

> In 1930, in the early May, I dreamed one night that I was on the north side of an east-west road in Wisconsin. And I stood there knowing that I was Dr. Erickson. And I was looking at a small boy who is running up and down. By the grading on the side of the road, by the hills, was a maintenance crew. A fence on the top of the grade and barbed-wire fence. Hazel bush, an oak tree, a wild cherry tree. And I saw that barefoot boy with overalls curiously probing the fresh graded ground, and excavating around the cut ends of the roots and looking at the oak tree, and looking at the wild cherry tree. And then examining the cut ends of the roots, trying to determine which roots came from the wild cherry tree and which came from the oak tree. The little boy was sure none of those roots came from the hazelnut bush. I approved of that boy. I could see him plainly. . . . I recognized him as little Milton Erickson, but he could not see Dr. Erickson. He didn't even know I was on the other side of that east-west-bound road. And I enjoyed watching that little boy and thinking that how little appreciation he had of the fact that he was going to grow up and become Dr. Erickson . . . and I was still a little boy, a barefoot boy. I had long forgotten that, but my unconscious mind had remembered it (Erickson & Rossi, 1976)

## ADDITIONAL COMMENTARY

In reviewing this paper, Michael Geis, M.D., of the Family Therapy Center, San Francisco, made the following observations for which I am grateful.

There are parallels in all three stories: the woman's seizures, my interactions with Erickson, and the fighting couple. In each there is a twofold action: 1) A secure background is introduced which relaxes and reassures and 2) there is something arising out of that background available for identification and change.

For the first woman there is the quiet, calm pond which is her secure place that is background. There are also trees whose stability is there for identification of a reliant, flexible part of the self. For me, there is the background of a father who takes pleasure in his child's successes.

Arising from that is my re-identification with the self of my reverie-filled tree-climbing days. For the couple, there is the background of the circus and its cooperative family of performers. In the foreground for identification is the team of trusting members of a trapeze act.

The very act of creating a secure background itself creates change. Rather than convulsing, the woman listens to my story; rather than "observing" Erickson from the outside, I am at free play inside his story; rather than bicker with each other or me, the last couple shares listening to me.

The therapist in each situation acts to answer two questions. First, "Who do I need to be, and what do I need to do in order to provide a safe place for change?" and second, "What shall I put there to be found that might produce specific change?"

## REFERENCES

Bachelard, G. *The Poetics of Reverie.* Boston: Beacon Press, 1969.
Erickson, M., & Rossi, E. *Hypnotic Realities.* New York: Irvington, 1976.
Winnicott, D. *Playing and Reality.* New York: Basic Books, 1971.

PART VIII

# *Case Studies*

*Leo Alexander, M.D., is a lecturer in psychiatry at Tufts University and Medical School. He has published extensively in the areas of hypnosis and analytic psychotherapy and is past president of the New England Society of Clinical Hypnosis. Erickson and Alexander were longtime colleagues. In fact, of all the people in attendance at the Congress, Leo Alexander knew Erickson the longest; they worked together in the late 1930s at Worchester State Hospital.*

*The case Alexander describes occurred when Erickson lectured and demonstrated at the Boston State Hospital for a program that Alexander organized. Erickson used Alexander's nurse as a demonstration subject, and under the guise of merely demonstrating hypnosis, Erickson actually provided potent psychotherapy.*

*Erickson also described this case, and his description was published in the book* A Teaching Seminar with Milton H. Erickson, *which I edited. However, Erickson's recollection of the case differed substantially from Alexander's. In June 1979, Alexander was invited to speak at the Congress. He replied that he wanted to discuss Erickson's 1956 demonstration case. I explained that I had transcribed the case in my book, and I sent him a copy of Erickson's description. After receiving Erickson's report, Alexander informed me that Erickson's recollection substantially differed from his own.*

*Subsequently, I called Jan Kropenick, the nurse who was the subject of the demonstration, and asked her to send me her impressions of the 1956 demonstration. Just before my phone call,*

*Jan had attended a workshop on Ericksonian psychotherapy led by Stephen Lankton. Steve had discussed Erickson's case report, and Jan became aware for the first time that Erickson did not remember the events in the same way that she did.*

*Alexander corresponded with Jan before the Congress, and when it became evident that she would attend the Congress, Alexander invited her to be a discussant for his paper. O. Spurgeon English, M.D., the moderator of the panel, Leo Alexander, and Jan Kropenick discussed Alexander's paper after its presentation. Their edited commentary is included as an appendix to Alexander's chapter.*

*The reports from Alexander and Kropenick are basically similar. There are two possible reasons for the discrepancy between their report and Erickson's. First, Erickson may have confused cases and mixed facts from two separate cases into his report. Second, Erickson was concerned mostly with the effect of his communication on the students at the seminar, i.e., he was interested in having personal and professional impact on his students. Therefore, he may not have been concerned that the case report was completely accurate. In fact, Erickson commonly changed details of his teaching stories to fit the needs of the group. However, at his teaching seminars, Erickson would follow most of his case reports by displaying a picture, letter, or gift from the patient to "prove" that the case report was factual and not just made up for teaching purposes.*

*Paul Sacerdote, M.D., Ph.D., has practiced and taught hypnotic techniques for over 25 years. He has authored more than 30 papers on hypnosis, mostly in the areas of pain control in cancer and the induction and utilization of dreams. Dr. Sacerdote is past president of the Society for Clinical and Experimental Hypnosis and wrote* Induced Dreams.

*Sacerdote's chapter summarizes his use of a succession of hypnotically induced dreams. The chapter outlines a typical session, including the actual suggestions that Sacerdote frequently uses. The paper on hypnotically induced dreams was actually presented at a pre-congress workshop, but since it contains new and relevant information, it is included here.*

*David Calof conducts a private practice in hypnotherapy in Seattle, Washington, where he is codirector of the Seattle Strategic Therapy Institute. Calof has lectured extensively on the topic of hypnosis in the United States, Canada, and Australia. Calof's position as a strategic therapist is in line with the admonition of the Greek author, Nikos Kazantzakis, that "The ultimate, most holy form of theory is action." Calof's case study is noteworthy for the cleverness he shows in devising a strategic family therapy intervention. However, his primary purpose in presenting this case report on adolescent enuresis is to emphasize the flexibility needed in selecting treatment approaches.*

*Ericksonian techniques of habit modification are powerful because they are tailored to the individual. Individualizing techniques requires a unique approach to diagnosis. Special attention is placed on both thorough diagnosis of the habit pattern and diagnosis of the individual patient's values. In my own presentation, case reports elucidate Ericksonian approaches to diagnosis and treatment. Indirect techniques follow from the diagnosis.*

*Moris Kleinhauz, M.D., is a psychiatrist specializing in psychotherapy and hypnotherapy in Israel. Dr. Kleinhauz is director of the Community Mental Health Center at Yaffo-Tel Aviv and a lecturer at Tel Aviv University.*

*Kleinhauz presents a case where psychological trauma was suffered after the subject had taken part in a stage hypnosis demonstration, illustrating that one must realize the potential dangers in the use of hypnosis.*

*Kleinhauz reports his Ericksonian style of intervening in this case. He also provides theoretical explanations regarding the possible causes of psychological trauma following an authoritarian, routinized approach to hypnosis. Self-determination is an important human drive, and authoritarian manipulations for the hypnotist's personal gain may cause harm. Erickson's position was that therapeutic manipulations would be effective only if they were done with an attitude of benevolence and directed to the needs of the individual.*

Chapter 18

# Erickson's Approach to Hypnotic Psychotherapy of Depression

*Leo Alexander*

The use of the dynamic meaning of a symptom or symptoms under hypnosis, which had become the point of departure of the psychoanalytic approach, was reincorporated into hypnotic psychotherapy as early as 1897 by Renterghen (1897). Suggestions were formulated in terms of the dynamic meaning of the symptom revealed by the patient during the trance, rather than in terms of the superficial manifestations of the symptom. Further development of this approach was implemented by Hadfield (1920), Erickson (1943), Wolberg (1948), and has become an important concept in psychiatric hypnotherapy. A more recent addition is the technique of the induction of experimental (better termed "artificial") conflict or symptoms by Luria (1932) and Erickson (1935) so that the awareness and subsequent removal of the symptom or conflict may be made to generalize to the patient's real and more severe problem. Erickson's genius included the ability to bring into action a chain of mutually conditioning and reinforcing suggestions, which following one upon the other exert a powerful, in fact inexorable, effect in motivating and driving the patient toward health. I have seen Dr. Erickson relieve a patient from a severe suicidal depressive reaction, by producing and subsequently removing a suggested physical pain. Its relief generalized to the depression by the emphatically worded suggestion: "No pain lasts forever" (Alexander, 1965). Dr. Erickson's powerful capacity to bring about the generalization of suggestions had impressed me, but this particular treatment, which he performed on September 29, 1956, surpassed anything I had seen him or anyone else do in its elegance, specificity, and sure-fire lasting effect.

The occasion was the Fourth Annual Institute of Psychiatric Treatment, in Boston, on September 27, 28 and 29, 1956. The Annual Institute, founded by Dr. Robert Arnot and myself, involved teaching sessions at the Boston State Hospital, at which innovations in various methods of treatment in our field were presented by the originators. Nineteen lecturers participated on this occasion and 68 neuropsychiatrists from all over the United States had subscribed.

On the last day of the course, from 3:00 to 5:00 P.M., a lecture and two demonstrations by Erickson were scheduled. For his first demonstration, Erickson had brought a former patient of his whom he age regressed to age two; he also wanted to present a volunteer whom he had never hypnotized before. One very able, intelligent and personable nurse, Janice Pond, signed up for this demonstration; she was the treatment room nurse, who also assisted me with demonstrations of treatment techniques, and with demonstrations of lantern slides and electrical current patterns. The day before the demonstration, when it became known this nurse had offered to become Erickson's volunteer, the assistant superintendent of the hospital came to see me to discuss his concerns. He and I knew that she had been severely depressed. We had discussed her potential treatment needs before, and she was receiving analytically oriented psychotherapy. Her depression had begun after she had been deserted by her fiancé. The assistant superintendent, Dr. John McKenzie, had suspected that this very attractive, intelligent nurse might be potentially suicidal and suggested that I should discuss this with Dr. Erickson, preferably to dissuade him from using her as a demonstration subject, but in any case to warn him so that he would be aware of the danger of inadvertently subjecting her to a treatment that might trigger a dangerous response. I spoke to Dr. Erickson that evening and informed him fully. He listened to me patiently, smiled gently in his enigmatic way, and said, "I think there will be no difficulty."

The next morning, an hour before the teaching session, Ms. Pond and I were setting up the electrical equipment for the morning's demonstrations. About half way through these preparations, Dr. Erickson walked in, greeted us, and asked me whether I could spare Ms. Pond for a few moments. He took her to the library next door to the lecture hall. I continued with my preparations while she was absent for what seemed to be about two to three minutes. She then returned and resumed helping me. Shortly after her return, however, she told me that she could work only with her left hand because a severe pain had developed in her right arm, and that she could not freely move it. I did not connect this pain with her brief visit with Dr. Erickson in the library. I merely told her to be careful with her right arm and not to overstrain it, expressing the hope that the pain would soon pass. Ms. Pond assisted me effectively throughout the subsequent demonstrations, but she did not use her right arm. I did not see her at lunchtime, but I noticed that she was in the lecture hall during the early afternoon program.

Dr. Erickson's lecture began at 3:00 P.M., and his demonstrations were to begin at 4:00 P.M. After an excellent lecture on the general subject of hypnosis, he presented a patient of his who happened to live in Boston, whom he age regressed to age two. It was a very effective demonstration. At the completion of his demonstration, Dr. Erickson announced, "Will the other person who is already in a trance please come forward to the podium." Ms. Pond rose and then, in a somnambulistic manner, without turning her head to the right or left or moving her arms, walked straight to the stage. Dr. Erickson welcomed her, handed her a writing block and a pen, and said, "Will you please sign your name." The patient struggled to bring her right arm up but could not. Dr. Erickson then told her, "It is perfectly all right to use your left hand." Since I was sitting in the first row, I could not help noticing that her face lit up blissfully as he spoke these words, and with an ecstatic smile, she lifted her left hand, took the pen, and signed her name. He then told her, "No pain lasts forever; after the rain comes the sunshine." Immediately Ms. Pond lifted her right arm without any apparent discomfort and waved it about with a serene and smiling facial expression. Dr. Erickson then thanked her, and she went back to her seat.

The apparent simplicity of these suggestions was in striking contrast to their profound and far-reaching effect. I was also impressed with Dr. Erickson's extreme discretion and respect for his volunteer patient's privacy. As far as the uninitiated audience was concerned, they had merely seen the rapid relief of a severe state of pain by hypnosis. I did not have to wait long to appreciate the enormous depth of the change that had occurred in Ms. Pond. That evening, the last day of the three-day course, I dined with the staff members who had participated in the course, in a private dining room of a restaurant in the vicinity. I had seated Ms. Pond to my right, while Dr. Erickson was seated at Mrs. Alexander's left. As we sat down, Ms. Pond, in a whisper, thanked me for having given her the opportunity to be treated by Dr. Erickson. She said, "I believe Dr. Erickson saved my life—I had planned to commit suicide tonight since I did not want to do it before the course was over, but nothing is farther from my mind now!" To the great surprise of the hospital staff who knew her intimately, Ms. Pond's recovery remained a sustained one. One and a half years later she accepted a nursing position elsewhere.

I mentioned this remarkable accomplishment of Erickson in a paper (Alexander, 1965) to which Dr. Erickson added the following footnote:

> This patient had been under psychoanalytical therapy because of depressive reactions. She had set the date for her suicide in the next month and had already written her suicide notes. When Dr. Erickson asked her to act as a demonstration subject for his afternoon lecture, she consented, feeling only that she might as well, since things were all finished for her. Much pressure was privately put on Dr. Erickson not to use her as a subject but he was adamant, asserting that the girl had nothing to lose and everything to gain. The girl asserted she had nothing to gain, that all was lost, so why not do just one thing more before she died.
>
> She gave a remarkable somnambulistic demonstration of hypnotic phenomena, during the course of which Dr. Erickson made casual, indirect psychotherapeutic suggestions, difficult to recognize as such, and often of a general character such as, "No pain can last forever," "After the rain, the sunshine," etc. The patient obviously began to enjoy herself, and her rapport with Dr. Erickson was excellent.
>
> This was in the latter part of September, 1956. Approximately a week after this occasion, Dr. Erickson received a postcard from the patient stating that "All is well and I have discontinued all therapy." She left the hospital where she worked in 1958, and today, late 1964, is married to an officer of a large organization, is the mother of two fine, healthy children, and she reports that she is exceedingly happy and well-adjusted.
>
> Yet, for months after that one hypnotic session, her fellow employees at the state hospital fearfully expected the worst. During this time, she sent Dr. Erickson an unsigned postcard (the handwriting and postmark indicated that she had sent it), reading, "They can't understand. They still expect the worst. Thanks."

Eight years later, on September 9, 1972, Dr. Erickson sent me the following letter:

> I think you will always remember Janice Pond, that suicidal nurse that I rashly used as a hypnotic subject. Last June Janice called me from Florida and said she was thinking about all the nice things that had happened in her life and she thought that an acknowledgment to me was long overdue. I know this information will please you too.

> You might summarize matters by saying that not only is the therapist rewarded by the privilege of being there and demonstrating hypnotic phenomena, but to serve as a subject is so rewarding that an entire life pattern can be changed.

He enclosed the copy of a letter that Janice had written to him a few days before, detailing the news about her husband and children, their happy family life, and also about her continuing work as a nurse. Now, another eight years later, a total of 24 years since her one-day treatment, the news about her life remains excellent. She remains happily married to this day (1980) and is the proud mother of five children, ages 18, 17, 15, and twins age 13 years.

This very effective treatment is a classic example of Dr. Erickson's genius in allowing minimal clues and suggestions to acquire powerful and effective proportions. I have discussed this remarkable strategy with him a number of times. In the few minutes in the library he had apparently discovered that Ms. Pond was left-handed but had been retrained to use her right hand. It was, therefore, likely that she would experience encouragement to use her left hand as a powerful source of acceptance of the way she was rather than the way she was brought up to be, and also as a potent method to make her feel that she had more powerful resources within her than she had previously been aware of. Acceptance of the use of her left hand clearly had a liberating, refreshing, and strengthening effect upon her, once her learned resource, namely, the use of her right hand, had been temporarily obstructed. In the meantime, she had been able to identify pain with her depression. It was one of those remarkable feats of generalization in which Dr. Erickson was so skillful: to let the patient identify pain with depression and allow the generalization of the relief of pain to affect the much more profound and deeply disturbing depression.

The ability to stimulate patients to generalize from less important problems to the crucial one is one of the most striking manifestations of Dr. Erickson's therapeutic-strategic genius. I can never remember this particular event, the treatment of Ms. Pond's depression, without feeling deeply moved by the effectiveness of the result mediated by a remarkably small chain of decisive steps.

*O. Spurgeon English M.D. (Moderator of the panel):*

Thank you, Dr. Alexander. It is not often that we have the privilege of seeing the person after therapy, and so we are fortunate today to have Mrs. Janice Kropenick here who will make some remarks and discuss Dr. Alexander's paper.

*Mrs. Janice Kropenick:*

I don't like the name, Janice, because the other day I removed the "ice" out of my name and I'm "Jan." It is exciting to sit here and talk of past events and what Dr. Erickson did for me.

What is in the *Teaching Seminar* book (Zeig, 1980) is not true in one sense. If it were written the way that it happened, no one would understand it. Also, the way that Dr. Alexander perceived it was not the way that I perceived it. Consequently, I must take you back very rapidly to September 1956 when Dr. Erickson, sitting across the desk, asked me to sit down. Of course, he observed that I used my left hand a great deal. He asked me if I would volunteer, and I said, "Well, I'm very apprehensive." After all, in front of 60 psychiatrists, I felt I might be on the brink of tears. Besides, I might reveal what I intended to do and that might take away my last bit of courage to end my life. Anyway, I said, "Well, could you just try to hypnotize me?"

He asked me to relax, if I wanted to, and after I relaxed, my hand might touch my face, and then my eyes could close. Then he told me, "And now you fix the pencil in your right hand to a piece of paper, and you are going to write your name as you did as a little girl for the first time and you are going to receive the same gratification." I didn't realize until two days ago how Dr. Erickson immediately put me in a double bind. He put me in a double bind in the sense that I always considered myself a failure. Now he couldn't hypnotize me because I couldn't write with my right hand, but was I the failure or was Dr. Erickson the failure? He didn't hypnotize me, at least I didn't think he did. But did he? Was I going to allow him to be a failure and for me to be successful? I never knew this, but it was already in my unconscious mind, so I had learned it.

I opened my eyes and told Dr. Erickson, "I'm sorry that you can't hypnotize me because I only use my left hand. And, well, Dr. Erickson, you know, as a little girl, this was such a problem. My first-grade teacher, my second-grade teacher, my mother—all said that I *must* use my right hand, and I just cannot use my right hand." He said, "All right." Then he looked over the desk, and he said, "And will you show me how, with only your left hand, that you tie your shoe laces?" I looked down at my foot, and I said, "Oh, my goodness. How do you do it with only the left hand? I have to use my right hand. I never noticed that I used two hands."

Now that really put me in a bind. That was confusing. He said, "Now, if you want to be a volunteer this afternoon, I only have two stipulations. You must hear every word I say, and you must sit where you can see me at all times."

Of course, I didn't realize that if I sat where I could see him, he could also see me at all times, too. I didn't know that, but it was all right. I did recognize that my right arm ached. I even gave up my lunch; I wanted to write with my right hand, and so I spent most of my lunch hour trying to write with my right hand. I could only scribble, and the pain kept getting worse. As Dr. Alexander was talking about it just now, my arm did ache again like that day.

Dr. Erickson gave his lecture, and hypnotized Sally. He had Sally review the movie *Carousel* in full technicolor in three minutes. He regressed her to age two and had her creep along the floor and read the headlines of the Boston paper on the floor so if anyone questioned that they could go to the newspaper and check the headlines of that paper.

In Dr. Erickson's way, he did not ask me to come forward. He just asked Sally if there was somebody there to the right and if there was someone in the back. Then he moved over and, of course, if I saw him, he could see me.

He said, "Is there anyone in the back who thinks they are hypnotized?" He didn't say that I was hypnotized. He said, "If you *think.*" I just stood up and walked down in front of everyone, and a beautiful veil came over everyone so that I could talk directly to Dr. Erickson.

Dr. Erickson said, "And what would you like to do?" I said, "I'd like to write with my right hand." So he asked Dr. Arnot to give me a piece of paper and a pencil, and I wrote my name. I wrote Janice E. Pond with my right hand. He then said, "Which hand would you like to use?" I passed the pencil back and forth in my hands, and there was such an overwhelming pressure. I put my hands to my forehead, and he said, "You know, I'm your friend, not your schoolteacher." I immediately took the pencil in my hand and wrote with my left hand. It was an exciting feeling. I then returned to my seat. I had to hold onto the chair because I wanted to go back to be with Dr. Erickson.

After the lecture was over, I was able to tell Dr. Erickson, "You know, when I put my hand to my forehead, I was about to cry." He said, "Yes, I knew that." Then he said, "You know, in a moment's time, you experienced the same feelings you have had for three or four years, and you lived through that experience. You can live through this." And I did.

The next year I was going to get married to a millionaire. I had moved my clothes into his 26-room house. I had a horse, and he had ordered me a custom-made English riding outfit. We were going to have a civil service wedding at approximately 6:30 o'clock in the evening. By 7:30, I realized he was not going to show. I had to wait until morning and call the director of nursing and say, "You know, I resigned my job, but may I please have my job back because I need it and I love nursing. May I go on duty tomorrow morning and announce to the entire staff in the building that I am not married and I will probably never marry this man. I want the next day off so that they can discuss it freely without me in the building. Then the next day, I promise I will start back to work." It was that easy and that simple because I had lived through it and I could handle it, and I can look at any challenge in life. I may not like it, but I can make it a moment of my lifetime.

*Dr. English:*

You didn't mention Erickson's remark, "After the rain comes the sunshine." Also, you said that you had always felt that you were a failure. Was the failure tied up with the fact that you were not very good or very right if you are left-handed? A left-handed child cannot do a lot of things right and often may do things wrong. I would like you to comment on those two things: Were your feelings of unworthiness linked up with the fact that you were disapproved over being left-handed, and do you remember the words, "No pain lasts forever. After the rain comes the sunshine"?

*Mrs. Kropenick:*

Dr. Erickson, as far as I know, never said those words to me. He only told me that I could reflect back to the feelings that I had and recognize that I could live through three years of this experience.

I read Jeff's book, and it was nice for me to read a mystery story. If Dr. Erickson had had the time, he would have told me exactly what Jeff has in the book. And I know that many of you don't understand it, and it is all right—you will.

Dr. Erickson allowed me to find where the sun was and what it feels like, and I feel that he allowed me to discover it myself. You are absolutely right. If you only do something with your left hand, how can you be right. My mother had described me as a poor child with an inferiority complex, and I was a good girl most of the time, so I complied. Also, when you are growing up and you weigh about 180 pounds and you have glasses on your nose, you just don't fit into any particular picture. How can you see yourself in a picture? So, consequently, I never did.

*Dr. English:*

I want to make a comment because I was privileged to hear Jeff Zeig, Dr. Alexander, and Jan discuss their versions of this particular episode. For me, the individual differences and perceptions are extremely interesting. However, the most important lesson that I have learned is that a little change can start a whole train of events, of reinforcements, that enable the individual to keep growing 26 years and for an infinite number of years. We are all privileged to have a longitudinal study and learn that even a brief interpretation such as "I'm your friend, not your teacher," may really free the individual in the right atmosphere, if you will, to continue growth indefinitely.

## REFERENCES

Alexander, Leo. Clinical experiences with hypnosis in psychiatric therapy. *The American Journal of Clinical Hypnosis,* 1965, *7,* 190-206.

Erickson, M.H. A study of an experimental neurosis hypnotically induced in a case of ejaculatio precox. *British Journal of Medical Psychology,* 1935, *15,* 34-50.

Erickson, M.H. Hypnotic investigation of psychosomatic phenomena. A controlled experimental use of hypnotic regression in the therapy of an acquired food intolerance. *Psychosomatic Medicine,* 1943, *5,* 67-70.

Hadfield, J.A. Functional nerve disease. London: H. Frowde, 1920.

Luria, A.R. *The Nature of Human Conflict.* New York: Liveright, 1932.

Renterghen, A.W. von. Ein Fall von Muskelkrampf (Tic rotatoire). *Ztschr. f. Hypnotismus.* 1897, *4,* 259-263.

Wolberg, L.R. *Medical Hypnosis. Vol. I. The Principles of Hypnotherapy. Vol. II. The practice of hypnotherapy.* New York: Grune & Stratton, 1948.

Zeig, J.K. (Ed.) *A Teaching Seminar with Milton H. Erickson.* New York: Brunner/Mazel, 1980.

Chapter 19

# Hypnotically Induced Dreams: Theory and Practice

*Paul Sacerdote*

Almost 30 years ago, Milton H. Erickson (1952) described dream induction among his strategies for achieving satisfactory deep trance, stating:

> Still another form of this technique [the rehearsal technique] has been found useful in inducing deep trances and in studies of motivation, association of ideas, regression, symbol analysis, repression, and the development of insight. It has proved a most effective therapeutic procedure. This technique is primarily a matter of having the subject repeat over and over a dream, or, less preferably, a fantasy, in constantly differing guises. That is, he repeats a spontaneous dream or an induced dream with a different cast of characters, perhaps in a different setting, but with the same meaning. After the second dreaming the same instructions are given again, and this continues until the purposes to be served are accomplished.

Erickson warned that the therapist should use dreams of a pleasant character. If this were not possible, he should implant an artificial complex to limit the range of unpleasant emotions, and this methodology should be discontinued if it appears to lead to a situation beyond the hypnotist's competence.

I am trying to reconstruct, to the best of my recollection, my thinking processes in the late 1950s, at a time when I was already deeply involved with the theory and practice of hypnotherapy. I began experimenting with Erickson's approach to the use of spontaneous and induced dreams. At the beginning, I probably adopted this type of rehearsal technique for the primary purpose of having more of my patients reach somnambulistic levels of trance. I soon recognized that the therapeutic value of such an approach went well beyond the deepening of the trance. Many patients with low hypnotic talent or extreme resistance to deepening became amenable to hypnotherapy after I had suggested that they may have a succession of dreams in the course of one or more nights. In fact, many patients started to recollect more and more of their dreams and to understand them as the symbolic expression of important conflicts and other problems. Often, the successive dreams comprised a testing of possible solutions.

Almost every patient, including the ones who had only reached an hypnoidal state or simply achieved a state of concentrated attention, was capable of responding to my suggestions for useful dream activity. The response often involved subjects' gradually learning to remember entire dreams or parts of them, when they had previously stated, "I never dream," or "I seldom dream," or "I never remember any of my dreams."

Eventually, I found myself tying together Erickson's experiences, Freud's (1933) interpretation of dreams, and Jung's dream theories with clinical utilization and with the (then new) discoveries of Dement (1960) and Kleitman on the relation between eye movements, body motility, and dream activity (1957a, 1957b).

From the very beginning, I was pleasantly surprised with the profusion of nocturnal dreams produced even by those subjects who had been unable to "dream" during several hypnotic trances. Consequently, I began to utilize induced dreams through a methodology significantly different from orthodox analysis. Essentially, while basically agreeing with Freud's postulate that, "Dreams are the royal road to the unconscious," I became impressed with the obvious fact that it was not necessary to have the patient laboriously tying associations to a word, or a statement, or an image, or a certain realistic or symbolic activity in his dreams. Each new dream or part of a dream represented a free association to general meanings or to elements of a previous dream.

In some cases there was progress from more abstract or symbolic dream imagery to more realistic presentation, often with deeper insight. Sometimes therapeutic solutions were tested, and became evident. In other cases, the succession of dreams tenuously or strongly associated with each other represented but a small step in the progress of therapy.

I also realized that the term "hypnotic dream" was used rather loosely by a number of experimenters and clinicians. It was necessary, at the very least for clarity of description, to give an operational definition of "hypnotic dreams." For many clinicians, experimenters and theoreticians, any kind of imagined or visualized scene or activity in the course of induced hypnosis or self-hypnosis is called dreaming (e.g., dreaming is one of the items in the Stanford Profile Scales of hypnotic susceptibility (Weitzenhoffer & Hilgard, 1967).

For the purpose of definition, dreams during or under hypnosis are hallucinated visual and multisensory experiences which occur *after sleep-suggestions* given during hetero-hypnosis *have been executed* and within the period of suggested sleep.

I am now ready to briefly bring together some of the facts and experiences, as well as some of the assumptions, which constitute the basis for my methods of utilizing induced dreams. Reviewing the thousands of studies resulting from the monitoring of sleep and dream states which have been published in the last 20 or more years, I have concluded that "natural dreaming" appears to be a necessary physiological activity which occupies a significant part of our sleeping hours. In spite of some recent papers which attempt to deny any intellectual or psychological meaning to our dreaming, I feel that "natural dreaming" also represents a useful and probably indispensable psychological entity.

My experience forces me to accept the hypothesis that oneric activity serves important intellectual and psychodynamic functions. This is true even for the numerous individuals who usually do not remember dreaming, or who deny that they ever dream. Freud himself, while postulating that "dreams are the protectors of sleep," also implied that they represent a particular attempt by individuals to deal with problems, to communicate with themselves and (in analysis) with the therapist. I also believe that dreams provide us opportunities for dealing, at different levels of awareness, with problems and conflicts which have not been resolved while awake, for lack of time, patience, insight, or ego strength. Viewed within this frame of reference, one of the functions of sleep, and in particular of stage I sleep, is to provide the proper physiological state for dreamwork. I assume, therefore, that individuals who deny dreaming may either have an overwhelming need to repress insights achieved during dreaming or their dreamwork is so directly effective there is little need for communication of the results from the dreaming state to the awake state. I firmly believe that parts of those dreams which are totally or partially remembered represent communication, often in symbolic form, from the dreaming ego states to awake ego states. When not recollected, they can be conceived as internalized communications.

Dreams provide specific communication from patient to therapist during psychoanalytic or hypnoanalytic therapy. The purpose of analytical interpretation of dreams is to clarify for the patient those observations, discoveries, and conclusions that he has been struggling to achieve during dreaming, but which he does not yet clearly understand or accept in his awake state.

Orthodox analytical therapy purports to utilize "natural dreams." In reality, these "natural dreams" are "induced dreams," since the patient is subconsciously and consciously aware that the analyst expects and needs meaningful dreams for productive therapy. Positive transference and implied suggestion compel the patient to bring to his therapist the gift of a daily dream.

Let us accept the reality that dreams reported during analytical therapy are essentially induced dreams. It then becomes very natural to use hypnosis as a powerful tool for suggesting dreams, their possible contents, and desirable goals. It is interesting that a number of patients from the Caribbean Islands, whom I met in the outpatient clinic of a major hospital, routinely selected and suggested to themselves before bedtime the dreams they would have during the night.

A large proportion of patients referred to me have been able to produce successions of nocturnal dreams by post-hypnotic suggestion. Patients capable of deep hypnosis have little difficulty in producing successive dreams during hetero-hypnosis and even during self-hypnosis.

To avoid disturbing the doctor-patient relationship, I have avoided conducting dream-induction hypnotherapy with patients electronically connected to monitoring equipment. Therefore, I cannot unequivocally state that periods of apparently natural sleep and natural dreaming within the hypnotherapeutic hour are occurring within stage I sleep. The resulting dreams, however, are psychodynamically equivalent to nocturnal dreams.

Generally, after inducing at least a light trance, I use the following verbalization for inducing dreams in a hypnotherapeutic setting: "We all dream repeatedly for periods of 15 or 20 minutes during our nightly sleep. The dreams are the mind's creation. It is *your* mind that goes to work before and during the various stages of your sleep. In preparing, creating, and experiencing dreams you are, in reality, the writer who writes a story. In addition, you are the playwright who creates a drama, or comedy, or a musical out of the story, and the director who selects the scenery, backdrops and the props, then assigns the parts and supervises the actors. You act in one or more parts in the play, while participating at the same time as audience, and even as theater critic whose job is to understand and interpret the play's purpose and meaning, while evaluating the actors' performances. In such a capacity you may discover significant trends and ideas that, as author, you may have failed to recognize."

The above verbalization is generally the same, whether I prepare the patient for dreaming in my office or during post-hypnotically suggested dreaming at home. I inform the patient that the dream (show) that he will have could be the beginning of a series of dreams and that, as the series progresses, he will understand it better and discover new meanings. To avoid the onset of unnecessary and countertherapeutic defenses, I present the idea that dreams are pleasant, relaxing, interesting and instructive. I prepare the patient for the adoption, in his dreams, of symbols and stories of innocuous appearance. I also permit him to forget part or all of his dream experiences if they are too disturbing for his awake ego to handle, or if there is insufficient time during the session for working through of the material. Permission is also given or implied for withholding from me as much of his dream as may be needed consciously or subconsciously. The patient is free to deny that he was in hypnosis, or that he was asleep, or that he was dreaming.

Hypnotically elicited dreams and post-hypnotically suggested nocturnal dreams can at times permit age regressions (see also Fromm, 1965), which the patient had been unable to experience during hypnosis. Series of successive dreams in the course of one session or one night, or in successive sessions or nights, may begin with an apparently insignificant dream or with one that appears so completely nonsensical that the patient and I can at best recognize in it memory traces of some experience of the previous day. As the second suggested dream develops, one or more of the themes that were not previously recognizable in the first dream make an appearance. By the third or fourth dream, actions, images, metaphors and symbols direct our attention to problems or conflicts and to tentative solutions.

Obviously, with those patients who learn to dream during hypnosis there is opportunity for constant interaction between myself and the patient. Schematically, a one-hour session for induced dreaming during hetero-hypnosis is as follows:

1) Induction and deepening, which may require only a few minutes with a patient who is capable of deep trances.
2) During trance I suggest: "Shortly after I stop talking to you, you will awake comfortably and completely. You may feel like changing your position, maybe you will stretch and yawn; you will rub your eyes slightly, because they will feel quite heavy and drowsy; you will become progressively more drowsy and begin to sleep in a very deep

and easy natural sleep, while your head rests on the back of the chair."

3) Upon opening his eyes as suggested, the patient will spontaneously, or upon questioning, agree that he had a nice relaxing rest. Then, in all probability, he will adjust his position, stretch, yawn, rub his eyes and possibly remark that he feels quite drowsy. Before he realizes what is happening, he falls asleep.
4) At this point I suggest that, even while sleeping, he will continue to hear the following instructions: "Would it not be a very good idea to take advantage of this state of sleep and have an interesting dream, maybe even a strange one, with a very pleasant conclusion? Even better, the dream could deal with some of your problems, maybe even test some of the possible solutions." I then instruct him to wake up rested and relaxed as soon as his dream is finished. I ask him to clearly remember the dream and be ready to report it to me, unless part or all of the dream should not happen to be my business.

   During the period of dreaming, I can detect rapid eye movements (REMs) under the closed eyelids, while noticing changes in the pattern of respiration. Often seen are abortive motions in the fingers and the hands. As soon as I notice that the patient is about to wake up, I add the instruction that, as soon as he has finished reporting the dream, he will again feel very drowsy and his eyes will close. He will then begin to sleep again and, after a short while, to dream again about something or somebody connected with the dream just finished.
5) The responsive patient wakes up rather promptly at the end of his dream and spontaneously or upon questioning relates the dream he has just had. Occasionally, a patient will state that he did not have a dream, that he had only been thinking or visualizing. If this is his first experience with induced dreams, he may apologize about having fallen asleep again. At the same time he will already be stretching, yawning, changing positions, and falling asleep again in response to the last suggestion.
6) He will usually carry out most of the instructions received at the end of the previous dream period and again begin to show objective evidence of dreaming. Depending upon the contents of the dream, its manifest and latent meaning, and its possible connections with previous information that has surfaced during therapy, I may intervene with some comments. Before reawakening, post-hypnotic suggestions about falling asleep again and new dreaming can be given once more, if time permits.

Generally the alternating periods of sleeping, dreaming, and awakening have the effect of deepening the trance. At the same time, the dreams gradually change in character, at times becoming more realistic, at other times assuming all the characteristics of a naturally occurring dream, including symbolization, displacement, metaphors, puns, and so forth. By this time the patient may start to recognize the meanings of his dreams.

At the end of the third or fourth dream, the patient can be instructed to fall asleep, to dream and to *describe the dream while it is occurring,* with additional suggestions for remembering, understanding, and constructively utilizing parts or all of the dreams.

The above describes the basic conduct of a session with responsive subjects. Changes will be made according to the interactions between therapist and patient. For those subjects not yet able or permanently incapable of dreaming during hypnosis, I simply mention during trance that it is very natural, during the night or nights following therapeutic hypnosis, to have and recollect one or more dreams related to important personal problems and to the hypnotic experiences and expectations. I then instruct such patients to report any dreams at the time of the next visit.

In the second session, the patient is invited to talk about recent nocturnal dreams, to comment about them, and then, after hypnosis has been reestablished, to redream details of nocturnal dreams that have been forgotten. Encouraged to recognize meanings which he had missed, he may redream or refantasize his nocturnal dreams in different guises, different settings, and/or with different actors. Conflicts, motives, and concerns usually become more easily recognizable. A good part of this new information is continuously fed back to the patient while in hypnosis then discussed again when he is awake.

Induced dreams are for some patients the most important diagnostic and therapeutic tool. For others they are but a part in the overall therapy. Generally, I have found it useful to combine the diagnostic and therapeutic possibilities of induced dreams with other projective hypnoanalytical techniques like automatic writing (real and hallucinated), hypnography and hypnoplasty, or age regression and age progression (Sacerdote, 1969). I have often found both induced and spontaneous dreams (occurring at home during natural sleep or in the office during or following hypnosis) to be valuable diagnostic tools. Profound changes are often "forecast" in a series of dreams weeks or months before the changes become recognizable to therapist and patient. The therapist may find it is countertherapeutic to interpret such dreams to the patient. It may be wise not to use the "information" immediately, allowing the patient's subconscious to gradually convey the understanding to his conscious, rational mind.

## CLINICAL CASES

### *Case One*

The following is a sample of successive dreams by a 40-year-old woman at the beginning of her pregnancy. The only previous pregnancy, in her late teens before her first marriage, had been terminated by abortion. In this second marriage she had a love-hate relationship with her husband, who suffered from premature ejaculation, and who at times repelled her with vulgar language and behavior. She declared herself to be very happy to be pregnant. She was very eager to have her first and probably only child, but she was not quite sure she was happy that her husband was the father. Still, she had become pregnant by artificial insemination with her husband's sperm. She recently severed a relationship with a previous lover, and hoped that the birth of the child would improve her marriage. She was also very fearful that this pregnancy so late in life might result in the birth of a defective child.

During previous visits she repeatedly talked about her unhappy childhood due to the fact that her mother was in and out of psychiatric hospitals. Her mother had died at the age of 41 and she suggested several times that the same thing could happen to her at a time when her expected child would be only one year old. She also mentioned, as an example of her "craziness," a long-lasting episode of phobic behavior which started when somebody stared at her while she was eating. She had been unable to lift a spoon to her mouth for many months after that. During frequent periods of stress, she also developed acute episodes of colitis and was petrified by the presence of stools covered with bloody mucus.

In my office, one day after her first visit to a highly recommended obstetrician, she gave her impression of the doctor as "a very cold fish." The following is the first dream that she had in my office after her first OB visit. "I am holding this bottle that *must be prepared* for its first use. I've gone from building to building and no one seems to want to bother. I am bewildered: This is a service that all superintendents and concierges are happy to perform." The dream then continued with an apparently different set of characters and places: "I have just spread some

"Réplique" (perfume or cologne) on my arms. This is a stuff that they hate in Paris, but love here. There are puddles of it on my arms and I start to smear and spread this yellow, oily, brown stuff all over my arms. Then I see my friend E. Apparently she loves Réplique and I have brought her a huge bottle to thank her for taking care of my dog. I spray some Réplique on her."

Another dream developed during sleep on the following night in partial response to a suggestion to continue to have other dreams: "I am playing in a sandbox with my friend. He is making designs using sand and paint and this design is supposed to look like fancy hors d'oeuvres. I pick up one which looks like a centipede. I feel compelled to draw a horizon line using sand and paint. I make many concentric, overlapping circles, above and below the horizon line, with different colors accentuating each circle."

During hypnosis she realized that the bottle which must be prepared for its first use represented her womb, and that all the men that do not seem to want to bother represented her previous husband, present husband and various boyfriends, by whom she feels she has been rejected. At the same time, she also realized that the bottle in the same dream is a baby bottle. The Réplique she had in reality bought during a recent trip to Paris. In the dream it represented the blood-smeared mucus secondary to her colitis. While she was unable to understand the meaning of the centipede, she realized that the horizon line she was compelled to draw represented a need to set limits and controls upon her behavior and her reactions. She also saw the connection between the dream of the Réplique perfume smeared over her arms and the tubes of paint which are squeezed over the sand to make the overlapping circles.

She realized that the colors in the dream had important significance, but she was unable or unwilling to explain further. She mentioned, however, that she knew that concentric circles which appeared in the dream represented vaginas. She then went on to communicate her concern about the probability that her pregnancy would be terminated by Caesarean section. In further associations she talked about a cousin whose recent pregnancy ended with a stillbirth.

In further sessions, as we continued to use induced dreams to help her work through contradictory feelings and motivations, she learned to cope with her anxiety about the possibility of giving birth to a defective child and the fear of dying either during delivery or at the same age as her mother, leaving a helpless little orphan behind.

*Case Two*

The second case concerns Dr. F.R. who was referred to me after she finally decided she needed psychotherapy to free herself from recurrent problems of anxiety. She recognized that she was becoming progressively more dependent upon a Valium or a cocktail to escape tension or anxiety. Also, for many years, since college, she had used Dexamil for several successive days when exposed to stress or the expectation of stress at home or at work. Unsuccessful psychotherapy a few years earlier had been exclusively behaviorally oriented and supportive, with no attempt to explore and analyze the roots of her anxiety.

During childhood and adolescence, as well as during her years in college, she had been constantly exposed to the changeable moods of a mother who was the victim of a manic-depressive psychosis. The patient had found compensation in a brilliant scholastic career, which had culminated with a fellowship at an ivy-league university. When her mother had prevented her from accepting it, she had suffered a severe reactive depression.

Dr. F.R. and her husband had continuous problems with their daughter. Dr. F.R. feared she might be responsible for recreating the mother-daughter conflict from which she had suffered. In spite of these emotional difficulties, Dr. F.R. had achieved and maintained an outstanding position in a prestigious research institution.

At the time of her second visit we discussed her feelings about the possibility of utilizing hypnotherapy. She expressed considerable skepticism, as well as doubts about the probability of her experiencing hypnotic phenomena. She agreed, however, to test her responsivity with the conducted reversed right hand levitation methodology. A rapid and smooth trance developed, during which I induced a localized vaso-dilatation or constriction of the tips of her fingers. This experience with control of her autonomic nervous system prepared her to be open-minded about my suggestion that she may be able to regulate the production of her own amphetamine-like substances, without the occurrence of any side-effects. This would enable her to function effectively despite work and family stress, while experiencing the same joyful relaxation she habitually achieved when on vacation. This would permit her to discover different feelings and understandings in relation to her daughter, while becoming pleased about her talent. She could also develop a sense of humor in dealing with her daughter.

Upon emerging from this first trance experience, she expressed surprise and pleasure about her response. As it is my habit, I terminated the trance with the suggestion that she would come out of hypnosis calm and pleased with herself, and remain awake and alert for the rest of the day and evening until safely in bed for the night and ready for a good night's sleep with pleasant dreams. Some of the dreams would probably deal with various issues which we had discussed, including which kind of therapy she would require, whether goal-oriented short therapy or extended analysis.

During the trance, I had also casually remarked that for too long she may have saddled herself with problems and conflicts which were no longer meaningful or important in her present situation.

At the next visit she brought the remnants of two dreams from the first night following the first hypnotic experience. In the first dream she was at a train station where she had to change trains. She was undecided between boarding a slow train or the express train, and asked the conductor to advise her about which one was the best for her. In the second dream, which seemed to be a continuation of the first one, she was traveling some place and felt very light, suddenly realizing that she "had left the very heavy suitcase on the other side of the mountain." The meaning of the dreams became clear to her during the subsequent trance. She also realized how efficiently and pleasantly she had started to function without Dexamil, and with what equanimity she was looking ahead to the expected homecoming of her daughter.

## REFERENCES


Dement, W. The effect of dream deprivation. *Science,* 131, 1705-1707, 1960.

Dement, W. & Kleitman, N. The relation of eye movements during sleep to dream activity. *J. Exper. Psychol.,* 53, 339-346, 1957a.

Dement, W. & Kleitman, N. Cyclic variations in EEG during sleep and their relation to eye movements, body motility, and dreaming. *Electroenceph. Clin. Neurophysiol.,* 9, 673-690, 1957b.

Erickson, M.H. Deep hypnosis and its induction. In: L.M. LeCron (Ed.) *Experimental Hypnosis.* New York: Macmillan, 1952, pp. 70-114.

Freud, S. *Neue Folge der Vorlesungen zur Einfuhrung in die Psychoanalyse.* Wien: Internationaler Psychoanalytischer Verlag, 1933, pp. 9-44.

Fromm, E. Spontaneous age-regression in a nocturnal dream. *Int. J. Clin. Exp. Hypnosis,* 13, 119-131, 1965.

Jung, C.G. *Memories, Dreams, Reflections.* New York: Vintage Books, 1965.

Sacerdote, P. Some projective techniques in hypnotherapy: Induction of dreams, and real, versus hallucinated sensory hypnoplasty. *Amer. J. Clin. Hypnosis,* 11, 253-264, 1969.

Weitzenhoffer, A.M. & Hilgard, E.R. *Stanford Hypnotic Susceptibility Scale. Form C.* Palo Alto, Ca: Consulting Psychologists Press, 1967.

Chapter 20

# Shifting Therapeutic Paradigms: A Case Report of Adolescent Primary Enuresis

*David L. Calof*

## INTRODUCTION

The central premise of this paper is that it is useful for therapists to be able to shift conceptual models of problem maintenance and resolution, particularly for those cases which present as chronic or which are at impasse. Before elaborating more fully on this theme and its relevance to the particular case to be reported, I will offer an exemplary anecdote in the hope that it will begin to generate in the reader a personal, intuitive understanding of the theme.

Some weeks prior to the preparation of this paper, I was working at home with a friend who was helping me prepare another manuscript. Late into the evening, my friend, Michelle, discovered and called to my attention that she had run out of typewriter ribbons. This was critical since the chapter she was typing was due to be mailed the next day.

Responding to this crisis situation, both Michelle and I at once set our minds to the resolution of the problem as we understood it—namely, *to find a replacement ribbon for the typewriter in my study*, at that late hour. Our first move within the paradigm we had established was to phone a local variety store which we knew stayed open late each night. Though open, we learned that the store could not supply the specific type of ribbon we required.

Next, I recalled that I had picked up my office typewriter from the repair shop the previous day and that it was still in my car because I had forgotten to drop it off at my office. Toward the end of *finding a replacement ribbon*, I reasoned, and Michelle agreed, that we could check the ribbon in the machine in the car to ascertain if it was compatible with the typewriter in the study and then use it until we could obtain a replacement ribbon during business hours the next day.

We each painstakingly made visual estimates of the size and shape of the ribbon in the machine in the study. Armed with this frame of reference, we trouped down to the cold, rainy parking lot to compare our mental estimates with the dimensions of the ribbon in the typewriter sitting on the back seat of my car. Our hopes were dashed, however, when we discovered that the typewriter in the car used a ribbon configuration *which was not compatible with the typewriter in the study.*

We rushed back to the house still frantic, albeit somewhat relieved to have exhausted yet another possible move (within our paradigm) so that we might get on to other problem-solving moves. Our next move was to examine the typewriter in the study even more closely than before. We were mindful that useful clues might have been overlooked in our frantic zeal. We wished not to let any possibility escape us in *this matter of locating a replacement ribbon.* As a result of our closer scrutiny, we discovered a small tag on the machine (previously regarded as "meaningless" data) which gave the name and address of the firm from which we had rented the typewriter. The tag advertised a full line of typing accessories. Although it was 9:30 P.M. on a Monday night, our desire to exhaust every "conceivable" possibility was ardent. We decided to call the shop.

I dialed and much to my surprise a male voice promptly answered the phone with a drunken "Hello!" The sounds of a party were evident in the background. I inquired if I had reached the typewriter shop. The man responded barely intelligibly, "Well, it was until 6:00 P.M. We're closed, but we're having a helluva party now!" I explained my dilemma to the man and finally convinced him to sell me the needed supplies. He stipulated, however, that I would have to be at the shop within ten minutes since he was preparing to leave and wasn't inclined to wait for me.

Now elated, Michelle and I ran to my car and raced off to the typewriter shop making the usual 15-20 minute drive very nearly within the allotted ten. (Ironically, during one rather severely executed turn, I felt a twinge of caution out of some vague recollection that I had placed something fragile in the back seat earlier that day.) After purchasing the ribbons, Michelle and I made our way slowly back to my house feeling triumphant that our quick thinking had saved the day.

Only after returning to my house and reinitiating work did both Michelle and I independently realize that we had overlooked the "obvious" option of using the office typewriter which still sat coldly in the back seat of my car, complete with its own fresh ribbon.

This vignette exemplifies a phenomenon which occurs frequently in daily living. The eyeglass wearer who "loses" his spectacles on his head, and the structure of many so-called "brain teasers" are each commonplace examples of the same phenomenon. In other words, the conceptual model or paradigm adopted to solve a particular problem will dictate what shall be construed as meaningful data, sometimes to the exclusion of both valid data and problem-solving strategies.

In order to understand this principle as it applies to the field of psychotherapeutic change, it will be helpful to describe the therapeutic interventions in terms of four separate (yet overlapping and frequently simultaneous) components:

First, the therapist must select a paradigm and formulate a model of problem formation and resolution. Many divergent points of view exist in the field. They range from the postulate that problems develop and are maintained from the "karmic effects" of some remote "past life" to the position which argues that problems form and are maintained solely through their selective reinforcement. The reader is undoubtedly aware of the plethora of contradictory models which are currently proffered as "truth."*

Second, from within the adopted model of problem maintenance and resolution the therapist must develop a theory or hypothesis that related the model to the particular patient problem to be addressed. For example, let us say that the adopted model suggests that human problems are originated and persist as a result of the patterns of interaction within

---

*Adherents each model suggest that their model is the ultimate "truthful" view. Such beliefs are similar to those which Newtonian physicists made when they moved from a metaphorical view of the universe as a "great machine" to a stance which suggested that the universe *is* a great machine. Much of the work of quantum physics over the last 50 years has been to reinstitute the notion that our views of the universe are metaphoric rather than absolute. The difficulty with attempting to prove the veracity of a model is that adequate criteria cannot be adduced. The criteria must either be a part of the "language game" that defines the model itself or they must occur in a model which subsumes the model being studied. In the former case, nothing is proved except the logical consistency of the model to itself. In the latter case, the investigator will still be faced with the inherent limitation of the former case but in ever-widening (infinite) spheres of discourse.

Lastly, while investigating the nature of what it means to be human is an interesting and, I believe, important task, it is not the task of the therapist whose job it is to help people change. Consequently, the therapist who has available alternative paradigms will have more options for this job. Similarly, when physicists decided that the question of whether light was "truthfully" a particle or wave phenomenon was formally undecidable, they freed themselves to construe light as waves for the purposes of certain experiments or tasks and as particles for others, thereby increasing their options.

a system of people. As an example, in a case of adolescent anorexia nervosa, the therapist might adopt a hypothesis which states that anorexia is the way in which spouse conflicts become diffused or detoured through the anorectic child. This would suggest that the job of the therapist in this example would be to intervene in this triangulation and remove the child from her functional position in the spouse subsystem of the family.

Third, the therapist must (be able to) select from a variety of techniques, e.g., psychosocial, medical, etc., those appropriate to carry out the indicated intervention.

Fourth, the therapist must be able to select from a variety of communicative behaviors those appropriate to implement the chosen technique(s).

The job of the therapist is to select a model which is most *useful,* i.e., one which will lead to a definable (and testable) hypothesis of problem formation and resolution that will, in turn, generate clear options for effective intervention. The utility of the model for explaining etiology is of lesser import. It does not matter, for example, whether manic-depressive "disease" is, "in truth," a chemical imbalance or a consequence of certain interactive patterns of intrapsychic processes and interpersonal transactions. What matters from the standpoint of the treatment provider is whether the model and hypothesis chosen will facilitate or hamper effective therapeutic change.*

The therapist who recalcitrantly suggests that each case of manic depression can only properly be understood in psychosocial terms and therefore will never prescribe lithium for his therapeutic failures commits the same error as the therapist who must treat every chronic pain patient within the medical model while ignoring such factors as "secondary gain." Unfortunately, much of the current training in psychotherapy stresses technique and etiology without also supplying complementary tools of critical thought. As a result, a typical move which is made at therapeutic impasse is to hold to one's assumptions dearly and then adjust only one's technical or implementation strategies.** While this move can, at times, lead to a resolution of the impasse, it can also result in the therapist proverbially "doing more of the same only longer and louder" with an apparent lack of regard for undesirable outcomes.

---

*It may be apparent to the reader that the difficulties of determining a useful change paradigm will also be present in constructing criteria of what constitutes an "effective" intervention.

**The Chinese character for physics is Wu Li, which also has several alternate meanings, including "nonsense," "enlightenment," and "I clutch my ideas."

In my personal anecdote, the reader will recall how I persisted in my assumption that my task was *to find a replacement typewriter ribbon* and how I consequently made various tactical moves while clutching this assumption. Fortunately, after a number of moves which can retrospectively be construed as "the same only longer and louder," I was able to solve my problem. The reader can also appreciate that I might have exhausted all the available moves within my initial formulation and not have reached resolution because of my unwillingness to shift my task to that of *finding a replacement typewriter.*

When therapists have reasonably exhausted the available tactical moves suggested by a paradigm, they have a number of choices: 1) They can blame the client; 2) they can declare the client to be unable to change; 3) they can persist doing the same thing only longer and louder without regard to outcomes; or 4) they can reexamine their assumptions and shift paradigms.

In the case report which follows, the reader may glean that I opted for each of the above choices at various times. Only by embracing the fourth option, however, was I finally able to bring about lasting therapeutic change in my patient.

## CASE REPORT

I received a phone call from a woman who was seeking hypnotherapy for her 12-year-old son. Mrs. Smith explained that Billy had suffered from nocturnal enuresis continually since infancy in spite of a multitude of corrective measures she and her husband had employed over the years. Since Billy was to enter junior high school in three months, both he and his parents had grown increasingly anxious and frustrated about his problem since progressively it had eroded his confidence. It had even begun to interfere with what had been an above-average achievement record in school. On the advice of their family physician, Mr. and Mrs. Smith had decided to seek hypnotherapy for their son since, in Mrs. Smith's words, "We've tried everything else and nothing seems to have worked."

I told Mrs. Smith that hypnotherapy often worked in cases like Billy's where other "conventional means" had proven futile. I then asked her if she had discussed with Billy the prospects of seeing a hypnotherapist. She replied that both she and her husband had discussed this with Billy and that he had seemed "very eager to try it." She further related that Billy viewed hypnosis as "a kind of magic" that would be far more powerful than any of the measures previously applied. As an afterthought, Mrs. Smith volunteered that Billy had proudly announced his intentions to be hypnotized to his two younger sisters (ages eight and six). An appointment was scheduled for two weeks. *Mrs. Smith asked if I wished for the whole family to come to the first session. I replied that I could think of no reason why it would be necessary to see the whole family.*

In retrospect, I am aware that at this point in my interaction with the Smith family I had already unconsciously selected a model of problem maintenance by which to understand Billy's bed-wetting. I initially viewed the problem as an intrapsychic phenomenon. I assumed that the problem was being maintained by a set of unconscious cognitive structures (e.g., self-statements, imagery, expectations, associations, etc.) which were being triggered by certain internal and/or external events (e.g., bladder pressure sensations, sleep, cognitions, etc.).

The reader will recognize this model to be the assumptive basis which underlies most behaviorally-oriented hypnotherapeutic approaches to adolescent enuresis. The usual role of the treatment provider within this paradigm has been to help the child modify his cognitions and information-processing strategies regarding the problematic behavior. For example, the child might typically be instructed in a trance, "Now, you will begin to imagine yourself having more and more dry beds each week. At night, just as you go to sleep, you will imagine yourself waking up in a dry bed feeling very pleased. When you have to pee during the day time, you know exactly what feelings and thoughts remind you to go the bathroom. From now on, if you get any of these same thoughts or feelings when you are asleep at night, a part of your mind will automatically awaken you and you will go to the bathroom and pee. As soon as your head touches your pillow again, you'll instantly fall fast asleep again." The child may also be instructed both to avoid excess fluids immediately before retiring and to sleep somewhat less deeply until the new cognitive and behavioral patterns are automatic. These instructions, when coupled with directed, ideosensory experiences and tempered with the creation of an expectancy for slow, steady progress, often constitute the total intervention necessary for a complete resolution of adolescent, primary enuresis over a course of several weeks. These approaches have been described by workers such as Crasilneck and Hall (1975), Hartland (1971), Cheek and Le Cron (1968), Erickson, Hershman, and Secter (1961), Wolberg (1948), and Meares (1960).

This, then, was the intervention (*based on the paradigm which I assumed*) I expected to use with Billy at his first session.

Because of my unconscious selection of this specific paradigm, I disregarded certain "obviously" insignificant data. Retrospectively, four particular pieces of information supplied by Mrs. Smith were ignored: 1) *Mr. and Mrs. Smith's growing concern;* 2) *Billy's announcing to his sisters his plans to seek hypnotherapy for his problem;* 3) *the sheer multitude of attempted remedies;* and 4) *Mrs. Smith's volunteering for the whole family to come to the initial interview. From my perspective as a hypnotherapist,* these data simply were dismissed as *conscious attempts to solve an unconscious problem.*

Mrs. Smith accompanied Billy to the first interview. I initially encountered them laughing and joking in my waiting room, and invited them both into my office. After introductions and some light discussion of the weather and several items of memorabilia in my office, I asked Billy if he knew why he had been brought to see me. He replied that *he and his parents were quite concerned about his constant bed-wetting* and now hoped that hypnosis could solve it *in spite of their many, unsuccessful remedies in the past.* With a mind toward developing an even greater motivation and desire for hypnotherapy in Billy, I asked him to recount each of the unsuccessful measures. With periodic correction and coaching from his mother, Billy recounted the following list of tactics: 1) verbal and physical punishment and ridicule; 2) positive and negative behavioral consequences (e.g., granting and suspension of privileges); 3) the use of various aids and appliances such as rubber sheets and pants, and moisture-activated bed alarms; 4) change of sleeping locations; 5) modification of sleeping hours; and 6) "forced" elimination prior to retiring.

As Billy and his mother recounted these various measures, I construed each to be an example of an unsuccessful, conscious mind approach to problem resolution, further substantiating my hypothesis that Billy's unconscious cognitive structures needed to be modified through hypnotic technique. Again, *neither the sheer magnitude of the Smith family's attempts to seek a solution over nearly eight years of effort nor the exactingly serious and precise nature of Billy and his mother's account were considered significant.*

I then interviewed Billy extensively regarding his understandings of hypnosis and how it might potentially help him. His beliefs about hypnosis and hypnotherapy largely coincided with my planned strategy. Billy's mother apparently had briefed him quite extensively after her phone conversation with me in which I had outlined the general strategy I expected to use. *Mrs. Smith's frequent corrective intercessions to Billy's account during this phase of the interview were also considered insignificant.*

With Billy's consent, I then dismissed his mother from the room. Using a direct eye catalepsy approach, I was able to rapidly induce a deep trance in the boy. Once this was obtained, I gave him the "standard" suggestions as described above. After each suggestion, I asked for and obtained Billy's verbal agreement that he understood the suggestion and intended to follow it. I then awakened him. Upon awakening he manifested a total, spontaneous amnesia for all of his trance activities and could not account for the 20 minutes he had been in trance. He seemed not at all perplexed by this and asked if we were done for the day. I replied that we were and pointed out how interesting it was that he could lose so much time unexpectedly and how it would be "just as easy to lose some other things just as surprisingly." With that, I walked him to the waiting room to rejoin his mother. Upon seeing us, Mrs. Smith smiled broadly and said, "Well, Billy? Did you enjoy it? Did it work?" Billy was nonplussed by this remark and began to exhibit trance behavior. Responding to this, I quickly directed the conversation back to a pretrance subject in order not to disrupt Billy's amnesia. I then said, "Mrs. Smith, Billy's worked hard. I think you should let him think some things over for himself until he's had a chance to dream a pleasant dream tonight." Mrs. Smith replied, "Sure. He's a good boy and we're all expecting great things." Subsequently, an appointment was made for two weeks to "find out how well Billy is progressing" and the pair was dismissed. *Neither Mrs. Smith's remarks to me or her son were construed by me as particularly noteworthy.*

*Billy was accompanied by both his parents to his next appointment.* I met the trio in the waiting room and was introduced to Mr. Smith by Mrs. Smith. After shaking hands with me, Mr. Smith asked if he and his wife could speak with me briefly in private before I saw Billy. I consented to this.

Once in my office, the couple related that Billy had improved significantly for nearly one week following the first appointment but that the progress had substantially eroded in the second week. In describing Billy's behavior of the second week, Mr. and Mrs. Smith frequently contradicted each other's renditions and at one point engaged in a rather heated exchange. *Based upon my previously adopted frame of reference regarding Billy's problem, I considered the relative decline in Billy's progress as significant, and I was virtually oblivious to the manner in which his parents had communicated this information.*

Convinced I needed to "do the same thing only longer and louder" with Billy, I interpreted Billy's behavior to his parents as "normal and even somewhat expected." I explained that progress was generally labile at first and that with additional time and reinforcement, it usually stabilized. My explanation reassured Billy's parents and they both consented to withhold judgement about the effectiveness of the hypnotherapy for two more weeks following a "booster" which I would give Billy that day.

My hypnotic work with Billy that day was virtually identical to that which I had done with him in the first session. However, there were two exceptions. At the end of the suggestive phase, I questioned Billy in trance as to whether he knew of any objections he or any members of his family had to his getting over his problem. I also inquired about his attitudes regarding his progress over the previous two-week interval. Billy could think of neither a personal nor family objection to his improvement and expressed the belief that he would improve *"if we all just keep trying real hard."* Billy's remarks were construed by me as further evidence that my conceptual map of the case was correct and only required more time to come to fruition. Billy was then awakened, again manifesting a total, spontaneous amnesia.

Billy and I then joined his parents in the waiting room who apparently were still debating over their respective interpretations of Billy's problematic behavior during the previous two weeks. I made an appointment to see Billy in three weeks, explaining to his parents that "due to the labile nature of change of this sort we should probably let it go a while longer to get a baseline on Billy's progress." The trio left with Mr. Smith offering the concluding remark, "Please let us know if there is anything we can do. Even Billy's sisters are willing to help in any way they can." I thanked Mr. Smith for his "helpfulness" and made a mental note that I might call upon Mr. and Mrs. Smith to reinforce my hypnotic interventions at home through the use of prepared scripts if Billy did not show significant improvement by the time of the next session.

Several days later, while reviewing some of the literature on structural family therapy, the Smith case came to mind. I was particularly intrigued over some theorists' views that psychosomatic children could be construed as functionally included in the spouse subsystem. Several authors wrote of the phenomenon of marital conflicts being detoured through a symptomatic child. The more I read, the more I reconsidered my assumptions in the Smith case.

As a result of my reconsideration, I became aware of a wealth of data that I had previously regarded as insignificant to my understanding of the case. This data now seemed to support a view that Billy's enuresis could be construed as a function of a triangulation between Billy and his parents. The significant data seemed to be: 1) Mrs. Smith's offering to bring the family to the first session; 2) Mr. and Mrs. Smith's "growing concern" as reported by Mrs. Smith; 3) Mrs. Smith's somewhat obtrusive behavior toward her son in the conjoint interview; 4) Billy's multiple references to "we" (he and his parents) in conversations; 5) the rapid decline of Billy's progress following the first interview; 6) Mr. Smith's surprise presence at the second session; and finally 7) the heated manner in which Mr. and Mrs. Smith argued over Billy's improvement.

I consequently decided that rather than continue to make various technical moves within my originally adopted change paradigm and hope for the curative effects of time, I would instead change paradigms. The value of the systems paradigm and hypothesis of triangulation now seemed so correct to me that I was astonished at my earlier short-sightedness.

Billy was accompanied to his next appointment *by his parents and his sisters.* I excitedly construed the presence of both parents as validation of my new frame of reference. *The presence of the daughters was considered insignificant.* When I encountered the family in the waiting room, Mr. Smith introduced me to his two daughters, explaining that they were concerned about Billy and had come "to lend their moral support and help in any way they can." With my "new set of eyes" I interpreted the daughters' presence and Mr. Smith's comment as an attempt by the family to focus away from an assumed marital conflict. When Mr. Smith again asked for private time for he and his wife, I felt further reinforcement for my interpretation. I refused Mr. Smith's request and said, "I think I should see the three of you (parents and son) because there is something important we need to discuss." Mr. Smith readily replied, "Well OK, if you think that would be helpful. We're willing to do whatever you think will be helpful."

I was somewhat taken aback by Mr. Smith's apparent willingness to consent to a conjoint interview. When Mrs. Smith gave her nonverbal support, I was able to construe the parents' behavior as an overcompensation against admitting any marital conflict. I was mindful of Salvador Minuchin's claim that psychosomatic families often exhibited a rigidity, not as the rigidity of a stone, but rather as the ebb and flow of water (Minuchin, Rosman, & Baker, 1978, p. 105)

I opened the conjoint interview by blatantly and confidently stating, "Billy has not improved. Now, you two must help him." Mr. and Mrs. Smith were obviously nonplussed by my remark. After several seconds of silence, Mr. Smith finally said, "Well, you're partly right. Billy isn't as good as he was the first week but he's done a little better, though." (The reader is reminded that my objective in this conjoint interview was to "de-triangulate" Billy from his parents' marital conflicts.) I replied, "Well, what do you attribute Billy's slight progress to?" Mrs. Smith now replied (and this was taken as further "proof" of the triangulation),

"Well, we're not sure. We've thought about what you said about this taking time so we've just pretty much left it up to Billy." This remark was accepted as a further metaphoric reference to the detour of marital conflict through Billy.

Then, certain that I was at last on the right track, I wove an intricate frame of reference which viewed Billy's symptom as symbolic of his unconscious concern that one or the other of his parents might abandon him. I explained that this was an unusual developmental feature for Billy's age. In response to this explanation, *both parents eagerly asked what they could do to help Billy.* I explained that what they needed to do was twofold. First, they needed to demonstrate for Billy, even better than they had previously, the strength of their marital union. Second, they needed to show Billy that, even if he was excluded from some of his parents' activities, they would still be together without threat of one or the other abandoning Billy. I further explained that these "trial separations" from Billy would begin to foster a greater, age-appropriate independence in him. I suggested that Billy might even babysit his sisters so that Mr. and Mrs. Smith could have further opportunities to demonstrate the strength of their union and allay Billy's "unconscious overconcern."

My intention here, of course, was to provide a frame of reference in which I wouldn't need to comment directly on any marital conflict but which would tend to strengthen the spouse subsystem and begin to exclude Billy as a functional member of that subsystem. With only minor protestations, both parents accepted the frame of reference *while excessively reassuring me that they would do whatever was necessary to continue to help Billy.* I told them that as long as they began to behave according to my prescription, they could continue to give Billy support for solving his problem. After this, I made an appointment for the three of them to return in three weeks and quickly dismissed them.

*The entire family once again reported to the next appointment.* While greeting them in the waiting room, the six-year-old said to me, "Billy's sad. Dad says we [indicating her sister] can help him, but we don't know how." She then began to cry and was comforted by all the other family members. *With the exception of the parent's united effort toward her, the incident had no meaning within the paradigm in which I was functioning.*

After the daughter had been sufficiently calmed and reassured, Billy and his parents accompanied me to my office. In response to my inquiry about the interviewing period, Mr. Smith reported (and Mrs. Smith agreed) that they had done a good job of implementing the prescription I'd given them but *in spite of the unified support they'd given Billy, he had not had a single dry bed since the last session.*

This report was shocking to me. I needed time to sort out my thoughts and feelings. I told Billy and his parents that I had an idea of something I wanted to do but I would need a few minutes to prepare in privacy. I asked them to go temporarily to the waiting room where they could check on Billy's sister.

Once I was alone in my office, I reviewed the case again from my notes and recollections. The daughter's face kept appearing in my thoughts and I kept hearing myself saying, "What have I missed here? What am I not seeing?" Suddenly, a sequence of visual and auditory recollections occurred as I sat at my desk with my face buried in my hands. These were: 1) Mrs. Smith's volunteering to bring the whole family to the first interview; 2) Mrs. Smith's report of her husband's and her "growing concern"; 3) the sheer magnitude and tenacity of the family's history of attempted remedies for Billy's enuresis; 4) Billy's and his mother's exacting rendition of the attempted solutions; 5) Billy's multiple references to "we"; 6) the decline of Billy's progress in the face of his parent's "support" and increase in the face of diminished "support"; 7) the increasing numbers of family members reporting to each successive appointment; 8) the obsessional quality to the parent's requests to be helpful; and finally 9) the sheer desperation of Billy's sister.

This last image finally revealed for me the missing element. Billy's problem had been a family concern well before his sister was born. The desperation she had manifested in the waiting room stemmed from a lifetime of being an actress in the family drama of curing Billy. Her desperation was symbolic of the family's preoccupation and consequent frustration relative to the problem. *They were purely and simply trying too hard! Their best intentions and attempts to solve the problem had, over time, become the problem.*

By using the various change paradigms I had adopted in the case, I had ignored the crucial feature. The evidence for my new hypothesis simply had been meaningless in each of the frames of reference I had previously adopted.

Based on my hypothesis that Billy's problem was being maintained by his family's best intentioned efforts to solve it, I realized that any subsequent intervention must contain the following features: 1) It must deemphasize the severity and chronicity of Billy's problem both in his mind and in the mind of each of the family members; 2) it must recognize and utilize the tremendous amount of energy the family wished to direct toward solving the problem; and 3) it must create an attitude of expectancy in each of the family members that Billy was progressing.

I walked to the waiting room and, in the presence of the entire family, I addressed the six-year-old daughter, "I know what you and Robin (her sister) and mommy and daddy can do to help Billy. But I must be sure that each of you love him enough to do it. Now, I'm going to talk with Billy for a while and then I'll be back and talk to the rest of you and find out if you love him enough to do what I'm going to ask you to do."

Without allowing time for any of the family members to reply to my remark, I turned quickly and headed back for my office, gesturing for Billy to follow. Once Billy and I were seated in my office, I slowly and deliberately said, "Well, things aren't going too well for you. I'm sure you're even beginning to wonder if you can ever get over this nasty old problem. In fact, you might not even believe me *until you wake up one day and realize it's been gone for a long time and wonder where it went.* Now, you know what hypnosis is and you've done very nicely in hypnosis before, so you can go into hypnosis now thinking about what I've just told you and prepare to do exactly what I'll tell you to do only if you're really ready to wake up some day and wonder where your problem went." At this point, Billy's eyes closed and he slumped in his chair in a pose characteristic of his past trance behavior.

I continued, "Now, go even deeper than you've ever been before only because you're ready, and then listen very carefully." Billy slumped even further in his chair.

I continued in a slower, measured cadence, "Now very deeply asleep and the back of your mind listening to me and prepared to do exactly what I'll ask you to do, you can believe everything I tell you to be absolutely true. From this moment on, you will forget that you ever had that nasty old problem. You will be able to remember anything else you want from your memory except the wet beds. You will also completely forget that anyone has ever tried to help you with that nasty old problem. You will know that your family loves you and has helped you in many ways, but you will forget any help they have given you about the old problem. Do you understand what it is that I am asking you to do and how this can help your family to stop worrying about you?" After several seconds, Billy nodded his head and said, "Yes."

I further instructed Billy, "Now, some mornings over the next weeks or even months you will wake up and know that you must change the sheets on your bed. You will do this by yourself, putting the old sheets with the other laundry, and as you do you will know you are helping your mother for all the love she has given you. After some time, you will find other, different ways to help her.

"If your mother or father or either of your sisters ever asks you about your changing your sheets *or anything about that,* you will explain that you are simply helping your mother. Then you will find yourself talking about something totally different.

"One day in the future, weeks or months from now, you will wake up and suddenly realize that you used to have a problem but somehow or another you lost it and you won't care how. This will make you feel very proud and confident and you will feel very good about yourself and your family.

"Now do you understand completely and exactly what I want you to do and will you do it for you and your family?" Again, after a few seconds, Billy nodded and said, "Yes."

I then explained to Billy that he would wake up without remembering anything of the session "losing the time you have been with me completely—just as completely as you will lose that old problem some day."

I then told Billy that after I awakened him, he would feel "incredibly sleepy. In fact, so sleepy that you just won't have enough energy to talk with anyone in the car on your way home. When you get home, you will immediately go to the bathroom and pee and then you will go to bed and sleep deeply until tomorrow morning [the time was 7:45 p.m.] and have many pleasant dreams about how you and your family will be very happy some weeks or months from now."

With that, I awakened Billy and escorted him to a vacant office to wait for his family. He acted quite sluggish and groggy. I then walked into the waiting room to the rest of Billy's family. Addressing the younger daughter I said, "Well, what's your answer?" She replied between sobs, "We do love Billy! We do!" I responded, "I know you do, sweetie, and now I'm going to tell your parents how they can help Billy and then I'll tell you and your sister. OK?" The girl smiled and chirped brightly, "OK!"

I motioned for Mr. and Mrs. Smith to accompany me to my office. Once seated, I declared that I was now certain that Billy would demonstrate progress over the next several weeks, but that he would require "a very special kind of help" from them in order to do so. I expressed that they had done so much for Billy already that I was hesitant to ask them for what would surely be a further, significant sacrifice. Both parents strongly assured me again that they were willing to do anything to help their son. In response to this, I told them that before describing what I wanted them to do, I would explain how I viewed their son's status (thus creating an even more powerful motivation to follow my prescription.)

I explained that Billy carried considerable guilt about disappointing his family in their loving offers of assistance over eight years and that was standing in the way of the hypnotic suggestions working properly. I further elaborated that the only way for Billy to be able to successfully follow the suggestions would be for him to believe that he had changed on his own. This, then, would constitute his "restitution." I cautioned them that any attempt on their part to confront Billy about his guilt would only meet with his denial and could potentially increase his guilt and thus make his progress more difficult.

Both parents acknowledged the probable truth of my explanation and again begged me to tell them what they could do that would be effective. I reluctantly told them that I wanted them to behave around Billy "as though he doesn't have the problem now nor did he have it at any time in the past." They were to expect that Billy would change. I also told them that I had instructed Billy to change his own sheets "as a part of his restitution," but that neither parent was to comment on this directly unless Billy brought up the subject. I explained that if Billy did raise the subject, they were only to respond with gratitude for Billy's "willingness to help with the household chores." I then obtained both parent's agreement that they would follow my instructions exactly for a period of at least 90 days, recognizing that it would take "at least that long for Billy to work off his guilt."

Both parents were greatly relieved that what I had asked them to do seemed quite minor in comparison to their past efforts. I assured them that their role might seem minor to them but that it would "surely make the necessary difference for Billy." I then asked the parents to bring the daughters into the office so I could explain their "helping role" for the next 90 days.

Once the parents and daughters had gathered in my office, I expressed that I was quite moved by their love for Billy and was most certain that they would do whatever I asked of them even if they didn't understand it well. I stated that mommy and daddy were certain that I wanted to help Billy and knew I would help because I had gone to special schools to learn how to help children like Billy.

I explained that while helping Billy, the rest of the family could have fun because they deserved to after all their loving help. I then announced that the four of them were to have a "contest" and that the winner would be recognized by the other three as being the most unselfish helper toward Billy. I described that the contest would be to see which of the four of them could best "pretend" that Billy didn't have a bed-wetting problem now or at any time in the past. I added the cautionary note that the person who did the worst in the contest might end up hurting Billy's feelings by accident. I conceded, however, that there was a possibility that the contest could end in a tie but that would be okay since in that event it would be even more helpful to Billy. After obtaining each person's agreement to be a part of the contest and stressing the importance of the four of them keeping it a secret from that moment on, I dismissed them. As they were preparing to leave, I told the parents to call me in 85 days to report to me on who seemed to be winning the contest at that point in time.

I received a phone call 135 days later from Mr. Smith, who apologized for not calling sooner, reporting that the telephone call had slipped both his and his wife's minds. He reported that based on Billy's use of linen his problem began to subside within a week of the last interview, and that "with rare exceptions" it had virtually disappeared altogether by the time of the call. He also reported that the daughters had lost interest in the contest within 30 days and had not mentioned it since.

At the time of this writing, which is nearly a year after the last session with the Smiths, I called Mrs. Smith to obtain a follow-up report. She related she was fairly certain that Billy had had "less than a handful of wet beds," since my phone conversation with Mr. Smith.

## REFERENCES

Cheek, D.B. & Le Cron, L.M. *Clinical Hypnotherapy.* New York: Grune & Stratton, 1968, pp. 210-211.

Crasilneck, H.B. & Hall, J.A. *Clinical Hypnosis: Principles and Applications.* New York: Grune & Stratton, 1975, p. 132.

Erickson, M.H., Hershman, S., & Secter, I.I. *The Practical Application of Medical and Dental Hypnosis.* New York: The Julian Press, Inc., 1961, pp. 244-245.

Hartland, J. *Medical and Dental Hypnosis and Its Clinical Applications.* Baltimore: The Williams & Wilkins Company, 1971, pp. 213-215.

Meares, A. *A System of Medical Hypnosis.* New York: The Julian Press, Inc. 1960, pp. 334-335.

Minuchin, S., Rosman, B.L., & Baker, L. *Psychosomatic Families—Anorexia Nervosa in Context.* Cambridge, MA: Harvard University Press, 1978.

Wolberg, L.R. *Medical Hypnosis: Volume I—The Principles of Hypnotherapy.* New York: Grune & Stratton, 1948, pp. 394-396.

Chapter 21

# Ericksonian Approaches to Promote Abstinence from Cigarette Smoking

*Jeffrey K. Zeig*

A recent review (Holroyd, 1980) indicated that hypnosis is an effective technique that can be used to help people quit smoking. Holroyd suggested that the hypnotic treatments reported in the literature can be divided into two types: those that provide standardized suggestions and those that provide individualized suggestions. Many standardized approaches to smoking control are often limited to one session. The most popular standardized approach is the one developed by Herbert Spiegel (1970). Termination rates of 20 to 25% are reported in Spiegel's data and in replications by other authors (Holroyd, 1980). The approaches that provided individualized suggestions consistently show a higher rate of success than the standardized suggestions. With individualized suggestions, success rates of up to 88% have been reported (Kline, 1970). Holroyd (1980) concluded that four therapeutic factors increased the percentage of abstinence: 1) an intense personal interaction; 2) suggestions designed to capitalize on the individual's motivation; 3) adjunctive counseling or telephone contact; and 4) several hours of treatment.

It is not surprising that individualized suggestions would be more effective than a rote procedure. If controlling the urge to smoke is an art, then the therapeutic treatment should also be an art. Erickson, of course, was adamant about the importance of individualizing one's therapeutic approach. He did not look with favor upon cookbook approaches. In fact, he compared such approaches to an obstetrician's using forceps for *every* delivery (Note 1).

Individualized approaches work better because each personality is unique and because symptomatic behavior occurs for idiosyncratic reasons. The purpose of this chapter is to speak to techniques of individualizing treatment. I will offer suggestions to help clinicians conceptualize how they can make their techniques fit the particular motivations and potentials of individual clients. The indirect techniques developed by Milton Erickson, including his interspersal approach (Erickson, 1966), are emphasized. The case studies illustrate the use of hypnotic techniques without the necessity of formal induction. Additionally, I will describe one couple's therapy that centered on stopping cigarette smoking.

## DIAGNOSIS

To individualize one's approach, you must pay attention to salient personal factors. The standardized approaches give minimal attention to individual differences; hence diagnosis is considered superfluous. Spiegel spends very little time getting diagnostic information from his patients. He commonly asks his patients why they want to quit smoking and if they have quit for any substantial time in the past. However, in practice, Spiegel does not follow up to any great extent on the information that he receives.

To diverge momentarily, I want to point out that Spiegel's approach includes many clever and effective aspects. I have successfully used some of Spiegel's methods in my own work. However, I often modify suggestions to fit the individual client, and I use only portions that can be predicted to lead to a positive effect.

Usually, in the first session with a new client, I concentrate solely on information-gathering, and often no overt therapy is undertaken. During the first session, at times I will just get diagnostic information so that I can plan subsequent treatment. Sometimes the first session will be brief, and the patient is charged accordingly. Sometimes, however, all of the therapy can take place in the first session. Diagnosis is critically important since the diagnosis is implicitly a plan of treatment. A standardized medical/psychiatric diagnosis is not necessary, but one should evaluate the patient's specific characteristics around which effective treatment can be organized. Diagnosing motivation is crucially important.

Much diagnostic information is gathered on a nonverbal level. During one of my early sessions with Erickson in 1973, he drew three lines on a piece of paper—one vertical, one horizontal, and one diagonal—and asked me what the lines meant. I pondered his question, looked at the paper, and tried to find symbolic meaning in the designs. Finally, I told him I was stumped. Erickson then pointed out that people commonly move their heads in one of those three orientations. We shake our heads "yes," nod "no," or cock our heads to the side to show uncertainty. Erickson's point was that you note your patient's verbal response to your question and look for confirmation from the nonverbal response.

Unconscious head movements provide diagnostic information. When a patient comes in for therapy, you can ask in a general and interested way why he sought out consultation and then reflect back his words, e.g., "You are here to stop smoking." Notice the patient's nonverbal response. Is he nodding his head? Shaking it? Or holding his head diagonally? This is often valuable information about the patient's motivation and unconscious reasons for wanting therapy.

Implicit in this initial diagnostic approach is a point that is rarely stressed in the literature on hypnotic approaches to achieving abstinence from smoking. Most therapists realize that the presenting problem is not necessarily the point where the therapy should be applied. Often, the presenting problem is a smoke screen for underlying issues or an unrecognized rationalization that provides an acceptable reason for seeking out treatment.

For example, once a woman came asking for therapy to help her husband quit smoking. The couple were Eastern European refugees who had come to the United States during World War II. Both the husband and wife were extremely intelligent. The man had earned a law degree before the war but was never able to practice in the United States. He worked in a steel mill after immigrating to America, subsequently earning a master's degree and then working in a semiprofessional field before retiring. The wife also had graduate degrees and similarly was retired. It was really the wife's request that her husband stop smoking. She brought him into therapy so that I could "make him stop smoking."

After talking briefly with both of them, I interviewed the husband alone. I asked him what he liked about smoking. He replied philosophically, in an old-world accent, "Life is like smoke, and I just like to see the smoke as it rises." He made it clear early in the session that he was not really interested in stopping smoking. His stopping smoking was more important to his wife than it was to him. However, he had quit smoking in the past after one session of hypnosis. When I asked about his pattern of smoking, he replied that he smoked six cigarettes a day and never went over that amount. Not only did he limit himself to six cigarettes a day, but he didn't inhale any of them. Clearly the problem had more to do with the interaction between the couple than it had to do with the habit of smoking.

The wife was interviewed alone. She was absolutely adamant that her husband stop smoking. She stated, "He is the only thing that I have in life. If he dies, I won't have anyone. All of my people are in the old country." I asked about her attempts to get her husband to stop smoking. She said that she had tried both badgering him and not pushing. She said that if she didn't prod him about stopping, she would feel that she did him a disservice.

The actual therapy for the couple was rather direct. I explained to the wife that I was one of the most eminent practitioners of smoking control therapy in Arizona. If I couldn't help her husband, clearly no one else could. I would give her husband hypnosis, and if he responded that would be fine. If he didn't respond, she could finally rest assured that she had done her best. The husband agreed with the therapeutic contract. They scheduled a second session for the hypnosis. After the hypnotic therapy was presented, no follow-up was requested. Actually, follow-up was unnecessary. The man's smoking habit was minimal and really could not jeopardize his health. The therapy was directed to the dynamics of the relationship between the couple. The fact that the therapy ostensibly centered on smoking control was incidental.

In diagnosing motivational factors, it is important to realize that individuals have unique reasons both for smoking and for quitting. Some people need to quit smoking for health reasons. Some need to stop smoking for social reasons. Some people continue to smoke because it is an unconscious pattern and they have limited conscious realization of their actions. Others smoke to release stress. The therapeutic approach needs to be geared toward the motivation. An approach that would be successful for the person who smokes for stress reduction should differ from the therapy for the person who needs to stop because of health reasons.

Another crucial issue in the therapy of habit control problems is one of getting enough leverage to demonstrate to the patient that a minimally strategic change can be made in his pattern (cf. Watzlawick, Weakland, & Fisch, 1974). Erickson pointed out that therapy consists of anything that alters the habitual pattern of behavior. In which direction the change proceeds does not matter. Once the person's particular pattern and motivations are established, the therapist can begin to use the diagnostic information to promote minimal change. In their training seminars, Fisch and Weakland use the concept of "hooks," values to which a patient is attached. For example, one person may value being unselfish, and his therapy can be directed (hooked) to that value. That patient can be encouraged to change purely for others. For a selfish person, the therapy can be framed as purely for personal gain. You use hooks to promote minimal strategic change.

In gathering diagnostic information, I often ask questions that are designed not only to elicit information but also to "seed" the idea that change will happen. Questions can be formulated to increase motivation and to elicit associations that demonstrate to the patient that he has the resources in his own history to overcome his problem. Many of the initial questions seem to be oriented to garnering factual information. I frequently ask patients, *"What brand of cigarettes have you been smoking?" "How long have you smoked?" "How much have you been smoking?" "How many cigarettes do you currently have in your possession?" "Why have you decided to stop smoking now?" "Have you ever quit smoking before?" "Have you ever had previous therapy to help you quit smoking?"* These questions provide information and, on a covert level, they convey implied messages. I ask, "How much *have you* been smoking?" (implying up to this time), rather than "How much do you smoke?" (which implies continued smoking). Subtle linguistic tools, in and of themselves, may not promote change, but when they are used repetitively, the positive effect is multiplied.

Patients are commonly asked, *"What other habits have you overcome and how have you done that?"* I pay special attention to the strategy that they used to surmount other habits since the same strategy can be applied to the current habit problem.

I frequently ask patients, *"What have you enjoyed about smoking?"* If you can find out what has been pleasurable about the habit, a hypnotic strategy can be devised to supply the same sensations. If a patient smokes for relaxation, then self-hypnosis can be substituted. If the patient enjoys any other sensory sensation when smoking, that sensation can be recreated through hypnotic hallucination.

Questions can be asked with aversive connotations. For example, *"What have you enjoyed about the mechanical act of smoking?" "Have you enjoyed the puffing?" "Have you enjoyed the feeling of the smoke hitting the back of your throat?" "Have you enjoyed the feeling of it filling your lungs?" "Have you enjoyed blowing the smoke out of your mouth?"* and so forth. The therapist's nonverbal communication while asking these questions is geared at projecting warmth and curiosity, not confrontation. The idea is to subtly create a negative connotation. This technique uses the patient's consciousness as a tool to fight an unconscious habit. With this sort of questioning, the therapist can make the patient *painfully* aware of what he has been doing, thus promoting minimal strategic change. The idea that the habit is personally aversive can be developed from within the patient.

In working with all kinds of habits, another therapeutic strategy is to promote pattern disruption. You should find out as much information as possible about the patient's habit. Usually the habit is circular in nature; the pattern results in more of the same behavior. However, by delineating the pattern through careful questioning, the therapist can find the weakest link and use hypnotic techniques to disrupt the pattern at this point. Frequently, a smoking habit pattern can be disrupted by applying therapy at the point in the pattern at which the patient feels an urge to smoke. Often the urge to smoke is the first point that the patient is aware of in the pattern. However, careful questioning will usually reveal other unconscious or preconscious factors that precede the actual feeling of desiring a cigarette.

I often ask my patients, *"Will you describe the urge to smoke in detail?"* Frequently they have difficulty doing this task. I then explain that all feelings are bodily sensations, and I illustrate and talk about a particular feeling. Commonly, I will use the negative feeling that I think the particular patient feels most often. With a patient who projects depression, I will describe depression, "You know what the feeling of depression is like. When you are feeling depressed, your shoulders are heavy, your body is heavy, you may have a tight feeling in your chest or a heavy feeling in your stomach, etc." I will then ask the patient again to describe his urge to smoke. Invariably the response will be a vague metaphor, e.g., "Well, it is like a pressure." I forcefully demand a specific response, "Is it a burning feeling? Is it a tingling feeling? What has it been like?" Rarely can a patient give an accurate physical description of the urge to smoke, but the effect of this questioning is to make the patient consciously think about the urge in order to promote pattern disruption. The patient is encouraged to become overly self-conscious, and a conscious strategy is thus used to disrupt an unconscious pattern. For more indirect pattern disruption I might ask the patient to compare the urge to smoke to another (negative) feeling such as anger, fear, etc., thereby attaching more negative affect to smoking.

I often will explain to the patient that there is some sensation that is a "trigger" that leads to smoking. I ask, *"Just before you reach for a cigarette, what is going on?"* Such questioning is useful in finding out the minute detail of his pattern. The more detail that can be gleaned, the easier it is to seed possibilities for change.

Often, I will explain to the patient that there are two opposing parts that need to be recognized: One part is definite about stopping smoking. The other part has been holding back. There is a part that has enjoyed smoking, and there is another part that doesn't like it. I ask the patient to quantify the parts: *"If you had a 100-point scale, how much would you ascribe to the first part and how much would you ascribe to the second?"* Most often the patient will give numbers such as 80/20 or 75/25. Rarely have I had someone go as low as 50/50. This information is useful in assessing the patient's motivation. Additionally, the dissociative technique serves as a seed that can be used later.

You can ask a patient, *"How long will you have to stop before you realize that you are permanently free?"* I want the patient to commit himself to some period of time. Most people feel that they will need two to three weeks. In this way, the patient is given a target, and he has subtly committed himself to a time limit for his struggle.

Either of the last two questions can be followed by asking the person, *"Will you describe in detail all of the reasons that you can think of for not taking a first puff after you have stopped smoking?"* With some patients this procedure of making a list has been quite ceremonious. Once a person verbalizes a reason, it becomes more difficult to use that reason to rationalize maladaptive behavior.

The patient can be asked, *"How will you tell people that you have stopped smoking?"* This question presupposes change and orients the person to a positive future. If the patient does not have a ready response, I often give him an anecdotal illustration. I explain that I had a delightful experience with my own family. I went home one Christmas after growing a moustache for the first time in my life. My parents and my youngest sister greeted me at the airport. They couldn't help but notice my moustache. The next morning my mother was the only one at breakfast, and she noticed that I had a Cheshire-cat grin on my face. She asked me what was going on, and I replied "Nothing." She didn't stop questioning me, and I couldn't stop my Cheshire-cat grin. Finally I pointed to my lips, and my mother noticed that I had shaved off the moustache that morning. A few minutes later my sister joined us. I had control of my grin, but this time my mother was smiling. Edye asked what was going on, and finally my mother pointed to her upper lip. Edye then realized what was going on. Three days later over dinner we told my father. It was a delightful learning experience.

People often view quitting smoking as a life-or-death struggle. The idea of quitting can be reframed so that more positive feeling can be attached to the process. Additionally, quitting smoking is something that can be a process of getting "one up" on other people. There is no amount of social reinforcement that a patient can get that will match the energy it takes to stop smoking. The process can be reframed as a game that the patient can control in his/her social context.

Two other parts of my technique need to be noted here: 1) I write down all of the patient's answers as exactly as I can so that I can learn the patient's linguistic style and use his own rephrased words to create therapeutic suggestions during the induction of hypnosis. 2) I am careful to maintain an attitude of expectancy in regard to change.

There is a story that may be apocryphal about a research experiment. The experimenter asked a graduate student to conduct the research. The graduate student was told to go into a small room in which he would find two undergraduates. He was instructed to give one of them a dime and the other a dollar. No other information was provided. Unbeknownst to the graduate student, the experimenter had met with each of the students individually before the experiment. One of the students was told that the graduate student would come in and give him a dime. The other student was told that the graduate student would come in and give him a dollar. Of course, the result was that frequently the student who expected the dollar got the dollar and the student who expected the dime got the dime.

Even if no direct therapy has been attempted in the first session, patients invariably report a decrease in smoking at least for a few days after the first session. By monitoring this decrease, I can learn something about the patient's responsiveness to the indirect techniques presented in the first session. Further, I can point out to the patient that his unconscious mind has demonstrated that he is really motivated for change.

## INTERSPERSAL TECHNIQUE

In traditional hypnosis the therapist applies an induction (usually standardized), followed by a deepening technique, which is followed by the therapy. During the therapy, usually a direct negative or positive suggestion is supplied, e.g., "No longer will you want to smoke. Cigarettes will taste terrible to you, etc."

Erickson blurred the distinction between induction, deepening, and therapy. Therapy can take place during the induction as well as the deepening phase of hypnosis. Suggestions can be interspersed when the patient is least expectant and less mobilized to resist. For example, during an induction, you can explain to a patient, "There is no need to do anything, no desire to do anything; you can just be comfortable in sitting and listening, and there is no need to have any other experience but to pay attention to the developing comfort." This communication is ambiguous in that it can be interpreted on a number of levels. The patient is being instructed about hypnosis; however, at the same time he is there to stop smoking. Suggestions about "no need" and "no desire" can apply either to the state of hypnosis or to the urge to smoke.

Erickson often demonstrated that symbolic techniques during the induction could be used for the dual purpose of promoting hypnosis and promoting psychotherapy. For example, while doing an arm levitation, the patient can be directed to notice the pleasure of his hand reaching up to his face. "It can be very pleasant when your hand comes near your face, and although you haven't recognized it there is no urge to cheat . . . because your head hasn't moved down to touch your hand. Your hand has only moved up to your face." Again the suggestions occur on several levels. By interspersing them, suggestions are stacked to a particular goal at a time when a patient's conscious attention is distracted.

Psychotherapists often talk to their patients about the importance of not trying to control an urge directly. They speak to the importance of indirect control. However, therapists often give patients direct techniques to establish indirect control. In using an Ericksonian interspersal approach, indirect techniques are presented to promote unconscious learning and to demonstrate to the patient that such control is possible.

## SYMBOLIC TECHNIQUES: A CASE REPORT

Symbolic techniques are not circumscribed to the induction period. Sometimes the entire therapy can revolve around symbolism (cf. Zeig, 1980, p. 149).

A retired woman sought psychotherapy to overcome a delayed grief reaction. She responded well to symbolic rituals, and these techniques were used to absorb the grief of the loss of her husband. Then she referred her daughter for psychotherapy. Among other problems, the daughter wanted to stop smoking. I asked her about the techniques that her mother had used to quit smoking. Her mother had bought a reduction filter. When she got down to the last filter, she lost it and decided to just quit. The daughter also used a filter when she smoked, so I gave her an assignment: "I want you to take your cigarettte filter on a round trip up Squaw Peak (a local mountain that people commonly climb for health reasons and for the spectacular view of the valley). In order for this assignment to be therapeutic, when you are down at the bottom of Squaw Peak, I want you to look up at the top and say, 'Sometime in the next few hours, I am going to be there.' Bring the cigarette filter up to the top, and when you get back to the bottom, you are *free* . . . to do anything that you wish with it."

The daughter was elated when she came back for the next session. She had quit smoking. She said, "I brought that cigarette filter up to the top of Squaw Peak. I brought it down to the bottom, and somewhere between the bottom of the path and the parking lot, I lost the filter. Did you suggest that to me?" I replied that I hadn't. The daughter could use a pattern that was similar to the one used by her mother. No hypnosis was used formally, but hypnotic techniques of suggestion were apparent. The psychotherapy was effected through use of a symbolic ritual.

## HYPNOTIC TECHNIQUES WITH COUPLES

When a patient initially inquires about therapy for smoking problems, I will often ask if there is anyone else in the family who currently smokes. A spouse or child can be brought into the session if he or she is also interested in quitting. Often, habits result from maladaptive patterns within a relationship. Also, dynamics inherent in the relationship can be used as additional leverage to promote change.

Additional diagnostic questions are pertinent when working with couples. In individual interviews, I ask, *"Who has typically smoked first? Who has it been who has reached for a cigarette first?"* Many times, one member of the couple has initiated the smoking behavior, and the other member has responded to that external cue. Such external responsiveness is especially the case with people who are highly responsive hypnotic subjects and thereby highly responsive to social cues. Typically, such people will quit smoking easily because of their capacity to be responsive to treatment. However, when sent back into their home environment, they relapse. Often, the responsive smoker is the better hypnotic subject. Open discussion of this dynamic makes the responsive smoker more self-conscious because many times he doesn't like the idea that his habit pattern has been dependent on an external cue provided by his spouse or parent.

Sometimes it is impossible to effect change by working with the more responsive member of the couple because of particular relationship patterns. Then the other factors in the relationship can be used for leverage.

### *Case Report*

A man phoned and said, "I have been smoking for 30 years. Can you help me to stop?" I asked if anyone in his family smoked, and he said that his wife had also been smoking for 30 years. She was also interested in stopping, and so she was asked to come to the consultation.

The husband was a rather insecure man who projected the image of being "macho" and in control. One of his first comments was, "Listen, you and I both know that there is nothing that you can do or say that is going to stop me from going out of here and having a cigarette." I replied, "You know, you are absolutely right. There is nothing that I can do or say that will stop you from having a cigarette when you get out of here." He found out that I was a sensible person with an intelligent understanding of the situation.

I met with the couple together and got some diagnostic information and then met with them individually. In meeting with them together and individually, I wanted to find a usable hook. The husband was competitive, and I thought that competition could supply leverage because the wife seemed to be a more responsive hypnotic subject. My initial thinking was that the wife would respond to hypnosis, stop immediately, and then the husband would have to stop to retain control. I presented this idea to her when I met with her individually. She felt that it would not be a workable solution, stating, "I have stopped smoking before, and whenever I have, he subtly sabotages it. He doesn't mean to. He really loves me, but he leaves cigarettes around, smokes in my presence, and subtly does things to sabotage my efforts to stop."

I then asked her if there were things that her husband didn't like to do. She thought for a moment and said, "You know, we have been married for over 30 years, and during that time we have never taken a separate vacation. He will never allow me to go anywhere on my own." This bit of information supplied the hook around which the therapy could be organized. The wife and I agreed on a plan of action. The couple was given an appointment to come back the next week for their hypnotic treatment. It was agreed jointly that the husband would have to lead the way as far as the therapy was concerned.

During the drive home, the couple had a cigarette. After they finished the first cigarette, the wife said to the husband, "You know, it is really not going to mean anything if you stop smoking because of Dr. Zeig's hypnosis." The husband agreed, and the wife continued, "It's really something that you need to do on your own." Again, her husband agreed. She then said, "So, what I'm going to do is I am going to visit the kids in California while you stay here and come to grips with the smoking problem." He said, "Now, wait a minute!"

A few days later, the wife called back and cancelled their appointment. She said that there was no need for an appointment because they had both stopped smoking.

Her husband would do anything rather than have his wife go on a vacation alone—including stopping smoking. He had his one cigarette after leaving my office although he didn't realize how concrete his responsiveness was.

## USING HOOKS: CASE EXAMPLES

The following cases are complex and illustrate many interventions. They provide examples of using hooks and "seeding" technique.

### *Case One*

A woman presented with problems involving alcoholism. During the initial session it became clear that marital problems were primary, and her husband was asked to come into the second session. This was a very intelligent professional couple. The husband also had a problem with excessive use of alcohol. When he was interviewed, it was clear from his nonverbal behavior that he really was not interested in stopping drinking. The wife desperately needed to stop drinking.

The couple was given the symbolic assignment of taking small plastic containers of alcohol on a round trip together up Squaw Peak. The ritual was conducted in a very ceremonious manner by the wife. It really meant something to her, and after coming down to the bottom of the mountain she poured out the alcohol and stopped drinking completely for a period of time. The husband continued to drink.

In the meantime, marital therapy was initiated. I suggested to the husband at one time that he might want to stop smoking. He replied, "Well, I guess so. I'm not really motivated to stop smoking. I have tried to stop a couple of times before when I have been motivated, but I wasn't successful." I replied, "This may be a better time because there is no pressure."

An individual session was scheduled for this purpose. I identified four hooks: 1) He liked to gamble. 2) He explained that when he was driving in a car, he wouldn't smoke. 3) There was a captain's chair that he wanted to purchase for himself. 4) He did a lot of professional work with children.

He was asked how much he wanted to quit smoking, and he replied that his positive motivation was about 75%. He was going on vacation the next weekend, the couple would be taking a long drive. The therapy was timed so that he would not stop smoking until he began his vacation. I told him to clean out the ashtrays in his house and in his car the night before leaving. Hypnosis was employed, and I talked with him metaphorically about controlling urges. By way of illustration, I told him an anecdote while he was under hypnosis.

I explained that I saw an interesting event happen while I was in the Driver's License Bureau. I saw a five-year-old boy sitting on his mother's lap. The five-year-old boy was agitating; he wanted something—he wanted down. The mother put the boy down. She held him by the shoulders, looked him straight in the eye, and said, "Okay, you can get down, but you stand right there!" That caught my attention because it was said with such force. The little boy looked up, took a step back, and then looked up and took a step back again. Within 30 seconds, he was at the end of the corridor yelling for candy. The mother collected the little boy and put him back on her lap. A few minutes later, he was agitating again. He wanted down. The mother took the little boy again, held him by the shoulders, and looked him in the eye. She said, "All right. You can get down, but this time you stay right there!" Again, the little boy looked up, took a step back, looked up and took a step back and within 30 seconds was at the end of the corridor yelling for candy. I then said directly to my patient, "You know, that mother was 75 percent smarter than the little boy, and that mother was 75 percent stronger than the little boy. But when that mother told him what to do directly, the little boy showed how strong 25 percent could be."

After bringing the patient out of hypnosis, a follow-up appointment was made. I explained to the patient that he was to give me a check for the follow-up appointment which was to be held in two weeks. If he were not smoking, I would give him back the check, and the follow-up session would be free of charge. The man was a gambler, and he liked the idea of having some money involved. I further explained to the patient that he and I, two strong men, could not hold that five-year-old in one spot without putting out an enormous amount of energy.

When the man came back for the follow-up session, he had stopped smoking. We agreed that he would buy himself the captain's chair as a gift for two weeks of being free of smoking.

Smoking control was really not the major issue in the therapy. Controlling smoking was a metaphor. If the man could control one habit, he could control another. I expect that sometime in the future this patient will want to stop drinking and then will come back for therapy. He controlled his hand movement in relation to one habit, and sometime in the future he should be able to control his hand movement in regard to another habit.

Subsequent follow-up indicated that the husband continued abstinence from smoking for over a year.

*Case Two*

A 37-year-old male named Ralph, who was in a social service occupation, was referred to me by Erickson after Erickson had retired from private practice. The patient requested treatment for smoking control. He explained that he had had one session with Erickson years ago that also centered on smoking control. Erickson's therapy made him feel like it would be so easy to stop smoking that he didn't feel like he had to really try.

When asked about his smoking pattern, the patient explained that he could control his cigarette smoking in many situations but not in all situations. The patient added that he didn't like to be "known as a smoker" in front of his family, colleagues, and friends. Additionally, he did not smoke in front of people because it made him appear weak-willed.

The first session was reserved for taking history. Hypnotic psychotherapy was started during the second session. Before the second session the patient explained that he had smoked less during the previous week. In hypnosis, suggestions of relaxation were given. The patient was reminded of his reasons for wanting to quit smoking. His own reasons and concomitant verbalizations were restated and presented as suggestions. Interspersal techniques were also used; in hypnosis it was suggested that the patient could experience a sense of weight (wait) in his hands. Basically, the indirect suggestion was that the kind of relaxation that he experienced in hypnosis could be used to deal with anxiety in tense situations.

At a follow-up session the patient revealed that he had stopped smoking for a short time after hypnotic session, but later resumed smoking. As part of the therapy, the patient agreed that after this session any smoking would be punished by two weeks of smoking regularly in front of other people. I explained that his smoking was a childish habit and that a childish habit could respond to punishment. Hypnosis was again used, and suggestions of relaxation were supplied. Additional techniques of dealing with the urge to smoke were suggested.

Two weeks later the patient returned for a follow-up appointment. He explained that he had stopped smoking for ten days and then began again after he unexpectedly encountered some frustrations. The fourth session ended after a brief interview. The patient was instructed to proceed with our agreement. He was to smoke regularly for the next two weeks in front of people. He was obviously upset with the assignment.

Two weeks later the patient returned, and again hypnotic therapy was offered. Previous themes were reinforced and elaborated upon. Subsequently, the patient has stopped smoking and has not restarted again for two years.

One of the patient's hooks was his need for a challenge. Therapy was effected so that the patient could both have and surmount the challenge that he required. In this case, the symptom (smoking) was used as punishment to provide leverage for overcoming the symptom.

## CONCLUSIONS

Individualizing suggestions is an important technique in increasing therapeutic effectiveness in hypnotic approaches to smoking control. Patients' characteristics (hooks) should be diagnosed and used to individualize the therapeutic approach. The cases illustrate the use of multilevel communication and naturalistic hypnotic technique. Although I have concentrated on the issue of smoking control, these techniques should also be applicable to other habit control problems, including obesity and alcoholism.

## REFERENCE NOTES

1. M.H. Erickson. Personal Communication, 1979.

## REFERENCES

Erickson, M.H. The interspersal hypnotic technique for symptom correction and pain control. *American Journal of Clinical Hypnosis*, 1966, *3*, 198-209.

Holroyd, J. Hypnosis treatment for smoking and evaluative review. *International Journal of Clinical and Experimental Hypnosis*, 1980, *28*, 341-356.

Kline, M.V. The use of extended group hypnotherapy sessions in controlling cigarette habituation. *International Journal of Clinical and Experimental Hypnosis*, 1970, *18*, 270-282.

Spiegel, H. A single treatment method to stop smoking using ancilliary self-hypnosis. *International Journal of Clinical and Experimental Hypnosis*, 1970, *18*, 235-250.

Watzlawick, P., Weakland, J. & Fisch, R. *Change: Principles of Problem Formation and Problem Resolution*. New York: Norton, 1974.

Zeig, J.K. (Ed.) *A Teaching Seminar with Milton H. Erickson*. New York: Brunner/Mazel, 1980.

Chapter 22

# Ericksonian Techniques in Emergency Dehypnotization

*Moris Kleinhauz*

These insightful words of Milton H. Erickson that appeared on the Program for the Erickson Congress can also serve as the theme for this lecture:

> Each person is a unique individual. Hence, psychotherapy should be formulated to meet the uniqueness of the individual needs, rather than tailoring the person to fit the Procustean Bed of a hypothetical theory of human behavior.

The primacy of the uniqueness of the individual and his needs is an important theme that not only underlies psychotherapeutic relationships, but also ensures that significant interpersonal relationships will develop harmoniously and successfully. The principle, stated so succinctly by Erickson, should guide the design and performance of all "manipulative" encounters, including formal and informal hypnotic inductions and the application of dehypnotization procedures.

Psychopathological disorders may be expected whenever an intimate or significant interpersonal encounter is not based on the uniqueness of the individuals involved. At a minimum, we should not be surprised when psychopathology follows a routinized encounter. Since stage hypnotists use a stereotyped approach designed to create a situation that they can then exploit for entertainment, they are not interested in their subjects' uniqueness. Rather they want to induce a quick and deep hypnotic trance in which they can manipulate the relationship. Thus,

---

I wish to thank Mrs. Barbara Beran for her assistance in the preparation of this manuscript.

for the subject, this encounter may be viewed as epitomizing the diametric opposite of the principle outlined by Erickson.

There may be no apparent trauma after stage hypnosis for some subjects. Many people may have repressed exhibitionistic impulses. For them, the chance to act on stage could meet prior needs and be experienced as a wish fulfillment experience. Others may be able to mobilize adequate ego-defense mechanisms and thus defend themselves against the insult.

On the other hand, some subjects may experience trauma and psychopathologic manifestations triggered by the stage-hypnosis experience. Any aspect of the hypnotist-hypnotized interpersonal relationship ("rapport") and any specific suggestion given to the subject may have symbolic "adequacy" to be "adopted" metaphorically by the subject and to become a neurotic resolution for repressed conflicts. Psychopathological manifestations may also be aroused by the reawakening of forgotten traumatic experiences and their repressed emotional connotations. A clear example of the latter mechanism may be found in a case I have reported previously (Kleinhauz et al., 1979). Stereotyped procedures by the stage-hypnotist, his failure to identify and meet the specific emotional needs of the subject, and his failure to recognize and deal with distress in its early manifestations, may lead to a psychopathological manifestation, or to difficulties in dehypnotization.

Surprisingly enough, we do not find many post-stage-hypnosis psychopathological casualties reported in the scientific literature. Nor is this type of problem salient in the experience of physicians, possibly because of faulty diagnostic procedures. Also, lack of awareness of the dangers of stage-hypnosis and misconceptions in general, both by the public and by the medical profession, may cause the patient to fail to report the stage-hypnosis experience since he does not consider it as significant. If he does report it, the medical professionals may fail to understand its significance. Obviously, the patient may repress the hypnotic events and experience amnesia for them (as usually happens following deep hypnotic procedures). Therefore, instead of dealing with the underlying experience, physicians may use other treatment modalities in vain.

I would like to discuss one extreme case of post-stage-hypnosis psychopathology that is both dramatic and interesting from a medical and psychological point of view.

A girl in her mid-teens, P, naively participated in a hypnotic entertainment program during a holiday party. Among other demonstrations, the suggestion was given that her body would become "as hard as a steel rod." She was then suspended between two chairs, and the hypnotist stood on her abdomen to demonstrate the efficacy of the suggestion. Following this, he suggested that "she would wake up feeling like a good, nice, and happy girl." Her companions informed the hypnotist that she felt drowsy and unwell. He responded that "she should go home and sleep it off for a few hours and then everything will be OK." On her way home, still feeling drowsy and unwell, she was taken to a first-aid clinic where she received an intramuscular injection of diazepam 5 mg. This did not help, and 30 minutes later at home her condition worsened, and she gradually fell into a stuporous state. Her family physician referred her—as an emergency—to the regional general hospital.

The hospital admission report stated that she had participated in a stage-hypnosis performance and that it had not been possible to arouse her. Questioning of P's parents and family revealed no previous signs of physical or emotional disorder or particular problems in her behavior, although she was rather shy, passive, and strongly attached to her home and family. About one month previously, she had experienced an episode of urinary retention for two days during her father's hospitalization for fainting during a febrile illness. Catheterization was performed, and the problem disappeared.

Upon admission to the emergency room, she was lying with tightly closed eyes, and although responding to simple commands, she would not answer questions and remained mute and rigid. Vital signs were within normal limits, and all clinical examinations, including neurologic assessment and routine laboratory examinations, showed no pathological findings. A diagnosis of "probable hysteria" was made.

At this point, the stage-hypnotist was summoned. He assumed a harsh authoritarian approach and succeeded in temporarily partly arousing her to a confused and incoherent state. An intravenous infusion was started, and since urinary retention developed, she was catheterized. Chlorpromazine 25 mg and diazepam 10 mg were given intramuscularly.

On the second day, another hypnotist, in response to news reports, volunteered to attempt to "awaken" her. This attempt included shouting and pricking her with pins. She did rise from her bed and took a few steps. However, she walked discoordinately, with closed eyes and after a few minutes went back into her stuporous state.

Since P did not respond to treatment, acute organic brain syndrome was considered. Negative results from a full neurological examination, including EEG and lumber puncture, eliminated this diagnosis. On the third day she was given methylphenidate 10 mg intramuscularly in a vain attempt to awaken her. Further psychopharmacological approaches included haloperidol 2.5 mg and promethazine 10 mg, with no results.

Four days went by. The hospital records stated that she was aimlessly turning her head and rolling her eyes. She did not respond to stimulation, including pain, sound, smell, or light. Further from the records: "She is negativistic and in a completely dissociated state, that seemingly has no direct connection with the post-hypnotic state." In the evening, in order to induce physiological sleep and normal awakening, pentothal 150 mg was given intravenously. Again there were no results. By the sixth day of hospitalization, P had developed secondary complications including a urinary tract infection for which antibiotic therapy was prescribed. As a last alternative, electroconvulsive treatment was contemplated.

I was called in on the seventh day because of my status as a psychiatrist practicing hypnosis. I found P's condition as described, rigid, nonresponsive, mute. Her eyes were closed, but there was the discernible fluttering of her eyelids so commonly seen in hypnotized subjects. I immediately began to introduce myself into what I assumed to be her disrupted hypnotic "rapport." I raised and lowered P's arm in an attempt to indicate my physical presence and reassurance. In a soothing and monotonous voice I said, "I am a doctor and a very good hypnotist too. I know that you were hypnotized. I am a much better and stronger hypnotist than the man who hypnotized you. If you are willing to let me help you, I will. I am able to help you. If you want me to help you, you can hear me. I will help you." At this stage, I decided to use the fluttering of P's eyelids as a starting point for communication. I continued, "Are you willing to let me help you? If yes, please try to open your eyes, and if no, try to close them tightly." I was trying to connect opening her eyes with "being awake" and closing them with her stuporous condition. She responded by lifting her eyebrows, and I continued, "Good . . . very good . . . . . . now we, together, will try to open your eyes." I explained that, for the time being, she could respond to my questions by a "yes" or "no" answer by means of her eyebrows. I proceeded to cover her right hand with mine and closed it while saying to her, "Now I shall close your hand, the hand closest to me . . . . Now I have closed your hand . . . . your hand is closed . . . is tightly closed . . . as tightly closed as your eyes . . . . In a while I shall open your hand . . . . when I open your hand, your eyes will also open . . . . Now I am opening your hand, and your eyes are opening . . . . Now your hand is open . . . . Now your eyes are open." She opened her eyes, but the eyeballs were rolled up in the sockets, obviously failing to see anything. I went on, "Fine . . . very good . . . you are able to open your eyes . . . . Now I am closing your hand again . . . . When I open your hand, you will open your eyes again and you will see something . . . . I do not know what you will see. . . but you will see something." When I opened her hand, she focused her eyes and looked at me.

"Now I shall close and open your hand again, and when I do so, you will be able to answer me in words . . . in your own voice . . . do you agree?" Her eyebrows showed a positive answer. I then proceeded to very slowly close and open her hand while saying, "Do you hear me?" She responded, first faintly and then audibly, "Yes." I reacted, "Very good . . . from now on, after I close your hand, you are going to be able to open it by yourself," and then "Now . . . when you open your hand, you again will see something . . . good . . . . What do you see?" She replied, "Your eyeglasses," and from there to "Eyes," "nose," "mouth," and finally "your face." Soon I gave her also the control of closing her hand, so that my control gradually was totally transferred to her. I also established her control by always asking "Do you agree?" and "When?" before any suggestion was put into effect, and I never used the imperative case. P's sight was completely restored in several steps, and in the same tedious step-by-step procedure she was led to the recovery of hearing, touch, and smell, and her speech was broadened from the simple one-word answers to the conversational dialogue. P complained that she did not feel her body, so body and proprioceptive perception were restored. This step was accompanied by bodily relaxation, movements, and clear signs of pain. Suggestions were given to alleviate her discomfort and pain. She refused at first to eat or drink, saying that she felt no need. After seven days of fasting, clearly her senses of thirst, hunger, and taste had to be aroused. Once this was done, she was able to drink and eat, and shortly the intravenous feeding and catheterization were discontinued.

These steps required four hours of uninterrupted contact. An essential part of the dehypnotization treatment was to reestablish her injured sense of self-control. Thus, I let her set the pace and assume control of what was happening to her. After a short break, we went back to work. It became apparent that P was suffering from total amnesia; she refused a reunion with her family and explained that she could not remember them, her name, address, neighborhood, or anything about herself and her past. Again I applied the same technique, but by now I was giving only directions. All the "closing-opening" of her hand was voluntary, and only occasionally, at her request, would I "help" her. Her requests for help were interpreted as a need for contact and reassurance when she had to deal with more traumatic events. After her memory of self, parents, and past events was restored, it was necessary to restore her memory of the hypnotic experience itself. The process proved to be quite difficult since the experience had been traumatic, as was the hospitalization. After about eight hours of intense interaction, the session ended with a successful reunion with her family.

Over the next three days, long daily sessions were held with P. She tried to prolong and turn them into friendly chats while avoiding any direct discussion of her problems. This attitude and her coquettish behavior showed a transferential relationship toward me. Although the need for further therapy to deal with P's transference and conflicts was obvious, she acknowledged the pragmatic difficulty of continuing treatment in face of the geographical distance (85 miles each way), and the high expenses involved, which she could not afford. Despite her feelings of rejection, P agreed to be referred to a local psychiatrist for further therapy.

P was released from the hospital on the tenth day. Three months later she requested to see me for difficulties in concentration, irritability, weakness, and general distress. The day before she was to see me, she relapsed into her previous stuporous condition and was rehospitalized. Therapeutic procedures were directed as before, but recovery this time proved to be more difficult; for some time she "refused" to regain her sight. I took a more firm and directive approach. After three days P was released from the hospital and this time decided that in spite of the practical difficulties it was essential to find a way to continue therapy. A supportive-dynamic psychotherapeutic relationship was continued for six months on a once-a-week basis. During this period, a full psychological evaluation was carried out, including Bender, WAIS, Rorschach, and TAT. The evaluation described an introverted girl who was closely attached to her family, rather quiet, with few outside interests, of average intelligence, and with tendency to be concrete. She was described as passive in interpersonal relationships and avoiding possible sexual interpretations and meanings. She dealt with inner feelings of anger and aggression, when aroused, by negativistic behavior and by "closing off" from the outside world. Repression was her main ego-defense mechanism.

After six months, P was feeling better and functioning, so we discontinued therapy by mutual consent and agreed to maintain contact through sporadic follow-up sessions and letters, depending on her needs. Follow-up contact was maintained for five years. On our last contact, although complaining of some irritability and difficulty in concentration, she happily announced that she was to be married.

*Discussion*

Even before actually seeing P, I had a few preconceptions. On the basis of medical reports I knew that

- She was in stuporous condition, rigid and unresponsive.
- Immediately preceding this condition, she had participated in a stage-hypnosis performance, and she felt drowsy and unwell afterwards.
- She had been hospitalized for seven days.
- All clinical and laboratory examinations performed showed no pathology, and psychopharmacological treatments were not successful.
- She was reported to be rather shy, obedient, and strongly attached to home and family, and one month previously she had suffered an episode of urinary retention requiring catheterization during her father's hospitalization.

On the basis of such limited information, I speculated that deep and strongly repressed conflicts had been triggered by the stage-hypnosis experience. These, in addition to iatrogenic factors, could have been responsible for P's condition, which seemed to be a self-reinduction or continuation of the hypnotic experience.

Through her main ego-defense mechanism—repression—and by the reaction of negativism and withdrawal as a response to strong feelings of anger and aggression, this rather dependent girl had maintained an homeostatic balance that allowed her to function more or less smoothly and without overt symptomatology, except for that incident of urinary retention, which does hint of some specific conflict. The explosively charged symbolism of the stage-hypnosis experience in a passive-aggressive personality, strengthened by the associations, feelings and connotations aroused by the hypnotist standing on her abdomen, aroused in P an intense and mounting anxiety. Furthermore, the hypnotist's unconcerned response when asked to take care of her because she was feeling drowsy and unwell aroused deep feelings of frustration and rejection and, consequently, mounting anger, aggression, and rage, feelings that she could not express. There was also a complex transferential relationship with the hypnotist, so that his faulty and incomplete dehypnotization procedures and her weakened ego-defense mechanisms created optimal conditions in which her repressed wishes, past experiences, feelings, and conflicts threatened to "break through." Under such circumstances, the suggested rigidity, with both its real and symbolic meanings, became an extremely appropriate suggestion for the resolution of the intricate emotional situation. She adopted the suggestion of "being an iron rod" in a reified way. By doing so she could strengthen her repression and mobilize her negativism and "closing-off" reaction from the outside world to defend herself from the impending threat to her ego integrity.

These psychodynamic factors plus the influence of iatrogenic elements such as faulty evaluation of the stage-hypnosis experience, psychopharmacological treatments, the atmosphere of the emergency room, and the outspoken reaction of the medical staff to the unsuccessful attempts to treat her and to the news reports created in P a vicious circle of anxiety and further mobilization of her defense response. These combined factors may explain, at least partly, the prolongation of her reaction.

Returning to her community was difficult for P to cope with. Her case had been widely publicized for ten days, and she found herself to be a figure of notoriety in her home town. Friends, teachers, storeowners—the entire web of her past social networks—all knew and responded to her as a figure of the mass media. She could not fit into her past role relationships, and she was unable to build a new therapeutic relationship after the "broken" unresolved transference with me. All this frustration, anger, and aggression combined to raise her distress and anxiety to an overwhelming point. Three months after her release, she overcame her reluctance and asked for an interview with me. Immediately before her appointment, she used the former psychopathological reaction that she had now "learned," in order to cope with the mounting strain. She simultaneously communicated her feelings of anger and aggression and tried to punish and control me and ensure the renewal of our disrupted relationship.

In order to change her patterns of coping with the stress of her daily life and to encourage a new homeostasis, I adopted an eclectic psychotherapeutic approach. Her reaction to the community behavior required supportive and behavioristic approaches and techniques, and her inner conflicts and consequent transferential relationship had to be "worked through" by an interpretative-dynamic approach before we could—by mutual consent—end the psychotherapeutic relationship.

In conclusion, it seems to me that this case clearly shows the need for flexibility in adapting our psychotherapeutic strategies to the individual patient. P's treatment was characterized by the use of a step-by-step technique and by the fluctuating use of suggestive, supportive, behavioral, and psychodynamic techniques in a developing psychotherapeutic relationship.

## REFERENCE

Kleinhauz, M., Dreyfuss, D.A., Beran, B., Goldberg, T. & Azikri, D. Some after effects of stage hypnosis: A case study of psychopathological manifestations, *The International Journal of Clinical and Experimental Hypnosis*. 1979, *27*, 219-226.

PART IX

# *Ericksonian Approaches in Medicine*

*David B. Cheek, M.D., an obstetrician and surgeon in San Francisco, is a past president of the American Society of Clinical Hypnosis. Cheek has published numerous articles on the topic of hypnosis and co-authored a text with Leslie Le Cron entitled* Clinical Hypnotherapy. *Cheek is one of the world's leading authorities on medical hypnosis and has written extensively about the ability of surgical patients to hear and be aware of what is happening in the operating room even though they are under anesthesia. Through hypnosis, ideomotor finger signals can be used to retrieve information heard by the anesthesized patient.*

*John Corley, M.D., is a professor and chief of the Division of Education, Department of Family Practice, Medical University of South Carolina. A Canadian, he practiced general medicine in Calgary for 25 years before accepting a faculty appointment in South Carolina. Corley has been a friend of the Erickson family for almost 30 years.*

*Therapy should center on eliciting adaptation from within the patient. This is a philosophy that must permeate medical practice; it is not a principle to which one should just pay lip service. The therapist should be cognizant of the patient's capacity to respond to appropriately presented ideas.*

*Chong Tong Mun, M.D., has conducted a general practice in Singapore since 1958, and is a clinical instructor at the University of Singapore. Chong has used hypnosis in his practice for almost 20 years.*

*Chong delineates principles of Ericksonian practice that are important in general medicine and provides case examples of successful use of Ericksonian techniques. The general practitioner should be cognizant of the crucial importance of psychological factors in promoting healing and of the plethora of possible uses of hypnotic technique in medicine.*

Chapter 23

# Some of Erickson's Contributions to Medicine

*David B. Cheek*

Erickson lives on. He has influenced all of us who have been ready to recognize the value of hypnosis in the healing arts. That influence will continue through his writings and the vivid imprintings he left with the students lucky enough to have had personal contact with him through the years.

Erickson was a shining example of the Hippocratic ideal: "In order to cure the human body it is necessary to have a knowledge of the whole of things."

He spent minimal time searching for causes. Among his gifts was a genius for inventing interesting ways to help people overcome old problems. He was delighted when his patients succeeded, but he respected their right to fail when this seemed necessary.

His powers of perception led many of us to feel he was clairvoyant. Erickson denied such a ridiculous idea.

## HIS CONTRIBUTIONS: GYNECOLOGY, OBSTETRICS, UROLOGY

Erickson helped women recognize their right to sexual responsiveness and men overcome sexual fears (1958).

He taught women ways to stop abnormal uterine bleeding due to anger and depression at a time when most obstetricians and gynecologists were ignoring emotional causality (1960b).

Erickson showed pregnant women how they could sit across the room and, employing imagery, watch their physical body have uterine contractions. He taught them that they need not be uncomfortable with labor, that they could center their attention elsewhere, to sequential events of the past. He recognized the ability of the mid-brain reticular activating system in attending to one set of experiences while ignoring another. He never claimed a parochial right to discovery in his methods, being familiar with world literature and recognizing that children are masters of this art. Finally, like Grantly Dick-Read and Frederick Leboyer, Erickson believed childbirth should be considered a natural process, not a disease. Babies have a right to enter the world without feeling guilt over a mother's discomfort.

## ERICKSON AND BODY IMAGE

Erickson recognized the importance of healthy body imagery. He used hypnosis to help at least two young women allow their breasts to grow in response to their own hormones. They had previously inhibited such interaction, considering themselves unfeminine and unattractive (1960a).

In 1960 he told me about a 20-year-old man who grew 12 inches in height in the span of one year. In hypnosis, at the start of therapy, this stunted young man looked out on his world as though unwilling to grow, a modern-day Peter Pan. For example, he described a room as though he were standing beneath a table. Similarly, a cow on his farm was visualized as though it were ten feet tall; his eyes were on a level with the cow's udder. Growth began to take place when Erickson encouraged the man to hallucinate his world as though he were standing part way up a staircase.

I said, "Why have you kept this report out of the literature?"

Erickson smiled and said, "No respectable editor of a scientific journal would publish such an impossible thing."

"Dr. Erickson," I answered, "You are the editor of a respectable journal."

He smiled again and said, "I would like to keep my job."

## SPONTANEOUS HYPNOSIS WHILE REMEMBERING SEQUENTIAL EVENTS

In my opinion, one of Erickson's greatest contributions to the broad field of medicine was his early observation that people go into hypnosis when they attempt to remember sequential experiences (1961). This realization allowed him to go directly to the task of healing without wasting time with formal induction methods. Utilizing this insight has permitted many of us to continue our use of hypnosis when others have abandoned hypnotherapy, believing it to be too time-consuming to be practical.

## SPONTANEOUS HYPNOSIS TO CARRY OUT POST-HYPNOTIC SUGGESTION

Betty Erickson shares credit with her husband for recognizing that people carrying out post-hypnotic suggestions reenter trance in order to satisfy the request (1941). What a help this concept has been in facilitating the use of hypnosis during subsequent interviews!

## ERICKSON AND AWARENESS UNDER ANESTHESIA

In 1954 I heard both Erickson and Le Cron say that surgeons and anesthetists should be careful about what they say in the presence of an anesthetized patient. I had been concerned about this possibility, stemming from personal experience with an operation while in college, but all my efforts to explore this matter with hypnosis had failed. While assisting Le Cron in another workshop, I accidentally discovered the reason for those previous failures (Cheek, 1959).

I presented this accidental revelation to Milton. He then casually and gently introduced me to his classic paper of 1937 reporting interviews with a man who had been drugged and beaten into unconsciousness. There was no conscious memory of the experience or the events leading to his period of unconsciousness. Through repetitive subconscious reviews of the events preceding the period of unconsciousness, the man remembered steps along the way and finally relived the period of unconsciousness.

In his study with this man Erickson was working at a conversational level, but he was also forcing his subject to subconsciously review the sequential events preceding his comatose state. My accidental discovery in 1957 was that the process of repetitive subconscious review could be carried out in a very short space of world time if the hypnotized subject was restrained from making any effort to recall events at a talking level of memory. I could see the start and the finish of the review indicated by unconscious movements of designated fingers. Other factors involved accelerated retrieval of events during unconscious states as follows:

1) I must choose words which confidently project the idea that memory is possible and expected.
2) I must keep my subject from prematurely talking about an event before he recognizes a finger has lifted unconsciously, signalling he is ready to remember.
3) I must ask for and obtain permission for him to know consciously, and to tell me what he has learned.

4) Every repetition of a traumatic experience at a subconscious level of awareness diminishes its emotional impact, apparently pushing it progressively into the past.

Adhering to these rules, it is possible to learn very quickly (within five minutes of training the patient to use ideomotor signals) whether or not an experience under general anesthesia has been stressful, and whether or not its influence has been damaging.

Interview time with traumatic experiences will vary from minutes to hours depending on the gravity of the experience. When the impact has become too great to handle at conversational levels of awareness, it is sometimes possible to have the patient invert the experience by reporting the operation as if all the *right* things had been said and done to make it a pleasant experience. This strategy has proven therapeutic. The patient can be urged to let this recreated experience replace the real one, a method I have found very helpful for correcting harmful imprintings at birth.

Erickson explained to me that his interest in continued hearing ability during general anesthesia resulted from a very stressful experience which he later documented (Erickson, 1963). He said that his personal experience and his findings with patients led him to believe that anesthetized people are aware of everything around them, yet they pay great attention only to what they consider *meaningful* at the moment. This could be something frightening or reassuring. Even silence at a critical moment could be meaningful.

The word *meaningful,* therefore, became an important part of the title to my first paper on the subject of continued hearing.

## ERICKSON THE JOURNAL EDITOR

Part of my homage to Milton Erickson concerns his open-mindedness as first editor of the *American Journal of Clinical Hypnosis* from 1958 to 1968.

He both stimulated me to explore continued hearing ability and led me to present a paper on this subject at the First Scientific Meeting of the American Society of Clinical Hypnosis in 1958. He then mildly coerced me into writing it up for publication at a time when I know no other journal reporting on findings relating to surgery or anesthesiology would have given me encouragement or space.

Erickson published corroborating papers by Wolfe and Millet (1960),

Hutchings (1961), Pearson (1961), Brunn (1963) and Kolouch (1964). He went on to publish six other papers of mine on this subject (Cheek, 1960, a, b, 1962, 1963, 1964, a, b).

During the 21 years since publication of my first paper on anesthesia awareness, there have been various reports by nonhypnotically oriented anesthesiologists. Some of them have limited themselves to asking patients on awakening whether or not they heard anything or "dreamed" anything during the operation. These authors were satisfied that any "awareness" that could be reported verbally was related to inadequate amounts of anesthetic agent or faults within the equipment used.

A study by Terrell, Sweet, Gladfelter and Stephen (1969) showed that anesthetized persons were unable to hear. Of researchers using prospective tests with sounds transmitted to patients during surgery, only Wolfe, Hutchings and Levinson (1965, 1969), have respected the meaningfulness of information and timing. Retrospective studies have shown that persons under general anesthesia are troubled by earphones that keep them from attending to sounds in the operating room. Generally, patients are attuned to the voices of the surgeon, his assistant and the anesthetist, but they are tuned in at understandably selective moments.

Until the incision is made and after the incision is closed patients are attentive to the anesthetist. The rest of the time attention is directed toward surgeon and assistant. To expect anesthetized people to care what is said by an unknown voice on a tape recording transmitted through earphones is to underestimate the reticular activating system of the midbrain. Certainly no commonly used anesthetic obliterates ability of the primitive brain to continue its contact with the outside world. All sensory input comes into the brain stem regardless of what is happening to the much more vulnerable cerebral cortex.

In addition to my thanks to Milton Erickson, I would like to thank anesthesiologists David Scott of England (1974), Bernard Levinson of South Africa (1965, 1969) and Jean Lassner of France, who very kindly translated my first paper into French. Each of these men has helped spread the idea that people under anesthesia are listening, that their understandings are literal and childlike, that what has been frightening to them during a period of unconsciousness is not resolved by reassurance or contradiction after they have regained consciousness.

I will be forever grateful to Milton Erickson for his friendship, encouragement and wisdom. I am not alone in expressing gratitude to this great teacher, writer, editor, and humanitarian.

## REFERENCES


Brunn, J.T. The capacity to hear, understand, and to remember experiences during chemo-anesthesia: A personal experience. *American Journal of Clinical Hypnosis*, 1963, *6*, 27-30.

Cheek, D.B. Unconscious perception of meaningful sounds during surgical anesthesia as revealed under hypnosis. *American Journal of Clinical Hypnosis*, 1959, *1*, 101-113.

Cheek, D.B. Use of preoperative hypnosis to protect patients from careless conversation. *American Journal of Clinical Hypnosis*, 1960(a), *3*, 101-102.

Cheek, D.B. Removal of subconscious resistance to hypnosis using ideomotor questioning techniques. *American Journal of Clinical Hypnosis* 1960(b), *3*, 103-107.

Cheek, D.B. Importance of recognizing that surgical patients behave as though hypnotized. *American Journal of Clinical Hypnosis* 1962, *4*, 227-236.

Cheek, D.B. Physiological impact of fear in dreams: Post operative hemorrhage. Case report. *American Journal of Clinical Hypnosis*, 1963, *5*, 206-208.

Cheek, D.B. Surgical memory and reaction to careless conversation. *American Journal of Clinical Hypnosis*, 1964(a), *6*, 237-240.

Cheek, D.B. Further evidence of persistence of hearing under chemo-anesthesia. Case report. *American Journal of Clinical Hypnosis*, 1964(b), *7*, 55-59.

Erickson, M.H. Development of apparent unconsciousness during hypnotic reliving of a traumatic experience. *Archives of Neurology and Psychiatry*, 1937, *38*, 1282-1288.

Erickson, M.H. Naturalistic techniques of hypnosis. *American Journal of Clinical Hypnosis*, 1958, *1*, 3-8.

Erickson, M.H. Breast development possibly influenced by hypnosis. Two instances and the psychotherapeutic results. *American Journal of Clinical Hypnosis*, 1960 (a), *2*, 157-159.

Erickson, M.H. Psychogenic alteration of menstrual function. *American Journal of Clinical Hypnosis*, 1960 (b), *2*, 227-231.

Erickson, M.H. Historical note on the hand levitation and other ideomotor techniques. *American Journal of Clinical Hypnosis*, 1961, *3*, 196-199.

Erickson, M.H. Chemo-anesthesia in relation to hearing and memory. *American Journal of Clinical Hypnosis*, 1963, *6*, 31-36.

Erickson, M.H. & Erickson, E.M. Concerning the nature and character of post-hypnotic behavior. *Journal of General Psychology*, 1941, *2*, 95-133. (Reprinted by Kuhn, L. & Russo, S. *Modern Hypnosis*. Wilshire Book Company, Hollywood, 1958, pp 105-142.)

Hutchings, D.D. The value of suggestion given under anesthesia: A report and evaluation of 200 consecutive cases. *American Journal of Clinical Hypnosis*, 1961, *4*, 26-29.

Kolouch, F. Hypnosis and surgical convalescence: A study, of subjective factors in post-operative recovery. *American Journal of Clinical Hypnosis*, 1964, *7*, 120-129.

Lassner, J. Memoire auditive sous anesthesie generale revelee par l'hypnosis. *Cahiers d'Anesthesiologic*, 1965, *13*, 105-127 (translation of Cheek, 1959, Unconscious perception, etc.).

Levinson, B. States of awareness under general anesthesia. *British Journal of Anaesthesiology*, 1965, *37*, 544-546.

Levinson, B. An Examination of States of Awareness During General Anaesthesia. Monograph, Doctoral Thesis, 1969, Unpublished.

Pearson, R.E. Response to suggestions given under general anesthesia. *American Journal of Clinical Hypnosis*, 1961, *4*, 106-114.

Scott, D. *Modern Hospital Hypnosis*. Chicago: Year Book Medical Publishers, 1974, pp. 143-148.

Terrell, R.K., Sweet, W.O., Gladfelter, J.H. & Stephen, C.R. A study of recall during anesthesia. *Anesthesia & Analgesia*, 1969, *48*, 86-90.

Wolfe, L.S. & Millet, J.B. Control of postoperative pain by suggestion under general anesthesia. *American Journal of Clinical Hypnosis*, 1960, *3*, 109-112.

Chapter 24

# Ericksonian Techniques with General Medical Problems

*John B. Corley*

In the fifties I was introduced to hypnosis when I attended a workshop in Banff which was presided over by Milton Erickson. I then belatedly perceived that hypnosis was a neglected medical modality with broad applications in general medicine.

Milton eventually became a friend, a teacher, and a tutor. For years, we maintained a continuing correspondence, Milton utilizing the secretarial services of Roger (the canine member of the Erickson family). Late at night, Roger would write voluminous letters on a yellow pad, his handwriting bearing a curious resemblance to Milton's. He would describe patients his master had encountered that day, how the problems had been approached and the difficulties and the successes that had ensued. My replies to Roger were in a similar vein and Roger would subsequently comment upon difficulties I had encountered and suggest alternative approaches that I might consider. While I never came even close to developing the unique skills that my friend and preceptor possessed, I did become comfortable with the utilization of this neglected modality as I continued to deal with general medical problems. As a practicing physician, I would have been as lost without my ability to utilize hypnosis as I would have been had I lost my stethoscope.

What were the Erickson techniques that I found so applicable to general medicine? I do not favor the term "techniques." I was never able to learn how to implement many of Milton's specific techniques. For instance, he spent a morning in my home trying to teach me his celebrated "confusion technique." I comprehended the principle but I was never able to learn how to apply it. Whenever I tried, I wound up as confused as my patient. Rather than the term "techniques," I prefer to speak of principles and practices which Milton taught and which have stood me, and will stand all of us, in good stead when we wish to utilize the medical therapeutic modality of hypnosis. I can illustrate one principle with a story:

The first day I spent with the Ericksons in Phoenix, many years ago, I sought Milton's help in trying to comprehend, "What is hypnosis?" I asked him that question early in the afternoon and he hummed and hedged and refused to answer. I was a little turned off by this obvious refusal. That evening the Ericksons took my wife and I out to dinner. During a lull in the conversation, I repeated my question. Again Milton beat around the bush and refused to answer. This time even Betty became annoyed and for the first time, and the only time in my presence, sharply scolded Milton. "John asked you a straightforward question. He is entitled to a straightforward answer." Betty got no further with him than I had and there was a momentary strain around the dinner table until my wife tactfully inquired about the Erickson children. Milton could never refuse that bait. The tension broke, we all relaxed and had a pleasant evening—but my question remained unanswered.

During the following days, I observed Milton working with his patients. Various behaviors would be evoked—profound relaxation, anesthesia, amnesia, age regression, acquisition of new insights, etc.—and then Milton would turn his quizzical eyes on me and ask, "Is that hypnosis, John?" I slowly appreciated that Milton—in his own way—and, in the only possible way, was answering my question, "What is hypnosis?" Milton had no intention of becoming involved in unprofitable metaphysics or quasi-scientific definitions. The patients were real. They presented personal problems. As a physician, Milton accepted the responsibility of helping them cope better with problems. He made no pretense of being a magician. He had simply learned that patients could be assisted in managing their problems more effectively by eliciting and experiencing the behavioral responses which we, for lack of a more precise definition, call hypnosis.

This refusal to play games and to pretend to know that which nobody truly knows is well illustrated in *Hypnotic Realities* (Erickson, Rossi, & Rossi, 1976). In the discussion of "Rapport in Mutual Hypnosis," Erickson noted that patients often look right at you without really paying any attention to you. Ernest Rossi was quoted as saying, "Yes, they will have a faraway look in their eyes," and Milton then asked "But can you define that faraway look in their eyes?" Again he was addressing the issue of defining hypnosis. Rossi, as you may remember, replied, "That would be difficult. You are really saying, Milton, that this comes only with experience until it becomes almost unconscious intuitive knowledge on your part." Milton simply replied, "Yes."

This was the first principle that I learned from Milton, namely, *one does not have to define consciousness to recognize conscious behavior.* One does not have to define sadness or pain or distress to recognize sadness or pain or distress in a patient. As a physician, Milton was saying, you must work diligently to acquire the intuitive skill to recognize the character and nature of the presenting problem and learn to respond to the patient's implicit (if muted) plea for help and support. Don't be distracted by your failure to explicitly define the precise character of the plea. Be content to learn to recognize it and to respond appropriately.

What else did Milton teach me as I struggled to incorporate hypnosis into my practice of general medicine?

Next is a complex truth which, in its complexity, expresses a very simple observation: *"Patients are thinking, feeling creatures, possessed of an innate capacity to formulate ideas and understandings and capable of integrating them into their total experiential comprehension"* if only the physician will—as Milton always tried to do—provide the requisite guidance. Milton carried these observations further by reminding me that while all of us possess this capacity of formulating, comprehending and absorbing new concepts and deeper understanding of ourselves, "We only can do this in accord with the actual functioning processes we ourselves possess." It was Milton's unique skill to recognize intuitively "the actual functioning processes" which each individual patient personally possesses, and then to utilize the patient's own resources in therapy. Obviously, Milton could not impart his intuitive skills to others, but he could and did teach us to appreciate what he taught, and he did inspire us to struggle to do, as best we could, what he did intuitively and with consummate skill.

Another of Milton's cardinal principles was that *physicians must respect, and continually acknowledge, a patient's right to be a person.* One day Milton was teaching a young woman how to cope with dysmenorrhea. He had succeeded in teaching her how to have her menstruations with minimal discomfort. She was very grateful. It was their final formal session. She had quickly entered a hypnotic trance and she and Milton were discussing what she had accomplished: "You now know how to experience your menstruation with little or no discomfort. But remember, if at any time you feel your husband or your children are making unreasonable demands upon you or are taking you far too much for granted—and you believe you deserve and need a little more attention, you are perfectly free to suffer a little misery and so gain the attention you need. But, do the cramps have to be so severe?" Even in the deep trance she was in, it was apparent the young lady appreciated Milton's statement, and acknowledged that she did, indeed, retain that privilege and that right. Milton simply gave her his unconditional permission to exercise her rights as a person, in accordance with her needs. But the implication was clear, to the three of us, that it was not likely that she would find it necessary to exercise *that* right because of what Milton had helped her learn about herself and about her own capabilities as a "thinking, feeling creature" in her own right.

Another truth that Milton vividly illustrated many times was that, even in a deep trance, *the patient and the hypnotist are continually communicating with one another.* The doctor's communications tend to be quite obvious, even when nonverbal. The patient's communications will necessarily be subtle—a fleeting quiver of the lips, a brief muscular contraction of a finger, etc.—but the communications will be there if one is trained, as Milton was, to be intently observant of the slightest nuance of a patient's reaction to a word, a phrase, a suggestion. The applicability of this truth in general medical practice is universal whenever a physician-patient encounter occurs. How many times does the doctor remain blissfully unaware of even very obvious communications? How often do patients struggle to express a need as the physician talks and talks—totally absorbed in the sound of his own voice and tragically insensitive to responses and reactions of the patient? These basic truths have everyday applicability to the general practice of medicine, quite apart from their specific utilization in hypnotherapy.

In summary, these are a few of the principles that Milton taught me which have applicability to general medicine:

1) It is not necessary to be able to define a concept in order to recognize the behavior. The physician must train himself to recognize intuitively the real nature of the presenting problem with which the patient needs help.
2) Never underestimate what a patient is capable of understanding, comprehending, and learning but stay within the framework of the patient's personal functioning processes.
3) Respect each individual patient as a person with every right to be himself—to be a person according to his values and his needs. Never judge. Never preach. Learn to tactfully offer suggestions and alternatives that are within the patient's capacity to comprehend, initiate and activate for his, not your, benefit.

4) Remain eternally alert to the fact that, regardless of the apparent depth of a trance, the patient and you are continually communicating with each other. Be sensitive to subtle communications. They will be present. Recognize them and learn to respond appropriately to them. This is your obligatory responsibility.
5) Formal hypnotic inductions are rarely necessary when working with patients. Should it be appropriate to induce hypnosis, use whatever is already happening between you and the patient to promote your goal of teaching the patient what he is capable of achieving. If the patient is in tears you may be unaware as to precisely why this patient is crying, but that, at the moment, is irrelevant. Therefore, one might slowly say, "It is good sometimes, isn't it, to cry. It really helps, doesn't it, sometimes to just let go. And it is a good feeling, isn't it, when you do let go. How easy it really is to truly let everything go and slowly then, just to become relaxed. Tears are good, tears are healthy, tears really help, but perhaps now is the time to let the tears dry up."

## REFERENCE

Erickson, M.H., Rossi, E.L., & Rossi, S.I. *Hypnotic Realities: The Induction of Clinical Hypnosis and Forms of Indirect Suggestion.* New York: Irvington, 1976.

Chapter 25

# Ericksonian Approaches in General Practice

*Chong Tong Mun*

I personally believe that all therapies, whether chemotherapy or psychotherapies with or without hypnosis, and possibly even surgical procedures, must be presented to the patient "in such a fashion that he will be most receptive to the presented therapies and thereby motivated to explore his own body's potentials for a successful outcome." Erickson (1965) stressed that in all therapies, "It is important for the patient to be receptive of the therapies and cooperative in regard to them. Without the patient's full cooperativeness, therapeutic results are delayed, distorted, limited or even prevented" (p. 57). I fully agree with Erickson. In my practice, I always stress to the patient that the injection he is to receive or a certain pill given to him will relieve his symptoms. It really does not matter whether the medication was actually specific for these purposes so long as the beneficial results desired are stressed emphatically and confidently. One cannot depend on the pharmacological action of the drug alone. We all know that the pharmacological action of a drug can be potentiated, inhibited, altered, or even reversed by many factors (Claridge, 1970).

The patient's needs, cultural background, and belief system are of great importance. Wolberg (1972) cited the case of a psychiatrist from an African country, who was the son of a chieftain in a primitive part of that country. He had been educated in England both as a physician and as a psychoanalyst. His objective was to go back to the locale where he had been raised and bring scientific, non-magical psychiatry to the native population. He did so. He found that he was almost completely ineffective. When a tribesman became depressed or developed anxiety or a phobia, he was likely to react favorably to a witch doctor, who diagnosed the type of spirit infestation and then prescribed appropriate rituals accepted by the group to be specifically designed for his trouble. However, when the doctor tried to apply what we would call scientific psychiatry to the problems of his people, it resulted in failure. There was no traditional acceptance of his methodology. The natives could not relate to what he was doing.

There is a common belief in certain Chinese sections of Singapore that it is better to consult a "traditional doctor" than one trained in modern medicine when one suffers from nasal obstruction or discharge, since the former skillfully extracts "the dragons in the nose," small bloody pieces of tissue, and presents them to the patient, who experiences dramatic relief. Histological studies made of such tissue have disclosed them to be lymph tissue from slaughtered hogs (Shanmugaratnam, 1962). The therapeutic suggestive effects, however, were valid.

Hence, it is not surprising that vasomotor rhinitis based upon emotional states may respond better to suggestion than to chemotherapy not directed to the causative effect. It is for this reason that conventional medical procedures often fail to meet the personality needs of the patient and thus make the public in part dependent upon the charlatan or the unscientific practitioner who satisfies the individual as a personality. Thus, I often oblige a patient with an injection when he demands an injection for his condition. It may not matter what you give him. I find vitamin injections just as effective in such cases where the patients are convinced that nothing short of an injection could cure them.

The most frequent symptom that brings a patient to the doctor is pain. Many factors influence the entity called pain. Some of these factors are emotion, attention, distraction, fear, etc. Erickson (1967) said that "there has been built up within one's body, although all unrecognized, certain psychological, physiological, and neurological learnings, associations and conditionings that render it possible for pain to be controlled and even abolished." He exploited these factors to help his pain patients.

I find this approach for pain patients most useful in general practice. I seldom need to give my patients many analgesics. I usually use less than half the usual dosage. For example, during a mass inoculation of children because of a cholera outbreak, my practice in administering inoculations was to emphasize by emphatic assertions of "no pain, no pain" the painless character of the experience, taking care to begin with the largest child, since, should one begin with the youngest and he should cry, then all the rest would, too. The good response of the larger child favorably influenced the smaller children. Shouting "no pain, no pain" served to distract and to suggest as I quickly plunged the needle into the patient.

I use the same technique to stitch a small wound or to lance an abscess to drain the pus. I do not use local anesthetic in these cases because the injection and infiltration of the anesthetic substance would cause more pain to the patient. For patients coming to me with renal, intestinal, or biliary colic I often find that just treating the underlying infection by an injection or pills would be sufficient without giving any analgesics. In these cases I often tell the patient that the injection or pills he is to receive will also aid in relieving the pain. This must be stressed emphatically and confidently to the patient. In 10 years of obstetric practice in the 1960s I seldom needed to use more than 50 mg of pethedine for pain during childbirth. Episiotomy and simple perineal repairs requiring only one or two stitches were often done without any local anesthetic.

In the management of the cancer patients with intractable pain Erickson's (1967) hypnotic procedures in pain control are often used very successfully. For example, I treated a 40-year-old man who had pain and swelling of his inguinal gland. Biopsy revealed a malignant metastasis from an unknown maligant melanoma. He was given five weeks of deep x-ray therapy followed by chemotherapy with no results. The gland became larger and ulcerated and his thigh became swollen. He suffered from severe intractable pain radiating down his whole leg. He also had headaches, vomiting, and insomnia. Three attempts of subarachnoid injections of alcohol failed to give him any relief. For many weeks preceding hypnosis, he had been kept in a narcotic semi-stupor, since this was the only way to control his pain, enable him to sleep, and enable him to eat without excessive nausea and vomiting. The patient was taught autohypnosis, hallucinations, analgesia and anesthesia, time distortion, amnesia, body disorientation, and dissociation. His narcotic requirement became dramatically reduced. Although bedridden for the last few weeks he continued quite comfortably with minimum narcotics and a complacency and acceptance rarely seen except in the well conditioned hypnotic subject (Chong, 1968).

Another Ericksonian approach is the utilization of the patient's behavior, emotion, and experiences. This approach is useful even in emergency situations. For example, an old man upon whom I made an emergency night call complained of severe pain and vomiting due to a strangulated inguinal hernia. The patient desperately feared the emergency operation that I advised. Instead, he requested injections to control his pain. An explanation was given to him that if he would cooperate fully, the hernia could be reduced, thus rendering an operation unnecessary. He cooperated well. A deep trance was obtained and the hernia was reduced without subsequent complications.

Another example was a case of excessive bleeding that had continued throughout the day, following a dental extraction in a 14-year-old girl. Induction of hypnosis was easily achieved by just asking her to sit on a reclining chair, close her eyes and view her favorite TV program. The girl's state of fear was alleviated and instructions not to suck at the wound nor to prod it with her tongue were given. The patient's relief from her symptoms and absence of fear reactions were most pleasant to behold.

A very painful injection could be made more effective by admitting that it is a very painful injection and a very powerful one. Some injections give an immediate odor after administration. This subjective experience of the patient can be advantageously exploited to increase the therapeutic efficacy, pointing convincingly to the patient how fast the medicine acts.

In medical practice, much depends on how the doctor presents ideas and understandings to the patients. Cough is a common complaint seen in general practice; moreover, the majority of patients presenting cough have no lung pathology. It is often initiated by upper respiratory infections and the cough often drags on for weeks and even months for reasons unknown, perhaps due to emotional or psychological factors. Prolonged coughing in children often leads to bronchial spasms and many of them become asthmatic (Chong, 1969). Because of my success in treating cough, particularly in children, I have a good number of mothers bringing their children to me for this complaint. Often after a few visits, if their cough still persists, I would suggest to the mother in the presence of the child that should the cough not be cured with the present medication, I would use an injection at the next visit. This tactic often accelerated recovery.

The causes of bronchial asthma are multifactorial, and in the majority of cases psychological factors play very important roles in the causation and maintenance of the condition. Attendance to these factors will lead to a successful outcome (Chong, 1977). Usually, the asthmatic patient has a long history of suffering and has sought help from various sources, often to no avail. Such patients by the very nature of their illness are anxious, fearful, and highly motivated in their search for help. Consequently, they are usually good subjects and develop deep trances easily. From my experience hypnotherapy is the treatment of choice for these chronic asthmatics.

Every asthmatic is taught self-hypnosis and exhorted to practice it at least three times daily. In addition, they are taught how to abort an attack. The patient is conditioned under hypnosis that when he feels an attack developing he will sit down or lie down, close his eyes, breathe deeply, then hold that breath deliberately for a brief while; then slowly and comfortably he will exhale with ease and comfort and without fear. This procedure is to be repeated at least five times and has the immeasurable effect of reeducating the patient's breathing attitudes and relieving his fears and tensions; it also tends to abort the attack. Thus, the patient is given the confidence of a ready and sufficient remedy in times of need. In deep trance subjects, it is easy to induce an asthmatic attack and then abort the attack. This will convince the patient of the efficacy of the procedure.

In the management of serious illness, it is important to deal with the psychological component of the illness and to stimulate "the will to live" in the patient. Psychological implications not only hinder but also delay recovery in any illness. Actually, recovery from any illness depends on the patient's ability to restore his own homeostasis. Doubts, fear, apprehension, anxiety and depression act adversely against the patient's defenses and his ability to restore his own homeostasis. Sir William Osler declared, "What happens to a patient with tuberculosis depends more on what he has in his head than what he has in his chest." This is true with all illnesses, for every illness has a psychological overlay.

Even Plato in his day lamented, "For this is the great error of our day . . . that physicians separate the soul from the body." The fact that the mind rules the body, no matter how much it was neglected by biology and medicine, is the most fundamental fact which we observe continuously throughout our lives. All our emotions are expressed through physiological processes: joy by laughing; sorrow by weeping; shame by blushing; despair by sighing; fear by palpitation; anger by increased heat beat, elevation of blood pressure, and a change in the carbohydrate and cholesterol metabolism; and so on. The following two cases of cancer will provide illustration (Chong, 1979).

A 37-year-old man was very much distressed when he was diagnosed as having carcinoma of his stomach requiring surgery. He was very depressed, fearful, and unable to sleep. Two hypnotic sessions turned him from a state of complete despair to one of confident hope. His surgery was also facilitated. He required no sedation before surgery; the amount of thiopentone used was much reduced; he needed only one single injection of omnopon after the operation, and his post-operative convalescence was remarkable. The operation was done in 1964. The pathology report showed poorly differentiated adeno-carcinoma of the stomach, showing considerable areas of carcinomatous simplex appearance. There was right regional node involvement. He is still alive and very happy and fit, although the operating surgeon told his relatives that he had only 12 months to live.

The case of the second patient is equally illustrative. A staff-midwife told her doctor-employer that her father, age 55, had painless hematuria and had consulted a general practitioner two times. He was immediately sent for IVP which showed a hypernephroma of his right kidney. He was persuaded to go for an operation to "cure him" of his condition. He accepted the advice and was soon operated on. Immediately after the operation he was told that he had been "successfully operated upon." He had an uneventful post-operative convalescence and underwent a course of deep x-ray therapy. The pathology report showed "clear cell" renal carcinoma, with chronic pyelonephritis in the adjacent renal tissue. There was an embolus in the renal vein. The operation was done in 1971. He is still alive and well. No formal hypnosis was used in this case. The idea of "cure" and "successfully operated" had been communicated to him both consciously and unconsciously.

Most patients, especially when they are in hospital for surgery, are in a hypersuggestible state and may be treated as though already in a hypnotic state. That psychological intervention in these two cases had helped in their favorable outcome cannot be asserted dogmatically. It is probably that through psychological intervention their belief systems were altered and they did not want to die just yet. Further research should be in the direction of a better understanding of the role of normal and abnormal emotional factors upon the defensive mechanism of the body.

## REFERENCES

Chong, T.M. The use of hypnosis in the management of patients with cancer. *Singapore Med. J.*, 1968, *9*, (3), 211-214.

Chong, T.M. The study of bronchial asthmas in children in Singapore and their management by hypnotherapy. M.D. thesis, Faculty of Medicine, University of Singapore, 1969.

Chong, T. M. The management of bronchial asthmas. *J. Asthma Research*, 1977, *14*(2), 73-89.

Chong, T. M. Psychological intervention in patients with cancer. *Singapore Family Physician*, 1979, *4*(1), 20-25.

Claridge, G. *Drugs and Human Behavior.* Harmondsworth: Pelican Books, 1970.

Erickson, M.H. Hypnosis in painful terminal illness. *Amer. J. Clin. Hyp.*, 1959, *1*, 117-121.

Erickson, M. H. The use of symptoms as an integral part of hypnotherapy. *Amer. J. Clin. Hyp.*, 1965, *8*, 57-65.

Erickson, M.H. An introduction to the study and application of hypnosis for pain control. Proceedings of the International Congress in Hyp. and Psychosom. Med., Paris 1965. New York: Springer-Verlag, 1967.

Shanmugaratnam, K. "Dragon in the nose," an investigation of tissues removed from the nose by unqualified persons in Singapore. *Singapore Med. J.*, 1962, *3*(1), 16-19.

Wolberg, L.R. Some psychiatric and hypnotic considerations of acupuncture. Proceedings of the First Acupuncture Workshops at the Postgraduate Center for Mental Health, New York, June 3, 1972.

PART X

# *Ericksonian Approaches with Children and Adolescents*

*David Rigler, Ph.D., is a clinical psychologist practicing in the Los Angeles area. Formerly he was a clinical professor at the Medical School at the University of Southern California. He also served as the chief psychologist at Children's Hospital in Los Angeles. Rigler discusses the use of Ericksonian techniques as they were practiced at the Children's Hospital and gives examples of ways in which he and his staff made use of hypnosis with medical pediatric patients.*

*Franz Baumann, M.D., is a pediatrician in private practice in San Francisco. Dr. Baumann is the past president of the American Society of Clinical Hypnosis. He is a noted authority in the area of pediatric hypnotherapy and has special expertise treating enuresis.*

*Baumann illustrates the use of naturalistic Ericksonian techniques in pediatric practice. He emphasizes understanding the child's vantage point and using it to elicit adaptive responses. He places special emphasis on symptom utilization, "double bind," and confusion techniques.*

Chapter 26

# Ericksonian Techniques in a Pediatric Hospital

*David Rigler*

When I was invited to submit this paper, my plan was to abstract from the principles and methods taught by Dr. Milton Erickson those especially applicable to a pediatric hospital and to illustrate these principles by means of case examples. I also intended to describe the training program we initiated to train our psychological interns and others in these useful methods.

Events that occurred subsequent to submitting the initial abstract seem almost to require that I revise that plan, and that I begin with an account of circumstances that led me originally to an interest in hypnosis and to the work of Dr. Erickson. And with this I would like to share with you some of the events that followed.

In his foreword to Erickson and Rossi's Casebook, Dr. Sidney Rosen quotes Erickson: "There is nothing more delightful than planting flower seeds and not knowing what kinds of flowers are going to come up." At first glance Erickson seems to be talking about the pleasure of the surprise of seeing the flowers come up. But Erickson frequently distinguished between a process and the end result of that process. Thus, planting seeds can be an interesting activity and important in its own way, irrespective of outcome. Without delving too deeply into the Freudian implications of that observation, consider that seeds may mature into loco weed, stinkweed, poison ivy, or even into sour grapes. What follows in this paper is a brief account of the initial state of the garden patch, the activity of seeding, and the complicated but incompleted harvest.

Let me describe the setting. The Children's Hospital of Los Angeles is a nonprofit community institution affiliated as a teaching center with the School of Medicine of the University of Southern California. It provides primary and advanced medical care for large numbers of children and adolescents in Southern California. Instruction and training are offered there for medical students, residents and advanced fellows, as well as for several health-related disciplines. There is a strong tradition of clinical research, and the hospital has an international reputation as an academic center. Many of the pediatricians who practice in the greater Los Angeles community belong to the hospital's professional staff, but much care is rendered by a full-time faculty and by the resident staff. Although Children's Hospital has a deserved and enviable reputation for being at the forefront in applying up-to-date pediatric knowledge in traditional spheres of medicine and surgery, I think it is fair to characterize its commitment to psychological aspects of patient care as ambivalent, uneven, and of lower priority. In this respect, it should be noted that the children and adolescents seen here present physical problems. Although psychiatric patients are seen in outpatient care, no beds are reserved for psychiatry, and patients with neuropsychiatric disorders who require restraint are precluded from admission by the rules of the professional staff.

As might be imagined, this policy generates problems. First, patients are not always so accommodating as to limit their pathology to physical disease only. Thus, patients with cancer, diabetes, or juvenile rheumatoid arthritis may also present symptoms of psychiatric disease. Second, physical diseases are not uncommonly reflected in behavioral manifestations that cry out for appropriate management. Third, serious illness and hospitalization are frequently associated with separation, fear, mutilation, pain, and the shadow of life threat, resulting in a potential for acute and chronic psychological problems. Fourth, surgical and medical intervention for diagnosis and treatment may itself intensify mental stress, as for example when it results in loss of hair, delay in growth rate, and change in life-style. Fifth, but by no means finally, physical symptoms and psychological states have long been known to interact with each other, as in the so-called psychosomatic diseases.

It was to this setting that I came in 1969, eclectically trained in clinical and developmental psychology, and interested in developing a training program in the then new field of pediatric psychology. I came as chief psychologist in the hospital's Division of Psychiatry, and as professor in the affiliated USC School of Medicine. What little I knew about hypnosis at the time was prejudiced by my feelings that it was unscientific, mystical, not effective, not relevant to children, and especially that it was not accepted practice in a traditional, conservative academic setting. On the positive side, I was curious.

Consequently, I did attend some lectures, and I invited two hypnotherapists to present demonstrations to my interns. And then I was profoundly impressed by a demonstration at the local hypnosis society by Dr. Clara Younger, a local pediatrician who was not on our staff. Dr. Younger demonstrated with a young asthmatic patient and described her work in the emergency room. I felt we were overlooking something of value, but I did not know how to introduce this.

However, my most interesting lesson and opportunity was provided through the admission of a 14-year-old boy with the life-threatening diagnosis of acute myelogenous leukemia. More assertive in expressing his fear of and resistance to invasive diagnostic procedures than most, this young man tried to negotiate a contract with his physician that he would not be stuck with any needles. Bone marrow aspiration is a common evaluative procedure in such cases, involving insertion of a large needle into the hip bone. So frightening was this to him that it was initially carried out under general anesthesia. Now, when another specimen had to be obtained, and the risk of anesthesia was deemed unacceptable, a search for alternatives became imperative.

The Children's Hospital is located on Sunset Boulevard, at the eastern edge of Hollywood. Beyond Hollywood to the west lies the entertainment zone known as Sunset Strip, comprised largely of restaurants, bars and nightclubs. In one of the clubs a hypnotist often performed. Known to the patient's family, this hypnotist volunteered to assist. The information was relayed to me by the psychology intern assigned to the case. A small dilemma was created by the prospect of inviting professional assistance from a nightclub performer who lacked formal credentials and training. What kept the dilemma small was the absence of awareness on the part of most of the staff. A crisis was averted when we realized that as a family friend, the hypnotist could make a social visit. Naturally, the visit was timed to coincide with the scheduled procedure. Just in case, a strong-arm crew was kept waiting, prepared if necessary to wrestle the patient into submission. But the hypnotist prevailed, the patient accepted the invasive needle, the marrow sample was obtained, the strong-arm crew retired, and the hematologist was heard to complain that, in his opinion, the patient had not really been hypnotized anyhow. A door had been opened.

The show business act was followed by those with more orthodox credentials, and staff and students enrolled in workshops and developed skills. When new staff with skills came on board, we began to use hypnosis to help children to cope with fear and pain.

With Dr. Lonnie Zeltzer, a physician then on staff, we applied for and received a grant for a project that became known as the Adolescent Self-Help Program. Among its goals was teaching adolescents with cancer to utilize hypnosis and self-hypnosis to cope more effectively and more autonomously with their disease and its treatment, especially to reduce pain and discomfort associated with medical interventions. To our surprise and delight, Dr. Erickson agreed with enthusiasm to assist in training the project's staff. We made a pilgrimage to Phoenix.

I cannot speak for my colleagues, but as I entered Dr. Erickson's office, I was in awe. He began, as he often did, by circulating a blank sheet of paper to each of us, sternly instructing us to write our names, our ages, all the schools we had attended and their locations, our marital status, whether or not our parents lived, whether we had grown up in the city or in the country, and many other items too confusing to keep in mind. While we struggled, he circulated some newspaper cartoons, and then posed the question about the number of ways by which one might pass from his reception room to his office. Erickson's methods of teaching were unique. He posed riddles, told stories, and he demonstrated hypnosis with those present. Perhaps because we were from a pediatric setting, more of the stories than usual may have been centered on the eight children who grew up in the Erickson household. For the same reason he may have demonstrated with us more age regressions to childhood than usual. At the end of the four days, I returned to Los Angeles still in awe, perhaps in trance as well, and wondering just what it was that we had learned.

Erickson was a good teacher. The Children's Hospital offered endless opportunities for those he trained on that visit and on subsequent visits to apply their skills. An adolescent girl with cancer had been bedridden for days and was unable to keep food down following each month's course of chemotherapy. After hypnosis she found herself with an appetite on the first afternoon, and going to a party on the following evening. A young man who suffered nausea so severely that he sought to avoid treatment, and who suffered great pain from the injections of chemotherapeutic drugs, learned to enjoy and elaborate trance states that helped him with both these problems. A patient with sickle cell disease had been a heavy user of drugs that he begged from every physician with whom he had contact. He was known to seek them as well on the street. With the aid of hypnosis he learned to increase his own peripheral blood flow and skin temperature when threatened with an attack. Flushing more blood through his capillaries reduced his experience of pain sufficiently so that he was able to take on employment without need of drugs.

A 12-year-old boy had suffered from abdominal pain of unknown etiology for two and a half years. He had undergone many tests without resolution. He was terrified at the prospect of gastroscopy, and the pediatrician referred him to help overcome that fear. The boy's family believed the pain was in the boy's head; for the boy that only made the problem worse. Both multigenerational family therapy and hypnotherapy were integrated, with the effect that the pain diminished and then disappeared.

A 15-year-old with rheumatic heart disease was required to get a monthly antibiotic injection. His fear of the pain that he associated with that injection was so great that it was difficult to say whether the procedure was harder on the boy or on the nursing staff who had to hold him. He was hypnotized, given his shot and then expressed incredulity that it was over.

In a final example, a four-year-old patient of the Dialysis and Transplant team required crisis intervention in the midst of a violent tantrum, during which there was danger that he would pull a shunt from his arm. To calm him enough to carry out hemodialysis he was being tranquilized, but this too was a threat to his health. Using principles learned from Erickson, the psychologist interrupted the tantrum and then helped this child to achieve more effective control by teaching him how to hypnotize his doll.

Each of the foregoing examples might with interest and value be described more fully, but for the purposes of this paper it may be of even greater usefulness to understand what are some of the features common to these and similar interventions.

In his well-known paper on pediatric hypnotherapy, Erickson dealt with the emergency needs of his three-year-old son. Robert's lip was gushing blood following a bad fall, and the little boy was screaming. In the brief moment it took for Robert to draw a new breath so that he could continue to scream, Erickson interjected, "That hurts awful, Robert. That hurts terrible." In the pauses that followed Erickson pointed out that it would go on hurting, that Robert wished it would stop, that perhaps in a little while it would stop, in a minute or so, perhaps it would stop hurting. As they achieved agreement on this likelihood, attention was redirected from hurt to the amount, quality, and color of the blood, and on its change to pink as it was diluted by the wash water. Ultimately, Robert was consoled for the fact that only seven stitches were required to close the wound (his sibling had had more), by virtue of the interesting geometric pattern in which they were arranged. Starting from an attention-getting remark, Robert was led to an awareness that change could occur, and then to commitment to achieve that change. The move had been from pain and anguish through hope to intellectual curiosity and then to emotional growth.

This case has received much attention, and I have used it many times as a teaching example. My students have suggested that no hypnosis was involved. Erickson himself poses and then answers the same question: "Actually hypnosis began with the first statement to Robert and became apparent when he gave his full and undivided interested and pleased attention to each of the succeeding events that constituted the medical handling of his problem." While Erickson is clear that this was hypnosis, it is of interest that he makes no reference to the induction of trance. The questioning of my students may be interpreted as asking how could it be hypnosis if there was no induction. Indeed, had we not already known that Erickson was the author of this account, we might have understood it as the behavior of an intuitive parent who kept calm in the face of an injury to his child. Is this not something to which any concerned parent might aspire?

I have listed the three steps that seem to contain the essence of the method as I have observed it in the work of Erickson as well as in our own work. Stripped of jargon, the method is deceptively simple: 1) *Get the patient's attention;* 2) *communicate to the patient's satisfaction that change is possible; and* 3) *enlist the patient's commitment in the service of positive change.* The means by which attention is captured may vary greatly and may involve any or all of the sensory modalities, or they may be cognitive and embedded in the meaning of verbal communication. Awareness of the possibility of change (hope) may already exist, but if it does not, it is the therapist's task to bring it about. Actually, many patients alternate between helplessness and hopefulness. The third principle is to enlist the patient's motivation to achieve positive change. Unless the patient joins in and commits him or herself to the change, the goal will not be reached. The application of these principles may be infinitely elaborated, and may require creativity, empathy, artistry, and genius. Nevertheless, these basic elements appear and reappear in Erickson's accounts of his work. They appear as well in our retrospective look at our own work.

Trance induction may be present or not. Erickson gives another example of crisis intervention with a bleeding child (Erickson, 1959). Seven-year-old Allan was frightened by pain and by the blood from his lacerated leg. When he swabbed his blood with a towel,

> He was urgently told, "Wipe up that blood; wipe up that blood; use a bath towel; use a bath towel; use a bath towel; a bath towel,

> not a hand towel, a bath towel," and one was handed to him. He dropped the towel he had already used. He was immediately told urgently and repetitiously, "Now wrap it around your leg, wrap it tightly, wrap it tightly."

Again we can see the successful effort to gain attention, the communication that change was feasible, and elicitation of the patient's motivation to effect change. Allan was given the responsibility for overseeing restorative steps, including counting to make sure that the proper number of sutures would be utilized. Confirmation of this schema is provided by Erickson in his summary statement.

> No mention of pain or anesthesia was made at any time nor were any "comforting reassurances" offered. Neither was there any formal effort to induce a trance. Instead, various aspects of the total situation were utilized to distract Allan's attention completely away from the painful considerations and to focus it upon values of importance to a seven-year-old boy in order to secure his full active cooperation and intense participation in dealing with the entire problem adequately.

Arnold was the four-year-old dialysis patient alluded to earlier. He was seen by Dr. Bruce Bongar, then a member of the Children's Hospital staff. Bongar interrupted Arnold's tantrum by ostentatiously and slowly removing his necktie, wrapping it around a blood pressure cuff, and pointing to the oscillating mercury level as he inflated the cuff. Having captured his attention he used some intriguing verbal nonsense to sustain it, again moving to gain Arnold's cooperation.

Why was trance not induced? The master of trance induction was equally the master at using naturalistic behaviors in the service of hypnosis. In 1962, Erickson published a paper entitled "Basic Problems in Hypnotic Research." He pointed out in that paper that hypnosis is a process of behavior that, like physiological sleep, can occur under a great variety of circumstances. Although sleep is most likely to occur while lying in bed, it can happen while driving a car or sitting in a lecture hall. From a scientific point of view it is what occurs during physiological sleep that is of primary interest, not where it takes place. So it is with hypnosis. Attempts to study hypnosis in relation to eye fixation or body relaxation are confusing in that they are like trying to study physiological sleep in terms of the hospital bed or the studio chair in which it takes place.

Defending the notion that hypnosis is not dependent on formal trance induction may seem like proving the obvious, at least to those already familiar with Erickson. But there is a special manifestation of non-trance hypnosis, one that occurs in real-life situations, that appears to have special relevance to a children's hospital. I refer here to that which is usually thought of as "conditioning." Let me again give some brief examples. In the last cited paper by Erickson on problems in hypnosis research he tells us about Ann, who at the age of eight was taken to see the dentist:

> She was a frightened little girl, and she was squalling and yelling because her parents were the type of people whose children would cry when they went to see the dentist. The dentist believed in the wet towel method of handling crying children. He slapped her face with a wet towel, picked her up and put her in the chair, slapped her face again and told her, "Shut up and be a good girl." So she was! At age 21 Ann walked into another dental office and said to the receptionist, "I want to talk to the dentist. Tell him I'll be out in the hallway." The receptionist told the dentist about it as he went out in the hallway where Ann was standing fearfully. "You won't slap me, will you?" she asked pitifully. Ann was a college graduate, an intelligent girl, but such was her uncontrollable fear that she had to make absolutely certain that she would not be slapped. It was impossible for her to believe otherwise at first, and the dentist had much work teaching Ann that brutality was not a part of dentistry. Ann had never been to a dentist since that childhood experience; she had been thoroughly conditioned in one single experience. The dentist had to be most laborious in his deconditioning of the girl, who now wears complete dentures as a result of that original experience.

Reading that account reminded me of another example, one that may or may not have been published. I give it from a somewhat fallible memory as it was described by Raymond LaScola, M.D., in the course of a seminar.

A young woman consulted him when she found herself overburdened by work imposed on her by her fellow workers. She was constantly called upon to do extra work as a favor and for no compensation. Worse yet, this young woman had great difficulty in getting gasoline for her car. When she drove into a service station, she might be propositioned by the attendant, and find herself unable to refuse his sexual advances.

He would relay what had happened to his colleagues, who would approach her on her next visit, and again she could not refuse. So she was constantly needing to find a station where she was not yet known. In the first session LaScola did an age regression, returning her to the age of three where she was engaged in noisy play at a time when her mother was trying to talk on the telephone. Her mother scolded her to no avail. Finally, her mother asked her whether she would stop. She glared defiantly at the mother and said, "No." Her mother slapped her face sharply, shouting, "Don't you ever say 'no' to anyone again." I would like to suggest that in both these illustrations the same three elements of attention getting, prospect of change, and enlistment of the patient's cooperation were present at the time of the original conditioning, and that these events cannot be distinguished from hypnosis as we have utilized it. In a pediatric setting the possibilities for good or evil for similar conditioning are evident every day.

Let me return to my account of the beginning of hypnosis as I observed it at Children's Hospital, and to the metaphor of planting seeds. I would like to tell you that we now have some beautiful flowers. As a function of economic and administrative difficulties, on July 1, 1980, most of the psychologists on the hospital's staff had undergone separation. My own position as chief psychologist and professor was eliminated, and the Division of Psychiatry was essentially dissolved. The training program was eliminated. A small group of psychologists, mainly those associated with the Division of Hematology-Oncology, remain at this time, perhaps to be more successful in planting seeds.

## REFERENCES

Erickson, M.H. Pediatric hypnotherapy. *American Journal of Clinical Hypnosis*, 1958, *1*, 25-29.

Erickson, M.H. Further clinical techniques of hypnosis: Utilization techniques. *American Journal of Hypnosis*, July 1959, *2*(1), 13-14.

Erickson, M.H. Basic problems in hypnotic research. In: *Hypnosis: Current Problems*, G. Estabrook (Ed.), New York: Harper and Row, 1962, pp. 207-223.

Erickson, M.H. & Rossi, E.L. *Hypnotherapy: An Exploratory Casebook*. New York: Irvington, 1979, p. xii.

Chapter 27

# Hypnotherapy with Children and Adolescents: Some Ericksonian Ideas

*Franz Baumann*

One of the stories told about Milton Erickson's childhood centered on a question his father asked him, namely, "Would you rather slop the hogs and feed the chickens before breakfast and then milk the cows and sweep the yard, or would you rather sweep the yard first, milk the cows, have breakfast and then slop the hogs and feed the chickens?" Young Milton was given a choice. In later years, that form of communication became one of his therapeutic techniques. It is called the double bind. Neither answer would have kept the work from being accomplished. I expect to give you a few examples of how this and other Ericksonian approaches are applied in my pediatric practice.

Perhaps you can recognize Erickson's influence in the way shots are given in my office. The antiseptic is applied to 15 or 20 different parts of the body. The patient has had his arms and legs rubbed as well as his neck and forehead. Then the following statement is made, "I don't really know where you would like this injection." (We don't call it a shot, we call it an injection.) Next, the child is given the cotton to hold, and he is asked to smell it. While he does that, he gets the injection somewhere in one of those cleaned places. At this point he might say, "When am I going to get the shot?" "Oh, you already had it. You had it here in your arm." And then the child might say "Ooooh." I might reply, "If you don't like it there I'd be happy to move it some other place where you would like it better." Most of them say, "No, I like it right where it is." And that settles that. So utilization, confusion, and other techniques can be applied every day in a naturalistic manner.

What is the proper age for hypnosis? Children can experience hypnosis at any age. Just doing more than one thing at a time may induce the state. Recognizing the patient's feelings, respecting them, and describing them will help. When a small child is dragged into the office frightened and screaming, how do we handle that? We pick the child up and give him or her a big hug and say, "I bet you *were* scared, weren't you?" That is recognizing the feeling right now, respecting it, speaking about it, and yet putting it into the past tense. "You *were* scared, *weren't* you?" Sometimes children draw a deep sobbing breath and say, "How did you know?" Sometimes they just calm down and feel comfortable. Touch is provided and communication is established. Adults and children alike can tolerate more when they feel understood.

Another Ericksonian approach with small children who are crying and fearful is to simply admire their tears. We blot them off and hold up the tissue against the light and notice how very beautiful and clear those tears are and say, "Could we please have some more?" The child looks up and after a while is very proud of the tears but won't give us any more because the natural tendency is to resist an order, to negate a command. Then we invite him to *please* cry a little louder so everyone can hear it very well. That kind of approach leads to the decision, "I will not!" Calmness is thereby restored. Naturalistic techniques consist of the utilization of what exists and what the patient brings to you.

One of the numerous techniques Erickson taught was to utilize the symptom. We illustrated that by prescribing the crying and the tears. Another approach is to project around the symptom, around the present, around the frightful episode, and discuss the future. One might say, "When you get home, will you please turn on the kitchen light?" Or, in older children, a different approach might be used, such as when seeing an acutely ill teenager who expects to die from mononucleosis and who feels depressed and exhausted. In this case one might well shake hands as he leaves and say, "I wonder if you will give me a ring a week from next Monday after school and let me know how much better you feel." This is the implied suggestion that there will be an end to the discomfort he presently feels. This may seem naive, but it is listened to and registered. Of course, the physician knows that recovery is spontaneous, but now the patient knows it also.

The confusion techniques as described above with injections work in many other situations. For example, the child may find me examining the left leg when the right leg hurts. The child may become so totally absorbed with the stupidity of the physician that he forgets his personal distress. After a while he might work up enough courage to say, "You know, Doc, that is not what I am here for." At this point I might say something about that leg that I was looking at such as, "Really, that is a very good leg!" He may repeat, "But that is not what I am here for, I am here for *that* leg!" I might at this point say, "Where is *that*?" This may seem a ridiculous trance induction, but it works and others have found similar techniques to be useful.

When working with children old enough to have homework that they don't want to do, one can make the following statement, "I'd like you to really think about the fact that everyone needs recreation; it is important for all of us, and I would like you to make *your* plans for homework right now with the idea in mind that you are *leaving enough time for recreation.*" "Leaving," of course, is the indirect suggestion in that he has to do his homework *first.* Furthermore, he will enjoy his recreational activity more because he has done his homework.

The double bind that young Milton Erickson experienced with slopping the pigs before or after breakfast can be utilized if you are a medical person who has to perform an examination on a youngster, e.g., "Would you like to have me lift you onto the examining table or would you rather climb up there all by yourself?" The result, of course, is the same. He is going to be there when you need him there.

Another application of Ericksonian approaches might be to say to a high school student at a time when he is contemplating dropping out of school, "I really don't know which college would be best for you." When you say that to him, the indirect suggestion is that you are convinced that he *can* go to college. This would mean that he has to graduate from high school and this might be the first time in his life that he has thought of himself as college material. Again we have direction by indirectness.

It has been noted in studying Erickson's approaches that he sometimes took sides. This was an attention-getting mechanism and thereby "hypnotic." There was the case of a youngster who came to Erickson and was dragged into his office because of bed-wetting. Erickson said, "Your parents have no right to drag you here and *make me* work with you. I don't really think it is appropriate." There you see confusion and ganging-up, identifying with a patient and taking sides against the parents (who, by the way, usually have been informed in advance).

You probably remember the case of the thumbsucker, the adolescent girl who was dragged to the office because she was sucking her thumb. The parents first were told not to interfere with the doctor's suggestions, no matter what! They had to agree to his method. The parents were then sent out of the treatment room and the youngster was told, "I don't want them here right now. I just would like to talk to you . . . . Now, you don't understand this but I think that you should suck your thumb good and loud and thoroughly for a long, long 20 minutes every night when your father reads the paper and really, really let him know, and when you are through doing that, then I would like you to go to the old lady and annoy the hell out of her." (This girl, by the way, had been prayed for in church to stop her thumbsucking. Theirs was a very religious family. Consequently, when Erickson used the term "to annoy the hell out of her," that was in a sense a hypnotic induction. It fixed her attention because she knew that it was inappropriate for a physician to use that kind of horrible language). The youngster faithfully followed Dr. Erickson's instructions and within a month cut down the length of time from 20 minutes to 15 and then to 10 and finally to 5. She resented terribly having to do things that she didn't really like and so she stopped. In the meantime her parents were told not to react in any way and not to make any comments. For a month they went through the tortures of

Prescribing the symptom is an Ericksonian technique of great value. He used it for the treatment of habit disorders such as nail-biting. Erickson looked at one nail biter and saw that all the nails had been bitten down to the quick. He said, "You know, I really feel sorry that you never had the pleasure and joy of sinking your teeth into a full grown nail." The same approach can be applied to stammering, whereby the practitioner could prescribe deliberate stuttering.

Long before the American Society of Clinical Hypnosis was founded and Erickson was still teaching with the Seminars on Hypnosis group, I was seeing a delinquent teenager who was in lots of trouble. I had not gotten anywhere with him. So I told him Dr. Erickson would be in San Francisco the following month. Each week I reminded him that Erickson's visit was one week closer. Finally the seminar came to San Francisco and the boy was walked into the large, crowded meeting room, between all kinds of tables; then he had to get behind the speaker's table, which was very close to the wall. He actually had to worm his way through and then a speaker had to get up so that my patient could sit down. He was terribly embarrassed and blushed uncomfortably and obviously was in hypnosis. Dr. Erickson looked at him at great length and then he said, "Dr. Baumann tells me you are having lots of trouble." The boy answered "Yeeesss," and Dr. Erickson said very slowly, "And I don't know *how* you are going to change *your* behavior." *That was all!* That delinquent teenager is now a well-known attorney.

PART XI

# *Pain Control*

*Bertha Rodger, M.D., practiced anesthesiology for many years in New Jersey. Subsequently, she retired to Florida. Dr. Rodger continues to be active in teaching hypnosis and travels frequently to present workshops at various locations in the United States. She is a past president of the American Society of Clinical Hypnosis.*

*In her chapter, Rodger presents and discusses transcripts of her approach in using hypnosis in pain control and tension reduction. This fascinating paper includes not only the transcript but also Rodger's comments on her own technique. This is an opportunity to experience her induction language directly. She offers interesting and practical approaches and emphasizes naturalistic methods. Some of the case examples include previously unpublished material that Erickson used in his early teaching seminars.*

*Joseph Barber, Ph.D., is a clinical psychologist with considerable expertise in the area of hypnotic pain control. He was an assistant professor at the Department of Anesthesiology and Oral and Maxillofacial Surgery at UCLA and worked at the UCLA Pain Management Clinic. Barber, who is editing a volume on techniques of pain control and conducts a private practice of psychotherapy in Los Angeles, frequently conducts workshops on hypnotherapy and hypnotic approaches to pain control.*

*Barber's chapter speaks to the importance of using indirect techniques to modify sensations of pain. Traditional approaches to pain control use anesthesia (no sensation) and analgesia (diminished sensation). However, additional techniques that insure that most patients can learn to modify their pain are available. Barber suggests a framework to help the practitioner decide how to approach a pain patient. Case examples illustrate the technique of reinterpreting pain sensations, present a novel use of Erickson's interspersal technique, and illustrate the importance of attending to the subtle nuances inherent in the patient's communication.*

*Sacerdote reviews Erickson's general approach to pain control. Principles of hypnotherapy for pain control are the same as those used in psychotherapy. Previously unused potentials are elicited; each person has, within his or her own history, resources that can modify pain sensations. In general, the patient is set on a train of thought or action that induces modification of pain. The change in pain sensation can begin during the diagnostic process.*

*Additionally, Sacerdote reviews the pain control techniques that Erickson described in 1965 at the International Congress for Hypnosis and Psychosomatic Medicine in Paris. Sacerdote's understandings of Erickson's methods are not just intellectual and academic. He presents a case in which he uses Ericksonian methods with a patient suffering from cancer pain.*

Chapter 28

# Ericksonian Approaches in Anesthesiology

*Bertha Phillips Rodger*

The aim of this paper is to demonstrate some of the principles of anesthesia which Dr. Erickson taught—often pioneered—and the way adaptations can fit the particular style of the anesthesiologist, as well as the needs of the patient and the situation. These procedures take no time beyond that usually spent with the patient and replace the superficial conversation so often wastefully used in the attempt to distract and reassure. The time it takes to acquire this mode and make it habitual is well worthwhile. It saves time in the long run and cuts down markedly on the amount of medication needed.

Imagine, if you will, that you have just been in some kind of an accident which happened so fast you are still not sure what it's all about. You find yourself in hospital surroundings with strange people insistently asking, "What's your name?" "Where does it hurt?" "Who is your next of kin?" Suddenly a quiet, caring voice comes through with the startling, "You won't *mind* being *comfortable* while we work, will you?" It's enough to concentrate anyone's attention—and this is its main purpose, for, according to Milton Erickson, attention can as readily be fixed on an idea as upon a spot on the wall, thereby facilitating trance induction and use. In a situation already fraught with confusion, this clear redirection of thought, firmly presented, is in accord with the patient's needs and leads rapidly toward the development of trust and cooperation.

The gentle voice persists, as kindly eyes continue to observe keenly and unobtrusively: "You *know* anything *hurts less* when you can relax even a little bit, or when you begin to distribute some of your attention elsewhere." No one can argue with this. The truism initiates positive response, the important "yes-set" of mind. "You *know* the pleasant sensation of warmth on your skin when you stretch out in the sun in a favorite spot. You have *time* now to think about such things, to *let your mind wander* . . . and *wonder* . . . as you wander. You don't even have to pay attention to what I am saying. The deep part of your mind can listen to the voice speaking directly to you. All other sounds can deepen that sense of comfort that comes as you relax and rest so pleasantly."

In this brief example, a number of Dr. Erickson's teachings are applied. Many of them are better caught than taught, like his characteristic way of saying, "Tha-at's ri-ight!" as he accepts with delight whatever response the patient makes to his suggestions, giving ratification to it as part of trance behavior and therefore useful. All the devices of communication come into play in addition to the carefully chosen words. Manner, gestures, facial expression, the infinite nuances of voice inflection, tone, pauses, emphasis on key words—all have significance. Dr. Erickson was master of these, insistently calling attention to their importance, working incessantly to get these details on paper or on tape for better sharing. Bringing such minutiae to awareness enables fuller utilization.

The confusion of that apposition of opposites, "You will, . . . won't you?" joggles attention too long tied up in apprehension and distress, guiding it to the idea of being comfortable which is so far from the mind at that moment. The anesthesiologist continuously reassesses the patient's needs, seeking to meet them with respect for the *total person.* At first glance it may sometimes seem bizarre to the onlooker, but the patient responds in a way that proves therapeutic.

"Let your mind wander . . . and wonder . . ." starts a depotentiation of the conscious mind by "not-doing, not-knowing." This frees it from a locked-in negative approach, allowing inner resources to come forth. Listening only to the voice that speaks directly is a great help in tuning out static sounds. Those which might disturb are transposed to signals for deepening this comfortable state of trance. The broad statements about sensations of warmth in a favorite place give free rein to the patient's own imagery.

## ANALGESIA BY INDIRECT APPROACH

The following verbalization is a mosaic which also illustrates a number of Erickson's teachings. Most ideas are drawn directly from Seminars on Hypnosis* or other workshop notes. Many have filtered through the

---

**Editor's note:* The Seminars on Hypnosis were workshops led by Erickson and others in the 1950s. The American Society of Clinical Hypnosis was founded as an outgrowth of the Seminars. For additional information, see the chapter by Irving Secter in this volume.

lectures of others trained by him. It is no longer possible to sort out the sources of such contributions. Words, phrases, and approaches come spontaneously into use after long steeping in them.

A patient referred for learning hypnoanalgesia was somewhat diffident and apprehensive about hypnosis. Hence it seemed best to separate trance development from its use, as Erickson so characteristically did: "I really cannot hypnotize you. But at some time in the future when *you* are ready to learn to go into a trance, I can help you do so. Then you can learn to use it . . . and go on doing so all the rest of your life."

It is made clear that the patient, not the facilitator, "does the hypnotizing," retaining control. Appearing to put it off to the nebulous future decreases its threatening aspect. Yet it leaves the matter open for change as readiness for it comes.

The anesthesiologist continues: "Meanwhile, there are some very interesting things you can learn that will help you. We can forget about hypnosis until you understand more about it and want to work with it [She did this at the same session!]. There are certain things you already know about dealing with discomfort or pain that you can put to use right now—like the distraction that occurs when you give your full attention to a TV program, tuning out everything else. You may even get so absorbed in what is going on that it seems as if you are really there, participating in the action. This is called 'dissociation.' It is just a matter of degree. So you have the choice of concentrating on the hurting—or turning to something more interesting. The more you do the latter, the less anything bothers you."

This falls within the realm of setting the stage for increasing collaboration. To go on with demonstrating a point is vastly more effective than remonstrating. It gives a firm basis upon which to build: "Tightening muscles seems to set nerves on edge so that discomfort increases. Tension always aggravates pain and can even cause it. Yet as much as 40 percent of pain is relieved by simple relaxation. You can test this out for yourself. Double up your fist and hold it very tightly. Pinch the back of your hand to discover how sharp it feels. Now make your hand go as limp and floppy as a Raggedy Ann doll and note how little a pinch bothers it now."

It's a little difficult to record on paper the grimace that accompanies the first pinch and the smile that goes with the second. Both are important. With the fact verified that helpful information is indeed being supplied, it is easier to proceed. This time a certain vagueness is introduced, producing slight confusion. Communication techniques use multiple levels of verbal content, voice variance, and nonverbal demonstration. All of these reinforce the changes in awareness and provide guidance.

To continue: "Turn your attention to the wealth of sensations you can sense in your hand . . . and to their changes. Just which part is the heaviest? Is it in the fingers? In the palm? Near the wrist? Where does it feel lighter? As if it might like to lift? To float upward? Does that tingly feeling start first in your fingers? Or the back of your hand? Is there a bubbly feeling along with this? Or does it feel stiff . . . as if it is made of wood . . . feeling only a slight vibration . . . if anything? *Notice* where it feels most comfortable of all . . . where nothing bothers it . . . nothing disturbs it. And that feeling of comfort is so pleasing . . . you wonder . . . how long it really needs to take . . . to spread even further . . . and deeper . . . through that whole area . . . and even beyond . . . for an extra margin . . . and how well it can remain . . . to keep you entirely comfortable. The comfort can stay as long as normal healing is going on. Your body knows how to heal. As you keep yourself comfortable . . . all the energy goes to the healing process. It's so good to be able to work so nicely with your body."

Numerous techniques are effected including: conviction of her ability to develop and retain comfort; raising her expectation of something desirable happening; showing her the creative choices; and focusing on the goodness of her body. All lead her to an experience of better functioning by her own skills. She readily developed a pleasing analgesia so that she did well during the surgical procedure that followed.

## ATTENTION TO DETAIL

Erickson emphasized in his seminars the importance of giving attention to small details. Speaking of an amputee returning home for a first visit after acquiring his prosthesis, he would ask, "What do you suppose will be most difficult for him?" Answers would come about major problems, getting used to being without a meaningful part of the body, to people staring or studiously avoiding any recognition of the loss, etc. The desired answer had to do with the seemingly minor problem of being greeted enthusiastically by the two-year-old son who hugged him around both legs, tipping him over unceremoniously. The humiliation would have been hard to bear.

Erickson would have agreed with the wit who declared,

It's the little things that bother us
And keep us on the rack.
We can sit upon a mountain,
But not upon a tack!

His attention to infinitesimal detail is seen in the famous "handshake induction," by which Erickson would turn a normal handshake into a nonverbal confusion induction leading to arm catalepsy. The signals given to allow the hand to remain as if suspended in midair are so minute as to be received on an unconscious level and the response is made out of awareness. This type of touching can communicate much reassurance in other applications. Notifying first by lightly brushing the sleeve, or delicately moving the sheet, or momentarily holding the hand poised over the skin so its warmth is sensed avoids startling and denotes a respect that builds trust. In applying the blood pressure cuff or placing the arm on a support prior to starting an infusion, taking the hand as if to shake hands and giving the same kind of delicate signals used in the handshake induction set the stage for procedures to be a friendly, cooperative effort rather than an invasion of the privacy of the body or a mechanical act.

At one seminar, Dr. Erickson suggested saying to a patient with a fractured wrist. "Let's find just the right position for your *elbow*—and *even your little finger*!" Beginning with the index finger, he would then continue to develop analgesia upward over hand, wrist and forearm. Concern for elbow and "even the little finger" reassured the person far more than words could.

Simultaneously, it is essential to pay attention to the patient's expectations. One who expects to feel *nothing* during treatment may be quite upset to feel *something*, interpreting any sensation as *pain*. Anticipating this is part of paying adequate attention to detail. It might be explained in this way. "*Analgesia* is like turning down the rheostat, the dimmer, to where sensation is tolerable, even comfortable. *Anesthesia* is like turning off the switch. It's possible you might feel a *little* something. *If* you were able to feel the incision, it would feel like a fingernail drawn lightly across the skin—a tickle or a trickle." Demonstrating this so lightly as to tickle makes it clear. The alliteration introduces a bit of levity that favors acceptance. Emphasis is of prime importance. It is one thing to put emphasis on the "if," quite another to land heavily on "feel the incision."

## COMMUNICATION BEFORE, DURING, AND AFTER OPERATION

Preoperative preparation alleviates much anxiety. This is also the best time for dealing with postoperative complications by giving clear, positive, brief suggestions as to what to expect and how to respond. It is essential to give adequate leeway to allow for unexpected changes that might otherwise negate too specific a sequence. Complications can be averted by such generalities as: "You can recover quickly, completely and comfortably." "You can be pleased to find how easily you can pass water, move your bowels, breathe deeply . . . how much you enjoy food and fluids . . . how soon you feel like yourself again!" Open-ended and class suggestions are well received. Not only are such ideas helpful before operation, but during it they can be reinforced, for hearing is still present even during deep chemical anesthesia.

Melba Vickery (Sr. Teresa) (1963), a nurse-anesthetist who had the advantage of extensive acquaintance with Dr. Erickson, preserved for us the title he gave for an anesthetic which should have consistent use. It is "VRA," standing for "Verbal Reassurance Anesthesia." It consists of "the air that passes between the vocal cords of the anesthetist communicating with the patient in a reassuring manner." One of the most potent of agents, it acts synergistically with any chemical one, decreasing the quantity needed of the latter as well as making it safer. There are no adverse effects. In fact, it can even counteract such destructive remarks as: "She won't be able to sit down for a week!" made by one obstetrician suturing an episiotomy. "With all this wire in his belly he'll not only hurt, he'll feel as if he has to shift gears every time he moves!" according to a surgeon repairing a wound dehiscence with wire.

In such instances a carefully chosen, perhaps seemingly facetious remark made earnestly by the anesthesiologist may correct the error, "Won't the good doctor be surprised when this patient *doesn't mind* at all those sensations that are a reminder that the area is securely put together again!" Fortunately, people most often choose the comfortable alternative when both are presented confidently.

It behooves the anesthesiologist, surgeon or family physician to make the effort to write out a series of well-worded suggestions for use pre-, intra-, and post-operatively for routine use with modifications to meet special situations.

Throughout his teaching, Erickson ratified and amplified the value of talking to patients as if they were in a trance. The person in low stress will go into trance as the voice slows, as significant use is made of pauses and other communication devices that facilitate the comfort of that state. This is true also as ideas are conveyed that relieve anxiety or inform about the wonderful healing abilities of the body. Many patients in the anesthesia-surgery situation are already in a trance as attention is narrowed by anxiety engendered by the unfamiliar surroundings, happenings, and people or by worry over the consequences of the procedure.

This makes them ideal responders to VRA, which provides a healthy answer to the ever-present, now intensified, human dependency need.

## DISSOCIATION AND TIME DISTORTION

The tediousness of waiting tensely for transport to the operating room, dozing fitfully, being bored or groggy during operation or any feared procedure, can be alleviated by dissociation which is readily induced: "Your medication (or moving onto the carrier) can be a signal for you to start a pleasant daydream going . . . of some activity you really enjoy . . . in a special place . . . where you feel safe, secure, and contented. You might be pleased to find how quickly time passes until you are back in your room again."

What happens in the operating room is likely to be of little interest to the person happily ensconced elsewhere in a daydream. This incorporates the concept of time distortion, which can be deliberately taught. Time can be contracted or expanded as desired. This technique is helpful in dealing with pain. For the patient in labor a sample verbalization could be: "You can let the time of the contraction seem to go by like a flash . . . so fast you hardly notice it except for timing it. The time between contractions can seem like a nice long time. So you have plenty of time to rest, relax and enjoy whatever you wish." Indeed, patients report liking this aspect especially: "I knew it was two minutes by the clock for my husband was timing contractions. To me it seemed like 20 minutes. I felt so rested and comfortable afterward. It wasn't at all like my last delivery when I was so exhausted!"

This applies equally well to the episodes of pain of a person with recurring pain from cancer or other source. The time between episodes can be expanded so they have time to enjoy family and friends, tidy up affairs, etc.

## COPING WITH PAIN

Few have anything near the equivalent of Dr. Erickson's firsthand understanding of pain or his vast professional knowledge or the ability to use resources so creatively. Eternally curious, he always gleaned learning from every part of his own experience, from patients and from colleagues. Finding from his own sufferings how overwhelming it can be to try to cope with pain, he advocated nibbling away at it a fragment at a time in a multiplicity of ways.

When it occurs, pain takes nearly total attention. Emily Dickinson expresses succinctly what it is like,

Pain has an element of blank;
  It cannot recollect
When it began, or if there were
A day when it was not.

It has no future but itself,
Its infinite realms contain
Its past, enlightened to perceive
New periods of pain.

Past pain, including any painful thinking about the condition, can be symbolically locked up in a safe place until it is truly needed. Then any portion can be extracted. The same is true of future pain, surely not needed during this interesting session. This leaves present pain to stand alone for more ease of handling. Developing amnesia for pain is a way of fragmenting it as well.

Erickson pointed out that when a child is hurt, it is in his entirety. Narrowing down the area to where the pain is actually felt and recognizing that all the rest of the body is free from pain enables easier management. Now a desensitization process can whittle away at it further. It is more readily accomplished a bit at a time, dimming sharpness, turning "dull misery" into "a wonderful weariness," even a "lovely lassitude" as that feeling is slowly attenuated. The "red hot poker" effect can be cooled through "real hot" to "still too warm," which is like moving away from the hot fireplace until it becomes "comfortably warm" or "pleasantly cool" or even "numbingly cold."

This gradual weaning is both simpler to produce and more helpful to the patient since it allows for re-education of the factors involved in problems behind the presenting one. Pain can be decreased in intensity, in duration, in frequency of occurrence, and spaced with longer intervals between episodes. During this procedure ideas can be interspersed for "not minding" sensations, for re-interpretation as to their meaning and for separation of the actual stimulus from the signal for it. As attention is directed to rove from, "the feeling of the shoes on your feet . . . to the watch on your wrist . . . or the glasses resting on your nose and ears. . . ," it is diverted from its focus on the hurt. This also proves the point that one really does know how to develop an analgesia by "forgetting" one sensation while paying attention to another.

## GIVING VERSUS TAKING

Pain belongs to the patient with all its meanings. The doctor has no right to take it away. It is better to teach the patient how to give it up as little at a time as he is willing to let go. Dr. Erickson might suggest, "At first this might be imperceptible, well within the range of error of perception. If .01 percent were to drift off in the next hour you certainly wouldn't notice it . . . and .02 percent in the next hour . . . and .04 percent in the next . . . and .08 percent . . . and .16 percent . . . and so on. You will be very pleasantly surprised when you notice some of the pain has disappeared . . . and will like feeling the warmth and pleasure of achieving something you did not know you could do!" Note the deliberate shift of tense to the more definite "you will be . . . very pleasantly surprised."

## THE MONOLOGUE

Starting with what appears as just conversation, Erickson was apt to wander into a prolonged monologue. It might even have seemed somewhat boring at times, but it was actually purposeful, with intermittent phrases, statements, or references to pertinent interests of the listener. He spent much time thinking through exactly how to present such an approach, perhaps writing it out at length, planning words, phrases, intonations, pauses, gestures—all the tiny details that made every contact so deeply meaningful. Then he might well condense the plan to its essentials. Always he stressed that those he was teaching could do the same things he did. It was not "magic" but meant learning the patient's language of body as well as speech and his way of perceiving so needs could be answered accordingly. The following is one of my own attempts to transpose his example to fit my abilities:

## SOLILOQUY ON PAIN

"Give your full attention to your pain. *Try* not to let your mind wander from it—even for a moment. Find out *exactly* where it is located, exactly how it feels. Keep your mind fixed on it so you won't miss anything significant about it." Starting with what the patient is already doing, giving full attention to his pain, the task is made more difficult by the effort it takes to keep such intense concentration. A point of no return is soon reached, after which the harder one tries, the less he succeeds. Erickson long ago observed that when he spotted an acquaintance walking ahead of him, he could catch up, get in step, then as he slowed his steps, speeded them, turned right or left, the other would go along with his assumption of leadership quite out of awareness. Such minute observation fostered his unique communication by indirect ways which avoid resistance.

Now mental imagery is introduced, "There is a building in Boston containing a circular room with a bridge across its center. Standing on the bridge is like being on the inside of a globe, with colored maps of the world on the surrounding walls. Imagine walking into such a globe with a map of your pain on its walls, lighted from outside so you get a really good look at it. The color in the area of pain shows the intensity and concentration as well as the exact area covered." A vivid picture, painted "in living color" is easily held, easily changed with the speed of thought to stir helpful associations. It allows a search for meaning or causation without bringing material to consciousness unless the patient is ready to do so. Mental energy is thus accumulated and directed usefully.

The soliloquy continues, "Watch what happens now, as a diluting color is put into the one representing pain. It begins to fade a little, turn paler. Some neutralization seems to be occurring, as if it's being suctioned out, washed out further, rendered more harmless. It looks better. You can see more clearly what was beside it, beneath it, behind it, around it, within it. You can also see relationships of timing . . . when it began . . . when it recurs . . . in relation to what . . . and to whom." Putting the picture into a different frame allows broader vision, possibly the taking of a new road instead of continuing in the same old rut. Yet this is done without meddling. The patient can find his own meaning when he is ready, encouraged by this understanding support.

Continuing: "You wonder how long its duration really needs to be . . . to fulfill its purpose as an alerting signal . . . that something is going on that might need attention . . . some care. It's like when a hot potato is tossed to you, you find that tossing it back is better than burning your fingers. . . . It cools in the process enough to be handled comfortably.

"You tell me you have pain . . . and I know you really do have pain . . . and you know it hurts less when you relax. You *know* how to hurt. No one has taught you how *not* to hurt. I can do that. Simple relaxation can deal with as much as 40 percent of pain. That's almost half. As you learn to let the area go as soft, limp and floppy as a Raggedy Ann doll and keep it that way, you can *have* the pain or you can *halve* it!"

Thus the patient is led away from being steeped in negative thinking and responses with alternatives couched in broad enough terms to allow for individual adaptation. He can learn to part with pain a little at a time or to trade it for a sensation less disturbing, less restrictive of function. While this re-education is going on, he has the option of *having* or *halving* the pain.

## PLAY ON WORDS

Erickson's facility in making use of a play on words was adapted to meet the needs of a cancer patient whose family was adamant that she not be informed of this diagnosis. As a consequence of their attitude, she insistently tried to find out from everyone coming near whether her pain was due to the cancer she feared. The referral was made with the strict injunction that the family's desire for silence be respected. My voice wandered to her, "You *know* you have pain . . .and many painful feelings too. And this pain . . . and the painful thoughts that go with it . . . can so fill your mind . . . as to drive out all other thoughts. You *know* you have pain . . . and you *know* that you know it . . . and *no* one can tell you any different. What you do *not know* . . . is that you also have areas of *no pain* . . . and you can *know* this *no-pain* . . . and the *time* of *no-pain* . . . can get *longer* and longer. . . . The *area* of no-pain can get *larger* and larger . . . so you have more and *more* no-pain . . . until you are entirely free!

"You would like so much to say *no* to *all* pain. . . . You want your no to be a *good* no . . . the *right* no. There are many things *you* know . . . and you know others know them . . . and sometimes they *do not want* you to know *they* know them. So you do not let them know that you know them . . . to protect their feelings. There may be one person with whom you can share what needs to be shared . . . without distress to anyone. There are so many things you *do* know that will help you to say the *right no* . . . and let you become more and *more aware* of no-pain . . . until you consistently *feel no pain*!"

This proved to be a great relief to her. She did find an opportunity to talk with her clergyman about some of the things that bothered her and to learn some helpful ways of proceeding. Various adaptations have likewise afforded aid to other patients.

## NATURALISTIC APPROACH

The naturalistic and the utilization approaches were pioneered by Erickson. The idea of helping the patient to do better what he is already doing provides a good way of handling such emergencies as excitement on emergence from anesthesia or the building panic of a frightened person, adult or child.

In the recovery room a patient was wheeled in from the operating room tied to the stretcher by twisted sheets as well as the usual safety straps and held by extra attendants as he struggled to sit up. A voice spoke close to his ear from behind his shoulder, "That's a terrible program, isn't it? So noisy! Wouldn't you rather watch the ballgame? Would you like me to change the channel? Just lean back and get comfortable!" He did just that, to the astonishment of the attendants. Again, this was a getting in step, then using communication like a hinge to turn him in a more helpful direction.

A frightened patient just admitted to labor room was on the verge of panic, becoming unmanageable. Grasping both her hands in the manner of a handshake, I spoke firmly to her, "If you *really* have to panic, you ought to do a good job at it! Come on . . . I'll help you . . . . Get your heart beating *faster* . . . pumping *harder* . . . *much* harder . . . and faster . . . and *breathe* in little spasms . . . deeper . . . faster . . . get that *blood press*ure up higher. . . . It's so *very uncomfortable,* isn't it? So why don't you *stop halfway?*

"Wouldn't you really rather just let your eyes close? And snuggle down . . . just listen . . . to the voice that speaks directly to you . . . to tell you just what to expect . . . and how to respond . . . so as to keep yourself quite comfortable. . . ."

The novel idea of stopping halfway is a bit of a shocker that consistently gets attention, as does the unusual way of clasping both hands as if for a dual, friendly handshake. It's bewildering. Being urged to panic better is just too much—as is the alternative Erickson often advocated of putting it off to a more convenient time, with the offer of help—*if* panic was still necessary! The switch to talk of comfort and release from the unknown is apt to be welcomed and instructions followed well.

## SUMMARY

It is indeed both possible and profitable to make direct use of or to alter as needed Milton Erickson's ingenious approaches and teachings in everyday situations. Watching his demonstrations, wondering how he evoked phenomena, listening to his innovative ways, feeling awed by the subtle cues, responses and interactions, one often had the impression that this was wonderful to watch, yet impossible to imitate. However, he consistently encouraged those he was teaching to try out what they did learn for themselves, insisting this really was possible. The many people who have interpreted his work, picked it apart and commented on it, especially those with whom he collaborated at length in this effort, have made it available so that much is widely applicable in routine use, as well as in dealing with more difficult and spectacular situations. Patients and physicians alike are eternally grateful for his enormous and unique contribution.

## REFERENCES

Sister M. Teresa, C.R.N.A. (Melba Reis Vickery) Every patient needs this anesthesia technique, *J. Am. Assoc. Nurse Anesthetists,* April, 1963, *31,* pp. 114-121.

Chapter 29

# Erickson's Approach to Pain Control: Therapeutic Alchemy

*Joseph Barber*

When I think of Erickson's work with pain, it is not merely magic, but *alchemy* that comes to mind. One would expect a magician to deal with pain simply by making it disappear. But an alchemist works differently, by changing one thing into another, and presumably changing something that is worthless or of questionable value into something better—as, for example, changing lead into gold, or changing pain and suffering into something perceptibly more tolerable.

Erickson was sometimes an alchemist in his approach. Erickson, like other good psychotherapists, was able to use himself as a model from which to empathize with other people. He knew what pain was, and he knew how to make the most exquisite discriminations between sensations in order to distinguish between various subtle degrees and kinds of pain. As you realize, being humans who have had pain from time to time, pain does have subtle variations in the way it manifests itself in your own experience. As therapists for pain patients, you can use your own experience with great benefit. It is difficult simply to take away someone's pain, but there are fascinating ways in which you can change various aspects of that pain to make it a more tolerable experience.

I have watched people perform imitations of Erickson in the hope, presumably, of doing a fine job of psychotherapy—trying to imitate his voice and his pacing, his inflections, his sometimes very strange and mesmerizing body movements. However, I want to cast a vote for *not* imitating Erickson or anyone else. I have observed that people are able to imitate only the superficial qualities, and somehow they come out empty. You can't properly imitate Erickson unless you're willing to have

I would like to thank Cheri Adrian, Ph.D., for her indispensable conceptual guidance and editorial miracles.

polio twice, unless you have asthma, unless you have the pain of polymyositis, unless you have color vision deficits, dyslexia, and tone deafness—and have good things, too, like Betty for a wife.

However, we can identify principles in Erickson's work that will allow us to learn from, not simply slavishly imitate, his techniques—and perhaps ourselves perform a little alchemy. We notice his empathy and observation—principles of any good psychotherapy—but his powers of observation were legendary and his power of empathy was amazing. There is power in an ability to empathize with another person's experience of suffering. Empathy in itself opens the way to transforming that experience from suffering into something else. From the patient's point of view, since misery loves company, it's nice to have someone else be there, even if—and here is the key—that person's empathy may begin transforming that misery into some other quality.

When I'm working with a patient I ask myself: What is the meaning of this pain for this patient? What does it mean for this patient that he is perhaps disabled by this pain, that he is prevented from experiencing pleasure, that he is interrupted in social and occupational activities? If I conceptualize the misery that this patient experiences in his life as being focused into a pain complaint, might that help to treat the patient? How does the concept of time affect this patient's experience of pain? How much does memory of past pain and fantasy of future pain influence the present experience of pain? If the memory of past pain—perhaps the resentment of past pain—becomes important to the patient, how might we help him to discriminate between what was past and what is present? If he fears future pain, how might we help him distinguish between what isn't yet and perhaps may not be and what is now? Now is merely now, and pain for just a moment is only a moment's worth, unless we add to it the memory of past pain and the fantasy of future pain.

Most people are aware of Erickson's case of the woman who was terminally ill, experiencing a great deal of pain. Erickson told her, "If you looked over at the door and saw that there was a large, hungry tiger staring at you, how much pain do you think you'd feel?" Now that's a different way of treating someone's pain than anyone had used before. Historically hypnosis had been used for the treatment of pain in a straightforward fashion, such as inducing a sense of anesthesia in the painful area or reducing the pain in a direct manner. But knowing from personal experience that some pain is not so simply made to disappear, Erickson developed more subtle ways of altering experience, including changing certain sensations into other sensations.

He taught that if a patient is going to be having pain for a long time, for example, because of a neurologic lesion, you cannot simply presume that the painful stimulus can be ignored all the time. However, that stimulus can be reinterpreted. If a man, for instance, is suddenly racked with excruciating pain throughout his body and feels that pain as a kind of buffeting, writhing agony, this is very hard to tolerate. But what if those sensations of being buffeted, those sensations of being pushed and twisted were not the result of pain but instead simply the result of enduring a 30-mile-an-hour desert wind? Now that might be annoying and it might be tiresome to have to put up with a 30-mile-an-hour desert wind blowing through your bedroom, but at least it's something one can tolerate. One can always take a nap, or watch television, or talk with friends, and one doesn't have to suffer. There is a tremendous difference between having pain you suffer with and having a sensation that is very annoying.

Erickson stimulated my interest in finding alternative perceptions for patients, in taking a particular stimulation that a patient is experiencing and offering an alternative way of experiencing it. For instance, if a man has pain in his arm, and if that pain is also associated with shaking of that arm, it would be more comfortable for that man if he were able to focus on the shaking movement, rather than the pain. The pain impulses could become more impulses, more energy for the movement, so that what he noticed was how much his hand was shaking. Now that can be annoying and that can be unpleasant, but it is not agonizing.

I had a 33-year-old patient some years ago who was a musician and suffered from lupus erythematosis, a cruel rheumatologic disorder. She played cello in an orchestra, and her husband was also a musician. As fate would have it, the pain that the lupus gave her was increased by vibratory stimulation, by any subtle vibrations in a room. Walking on a wooden floor, for instance, caused enough vibration for her to experience an agonizing, burning pain. Musical vibration caused really excruciating pain. It's a tough kind of experience for a musician, and she felt hopeless about it. I must say, at the beginning I felt pretty hopeless about it, too.

Then I realized that she kept describing the pain as "burning." The burning was the most significant part of the sensation. I remembered when I was a kid, I used to like to play with dry ice. Dry ice is very cold stuff, but it doesn't feel cold when you hold it in your hand. It burns. There is often interesting confusion in thermal sensations between something that is hot and something that is cold. If you have your hand in cold water and then you put it in very hot water, there is a funny kind of confusion in your hand about whether it is feeling burning or cold.

I talked with this patient while she was in a trance about my experiences with cold and with hot. I didn't talk about her pain specifically. I just talked about how confusing it can be sometimes to discriminate between burning and cold, and that we don't always have to know the difference, we just have to know that it doesn't matter too much. I talked to her a long time about the lack of need for being really clear about that distinction. Do you really need to know for certain whether what you're feeling is cold or hot? And if it isn't hot, does it really matter that much?

When she came to see me the next week she said that she had noticed a change in the feeling in her back. She said it felt as though she had a funny kind of hallucination that she was eating mint ice cream. I never would have imagined that eating mint ice cream would have in any way been related to what we had been talking about. But now, when she was beginning to have back pain, when she thought her back was beginning to burn, she would have a memory of eating mint ice cream, and that funny feeling in the roof of her mouth, which was a kind of burning, tingling feeling. She wasn't sure whether it was hot or cold, it was just a funny kind of sensation. Now, instead of an excruciating burning feeling, she experiences, oddly enough, a cool minty feeling in her back. This is sometimes annoying for her, and she sometimes has to wear a sweater in order to be warm enough, but she doesn't have to suffer with that excruciating burning feeling in her back, and she doesn't have to avoid music. She is able to play music and she's able to listen to music.

I never would have guessed mint ice cream as the "right" choice. But then I didn't need to guess that. And since I didn't tell her anything specific that she ought to feel, that left her free enough to find her own way to feel. That kind of alchemy is one of the most exciting ways that hypnosis can be used in the treatment of chronic pain. I'm no longer dependent upon being able to take away someone's chronic pain by creating a feeling of numbness or by suggesting to him/her that the pain that he or she has had for a long time is going to go away.

Erickson's paper, "The interspersal hypnotic technique for symptom correction and pain control" (1966), has been most helpful to me in dealing with hypnosis and pain. It taught me that there are strange and wonderful ways of talking with someone about pain without ever having to talk about the pain. It illustrates that you need not accept ordinary limits to what you can do with someone if you are willing to be with him in the way he needs, if you're willing to tell someone a story that's interesting to him, if you're willing to talk to a man who grows flowers about the growth of a tomato plant.

During the course of treatment of one of my patients who had chronic pain, his father was diagnosed as having cancer and as having only a few months to live. His father had severe abdominal pain. My patient asked me to help his father. I was aware that this fellow and his father had a fine relationship and had a history of being able to help each other. It occurred to me that probably my patient could help his father better than I, if he knew how without having to wonder whether he could. While my patient was in a trance, I read him the story that Erickson told his patient about the tomato plant. I suggested to him that he wouldn't have to remember the details of the story I told him, that he wouldn't have to remember even that I had told him the story, but that when he went home in the afternoon he could be confident that he could sit down with his father and simply talk with him and maybe even tell him a story and allow his father the opportunity to find ways of feeling comfort for the rest of his life. He called me the next day and told me that I wouldn't need to help his father because he had learned a way to help his father himself. He said, "I think that I learned how to hypnotize my dad last night." I said, "How did you do that?" He said, "Well, we just sat down to talk and it occurred to me that we could talk about our garden, and I don't know why, but I began talking to him about the tomato plant in our garden, and my dad started feeling better and then he just went to sleep. And the next morning he asked me if I would tell him that story again." Every evening my patient would sit down and tell his father that story, which he remembered in detail. His father would go to sleep comfortably, spend the night and the next day comfortably, and ask him again, "Would you tell me that story?" The father lived comfortably for the next six months and felt very close to his son. He didn't need narcotics and he didn't need anyone else to tell him that his pain was going to go away. He and his son found their own particular way of doing that.

Altering pain experience through reconceptualization or recontextualization is, like any approach, not always necessary or desirable. Erickson taught us above all to observe, to attend to the patient. At the end of my first session, an assessment interview, with a functioning schizophrenic who had a history of headaches with no known physical explanation, the patient told me that his headache had gone away. I asked, "Why do you think your headache went away?" He said, "Well, it wasn't anything we talked about." And I said, "Well, what do you think it might have been that we didn't talk about?" Then he began to tell me about a particular problem that had been plaguing him for years and which he could not tell anyone about, because it was too embarrassing.

He said he would like to tell me about it, but he first had to find out whether or not I could keep a secret. He finally felt confident that I would keep the secret as long as it did not violate the legal requirements of my profession. He told me the secret and he talked about his problem. It was a problem which could be dealt with.

Suddenly he said, "You know, my headaches are not organic." (I still hadn't made that leap.) I said, "What makes you think so?" He said, "Because they're caused by pressure between my ears." I said, "Well, what sort of pressure between your ears?" He answered, "Well, what we've just been talking about, this problem of mine, creates such pressure between my ears because I can't let it out, but now that I'm letting it out with you, I think it's going to make a big difference." This reminded me that often we don't take a simple explanation for a patient's pain as a possible one. He simply had a secret that was bursting within him and that made him have headaches. The patient has had a significant decrease in headaches since that time, so I think I'll believe him.

Careful attention to the way a patient describes and accounts for the pain experience is the first step in the process of therapy. When seeing patients who have pain, any kind of pain, we need to take everything that they are giving us visually and auditorially and be willing to see and hear all of it, including things that may not fit our initial hypotheses. In finding ways in our own minds to transform one experience into another and, hopefully, an unpleasant experience into a pleasant experience, we find ways to integrate our own style of being and our own style of therapy. We can take some of the ideas we learn from Erickson and other teachers, but each of us must find our own way of allowing in each therapeutic situation just the right kind of magical transformation to happen.

## REFERENCE

Erickson, M.H. The interspersal hypnotic technique for symptom correction and pain control. *American Journal of Clinical Hypnosis*, 1966, *3*, 198-209.

Chapter 30

# Erickson's Contribution to Pain Control in Cancer

*Paul Sacerdote*

Hypnosis is a successful tool for learning to control pain of organic origin, as well as pain with predominantly psychological components. Cancer, more than any other illness, is associated in our thinking with the image of severe, recurrent, protracted pain and painful death.

Experimental studies and clinical experience have demonstrated that hypnotic pain control results from something more than reduction of anxiety or "placebo" effects. Probably mechanisms similar to the ones proposed and described by Melzack and Wall (1965) in their "gate-control" theory become more easily activated under hypnosis. In clinical practice hypnotic approaches can be utilized for modifying, modulating, and generally controlling the intensity, quality, and duration of the pain experience, and the areas involved, while reducing anxiety and expectations of suffering.

While Hilgard and Hilgard's (1975) distinction between pain and suffering is a valid one, I cannot accept totally their implications that hypnotic anesthesia and analgesia are less authentic than that obtained by chemical means.

In Erickson's conception, hypnosis is an effective means for conveying to the patient ideas and understandings. Hypnotic trance is a state of special receptivity which increases the effectiveness of the therapist's communications. Erickson used hypnosis to motivate the patient to *translate* verbally and nonverbally expressed ideas into physiological, behavioral, and emotional responses.

Although the average person (including the physician with limited experience of hypnosis) views pain as a distressing and intense experience over which the individual has no control, Erickson devised and taught patients to make use of previous psychological and neurophysiological learnings to reduce or abolish pain. For instance, he often gave the example of the severely injured soldier or civilian who was unaware of pain for minutes or hours because his focus of attention was directed away from the injury. He stated (Erickson & Rossi, 1979), "by such experiences as these in the course of a lifetime, be they major or minor, the body learns a wealth of unconscious psychological, emotional, neurological and physiological associations and conditionings. These unconscious learnings, repeatedly reinforced by additional life experiences, constitute the source of the potentials that can be employed through hypnosis to control pain intentionally without resorting to drugs."

Erickson's clinical successes in a variety of psychotherapeutic situations, including pain problems and especially pain related to cancer, were based upon principles of universal validity which went beyond the skillful use of hypnosis. His approaches were painstakingly calculated to bring the patient into contact with previous meaningful life experiences and to mobilize actual or potential talent, while meeting and satisfying the subject's conscious and unconscious needs. Every therapeutic move in his strategic and tactical interventions was deliberately planned, executed and modified according to the patient's positive or negative responses.

In learning to achieve maximum success with cancer patients, we must thoroughly understand Erickson's approach to the patient, his problems, and his pain. Necessary first steps include a very careful look at the patient's appearance, behavior, facial expressions, and speech, and thorough gathering of information from the patient, family and friends. Also examined are family composition and reciprocal relations, friends, work, hobbies, present and past places of residence, and all possible areas of particular interest, including religious and political beliefs, education, and biases. Erickson utilized his extensive personal experience and his "many ears" as a clinician to almost intuitively discover and uncover the patient's expressed and unexpressed expectations, fears, anxieties, and doubts, and his conceptions of his illness and his pain. This systematic preparation allowed Erickson to assess physical, intellectual, and emotional capabilities well before actual initiation of hypnotherapy.

In all his therapeutic and hypnotherapeutic work, Erickson exposed the patient—gradually through anecdotes, symbols and metaphors, or suddenly through a surprise technique—to unexpected ways of looking at reality. He guided and forced the patient into restructured frames of reference. In the case of cancer pain, this included the acceptance of altered sensory-perceptual processes and responses. When a surprise approach was introduced, the patient had usually been prepared through subliminally interspersed suggestions for new physical, intellectual, and emotional discoveries and responses.

Basic to Erickson's approach was the construction of positive rapport to facilitate response attentiveness (receptivity) and positive expectations.

General and specific therapeutic suggestions were generally defined by Erickson as the "presentation of ideas." These were often deliberately interspersed during apparently aimless conversation or while reminiscing about some personal experience. Subtle variations in the volume, the tonality, and the speed with which ideas were presented subliminally conveyed to the patient's "unconscious" unexpected choices, indirect directions, or permissive commands. Often suggestions were so presented that the patient failed to notice the double or triple bind into which he had been guided and any response inevitably became a step along the path that Erickson created for mobilizing the patient's talents and for restructuring or discarding habitual, repetitive, or limited ways of perceiving, experiencing, and responding.

Erickson deliberately steered away from the simplistic view that pain was a "sensation" that should be eliminated. He acknowledged that there was indeed a physical component to pain, which was present even when conscious awareness was absent, e.g., in certain stages of sleep, in deep narcosis, in specific types of chemical anesthesia, etc. But, he dealt with pain essentially as a conscious and subjective phenomenon with disturbing, threatening, or dangerous connotations. Following careful preparation, the hypnotherapeutic approach appeared sometimes to solve the problem with unbelievable ease, even in cases where the pain was intense, protracted, and recurring. Still, Erickson recognized that for some patients, pain stubbornly resisted full modification.

Erickson did not isolate a physical component from psychological suffering; rather he noted that pain was not identical with a simple and uncomplicated noxious stimulus and that cancer pain was an entity characterized by differences in the parameters of time and space, an entity with psychological associations, based upon intellectual and emotional *body memories*. He also guided the patient to recognize that pain was a constructive motivational force in life. More than any other physical sign or symptom, pain serves, or has served in the person's past, a defensive or protective role in the integrity of the patient's body and identity. Concrete examples were used to illustrate the basic purpose of pain—to protect against more extensive damage. Recognizing that, for the patient, the memory of yesterday's pain contributes to today's pain perception and to tomorrow's expectations of still stronger pain, he utilized time distortion and memory manipulations to effect change.

The patient's attitude towards pain (Does he feel it as transient or persistent, unique or recurrent, acute or chronic?) suggested different, appropriately tailored, hypnotic approaches. Erickson pointed out that pain persisting in the same area of the body for a long time may result in the patient's attributing a painful character to any other sensation arising from that area; pain now becomes a habit which leads to other painful disturbances.

Illness and pain can originate or increase through the physician's conscious or unconscious attitudes and projections. Optimistically, it can be deduced that, if pain and illness have developed or become magnified iatrogenically, they can also be reduced or eliminated by the physician capable of using hypnosis.

Well in advance of more recent therapists who ask for the color and appearance of the pain, Erickson endeavored to extract from the patient a description of the pain. Was it dull, heavy, dragging, or sharp; cutting, burning, stabbing, biting or lancinating; was it twisting, nagging, grinding, or throbbing and gnawing; cold or hot? Realistically, he often limited himself, at the beginning of therapy, to eliciting minor modifications in the complex somatic and psychological pain-complex, as a first step toward gently and radically changing the total pain experience.

Among various hypnotic procedures for pain control, Erickson described *direct hypnotic suggestion* for total abolition of pain. A wonderfully simple approach, it, unfortunately, is effective with only a limited number of patients, and if unsuccessful, risks discouraging the much larger group of less responsive subjects, depriving them of the further use of hypnosis. Consequently, Erickson found *permissive indirect hypnotic abolition* of pain more conducive to receptiveness and responsiveness. He also promoted a *total or partial amnesia* for some of the subjective qualities which the patient attributed to the pain complex.

Another hypnotic procedure involves the development of partial, complete, or selective *hypnotic analgesia*, where the pain experience is reduced without the loss of other normal useful sensations of tact, pressure, temperature, position, etc. Even if the resulting analgesia is far from complete, the patient gains satisfaction, relief, and a sense of mastery.

*Hypnotic anesthesia* can preferably be indirectly achieved by the creation of psychological situations which are contradictory to the pain experience, so that the anesthesia can more easily be continued as a posthypnotic suggestion.

In some cases, Erickson found it feasible to suggest to the patient the *replacement or substitution of sensations.* He spoke of a cancer patient who accepted the idea of an incredibly annoying itch on the sole of one foot. In a weakened state, she could not reach down to scratch the bottom of her foot, and the suggested itching diverted her attention from the pain. Later on, he induced feelings of heaviness, numbness, or coolness to a number of painful areas, thus successfully replacing the original, intractable pain. *Displacement of the pain* from the affected area to a smaller, different area represents still another approach. Whenever feasible, Erickson prepared his cancer patients to experience *hypnotic dissociation* and *time or space disorientation,* which could be maintained after the termination of the hypnotic trance. By reorienting to a time before his illness and pain (actually an example of age regression), the patient is dissociated from his present painful condition or his pain loses some of the subjective qualities. *Space and body disorientation* permit a responsive patient to experience himself "apart from his body," leaving his sick body in one place and experiencing himself in another place or time.

For other patients, a useful hypnotic procedure is the *reinterpretation of the pain complex* as a feeling of heaviness, or of profound relaxation, warmth, and inertia. A stabbing, biting pain is hypnotically reinterpreted as nothing more than a sudden, startling reaction, very short and hardly painful. *Time distortion* was utilized by Erickson to transform the perception of four long hours (between narcotic injections) to that of a few short minutes. Or each attack can—because of suggested amnesia for the pain experience—come as a complete surprise and trigger a profound trance of 10 to 20 seconds duration. Erickson would utilize deep trance to suggest even fuller amnesia for all past pain attacks and the patient emerging from the trance would have neither awareness of having been in hypnosis nor recollection of suffered pain. Still another approach is the suggestion of an *inperceptible gradual diminution* of pain, continuing hour after hour and day after day.

It would be impossible to describe in detail all the possible variations in Erickson's use of hypnotic intervention for the purpose of modifying the pain experience. A careful and fairly complete description would indeed require a presentation of numerous cases and the explanation of why certain actions, comments, or words elicit certain verbal or nonverbal responses in the pain-afflicted cancer patient. Such detailed descriptions can be found in his numerous papers and in the books by Erickson and Rossi (1976, 1979) and by Haley (1967). I can only wish that every clinician who is using or intends to use hypnosis for the relief of pain, especially cancer-related pain, would carefully read and understand Erickson's use of innumerable roads to hypnosis, therapy, and the relief of pain.

## ADAPTATION OF ERICKSON'S APPROACHES TO PAIN CONTROL IN CANCER

I advocate a careful reading, rereading, and understanding of Ericksonian hypnotherapy, but feel it would be an error for any of us to attempt to copy, step by step, Erickson's clinical approaches. It is important to clearly understand how he selected the goals, then planned and adapted the therapy to each patient, using cognitive and intuitive appreciation of the individual's conscious and subconscious needs. His conception of memory involves and includes body-memory, inseparability of body and mind. The neurophysiological and biochemical substratum which underlies all physical and mental functions is implied in his attitudes and verbalizations. Erickson's *unconscious,* quite different from the Freudian id (it may be closer to a Jungian "archetype"), has attributes of basic wisdom which include the capacity of the body's organs and cells for producing physical and mental healing.

Each one of us in clinical hypnotherapy has evolved his own style for inducing, deepening, and utilizing productive hypnotic trances. The following is an example of Ericksonian principles and techniques for a cancer-related case of "phantom-limb pain," still in the process of active therapy.

Mrs. C.R., an ex-elementary school teacher, is 71 years old. Eighteen years ago an "inoperable" cancer of the right breast was treated with Betatrom at one of the best known hospitals for the treatment of malignant diseases. A few months later, she was able to resume her teaching career. But within three years, pain developed in the right shoulder, leading to the discovery of a metastatic lesion and treatment with radioactive cobalt. Four years later, she was forced to retire from teaching because of increasing pain and gradual functional impairment of the right upper extremity; hand and arm became progressively more edematous. From that point on, in spite of many therapeutic interventions (physiotherapy, exercises, intermittent rhythmical pressure, acupuncture, nerve-stimulation, novocaine and alcohol injections, and finally biofeedback), there was progressive deterioration and intolerable pain, which was not relieved by rhizotomy (1977).

In January of 1979, onset of progressive gangrene had forced Mrs. C.R. to accept amputation of the arm and hand. In spite of assurances that she would be quite comfortable within a couple of weeks of surgery, pain persisted, increased in intensity, and "localized" in the small finger, the palm of the hand, the wrist and the forearm of her amputated extremity, with the pain reaching maximum intensity three months after surgery (March of 1979).

The accurately constructed prosthesis was delivered, by coincidence, on the eve of her wedding anniversary. She tried it on, then took it off, and put it down on a chair and suddenly realized: "Part of me was on that chair. . . . I felt more at ease without the prosthesis than I was with it." To make things worse, while she had been told that hardly anybody would even notice, the plastic material of the hand became stained by the print of the Sunday paper. The stain remained indelible, forcing her to use a glove. This episode signaled the onset of a severe depression, which was aggravated when her intolerable pain was labeled "phantom-limb pain." Psychotropic medications and active treatment at a major pain clinic relieved the depression, while biofeedback achieved some temporary results in pain relief.

At this time she was referred for hypnotherapy. Therapy consisted of a reversed levitation induction using the left hand, followed by progressive eye closure and deepening, with dissociated motions of the fingers leading to beginning levitation.

During the period of trance, I conveyed the following ideas: that it was perfectly all right to let the "right hand" *sense and move like the left one,* even while perceiving pain in the small finger, in the palm of the hand, the wrist, and in the forearm muscles. I also mentioned, "It is not too difficult to learn to relax, and to stay relaxed even when not in hypnotic trance." The more relaxed you are, the less you feel." I also suggested her unconscious mind might begin to think about letting just 5 to 10 percent of the pain disappear, following each trance.

In spite of very horrible weather, the following three days were very comfortable; she felt very little pain. But the pain reappeared on the fourth day and required the use of Tylenol. In the meantime, feeling much more comfortable, she had stopped the antidepressant medication (Elavil). Part of the second visit was dedicated to a slow, lengthy discussion of brain-memory and body-memory, and it was stressed that she had the need and the right to "keep her painful right hand and arm," rather than to accept as her own a piece of sculptured plastic. After formal induction by repetition of conducted-reversed-left-hand levitation, I presented her with the suggestion that she could choose among retaining her right hand with full pain—if really necessary, renouncing all of the pain, or eliminating only another 5 to 10 percent. She might also choose to have recurrence of pain shortly before each visit to my office. Two weeks later, before the third visit, she had been surprised upon awakening in the morning by the total absence of pain. Afraid that pain would return upon getting up, she had remained in bed for several more hours, perfectly comfortable. This third visit was dedicated to the learning of self-hypnosis. This included the instruction of possibly "losing the habit of pain" without having to renounce the memory of her hand.

One day before the fourth visit, there was a recurrence of very intense pain. This she attributed to the weather (an early snowfall) and to the physical and emotional stress of having her apartment repainted. Before that recurrence, she had been able to practice self-hypnosis twice daily with fairly good success. During this visit, she became involved with multiple, probably significant, spontaneous free associations. These included the sensations of the rings which she used to wear on her right hand and of her brother's death in a plane accident in Europe, which had happened on the same day her father had died in a nursing home in New York. During his last few months in the nursing home, her father had developed the habit of kissing her right hand, the first and only outward sign of affection which he had ever shown. The recurrence of intense pain had coincided with her attending a funeral ceremony in the same chapel where the services for her brother's death had taken place, 20 years earlier. She also mentioned, rather casually, "I just happened to remember that back in 1959, when the pain had started to be rather severe and continuous, I had been able to "separate" myself from the pain between 9 A.M. to 3 P.M. every school day while teaching."

Following induction of hypnosis, I told her, "You still need to feel your hand . . . you may feel your hand on the cheek of a child, . . . or holding a piece of chalk, or wiping the blackboard, . . . or turning the pages of a book, . . .or you may feel the hand immersed in tepid water." I also speculated aloud about whether it would be easier for her to keep her hand with many, many pleasant memories or to become prepared to have no sensations of that hand and arm.

She attributed some difficulty in concentrating on her left hand and in achieving self-hypnosis during the following week to her doubts about permanence of success: "I always become enthused at the beginning of a new treatment. Then I gradually question whether I am really getting well or if I do this to myself?" The rest of this session is reported below, almost verbatim:

Dr.: "Do you think this happens because you *need* to have doubts that the pain will really go away? Look, this time, at your *right hand*—not at your left hand—and think more, understand more, and *know more of this pain in the right hand and the right arm.* Think more, understand more and *NO MORE of this pain in the right hand and right arm."* Every five to ten seconds, I repeated the same sentence with gradually increasing emphasis on the *"KNOW (NO) MORE* of this pain in the right hand and right arm." I observed an intense, but silent, abreaction, while I continued to repeat, "Think deeper and deeper, understand more, *need know (no) more of this pain in that hand and in that arm.* . . . Already you understand more, and know (no) more of this pain in your right hand and in your right arm, every second you continue to think very very deeply and understand more and *need know (no) more of this pain."*

At this point she "wakes up" spontaneously, states she has *no more* pain in the right arm, but has been unable to shake off completely the pain from her right hand.

Reinduction follows:

Dr.: "Look at that right hand again and *NOW* you understand more and *know (no) more of that pain."*

Again she emerges spontaneously from hypnosis.

Reinduction follows:

Dr.: *"Now* look at *THAT HAND* without any effort, without any concentration, maybe for just a few seconds, or just a few minutes, and *(NO) MORE* of that pain." She "awakes" again and remarks: "The sharpness is gone," and I continue, "Because every day you think more, you understand more, you *KNOW (NO) more,* and you realize and you recognize many things. You succeed better and better, you increase your understanding and you increase your acceptance better and better, and *KNOW (NO) MORE* of that pain."

At the termination of the trance we agree that she and I have an *ideal goal* and that we are pursuing a *practical goal.* The two lines are moving toward the same point, but they are not yet at the point of perfect convergence.

Six weeks later therapy was resumed and continued for a total of three more visits. She was trained to achieve full somnambulistic trances, which she liked to define as "aware-awake hypnosis." During such trances she spoke freely, while well aware that she was really in "very deep hypnosis." During one such period of therapeutic interaction she accepted the possibility of changing the now rare bouts of pain from fiery-red to orange, then to yellow, and finally to normal skin color.

She was also given the choice to feel, at any one time, either a right *normal* hand, or nothing at all.*

*Patient had been comfortable immediately upon leaving the hospital, following the amputation, quite adjusted to the feeling of her right empty sleeve. It was only after first seeing the brand-new prosthesis on a chair that the phantom-limb and the intolerable pain had made their appearance.

She started to notice that at social gatherings, in the company or presence of other women she became totally unaware of her prosthesis, and felt absolutely no pain. At this time she learned to recognize and trust the reality of her experiences of self-hypnosis. This made it feasible for her to accept the idea of "putting pain on the inactive file," starting with the second anniversary of her last hospital admission.

She was contacted eight months after the last visit. She reassured me that she had maintained all of the therapeutic gains achieved during hypnotherapy, and was finally leading a normal and comfortable life.

## REFERENCES


Erickson, M.H., & Rossi, E.L. *Hypnotic Realities.* New York: Irvington Publishers, 1976.

Erickson, M.H., & Rossi, E.L. *Hypnotherapy: An Exploratory Casebook.* New York: Irvington Publishers, 1979, p. 95.

Haley, J. *Advanced Techniques of Hypnosis and Therapy. Selected Papers of Milton H. Erickson, M.D.* New York: Grune and Stratton, 1967.

Hilgard, E.R., & Hilgard J.R. *Hypnosis in the Relief of Pain.* Los Altos, CA: Kaufman, 1975. pp. 86-102.

Melzack R, & Wall, P.D. Pain mechanisms: A new theory. *Science* 150, 971-979, 1965.

PART XII

# *Law Enforcement and Coercion*

*Martin Reiser, Ed.D., is the director of the Behavioral Science Service of the Los Angeles Police Department and a coordinator and a consultant to the investigative hypnosis research program of the Los Angeles Police Department. He is president of the Law Enforcement Hypnosis Institute, Inc., and is the founder of the Society for Investigative and Forensic Hypnosis. Reiser has authored numerous articles on policy psychology and also has written three books:* The Police Department Psychologist, Practical Psychology for Police Officers, *and* The Handbook of Investigative Hypnosis.

*In his chapter, Reiser discusses the forensic uses of hypnosis. Recently, there has been considerable controversy regarding the use of hypnosis to elicit memories from victims and witnesses of crimes. Some experts theorize that hypnosis can be used improperly on a witness, thereby forever damaging the witness' testimony. Some lawyers theorize that hypnotic testimony infringes on the defense counsel's right and ability to conduct cross-examination. Ethical issues are also involved; both the American Society of Clinical Hypnosis and the Society for Clinical and Experimental Hypnosis deem it unethical for members to instruct nonprofessionals (including police officers) in hypnotic technique. Erickson believed that hypnosis could be used by trained investigative officers to enhance recall of victims and witnesses of crimes. Erickson provided training in forensic hypnosis to Reiser and also his investigative police officers and trained investigative officers of the Phoenix Police Department.*

*Reiser discusses some of the concepts that Erickson taught in a 1978 workshop on investigative hypnosis. He provides historical background on the use of hypnotic technique by investigative agencies and discusses controversial issues in the field. Reiser presents strong arguments for the use of hypnotic technique by the use of trained police investigators.*

*Jacob Conn, M.D., is an assistant professor emeritus of the Johns Hopkins University Medical School. He is a life fellow of the American Psychiatric Associate and diplomate of the American Boards of Psychiatry, Child Psychiatry, and Medical Hypnosis. Dr. Conn is past president of both the Society for Clinical and Experimental Hypnosis and the American Board of Medical Hypnosis.*

*Conn eloquently presents his position that hypnosis cannot be misused to unduly influence a subject to commit antisocial acts. Some experts have disagreed with Conn's position. Conn presents the history of the controversy and cites evidence to support his position, including personal communication from Erickson, who believed that hypnosis could not be used to promote antisocial acts and was, in fact, a handicap to producing such behavior.*

*Unfortunately, Reiser and Conn were unable to attend the Congress; both submitted videotapes of their presentations.*

Chapter 31

# Erickson and Law Enforcement: Investigative Hypnosis

*Martin Reiser*

Erickson had a long-term interest in the use of hypnosis in relation to crime and was frequently called upon by law enforcement agencies for advice and assistance. He considered hypnosis to be "a most valuable tool in investigating the problems involved in securing correct information from witnesses and victims of crime (Note 1). In January 1978, Erickson accepted the first honorary membership in the Society for Investigative and Forensic Hypnosis.

Erickson made significant contributions in the areas of hypnotically-induced memory, amnesia, and hypermnesia. He differentiated conscious and unconscious memories, addressed the possibility of clinically dissociating the affective and cognitive elements of a traumatic experience, and ingeniously demonstrated the hypnotic process of transferring memories from the unconscious to the conscious mind (Erickson, 1955, 1965). This pioneering work presaged the possibilities of hypnotic recall in major crime cases.

During a workshop on investigative hypnosis in Phoenix on August 19, 1978, Erickson reiterated several useful concepts in working with witnesses to crimes, e.g., have the subject tell you the "least important" detail involved in the incident in question, then circle inward toward the important details; depersonalize the subject as an onlooker; have just the emotional content remembered; place the subject out of hypnosis and then back in; and put the little bits and pieces together to develop the whole picture. Also, the subject can be told, "I want you to be sure not to tell me anything you don't want to tell me." In regard to recalling license numbers (one of the more difficult tasks for witnesses), he pointed out that the hypnotist can suggest that the subject see the bottom part of a number, the top of another, the bottom of another. "You know a lot of numbers, some of them are not important here, so when you see these numbers, they will stand out a little bit more."

Dr. Erickson was a strong supporter of training police officers in investigative hypnosis techniques. He recognized the clear distinction between hypnotherapy and the specialty of forensic hypnosis (Note 2).

## BACKGROUND

Historically, hypnosis had been used only occasionally by police agencies for investigative purposes. In a few special cases, the services of a stage hypnotist, a "lay" practitioner, or a mental health professional had been engaged to assist in memory refreshment. In the mid-1950s, an effort was made to train police for in-house use of investigative hypnosis; however, the time was apparently not right and these attempts were not successful (Arons, 1967).

The growth and development of investigative hypnosis over the past five years has made a significant impact both in law enforcement circles and in the larger community by providing a viable tool to enhance the recall of volunteer witnesses in major crime cases (Reiser, 1979).

In the early 1970s, while I was using hypnosis clinically in my role as Department Psychologist at the Los Angeles Police Department (LAPD), I was asked by detectives about the efficacy of hypnosis for eliciting repressed memories of a witness in a homicide case. This successful experience led to increased requests for hypnosis interviews. By 1974, requests for investigative hypnosis exceed my ability to provide service.

In order to make investigative hypnosis available throughout the Department and to provide requested service, I designed a one-year demonstration research project to train selected, experienced investigators. This decision was based on the impression that it was not only feasible but also likely to be cost-effective (Reiser, 1976).

With the assistance of a panel of well-known consultants in hypnosis from local universities and the community, in June 1975 a 48-hour training program was conducted at the Police Academy. Eleven lieutenants and two captains were selected for training based on experience, ratings, interest in the program, and communication skills. In addition to hypnotic induction techniques, there was instruction in areas of information-gathering, professional and ethical practices, legal constraints and considerations, and handling of special emotional problems.

In the second phase of the program, the investigative hypnotists worked in pairs along with a consultant on cases assigned by the project director. Toward the end of the project year, the trainees were working autonomously, with consultants available on call as needed.

In approximately 77 percent of the cases during the project year, witnesses hypnotized by the investigative hypnotists were able to recall information of importance that was not available on routine interview. The solution of 16 percent of these cases was attributed essentially to the hypnotic information since no viable leads were available prior to the hypnotic session. Similar data have been reported by the F.B.I. and the Los Angeles County Sheriff's Department (Ault, 1980; Stratton, 1977).

In December 1977, the project was given the American Express/International Association of Chiefs of Police Award as the outstanding contribution to police science and technology (*Police Chief*, 1977). The program at LAPD is now in its sixth year. In appropriate cases hypnosis is considered a standard tool available to the investigative process.

During the five-year period from June 1975 through May 1980, data tabulated on 519 cases, mostly homicides, rapes and robberies, handled by the investigative hypnotists at LAPD revealed the following: In 80.6 percent of the cases, additional information was elicited with the use of hypnosis. Sixty-six percent of this information was considered of value by the case investigators. In approximately 50.5 percent of the cases where new information was obtained, accuracy was unable to be determined. In the remaining cases, the information was found to be accurate in 90.7 percent and inaccurate in 9.3 percent of the cases. In 65.6 percent of the solved cases, the hypnosis information was considered of value. To date, there have been no instances of harm resulting to the volunteer witnesses undergoing investigative hypnosis sessions. A large number of subjects report benefitting from the experience in a variety of ways, including sleeping better, having fewer nightmares, having less fear and anxiety, and experiencing improved relationships with significant others (Reiser, 1979).

A case example can be used to illustrate salient points. A homicide occurred while a woman was present in her boyfriend's apartment. Because of extreme intoxication, she could not recall any of the details of the murder of her friend, though she thought someone had entered the apartment. In spite of her desire to be helpful, she could not remember anything, because, as she put it, "I was bombed out of my skull."

During the subsequent hypnosis session, she was able to remember considerable detail about a suspect, including physical description, clothing, conversation, and a drug transaction involving her boyfriend. The composite drawing made by the police artist during the session turned out to be an accurate depiction of the suspect, and the other details obtained from the witness in hypnosis were also corroborated (Reiser, 1974). This case added confirmation to the hypothesis that dual perception and encoding of information occur at both conscious and subconscious levels simultaneously. Aspects of this phenomenon were later studied in the laboratory and discussed in detail as part of the concept of the "hidden observer" (Hilgard, 1977).

Another important finding involved two homicides that were committed 10 years previously. Hypnosis facilitated recollection of important information. Memories do not necessarily fade over time and hypnosis can be employed long after the actual event has occurred (Reiser, 1974). More recently, a North Carolina case involved the hypnotic recall of a homicide committed 35 years earlier. Subsequent corroboration was made by exhumed physical evidence and a confession (*The Washington Post*, 1979). The fact that detailed original perceptions can remain encoded and stored in long-term memory under repression available for possible retrieval with the aid of hypnosis is an important confirmation for investigative hypnosis practitioners.

Because of a strong interest in keeping investigative hypnosis on a sound professional level, the investigative hypnotists at LAPD formed a new international society. The Society for Investigative and Forensic Hypnosis, which now has over 600 members nationally, including behavioral science professionals, requires its members to have specialized training in investigative hypnosis and to adhere to stringent ethical and professional guidelines.

## CONTROVERSIAL ISSUES

The development of the new specialty of investigative hypnosis has not been without controversy. Two major clinical hypnosis societies have passed resolutions declaring it unethical for their members to train, collaborate, or consult with police who use investigative hypnosis (*International Journal of Clinical and Experimental Hypnosis*, 1979). Additionally, these groups have pressured affected members into recanting or resigning (Note 3). The Society for Investigative and Forensic Hypnosis has issued its own resolution deploring the stance of the two clinical societies and has raised questions about the motivations and ethics of those groups (*Newsletter*, 1980).

It is interesting to note that, while declaring it off-limits for their members to consult with police practitioners, these same clinical societies are attempting to establish legal guidelines which would limit investigative hypnosis to only licensed health professionals, most of whom have no specific legal training or experience. The rationale appears to be that all hypnosis is defined as medical or psychological. Nonlicensed health professionals are labeled as "lay" persons. Defining members of an out-group as "lay" is an old political ploy often used to maintain proprietary guild interests.

A related issue concerns disqualifying police from doing investigative hypnosis because of their alleged ignorance of basic scientific facts about hypnosis or purported tendencies to coerce or influence witness responses. The assertion that police think hypnosis is a truth detection technique is unsubstantiated. Persons untrained in investigative hypnosis from any professional area may hold that mistaken notion. The belief that the investigative hypnotist will suggest answers or cue the witness is belied by the fact that there are no suspects or answers in most of the cases in question. It is essentially for the purpose of obtaining new leads that one resorts to hypnosis. The idea that hypnosis is dangerous when done by law enforcement professionals is akin to the myths of mind control and of precipitating psychoses which were laid to rest years ago (Conn, 1972). In any case, the basic concerns really involve the questions of professionalism and ethical practices on the part of police, rather than the nature of hypnosis.

Another controversial issue involves the assertion by opponents of police investigative hypnosis that confabulation, distortion, and fantasies are a regular byproduct of witness hypnosis sessions. Experimental laboratory studies using nonsense syllables and poetry, or clinical therapy vignettes are cited as authority (Stalnaker & Riddle, 1932; Orne, 1979). These studies are basically irrelevant and do not deal with real-life situations involving traumatized witnesses to major crimes.

Corroboration in a significant number of crime cases where hypnosis was used shows that, if anything, accuracy is increased compared to normal eyewitness testimony (Buckout, 1974). The asserted loss of judgment and discrimination by the witness generally doesn't occur when hypnotist demand characteristics are handled properly (Orne, 1965; Reiser, 1980).

That hypnosis forever ruins a witness' credibility is another claim put forth by opponents of forensic hypnosis (Diamond, 1980). If anything, the investigative hypnosis process allows almost microscopic scrutiny and extensive review of procedures by way of witnesses, tapes, transcripts, expert testimony, and cross-examination.

Controversy exists about what theory of memory is relevant for investigative hypnosis cases. Opponents denigrate the cybernetic model, claiming the reconstructive one is obviously proven. Scant attention is paid to possibilities of Pribram's holographic hypothesis or to parallel processing theories (Penfield & Perot, 1963; Pribram, 1969). The state of the art regarding memory clearly reveals there are no completely validated and consensually accepted processes (Nilsson, 1979). Definitive experimental and theoretical work needs to be done (Baddeley, 1976). Investigative hypnosis can make an important contribution to establishing accurate models of human memory.

## LEGAL STATUS

Currently, relatively few states have made appellate decisions in regard to investigative hypnosis. In general, if the hypnosis session has been conducted properly with adequate cross-examination possible, the question goes to weight of the testimony rather than to its admissibility (Reiser, 1980). In helping to refresh a witness' memory, hypnosis is considered in the same category as a photograph, a song, or written material. It is the witness' present memory, refreshed, weighed by the trier of fact, that is important.

Strong efforts are being made to convince the courts that investigative hypnosis routinely produces confabulation and forever ruins the witness' credibility (Orne, 1979; Diamond, 1980). However, the so-called experts making these claims have no proof or relevant data from major crime cases where hypnosis has been properly conducted by a trained investigative hypnotist. Artificial laboratory research with college students or clinical anecdotes with disturbed patients are not adequate evidence (Neisser, 1978).

## THE FUTURE OF INVESTIGATIVE HYPNOSIS

Law enforcement administrators are pragmatic people. Investigative hypnosis is being used widely by criminal justice agencies around the country because it works. Initial skepticism related to the old Svengali image and the myth of mind control is giving way to the awareness that this tool can often help solve serious crime cases. The few examples presented of the misuse of investigative hypnosis are overshadowed by the many publicized and unheralded instances of success (Reiser, 1980).

Milton Erickson lent his knowledge, his approval, and his support to the use of hypnosis in law enforcement. It is likely that investigative hypnosis will continue to be used effectively and will make a significant contribution to society.

## REFERENCE NOTES

1. Bloom, P. Personal communication, June 9, 1980.
2. Erickson, M.H. Personal communication, January 16, 1978.
3. Erickson, E. Personal communication, July 8, 1980.

## REFERENCES


Arons, H. *Hypnosis in Criminal Investigation.* Springfield, Il: Thomas, 1967.

Ault, R. Hypnosis: The FBI's team approach. *FBI Law Enforcement Bulletin,* January, 1980, 5-8.

Baddeley, A.D. *The Psychology of Memory.* New York: Basic Books, 1976.

Buckout, R. Eyewitness Testimony. *Scientific American,* December, 1974, 23-31.

Conn, J.H. Is hypnosis really dangerous? *International Journal of Clinical and Experimental Hypnosis,* 1972, *20,* 61-79.

Diamond, B.L. Inherent problems in the use of pretrial hypnosis on a prospective witness. *California Law Review,* 1980, 68, 313-349.

Erickson, M.H. Self-exploration in the hypnotic state. *Journal of Clinical and Experimental Hypnosis,* 1955, *3,* 49-57.

Erickson, M.H. A special inquiry with Aldous Huxley into the nature and character of various states of consciousness. *American Journal of Clinical Hypnosis,* 1965, 8, 14-33.

Gilbert, J.N. *Criminal Investigation.* Columbia, Ohio: Merrill Publishing Company, 1980, 117-119.

Hilgard, E.R. *Divided Consciousness.* New York: Wiley Interscience, 1977.

*International Journal of Clinical and Experimental Hypnosis,* October, 1979, 452-453.

Kroger, W.S. *Clinical and Experimental Hypnosis, Second Edition.* Philadelphia: Lippincott, 1977.

Neisser, U. Memory: what are the important questions? In: *Practical Aspects of Memory.* Gruneberg, M.M., Morris, P.E., and Sykes, R.N., Eds. New York: Academic Press, 1978, p. 5.

*Newsletter,* Society for Investigative and Forensic Hypnosis, February, 1980.

Nilsson, L.G. (Ed.) *Perspectives on Memory Research.* Hillside, New Jersey: Erlbaum, 1979.

Orne, M.T. The nature of hypnosis: artifact and essence. In: *The Nature of Hypnosis.* Shor, R.E. and Orne, M.T., Eds. New York: Holt, Rinehart and Winston, 1965, 89-123.

Orne, M.T. The use and misuse of hypnosis in court. *The International Journal of Clinical and Experimental Hypnosis,* 1979, *27,* 311-341.

Penfield, W. Memory mechanisms. *Archives of Neurology and Psychiatry,* 1952, *67,* 178-198.

Penfield, W. & Perot, P. The brain's record of auditory and visual experience. *Brain,* 1963, *86,* 595-696.

People V. Biehler, Crim. No. 30781, Second Dist., Div. One, March 5, 1979.

Pribram, K.H. The neurophysiology of remembering. *Scientific American,* January, 1969, 73-86.

*Police Chief,* December, 1977, p. 22.

Reiser, M. Hypnosis as an aid in a homicide investigation. *The American Journal of Clinical Hypnosis,* October, 1974, 84-87.

Reiser, M. Hypnosis as a tool in criminal investigation. *The Police Chief,* November, 1976, 36-40.

Reiser, M. Hypnosis and its uses in law enforcement. *The Police Journal* (British), January-March, 1978, 24-33.

Reiser, M. Investigative Hypnosis—A Developing Specialty. Presented at the Annual Conference of the American Society of Clinical Hypnosis, San Francisco, November 16, 1979.

Reiser, M. *Handbook of Investigative Hypnosis.* Los Angeles: LEHI Publishing Company, 1980.

Stalnaker, J. & Riddle, E. The effect of hypnosis on long-delayed recall. *Journal of General Psychology*, 1932, *6*, 429-440.

Stratton, J. The use of hypnosis in law enforcement criminal investigations. *Journal of Police Science and Administration*, 1977, *4*, 399-406.

*The Washington Post*, December 16, 1979, A 4.

Chapter 32

# The Myth of Coercion Under Hypnosis

*Jacob H. Conn*

Milton H. Erickson was a brilliant innovator, a scrupulous investigator, a superb, dedicated teacher, and the outstanding leader in American hypnosis.

In 1949, I wrote, "Erickson, probably is the most ingenious and clinically astute hypnotist of our time, who repeatedly has stressed the great need for the patient to participate actively in any reorganization of his psychic life." He has admonished the hypnotist "to use that technique, which permits him to express himself most satisfactorily and effectively in the special relationship, which constitutes hypnosis." Over the years I have kept these pertinent clinical observations as the core of my therapeutic endeavors.

My interest in the possibility that hypnosis can be used for antisocial purposes was alerted when in 1970 I read Glasner's (1955) paper, in which he severely criticized Erickson (1939) for "not employing proper techniques by which definitive antisocial acts can be obtained." I was especially aroused by Glasner's accusation that, "anyone familiar with the highly sophisticated techniques, which Erickson uses in most of his experiments, must be struck with the unimaginative planning and impoverished methodology, which he used in these experiments on the antisocial use of hypnosis" (p. 33).

When I reread Glasner's forthright statement in regard to improper techniques and "impoverished methodology," I recalled Erickson's (1962) critical question, "Why should anyone assume that hypnosis is of necessity a matter of distorting reality? . . . One could equally well say that hypnosis is a state of readiness to utilize learnings . . . and abilities" (p. 340). Since I needed further clarification, I wrote to Erickson, who replied, "The fact is that I wanted to know, if in some way, I could actually get a hypnotic subject to perform antisocially, and also was willing to employ a variety of techniques easily overlooked. I earnestly wanted my subjects to perform antisocial acts." (Note 1).

Thirty years after the publication of Erickson's (1939) paper on "An Experimental Investigation of the Possible Antisocial Use of Hypnosis," he still was of the same opinion, that:

> An antisocial act has to be antisocial. It just cannot be a laboratory performance. You don't need hypnosis to induce antisocial behavior. In fact, hypnosis is a handicap in inducing antisocial behavior. Anybody doing something antisocial wants to know where he is, and who is around, and what time of day it is, and the possible consequences. Hypnosis constricts awareness of our surroundings and this constriction defeats our efforts (Note 1).

Erickson's informed, critical comments may explain why professional criminals have avoided using hypnosis to expedite major crimes. Hypnosis cannot be used to augment antisocial behavior; in fact, as Erickson maintained, hypnosis would handicap efforts to carry out antisocial behavior.

However, during the past three decades, Kline (1972), Levitt, Aronoff, Morgan, Overley, and Parrish (1975), and Watkins (1947, 1972) have expressed statements, that conceive of hypnosis as being a powerful tool which can be used to coerce a subject to perform antisocial acts. Thus, Watkins (1972) is convinced that, "a hypnotist of evil intent could . . . mobilize harmful and destructive forces within his subject. If we can anesthetize an arm to remove pain, then we can anesthetize a superego to remove guilt" (pp. 97-98).

There are several basic errors upon which Watkins' thinking is predicated:

1) The above reasoning assumes that the hypnotic process is a powerful state relationship which can be manipulated at the whim of the hypnotist. However, hypnosis is not a "power" which can be used to overcome the "will" of a subject. It is often role-playing, a folie á deux, an alibi, a neurotic compromise, a rationalization of motivated helplessness, or a legitimatization of behavior, as well as being a genuine automatization and a dissociative, regressive experience.
2) It is not a part of a body which is being hypnotized but an integrated person with his motivations, expectations, attitudes and willingness to be hypnotized.

3) The superego is a hypothesized concept. As Erickson (1962) aptly has stated, "The ego [or superego] is a helpful and convenient concept, but that is all that it is. The term ego [or superego] is a verbalization to permit better communication of abstractions employed in conceptualizing. Then, to speak of the strength of the ego [or of anethesizing the superego] as a reality attribute serves only to lead scientific thinking further afield" (p. 340).

Moreover, as Erickson emphasized repeatedly, a trance state is unique and personal but belongs only to the subject who uses it as he wishes in accordance with his basic needs. Erickson (1962) suggested that hypnosis is not a state " . . . in which one person, the operator takes responsibility for another, the subject, or an interpersonal relationship in which the operator restructures the perceptions and conceptions of the subject" (p. 340). He conceived of hypnosis as being a form of *normal* human behavior.

Is a subject *always* in a "state" of hypnosis, or does a hypnotic "relationship" develop *every time* a subject stares at an object, closes his eyes, remains immobile, and/or maintains his arm in a fixed position? Is suggestibility or even hypersuggestibility the only or chief criterion? Should we not expect to obtain a subjective report of alterations of consciousness, changes in the body image, memory, time-sense, and an augmented capacity to tolerate logical inconsistencies?

Also, before we can begin to think of hypnosis as being the crucial, necessary, and sufficient factor in the production of antisocial behavior, the ubiquity of the simulation response must be scrupulously evaluated. Kubie (1972) has pointed out,

> It is equally certain then that all of us are vulnerable to an unwitting simulation of the hypnotic state, sometimes without knowing, that in part at least, we may be shamming. This is one of the confusing and disturbing facts about the whole range of research in hypnotic phenomena, i.e., that we do not have absolute criteria or precise tests to differentiate between consciously simulated hypnosis, preconsciously simulated hypnosis, and automatic or involuntary hypnosis, itself (pp. 209-210).

Therefore, it is probable that many of the reported cases of antisocial behavior under hypnosis include subjects who were not really hypnotized but were "shamming" or role-playing.

Furthermore, Haley (1963) has indicated that from a communication point of view the subject acts as if he is helpless, in order to force someone to take charge of him. The subject's behavior can, therefore, be considered as being a nonverbal communication. Van der Walde (1965) contended the trance state is actually the result of a subject's needs, motivations and willingness to be hypnotized, and is not due to the hypnotist's "power." As Orne (1972) has emphasized, "It is not the command quality of the instructions, which the subject receives directly, but the cue quality, which is implicitly communicated, so that regardless of appearance, it becomes apparent, that it is safe for the subject to proceed."

Therefore, Erickson was scientifically correct when he concluded that, "Laboratory crimes are impossible, because the perpetrators are in a completely protected situation," and that, "the entire performance is nothing but make believe" (Note 1).

Nevertheless, a vast literature exists which attempts to demonstrate that crime and seduction are possible under hypnosis. By 1860, Charpignon had collected many alleged examples of antisocial behavior following hypnotic induction. By 1887, Bjornstrom could admonish his readers that, "The unconsciousness and loss of will, which are so easily caused in the hypnotized, can of course, with the greatest facility, be used for immoral purposes." Bjornstrom was certain that rape, murder, robbery and abduction were easy to accomplish through hypnosis. He concluded that, "There would be no difficulty in making away with an enemy, in a manner, which would not betray the originator of the crime. It is only necessary to hypnotize the victim, and to give him the suggestion that he will commit suicide, which he could not resist." He cited A.M. Liégois, a professor of jurisprudence at Nancy, who had a special gift for making women believe that they owed him money, adding that, "*He does not even need to hypnotize them* in order to convince them of it." Thus, Liégois (cited in Ellenberger, 1970) was able to *suggest* to Miss E, who "apparently was in a *wakeful and normal state,* that she had stabbed her best friend, and that the body was still lying in the victim's home."

The lack of concern in the laboratory situation for the difference between normal wakefulness and the hypnotic state was based upon Bernheim's concept of the nature of suggestion. His major interest had been only in classifying individuals as being "more or less suggestible with only minimal concern about the nature of the relationship which develops between the hypnotist and his subject" (Ellenberger, 1970, p. 761). But, as Haley (1963) has also properly emphasized, "Hypnotic behavior is responsive behavior *only* in a relationship, rather than being an aspect of a person's character" (pp. 38-39).

In the 1880s there already were marked differences of opinion in regard to the probability of coercion under hypnosis. The Salpêtrière School led by Charcot denied the possibility of such crimes. The disciples of The Nancy School, whose chief protagonist was Bernheim, maintained the opposite point of view. These contradictory opinions led to frequent legal disputes between the experts of the two schools (Ellenberger, 1970).

Bernheim (cited in Ellenberger, 1970) believed in the existence of an "enhanced suggestive state." Nevertheless, he maintained that, "Hypnosis was nothing, but the effect of suggestion." He, therefore, could conclude that a woman had been "hypnotized," because she had acted "under the suggestion of her paramour, when she lured a bailiff into her apartment, so that her lover could strangle and rob him."

This type of theorizing about anecdotal data became the basis of the hypothesis that considered "hypnosis" to be an external "force" which could weaken or overcome the "willpower" of a subject. This belief in the overwhelming force of suggestions was fostered by the theories of faculty psychology promulgated by Thomas Reid (1710-1796) and his chief popularizer, Dugald Stewart (1753-1828). Their ideas became an integral part of Gall's phrenology (1758-1828). It was Braid's acceptance of the tenets of faculty psychology, which led to his belief in the existence of Phreno-Hypnotism. Braid was convinced that he could demonstrate its scientific validity by touching a cork, which was placed over the area or organ of "Veneration," and then hypnotize the subject. After "about a minute and a half" the subject would begin to clasp his arms in adoration, and kneel as if engaged in prayer" (Braid, 1960). No investigator in the present era has been able to replicate the phenomena of Phreno-Magnetism. Therefore, it would appear that Braid's subject must have had a conception of the theories of faculty psychology, was convinced of the existence of the organ of Veneration, and had *expected* to behave as he did (Conn, 1967).

It was this type of folie á deux that led Orne and Evans (1965) to begin working with simulators. These investigators replicated Rowland's (1939) findings in which a hypnotized patient carried out the suggestion to throw "acid" at an experimentor. They demonstrated that "similar apparently antisocial behavior could be elicited in control groups treated in an identical fashion to a group of hypnotized subjects. Furthermore, the frequency rate of compliance was highest for the simulators, and lowest for the waking controls with the hypnotized subject's compliance ranking after simulators." Orne and Evans (1965), therefore, concluded that "hypnosis may be capable of inducing antisocial, dangerous, or self-destructive behavior, but this is difficult to demonstrate since such acts may be elicited *without* hypnosis."

Our predecessors and pioneers in the development of mesmerism, the early magnetizers, were, in my opinion, better "psychologists" and clinicians than those modern hypnotists who still maintain that the hypnotized subject cannot defend himself and that his "willpower" can be surrendered to an "all powerful" hypnotist. Thus Puységur (1755-1848), the discoverer of magnetic somnambulism, could affirm in 1784 that "all of his patients had declared to him that they preserved, in that (mesmeric) state, their judgment and their reason, that they perceived very quickly the designs of the magnetizer, and that these could readily cause them to awaken" (Puységur, 1850).

Braid, who first used the term hypnosis in 1843, was of the opinion that perception and judgment were not abolished in hypnosis even in the "deep" stage. He believed, "If anything were done, which was opposed to their moral sense, they at once passed into the "alert" stage, and were capable of defending themselves, as when they were in the waking condition." Braid therefore concluded, "It is not the hypnotist's power, but the consequence of the patient's *self-suggestion,* by which he made himself believe, that hypnosis could be a condition of helpless automatism" (1960, p. 168). Also, Bramwell (1913) has stated, "Personally, I have never seen a single somnambule, who did not possess or exercise the power of resisting suggestions contrary to his moral sense." He, like Braid, concluded that, "If a subject believed that hypnosis was a condition of helpless automatism, then harm would result, *not through the operator's power,* but in consequence of the subject's *self-suggestions*" (p. 425).

In the present era, Wolberg (1948) also has maintained that the hypnotized patient may be "uncooperative and negativistic to the point of mutism, which may persist even in deep hypnosis. He may lose his motive for being hypnotized, and resist entering trance states. . . . The patient is an active agent, whose defenses are not obliterated. The capacity to reflect and synthesize remains unimpaired. The patient is very much aware, whether he is being investigated, or being treated in accordance with his basic characterlogic needs."

Gill and Brenman (1959) have asserted,

> It is a myth to believe that the hypnotic subject loses all of his normal capacity to appraise outer reality and to maintain his capacity for choice. . . . The defensive operations are by no means abolished in the hypnotic state, and . . . there is the freedom to act according to the hypnotic subject's needs.

More recently, Perry (1979) has reported two women who had sexual relations with a lay hypnotist. Both women stated there never had been any degree of coercion. Also, there had been no close relationship between the hypnotist and the two women, and there was no attempt to distort their perception of reality. Perry concluded, "Hypnosis per se was not involved in overcoming these patients' willpower." He presented two alternative hypotheses: 1) There is the possiblity of a "motivated helplessness." This could be a rationalization in retrospect, as a means of disowning responsibility for one's own behavior (Conn, 1972). 2) A "self-fulfilling prophecy" (Orne, 1972) is present or a "belief in efficacy" (Johnson & Barber, 1978) may occur, "when the patient believes that being in hypnosis means that all initiative and self-determination are surrendered to the hypnotist." This is only an apparently new point of view, since it is actually a corroboration of Braid's (1843) earlier conclusion that the significant factor is self-suggestion.

Investigators who believe that hypnosis per se can be used to obtain antisocial behavior have overlooked Erickson's pertinent observations. In his letter to me, Erickson (Note 1) wrote,

> Masters and Johnson would have been defeated in their studies of sexual behavior had they tried to use hypnosis. The person would want to be fully aware and as self protected as possible. . . . If a nurse were placed in a state of hypnotic trance and given suggestions that she go about her duties as if she were wide awake, and without her knowledge, a poison was placed in the milk in the refrigerator, and if she were to give the patient a glass of that poisoned milk, the result would be called, "The Use of Hypnosis in Producing Antisocial Behavior."

Erickson was adamant that "the hypnotic subject has to have knowledge of what he is going to do. He has to be aware that a crime is to be done, and any misconception of what his acts are abrogates any antisocial behavior." Indeed, he wrote, "If you were to alter a subject's perceptual awareness in order to bring about a crime, you would have the added problem of altering your own subjective behavior" (e.g. of asking a hypnotized subject to fire a loaded revolver). Erickson also related a number of examples of skilled hypnotists who "repeatedly failed in attempts to have sexual relations in the trance state with their wives or mistresses. In each case their sexual partners had refused, while hypnotized, but resumed sexual relations in the waking state, because they felt deprived by being in the trance state." Therefore, he correctly concluded, "For a real crime or genuine antisocial behavior, there has to be a knowledge of it, and an intent. Such knowledge and intent bring forth self-protective behavior" (Note 1).

My own experiences vindicate Erickson's denial of the possibility that antisocial behavior can occur under hypnosis. Two representative cases from my own practice illustrate why hypnosis per se cannot explain why certain females are readily seduced by their hypnotists. In each case the woman was married and stated that she "loved" her husband, was initially "puzzled" by her sexual compliance, insisted that her sex behavior was "unnatural" and that it had been "forced" upon her by a "skilled" hypnotist. Later, however Mrs. A said, "This hypnotist happened to be the one who came along—any other man would have been the same. He didn't need hypnosis." Mrs. B said, "I wanted to do the same thing my husband did; then I couldn't accuse him [of philandering], and I couldn't be hurt again." What is of particular interest is that Mrs. B on repeated attempts was not able to become more than lightly hypnotized by clinical or standardized scale criteria, thus making it difficult to posit hypnosis as the critical variable.

Bieber (1953) has described a masochistic maneuver in which patients who are "unable to fulfill a basic need to give love and be loved must seek gratification for these frustrated needs to be fully loved as they have been as children." They therefore endow the hypnotist with "magical power" and think of him as being a parent surrogate. These patients rationalize that they are being impelled to give in to what the hypnotist wants, when, in fact, it is what they themselves need.

Both of my patients had complained of having been rejected and "unneeded" by their husbands. Both had described their relationship to the lay hypnotist as being that of "a child to a kind, understanding father," and both had transformed their hypnotists into omnipotent lovers and father surrogates. Mrs. B stated, "I had a mission to perform. I *knew* what the hypnotist wanted, and wished to get it over with as soon as possible." She was not compulsively pleasing the hypnotist, but said that she had wanted to experience the "guilt" associated with her adultery, so that she would no longer be hurt by her husband's need for "freedom" (and philandering). Neither patient was a passive "victim" of a "powerful," highly skilled hypnotist; rather, each was actively seeking an erotic, masochistic, regressive relationship with a father surrogate.

If Erickson's conclusions are scientifically valid, and I believe that they are, how did the myth arise that hypnosis can be used coercively for antisocial purposes? Our cultural heritage of hypnosis includes the residues of demonology, magic, and the ubiquitous Evil Eye. Indeed, "the phenomenon of hypnosis has a close resemblance to that of witchcraft, which in societies that accept this belief exerts an awesome and destructive effect" (Orne, 1972). Many novels and plays have been written about mesmerized or hypnotized subjects who were totally controlled and compelled to perform suggested crimes by "diabolical" hypnotists who were well versed in occult lore. In almost every case the hypnotist is a stereotype who is described as having a "powerful will" and "piercing penetrating eyes," while the subject is said to be "very suggestible, humble, naive, and guileless" (Ludwig, 1963).

Other contributing factors to the myth of possible coercion are the illusions of stage hypnotists, who often "suggest" to selected volunteers that they should help them to put on a good show. These allegedly helpless subjects usually are role-playing and act as if they are totally deprived of "willpower."

If it is so easy to deprive individuals of their initiative and "willpower," why are there so few documented real-life crimes committed under hypnosis? Moreover, why don't crime syndicates utilize hypnosis to a greater extent? In a detailed review of the legal cases, Orne (1962) found not a single instance where hypnosis was used to induce antisocial or destructive actions without a longstanding and intense relationship with the hypnotist which was sufficient in and of itself to explain the events that transpired. He therefore concluded that, "when a subject carries out an action in hypnosis, it does not necessarily mean that he carries out the action *because* he is hypnotized. Careful evaluations of these situations invariably suggest that the distortion of perception or memory serve more to rationalize and legitimatize behavior than to act as *causal* behavior."

Watkins (1972) maintains that "we behave on the basis of our perceptions . . . if our perception of a certain situation can be altered, then our behavior in relation to it can be altered." However, since none of the controls that were utilized by Orne and Evans (1965) were employed by Watkins (1972), it cannot be concluded that the restructuring of a subject's reality is either a necessary or sufficient cause of antisocial behavior under hypnosis. Watkins' (1972) suggested antisocial acts, like his case of the hypnotized soldier who attacked a superior officer when he was described as being an enemy, occurred in the presence of an audience. Erickson (1967) indicated the qualitative difference that exists between laboratory and clinical hypnosis. Since Watkins' results occur in quasi-laboratory settings, the subject may believe that he is doing something for "science" or for himself and may attempt to discover the goals of the investigator in order to help him to achieve them.

How can we avoid such artifacts? Can we prevent our subjects from believing that all initiative and self-determination are surrendered to an "all powerful" hypnotist? This is a "shared illusion," and "the more widely it is understood that subjects retain the ultimate decision to comply with or refuse a suggestion, the less likely it is that the fiction of hypnotic power will be used in a manner destructive to the hypnotist and subject" (Orne, 1972).

The myth of coercion under hypnosis has been fostered by cultural lag, stage hypnosis, stereotyped science-fiction novels and plays about "diabolical" hypnotists, and more recently, by uncritical and misinformed investigators. It can be corrected only by the dedicated efforts of informed practitioners of the art and science of hypnosis. This is the epitome of the teaching of Milton H. Erickson who wrote (1948) that, "Direct suggestion implies that the therapist has the miraculous power of affecting therapeutic (and antisocial) changes in the patient, and disregards the fact that therapy (and change) results from an inner resynthesis of the patient's behavior achieved by the patient, himself."

I conclude, and concur with Erickson's conviction (1939) that "Hypnosis cannot be misused to induce hypnotized persons to commit actual, wrongful acts, either against themselves or others, and that the only serious risk encountered in such attempts is incurred by the hypnotists in the form of condemnation, rejection, and exposure."

## REFERENCE NOTE

1. Erickson, M.H. Personal Communication, 1970.

## REFERENCES


Bieber, I. The Meaning of Masochism, *Am. J. Psychotherapy*, 1953, *7*, 433-448.

Bjornstrom, F. *Hypnotism, Its History and Present Development*, New York: Humbolt Publishing Co., 1887.

Braid, J. *Braid on Hypnotism*, New York: Julian Press, 1960.

Bramwell, J.M. *Hypnotism, Its History, Practice and Theory*, London: W. Rider and Son, 1913.

Charpignon, J. Rapport Du Magnetisme Avec La Jurisprudence, *et la Medicin Legal*, Paris: Ballier, 1860.

Conn, J. H. Hypnosynthesis—Hypnosis as a unifying interpersonal experience, *J. Nerv. Ment. Dis.*, 1949, *109*, 9-24.

Conn, J.H. The clinical aspects of consciousness in hypnosis. In: *Psychodynamics and Hypnosis*, M.V. Kline (Ed.), Springfield, Il.: Charles C Thomas, 1967.

Conn, J.H. Is hypnosis really dangerous? *Int. J. Clinical and Exper. Hypnosis*, 1972, *20*, 61-79.

Ellenberger, H.F. *The Discovery of the Unconscious*, New York: Basic Books, 1970.

Erickson, M.H., An experimental investigation of the possible antisocial use of hypnosis. *Psychiat.*, 1939, *2*, 395-414.

Erickson, M.H. Hypnotic techniques for the therapy of acute psychiatric disturbances in war. *Am. J. Psychiat.* 1945, *101*, 668.

Erickson, M.H. Hypnotic psychotherapy. *Med. Clinics of North America*, 1948, p. 574.

Erickson, M.H. Basic psychological problems in hypnotic research. In: *Hypnosis: Current Problems*, G. H. Estabrook (Ed.), New York: Harper and Row, 1962.

Erickson, M.H. Laboratory and clinical hypnosis: The same or different phenomena?, *Am. J. of Clinical Hypnosis*, 1967, *9:* 3, 166-170.

Gill, M.M. & Brenman, M. *Hypnosis and Related States.* New York: International Universities Press, 1959.

Glasner, S., Social psychological aspects of hypnosis. In: *Hypnodynamic Psychology*, M.V. Kline (Ed.), New York: Julian Press, 1955.

Haley, J., *Strategies of Psychotherapy*, New York: Grune and Stratton, 1963, pp. 38-39.

Johnson, R.F.Q., & Barber, T.X. Hypnosis, suggestion, and warts, an experimental investigation—Implicating the importance of belief in efficacy. *Am. J. Clin. Hypnosis*, 1978, *20*, 105-174.

Kline, M.V. The production of antisocial behavior through hypnosis: New clinical data. *Int. J. Clin. and Exper. Hypnosis*, 1972, *20*, 80-94.

Kubie, L.S. Illusions and reality in the study of sleep, hypnosis, psychosis and arousal. *Int. J. Clin. and Exper. Hypnosis*, 1972, *20*, 205-223.

Levitt, E.E., Aronoff, G., Morgan, C. D., Overley, T.M., & Parrish, M.J.; Testing the coercive power of hypnosis, committing objectionable acts. *Int. J. Clin. and Exper. Hypnosis*, 1975, *23*, 59-67.

Ludwig, A.M. Hypnosis in fiction. *Int. J. Clin. Exp. Hypnosis*, *11*, 71-80, 1963.

Orne, M.T. Antisocial behavior and hypnosis: Problems of control and validation. In: *Hypnosis: Current Problems*, G.H. Estabrook (Ed.), New York: Harper and Row, 1962.

Orne, M.T. Can a hypnotized subject be compelled to carry out otherwise unacceptable behavior? *Int. J. Clin. and Exper. Hypnosis*, 1972, *20*, 101-117.

Orne, M.T. & Evans, F.J. Social control in the psychological experiment: Antisocial behavior and hypnosis. *J. Per. Soc. Psych.*, 1, 189-200, 1965.

Perry, C. Hypnotic coercion and compliance to it: A review of evidence presented in a legal case. *Int. J. Clin. Exper. Hypnosis*, 1979, *27*, 3:187-218.

Puységur, C. de, cited by Deleuze, J.F.P., *Practical Instructions in Animal Magnetism*, New York: Appleton and Co., 1850.

Rowland, L.W. Will hypnotized persons try to harm themselves or other? *J. Abnorm. Soc. psychol.*, *34*, 114-117, 1939.

van der Walde, P.H. Interpretation of hypnosis in terms of ego psychology. *Arch. Gen. Psychiat.*, *12*, 438-447, 1965.

Watkins, J.G. Antisocial compulsions induced under hypnotic trance. *J. Abn. Soc. Psychol.*, 1947, *42*, 256-259.

Watkins, J.G., Antisocial behavior under hypnosis—Possible or impossible? *Int. J. Clin. Exper. Hypnosis*, 1972, *20*, 95-100.

Wolberg, L.R. *Medical Hypnosis.* New York: Grune & Stratton, 1948.

## PART XIII

# *Transcultural Approaches*

*Erickson often admonished his students to study anthropology. His approach was based on modifying psychotherapy to the unique characteristics of the individual. Normality, psychopathology, and even response to hypnosis vary across cultures. Psychotherapists need to recognize cultural differences and maintain enough flexibility to respond to such differences in their patients.*

*Madeleine Richeport, Ph.D., is a visiting professor of anthropology at the Federal University of Rio Grande de Norte in Natal, Brazil, where she has researched ritual trance. Dr. Richeport also worked as an anthropologist at the School of Health in San Juan, Puerto Rico, where she studied mediumship and Puerto Rican spiritism.*

*Richeport was one of a number of anthropologists (including Margaret Mead and Gregory Bateson) who studied with Erickson and benefited from his expertise on hypnosis. In her chapter, Richeport applies an Ericksonian orientation to understanding ritual trance. Spiritist possession can be reframed as a socially acceptable way of explaining normal and pathological psychological aberrations. She describes a case in which spiritism was used to promote effective psychotherapy.*

*Gosaku Naruse, Dr. Med. Sc., is professor of psychology on the Faculty of Education at Kyushyu University in Japan. Previously, he served as Dean of the Faculty of Education at Kyushyu University.*

*Naruse's work in the field of hypnosis is well-known. For seven years, he served as editor of the* Japanese Journal of Hypnosis. *He has authored seven Japanese books on hypnosis and psychotherapy and has edited 10 additional Japanese books on hypnosis and psychotherapy. Additionally, he has written more than 60 professional papers on the topics of hypnosis and psychotherapy. Currently he is editor of the* Japanese Journal of Rehabilitation Psychology.

*Naruse presents the basic format for the application of Jiko-control, the psychotherapy that he originated and which is apparently one of Japan's most popular schools of psychotherapy. It is a systematic method of self-therapy based on physical as well as psychological interventions. Its approach includes having the patient take an active part in the training.*

*Michael Vančura is a psychotherapist who lives in Prague, Czechoslovakia. He has published and presented papers mainly in the area of schizophrenia and family interaction. Drs. Stanislav Kratochvíl and Jiri Hoskovec are leaders in the field of hypnosis in Czechoslovakia. Though both were invited to the Erickson Congress, they could not attend and suggested that Dr. Vančura present in their place. The paper coauthored by Kratochvíl and Vančura presents an overview of the use of hypnosis in major Eastern European countries. They discuss important researchers and practitioners along with their areas of investigation. The popularity of hypnosis in each of the Eastern European countries varies.*

Chapter 33

# Erickson's Contribution to Anthropology

*Madeleine Richeport*

Many anthropologists have benefited from Dr. Milton H. Erickson's commentary on their work with ritual trance, most notably Margaret Mead and Gregory Bateson in Bali, Jane Belo in Bali, Maya Deren in Haiti.

Trance states are of particular interest to anthropologists because they are such widespread phenomena. In a survey of more than 1000 cultures from all parts of the world, Bourguignon (1974) reported that more than 90 percent have some institutionalized form of trance, most commonly within a sacred context. She noted that this percentage is underrepresented; trance states are a universal human potential. As such they are subject to learning and molding.

When trance is present in religious contexts, children often grow up learning conscious and unconscious models for relationships with supernatural entities just as they learn about any other relationships. We know that trance states are also present in times of social stress and mediate between individual and social change (Pressel, 1973).

This chapter is limited to my own work on the anthropological study of trance during five years in Puerto Rico and nearly five years in Brazil. Ten years ago, when I was deciding on a project for my doctoral research, I lived in New York City and went into the homes of Puerto Rican patients with the Visiting Nurse Service. I noticed altars with saints' statues, African statues, and all kinds of strange substances. My investigation of the communication between these nurses and their patients revealed a great difference in their beliefs about illness and its treatments.

---

I want to thank in particular Hilton L. Lopez, M.D., in Puerto Rico, and David Akstein, M.D., in Brazil, for their patience, collaboration, knowledge, and encouragement in this study.

I began to attend public seances, which were conducted in Spanish (which at that time I did not understand) and saw people moving in a strange hyperkinetic way in a state that I had never seen before.

I wrote to Erickson, and he answered with a brief explanation of ritual trance. At the same time I was also fascinated by Navajo Indian culture and had to choose between that and the Puerto Rican beliefs for my research. Dr. Erickson talked to me about the difficulty of communicating with a Navajo, how I might have to sit on a bench next to the same Indian every day for a year before he might say hello to me. He also spoke about the easy communication and open expressiveness of Latin American culture. With this indirect suggestion, I began a study of Spiritist mediumship; my understanding of this state became more and more complex each year. Several years later, Dr. Erickson remarked casually, "Why don't you develop mediumship?" I still do not understand why he suggested that but I have tried to be a participant, rather than merely an observer. Entering trance has enhanced my credibility; it feels good and is beneficial. You cannot really learn about any kind of trance without experiencing it.

## SPIRITISM, A WAY OF LIFE

Spiritism is a religious philosophical system that integrates this world and other-worldly phenomena through gifted individuals, or mediums, who act as intermediaries between these spheres. In Latin America and the Caribbean, Spiritism may be viewed as a continuum of cults ranging from those richest in African traditions, such as Candomble in Bahia and Shango in Recife or Lucumi in Cuba, to the European brand of Spiritism codified by a Frenchman, Leon Denizarth Hippolyte du Rivail, alias Alan Kardec, whose books were readily accepted by intellectuals in Brazil and Puerto Rico in the late nineteenth century. The intermediate syncretic forms of Umbanda, which originated in Brazil, and Santeria, which originated in Cuba and are popular among Puerto Ricans today, blend African gods and goddesses with European spirits of the dead, equating their supernatural pantheon with Catholic saints, as well as blending some Amerindian elements.

Imagine living in a city where there are 40,000 registered Spiritist centers; where you can buy a Spiritist newspaper along with your daily paper; where radio and TV stations broadcast Spiritist messages; where legislators use their Spiritist affiliations to win elections; and where tens of thousands of residents perform Spiritist rituals on street corners and beaches from humble shanties to elegant avenues. In the downtown financial area you can ride the elevator of a skyscraper and glimpse a twentieth floor luncheon session where professionals receive hand passes and other treatments at a Spiritist Medical Society. This city is Rio de Janeiro. Spiritist practices reach from Porto Alegre to Manaus and are unified by regional, national, and international federations. Local groups support social and medical services, including hospitals, clinics, orphanages, and schools.

In other countries, such as Puerto Rico, Spiritism is more covert than in Brazil. Nevertheless, in some Hispanic neighborhoods in New York City, one can find on a single street as many as five *botánicas* selling Spiritist ritual paraphernalia. In spite of Puerto Ricans' fear of ridicule by North American health professionals, surveys in health clinics show that a high percentage of patients consult Spiritists for problems of health, work, and marriage (Garrison, 1977). Folklore, popular entertainment, and local humor contain Spiritist themes, which all support the assertion in Dan Wakefield's (1957) book, *Island in the City*:

> If you ever talk to a Puerto Rican who says he doesn't believe in the spirits, you know what that means? It means you haven't talked to him long enough.

The social welfare aspects of the Latin American Spiritist movement, initiated by an elite class in Puerto Rico during the late nineteenth century, have been supplanted by cosmopolitan medical and social services in Puerto Rico. However, such aspects are still strong in Brazil. Cruz-Monclova (1952) reported that Spiritists founded hospitals, as well as libraries, and orphanages, in the towns of Utuado, Mayaguez, and Aguadilla. None of these exist today.

In Brazil, Spiritist institutions complement overcrowded or non-existent psychiatric services. Spiritist hospitals offer more humanitarian treatment than public hospitals. Some have good medical reputations. The charity ethic of Spiritist institutions is even more visible when they are compared to some public mental institutions known in the vernacular as "factories for the insane." Spiritists also run specialized hospital services such as the hospital for *penfigo* (wild fire) disease where mediums devote their time and energy to patients who would otherwise go untreated. They also provide room and board to indigent northeasterners who travel from the interior to the city for medical treatment.

Even when psychiatric services are available, researchers report that patients often consult informal practitioners as a first choice or continue Spiritist treatment while consulting a psychiatrist (Akstein & Richeport,

1976; Manzanero, 1976; Poggi & De Souza, 1975; Souza Santana, 1977). In Puerto Rico, public psychiatric services are more accessible than in Brazil because of a network of Community Mental Health Centers. However, personnel report that many patients are in Spiritist treatment while attending the mental health clinics. It has been argued that these patients go to the clinic for medication and to the Spiritist for therapy (Wintrob, 1975).

The important point relevant to this study is that an overwhelming number of people enter possession trance each day in the context of Spiritist therapy. The cults number in the hundreds. I will only describe the most popular forms—Kardecian Spiritism, which emphasizes a static trance state, and Umbanda, a popular and widespread Brazilian religion that emphasizes a kinetic trance. Most people practice syncretic forms combining European, African, and Amerind elements.

*Kardecian Spiritism*

In contrast to the energetic activity of the Umbanda sessions, Kardecian Spiritism is always conducted around a table where the mediums are seated. It is referred to as "mesa blanca" (white table) in Puerto Rico or Spiritism "da mesa" (table Spiritism) in Brazil. Practices vary considerably from small family-style sessions in private homes to those in large public auditoriums organized into schools for mediums. The consistent aim is to develop mediumship by invoking spirits of the dead to provide tranquility and a feeling of well-being to clients who come to solve organic, psychological, and psychosomatic complaints.

Decorations include religious images of Christ, a bowl of water, and flowers. Sometimes soft music plays as the room is purified with incense. Each person is cleansed in turn, adding to the hypnogogic and mystical atmosphere.

Each center has a leader who directs the sessions and usually does not receive entities. In the first period, lasting from 30 to 40 minutes, participants read from the books of Kardec or other well-known mediums such as Chico Xavier, a Brazilian medium who used automatic writing to author nearly two hundred books. Mediums and clients concentrate; most close their eyes, lean their heads forward, with hands on the table facilitating muscular relaxation. The monotone voice of the reader, lack of movement, and the friendly and anticipatory atmosphere of focused attention (monoideism) on problem-solving facilitate trance induction.

Lights are dimmed. Mediums hyperventilate and receive their guides or protecting spirits. Some of these are very elevated spirits of dead illustrious individuals who may have been famous doctors, lawyers, or statesmen in their lifetimes. Mediums are identified with their guides, such as the famous surgeon, Dr. Fritz, who possessed Arigó, a Brazilian surgeon whose rusty knife baffled scientific experts because of the absence of infections (Fuller, 1974). Chico Xavier's books are authored by the spirits and do not bear his name.

Mediumship is classified on the basis of awareness during trance. A medium may describe his work as being done unconsciously, consciously, or semiconsciously. Mediums who claim to work consciously remember everything, and mediums who work semiconsciously remember selectively. If a medium receives a low spirit, the passive trance characteristic of Kardecian sessions with its lofty verbal messages, hand passes, and light massage may develop into seizure-type trance behavior. This is not desirable and is identified with "low Spiritism."

The leader generally asks those present if they have any messages to offer and at the end asks people to relate what they felt during the session. Mediums apply "magnetic passes" to those present, and a peaceful atmosphere is achieved.

### *Umbanda Religion*

Umbanda has been called the national Brazilian religion. It was founded by the middle classes in Rio de Janeiro in the 1950s and has spread throughout Brazil, with its major concentration in Rio and São Paulo. Its rituals, like those of *Santeria,* induce kinetic trances among its adherents who become possessed by prescribed entities. It is difficult to standardize the diverse styles of practice in the thousands of *terreiros* (Umbanda centers) where sessions (*gira,* literally "the turn-around") take place. They range from small family-style centers in private homes to large organized centers that accommodate thousands. For example, Caminheiros de Verdade is a well-known center with 10,000 members.

The *pai* or *mae do santo,* the spiritual leaders of the group, initiate their "holy sons and daughters" by teaching them the rituals required to develop mediumship or to adopt one of the other roles in the spiritual hierarchy. In addition to the spiritual hierarchy, a material hierarchy is led by a president who takes care of the group's organization and finances.

At the beginning of a session, mediums line up on either side of an altar that displays a mixture of Catholic and African sculptured images. Men and women are separated. Incense fills the room for purification, and an orchestra of drums and sometimes other instruments plays Umbanda music. Many of the sessions last through the night. However, people report that the same music is never repeated.

Mediums enter possession trances by rotating rapidly, arms out to the side with the head held either forward or backward in an unnatural position. They receive the principal Umbanda entities. Sometimes a night of the week is designated for a particular entity, or in some centers mediums may receive all of the entities sequentially in the course of the session.

Mediums may receive spirits of *caboclos,* dead Brazilian Indians who are known for being forthright, aggressive, and strong; they like cigars and rum. Clients line up to consult them and receive hand passes and *descarregos* (cleansing) with the tobacco smoke. A medium may have many *caboclo* guides. *Caboclo boiadeiro* (cowboy) struts around chanting loudly "reiah, reiah, reiah" with angular arm movements and strong and energetic passes.

Mediums also receive the spirits of *pretos velhos:* wise old Brazilian slaves who display patience and warmth and may scold in a fatherly manner. They take a position on a low bench, smoke a pipe, drink rum, listen, and cleanse the clients who consult them. Clients consult particular old slaves such as Pai Roberto or Pai Joachim, always giving them the traditional greeting and parting by kissing the medium's hand.

*Criancas* are the spirits of dead children, usually three to five years of age. These entities are ingratiating and helpful and are enjoyed by everyone. They skip around like children asking for candy and presents.

*Exus* are ambiguous entities representing both good and evil. Mediums may enact roles of the devil or guardian of the cemetery, assuming awkward postures and mean expressions. Female entities such as *Pomba Gira* and *Maria Padilha* are sensual pranksters who, like other *exus,* cry out in shrill laughter. Despite the negative connotations of these entities, they are relaxed and fun-loving and are enjoyed for their off-color humor, obscene gestures, and relaxation of moral behavior. *Exus* are characterized by puckered lips, special songs, and twisted fingers placed behind the buttocks. Although special sessions may be devoted to these spirits, they usually descend in many centers after midnight, only after the mediums have received the other entities.

On special occasions, Umbanda mediums receive the *Orixás,* Yoruban gods and goddesses. *Ogum* is the god of war and metal, who holds a sword to cut negative vibrations. He is characterized by a tense mouth and sharp cries. *Iemanjá* is the goddess of the sea and is seen in mass public rituals on beaches which are celebrated in different regions on different days of the year. In Rio, on December 31st, elegant Cariocas join humble shantytown dwellers in making offerings to the sea goddess on public beaches, partaking in ritual baths to the drums and lovely Umbanda chanting.

Possession is indicated by a hyperkinetic trance state that becomes much more controlled and stylized as mediums learn the characteristic behaviors of each entity. However, any violent seizure or crisis is interpreted as possession by a low or backward entity who can be educated or placated when "worked." For this reason, Akstein (1973) refers to mediumship as a desensitization process to the original emotional crisis accomplished through repeated experiences in kinetic trance; the crises diminish and are limited in time and space. Although Kardecian Spiritism emphasizes a static trance more similar to meditation, mediums may receive backward or prankster entities and enter hyperkinetic trances as well.

With an interest in the area of applied anthropology, I work as a Mental Health Consultant with the World Health Organization, identifying strategies to bridge nonmedical and medical healing. I have been studying the articulation of formal and informal healing systems. Informal medicine, sometimes called traditional, popular, lay, nonmedical, or local medicine, describes beliefs and practices that have been handed down through generations and are embedded in the world view of the communities in which they are employed. They are continuous with the structures of family life, kinship, political, and religious organization. Operationally defined, traditional medicine is "all of the practices of healers who have not gained entry to medical practice through graduation from allopathic institutions" (WHO, 1976).

Lessa and Rubim de Pinho (1971), reporting on their extensive background in psychiatry in Salvador, conclude: "Our experience has shown us that conventional medical treatments do not lead to positive results when the patient has magical religious manifestations of disease like trances, ecstasies, incarnations, and other 'spirit manifestations.' "

Considering the great many people who enter trance every day with mystical understandings of what they experience and considering the inadequacy of conventional therapy, it is important for therapists in these regions to learn to use trance and Spiritist practices.

Dr. Erickson referred me to various psychiatrists because of their astuteness in hypnosis. I call these psychiatrists "culture brokers" because they translate and integrate their scientific and subcultural knowledge, thus articulating alternative systems of healing (Richeport, 1979). In countries like Brazil, most people do not have access to formal psychotherapy but receive psychotherapy from different categories of healers. When a formal mental health system is implanted, trance or hypnosis may be considered a referential bridge. The purpose of the next section is to show that Erickson's approach to hypnosis leads to a more relevant psychotherapeutic technique in developing mental health programs.

## APPLYING ERICKSONIAN ORIENTATION TO RITUAL TRANCE

### *Hypnosis Is a Special But Normal Extension of Everyday Behavior*

> It is, in simple terms, nothing more than a special state of conscious awareness in which certain chosen behavior of everyday life is manifested in a direct manner, usually with the aid of another person. But it is possible to be self-induced. Hypnosis is a special, but normal type of behavior, encountered when attention and the thinking processes are directed to the body of experiential learnings acquired from or achieved in the experience of living. In the special state of awareness called hypnosis, the various forms of behavior of everyday life may be found—differing in relationship and degrees, but always within normal limits. There can be achieved no transcendence of abilities, no implantations of new abilities, but only the potentiation of the expression of abilities which may have gone unrecognized or not fully recognized. Hypnosis cannot create new abilities within a person, but it can assist in a greater and better utilization of abilities already possessed, even if these abilities were not previously recognized (Erickson, 1970, pp. 72-73).

I believe that a continuum exists between ordinary waking consciousness and trance states and that this continuum occurs in all people in all societies. The flow of social experience and self-awareness, of perceptions of the environment, and of memory associations that accompany thought and moods is more or less focused and selective. For instance, we experience amnesia when we forget things we think are impossible to forget. Many people become so absorbed in the theater or watching television that they lose their own identity and become part of the performance. They may even develop ideosensory responses, if, for example, the show is set in the Arctic, at sea, or in the Arabian desert. When the focus is intense, selectivity high and stereotyped, and memory altered, we observe the psychophysiological changes that define trance states (Michtom Richeport, 1975).

Viewing trance as a normal phenomenon is extremely important to the anthropological study of trance. Cross-cultural investigators often confuse trance with pathology, rather than seeing it as a meaningful element in the cultural system, part of the psychobiological heritage of the human race present in early archeological evidence. I will return to this problem of defining normality later.

Patients familiar with ritual trance often confuse hypnosis with supernatural control. Automatic drawing and writing are interpreted as spirit messages. Ideomotor and ideosensory responses are considered real supernatural possessions. Amnesia provides proof that another entity has incorporated into the body; disoriented and slow readaptive behavior during trance recovery confirms that mediums are returning from a spirit journey to the worldly sphere. Post-hypnotic suggestions mark the influence of the entities during possession. Because of these misconceptions commonly published in Spiritist literature, hypnotherapists in Brazil use strategies to separate hypnosis from mysticism.

### *Trance Is an Active State of Unconscious Learning That May Lead to Resynthesis*

The three-stage model used here to explain resynthesis through mediumship development is based on Ernest Rossi's (1973) article, "Psychological shocks and creative moments in psychotherapy."

#### *Stage one: Dissonance*

In order for an individual to change, there must be some motivation. Festinger's (1957) concept of "cognitive dissonance" may explain how Puerto Ricans and Brazilians become motivated in Spiritism to develop mediumship when natural mechanisms of the mind such as visions, dreams, fantasies, and other phenomena suddenly seem confusing and chaotic. Dissonance may take three forms when individuals embark on a mediumship career: 1) They must distinguish between mediumship phenomena and mental illness; 2) they must reconcile disparities between Roman Catholicism and Spiritism; 3) if they have middle-class orientations, they must differentiate themselves from lower-class practices.

Spiritism resolves the emotional and cognitive dissonance of stressful life situations by providing an ideology and set of ritual actions that encourage personal development and offer the possibility of achieving a prestigious role in the society. It views the unconscious mind as a positive, creative, integrating force in the personality. In a similar manner, some schools of professional psychotherapy utilize dreams and symbolic activity to cultivate personality transformation or psychosynthesis (see Assagioli, 1965; Progoff, 1963; Rossi, 1972; Sacerdote, 1967). Spiritism does not seek the highly cognitive understanding of "insight therapy" based on intense self-examination but instead emphasizes control over spiritual chaos. That the imagination can facilitate transformations without insight is well-known. For example, Carl Jung (1956, p. 235) called fantasies of intensely visual character, "something which in the language of the ancients would be called a vision," a useful form of "active imagination" that merges the self and unconscious processes and heals the disjunction of conscious and unconscious mental processes.

Positive assumptions concerning the imagination's capacity have been discussed in actual clinical studies that have utilized the imagination to facilitate transformations of the psyche (Erickson, 1967; Rossi, 1972). These assumptions form the basis of the second stage of the model, which explains the training steps leading to mediumship development.

*Stage two: Training*

Being in a trance state breaks the conflicted direction of habitual associations, allowing new learning in ritual contexts. Thus, one of the problems that Spiritists face is how to induce trance. Let us review the steps that individuals would have to experience in order to achieve trance.

*Functioning on multiple levels.* This natural mechanism usually enables people to look at themselves and to allow change to occur. If one operates at only one level, there is little possibility of acquiring another perspective. Spiritism offers a cultural explanation of possession trance as mediumship development in the form of role-playing dialogues within a religious context based on the Spiritist ideology. Initially, these multilevel communications are spontaneous, that is, the spirits or visions are not purposely induced.

*Learning signals to induce trance.* Hyperventilation, twirling, and symbolic associations are used to induce trance. Learning and practicing these signals facilitate control over entering trance. More importantly, these signals allow the individual to break down some of the directing functions of the ego and to discard habitual frames of reference. The ego still retains its observer function, but the learning that occurs in this state is experiential learning and happens autonomously.

*Learning greater control over the trance state.* In Spiritism, control or "free will'' is shown when mediums redirect their attention to particular goals, that is, to the guide or to supernatural communications or to the prescription for a client. Concentration on the other person allows maximum sensitivity to the individual, which may be interpreted as supernormal powers (see Birdwhistell, 1966). Greater control is also shown when the medium selects other selves, rather than passively acting as a vehicle for any entity.

*Cumulative change.* In many cases, the novice took a disturbing, painful, or ugly image and transformed it into a valued, sought after, and pleasurable one. In Spiritism, this process takes the form of recognizing a spirit guide. Once the individual can substitute a new behavior for a habitually patterned behavior or develop a new frame of reference, a domino effect may be set into motion, and other new behaviors and attitudes become possible.

*Rehearsal.* The belief that an action has already been achieved by symbolic actions provides a ''new psychological orientation of compelling force, effecting a new organization of thinking and planning'' (Erickson, 1967, p. 389). I have emphasized the use of possession trance as a ritualized means of defining attainable goals and of rehearsing behavior to achieve them. Individuals learn behavior and acquire attitudes in trance which they later transfer into real-life situations. Learning this orientation helps future mediums formulate and practice solutions to problems by adopting and changing guides or alternate roles. For the apprentice, mediumship trance is a self-healing mechanism. It may be aided by a trainer, but ultimate success depends on the medium's personal transformation.

We found that many of the behaviors that patients first expressed in mediumship trance—strength, aggressiveness, feminine liberation, freedom of expression—were expressed in the nontrance sessions and were later translated into their everyday lives. One phobic patient was able to feel strong enough to go outside alone, to express her dissatisfactions to her husband, to discipline her daughter, and to recognize that her dizziness was related to her phobia. Encourging mediumship trance in the clinical setting with Spiritist patients permits psychiatrists to utilize an important experience in their patients' lives and to allow a dialogue with alternate selves for increasing behavior change (Richeport, 1979, 1980).

### *Stage three: Resynthesis*

According to Erickson, ''the induction and maintenance of a trance serve to provide a special psychological state in which the patient can reassociate and reorganize his inner psychological complexities and utilize his own capacities in a manner in accord with his own experiential life . . . therapy results from an inner resynthesis of the patient's behavior achieved by the patient himself" (Erickson, 1948, p. 571).

Analysis of the Spiritist mediumship training process in possession trance showed that it leads to a "mazeway resynthesis" or cognitive transformation that creates new social and personal identities. According to Anthony Wallace (1969), the resynthesis combines preexisting configurations of cognition, often through hallucinatory trance experiences that are psychotherapeutic responses to stress. Wallace used the concept of "mazeway" primarily to deal with religious conversion movements, and I have used it to show how individuals change in the process of working to become mediums.

Wallace, Erickson, and Rossi emphasize sudden transformations via trance experiences. In the cases that I have studied, however, the transformations were always slow and gradual, and the restructuring of cognitive maps through training appears to need time. This slow resynthesis may be matched to Rodney Needham's (1963) comparison of an ethnographer who is "culturally blind" studying a strange people to a congenitally blind person who is given sight. Both first notice only disorder but slowly find order and meanings by classifying what they see. Like the blind learning to "see," the medium also learns to "see" things from a new perspective and to classify them in new and meaningful ways.

### *Channeling Behavior into a Socially Acceptable Area*

Erickson (Note 1) reported the case of a schizophrenic patient, Norma, who saw floating male nudes above her head. Although she was a school teacher, she could not hold a steady job. Erickson convinced her to put the nudes in his closet where she could check up on them; she did this and began to work steadily. One day Norma decided to move to another city where she had found a teaching job. She was afraid she would not be able to cope with her psychotic episodes. Erickson encouraged her to mail her psychoses to him in letters, giving them full identities. One day, she returned to his office and demanded to see the envelopes. He had saved them and showed them to her. When there was no hope for correction, Erickson channeled the behavior so that it did not interfere with living. Years later Norma became an alcoholic and died, but she functioned for 15 years productively and without being a burden to the state.

Encouraging mediumship development is a subcultural means to channel dissociation into a highly prestigious role in Puerto Rican and Brazilian society, possibly leading to personal and social transformation (Michtom Richeport, 1975). For a client who believes that spirits are responsible for his problem, channeling dissociation into a Spiritist seance is a socially acceptable modality for banishing the evil. Regardless of belief system, however, an American psychiatrist may channel the hallucinations of a schizophrenic patient when correction is impossible, thus enabling the patient to function in everyday activities.

Two important problems need clarification and further research:

*1) The normality or pathology of the medium or shaman:* Anthropological literature abounds with the controversy as to whether a shaman is crazy and directed into a prestigious role by the society, or is really astute and merely fulfilling cultural expectations. This question is relevant when formal mental health programs are implanted into countries like Brazil where an overwhelming number of people enter a hyperkinetic trance. Is this behavior to be considered pathogenic or pathoplastic? What are the behavioral limits acceptable within a particular culture? How much *hallucination* is acceptable?

Erickson did not look for labels but instead stressed how people function. His schizophrenic patient, Norma, functioned as a productive member of society for 15 years. An astute physician should use individual and cultural strategies to promote functional adaptation and survival for the patient.

Prince argued that "under conditions of stress, individuals have resorted to a repertoire of automatic self-healing mechanisms. The most important of these are so-called altered states of consciousness—dreams, dissociated states, a variety of religious experiences . . . " (1976). Prince used the point made by the Scottish physician, John Hunter (1728-93) that "an inflammation, rather than constituting a disease process in itself, was actually token of the body's attempts at self-healing." Freud, as quoted by Prince, applied this principle to psychiatric syndromes: "The delusion formation, which we take to be a pathological product, is in reality an attempt at recovery, a process of reconstruction" (1976).

Kinetic trances, although appearing pathological, constitute endogenous adaptive mechanisms to stress and have been reported to provide psychosocial equilibrium through psychomotor liberation leading to higher cortical activation. Psychiatrists who adapt these techniques utilize positive psychobiological human capacities within their cultural framework. The basic premise is that if the technique can work within its naturally occurring context, it would have even more positive results with clients when employed by a medically trained professional, who has the advantage of incorporating it as an adjunct to other recognized techniques.

*2) Is trance therapy useful with psychotics?* This question is another problem, especially among anthropologically oriented psychiatrists. Most Brazilian psychiatrists believe that ritual trance cannot benefit psychotics. Brody (1973), who studied mental illness in Rio de Janeiro, reported that consulting the informal system only delays treatment and leads to chronicity among schizophrenics and alcoholics. In Brazil the statement is often made that people are sick because they stopped working as mediums. Spiritist psychiatrists also disagree as to whether psychotics should attend Spiritist sessions, that is, whether a person in crisis should enter trance. If hypnotic and mediumship trances are analogous states, Erickson's use of hypnosis with psychotic patients opens an area for investigation in folk therapy and a basis for creating referral systems between alternate healing systems based on diagnosis.

There are medical doctors who accept Spiritist ideology and use Spiritist techniques without medication. This is a natural setting in which research could be done to determine the effectiveness of encouraging an experimental crisis in a patient already in crisis. The experimental crisis might serve to limit crises in random time and space. Erickson's description of Edward's case is relevant here:

> On the ward, Edward sat quietly in a chair. He would listen attentively when spoken to, but would never reply. However, about three times every 24 hours he became violently disturbed. He would rush wildly through the dormitory, crawling under and over beds, around beds, shoving them away from the wall. The disturbances would last from 10 to 20 minutes, whereupon, covered with perspiration, he would return to his chair, or, at night, to his bed. There was never a word of explanation received from Edward about these episodes. More than a dozen physicians endeavored repeatedly to interview the patient or to elicit some verbal response from him. Each interview was a failure—and this had been going on for three years (1970).

Erickson employed hypnosis, stimulating a crisis in this psychotic patient by asking him to redream his nightmares with a different cast of characters. Edward limited his crises on the ward, even when not requested by Erickson. In time, the patient was able to confront his problem related to his immigrant status. He left the mental hospital, married, and "is proud of his children. Through hypnosis, Edward learned the thing so vital to human living—how to communicate."

The following case history was described by Dr. Hilton L. Lopez (Note 2), a colleague and friend of Erickson's. The problem of normality and pathology, the use of culturally relevant therapy, and the use of trance therapy with a psychotic patient in Latin American culture are illustrated.

Dr. Lopez's client, Paul Lebron, is a 25-year-old schizophrenic, chronic undifferentiated type. His psychosis is manifested in the belief that he is possessed by a demon, which Paul defines as a low primitive entity that stays close to the ground. He first saw the demon when he was six years old as a face in his bedroom window. Shortly after this experience, his mother took him to a Spiritist who saw a black cloud in Paul's head and advised her to take Paul to a doctor. She relied on Spiritism until he was 23 years old when she first took him to a psychiatrist. Paul used the Spiritist's explanation of the black cloud to explain his feelings of detachment, nightmares, handwashing compulsion, and refusal to touch people. He dichotomized his world and the forces within himself into good and bad, with himself in the middle trying to keep the bad from predominating. To prevent the bad from taking hold of him, he walked compulsively for hours and had therefore never been able to hold a job. Until recently, he could not have sexual relations because the demon would take away his potency and make the woman into his mother.

After two years in psychotherapy, the psychiatrist felt that he could produce no further change and referred Paul to Dr. Lopez for hypnotherapy. Paul also requested hypnosis, saying that it would be a magical cure for his demon possession.* During his therapy, Paul also saw several mediums and continued to attend services in many churches—Catholic, Pentecostal, Rosicrucian, and others—because they symbolized goodness to him.

Dr. Lopez used hypnosis, behavior therapy, and family therapy before calling in a medium. Despite Paul's progress, including working part-time and returning to college, Dr. Lopez felt that since Paul was seeing mediums for help, he would use a medium to help banish Paul's demon.

---

*Some Spiritists express fear of hypnosis because they interpret dissociative behavior in trance states—hallucinations, visions, automatic writing, and other phenomena—as being controlled by outside forces. Paul did not fear that hypnosis would bring him under outside control; however, he insisted on a recognized physician.

According to Dr. Lopez, "as in any other therapeutic milieu, you use consultants. Through the Spiritist, Paul might be able to integrate in such a way that instead of working at three levels, the good, the bad, and the everyday, he could start working at two levels—an everyday personality and a good personality. Gradually, these two could integrate into a good person. When fantasies are mystical, this could work" (Note 2).

Carmen Sosa, an educated middle-class medium, worked with Dr. Lopez on Paul's case. Carmen was originally referred to Dr. Lopez by another psychiatrist for dysmenorrhea when she was 19. Her grandmother was a medium, and her family consulted Spiritists. When Carmen spontaneously became possessed by entities in Dr. Lopez's office, he encouraged her mediumship. He guided her into replacing unwanted spirit possessions with the suggestion that she might visualize her spirit guide. Rather than regarding this behavior as psychopathology, Dr. Lopez channeled her dissociation into a prestigious role where many opportunities opened up for her. Dr. Lopez's consultation with Carmen on Paul's case served to enhance her prestige and functioned as a practice session for her under his direction.

Dr. Lopez first asked Paul to give his history. Carmen went into trance and her guide, Lao-tzu, began to speak. Dr. Lopez welcomed the guide as he would welcome any person who entered the room. He assumed the role of the president of a Spiritist center who directs the seance. He asked the guide if he heard Paul's story. He transferred the direction to Lao-tzu who examined Paul's head and precordial area carefully. Lao-tzu concluded that Paul had made much progress and his mind was much clearer than he anticipated. Then the guide told Paul that he was only "confused," a less serious condition than "possessed," and with Dr. Lopez's help, through concentration, Paul could banish the confusion from his mind. Dr. Lopez agreed.

Carmen and Paul faced each other. Lao-tzu located the "evil" in Paul's left hand and the "good" in Paul's right hand. (This placement concurred with Paul's belief that he was "in the middle" of these two forces.) Paul appeared very expectant as Carmen clasped his hands together and then tore them apart sharply. Lao-tzu asked Paul to visualize these actions in his mind and asked Dr. Lopez to tell him when a half hour had elapsed. After ten minutes, Paul began to move his head from side to side and then shook and jerked his head against the pressure of Carmen's hands placed on his forehead. His left leg trembled. It was a contest between Paul's possessing entity resisting departure and Carmen's "vital fluid" working to push out the entity. Lao-tzu repeatedly suggested that Paul feel calm. He told the doctor that it would not be necessary to wait half an hour because the evil was gone. Reinforcing this idea nonverbally, Carmen clenched and opened her fists as if expelling something. Lao-tzu told Paul that he was "good, intelligent, and a normal man."

Before ending the session, Carmen said that she was very tired and needed strength. The others extended their hands and touched her forehead, forming a chain to pass energy from one to the other, as batteries in series increase the voltage.

Dr. Lopez resumed the direction of the interaction. As he thanked Lao-tzu for coming, Carmen, slowly recovering from trance, asked what happened. Dr. Lopez utilized the remainder of the time to allow Paul to verbalize how he felt and to reinforce the idea of the expulsion of the demon.

Today Paul has been working full-time for four years. He is completing a university degree. He has girlfriends and occasionally comes to see Dr. Lopez with one of them. He also continues to see mediums from time to time. Carmen is a prestigious medium and is invited to work with groups of doctors, professors, and businessmen; she stresses healing, philosophical discussions, and experiments with parapsychological phenomena. Through a member of the group she obtained a good job which she has held for the past three years. In addition, she has nearly completed her bachelor's degree.

Whether we are working in our own culture or in other cultures, Erickson's use of the client's behavior is of prime importance in his or her recuperation. The therapist's adaptations to the client's experience constitute a referential bridge that encourages acceptance. In this sense, every psychiatrist mediates between the client's immediate frame of reference and psychiatric training to motivate and encourage an acceptance set for resolving problems and developing additional options for organizing experience.

## HYPNOSIS AS APPROPRIATE TECHNOLOGY IN MENTAL HEALTH

I conclude by applying criteria for "appropriate technology" to the use of hypnosis in mental health. Today official psychiatric programs are opening up to more and more people who have never had access to psychiatrists but may have used other techniques applied by curanderos; one of the most important of these is trance. Any strategy for adapting ritual trance into the clinical setting by scientifically trained practitioners may be considered "appropriate technology." This concept, of great interest to the World Health Organization today, is defined as "the systematic application of knowledge (methods and techniques) from the health sciences in the solution of problems and practical tasks, . . . which do not provoke negative effects on the society, the economy, the culture, and the ecology where it is applied. It is based on the principle that the best technology is that which best adapts to the situation where it is used, recognizing that each society has its own technological tradition and that new technologies should adapt, grow, and develop within that tradition" (Grupo de trabajo subregional sobre tecnologia apropriada, San Jose, Costa Rica, 2-6 junio 1980). The criteria used for "appropriate technology" are discussed below.

### *Compatibility with Local Cultural Patterns*

Erickson discussed in many cases the problem of the cultural basis of personality and stressed the individuality of personality and cultures. I was interested in the cultural basis of trance behavior. During a group session Dr. Erickson said to me privately, "I bet Angela is Latin American." From her accent and physical appearance she did not seem Latin American to me. Upon questioning, Angela revealed that her mother was Mexican. I asked Erickson how he knew this, and he pointed out that her trance behavior was much more expressive than North American trance behavior.

Generally we think of the Latin American personality as being explosive and expressive of all emotions. However, for many people, hostility is expressed directly only as a last resort. Negative emotions and direct confrontations are avoided at all cost because they are incompatible with dignity, honor and shame. In terms of psychotherapy, this indirect expression of behavior offers a possible explanation for the popularity of spirit mediumship and ritual trance and suggests a culture-specific therapy. Role-playing of alternate selves in trance is in accord with this cultural pattern. Any therapeutic technique that uses indirect expression would also be more acceptable and culturally relevant and would create less resistance. Erickson's indirect approach to hypnosis, using indirect induction and suggestion, interspersal language, paradox, confusion techniques, and techniques such as "my friend John" or automatic writing would be more in accord with this cultural reality.

### *Using Local Resources*

Preventive medicine in developing countries must take advantage of local resources so that programs do not fail. Curanderos are already serving in various ways such as being trained (Mariz, 1978), working as collaborators, and receiving and referring patients (Harwood, 1977). Studying their techniques, which often employ trance together with an understanding of scientific hypnosis, can be an important contribution. Dr. Lopez's work with Paul and Carmen illustrates the way that a psychiatrist who utilizes Erickson's model can accommodate cross-cultural trance states in hypnotherapy.

Erickson's work has already fostered changing medical attitudes toward hypnosis. Applying his work to ritual trance opens an important bridge between alternative systems of healing. In the words of a Navajo medicine man when hypnosis was demonstrated in the Navajo Indian Medical School, "I'm 82 years old, and I've seen white people all my life, but this is the first time that one of them ever surprised me. I'm not surprised to see something like this happen because we do things like this, but I am surprised that a white man should know anything so worthwhile" (Bergman, 1975).

## REFERENCE NOTES

1. Erickson, M.H. Personal communication, December 1, 1976.
2. Lopez, H.L. Personal communication, December, 1971.

## REFERENCES

Assagioli, R. *Psychosynthesis.* New York: The Viking Press, 1965.
Akstein, D. *Hipnologia.* Rio de Janeiro: Editora Hypnos, 1973.
Akstein, D., & Richeport, M. *Study of Spiritism and Psychiatry.* Rio de Janeiro: Centro Integrado de Pesquisas Medicas (CIPME), 1976.
Bergman, R.L. Learning from Indian medicine. *Diversion Magazine,* 1975, Feb-Mar, 8-9, 35.
Birdwhistell, R.L. Research in exceptional phenomena. *American Journal of Clinical Hypnosis,* 1966, *8,* 237-244.
Bourguignon, E. *Culture and Varieties of Consciousness.* Addison-Wesley Module in Anthropology, 47, 1974.
Brody, E., et al. *The Lost Ones.* New York: International Universities Press, Inc., 1973.
Cruz-Monclova, L. *Historia de Puerto Rico* (siglo XIX). Puerto Rico: Editorial Universitaria, 1952.
Erickson, M.H. Hypnotic psychotherapy. In *Medical Clinics of North America.* Philadelphia: W.B. Saunders Co. 571-584, 1948.
Erickson, M.H. *Advanced Techniques of Hypnosis and Therapy: Selected Papers of Milton H. Erickson, M.D.* J. Haley, Ed. New York: Grune and Stratton, 1967.
Erickson, M.H. Hypnosis: Its renascence as a treatment modality. *American Journal of Clinical Hypnosis,* 1970, *19,* 71-89.
Festinger, L. *A Theory of Cognitive Dissonance.* Evanston: Row, Peterson, and Co., 1957.
Fuller, J.G. *Arigo: Surgeon of the Rusty Knife.* New York: Thomas Y. Crowell Company, 1974.
Garrison, V. Doctor, espiritista or psychiatrist? Health-seeking behavior in a Puerto Rican neighborhood of New York City. *Medical Anthropology,* 1977, *1.*
Harwood, A. *Rx: Spiritist as Needed.* New York: John Wiley & Sons, 1977.

Jung, C.G. *Active Imagination: Two Essays on Analytical Psychology*. New York: The World Publishing Co., 1956.

Lessa, L., & Rubim de Pinho, A. Afro-Brazilian mystique and mental disease. Paper presented at the World Congress of Psychiatry, Mexico City, 1971.

Manzanero, H. Articulacion de los sistemas formal e informal de salud y la participacion de la comunidad en la primera area IV Region de Salud, Caruaru, Pernambuco Consultor OPS, OMS, 29 de junio — 6 de agosto 1976.

Mariz, P., et al. Tentativa da utilizaeao do sistema tradicional comunitario de saude no Projeto Integrado de Saude Mental. Secretaria de Saude de Pernambuco, Brasil, 1978.

Needham, R. Introduction. In: *Primitive Classification*, Durkheim E. & Mauss M. (Eds.), Chicago: University of Chicago Press, 1963.

Poggi, M.T., & De Souza R. Situaeao socioeconomica da ilha de Itamaraca. Dept. de Planejamento da Secretaria de Saude do Estado de Pernambuco. FUSAM. Recife, 1975.

Pressel, E. Umbanda in Sao Paulo: Religious innovation in a developing society. In: *Religion, Altered States of Consciousness and Social Change*. E. Bourguignon (Ed.), Columbus, Ohio: State Univ. Press, 1973.

Prince, R. H. Psychotherapy as the manipulation of endogenous healing mechanisms: A transcultural survey. *Transcultural Psychiatric Research Review*, 1976, *13*, 115-133.

Progoff, I. *The Symbolic and the Real*. New York: Julian Press, 1963.

Richeport, Michtom. *Becoming a Medium: The Role of Trance in Puerto Rican Spiritism as an Avenue to Mazeway Resynthesis*. University of Michigan, Ann Arbor Microfilms, 1975.

Richeport, M. The psychiatrist as a culture broker: The hypnotic techniques of Hilton L. Lopez, M.D. *Svensk Tidskrift for Hypnos*, 1979, *5*, 16-19.

Richeport, M. O Uso do Transe Ritual na Clinica Hipnoterapica: Estudo de Casos em Psiquiatria Transcultural. *Revista Brasileira de Hipnologia*, 1980, *1*, 39-46.

Rossi, E. *Dreams and the Growth of the Personality*. New York: Pergamon Press, 1972.

Rossi, E. Psychological shocks and creative moments in psychotherapy. *American Journal of Clinical Hypnosis*, 1973, *16*, 9-22.

Sacerdote, P. *Induced Dreams*. New York: Vantage Press, 1967.

Souza Santana, V. Morbidade e Padrao de Assistencia Psiquiatricas num Bairro da Cidade de Salvador—Nordeste de Amaralina. Mestrado em saude publica, Dept. de Medicina Preventiva, Salvador, Bahia, 1977.

Wakefield, D. *Island in the City*. New York: Corinth Books, Inc. 1957.

Wallace, A. *Culture and Personality*. New York: Random House, 1969.

WHO Report on Traditional Medicine. Geneva, 1976.

Wintrob, R. Researchers study Puerto Rican folk healers. *Psychiatric News*, 1975, *10*, 22, 20-21.

Chapter 34

# A Systematic Method of Jiko-Control

*Gosaku Naruse*

## INTRODUCTION

In Japan, jiko-control is a systematic method of self-induced psychotherapy and a construct of self that is widely accepted both within the professional community of physicians, clinical psychologists, and dentists and also by patients and clients from the hospital, clinic, school or business fields (Naruse, 1969).

Although the Japanese word "jiko" is translated as "self" in English, jiko-control should not be confused with the self-control concept associated with behavior therapy. Jiko-control instead represents the view that all psychotherapy is essentially self-therapy, thereby differing fundamentally with hetero-therapeutic points of view such as psychoanalysis and most Western psychotherapies.

The concept of jiko-control in self-therapy involves two basic components: the active exercise of self-psychotherapy, and the subjective conscious and subconscious experience of living. The former involves the observing self, which works on the latter, which is the experiencing self of inner life.

## DERIVATION

Jiko-control grew out of the clinical practice of autogenic training (Schultz, 1932), which when combined with progressive relaxation (Jacobson, 1929) highlighted the existence of a common basis for self-activated change. Ultimately, Jacobson's concept of "self-operations control" (Jacobson, 1964) provided a theoretical foundation. Clinical study of autogenic training and progressive relaxation revealed the essential similarity to hypnotic treatment because both incorporate not only muscle relaxation but also a kind of trance. Characterized as a state of meditative concentration (Naruse, 1962), trance may be induced by hetero-hypnosis, self-hypnosis, autogenic training, or progressive relaxation.

I became interested in cases where subjects or patients developed familiarity with hypnotic trance after many experiences of repeated inductions in which the hypnotist was very passive or patient-centered in the induction process. It appeared that in such instances the patient entered into "pure trance" or "neutral hypnosis" in which he was not influenced by hypnotic suggestion nor affected by biased transference or the specific human relationship between patient and therapist. These patients reactivated gradually, recovering from hypnotic passivity independent of the hypnotist and on their own volition. In addition, it seemed that these patients exhibited both trance and waking state behaviors, selecting freely between both states. It may be thus hypothesized that in such a condition the patient is so free from waking-trance or conscious-unconscious distinctions that he behaves in an enlarged conscious state, with strengthened autonomy. Clinically this condition can be invoked through repeated hypnotic inductions; importantly, it also could be taught as a self-practice method, like autogenic training, progressive relaxation, or fractionation (Weitzenhoffer, 1957). In this way, the therapeutic value of self-striving can be used.

Following experimental research into conditioned imagery in the post-hypnotic hallucinatory state (Naruse, 1953), I incorporated hypnotic imagery into psychotherapy. Image therapy, as it has been named, successfully employs mental imagery in psychotherapy both with and without hypnosis. For some patients, mental imagery has proved to be a more valuable treatment tool than verbal communication.

Studying psychotherapy and zen-meditation, as well as yoga training, one realizes the important role that consciousness or awareness of one's body contributes to a patient's experience of his existential reality. The experience of self-existence may be divided into two phases. The first is self-body as a cognitive object, and the second is body-self as a subject to perceive or activate the self-body. For instance, in autogenic training, recognizing a feeling of heaviness or warmth is the content of cognitive experience of the self-body, and striving toward such a feeling through passive concentration is the activity of body-self. Similarly, in progressive relaxation, one experiences muscular relaxation as the cognitive phase of self-body, and striving toward this experience of relaxation or actually achieving complete relaxation is the activity of body-self. By distinguishing self-body from body-self, techniques of self-control as a treatment of subjective activity can be directed to control the self-body and can be used for objective content control of the self-body by the body-self.

## COMPOSITION

As an outgrowth of these clinical experiences and theoretical considerations, jiko-control was developed as a new systematic method of self-therapy, composed of the following five steps: relaxation, meditation, imagery, self-understanding, and action.

### *Relaxation*

Relaxation, the first step of self-control training, facilitates and strengthens the ability of the patient's body-self to work on his self-body through muscular relaxation. Patterned after Jacobson's progressive relaxation technique, there are, nevertheless, fundamental differences between Jacobson's method and relaxation in jiko-control. Jacobson treats each muscular group as a training unit, according to a physiological point of view. Jiko-control uses muscular groups to emphasize body awareness and psychological motor control by body-self.

1) Pre-practice. Initially, the trainee concentrates on experiencing and understanding the sensation of muscular tension. Lying on his back with his arms at his side, he bends his left hand back, following Jacobson's self-operations procedure (1964, p. 84), thus experiencing tension.
2) Practice schedule
   (a) Upper limb practice. The trainee, lying on his back, first observes sensations of finger tension by slightly bending both hands, then extending the tension into the palms. He then extends the sensation of muscular tension from the fingertips to the center of the body. For example, the wrists are engaged by slightly bending the hand forward; the elbows by bending the arms at the elbows; the armpits by tightening the arms at sides; and the shoulders by bending the shoulder blades forward. He can now feel the muscular tension of upper limbs as a whole. The trainee next releases tension from the upper limbs in the reverse order: shoulders, armpits, elbows, wrists, palms, and fingers.
   (b) Lower limb practice. A similar procedure is applied to lower limbs. To experience the feeling of tension, the trainee begins

bending his toes, then the soles of his feet. He stretches his ankles, bends his knees, and tightens his thighs and buttocks. After experiencing tension in the lower limbs as a whole, tension is released in the reverse order, from central to peripheral body parts.

(c) Trunk practice. Tensing and relaxing involves a simultaneous bending and tightening of upper and lower back—from the shoulder to the upper back, plus the back of waist, lower back, and central back.

(d) Whole body practice. The trainee practices body tension, incorporating both orientations at the same time, that is, tensing the fingers, palms, wrists, elbows, armpits, shoulder, and upper back to the central back, plus the toes and soles of feet, ankles, knees, thighs, buttocks, back of waist, and lower back to the central back. After tensing the body as a whole, he releases the tension in the reverse order.

*Meditation*

The second step of training involves the "warmth" exercise of Schultz's autogenic training, which incorporates self-suggestion. In learning meditation, self-suggestion of warmth at the left arm is extended to the right arm, left leg, right leg, upper trunk (including shoulders and neck), and lower trunk. Finally this passive concentration of warmth encompasses the whole body, excluding the head, face and upper neck.

When the trainee begins to feel body warmth through self-suggestion, activation of self by the trainee is twofold: suggested self and suggesting self. Activating the suggested self, he experiences his inner world more clearly, and the feeling of suggested warmth is strengthened through his passive concentration. Success with this passive concentration depends upon the suggesting self facilitating and encouraging the former self to experience the suggested warmth. As I discussed (Naruse, 1962), once the trainee consistently activates passive concentration, a state of meditative concentration results. Then the state of passive concentration is established more firmly and is less subject to disturbance. In addition, the trainee is freed from his usual patterns of feeling, cognition, thinking, or behaving. The practice of meditation enables the trainee to free himself from psychological restriction, and also allows him to work actively with the experiencing self or suggested self as a neutral observer, encourager, helper or strict controller of the suggesting self.

*Imagery*

The third step involves imagery. The trainee enhances his ability to experience mental imagery vividly and freely as an inner activity. This step usually follows meditation training; however, sometimes it is initiated without meditation or relaxation. Imagery training differentially enhances self-activity, that is, the observing self and experiencing self, suggesting self and suggested self, and controlling self and observed self.

Two training methods are commonly used. One utilizes the meditative exercise of Schultz's autogenic training. The other is a method of free imagination of landscape, scene, figures, things, stories, and so forth.

Schultz's procedure is composed of the following stages:

Stage 1. Static uniform colors,
Stage 2. Dynamic polymorphic colors,
Stage 3. Polychromatic patterns and simple forms,
Stage 4. Objects,
Stage 5. Transformation of objects and progressive differentiation of images,
Stage 6. Filmstrips,
Stage 7. Multichromatic cinerama.

The method of free imagination starts with a landscape of a field or seaside. When the trainee successfully images some scene, he then strives to see a more restricted part of the landscape, for instance, one house and garden. Next, he imagines even finer detail, perhaps two persons talking together in the garden. He then tries to hear or guess the topic of conversation, the identity of the characters, the actual content of the conversation, the theme of the scene, etc. When the trainee can successfully imagine a situation or scene, he strives to move further into the situation, developing a story, and he may deliberately introduce a particular person into the situation. Additionally, he can visualize an emotionally frustrating scene or a critical human relationship situation.

*Self-Understanding*

When training with relaxation, meditation, and imagery proceeds successfully, and the twofold activities of self are well differentiated so that each of them works suitably and specifically, the fourth step of training in self-understanding is initiated. The observing self learns how to work toward observing and understanding the experiencing self as calm, quiet, objective, and as clear as possible. The experiencing self learns how to feel, think, and behave as freely and as naturally as possible.

Self-understanding involves three stages of training: body awareness, self-image, and self-questioning.

1) Body awareness. To learn body awareness the trainee passively concentrates on his inner feeling of sensation and awareness of body. The entire body may be experienced through focus upon internal organs or muscular, motoric, or skin sensation using deep and complete relaxation and meditative concentration. The trainee strives to become aware, to clarify, intensify, and maintain the feeling or sensation of body.
2) Self-image. The trainee attempts to see and experience his own figure in imagery. Sometimes he may see only one figure, like a portrait without any background. Others experience themselves within a scene, for example, working in their business. Moving into a scene, the trainee develops a story or drama, according to his own inner theme. Subsequently, he tries to put himself into an imagined critical situation.
3) Self-questioning. With self-questioning training, the trainee learns to use imagery to answer questions about himself and sometimes for self-interpretation. Answering imagery is a kind of imagined response to the verbal, conceptual, or intellectual questions he has about himself. It may involve a process of interpretation in imagery, using emotional, intuitive, illogical, psychoanalytic, phenomenological, or even religious processes.

*Control of Action*

Finally, the trainee learns how to develop efficiency in action to improve performance in everyday life. He must first learn how to separate the activity of self into two parts, the acting self and the controlling self. The acting self is to be active, to behave, to strive for action. The controlling self can motivate, encourage, or control the acting self. Both must be understood and work in unison to promote effective action.

Training is divided into two parts: self-suggestion and mental control. Self-suggestion follows Schultz's autogenic training and is composed of two kinds of formulas: organ-specific formulas and intentional formulas. The latter include neutralizing, reinforcing, abstinence, paradoxic, and supporting formulas. Mental control is composed of five stages: mental warm-up, mental rehearsal, mental practice, thinking through imagery, and representation through imagery. All of them are characterized as an application of mental imagery for the purpose of promoting actions in everyday life.

1) Mental warm-up. An upcoming situation (e.g., a sports competition, a speech) is experienced in imagery, thus achieving an active preparatory set.
2) Mental rehearsal. Mental rehearsal includes inspection, overhauling, or refining of planned procedures for the upcoming situation through imagination. To imagine the scene in detail, clarify deficiencies, then remedy potential difficulties is to encourage and promote the positive internal theme.
3) Mental practice. Mental practice is a course of exercise to develop a skill or well-patterned behavior through mental imagery. It is similar to the techniques introduced by Drs. Cooper and Erickson (1954) as time distortion in hypnosis. They described cases of motor learning, nonmotor learning, mathematical mental activity, etc. I have successfully used these techniques with many champion athletes (Naruse, 1965).
4) Thinking through imagery. The trainee learns to use mental imagery and meditative concentration to encourage the activity of the experiencing self. To solve a problem, thinking through imagery is often superior to verbal or conceptual thinking, because image thinking does not follow usual logic, but rather specific logic in visual or pictorial form. Therefore, the trainee must rearrange or rethink the problem in verbal or conceptual logic for full understanding by the observing self.

   In Japan, this process has been used by businessmen as a valuable method for creativity training. For some teachers, this method is used primarily for teaching their pupils how to understand novels or science, or how to study effectively.
5) Representation through imagery. The trainee learns to represent the inner activity of the experiencing self through mental imagery. Compared to conceptual, verbal, or logical representation, it has been found that imaged representation is more free, natural, illogical, and nonstereotyped. The trainee is required to rearrange the represented imagery into a suitable form for the realistic and objective world.

   In Japan, school boys are learning how to represent ideas or the activity of the experiencing self through mental imagery in writing essays, drawing pictures, and in drama and artistic activities. A professional painter in Japan first learned how to use visual imagery 15 years ago, and he skillfully incorporated this imagery into wonderful and fantastic weavings.

## CONCLUSION

Jiko-control makes use of strivings for self-determination by maximizing patient input in the process of therapy. Training procedures have been used successfully in psychotherapy, sports medicine and promoting creativity in art and business.

## REFERENCES

Cooper, L.F. & Erickson, M.H. *Time Distortion in Hypnosis.* Baltimore: Williams & Wilkins, 1954.

Jacobson, E. *Progressive Relaxation.* Chicago: University of Chicago Press, 1929.

Jacobson, E. *Anxiety and Tension Control.* Philadelphia: J.B. Lippincott, 1964.

Naruse, G. & Obonci, T. Decomposition and fusion of mental images in the drowsy and post-hypnotic hallucinatory state. *Journal of Clinical and Experimental Hypnosis,* 1953, *1,* 23-41.

Naruse, G. Hypnosis as a meditative concentration and its relationship to the perceptual process. In M.V. Kline, Ed. *The Nature of Hypnosis.* Baltimore: Waverly Press, 1962.

Naruse, G. The hypnotic treatment of stage fright in champion athletes. *International Journal of Clinical and Experimental Hypnosis,* 1965, *8,* 63-70.

Naruse, G. *Jiko-Kontrol.* Tokyo: Kodansha, 1969 (in Japanese).

Schultz, J.H. *Das Autogene Training.* Stuttgart: George Thieme Verlag, 1932.

Weitzenhoffer, A.M. *General Techniques of Hypnotism.* New York: Grune & Stratton, 1957.

Chapter 35

# Hypnosis in Eastern European Countries

*Stanislav Kratochvíl and Michael Vančura*

For a long time, following the Second World War, hypnosis was under the influence of Pavlovian theory. This theory conceptualizes hypnosis as a state of partial sleep in which the hypnotist's word gains more influence than the real world. Later on, criticism developed in some countries, especially Czechoslovakia and Hungary, while the theory retained credibility in the Soviet Union. Today, even Soviet psychotherapy has rejected Pavlovian concepts as sufficient explanation for the various phenomena and types of hypnotic state. Hypnosis is now reconceptualized in Eastern Europe in constructs more similar to those of the Western world. A closer look at theory, methods, and practical applications of hypnosis in various countries highlights similarities and differences.

## CZECHOSLOVAKIA

In our native country, Czechoslovakia, the recent history of hypnotism started with the work of Ivan Horvai, a psychiatrist, and Jiří Hoskovec, a psychologist. Both investigated hypnotic phenomena, including age regression, visual hallucinations, and post-hypnotic suggestion. They were interested in whether those phenomena could be understood as genuine changes in perception and behavior or whether preconception played an important role. Findings supported the latter explanation. Horvai later published a text on clinical hypnosis and Hoskovec published one on the psychology of hypnosis and suggestion and another on theories of hypnosis. Hoskovec's position is an eclectic one with preference for Hilgard's and Shor's concepts.

Investigative research into hypnotic phenomena has been conducted at Kroměříž. Kratochvíl and his partner, Svoboda, dissatisfied with the conceptualization of hypnosis as a partial sleep state, have investigated the waking type of hypnosis which would not fit into this concept. Using highly susceptible, trained subjects, they developed two types of hypnotic trance, a passive one and an active one, which resulted in significantly different behavioral activity, as rated by independent observers. Kratochvíl and Svoboda sought to determine which factors were most commonly responsible for these varying degrees of activity in hypnotic subjects. First, it appeared that active hypnosis was more easily induced with highly susceptible subjects, while the passive trance could be easily achieved, even with low susceptibles. Another study, performed by Kratochvíl in cooperation with Nancy Schubat at Stanford University, demonstrated that subjects with a more active temperament exhibited a corresponding level of high activity in the hypnotic state. A third influencing factor, the preconception about what the hypnotic state would involve, was shown to be statistically significant by Kratochvíl and Zezulka. While the influence of the induction technique has not yet been demonstrated, it seems plausible that talking about sleep will result in a greater passivity of the subject.

An interesting spinoff, stimulated by this earlier work, is Kratochvíl's investigations into prolonged active hypnosis. Some subjects have been able to maintain a prolonged active hypnotic state for several days or even one week. They remained immediately responsive to hypnotic suggestion while preserving the normal waking-sleep rhythm, yet had full amnesia of what happened during the time spent in trance. While spending an academic year at Stanford, Kratochvíl studied sleep characteristics of the hypnotic state. Using EEG, he sought to determine which states of sleep permitted subject receptivity to hypnotic suggestions. These findings have been published in several articles in American hypnotic journals, as well as summarized in a Czech book on the nature of hypnosis and its relationship to sleep.

Various characteristics of hypnotic susceptibility and suggestibility have been examined at Koměříž. Situational factors have not been found to influence the hypnotic susceptibility of the average subject. However, some personality types appear more receptive to specific, personalized procedures (for example, "magic") while others respond to more common environmental stimuli of an impersonal nature. Hypnotic susceptibility correlated highly with hand clasp tests in the waking state and moderately with susceptibility to social influence (the work of Hájek, Holešovský, Vylídalová and others).

In Czechoslovakia, clinical investigations of hypnotherapy have been conducted with various neurotic and psychosomatic conditions. Associate Professor Milan Černý, his co-worker Věra Doležalová, and others from the Prague University Department of Psychiatry have developed a special technique of post-hypnotic suggestion using a signal activated by the subject. The method, briefly called "amulet," involved hypnotic training which was paired with a special signal the subject initiates himself. He might touch a particular object or simply press two fingers together to activate a specific post-hypnotic suggestion, for instance, that stage fright would disappear or that he would feel strong and self-assertive. This enables the subject to reactivate the post-hypnotic suggestion in situations in which he needs it. Černý has had good results with hypnosis in treating esophogeal spasms and other psychosomatic conditions.

The Czech Psychiatric Society formally adopted its hypnosis section in 1971, with Bouchal, Kratochvíl, and Hoskovec as the organizing committee. Meetings and workshops in both beginning and advanced hypnosis were organized for medical doctors and clinical psychologists. In the course of ten years, this educative effort has produced four hundred specialists, including many participants from Poland. Graduates have subsequently shared new insights and learning through papers presented at the meetings of the section. These interesting observations, experiences, and achievements can be summarized as follows: The most common induction method used is the verbal fixation method. Nevertheless, a growing number of hypnotherapists prefer to start hypnotic induction with directed fantasy, using various pleasant images and metaphors. This is a marked shift from the formerly directive, authoritarian "father-hypnosis" to a softer, protective "mother-hypnosis." This can be in some way associated with the growing number of female hypnotists, psychologists and doctors who combine independence and self-assertiveness with softness and tenderness.

It was Balcar from Prague who focused our attention on the individualized techniques of Milton H. Erickson. Teaching them in the advanced courses with great success, he emphasized the importance of the behavior exhibited at the beginning of the induction by the patient himself. He reinforced this, then he tried to manipulate it, shifting it a little bit in one direction or another to help the patient attain trance.

Schürer developed an interesting imaginative technique for children using the fantasy of a space flight for boys and various fairy tales for girls. Vyhnálek, using a Czech translation of London's Children Hypnotic Susceptibility Scale, demonstrated that children are more susceptible to suggestions of illusion and hallucination than to motor suggestion.

In stomatology, Kaiser used an imagined TV program to divert the attention of his child patients from the dental work in progress. Konečný induced hypnosis in very young children through an imitation technique. The child first lulled a toy doll to sleep, then participated in the same experience himself.

Less self-assertive hypnotists use autogenic training as a starting point in their hypnotic induction. With great success Machač from Prague developed a relaxation technique which combines and contrasts relaxation with an activation phase using images. Zikmund, of Bratislava, described positive results with hypnosis in polydipsia and Reynaud's disease and Doležalová with gynecological patients. Dostálová from Prague reported the positive influence of hypnosis on the psychic state of the patients with cancer. Many child psychologists have used hypnosis to treat bed-wetting, phobias and anxieties. Some psychologists claim positive results in treating alcoholism.

This brief overview points to hypnosis as a well-established method which, in Czechoslovakia, is incorporated into a more complex psychotherapeutic approach. Hypnotic states, hypnotic phenomena, and hypnotic susceptibility are continuing areas of interest for investigators especially in Prague, Brno, Kroměříž, and Bratislava.

## USSR

In the Soviet Union, the leading proponent of hypnosis is currently Professor Vladimir Evgenievič Rožnov, head of the Psychotherapy Department in the Institute for Postgraduate Education in Medicine in Moscow. For a long time Professor Rožnoz adhered to the partial sleep theory. In his practice, however, he developed an active technique of hypnotherapy called "emotional stress hypnosis," which he used especially in treating alcoholic patients.

Rožnov hypnotizes a group of about ten patients lying on their beds. After strong authoritarian suggestions aimed at the induction of deep hypnosis, he gives a suggestion of the smell of vodka. This is then associated with the suggestion of intense nausea and vomiting. These suggestions are given in a loud voice, while touching the patients. If they do not react appropriately, he puts cotton-wool drenched with vodka to their nose and the expected symptoms usually develop quickly.

Rožnov demonstrated his procedure with Czech alcoholic patients in the psychiatric hospital in Kroměříž and dramatically illustrated it when some of the patients actually began to vomit or cough. Results occurred in spite of the considerably less favorable attitudes of patients and present professionals than he had at his own ward.

In his work with neurotic patients, Prof. Rožnov uses a softer form of hypnotic induction and suggestion. In his research, hypnosis becomes a tool for investigating the reality of unconscious processes. For a long time unacceptable to Soviet psychology, the unconsciousness and unconscious processes are now popular topics in Soviet psychology. Professors Rožnov and Basin, both from Moscow, are among the leading researchers in this field. Prof. Rožnov uses post-hypnotic suggestions with amnesia, demonstrating that the subject can carry out actions without conscious awareness or motivation. In 1979, a special symposium in Tbilisi, Soviet Georgia, was devoted to the problems of unconscious psychic processes. There they tried to conceptualize unconscious processes as a phenomenon associated with the so-called "ustanovka" (set) of Prof. Uznadze.

Some of the Soviet psychologists from Moscow not directly associated with Rožnov, e.g., Prof. Tichomirov and Doctor Raikov, have analyzed age regression in hypnosis. When an early childhood age was suggested, marked desynchronization in eyeball movements and disturbances of eyeball location were determined. The appearance of child-like crying, sucking reflexes and Babinski's symptom were noted. The authors view these phenomena within the "genuineness hypothesis" rather than "role explanation" of hypnotic behavior.

Hypnosis as a psychotherapeutic method was very popular in Russia. In fact, about ten or 15 years ago, it was the primary method used, besides rational psychotherapy. Usage has declined in recent years in connection with the growing popularity of pathogenetic psychotherapy, the Soviet variant of dynamic psychotherapy. This now growing school uses Mjasiščev's conception of personality as a system of relationship-seeking to understand the development of the symptom and bring the patient to some insight into the intrapsychic and interpersonal cause of his neurosis. Nevertheless, hypnosis is taught in courses in the Institute of Postgraduate Studies. There are usually specially equipped rooms in most psychiatric hospitals for individual or group hypnosis. Daily sessions with six to ten patients in a darkened room last about 20 minutes. After the induction procedure and without testing the hypnotic depth, suggestions of calmness, general well-being and cessation of symptoms are usually given, sometimes with a fatherly authoritarian tone and at others with a mild mothering voice.

New textbooks on hypnosis keep appearing. Most recent is a textbook by I.P. Bul, an internist and hypnotherapist from Leningrad, who uses hypnosis extensively to treat various psychosomatic diseases.

## EAST GERMANY

The German Democratic Republic has traditionally used hypnosis. Gerhardt Klumbies, Professor of Internal Medicine, has been using hypnosis for the treatment of various psychosomatic conditions. In his book, *Psychotherapy in Internal and General Medicine,* he describes the positive disruption of disturbance and disease in almost every organ and system. He developed a special technique which he calls "ablative hypnosis," hypnosis without the hypnotist. He particularly recommends it for patients with chronic pain which has not responded to hypnotic or posthypnotic suggestion. He trains his susceptible patients to self-induce trance by means of various techniques which they can use by themselves without the presence of the hypnotist. For example, patients might stare at a special picture or listen to a tape of a hypnotic induction. After inducing trance they are trained to repeat therapeutic suggestions and then terminate hypnosis. Klumbies has described good results with patients with neuralgias, migraine headaches and so forth.

Alfred Katzenstein, Professor of Psychology in Berlin, uses hypnosis and autogenic training for patients with hypertension and myocardial infarction. He has edited two volumes on hypnosis, one oriented toward theory and research, the other toward psychotherapeutic practice. German and other Eastern European authors, as well as well-known Western authors, contributed to this volume. Katzenstein organized the first symposium of the socialist countries on hypnosis in Rostock in 1977.

Germany also has a section for hypnosis and autogenic training which exists as part of the Society for Medical Psychotherapy. The section has about two hundred members. It organizes courses in hypnotic techniques and autogenic training, which is also very popular in East Germany. A modern textbook on autogenic training has been published by Schaeffer, König and Dipol.

## POLAND

Up until the last ten years, hypnosis received little recognition in Poland. It was less popular in Poland than in Czechoslovakia or Germany. Now interest is growing very rapidly. Popular Western books on hypnosis, Lewis Wolberg's *Hypnosis—Is It For You?* and Leon Chertok's *Hypnosis,* have been translated into Polish language, as has Kratochvíl's comprehensive Czech textbook of psychotherapy in which considerable space is devoted to the professional use of hypnosis.

Jerzy Alekandrowicz, a leading psychotherapist from Cracow, uses hypnosis with neurotic patients as a treatment method. In theory, he emphasizes the emotional bond—the relationship between the hypnotist and patient. He argues that hypnotic susceptibility is correlated with the emotional involvement of the patient in this relationship, be it positive or negative. He expects that an indifferent attitude towards the hypnotist works as an inhibiting factor. Hypnosis as a state or hypnotic susceptibility as a stable personality trait is given less emphasis.

Several groups of psychologists in Poland are oriented towards experimental investigations of hypnosis. Jerzy Siuta from the Psychology Department in Cracow has investigated Rotter's locus of control concept in relation to hypnotic susceptibility. Another group of hypnotic investigators is at the University of Poznan, e.g. Pleszewski, Gapik, Domachowski and others. Overall, about 50 physicians and clinical psychologists use hypnotherapy at least occasionally in their clinical work.

A more general acceptance of hypnosis has been generated through courses on the understanding and usage of hypnotic techniques, presented by Zbigniew Pleszewski, Waldemar Domachowski, L. Gapik, and others. Besides general eclectic overview on hypnotic theory and reports of special investigations into the nature of the hypnotic state and hypnotic susceptibility, interested professionals are instructed in the practical application of hypnosis.

## RUMANIA

In Rumania the work of the psychologist Prof. Vladimir Gheorghiu is well-known. He investigated direct and indirect suggestions and developed many suggestibility tests, thereby making it possible to compare the results of the same type of suggestibility tests performed under direct and indirect conditions. For instance, the direct suggestion for falling backwards was compared with the expectation that a certain operation would have the effect that the subject would fall backwards. Another important investigation performed by Gheorghiu in Western Germany with Prof. Langen and Velek concerned amnesia and hyperamnesia in hypnosis. He published, in German, the results of his investigations in this area in his book on memory in hypnosis.

## HUNGARY

The Hungarian hypnotherapist, F.A. Völgyesi, has used various auxiliary techniques in his hypnotherapeutic practice to enhance the suggestive "magic" influence of his hypnotic sessions. One of them, which he called "Faraday's hand," incorporates electrical equipment to evoke faradic sensations in the subject when the hypnotist touches the patient's forehead. Without knowledge of the existence of the electrical circuit, the client is thus impressed by the hypnotist's power and falls more easily into the hypnotic trance. Völgyesi has also conducted animal experiments with hypnosis.

Researching the physiological correlates of hypnosis, Meszárosz from the Hungarian Academy of Sciences in Budapest has published a paper about evoked brain potentials in hypnosis. According to his findings, slight changes occur which suggest that the level of general activation is lower in hypnosis as compared to the waking state. Meszárosz also published a scientific textbook on hypnosis.

Eva Banyai, a psychologist from the same institute, has devoted much time and effort to the investigation of the active type of hypnosis. As an induction technique she used pedalling on a bike-ergometer and succeeded in hypnotizing subjects with their eyes open, while involved in a high level of activity. The performance of these subjects on the hypnotic susceptibility scales duplicated that of subjects tested under hypnosis which was induced with classical hypnotic induction techniques. This investigation was performed partly in Budapest and partly in Hilgard's laboratory at Stanford University.

## YUGOSLAVIA

Hypnosis also became quite popular in Yugoslavia, especially in the Slovenian part of this Federal Republic. Marian Pajntar, a gynecologist, is the most representative person of this group. At the recent second European Congress on hypnosis in Dubrovnik, in May 1980, there was a demonstration of the activity of the Slovenian hypnotist in the areas of both theory and practice. There is increasing application of hypnosis in various clinical areas. A special emphasis is on hypnosis in obstetrics and gynecology which, as yet, is less developed in other socialist countries.

## BULGARIA

In Bulgaria the development of hypnotic theory and practice was under strong influence of the Soviet Union and hypnosis was the most accepted psychotherapeutic method. The specific contribution of the Bulgarian psychotherapists in the area of hypnotherapy lies in the emphasis on abreaction, on the hypnocathartic aspect of the revivification of traumatic experience in the hypnotic state. It is expected that abreaction will relieve accumulated tensions and lead, as a causal therapy, to symptomatic improvement. A. Atanasov, Associate Prof. of Psychiatry in Sofia, uses group sessions with tape-recorded hypnotic induction and therapeutic suggestions. If, during this hypnotherapeutic session, signs of crying or sobbing are observed in some patients, they are taken from the common room to a separate room, where the hypnotist encourages full emotional release. Through suggestion, he stimulates the patient to reexperience the situation which is supposedly responsible for the onset of the symptoms. The patient is left for some time in the aroused state, then is encouraged to verbally express his experience. The sessions with hypnotic abreaction are repeated several times, until the strength of the affect is diminished. In some clinics in Bulgaria abreaction is used without hypnosis by means of imagination techniques.

## CONCLUSIONS

Hypnosis is currently quite popular in Eastern European countries. There are several common features and many specific differences in the different countries. The common feature is that hypnosis has traditionally been more authoritarian and manipulative than is presently found in the USA. The old stereotypes still persist, reinforced by the expectations of the patients that the hypnotist should possess almost god-like self-confidence and persuasive powers. Still, in some countries the alternatives, including mothering techniques or permissive imaginative techniques, are gaining popularity. A strong emphasis on Pavlovian "partial sleep theory," obligatory for a long time in the Soviet Union, leads some unsatisfied investigators, especially in Czechoslovakia and Hungary, to pursue an alternative, waking-alert active type of hypnosis.

In Eastern Germany hypnosis in the hands of both internists and psychologists, sometimes in alternation with autogenic training, is already traditionally employed as an important treatment tool with psychosomatic symptoms. Training in self-hypnosis has been developed as an auxiliary technique for chronic pain conditions. The specific contribution of Bulgarian hypnotherapy lies in the emphasis on the abreactive hypnocathartic technique. The Rumanians have contributed to the investigation of direct and indirect suggestions and of the influence of hypnosis on memory.

In Czechoslovakia, hypnotherapy reflects the theories, methods, investigations, and therapeutic uses of hypnosis practiced in most Western countries.

## REFERENCES


Aleksandrowicz, J. Interactional theory of hypnosis and hypnability. In: *Hypnosis in Psychotherapy and Psychosomatic Medicine.*M. Pajntar et al. (Eds.), Ljubljana: University Press, 1980.

Balcar, K. Individualized techniques of hypnotization: Contribution of M.H. Erickson. (Czech.) *Čs. Psychologie,* 1973, *17,* 468-476.

Bouchal, M., & Kratochvíl, S. Rationalization mechanisms in posthypnotic suggestion. *Am. J. Clin. Hypn.,* 1966, *8,* 181-186.

Bul, P.I. *Technika vrachebnogo gipnoza.* Leningrad: Medgiz, 1955.

Bul, P.I. *Osnovy psichoterapii.* Leningrad: Medicina, 1974.

Černý, M. et al. The physiological characteristics of emotional states induced by hyposuggestion. *Activ. nerv. sup.,* 1973, *15,* 59.

Černý, M. et al. An attempt to influence esophageal motility by hypnosuggestion. *Activ. nerv. sup.,* 1974, 16, 123.

Černý, M. Therapeutic use of posthypnotic suggestion evoked by autostimulation. (Czech.) *Čs. psychiatrie,* 1973, *69,* 11-16.

Doležalová, V., Černý, M., & Jirák, R. Relaxation and EMG activity in neurotics and patients with psychosomatic gastrointestinal disorders. *Activ. nerv. sup.,* 1978, *20,* 35-36.

Gheorghiu, V. *Hypnose und Gedächtnis. Untersuchungen zur hypnotischen Hypermnesie und Amnesie.* München: W. Goldmann, 1973.

Horvai, I., & Hoskovec, J. Experimental study of hypnotic visual hallucinations. In: *Hypnosis and Psychosomatic Medicine.* J. Lassner (Ed.), Berlin: Springer, 1967.

Horvai, I., & Hoskovec, J. Experimental study on some processes of visual perception influenced by hynotic suggestion. *Activ. nerv. sup.,* 1964, *6,* 72-73.

Hoskovec, J. *Psychology of Hypnosis and Suggestion.* (Czech.) Praha: Academia, 1967.

Hoskovec, J. *Theories of Hypnosis.* (Czech.) Praha: Universita Karlova, 1970.

Hoskovec, J., & Cooper, L.M. Comparison of recent experimental trends concerning sleep learning in the USA and the Soviet Union. *Activ. nerv. sup.,* 1967, *9,* 93-95.

Hoskovec, J., Svorad, D., & Lanc, O. The comparative effectiveness of spoken and tape recorded suggestions on body sway. *Int. J. Clin. Exp. Hypn.,* 1963, *11,* 163-166.

Katzenstein, A. (Ed.) *Hypnose. Aktuelle Probleme in Theorie, Experiment und Klinik.* Jena: G. Fischer, 1971.

Katzenstein, A. (Ed.) *Suggestion und Hypnose in der psychotherapeutischen Praxis.* Jena: G. Fischer, 1978.

Kleinsorge, H., & Klumbies, G. *Technik der Hypnose für Ärzte.* Jena: G. Fischer, 1961.

Klumbies, H. *Psychotherapie in der inneren und Allgemeinmedizin.* Leipzig: S. Hirzel, 1974.

Klumbies, G. (Ed.) *Hypnosetherapie.* Leipzig: S. Hirzel, 1981.

Kratochvíl, S. Sleep hypnosis and waking hypnosis. *Int. J. Clin. Exp. Hypn.* 1970, *18,* 25-40.

Kratochvíl, S. Prolonged hypnosis and sleep. *Am. J. Clin. Hypn.,* 1970, *12,* 254-260.

Kratochvíl, S. *The Nature of Hypnosis and Its Relationship to Sleep.* (Czech.) Praha: Academia, 1972.

Kratochvíl, S. Ausbildung von Hypnotherapeuten. In: *Suggestion und Hypnose in der psychotherapeutischen Praxis.* A. Katzenstein (Ed.), Jena: G. Fischer, 1978.

Kratochvíl, S., & Macdonald, H. Sleep in hypnosis: A pilot EEG study. *Am. J. Clin. Hypn.* 1972, *15,* 29-37.

Kratochvíl, S., & Schauerová, J. Messung der Hypnotisierbarkeit bei Varianten der Hypnosetechnik. In: *Hypnose.* A. Katzenstein (Ed.), Jena: G. Fischer, 1971.

Kratochvíl, S., & Shubat, N. Activity-passivity in hypnosis and in the normal state. *Int. J. Clin. Exp. Hypn.,* 1971, *19,* 140-145.

Kratochvíl, S., & Zezulka, K. The influence of preconception and induction techniques on active hypnotic behavior. In: *Hypnosis in Psychotherapy and Psychosomatic Medicine.* M. Pajntar et al. (Eds.), Ljubljana: University Press, 1980.

Machač, M. *Harmonizing Mental States and Performance.* Praha: Universita Karlova, 1976.

Meszárosz, I. *Hipnózis.* Budapest: Medicina Könivkiadó, 1978.

Pajntar, M., Roškar, E., & Lavrič, M. (Eds.) *Hypnosis in Psychotherapy and Psychosomatic Medicine.* Ljubljana: University Press, 1980.

Platonov, K.I. *The Word as a Physiological and Therapeutic Factor.* Moscow: Foreign Languages Publishing House, 1959.

Raikov, V.L. Theoretical analysis of deep hypnosis: Creative activity of hypnotized subjects into transformed self-consciousness. *Am. J. Clin. Hypn.*, 1977, *19*, 214-220.

Raikov, V.L. Specific features of suggested anaesthesia in some forms of hypnosis in which the subject is active. *Int. J. Clin.* Exp. Hypn., 1978, *26*, 158-166.

Rožnov, V.E. *Gipnoz v medicine.* Moskva: Medgiz, 1954.

Rožnov, V.E. Toward understanding the nature of hypnosis. In: *Hypnosis at its Bicentennial.* F.H. Frankel, & H.S. Zamansky, (Eds.) New York: Plenum Press, 1978.

Rožnov, V.E. (Ed.) *Rukovodstvo po psichoterapii. 3rd. Ed.* Taschkent: Medicina, 1979.

Siuta, J. Locus of control and hypnotic susceptibility. In: *Hypnosis in Psychotherapy and Psychosomatic Medicine.* M. Pajntar et al. (Eds.) Ljubljana: University Press, 1980.

Slobodjanik, A.P. *Psichoterapia, vnuschenie, gipnoz.* 3rd Ed. Kiev: Zdorovie, 197

Svoboda, M. Dimensions of activity and passivity in hypnosis and hypnotic susceptibility. *Am. J. Clin. Hypn.*, 1971, *14*, 44-47.

Tichomirov, O.K., & Raikov, V.L. An analysis of regression facts. In: *Hypnosis in the Seventies.* L.E. Unestahl, Örebro: Veje, 1975.

Völgyesi, F.A. *Hypnosetherapie und psychosomatische Probleme.* Stuttgart: Hippokrates, 1950.

Völgyesi, F.A. *Hypnose bei Mensch und Tier.* Leipzig: S. Hirzel, 1963.

PART XIV

# *Appreciation Papers*

*Kay Thompson, D.D.S., and Bob Pearson, M.D., have much in common. Both are past presidents of the American Society of Clinical Hypnosis, and both are exceptional teachers and practitioners of Ericksonian techniques. Both were longtime friends and colleagues of Milton H. Erickson (additionally, they are close personal friends), and they are both superb communicators. Theirs were among the most highly rated papers delivered at the academic assembly.*

*Kay Thompson has a part-time practice in dentistry. She teaches behavioral science at the University of Pittsburgh School of Dental Medicine and has a joint appointment in the medical school Department of Psychiatry.*

*Robert Pearson is a psychiatrist who resides in Northern Michigan. He is the Director of the Division of Adult Psychiatry at the Traverse City Regional Psychiatric Hospital.*

*Thompson and Pearson talk about some of the things that they learned from Erickson. Additionally, they present insights into Erickson's personality and style. As was the case with Erickson, Thompson and Pearson are not content to simply describe ideas; their presentations contain induction language and demonstrations of Ericksonian techniques.*

*Along with Ernest Rossi and myself, Thompson and Pearson were asked by the Erickson family to speak at Erickson's memorial service. Attending the Congress was an emotional experience for them. Erickson had been a major figure in their life, and they were acutely aware of their grief.*

*Peter Nemetschek conducts a private practice of psychotherapy in Munich, West Germany and works as a consultant for a preschool program on one of the German television stations. Before embarking on his career as a therapist, he studied fine arts.*

*Nemetschek's paper at the Congress was a slide presentation. He spoke of his personal experiences attending one of Erickson's teaching seminars and showed slides to provide his audience with a visual experience. It was important to Nemetschek that people see pictures of Erickson and his environment and how he worked with phenomena such as arm levitation. Nemetschek's presentation was flavored by his German way of speaking English. He explained: "To me it sounds natural when I think in English about Erickson's work and you get an authentic report of mine." For easier reading, his paper has been edited to take into account more common English usage.*

Chapter 36

# The Curiosity of Milton H. Erickson, M.D.

*Kay F. Thompson*

I learned a lot from Milton Erickson about the double bind, but my being here today may be, for me, the ultimate example of it. This tribute to him, with all his friends, but without his expected presence, just may be a magnificent demonstration of how he manipulates situations even by his absence. Many of us think that we must say something important here today, but all we can hope to do is contribute a little to something that began in 1901, and then rely on it to continue if it is meant to be.

This is not going to be a presentation for the lover of four-syllable words or erudition. Instead it is a statement of what I believe I've learned from Erickson, which I hope you will accept without interpreting it as religious fervor. There is a myth that if something is explainable in simple language, it is not valuable. The incestuous perpetuation of this myth mollifies the large group of people who need to convince themselves that they, their words, and their works are highly complex and therefore superior. I do not believe that myth, and neither did Erickson. I will try, in the simplest way I can, to tell you some of what I've learned about and from Erickson, and then rely on you to use that knowledge in your own ways.

It is curious how he knew, and I believe he did know, when he chose some of us for special attention, that we would try in our own ways, not his, to carry on the work he started. He did not expect us to be like him, and so he cultivated each of us according to our own needs. These encounter sessions over the years taught me many things, many of which I do not yet know I know. I do know that the mellowing and seasoning process is an important enrichment, for it does take time to begin to understand what you know. The power and the magnificence of Erickson 25 years ago is something I was privileged to enjoy and be part of, and I am sad for those who did not have that opportunity and for those who did but did not understand what was given to them.

It is amazing that so many people who thought they learned from him missed so much of the learning. There are those people today who maintain that they can explain Erickson. There are even some among them who will try to capitalize on his death now that it is safe to quote and interpret him without fear of refutation. But they fall far short of understanding Erickson the man, the curiosity.

No one should presume to explain someone who had so many facets. If a number of people look at a diamond from different angles and describe the light they see, they may all be accurate and yet all see a different light, with none of them being able to describe the whole or the source. I suspect that Erickson would want each of us to see the light first in our own way, and then to accept that our view is not the complete vision, but rather a glimpse of what might be possible. He did not want us to replicate his light; he wanted us to develop our own.

There are those who came to him but could not learn because he demanded that they respond to him as individuals. They went away with the need to explain the change in *them* by explaining *him.* They went away knowing what they thought he taught. Yet, they missed so much of the man who treasured humanity, who was so curious because there was always a new problem to solve in a novel way, because his aim was to help people by always learning new ways. Yes, he was a curious curiosity, but his curiosity led many others to be quietly curious on their own.

To stimulate the imagination of each individual about what he might be able to do, and to demand the patient's recognition of his fullest potential were both in Erickson's repertoire for growth and health. He was a very human and sensitive man who could accept hostility and abuse from his purported colleagues, and who persevered because he knew his methods worked. He must have understood that gradually the healing professions would learn the techniques incorporated in his work and occasionally even acknowledge his pioneering leadership.

Like the many sides of a diamond, the devil has appeared in many guises; Erickson was frequently a devil's advocate with his Machiavellian maneuvers, his manipulative machinations, and his occasionally outrageous therapy. But those behaviors were not Erickson; they were an essence of his methodologies to help the patient. It remained for his patients, in many instances, to be the ones to know that when he was manipulative he also took responsibility for teaching them how to handle the results of the manipulation. Anytime he was Machiavellian, the situation required it. Anytime that he was brutal, it was because the patient could not use sympathy but needed prodding to break through the walls restraining him from achieving his potential. One of Erickson's greatest satisfactions was to see an individual achieve that potential and know that he had had a significant role in opening that person's world. Although he was never content with anything less than the most, he knew and accepted that the limits of potential could vary widely. And always, along with his most outrageous behavior, there was respect and regard for the person. Gentleness and tenderness were always there. Many onlookers missed it, but his patients always knew, although sometimes only in retrospect. To be as vicious as he sometimes seemed to be, and to do it out of love, demands an infinite love for the individual, *just because* he is a human being!

Erickson helped people who had grown up intellectually to grow up emotionally. In doing so, he suited the treatment to the person, unorthodox though that might be. He was never afraid of behaving like a fool, because he did not rely on artificial dignity, and thus never was a fool. I wonder if that fear of foolishness is one which restrains so many therapists from reaching further than they do? He cared, and was not ashamed to care. Many therapists learn that they must remain objective and "uninvolved." But remaining objective need not exclude caring, and there are some people who can do both. Not so curiously, Erickson had this capacity for compassion. He taught the ability to accept caring: Patients could leave their wildest fantasies in his closet; he would provide a home for patients during therapy; he would keep a pet for them when apartment rules or travel regulations necessitated it; he went for drives with phobics; he went to dinner with people who didn't think they could; he did whatever was necessary without fanfare.

His teaching and his therapy were inseparable. One of his ways of preparing people to be receptive to change was to initiate confusion, to disrupt their conviction that any reality was fact, and to induce a shift in attention. He taught by parable, but often it would be years before the story would be recognized for the profound lesson it contained, even though previous to the recognition of Erickson's meaning the ideas had been implemented and accepted as the patient's own. Milton knew that the individual does not *need* to defend himself against stories, that he can listen to them as a child would, wondering and curious not only about the story, but also about why Erickson chose it especially for him. At the same time, the unconscious is listening to the multi-level messages, picking up nonverbal cues, and lulling the unsuspecting conscious mind with the recognition that this is, after all, only a story.

But the simplicity that Erickson *seemed* to present was the most deceptive thing for the people who came along in later years. It was the result of years of observation, learning, working, reformulating, practicing, and trying again and again. He learned to learn much by asking little, by seeming to ask innocuous questions, and by allowing intolerable silences. His final simplicity makes it difficult for us. We want to do it without work; our arrogance arises because he made it seem so simple.

There's another amazing quality that I'm not sure many of us have recognized about Erickson. He needed no credit from the individual. He did not need the person to come back and say, "Thank you; you did this for me." He was content for people to say, "Of course I can do this now." Few people have so little desire for credit or gratitude; yet this was a man who would laugh about having the biggest ego in the world. When you think about it, though, the meaning of ego depends on your orientation. It wasn't ego. It was hubris, that's the word—insolence in the face of the Gods! He had it. I think he earned it.

Some men climb mountains because they are there. Milton couldn't physically climb mountains, but he could help people to achieve the summit of their own private mountains. I realized this one day as I was sitting on top of an actual mountain. He taught me that it was only right to be myself, that I could dare to do whatever it was that I had inside me to do, that I could be the person I wanted to be. To dare is to risk the chance for change! Milton dared to challenge the present order to wonder about the future possibilities, and to take action to make the potential into the real. He had a curiously appealing and overriding quality of a child-learned faith that the world *ought to be* right and fair. Since it had to be your turn sometime, why not now?

The man was a clinician, a practitioner! But he had a sense of glee, a glad-to-be-alive curiosity about life. There was always some new toy to explore or an old one to look at in a new way—always with the wonder of a child. He retained the naïveté, the lack of inhibition of the child and merged these with the sophistication of the ultra-observant therapist, a disturbingly effective combination. He was always sincere as he communicated his wonder, his awe, surprise, and delight when one accomplished some new learning, even though many others had done it before. Like a parent watching his child learn to walk, he took pride and satisfaction in the marvelous achievement of each person's trying and accomplishing a new skill. And, like children who delight in their parent's excitement, Erickson's patients recognized his infectious pride and mischievous curiosity about their activities.

Erickson played with mood and feeling the way the sun plays with light and shadow on the peaks and valleys of the mountains. It really did not matter to him *why* a person had difficulty: All that was important was that the person could change! Explanation was irrelevant. In this, he differed greatly from "orthodox" therapy of the time, but times have changed, and insight is less essential now. The concepts he developed grow in strange and curious ways, through unlikely people in unusual places, as demonstrated by the variety of backgrounds represented at the Erickson Congress. As Erickson liked to explain, each oak tree spreads millions of seeds. Many will not grow, but enough will hit receptive soil to take root and grow tall and strong. I wonder whether anyone can guess how many of the thousands of seeds he planted will grow, each in its own way, none exactly like any one before it. Maybe this is why some of us were "allowed" to plant a tree for his seventy-fifth birthday. He knew we could not be like him, and did not wish us to be. He wanted to stimulate our thinking: to get us to wonder; to explore within our minds, without our minds, within our bodies, about our bodies; to be curious enough to want to learn. I wonder how many of us can permit ourselves to acknowledge what we began to learn from him. Too often we cannot give credit to those who gave us the glimmer of ideas, but I hope many of us can acknowledge the subtle learnings which originated with Erickson.

We can carry on the tradition of learning, of being open, of allowing each experience to be a new one that can enlighten. It can be done scientifically, if that is what some people need. But there will be those of us who go on in our own low-key way, learning to appreciate the people who permit us to teach them, and hoping that they will, in turn, teach others. So the third generation Ericksonians follow the second generation Ericksonians, and third generation people know whom they follow even though they may never have met him. I know one person who put off meeting Erickson during his later years. There were two possible reasons: first, the possibility that when he came face to face with Erickson, Erickson would see his inadequacies and frailties; and second, the possibility that when he came face to face with him, this person would see Erickson's inadequacies and frailties, and have to cry.

Back when I began my own experience with Erickson I could not have realized where I might be today. All I knew then was the fear, the sheer terror, the wonder, and the curiosity, even then, of the enigma named Erickson. Ted Aston was the reason this particular mouse came back to the Seminars On Hypnosis. Ted was a nice, comfortable man who, unlike Erickson, did not scare me. I had tried to stay clear of those eyes that could see inside my head (the "ocular fix," as Jay Haley described it), but then he singled me out for special attention, and the changing process began.

Erickson had the skill of the master teacher, who let us think we had discovered things for ourselves. It's curious but natural that his memorial service was attended, not by the people from the learned institutions, but by the people whose lives he enriched by having taught them that life is a game to be played the best way possible. He did not teach us what to expect . . . he couldn't. He taught us that we could handle the *un*expected, and that we would always have a response available. It might not be the perfect response, but it would be a response we could live with. As one of the people close to him was told, "Happiness is the endowment with value of all the things you have."

I have learned much from Erickson. As I improved in what he taught me about observation, formal induction techniques have evolved for me into informal trance with an emphasis on the recognition of the language of communication. Anything communicated in the therapeutic situation contains many multi-level messages. When a word or behavior charges out at me, I take the energy it has and utilize that spark from the person's polarity, offering positive potential even though sometimes in an apparently negative way. Just as I can generate a case for "pain interferes with healing," so too can I amplify one for "pain stimulates healing," depending on the circuitry the patient needs.

I've learned so much from Erickson that I cannot consciously teach, so others must learn from watching me. I have said for years that one of the most important things I learned from Milton Erickson was to trust in and rely on my own unconscious. My unconscious is more perceptive at times than I allow myself to be at a conscious level. Unconsciously, I absorb communications and then broadcast responses. When I am enthusiastic with these vibrations and people pick up on the smaller things, it means they can generalize to the larger, more significant messages, if they are worth it! (And if you were really paying attention, you aren't sure what I meant, because "if they are worth it" may refer to the "things," or it may refer to the "people.")

Maybe the true dreamer is the only true realist. We learn very early that reality never is what we think it is going to be, and so the dreamer can adapt to the unreal reality without its destroying his dreams. When we find genuine satisfaction in the growth of the present, we must know that when we get where we are going, we will recognize it again. The warm, creative influence of the imagination lends sensitivity, perception, and spontaneity to our vision. We are the momentary product of a lifetime of past memories and experiences. We are altered so that we can grow within the reflection of ourselves that we learn to see in our imagination, and because of this legitimate reflection of the dream, we are able to grow.

Milton was an actor who would do anything to accomplish his goal. His act was meticulously performed to enthrall his audience, to gain their attention, to get them caught up in the play. That a man so restricted physically could expand so many horizons for others was astonishing. He presented vivid proof that one need not accept any restriction, because restrictions need not exist in the mind. He would delight in defying the usual laws of order in order to break down the restrictions and patterns of life. He thought, he worked, he wrote, he practiced his lines and his movements for greatest effect, and then he threw himself into the performance like a director showing others how to act. His phenomenal sense of humor tempered the performance, keeping the melodrama from becoming too heavy, even when it was.

"Observation"—that was his philosophy. It's fun to wonder how he got started, out there on the farm. One might conjecture that his curiosity was one of the ways he compensated for all the things he did not have, and it led him to make better use of all the things he could develop. Instead of learning to look at colors, he looked at shades of people: He learned to distinguish subtle nuances of hue and saturation and what was apparent when no camouflage was possible. Since he could not hear any music in music, he distinguished people's tones as tunes, and learned to recognize "what the pitch was" in the voice and the inflection. For a man who suffered so much pain, he was intimately in touch with muscle and nerve control, reading nonverbal movements with accuracy. His illnesses taught him patience. He also knew that you could overcome physical disabilities by freeing the mind. His capacities were intimidating. His patients had to confront that intimidation, but once they passed it, the release of their own potential came so powerfully that it overflowed. The patient was then left waiting, and wondering, and wanting—more.

He knew that we could not be he, and that we could not really even be like him, no matter how much we liked him, but that perhaps it did not really matter, since that matter was not really matter. We would be what we must be, but we should be what we could be. He saw some seeds take root and grow, and he understood that people are beginning to understand, even though we stand under so many misunderstandings. When we stand away, we find that his standards stand alone. They only need to be, and to be used, and the effectiveness of the reality of their effect affects our own affectional effectiveness. He taught so that we were not always sure what we had learned, but so that we could use it. We go on, with the curiosity instilled in us still in us, to know where we go now—I wonder? Strange, or should I say curious, that those of us who are most curious about it are the ones who are most content to wait and see what the curiosity of that special curiosity that is Erickson will become. If I speak, as some say, the language of hypnosis, it is because he taught me how to get ready; how to listen to what the person is really saying; how to hear; and how, sometimes, to be able to communicate, to know that understanding is one of the greatest gifts we can give, even when we do not understand.

Solve your private puzzle, hear the puns, enjoy. George Santayana said "Life is neither a spectacle nor a feast. It is a predicament." Erickson saw it as a challenge, a puzzle to be solved, so the pieces could begin to fit. He even died between two birthdays and an anniversary, leaving us the puzzle of whether he did not want to spoil those days, or whether, in his own pixielike fashion, he wanted that day to be all his own. He would smile, as his daughter Kristi said in a letter to me, and say "Enjoy every day." He was unorthodox, innovative, creative, often in pain and lonely. He was also immersed in, and happy with, his family and extended family. There are those of us who miss him as a person, and that is all right, too. He was quite a guy! And all of that helped to accomplish some of this, so this and that mean that this is that, and that that is this, and that's that!

This poem is very special to me, and I wasn't sure I was willing or able to share it here. I offer it in the hope that those who do not understand may begin to see how we whose lives began to change from our encounters with Milton Erickson feel about what we have learned—that we can be. This poem, by Roy Croft,* is what I think I thought he taught:

I love you, not only for what you are,
But for what I am when I am with you.

I love you, not only for what you have made of yourself,
But for what you are making of me.

I love you for the part of me you bring out.

---

*From *Men Behind Boy's Fiction* by W.O. Lofts. London: Howard Baker Co., 1970.

I love you for putting your hand into my heaped up heart,
And passing over all the foolish, weak things you can't help
dimly seeing there

And for bringing out into the light all the beautiful belongings
That no one else had ever looked quite far enough to find.

I love you because you are helping me to make,
Of the lumber of my life, not a tavern, but a temple,

And of the words of my everyday,
Not a reproach, but a song.

I love you because you have done more than any creed could
have done to make me good,
And more than any fate could have done to make me happy.

You have done it
Without a word,
Without a touch,
Without a sign.

You have done it by being yourself.

Perhaps that is what being a friend means, after all.

Chapter 37

# Erickson and the Lonely Physician

*Robert E. Pearson*

There are several reasons why I chose this subject and title. One of them is a close parallel to Jay Haley's story* about Gregory Bateson's saying to him, "I think Dr. Erickson is going to manipulate me into coming to dinner." When Jay asked why he thought that, Bateson replied, "While I was talking to him on the phone he said, 'Why don't you come to dinner?' " I was manipulated in much the same way.

About a year ago Milton asked me what I was going to talk about at this congress. I responded by saying that he already knew the title of my presentation. Then he said, "Why don't you talk about me and you—as people—when we met—and things like that?" At the time I thought that it would be an enjoyable thing to do, with Milton sitting in the auditorium, grinning. Afterward we would have a hilarious time talking about the stories I had told. "Enjoyable" does not describe my feelings today.

Most presentations at this meeting have been about Milton Erickson's psychotherapy methods and various interpretations of them. This is proper for a congress; however, I am going to do as I was asked and speak of Milton as a person. It will not be in any way a scientific presentation—it will be more in the way of an admittedly biased remembrance. I will also relate some of the things I think I learned from him. So please forgive my liberal use of the first person singular—I don't know of any other way of telling you what I want to say.

He was a large part of my life for many years. As I said at his memorial service, he was certainly the most important male in it, and that fact doesn't take a single thing away from my father or any other of the fine men I have known.

---

*See Chapter 1.

I'm going to tell you my experiences by a series of anecdotes, Milton's favorite teaching method. I will not attempt to interpret the stories—I'll leave that to each of you. Those of you who understand what Milton was saying through the years will know that *all* our interpretations will be correct.

My title is "Erickson and the Lonely Physician." Lonely means to be alone—lonesome means to be dejected as the result of being alone.

I graduated from a very good medical school in the early fifties, a school dedicated to turning out well-rounded general physicians. The whole school was person-oriented. It was only later that I realized that one problem with the school was that the department of psychiatry was rigidly psychoanalytic in orientation. A short anecdote will characterize at least one of the professors. He came to lecture one day with a wide grin; he had had a man in analysis for a number of years and was happy to report that at that morning's session the man had been able to say "s-h-i-t" aloud. However, the professor *spelled* the word that the patient had spoken!!

While in medical school I occasionally heard tales about a maverick psychiatrist named Erickson who had left the university the same year I began my studies. It is safe to say that he had not been the most popular member of the department, at least among the professors.

In fact, the Department of Psychiatry at my medical school said terrible things about the man, e.g., "He didn't believe in insight!" or "He thought he could change people without knowing what was wrong with them!"

Marion Moore, in his paper at this congress, said that Milton "astonished" other physicians; however, a better word would have been "infuriated." He was saddened by that fury, but he did outlive a good deal of it.

At a meeting in San Francisco in 1963 I was outraged to learn that Milton was going to travel from San Francisco to Los Angeles and return the same day. In spite of being very tired and ill, he was to speak to a group of analysts. I met him at breakfast and told him in my usual gentle way that he was a goddamned fool to make such a trip in his condition. He listened politely, acknowledged that he felt terribly tired and ill, and said, "Bob, for so many years they wouldn't listen, and now some of them will."

After completing a rotating internship, I was to begin a solo practice in a small town in northern Michigan. Let me say in retrospect that general practice for 13 years is an excellent first residency in psychiatry. It was obvious from the start that, because of my relative isolation from the rest of the medical community and the universities, I would have to make a special effort to continue my education.

So one day I registered for a review course in general practice to be held at a downtown Detroit hotel. Immediately after the course began it was apparent that it was meant for a group that had graduated from medical school well before I did. It was too elementary for my needs. I was wandering in the halls of the hotel looking for something better to do, when I saw a sign that said, "Seminars On Hypnosis." I must admit that I have often since wondered whether or not that was a fortunate accident. The only thing that I "knew" about hypnosis was the dire warnings about it and Erickson I had heard in medical school.

Within a few minutes I had described my poverty to the lady at the desk, paid a reduced registration fee, and was listening to a man saying things that no one had ever suggested to me before—ideas that commanded my attention. Before long, I felt a little angry with my teachers for not telling me that some people thought this way. As far as I could determine, this man was not talking about hypnosis. He was talking about such strange ideas as patients participating in their own therapy, patients solving their own problems, therapists not doing things *to* people, or even *for* people, but doing things *with* people. I was fascinated by the man, his ideas, and the way he said it all. It was as if he were speaking directly to me on several different levels of meaning at the same time, some of which I thought I could grasp a bit. I was, if you will forgive the phrase, entranced.

I didn't find out until much later that this was *the* Erickson, the "crazy hypnotist who was chased out of town" by my medical school teachers.

That evening we had a practice session. I found myself trying to persuade a rational, intelligent human being sitting in front of me that he should raise his hand and forearm off his thigh and at the same time pretend that he wasn't doing it, and that if he did I would also pretend that he hadn't done it. After about 20 minutes of coaxing, I had made up *my* mind that if indeed that hand did have a mind of its own, it was a most stubborn hand and wasn't about to do as I asked it. It just sat there. If it could have smirked, it would have.

Then a voice behind me said, "And who is responsible for this?" Turning around, I found that the wife of one of the students, while listening to me trying to induce my partner, had gone into a very deep trance. Here was my very first subject, and I hadn't even known she was there! Milton had seen what had happened and spent the next few minutes demonstrating what the lady could do in a trance. He also carefully explained that she was free to do as she saw fit, that it was *her* trance. So I learned early and well that the trance belongs to the subject.

My own sense of entrancement deepened. I was hooked.

During that first workshop I learned some techniques for helping people to control pain. I went back to my practice in northern Michigan and found to my absolute astonishment that my patients could and would use the new techniques and that I could teach them to use them.

Deeper and deeper a-n-d d-e-e-p-e-r.

It was not easy for me to get to know Milton on a personal level, which I really wanted to do. That last remark is a gross understatement—for a long time I was convinced that he really disliked me or at best tolerated me because his wife and one of his daughters seemed to enjoy my company. But I wanted to go on. Therefore, I attended 11 more basic workshops, all the same, and learned things of value at each one. And Milton began to get used to having me around, and one day he even smiled when I walked into a room.

Deeper still.

An important aspect of Milton's personality was his sense of humor—how could he have survived his physical difficulties without it? He didn't always show his amusement; in fact, he often seemed to hide it. He delighted in carrying on a running private joke with one or two members of a group, leaving the rest to wonder what was going on. If the joke was really well done, the others didn't even know that anything unusual was happening.

He delighted in calling me "Sweet Old Bob," knowing that the initials have another meaning. He enjoyed passing around a picture of a field of boulders, saying that it was the saddest picture he had ever seen. It mystified anyone who was unaware of the fact that trolls who are accidentally caught in sunlight turn into rocks.

Milton and I enjoyed a number of private jokes about the original nationality of our families. He once wrote to me that he was extremely saddened to learn that an arsonist had set fire to the Swedish National Library and that both volumes had been destroyed. I, of course, responded by saying that the Stockholm police had ruled out the entire Norwegian nation, since as far as is known, none had as yet learned to read.

He enjoyed other kinds of private jokes, too. In 1973 a gentleman who is here and is known to you all came to me at a meeting on hypnosis, admittedly quite anxious about an appointment he had to visit Milton Erickson. He knew that I knew Milton and would I tell him about Milton—how to behave, what to say, what not to say, etc. He followed me around, not being unreasonable, but very anxious to make a good impression. I couldn't resist calling Milton and telling him what I knew about the young man. So the young man was absolutely astonished at what Milton knew about him at their first meeting. He thought that Milton was by far the most perceptive man he had ever known. Milton was unique in his perceptive powers, but this time he had prior knowledge. Incidentally, the protagonist of this story is Jeff Zeig.

The bola tie I'm wearing today was given to me by Betty and Milton. Also, they told me the story about how it was named. On his way to see Milton, one of his patients was wearing a Kachina bola. When he stopped at a restaurant, the hostess, mistaking him for someone who had made a reservation, asked, "Are there six of you?" He replied, "No, there used to be six of me, but my psychiatrist. . . ." As he went on, the hostess turned on her heel and muttered, "What can you expect from a man who wears a goddamned doll around his neck?" Ever since, this has been my goddamned doll.

Once Betty and Milton and I were flying back from a workshop, feeling good about the meeting, bantering back and forth. I turned to Milton and said, "Milton, some day I'll be the best operator in the world." He said, "And how do you account for that?" I said, "It's obvious—you're a number of years older than I, the odds are that you will die before I do, and that will make me number one." He thought for a moment and said, "And at that time, Bob, you will also have the biggest ego in the world." That is one prediction that didn't come true.

For several years Roger Erickson and Pepper Pearson carried on a spirited conversation by mail. Milton delighted in discussing the letters in front of a group to see how long he could manage to keep people from realizing that Roger and Pepper were dogs. One day a woman asked, in all seriousness, "You mean your dogs write to each other, really?" Milton only replied, "Of course!" I could not resist saying, "Well, that's not quite true, Milton. I must confess that Pepper doesn't write well, so he dictates to the parrot who lives next door."

Other personal encounters come to mind:

He taught me that I could save my life. When I learned that my head could not occupy the same space being occupied by a brick, I also learned that what Milton had been saying for years was true: *I* could use hypnosis, too. On hearing about it for the first time, and how well I thought I had handled the situation, he said simply, "I always presumed that you were at least as smart as some of your patients."

At one of the annual meetings of the American Society of Clinical Hypnosis, Milton used Kay Thompson and me shamefully. It was a political thing; something very important to many people had to be done. Milton's plan to bring about the desired change included deluding Kay and me into thinking that something else was happening. Our expectations were very different from the way things turned out. The machinations went on all week. During the last day, it dawned on me what really had happened. I turned to Milton and said, "I've been had, haven't I?" He responded by saying only, "Yes." After we had returned home, Kay and I came up with an idea. We composed a letter to Milton over the phone, which I typed as two originals on our individual stationery. Our names each have three letters, so the letters matched exactly, even to the same "typo" in each. We mailed them to arrive in Phoenix on the same day. It was a very angry letter—"How could you do this to us? We have every reason to believe that you love us. You cannot treat us this way. We are very hurt." Our only answer by letter came from Betty, who explained that if we were going to be part of the Erickson family, we had better get used to taking our licks and learning from them. Milton did not respond, but the next time I saw him I had to confront him. I said, "Milton, we're both still very angry; we have cried, *'How could you do that to us?'* " He was quiet for several moments, then said, "Bob, first of all it was very important that it be done that way, and secondly you are the only two people I could have done that to and know that the friendship would survive." How do you respond to that?

I once responded to a post-hypnotic suggestion given me by Milton seven years previously. When I expressed amazement at my unusual behavior, he cued my recollection of the original trance by simply naming the city in which it occurred.

At a meeting in Philadelphia in 1976, I had the opportunity to be alone with Milton for a "short while" while Betty Erickson and Kay Thompson did some shopping. He began telling me stories about cases he had treated. At first it seemed odd that he hadn't responded to my statement that my father had died two weeks earlier. He recounted case after case after case. *Three hours later* (I shall forever be convinced that he arranged it all) it suddenly dawned on me that he had been talking about me and my father all the time. Then he began to retell the first story he had told me three hours before. Well, I wasn't going to fall for that! I knew what that was about! After all, he had taught me that way to induce amnesia! I was insulted that he would expect that I would. . . . *I would what?* To this day I can't remember any of those stories, but I do know that in some strange, wonderful way I resolved the feelings about my father's death.

So what did I learn from Milton Erickson? Several years ago at a workshop here in Phoenix I introduced Milton by saying that everything of importance that I think I know about human behavior I learned either from him or by doing what he taught so many of us to do—*really* watch and *really* listen to other people. I have no reason to change that opinion now.

I learned that I could help an enuretic boy by not talking about bladders and urine, that I could talk about learning to play baseball, and running a little faster, and staying on the baselines, and how to pass a football, and learning to use those muscles exactly as you want to.

I learned that people could learn to do marvelous things, things that they had no idea they could do, like control their perception of and reaction to pain, and that I could teach them to do it. So I can remember a boy of about ten with a rather badly mangled tibia who was reassuring his crying father as I manipulated the fragments, saying, "I can hear the bones crunching, too, Dad, but honest, it doesn't hurt."

I learned to trust my unconscious and, even better, to trust my patients' unconscious. I could trust that they could learn to handle things that had seemed impossible to manage.

I learned to expect that patients could be creative without knowing it. They could resolve problems without either of us knowing how it happened, and that *neither* of us had to know the "cause" of the problem.

Concerning this business of high expectations on the part of the therapist, Milton once told me that he believed that people went into trances for him so easily because he had trained himself very early to continually express his astonishment and appreciation at his continuing good fortune to have such good subjects consult him.

I learned to do the unexpected. For example, remember the story of the screaming child that Milton quieted by screaming himself. For a long time I thought it a nice story, but certainly not something that I could or would bring myself to do. Then one day, faced with an angry and embarrassed mother trying, without success, to control her mildly injured child, I heard her shout, "Stop screaming and hold still." That provoked me to whisper to the child, "You scream just as loud as you want." The child stopped screaming while deciding whether or not to scream.

I also learned that there is no way I can know all I learned from Milton.

And now he is physically gone from us. He would have thought it stupid for us to try to imitate the things he did, because none of us is Milton any more than he was any of us. We can only integrate that part which was his into that which is each of us. We can modify our ways of dealing with the world, teach others to do it, and go on from there.

This is most of what I wanted to put on the record about Milton. I hope that you have some understanding of why I feel my life was altered that day when I became bored and began to look for something else. Milton changed the way I looked at the world. If he was sitting right down there and had heard that last remark, he would have grinned and said, "But you didn't say whether the change was for the good or the bad!" However, he knew.

So the physician of the title stopped being lonely a long time ago, but it now seems very unlikely that he will ever get over being lonesome for his dear friend.

Chapter 38

# 1201 E. Hayward: Milton H. Erickson, M.D.

*Peter Nemetschek*

By now we have many reports of Milton H. Erickson's work by himself and by others. Audio and videotapes allow us study what he said and did, but we don't know much about the inner process of his clients. I want to try to share briefly what I saw and experienced as a therapist, student, and client rather than as a scientist. When I quote Dr. Erickson, I give you what I remember; I don't quote from a transcript! I have never listened fully to the two taped sessions Milton did with me without going into a trance, and I don't want to disturb my continuing unconscious processes by analyzing everything.

Brief therapy and training in therapy with Dr. Erickson starts somehow the moment you become interested in his work. In the mid-seventies I heard more and more rumors about his work. I had training in hypnotherapy, I read books, and I was especially interested in Advanced Techniques. In 1978 his first books were translated into German. I decided to write Erickson a letter and asked to come for three weeks to learn with him. I wrote, "Listening to a tape a friend of mine took when he visited you in the States, I vividly imagine sitting in an airplane flying over, coming deeper and deeper in contact with my wish to visit you." I was born in 1937, and the earliest images of airplanes I can remember are those American flying fortresses moving like silvery fish in the sky toward the town. Three weeks later I had his answer:

> I was very much interested in your letter and pleased with it. I would be very glad to have you sit in on some of my training sessions. . . . If you come to the southwestern United States, I hope you will take advantage of your visit to spend some time seeing the beautiful sights of nature in this area. The northern part

> of the State is quite cold in the winter months, but the views of the Grand Canyon from the South Rim are open the year around.

Later I saw the piles of letters Mrs. Erickson had to care for each week.

I visited some colleagues and therapists on the west coast and came in to Phoenix by plane. Sitting in an airplane, looking at the mountains, some far-away clouds, and the desert from high above, was an excellent place for me to be in a sort of trance, preparing for the work with Dr. Erickson. As certain landscapes drifted away, my thoughts did as well. Then finally Phoenix appeared.

Somehow Milton H. Erickson made everything part of your unconscious work. Everything became meaningful. He sent me to the "Western Aire" Motel. The lady there told stories about him. Even in the social field I was constantly in contact with the purpose that I came with. He would even say things like, "Tonight when you go eating, you may go to this place or to that place." He knew we had to eat, so he made it part of the therapy and the training.

Every day you had to phone Mrs. Erickson to find out when the lecture would begin. There was always a little uncertainty, no routine. Some days Erickson was not in very good shape, and it took him hours to put himself in a state where he could communicate his experiences and demonstrate his approach. He was an absolute master at using his limited possibilities—breathing only with three ribs and one shoulder, talking with a dislocated tongue, paralyzed, colorblind.

When I first drove down 12th street, the taxi driver nearly passed the house of the famous Dr. Erickson; it didn't look extraordinary at all. When I looked closer there were the 10 plants in five rows, four plants in every row, and the inside was like a strange treasure box. My first meeting with him was a shock. I had thought I was so well prepared. A friend had even told me where to sit, that is, beside the front door so I would be directly in front of him and could watch everything and tape and take photographs. Mrs. Erickson pulled the wheelchair in. She put a purple rug under his feet. He looked directly in my eyes, very open, very free, and intense, with no social fear or restriction. He entered my personal space and asked, "You are Peter. What do think about these two societies?" That was the first of so many questions that I heard later, that for a short moment made you stop thinking. The story behind it was that Dr. Erickson had allowed some people in Munich to establish a Milton H. Erickson society and had asked them to use his name very responsibly, very humbly. Soon, however, there were differences, and two societies emerged. Fortunately, I hadn't joined either of them. I stuttered something, "I don't like it." With this one glance and this one question he had shot me out of my frame of reference: It is impolite to ask such questions in the beginning. Later he said, "My name is not a battleground." I hope it will not be one now when he is dead!

I had intensive training in hypnotherapy that had focused on the paradoxical and linguistic aspects of Erickson's approach. I recognized quickly that his work was far more complex than I had thought. I felt Erickson used a holistic approach. I was reminded of my experiences in Bavarian Baroque churches where every detail swings together with the whole: the paintings, the sculptures, the architecture, the organ, chorus, preacher, people. Milton was constantly in contact with his own unconscious mind or in a sort of trance in order to be able to describe his cases and at the same time communicate so personally with 10 or 12 people, putting some of them in a trance, demonstrating trance phenomena, teaching therapy, and, at least for me, doing deep therapy.

Most of the time he looked down to the floor, focusing on one point on the rug, swaying his head a little. One time I think (and I'm never sure, because I don't know how often I fell "spontaneously" into a trance) he described one case for one hour and started immediately on the next case, again for one hour, simply connecting both with an "and." When someone asked him a question, he never gave a theoretical answer but used the unconscious way of understanding by telling a story, reporting a case, or giving a metaphor. There were hours and hours of stories and then quick, brilliant questions to confuse my conscious mind. While looking down and speaking in that low, trance-like voice, he would give body signals long before the official demonstration. For example, he sat very still but shortly, before telling something about "going down the road," he would already have moved his feet. He described how a client "went down the road, turned to the right, and didn't know if it was right, so he turned to the left, . . ." and suddenly Milton's left hand moved directly toward the person who sat beside him in the "hot seat" or the "relaxing seat," penetrating into her personal space. I could feel the confusion this hand produced, coming out from nowhere into her visual field.

Erickson did very complex trance work, preparing someone's unconscious for the work, then putting that person into a very deep dissociated trance, bringing him partly out and in, back and forth. His confidence startled me; he was so sure of what he did. "Are you awake? Not the slightest doubt? How come I don't have any doubt?" And I could see and feel that he had no doubt! His late work was for me like the painting of the old Rembrandt, the fewest brush strokes—the deepest insight.

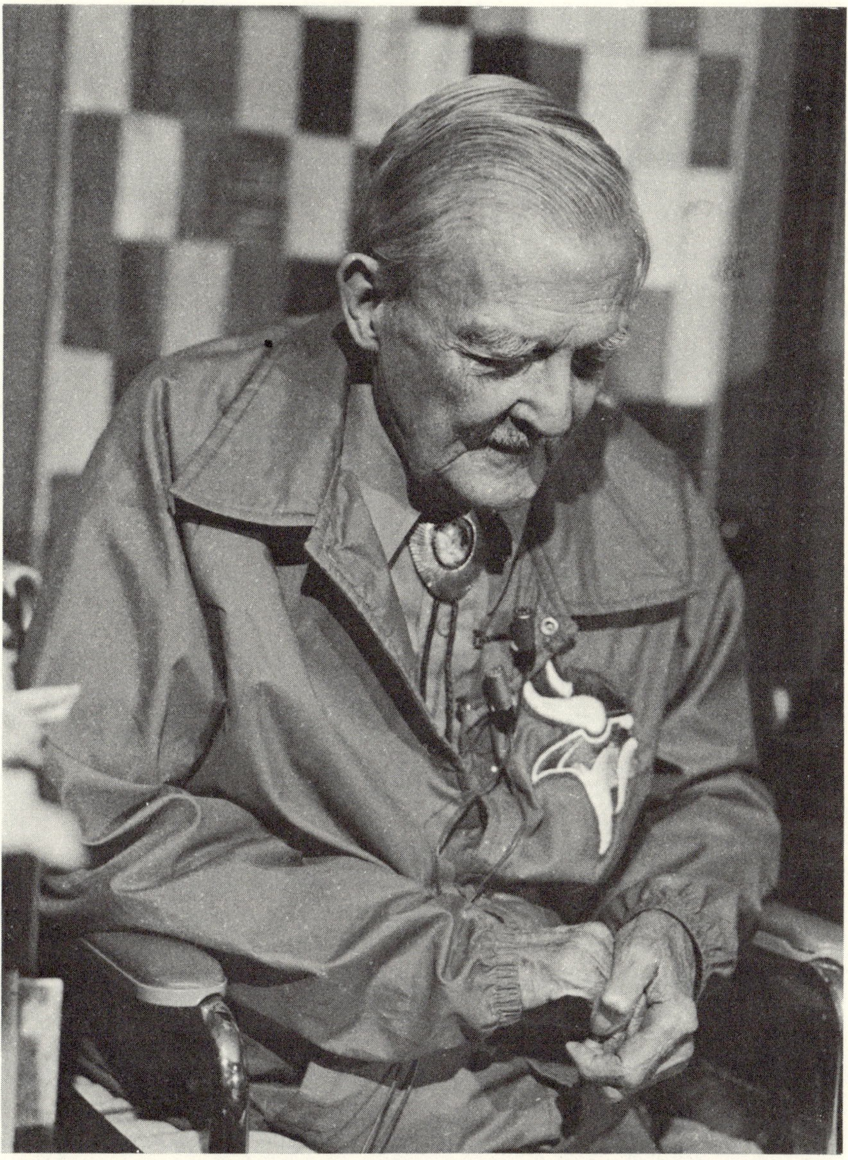

**Milton H. Erickson: Most of the time he looked down to the floor, focusing on one point on the rug, swaying his head a litte.**

To communicate with the unconscious mind, Erickson used everything—body language, facial expression (so vivid despite his handicap), stories, examples, and things to see and to touch. For every lecture he brought in some books, letters, or objects that he passed around. My attention was split between waiting till the object was passed to me, looking at it, and listening to his voice. His favorites were little gifts children had sent him as a thanks—an octopus or a purple cow that a child had sent him when she had no more temper tantrums or when the bed was dry. Probably the unconscious mind is very naive, like the world of a child.

He was ingenious in meeting his students at a very personal and special level. During each of the twelve sessions I attended, he mentioned something about Germany, very indirectly. "In English you say you get *on* the horse, in German du steigst *auf* das Pferd *auf*," or "How many ways can you go to the next room? I could call a taxi, go out by that door, drive down to the airport, fly to London, have a meal in Paris . . ." (I don't know if Milton mentioned Munich, but in my fantasy I saw him visiting my town) " . . . come back and enter the next room by that door over there."

Erickson used to start the daily demonstrations with a woman: it seemed they went easier into a deep trance. When he worked with men he used more complicated induction techniques. For example (pointing to one of the men), "Would you pass that book over to . . . (and now to Peter). Stop!" he said in the middle of his movement. "Was this a conscious or an unconscious movement?" Even as an observer I was very confused. He would indirectly mention some personal things to each person so that they had the feeling he was referring to them and only them. When he worked with a blonde woman, he would talk about a blonde lady who walked into his office one day. He would carefully watch how to catch a person's attention. For example, he knew one young woman was interested in photography because she had asked to take some pictures. So he let her look at a photograph that a student had sent him showing the stars circling round the Pole star, and used that as a way to have her go into a trance. In every demonstration he used hand levitation, partly to verify that your unconscious mind functions automatically and partly to fix your attention. When my arm lifted, I thought "Will it or will it not go up?" I was so fascinated by that idea that I didn't consciously hear what he said during that time. At times he would take a client's arm and do his famous fingertip confusion induction. Sometimes he would look very intensely at a subject's arm and then all the way up to where the arm should go. I realized that as

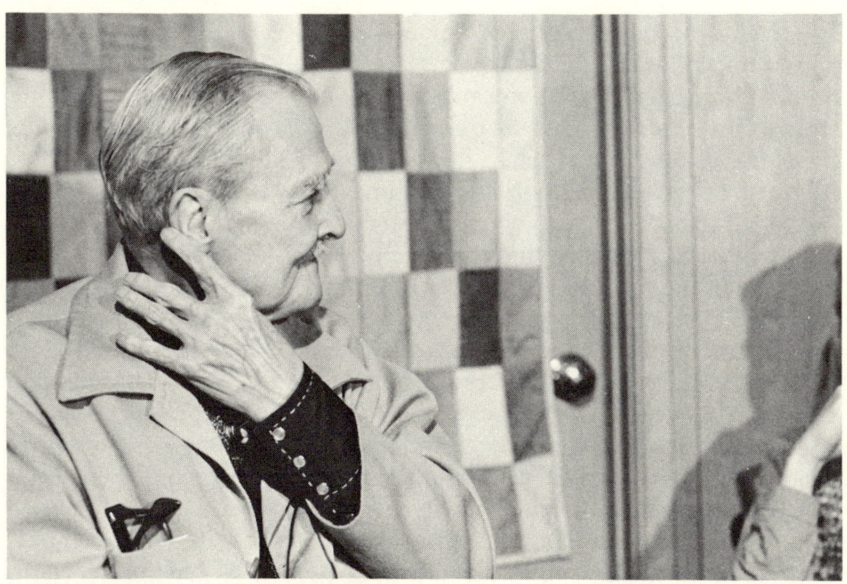

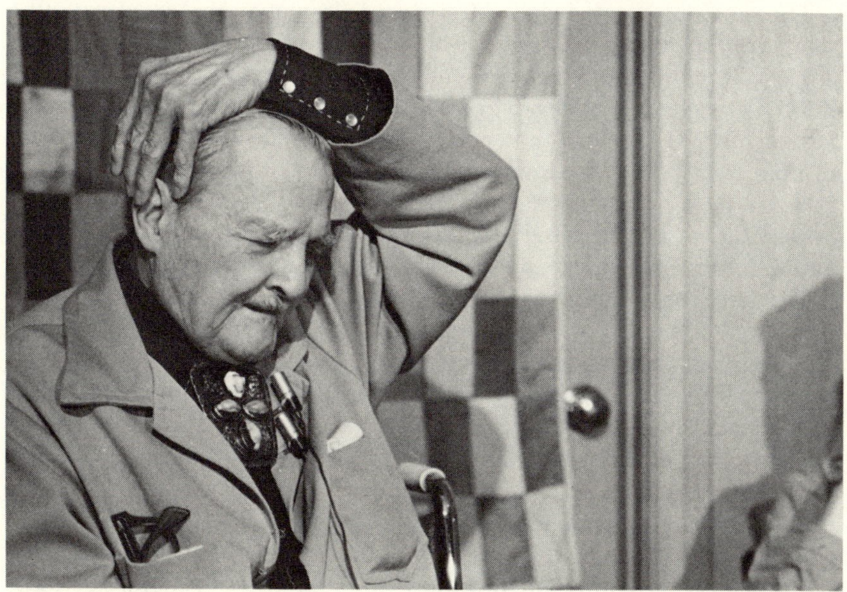

**Demonstrating the many possible ways there are to touch your ear.**

I watched I had lifted my arm "spontaneously." I looked around, and half of my colleagues had one arm "accidentally" up in the air. Milton prepared for every levitation carefully by telling stories and by making strange movements, such as demonstrating the many possible ways there are to touch your ear.

I think there is far more hidden behind how he used arm levitation. I have felt that a very deep body therapy was integrated with his mental therapy. Most of the time the left arm lifted first, and perhaps something happens in the right hemisphere. I'm not a scientist, but I feel certain that something happens right there with the arm rising. I was reminded of Feldenkrais' body therapy; he works with one side of the body and then lets you imagine this work in the other side. "Right" has double meanings, as does "left." For example, "If you put your left arm behind your back, which one is left?" (the right one!) Maybe it was only confusion, but when I watched the clients, I could see a change somehow. Not only the left and right hemisphere are involved, but the change goes deep down, literally in the "back of your mind," in the deeper part of the brain and the spine. I had a very (w)holistic feeling watching Erickson's arm levitations.

The sessions were deep, sincere, and dramatic. He asked a young woman what breed of dog was there in the corner? The corner was empty, and she had a positive hallucination of a dog out of her childhood. It was fun. I have watched a lot of therapists, but nobody so light. He seemed to work without any effort. Milton considered humor a fundamental part of the therapy. He liked to tell funny stories, to laugh, to make jokes. The unconscious mind is a fun place! At the end of the session he asked the blonde woman how she came to be in that chair and whether she came from her home mounted with two microphones. Integrating that humor was my biggest step forward in therapy. Since then I have much more fun inside and outside when I do therapy.

The group process was extraordinary. Every three days the people changed, but all the time I felt a warm human contact with all my colleagues. There was a lot of unconscious communication and serious talks and fun after the lecture. Somehow Milton communicated a deep human atmosphere. At the beginning of a group he asked you to write down some basic data—name, address, degree, age, birthdate, age of siblings, children, whether you were raised in an urban or rural setting. It was astonishing how much contact he could make by using this data. He could really talk to everyone in the group personally.

As far as I remember—you were never sure about some things, but Marion Moore took videotapes for Ernest Rossi to check—I sat for one day in the "hot seat." There were only two students. Milton talked, and at the same time I had the feeling he watched me very carefully. I don't remember if he put me officially into a trance, but I was not sure and that doubt is a good place for a change. Afterwards I looked at the tapes, but usually I went into the same trance when I looked at them. Milton demonstrated that phenomenon with a woman subject. She repeated exactly the same body movements! When he asked if she was fully awake and could step over "a certain line," she fell into trance in the middle of the room.

The next day Milton worked with me again. I remember the doubt and fascination of my arm lifting. Probably I was looking in the bright lights there for videotaping. He said something about diving. I remembered very vividly diving in the Mediterranean. I saw the sun reflecting on the surface of the water from deep below. (I was 19 then; my 42nd birthday came when I arrived in Phoenix. Did he chose that week because of that?) It was a marvelous feeling with all the sensations of being in the warm water. I floated like a bodiless mind in space and time. Later I remembered a scene when I was about five years old, rushing along with a free good feeling on a scooter with my little brother sitting on a seat I had mounted. I was very proud of how skillful I was. I could remember every important detail, including the rifts between the wooden planks of a bridge I passed . . . . When Milton asked if I could share some of my experience I could not recall the word for scooter ("Roller" in German) so I asked for a sheet of paper and made a drawing. I was sure that I was fully awake. After the session I looked at the videotape twice, and I remember saying, "Oh that's a five-year-old child's drawing." I must have still been in a trance because I made another one that turned out as a 10-year-old's drawing, as I later recognized. When I wrote this article a year and a half later, I drew the third picture in my usual quick style.

He never told me to do a certain thing. He simply said, "I wonder who likes to see sunrise on Squaw Peak and who prefers sunset." So I saw sunrise and sunset, and I was there in the afternoon. The first day I walked out of the office, looked around and walked toward the mountain I saw. I was not sure it was the right one. All the way I had that doubt, but I had to walk and climb. I felt that I worked something through deep inside. It was literally a mount(ain) of old problems, thoughts and feelings, and with every step higher, with every change of the perspective looking forward or back down, my inner perspective changed as well. I picked up a small black stone and carried it in my left hand. Then I looked for a white one and carried it in the right hand.

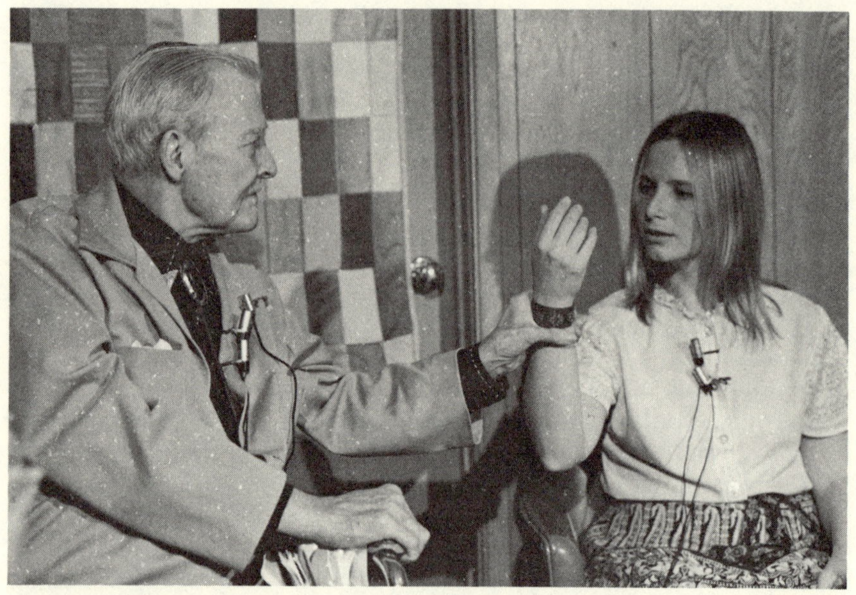

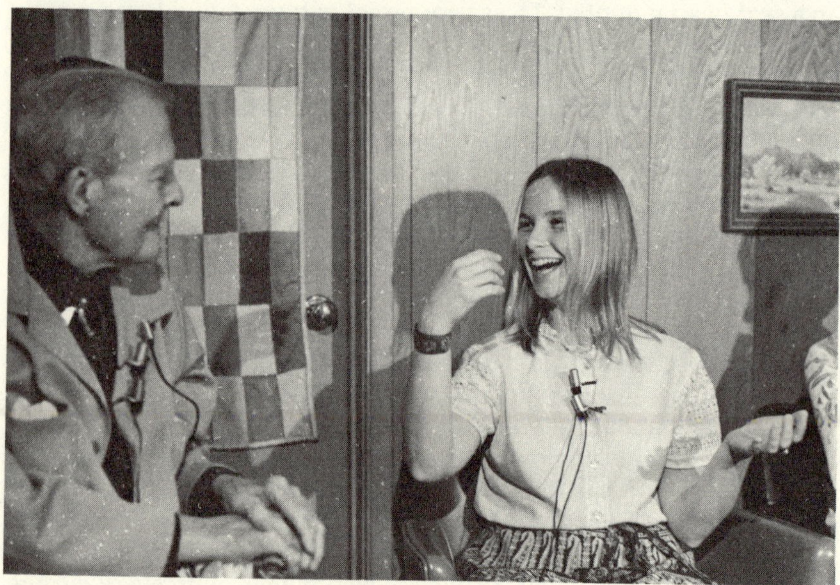

**Erickson demonstrating arm levitation.**

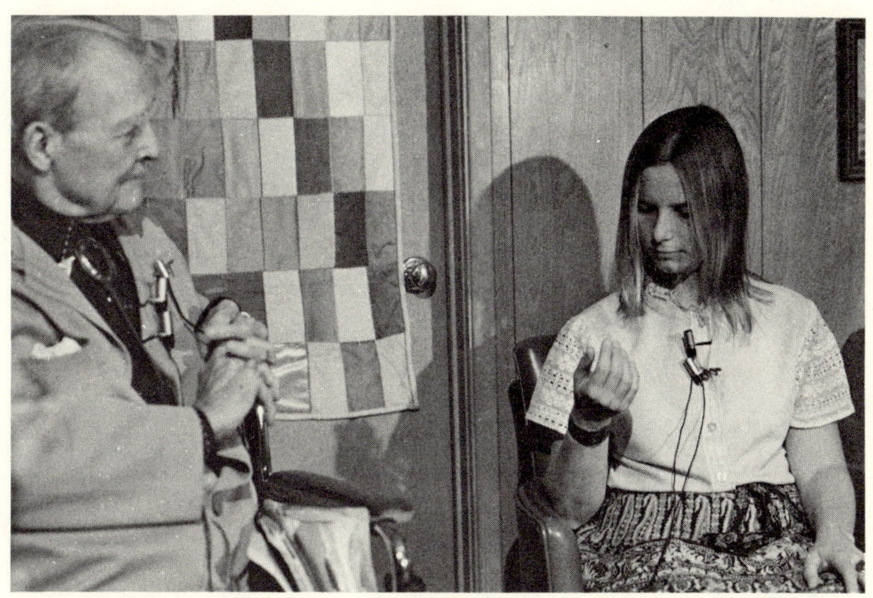

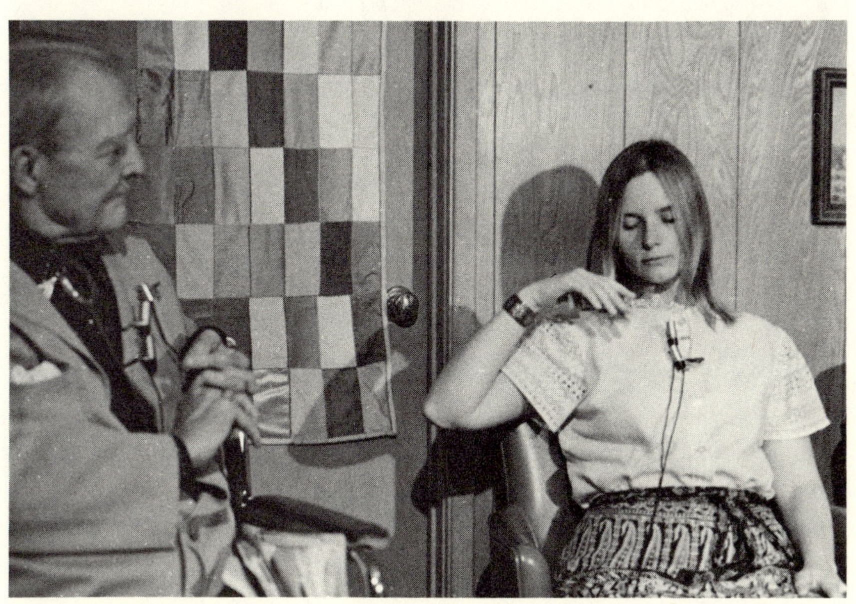

Later I picked up a red one and carried all three all the way up, changing them from one side to the other.

Changing the perspective seems to be one of Erickson's main principles, not only regressing but also seeing the scene from a different perspective. Climbing up Squaw Peak was perfect body therapy, deep breathing and relaxing, feeling, thinking. I had an inner dialogue with Milton the entire time. Finally I reached the official path up there, then the top. Was it Squaw Peak? I wanted to find out without asking somebody. I found a very small scratched bronze plague, hard to read: Squaw Peak. What a release!

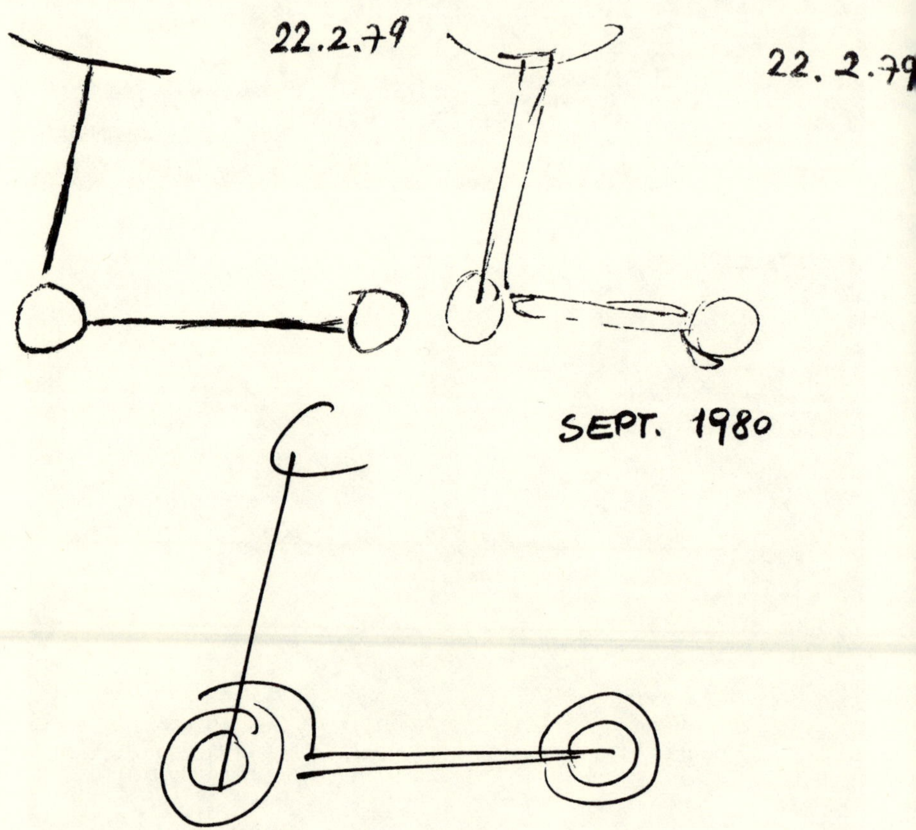


**Three drawings of a scooter.**

My sunrise experience pushed me out of my frame of reference too. "You limit your mind," as Milton said. I had imagined how it would be. Years before I had watched sunrise at the Grand Canyon. I went to Squaw Peak early in the morning with the blonde woman. When we reached the top, it was very foggy. I realized the gray became brighter by one thousandth of a grade when the sun finally rose. You may think a lot, but the experience is different.

Somehow Erickson or I kept myself working day and night. "Get your patient to do something, and when he does it, he will take this as a sign for change." I had very complex dreams; usually I don't remember them too often. In one I was drifting through lines of three-dimensional words that Milton had said, and every level of words had a different meaning. I could shift levels and focus on one level or on all together.

During the day I visited the places Erickson used so often as "projection-fields." At the Botanical Garden I was curious to find "the Boojum, that tree that isn't a tree, and you will recognize the creeping devils without reading the sign." I could sense the pain in my foot when I imagined stepping in those plants. I was impressed by all these forms and structures and strange plants. They all helped to widen my horizons. I went to the Heard Museum. There it was clear that Erickson had integrated out of his American background the Indian wisdom as well

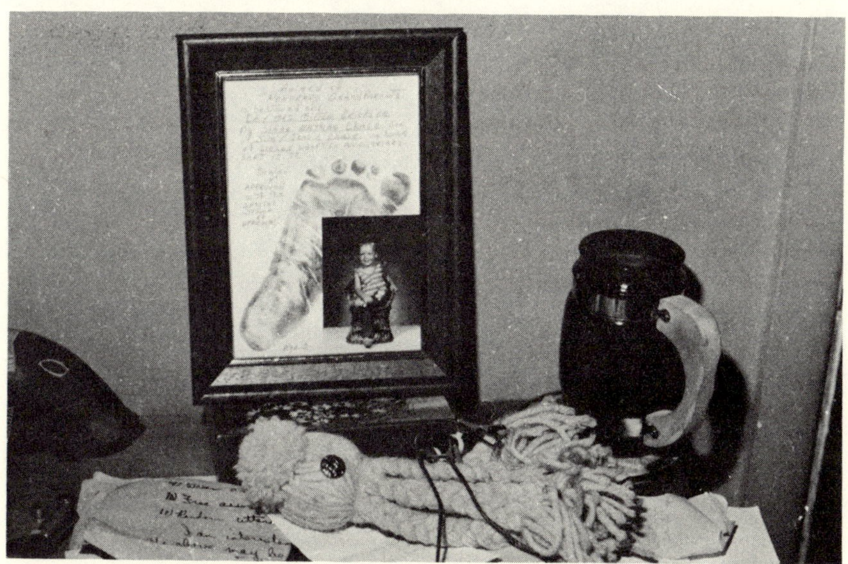

**Some of the objects used in Erickson's stories.**

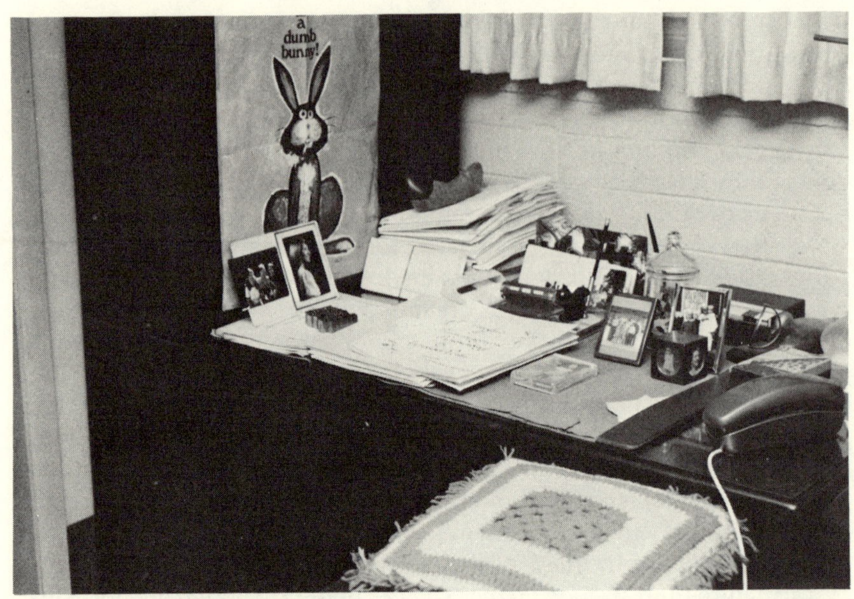


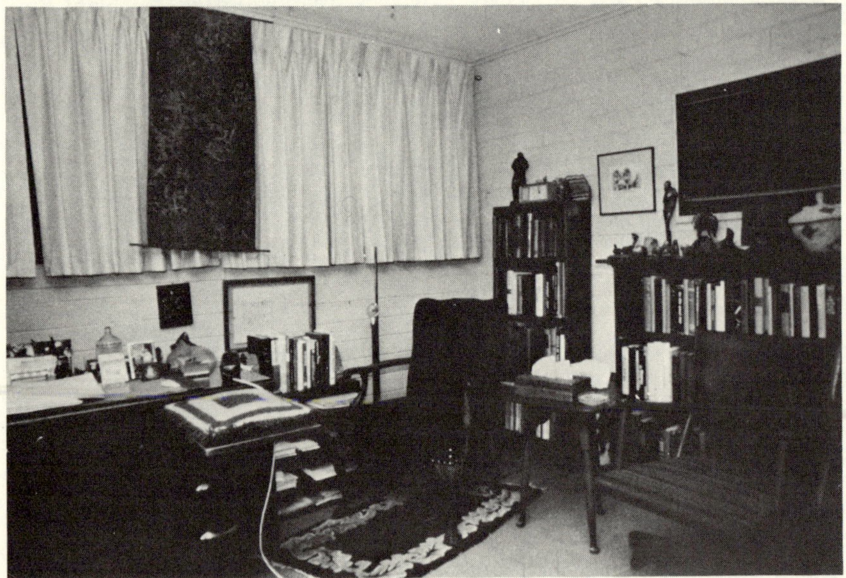

**Erickson's desk and a view of his office.**

as the European. His work had parallels with that of Rolling Thunder and other Indian shamans: great respect for every single creature, experiencing everything without bias or prejudice, believing in the power of the unconscious, talking in metaphors like Indians.

There was still his office with the purple telephone, the client's chair, the glass-paper weight he often used as a fixing point. He gave his lectures usually in the livingroom or the waiting room where there were many diplomas, pictures and strange objects. One automatically used them as projection material; these things spoke the language of the unconscious far better than any linguistically tricky sentences. "Watch that fish and pay attention it doesn't turn into a dracula." Milton liked to show you around. In his house he showed his "magic lamp," a hologram, "the schizophrenic mouse," all these confusing things that undermined how one thinks things are. What a surprise when I lifted up a small sculpture, and it was ten times heavier than I thought. It was made out of ironwood.

When I saw the livingroom, the kitchen, even his bedroom, I had the impression I literally could see the world of the unconscious mind. He always spoke the language of the unconscious in metaphors. "Peter, psychotherapy is: When I was young, a horse came to our farm and nobody knew to whom it belonged. So I mounted the horse and it started to go, and every time it went off the way and wanted to eat in the wheat I pulled a little, and when it went I let it go. When the way crossed, it turned to the left and later to the right. Then it went quicker, and I saw the farm where it belonged!"

His personal testament is deep in me, but he gave me some outer memories. He signed one of my books, "Your task is to fit your therapy to his individual needs and not to a hypothetical assumption of what they should be." And: "To Peter Nemetschek whom I value as a colleague and as a Student." And "It has been a great pleasure to meet you and I hope to have that pleasure again. Feb. 1979 Milton H. Erickson, M.D."

I didn't have the pleasure, and I knew I wouldn't. It would be against his way of living to be the middle of a congress. When I got the telegram, "Family and I regret to inform of death of Milton Erickson 3-25-80. December congress will be held in memoriam," I wept, and I was glad that he had taught me so much.

---

PART XV

# *About Milton H. Erickson*

*Irving Secter, M.A., D.D.S., is a professor of oral diagnosis emeritus at the University of Illinois College of Dentistry. He is a past president of The American Society of Clinical Hypnosis, and with Erickson and Hershman co-authored* Practical Applications of Medical and Dental Hypnosis.

*During the early 1950s Secter was a member of the Seminars On Hypnosis group. Erickson was the senior faculty member of the group that subsequently was instrumental in the formation of the American Society of Clinical Hypnosis in 1957. In his chapter, Secter discusses the format of the original seminars group and outlines the history of how the seminars group eventually became the ASCH. Secter wrote to leaders in the field of hypnosis and asked for their impressions of Erickson and his contributions to the early seminars. The replies include interesting and valuable insights into Erickson's personality.*

*Herbert Lustig, M.D., is a clinical assistant professor of child psychiatry at the University of Pennsylvania School of Medicine. He conducts a private practice of psychotherapy and hypnosis in the Philadelphia area. Lustig produced The Artistry of Milton H. Erickson, commercially available films of Dr. Erickson demonstrating his hypnotic technique in 1975.*

*Lustig presents a warm appreciation of Milton Erickson, tracing Erickson's professional and personal style to attitudes developed in his formative years. Anecdotes illuminate Erickson's attitudes about life. Additionally, Lustig provides a fine general description of Erickson's methods.*

*Sidney Rosen, M.D., a psychiatrist in private practice in New York City, wrote the Foreword to* Hypnotherapy *by Erickson and Rossi. He recently authored a book on Erickson's anecdotes entitled* The Teaching Tales of Milton H. Erickson. *As one of Erickson's closest collaborators, Rosen was in a unique position to examine Erickson's values and philosophies. Understanding Erickson's values gives a better perspective on his approach to psychotherapy. Rosen interviewed Mrs. Elizabeth Erickson to confirm some of his interpretations; however, most of Rosen's descriptions were gleaned from the personal contact he had with Erickson.*

*A special interaction hour was scheduled for the Congress and was to include Milton Erickson, Gregory Bateson, Jay Haley, and Ernest Rossi. After Erickson's and Bateson's death, Carl Whitaker, one of the keynote speakers, was kind enough to take part in the panel.*

*The special interaction hour was one of the most impressive events of the Congress. Almost the entire academic assembly of 2000 people was present. The speakers were insightful, warm and witty in their interaction with each other and the audience. Personally, I thought it was one of the premier events of the meeting.*

Chapter 39

# Seminars with Erickson: The Early Years

*Irving Secter*

Milton Erickson was a teacher. He shared his knowledge and experience with others until he had no more time to do so. A substantial part of his teaching in hypnosis was done as senior faculty member of what started in the early 1950s as Seminars On Hypnosis and which eventually became the workshops of the American Society of Clinical Hypnosis-Education and Research Foundation (ASCH-ERF). The last one of these ERF workshops in which he participated was held in Phoenix in January 1980. I, too, was a member of that faculty. To be listed on the same program with Milton was always a source of personal pride.

I came to Phoenix early to visit with Milton at his home and to discuss with him what he thought should be included in this paper. Our conversation was recorded. What follows is based on that meeting.

January 17, 1980 was a bright, cheerful sunny day in Phoenix. The sun was shining into my eyes as we talked. It was necessary to shift my chair so as to look at Milton without squinting. Images began to flash through my mind like high speed slides being projected on a screen.

As we talked the realization came to me that I had known this man for almost 30 years. (He had already lived a lifetime (50 years) when we first met, and it was in this earlier lifetime that he had already developed the knowledge and insights which, at the time of our first meeting, I was just beginning to glimpse.)

Hypnosis was a forbidden topic in medical school and college during the 1920s. Clark Hull was then Head of the Department of Psychology at the University of Wisconsin. He demonstrated hypnosis to a premedical class. Milton, who was in the audience, was fascinated by what he saw. He began to practice and experiment with fellow students. Hull encouraged him with his experiments during the spring and summer of 1923, and in September 1923, presented a seminar on hypnosis at which the psychological meaning of Milton's experiments was discussed. According to Milton, the Dean of the College of Arts and Sciences spent the next five years attempting to have him expelled from the university.

To get an internship, Milton had to promise not to use hypnosis or even to say the word "hypnosis." The internship was followed by a residency in psychiatry at Colorado Psychopathic Hospital. The Superintendent of the hospital had used hypnosis in his early years and had been thoroughly rebuked and punished for it. He approved of Milton's use of hypnosis and encouraged it. After Colorado he went to Rhode Island State Hospital where he again had to promise never to talk about hypnosis or use it.

Between 1930 and 1934 Milton experimented with and taught hypnosis at Worcester State Hospital, where he was appointed to the Research Service. Milton said:

> The medical profession looked down on me because of my work in hypnosis. They forgave me only because I was in the Research Service.
>
> Some years after I had left Rhode Island State Hospital, Superintendent Alfred Noyes invited me back to lecture and demonstrate. He was severely criticized for bringing in an outside psychiatrist to lecture on hypnosis.

From 1934 to 1948 Milton was Director of Research and Psychiatric Training at Wayne County Hospital in Detroit, Michigan. At the same time he taught in the Medical School of Wayne State University, was Professor of Humanities at Wayne State University and Visiting Professor at Michigan State University. He interested all of these institutions, as well as the University of Michigan, in hypnosis. Milton said: "I had a Civil Service job and couldn't be fired." Today hypnosis is much more favorably received. In large measure Milton Erickson's influence is responsible for this.

Milton was the star performer in several groups which undertook to teach hypnosis to practitioners in the therapeutic arts. In 1950 two of these groups merged into Seminars On Hypnosis. The original partners of the combined group were Erickson, Aston, Hershman, Kroger, LeCron and Secter. After some years Kroger and LeCron left the group to teach independently. The others traveled in this country and abroad, often sponsored by scientific academies, hospitals, medical and dental schools, and medical, dental and psychological societies. The interest developed by the Seminars led to the formation of the American Society of Clinical Hypnosis (ASCH).

Milton was the first president of ASCH. For the first ten years after its inception, he edited the *American Journal of Clinical Hypnosis* (AJCH), the official journal of ASCH and the Academy of Applied Psychology in Dentistry. He was also a charter member of the Society of Clinical and Experimental Hypnosis, which was formed about three years prior to the organization of ASCH.

The Seminars On Hypnosis were a fertile training ground for the development of teachers of hypnosis. In conjunction with the core group, more than 100 people served as faculty during the early years. Many of these were local people who subsequently stimulated a continued interest in hypnosis in their home community. These Seminars encouraged the growth of ASCH, as well as the formation of local societies.

On December 7, 1959, the Seminars were incorporated as a not-for-profit foundation named the Seminars On Hypnosis Foundation (SOHF). Erickson, Aston, Hershman and Secter were the original incorporators. Interested people contributed $50.00 each to form an endowment fund to support research and teaching in hypnosis. SOHF continued to conduct seminars until 1962. At this point in time the Seminars were operating at a financial loss. To preserve the endowment fund, which by this time had grown to about $40,000.00, Erickson, Hershman and Secter taught about 14 seminars during a period of a year and half without any remuneration.

Three years after its formation the SOHF articles of incorporation were amended to change the name to the American Society of Clinical Hypnosis—Education and Research Foundation. SOHF thus became the teaching arm of ASCH. Control of ERF and an intact endowment fund passed to ASCH with no strings attached. The ASCH Executive Committee elects the ERF Board of Trustees. The SOHF trustees at the time of change were Milton H. Erickson, Seymour Hershman, William T. Heron, Herbert Mann, Frank Pattie, and Irving Secter.

The flavor of the workshops and Milton Erickson's role in them may be captured from the following excerpts from letters by people who have shared seminars with Erickson in the early years.

Fredericka Freytag, a lovely person who happens to be a psychiatrist wrote:

> In the early days there seemed to be a greater degree of expectancy and excitement on the part of the audience—or was I projecting what I felt? You might check this with some of the old-timers. This

seems significant since all members of the panel presented the material in a way that definitely discouraged gullibility. All members of the panel were agreed on principles; it was in the presentation of the material that Dr. Erickson was unique.

In induction techniques Dr. Erickson used the presentation of ideas which the patient knew to be true or could verify instead of the direct suggestions so prevalent in other inductions. In psychotherapy he directed the patient's efforts toward becoming aware of his own potential and utilizing his learnings. Frequently he used humor, wit or anecdote and metaphor. For this to be effective it was necessary for him to be well-versed in analytic procedure though he did not use analytic psychotherapy directly. He left it to the unconscious to evoke the appropriate associations. Dr. Erickson's voice impressed his hearers. It was a soft, calming, soothing voice, pausing at intervals to permit unconscious association to take place. Where appropriate, there would be a word or a phrase with a question mark, mixed occasionally with a tinge of surprise. You will recall the first trip taken by the Seminar was a Caribbean cruise. The last night on shipboard some members wanted to have a gala affair. In this Dr. Erickson was to impersonate a voice because that is what the audience now called him.

In one of the earliest Seminars Dr. Erickson made a short statement: "Let the unconscious do the work." Only a simple statement, yet it is the "open sesame" to a well-structured human potential movement, sadly as yet unrecognized by the present myriad of alternative therapies.

William Kroger wrote:

I would say that Milton was a brilliant and intuitive therapist. He really was one of the first to use behavior modification in the form of the double bind. He was certainly an inspiration to all.

ASCH past president Lawrence M. Staples stated:

Milton Erickson was generally acknowledged to be the world's leading practitioner of clinical hypnosis. His writings and teaching on a wide variety of techniques in producing trance were phenomenal, and to the onlooker were accomplished with such uncanny simplicity and ease. This was due, I believe, to his ability to develop, almost spontaneously, a close interpersonal relationship by his attitude and manner, tone of voice, etc., in his approach to the patient, causing (the patient) to feel at ease and ready and willing to freely follow his suggestions. Erickson was the featured guest lecturer at each of our first four Boston workshops. Doubtless his inspiration was the impetus that carried us along over those early years. He exhibited enthusiasm for the fact that hypnosis was being taught in the Boston area. It was through the urging of Dr. Erickson that I was willing to accept the presidency of ASCH in 1968-69. Milton was still very active in the society and was indeed helpful in solving many problem situations that arose during my tenure of office.

David Cheek, another ASCH past president, referred to a seminar with Erickson in 1954.

What impressed me most was the permissiveness of Erickson's work. It was at this meeting that I heard both Erickson and LeCron talking about the danger of people overhearing conversation while under anesthesia. One of the anecdotes that I remember occurred during one of the workshops at the St. Louis convention many years ago. He invited me up to the platform where he was in his advanced course. In our exchange he asked me if I knew where he got his psychiatric knowledge. Of course I said, "No," and he said with his usual intonation, "From patients."

Gilbert Steingart contributed these anecdotes:

One time when he was our houseguest we were talking about selecting a likely subject for a demonstration. Instead of inviting an individual to come to the platform, he suggested requesting the person sitting next to the prospective subject to bring that person to the platform. This has been an effective approach for me. Another time I arranged to have one of my assistants serve as a subject for Milton. When he asked her if she would be his subject she accepted but stated that she did not believe that any one could induce her into hypnosis except me. Milton must have been suspicious that she had been set up to resist his efforts so he just asked her to show him how she went into hypnosis for me. She did and very nicely.

One of the questions that I had asked Milton was how he saw himself in relation to his associates on the faculty of the Seminars. He replied: "As senior faculty member." He agreed with my summation: "You were lecturer, clinician, and commentator, explaining to audiences what they were hearing and seeing from psychological, clinical, and medical points of view. On a personal basis you were our leader, friend, father, and guide."

Saturday afternoons at the Seminars were plenary sessions. All attended Milton's demonstrations and discussions of hypnotic phenomena. The observers were all enthralled and entranced. Milton demonstrated time distortion and described its uses for the terminally ill. We saw the effectiveness of the double bind wherein one had to choose between two courses of action, either of which contributed to the achievement of a desired goal. He demonstrated the ease with which a negative hallucination was developed by asking a simple questions such as, "Where did everybody go?" We learned how to make what the patient is thinking and doing the focus of the patient's attention so that auditory and visual images became subjective substitutes for objective environmental stimuli. We observed refractory subjects enter hypnotic states by visualizing and reporting on the hypnotizing of another person, the "my friend John" technique. We were amazed by the behavioral changes and recall produced by age regression. All the phenomena of the hypnotic state would come under scrutiny at some time or other. Betty Erickson's frequent participation as a subject in these demonstrations enhanced their effect and facilitated the learning process.

Although these afternoons were an opportunity for the rest of the faculty to get some time off, I seldom missed attending these sessions with Erickson. My own sophistication in hypnosis stems from the fact that I literally sat at his feet in over 100 seminars. Here the knowledge and experiences recorded in the writings of Milton H. Erickson came out in one form or another. (A complete bibliography compiled by Gravitz and Gravitz listing 147 publications appears in the July 1977 issue of the *American Journal of Clinical Hypnosis*. This issue honors Milton's 75th birthday and contains tributes and greetings from Margaret Mead and others important to ASCH and the Seminars.)

At the annual meeting of ASCH held in San Francisco in November 1979, most of ASCH's past presidents were still alive. Many of them attended this meeting. They met privately in two early breakfast conferences to reminisce about the early days. All the past presidents were regular or periodic faculty members of the Seminars. Milton Erickson's influence as teacher and clinician was acknowledged by all.

During our conversation in January Milton recalled the following with evident pleasure: "Wolberg introduced me as 'Mr. Hypnosis' in Chicago at a seminar. Raginsky also called me 'Mr. Hypnosis.' "

It is a joy to remember the three cruise conferences on hypnosis conducted by the Seminars group in 1955, 1956, and 1957. These were 14-day cruises in the Caribbean. They provided a relaxed atmosphere for learning. Sessions were held regularly on those days when we were not ashore. Betty Erickson recalled that she and Milton, his sister Bertha, my wife and daughter and I were assigned to the purser's table. Bertha loved to put us on by conversing with an imaginary character named Melvin. At first, this confused the staid old English purser. After about three days, he caught the idea and began talking directly to Melvin without using Bertha as an intermediary. It was on this cruise that Milton became known as "the voice."

Milton was proud of the fact that there were several physicians who switched to psychiatry in order to apply what they learned about hypnosis from him. Robert Pearson and Marion Moore readily come to mind as examples.

I deeply appreciate the help that Milton gave me in recognizing my own hypnotic experience and trance behavior. I demonstrated responses to post-hypnotic suggestion and did automatic writing upside down and backwards. His assistance was invaluable when, in 1958, during the Seminars, I conducted the experiments for my Master's thesis, "Hypnotizability as a Function of Attitude toward Hypnosis." The subjects were all seminarians who had previously been refractory to hypnosis. It was a great satisfaction to me that Milton saw fit to publish several articles based on these experiments in AJCH.

I am proud to be co-author with Erickson and Hershman of the book, *Practical Applications of Medical and Dental Hypnosis.*

In reviewing some of my old papers I found a copy of a letter from Milton recommending me for a faculty appointment to the University of Illinois College of Dentistry. His strong recommendation was, in my opinion, an important factor in the confirmation of my appointment. I am grateful for his backing. There are many others who benefited from Milton's advice and support.

Milton had the capacity for being a severe critic. At the same time he could demonstrate flexibility. I had incurred his displeasure and for several years I was persona non grata with him. In 1978 he was invited to attend my 50th wedding anniversary celebration. The invitation was accompanied by a note from me asking if he, too, was willing to let bygones be bygones. His response included the question, "Who's got time for bygones?"

1980 is an important year for me. It began at a seminar with Erickson. It ends at an Ericksonian seminar. "Mr. Hypnosis' " presence will continue to be felt by those who knew him personally and by those whom they will continue to influence.

Some of you remember the radio program in those early years entitled, "I Remember Mama." I will always remember Milton Erickson.

Chapter 40

# Understanding Erickson and Ericksonian Techniques

*Herbert S. Lustig*

When a truly gifted person creates his own art form, separating the creation from the creator sometimes obscures both. This is the dilemma we encounter in describing Milton Erickson's techniques in psychotherapy. Whatever he did in his office, he did in his home. Whatever was done with his family was done with his patients. Whatever attitudes and beliefs he embodied himself were imparted to others.

Milton was a pioneer farmboy. He was born in a frontier town in Nevada and raised on a farm in Wisconsin. His mother was a devoted and determined woman. His father was a responsible and industrious man who occasionally worked as a mental hospital attendant to support young Milton's family during the nonfarming months. As a child, Milton acquired the attributes of his pioneer parents: family loyalty, neighborliness, ingenuity, self-reliance, simplicity, curiosity, and a willingness to understand and use the varieties of phenomena in nature.

When Milton was 17 he contracted poliomyelitis and was confronted with his imminent demise. Instead of dying, however, he lapsed into a profound coma and awoke to discover that he was totally paralyzed. It was during the subsequent year of recuperation that he started to learn how every muscle in his body worked, how people communicated with words and how they communicated without using words.

As an adult, Milton conveyed to his patients and family many of the attitudes he developed during his formative years. These attitudes included respect, responsibility, creativity, resourcefulness, pragmatism, delight, curiosity, and confident anticipation.

Milton, above all, demonstrated a deep respect for himself, for others, and for his environment. His personal dignity and communicative power were remarkable. So, too, was his regard for others: their uniqueness as individuals, their personal lifestyles and values, their personal timetables, and their innate abilities. He understood that each person came to him with a unique background and with a different style of interacting with the world. He also appreciated that each of them had his own set of traits and preferences, his own tastes and customs, and his own schedule for the milestones and accomplishments of his life. Milton expressed an abiding faith in people's potential to manage their lives well, to solve their problems, to learn new skills, and to use their old skills in new ways. He also respected the environment, both the physical one in which he lived and the relational one in which he interacted.

Responsibility to self and others was something that Milton always stressed. He emphasized the importance of maintaining physical and emotional health and financial well-being, and of being accountable for one's own actions. He placed great stock in people fulfilling their obligations, in being trustworthy, and in being reliably available to the community. When Milton was a boy, he noted that if a farmer wanted to ensure that he would be helped by his neighbors to recover from a natural disaster that befell him or his property, he made sure that he helped his neighbors when such a calamity happened to them. That same responsible attitude was conveyed by Milton to his patients.

Milton enjoyed creativity and resourcefulness, and he enjoyed fostering it in others. He enjoyed telling stories about it—about the duality within each person of the conscious and unconscious minds, of the unconscious mind's ability to discover new ideas and new ways to handle situations, and of its reliability in making ideas and solutions available to the conscious mind. He taught his children to be imaginative when they were in difficult situations; he told them that their unconscious minds were faithful, dependable, and inventive. Milton also believed in dealing promptly and effectively with problems by utilizing currently available resources to develop solutions. It was not uncommon for his patients' formerly unappreciated physical characteristics to become valued assets, for their previously disregarded skills to become important resources, and for otherwise ignored social institutions to become bountiful reserves.

Milton was pragmatic and advocated practical approaches to problems. He believed that "less could be more" and that the simplest solution was the best. Whether the solution began with a word, a phrase, a story, or a gesture, Milton's goal was always the same: to produce the longest-lasting beneficial results within the patient from the briefest clinical intervention. It was the implementation of this attitude that created the distinctive elegance of his work.

To Milton, delight was the spice of life to which everyone was entitled. This attitude quietly pervaded all of his daily activities. He made certain that his current situations and relationships were continuous sources of pleasure to him, and that his future activities were similarly promising. Milton took particular pleasure from the little delights of the day. During one of my visits with him, he told me how much he had enjoyed eating a Pennsylvania Dutch breakfast meat specialty when he had been in Philadelphia. Scrapple, that specialty, was readily available in the Philadelphia area. However, most of it was frozen and sold in packages. Although distributors shipped it packed in dry ice to customers, they did not guarantee its hygiene after it had been shipped to hot climates such as Phoenix's. On my periodic searches at the supermarket, I had not seen scrapple in anything other than a frozen package. One day, to my delight, I found a can of it. Obviously, a can of scrapple was safe to ship anywhere. So I sent Milton a case of the cans. Several months later, when I had visited Milton again, I asked him how he had enjoyed the scrapple. He told me that he had been having a small slice of it cooked for breakfast and served with grape jelly every morning. I had never heard of anyone eating scrapple with grape jelly on it—maple syrup or ketchup, but never grape jelly. So I tried some. It was good! What a delightful way for Milton to have started the day.

Just as delight was the spice of life for Milton, so was curiosity the cornerstone of his living. He understood that learning was an active and experiential process, and that each day provided new opportunities for learning. Curiosity was the catalyst. In the process of acquiring knowledge, it was neither converted nor consumed, but was available at the end of the process for the next learning. Curiosity enabled Milton to learn how to use and enjoy his old skills in different ways, and how to acquire new ones.

When Milton's daughter, Roxanna, vacationed in South America with her husband for a few months, she left the family dog, Ernie, with her father. At that time in Milton's life, he was confined to a wheelchair. He spent his spare time sitting in his armchair in the livingroom while he watched television, talked with family and friends, and learned. His curiosity led him to wonder what new trick Roxanna's old dog could learn that would astonish his daughter when she returned home. He began to say the phrase, "Dad's dog," and reward Ernie with a dog biscuit whenever it sat to Milton's right. Soon, he could say "Dad's dog," and the pet would move to Milton's side from wherever in the room it had been sitting. Ultimately, Milton could say the magic phrase and the dog would interrupt whatever it was doing anywhere in the house and immediately run to Milton's side in the livingroom. One day, after Roxanna had returned from her vacation, she and her mother were sitting in the family room chatting, while Ernie rested nearby. Milton was sitting in his armchair in the livingroom talking with Roxanna's husband. During the conversation, Milton casually included "Dad's dog" in a sentence. Immediately, the dog leapt up, ran to the livingroom and sat by Milton's side. Roxanna was perplexed. Later in the day it happened several times more. Each time, her perplexity increased. It was only after she had become curious about her pet's strange new mannerism that she learned the secret of its genesis—much to her father's delight. What a lovely way for Milton to have occupied his spare time!

Another attitude that Milton conveyed to his patients was a confident anticipation of a benign future. He appreciated the fact that change and adaptation were natural parts of the daily evolution of all organisms. Because he understood that the passage of time allowed even insignificant changes to grow into noticeable differences, Milton exercised great patience with himself and with others. He also realized that people traveled on their own highways of life and that, potentially, everyone was able to do so comfortably, confidently, and competently.

When he worked clinically with people, Milton employed three principal methods: utilization, suggestion, and multi-level communication. Milton was a master at utilization, taking advantage of current conditions to achieve benefits for his patients. To foster clinical gains, he often utilized himself and his family, his patients' symptomatic behavior, and their natural human desires.

In working with patients, Milton frequently told stories about his own experiences and those of his family. He offered himself, the members of his family, and his family's functioning as models to which his patients readily could relate. When the Ericksons lived on Cypress Street in Phoenix, before they moved to the Hayward Street house, Milton's waiting room was the family livingroom. Rather than exclude his own family when he was expecting patients to arrive, Milton requested his family to use the livingroom as they would have normally. However, the children were instructed not to ask personal questions of patients. This allowed patients to maintain their privacy, yet observe and learn how families function, how children play and interact, and how parents parent.

One of the clinical methods for which Milton was most famous was his utilization of his patients' current behavior to control symptoms or problems. He knew that once the symptoms had been controlled, they were susceptible to being systematically transformed and eliminated. One of his methods for gaining control of symptoms was to induce a "symptom alteration" by asking his patients to change the symptoms' "who, what, where, when, how, or with whom." The "who" of the symptoms were the persons actively creating them; the "what" of the symptoms were the presenting dysfunctional activities or feelings; the "where" and "when" of the symptoms were their geographical locations and temporal relations; the "how" of the symptoms were their frequency, duration and intensity; and the "with whom" of the symptoms were the persons included in them.

Milton's other method for controlling patients' symptoms was "sequence interruption," i.e., disconnecting the behavioral and mental events that produced the dysfunctions. Once he had discerned the series of events that resulted in the symptoms or problems, Milton either added events or substituted events in the series to break the dysfunctional sequences and modify the symptoms. Similarly, he sometimes totally distracted his patients' attention from producing the symptom. For example, when a childless couple came to him to discuss their ruminations about whether to adopt a child, Milton told them to adopt two children at the same time. He then told them about the benefits they would derive in raising two infants together. The original question of whether or not to adopt a child was not raised by the couple again.

An additional utilization technique was to take clinical advantage of the patients' natural human desires: to acquire mastery, to obtain understanding, to have fun, to have certainty, and to have immediate results. People's desires to acquire mastery allowed them to learn new skills; their desires to obtain understanding allowed them to accept new frames of reference for defining themselves and their symptoms; their desires to have fun allowed them to discover enjoyable new experiences; their desires to have certainty allowed them to beneficially resolve clinically introduced paradoxes and double binds, and to favorably relieve clinically induced doubts and confusion; and their desires to have immediate results allowed them to welcome small successes.

Milton achieved great renown for his technical skills in making acceptable therapeutic suggestions to people. He did this both directly and indirectly. When Milton made therapeutic suggestions directly to patients, he did so straightforwardly, and offered them either acceptable solutions to their problems or acceptable first steps toward those solutions. However, the preambles to those direct suggestions were often elaborate, lengthy, and lulling .

When Milton made therapeutic suggestions indirectly to patients, he strategically inserted the suggestions inconspicuously into his conversations, anecdotes and metaphors. He frequently conducted conversations with patients that were covertly seeded with numerous acceptable solutions. In addition, Milton often told stories to his patients about how other people had handled situations that were very similar to their own. These anecdotes offered new ways to solve old problems. Occasionally, Milton used figurative language to create credible analogies to his patients' current dysfunctional experiences. These metaphoric equivalences subtly provided his patients with creative solutions to their problems and with new points of reference about them. He also regularly used patients' first successful trance experiences as metaphors for future learning and change.

The other clinical method that Milton employed, and the one in which he demonstrated unparalleled sophistication, was multi-level communication. Milton was the acknowledged master in transmitting more than one message to a person simultaneously, and in simultaneously transmitting different messages to the members of a group confidentially. He accomplished this by deliberately, systematically and precisely controlling his words, his voice and his body language.

Milton was very particular about the words that he spoke because he expected them to achieve the exact effect he desired. He was either very specific or very general in his word usage. When he wanted his patients to accurately receive a particular idea, he used very specific words; when he wanted his patients to customize his idea within themselves, he used very general words.

In clinical settings, Milton used his voice and his body similarly. By deliberately and systematically modulating his voice tone and tempo, and altering his body's position and movement, he was able to "train" his patients to receive subliminal messages that he was transmitting to them. It was not uncommon for patients to receive two messages simultaneously, sometimes even within the same sentence. The first message was sent with one particular vocal tone or tempo (body position or movement) and the second message was communicated with a different tone or tempo (position or movement). This complex technique was just an elaboration of the method that farmers had used to train animals back in Wisconsin when Milton was a boy.

One of the beautiful qualities of Milton's contacts with people was their enduring effect. In 1979 my wife and son and I were houseguests of Milton and Betty Erickson. During the visit, our ten-year-old son Jason had many opportunities to be with Milton and to chat with him.

He even conducted a private 30-minute interview with Milton for a school report.

This past March, I told Jason that I would be traveling to Phoenix for a few days to attend the memorial gathering for Dr. Erickson, who had just died. Nobody whom Jason had ever known had ever died, so he was appropriately curious. I explained that Dr. Erickson had passed on peacefully and that his family had been with him. Jason then asked, "How's Betty?" I replied that she was fine, and that he could write her a letter if he wished. Later that day, Jason went to his desk, took out his best "Snoopy" stationery and wrote her a lovely letter. At the bottom of the letter he affixed a shiny new penny and appended, "This is for good luck."

While I was away in Phoenix, Jason accompanied his mother to the neighborhood flower shop. He became attracted to a cactus plant that he had never seen before, and was able to convince his mother to buy it for him. It was a tall green plant covered by gracefully flowing silken white strands. He showed it to me when I returned home and asked, "Dad, would Dr. Erickson mind if I called this plant 'Milton'?" "No, Jason," I replied, "I'm sure that he would enjoy it." Several days later, we discovered the popular name for that particular species of cactus—the Old Man of the Desert.

Chapter 41

# The Values and Philosophy of Milton H. Erickson

*Sidney Rosen*

When we observe and examine the work of Milton Erickson, we must conclude that he was one of the most effective manipulators in the field of psychotherapy. Was he therefore a dangerous man—and are his admirers and followers likely to propagate harmful, self-aggrandizing movements? Most of us realize that it is not possible to be with others, psychotherapeutically or otherwise, without influencing them. The "value-free" approaches of psychoanalysis are obviously far from that goal. Therefore, we understand that therapists who do not consciously "manipulate" their patients are still influencing them and that the type of influence must be determined by the "kind of person" the therapist is—his manner, physical appearance, dress, and way of living. Under all of these attributes must lie his value system. Many therapists are not at all explicit about their value systems or even aware of them. In judging whether Erickson was dangerous or helpful, meddlesome or wise, we are not confronted with this vagueness. In over 150 papers, he was most explicit and accurate in reporting what he actually said and did with patients. We can review some of these papers and tape recordings of actual sessions and derive a rather consistent picture of his values and life goals. He was often explicit about his own values in his teaching sessions. I have had the privilege of discussing his values with him, with Betty Erickson, and with the Erickson children. Still, of course, any interpretations in this chapter are my own.

## UNIQUENESS OF THE INDIVIDUAL

Most philosophers, psychologists, anthropologists, and other scientists who examine the human condition, and even those who examine nature, have emphasized similarities and have grouped phenomena according to their similarities. For example, almost every psychologist or psychoanalyst has a theory of personality or character types. This tendency goes back to ancient days when the various temperaments were divided according to the elements as they were then seen: earth, fire, water, and air. In modern times, Freud grouped personality types (as later elaborated by Abraham) according to stages of psychosexual development into oral, anal, phallic, and genital types. Erich Fromm divided people into the marketing personality, the hoarding type, and others. His concept of the productive personality was equivalent to Freud's genital type. Karen Horney defined a morbid dependent type of personality, an arrogant-vindictive, and a detached type. Even in ordinary conversation we tend to type people—as geniuses, lazy bums, alcoholics, work addicts. Then, when we look at a particular person, we tend to see him in a narrow way.

Erickson's approach was different. He emphasized the differences between people, the uniqueness of each individual and even of each object. This emphasis is exemplified by his story of the allergist whom he told to sit in a field. After about three hours, the allergist returned to Erickson and said, "Did you know that every blade of grass is a different shade of green?" In telling this story, Erickson was pointing up the value of noting distinctions. Every person has different shades of any characteristic that we can define. Erickson encouraged us to treasure those unique shades.

In many stories, Erickson emphasized the value of his own differences from others, especially as manifested in his physical defects—color blindness, dyslexia, lack of sense of rhythm, and so on. Although most of us do not have so many obvious outer manifestations of difference from others, certainly we are all aware of thoughts and points of view that we assume are markedly different from the "normal." Erickson encouraged us to value these differences.

## OPTIMISM

He encouraged people to look at themselves and to treasure not only their differences from others, but also differences between their present and past behavioral patterns. This very emphasis on these latter differences, in contrast to others' emphasis on our tendency towards repetition, may be the prime factor leading to Erickson's optimistic view of life. For him, every day, every moment, offered an opportunity for new beginnings. This optimism is illustrated in his statement that in playing golf or any other game one ought to approach each shot as if it was the first one. Thereby one forgets previous attempts, previous tensions, previous failures, and even previous successes.

"Since we do not know what the next moment will bring, what tomorrow will bring," Erickson pointed out, "life is not something you can give an answer to today. You should enjoy the process of waiting, the process of becoming what you are. There is nothing more delightful than planting flower seeds and not knowing what kind of flowers are going to come up."

With regard to goals he said, "You encourage patients to do all those simple little things that are their own right as growing creatures. You see, we don't know what our goals are. We learn our goals only in the process of getting there." As his young daughter said once, when he asked what she was making, "I don't know what I'm building, but I'm going to enjoy building it. When I'm through building it, I'll know what it is!" "You don't know what a baby is going to become. Therefore, you wait and take good care of it until it becomes what it will."

This approach leads to looking at life with what I call the "innocent eye," with every moment being a potential surprise. Terms such as "surprise" and "delight" commonly were used by Erickson. With this way of looking at life's phenomena, one is more likely to feel optimistic than pessimistic. Certainly, pessimism is promoted by the conviction that we are bound to repeat the same destructive and boring patterns to which we have been conditioned, and Erickson was aware of both the value and the limitations imposed upon us by our conditioned patterns. Yet, more than most therapists he emphasized the positive.

## THE WISDOM OF THE UNCONSCIOUS

As Jay Haley pointed out in *Uncommon Therapy* (1973), "Unlike psychodynamically oriented therapists who make interpretations to bring out negative feelings and hostile behavior, Erickson relabels what people do in a postive way, to encourage change. He does not minimize the difficulties, but he will find in the difficulties some aspect of them that can be used to improve the functioning of a person or his family" (p. 34). Haley related this emphasis on the positive to the fact that "Erickson worked in a framework of hypnosis and that while others felt a distrust of those ideas outside of conscious and rational awareness, hypnotists made up another large stream of therapists who emphasized that the unconscious was a positive force."

In fact, if Erickson and his followers have any "religious" guide or belief, it must be in the wisdom of the unconscious. He believed that people can be guided by and can trust their own unconscious minds to determine what is best in any particular moment and in general. Even during hypnotic inductions he expressed this trust and belief by saying such things as, "Go as deeply into a trance as you *wish.*" He believed that people have the capacity and the resources to comfort and heal themselves. As he once advised a therapist who was treating an adult patient, "You can regress her to 11 years of age and then have her, as a separate person, comfort that 11-year old girl—as herself comforting herself." He felt there was always something constructive, even in the most foreboding or apparently sterile or destructive situation. He expressed this belief in an indirect hypnotic induction which began, "In my way of living, I often like to climb a mountain. I always wonder what's on the other side. On my side of the mountain may be meadows, hills, rivers and on the other side, there may be a desert, dark and foreboding." He concluded, "And I would know that however harsh and foreboding a desert was, I would in some way find something there of interest to me."

## IMAGINATION

Like Blake and Yeats, Erickson placed a high value on "imagination" or our capacity to form inner images. In modern times, the word "imagination" has become denigrated. We must go back to Blake and Yeats in order to understand the connection of this word with words such as "vision," "visionary," "imagery." Bronowsky (1978) writes, "In my view, which not everyone shares, the central problem of human consciousness depends on the ability to imagine" (p. 18). In his work with hypnosis, Erickson had discovered that by evoking imagery it was often possible to help patients change. Mere intellectual recollection often was ineffective. This emphasis on imagery, which after all is itself a form of experiencing, is connected with another value that Erickson emphasized, viz., *experience is essential.*

He would not want anybody to accept his philosophy or any of his statements because he had said them or because they were published in some book. In fact, he taught that "Therapy cannot be learned from books. It is learned from life." Erickson told me, "I received a letter from a woman last week which told about her daughter becoming six years old. The next day she did something her mother reprimanded her for and she made the remark, 'It's awfully hard to be six years old. I've only had one day's experience.' "

## PROTECTION OF THE PATIENT

Although he believed in the tendency of the unconscious mind to protect the conscious, Erickson felt that it is incumbent upon the therapist, who temporarily may be given the power to override this protective function, to himself protect the patient. He noted, "The patient does not come to you just because you are a therapist. The patient comes to be protected or helped in some regard. But the personality is very vital to the person, and he doesn't want you to do too much, he does not want you to do it too suddenly. You've got to do it gradually and you've got to do it in the order in which he can assimilate."

He would time his interventions according to the responses of his patient. When he said, "You've got to do it gradually," he obviously meant that you must allow the patient time and scope to move and grow, based on his own unconscious wisdom. He also felt that people's privacy must be protected against the intrusion of others. When he gave a demonstration, he would always ask his subject to reveal, "Only that which you can share with strangers." When I called him and asked him to coauthor our book, *Teaching Tales of Milton H. Erickson,* his first response was, "We must protect the individuals who are described."

Betty commented on her husband's desire for privacy: "Milton always took a dim view, and I have exactly the same feeling too, of having his biography written. He had a strong feeling of privacy—that there are things in your life, experiences, beliefs and relationships, that were just nobody's business." Betty recalled that he had said that if he wrote his autobiography he would either have to disguise or alter the things that he didn't think he would ever want written down or else he would have to make it so "wishy washy" that it would be uninteresting.

## ASSETS AND LIMITATIONS

We all know that Erickson believed strongly in utilizing whatever one had, including characteristics normally labeled as "handicaps." He also pointed out the importance of recognizing and accepting one's limitations. When I went to see him in 1970, asking him to use hypnosis to help me improve my memory for names, he made several comments to the effect that, "You know much more than you think you know." He then shared with me the information that he also had a poor memory for names and in fact for other information as well. He illustrated this with, "Here, in this office, I remember everything that is relevant about a patient. But, if I meet the patient outside of the office, I may not recall anything about him—even his name. The memory for this information belongs here—here in this office."

Later in that same session with me, he interjected an apparently irrelevant comment, "And at my mother's funeral, my father remarked, 'It was nice to have 73 wedding anniversaries with one person. It would have been nicer to have 74—but you can't have everything.' "

## ERICKSON'S IDEAS ON THE SUPERNATURAL AND ESP

Generally speaking, Erickson, like Houdini, dismissed so called supernatural and ESP-type experiences as being based on trickery, illusion, or highly developed observational powers. His attitude was summarized in a letter to Dr. Ernest F. Pecci, dated June 8, 1979, in which he wrote: "I feel that I should inform you that I do not believe that the field of parapsychology is scientifically established and I also feel that the so-called evidence for the existence of these faculties is based on false mathematical logic, misinterpretation of data, overlooking of minimal sensory cues, bias in interpretation and frequently on outright fraud. I have worked for over fifty years to disassociate the study of hypnosis from mystical and unscientific connotations."

He added, "Extensive experience and examination of evidence from a scientific perspective, likewise, makes me believe that so-called hypnotic regression to early infancy and to the womb are pure fantasy."

He liked to tell about the times when he had fooled fortune tellers. He accomplished this by feeding them false information—through the medium of subvocal speech! Apparently some fortune tellers, like Erickson himself, are able to read subvocal speech. He also told me about how he had deceived J.B. Rhine by looking at Rhine's cards from such an angle that he could see the light reflections on the back of the cards. He explained that the original cards were stamp impressed, and the diamond or star patterns could be seen if they were viewed from the right angle. He told me also about a patient who was able to identify cards by memorizing the very slight irregularities on the back of a regular deck of cards.

Erickson had developed his senses to the point that he could listen to a typewriter and often pick out the individual letters from their sound. He even learned to recognize the typing patterns of his various secretaries to the point that he could frequently tell whether the secretary was premenstrual, menstrual, or postmenstrual. He also could sometimes tell when a secretary had had intercourse the night before. When I asked him where he got the data for this last interpretation, he explained that he would check with the secretary's husband. If both he and his wife were in a good mood that day he would correlate this information and he would also correlate it with the typing patterns. "It's just that people are so expressive," Erickson commented, "Yet we are never trained to read these expressions."

When I asked Erickson for his opinion on so-called supernatural phenomena he said, "Well, there is a simple thing about religion, the soul, and mysticism. The cave man slept like you and I, and yet his daily life experience was very different. He fought with the bear, and in his dreams he fought hard and long with the bear. And in the morning there was no bear to be seen. It was a spirit bear! The *unexplainable* fits into the realm of 'spirit.' "

Betty told me, "Milton had the deepest respect for intellectual solutions and the sort of mind that can put together a problem, intellectually, and just cut through to the heart of it. But he was outraged by people who would call themselves scientists and yet would immediately accept the supernatural or paranormal explanations for something, without examining the possibility that the phenomena could be explained according to accepted laws of nature. He liked to refer people to 'Occam's Razor'; William of Occam stated that you don't postulate an explanation unnecessarily, when a phenomenon can be explained in terms of known relationships."

Betty added, "Milton felt that many people were far too gullible about things like healing by the laying on of hands." The sensations that some practitioners have reported, which have convinced them that some real energy is transmitted in this procedure, can easily be produced by autosuggestion.

Out-of-body experiences, Betty felt, can be explained by the loss of the background sensations that are present during normal consciousness and which used to be called "coenesthesia." These sensations often fade away when a person enters into a trance or when a person is in a precomatose state. The lack of coenesthesia at these times is interpreted as the spirit departing from the body.

## RELIGION

Before going to college Erickson was raised in an old-fashioned farm community, in the Methodist Church. When he broadened his knowledge of the world he moved away from conventional organized religion. As Betty told me, "His feeling was that you should lead as decent and productive a life as you could, and he didn't bother worrying about transcendental questions. These were matters that couldn't be answered definitely, so he didn't try to answer them." A patient of mine had been told by a Sufi teacher, who incidently had previously been a psychiatrist, that, next to the leader of his sect, the most spiritual person in the world was Milton Erickson. When I told Betty, she replied, "Milton would have been highly amused by that." Additionally, Betty pointed out that even though he was not religious in the conventional sense, "He never tried to dissuade anyone. His patients and students certainly felt free to express their own beliefs."

## LEARNING AND DOING

Even when he was discussing subjects such as death, Erickson would always instill the injunction, "Enjoy your life." He knew of course that not all things in life were enjoyable and would cite his mother's favorite quotation from Longfellow, "Into each life some rain must fall. Some days must be dark and dreary," but his main focus was on the enjoyment of life. He believed that two activities promoted this enjoyment more than anything else—learning and doing.

Learning about oneself and about the world, he felt, was good, pleasant, and satisfying. Learning new things about oneself is pleasing, so long as one is guided by principles of interest and curiosity. It need not be frightening or anxiety-provoking. In *Uncommon Therapy* (Haley, 1973), he stated, "I don't believe in salvation only through pain and suffering" (p. 282).

Along these same lines, curiosity and wanting to know are good. He once told a patient, "You had a dream with a lot of affect. Now I don't know if you want to find out the cognitive side of that today, tomorrow, or next week. Or perhaps later this year." He then explained that he had given her a choice, and he added, "I have human curiosity working for me."

The other great source of pleasure is *doing*. Erickson was not anti-intellectual. But he was certainly anti-intellectualizing. Especially with overly obsessive detached patients, he found it important to encourage them to get away from books and to *do* things. He would often say, "Get all of your hard work done as soon as possible so the last 40 years of your life will be happy." He might add, "You can have plenty of bad luck come your way, for free. If you want something in life, you have to earn it."

Erickson emphasized that it was not only important to do things but what one does must have social consequences. In his beautiful story of the depressed woman whom he encouraged to cultivate African violets (Zeig, 1980), he pointed out that his patient not only recovered from her depression, but that she always had African violets to *give*, as gifts for weddings, funerals, christenings, and other occasions. He concluded, "When she died, in her 70s, of natural causes, she was known as the African violet queen of Milwaukee. And she had an endless number of friends."

Erickson encouraged and arranged for productivity even in mental hospitals. Jay Haley (1973) tells of a patient in a mental hospital who believed that he was Jesus Christ. Erickson said to him, "I understand you have some skill in carpentry." When the patient admitted that he had, Erickson put him to work building bookcases. Subsequently, the patient was able to do other productive work and eventually to leave the hospital, free of delusions and self-supporting. Erickson was opposed to people's accepting welfare aid except temporarily and when it was absolutely necessary. Even then, his sense of fairness led him to believe that they should pay back in money or in some other way for any help that was received. He illustrated this with the story of a maid he had hired when he first came to Arizona. He said, "She was a widow with six small children. She had been in the hospital, having her sixth child, and her husband was killed. She went on welfare for a year. During that time she learned to read and write, and she then got a job as a maid. She paid back all the welfare money and supported her children."

I witnessed a session in which he told a patient that he would not charge her anything because she could not afford it. He also told her that she could not afford to stay in Phoenix and that she should return home immediately. She should insist that her child's father pay a reasonable child support, and she should work, even at such things as embroidery and typing, in order to support herself. He was very emphatic in his insistence that the only way she would get over her unhappiness would be to do things that were productive rather than wasting her time in self-examination and soul-searching.

## MANIPULATION

Erickson pointed out that he had often been accused of manipulating patients—to which he replied, "Every mother manipulates her baby—if she wants it to live. Every time you go to a store, you manipulate the clerk to do your bidding, and when you go to a restaurant, you manipulate the waiter. And the teacher in school manipulated you into learning to read and write. In fact, life is one big manipulation. The final manipulation is putting you to rest, and that is manipulation too. They have to lower the coffin, and then they have to get the ropes out—all manipulation. And you manipulate a pencil to write, to record thoughts. And you manipulate yourself, carrying around peanuts or cigarettes or Life Savers." In other words Erickson would equate what some people call manipulation with what others call exploration, experimentation, and mastery—of words, objects and situations. As I have mentioned above, in manipulating others he was always careful to avoid exploiting them, harming them in any way, or allowing them to harm themselves.

## RAISING CHILDREN

How did Erickson raise his children so that they could "manipulate" effectively? I believe that he accomplished this mainly by setting an example, especially in the handling of *them.* Betty Erickson agreed with my impression that Milton was a rather strict disciplinarian. She explained, "I think that is correct—that he was rather strict and believed when you laid down the rules, you enforced them. I think I suffered sometimes more than the kids did. But, I learned to just leave the room and keep my opinion to myself because, you know, his approach always seemed to work, even though it wasn't the way I would do it."

I'll give you one of my favorite stories, about his disciplining of two-and-a-half-year-old Kristi, as he told it.

"One Sunday, we were reading the newspaper—all of us—and she walked up to her mother, grabbed the newspaper, threw it on the floor. Her mother said, 'Kristi, that wasn't very nice. Pick up the paper and give it back to Mother. Tell her you are sorry.'

" 'I don't has to,' Kristi said.

"Every member of the family gave her the same advice and got the same reply. So I told Betty to pick her up and put her in the bedroom.

"I lay down on the bed, and she put Kristi beside me. Kristi looked at me contemptuously and started to scramble off. But I had a hold on her ankle. She said, 'Wet Woose!'

"I said, 'I don't has to.'

"And that lasted four hours. She kicked and struggled. Pretty soon she freed one ankle. I got hold of the other. It was a desperate fight, like a silent fight between two Titans. At the end of four hours, she knew that she was the loser, and she said, 'I will pick up the paper and give it to Mother.'

"And that's where the ax fell. I said, 'You don't has to.'

"So she threw her brain into higher gear and said, 'I will pick up the paper. I will give it to Mother. I will tell Mother I am sorry.'

"And I said, 'You don't has to.'

"And then she shifted into full gear. 'I will pick up the paper. I want to pick up the paper. I want to tell Mother I am sorry.'

"I said, 'Fine.' "

That is a beautiful illustration of the development of superego, isn't it?

Erickson showed the same kind of insistence in teaching his son to keep his word about taking out the garbage, repeatedly waking Robert up in the middle of the night, apologizing that he had forgotten to remind him to do this task during the day. Erickson emphasized that this kind of teaching of responsibility and limits is more easily done when the child is young. He would, however, treat grown patients in ways to ensure that they learned first to accept and then to incorporate authority. For example, we once asked him why he had insisted on sending a patient to climb Squaw Peak before he would do any other therapy with her. We wondered whether it was in order for her to get a feeling of accomplishment? Was it for her to get in touch with her own inner feelings of isolation?

And his answer was simply, "So that she would obey me." He had to establish obedience before he could direct her to do other things that would enable her to overcome the limitations of her phobic reaction.

Now, of course, we all know that authority can be misused, can be used cruelly, exploitively, insensitively, and destructively. We also know from the ways in which Erickson's patients have developed inner-directedness and productive ways of living that he did not misuse his authority with them. Certainly, his children have not turned out to be either overly compliant or overly rebellious. Any contact with them indicates that they are well-balanced, happy, productive, and healthy. They have learned to take responsibility for their own lives, and they have passed on these same ethics to their own children.

## MARRIAGE

In spite of some people's idea to the contrary, Erickson did not rigidly hold to the belief that marriage was sacred and had to be sustained, regardless of the unhappiness of the participants. Zeig (1980) recorded a story about a couple, both psychiatrists, who returned home from a visit to Erickson and immediately dissolved their marriage of more than

15 years. In addition, each one fired his or her psychoanalyst. Interestingly, the psychoanalyst (they were both being treated by the same analyst) *himself* came with his wife to see Erickson, and the two of *them* were divorced immediately after this visit. Erickson pointed out that they maintained very friendly, mutually respecting relationships after this divorce. *He* mostly was concerned that each person lead a happy life and that he make intelligent choices, taking responsibility for these choices.

## ATTITUDES ABOUT WOMEN

As Betty told me, "Erickson certainly felt that women should have every sort of opportunity and should be treated with complete fairness in the job market and elsewhere. He also felt very strongly that there is a basic biological and psychological difference between the sexes." He believed for example that there was a basic maternal biological urge. He would note that little girls in any culture who were not given conventional dolls would make them, even out of a stick of wood or from seaweed. He felt that this maternal behavior was so universal that, if it was learned, it was learned in the very earliest stage of life. He understood that later nurturing of children and caring for a home involved only a division of labor. This type of responsibility could be negotiated between husband and wife.

## RACIAL AND GENETIC DIFFERENCES

Erickson objected to the idea that racial or national characteristics were completely learned and cultural. He felt that in certain cultures anything that had definite survival value could have a basic biological substrate. For example, he noted that the Vietnamese child adopted by his daughter and son-in-law reacted to stress by withdrawing; she became rigid and silent and even shut her eyes. Erickson understood that for anyone, especially a woman, who lived in an area where for 400 years the group had to survive recurrent conflicts, there was survival value in fading into the background. There was the element of "survival of the quietest," and certain temperaments were likely to survive. Actually, Erickson felt that denial of genetic differences was not an effective way of counteracting prejudice; in fact, he loved the differences. He felt they should be heightened, not swept over, nor ironed out. Sometimes, of course, he felt that it was necessary for people to adjust to them.

Milton and Betty were very aware of the differences in their own children. For example, Allan from the time he could walk was a mathematician. When he was four years old, and the Ericksons were living at Eloise Hospital in Michigan, he decided to count the rails on the large iron rail fences on the grounds of the hospital. Betty told me that when she would send another child out to remind him to come home for lunch, he would put a stick in the fence to mark the place, then come racing home, with his eyes glowing, chanting the numbers. He is now a mathematician, working for the government.

## MARIJUANA

Erickson opposed the use of marijuana largely because he felt that evidence indicated that it was associated with loss of motivation. He also felt that we would not know for quite a while whether it is physically harmless. He recalled that when he was young, tobacco had been considered absolutely harmless. In fact, some studies had shown that people who smoked moderately were in better shape than people who didn't smoke at all. (This may have been due to the fact that people who were not in good health were not as likely to smoke.)

Aldous Huxley had worked with Erickson as part of his interest in altered states of consciousness. He had once remarked to Erickson that he felt at times that the insight gained with drugs could be compared to going down into a deep ditch and then climbing up onto a ladder. You felt that you were seeing very far, but, actually, you were still below ground level. Drugs elevate you from a very low level but not to a height that you could reach without drugs.

## ESTHETICS

Many people who have tried to imitate Erickson's approaches achieve some success even though they may apply them in mechanistic, programmed ways. However they usually miss a very important element—the element of poetry and of music. You see this feature in his stories, which contain a classical beauty and elegance in their form, rhythm, and tone. There is poetry and beauty in some of his posthypnotic suggestions. For example, he would say, "You will see a flash of color." I was reminded of this particular suggestion while reading Yeats' poem "The Lake Isle of Innisfree."

There midnight's all a glimmer, and noon a purple glow.
And evening's full of the linnet's wings.

I discovered, to my delight, that in the summer the linnet male has a bright crimson-red breast and crown. What a flash of color that would be!

## HUMOR

Anyone who has ever seen the twinkle in Milton Erickson's eyes, who has noted the secret smile on his face as he talked, or who has heard him chuckle about the many practical jokes that were played within his family knows the large role that humor played in Erickson's life. His own and his listener's laughter frequently punctuated his stories. His family shared his enjoyment of jokes, and they would often devote a great deal of time to the promotion of one of these jokes. After Erickson's memorial service his son Lance told me about some of the tricks and games Erickson would indulge in with his children, and Lance emphasized the fact that the family always liked to have fun. Of course Erickson carried his love of humor to his death bed.

## DEATH

During the two-week period before his death I told my acquaintances some of Erickson's stories about death and dying. My favorite was the joke that Erickson made in response to hearing that a former student of his had been concerned at the rumor that he was dying: Erickson had said, "I think that is entirely premature. I have no intention of dying. In fact, that will be the last thing I do."

I cannot summarize Milton Erickson's values and philosophy more concisely than author Gwynn Cravens did at our memorial service in New York, when she said, "There are thousands, if not tens of thousands of people, whom Erickson helped to discover the sweetness of everyday life, the joy of hard work, the use of the muscles, the senses, the heart, and the head." Salvador Minuchin wrote to Erickson after visiting him about a week before Erickson's death, "I was tremendously impressed with the way in which you are able to look at simple moments and describe their complexity and at your trust in the capacity of human beings to harness a repertory of experiences they do not know they have."

## REFERENCES

Bronowsky, J. *The Origins of Knowledge and Imagination*. New Haven: Yale University Press, 1978.

Erickson, M.H. & Rossi, E., *Hypnotherapy: An Exploratory Casebook*. New York: Irvington, 1979.

Haley, J. *Uncommon Therapy: The Psychiatric Techniques of Milton H. Erickson, M.D.* New York: W.W. Norton & Co., Inc. 1973.

Rosen, S. (Ed.) *My Voice Will Go With You: The Teaching Tales of Milton H. Erickson, M.D.* New York: Norton, 1982.

Zeig, J.K. (Ed.) *A Teaching Seminar with Milton H. Erickson*, New York: Brunner/Mazel, 1980.

Chapter 42

# Creativity: A Special Interaction Hour

*Ernest Rossi, Carl A. Whitaker, and Jay Haley*

*Ernest Rossi:*

Our presentation this afternoon will be very informal. It's rather unplanned, and for my part I'd like to think of it as a continuation of Jay Haley's keynote presentation yesterday afternoon. You will recall that his closing remarks were something to the effect that he is happy that he left the darkness of Milton H. Erickson unobscured. It is to that question that I would like to address our energies this afternoon.

Can we say something about the nature of Milton H. Erickson's creativity? Do we have any theories, any ideas? Do any of us here have mutual life experiences that can amplify and help us understand some of the darkness? To orient you, I would like to have you recall some of Milton H. Erickson's earliest experiences as a child. Some of these seem almost apocryphal by this time. All of you have heard many of the stories. I just want to repeat two or three to orient us to the subject at hand.

One of the most charming examples of Milton H. Erickson's early life was something he told me one afternoon. He said that when he was a young child going to school, he delighted in being the first one out into the fresh snow so that he would be able to make the first footprints. Instead of following the well-established sidewalks and roadways, he purposefully would make his fresh footprints into funny curves, long roundabout ways of getting to school, and he was always delighted when he came back home from school and saw that others had followed his circuitous path. Then, during the next few days, he would gradually change that path, cutting off one of the curves, then coming home and seeing how others now took a more direct route, and so on until finally there was the normal direct route. This was a young child at play. This was a game that he invented all by himself. What kind of an early consciousness was this?

There was another early memory that I could hardly believe when he told me. He was around five or six years old and from a farming family. His grandfather and other people apparently believed that planting should be done at a certain stage of the moon. You planted potatoes by the full moon or the new moon, I don't recall just which. This young lad chose to question it and planted some potatoes in his own private patch at the wrong time. He did his first scientific experiment and found that there wasn't any difference. However, when he tried to tell his grandfather about his results, he only got a frown and a disgruntled noncommittal response, his first bout with resistance. (*Laughter.*)

There is the charming story of his first use of what later became known as the double bind. His father was trying to pull a stubborn calf into a barn, and young Milton laughed at him. His father, still pulling the calf into the barn, yelled at Milton, "Do you think you could do better?" Milton went up and pulled on the calf's tail and, of course, the calf, to escape the worse of the two evils, immediately trampled over the father to get into the barn. Now this was a young lad, not yet in puberty—what kind of a consciousness was this?

The next thing I want to present is his first bout with polio at 17. I will review it briefly. Here was a young lad in a farm community stricken with a serious illness, and he overheard the doctor saying to his mother that the boy would not live through the night. Milton recalled that he felt great anger. He felt very indignant that a doctor should tell that to a mother, and he would be damned if he wasn't going to live through the night and not see another sunrise. With whatever energy he could muster, he asked his family to change the position of his bureau on which there was a mirror. They did not know why he wanted them to do that, but they did it. From the changed position of the mirror, he could see a reflection of the sunrise, and he did not die that night. He stayed up until he saw that sunrise, and then he lapsed into a coma for a number of days.

I am not sure of all my facts here, but as Milton told the story to me, he was completely paralyzed for at least six months. He was completely paralyzed, but his hearing was very acute and he could move his eyes. As he lay in bed all day he began to play mental games. He would listen for the barn door to close and then listen for the footsteps to reach the house. From the sound of just how the barn door was closed and how long it took to get to the steps and the sounds on the front steps, he knew who was there, what kind of a mood they were in and whether they might be either attending to him or not attending to him.

Apparently when he made bowel movements in the bed, it was trouble to clean up. So his family rigged up an apparatus with an old rocking chair. They cut a hole in the rocking chair and put a pot under there so there would be a little bit less mess. They would tie him into the chair. On one very critical day they forgot to untie him and put him back in bed. He was in the middle of the room, but wanted to be over by the window—at least then he could see out. He wished and he wished and then there was a very dramatic moment when, as he was wishing, he suddenly realized that the rocking chair was starting to rock. How did that happen? So the 17-year-old boy discovered by himself the basic principle of hypnosis, what we call ideomotor action—a wish, a thought, becomes translated into appropriate motor action autonomously, all by itself. Of course, he didn't give it any fancy language like that, but he began to wonder. "What if I tried to remember how I held a pitchfork?" He would watch his hand and imagine all the movements that his hand went through to grasp a pitchfork, to climb a tree, to open a barn door. He did that for days until, finally, as he was going through those real sensory memories—not imagination, mind you, not fantasy, but real memories of how he moved that finger—suddenly he saw a blip. One of his fingers did move. Aha! Again, ideomotor action: an idea of movement gave rise to a real physical movement. They did not have physical therapists around 60 years ago in that isolated farming community, but this is how Milton, the young lad, learned to heal himself. From then on, every day he worked with his sensory memories, gradually recovering most of his motor coordination.

I want to share one other observation with you. A number of times Milton—in a desperate effort, I think, to bridge the gap between our characters—was trying to tell me something. In my work with him, I was always a very gentle and quiet student. Perhaps that is why he did so much work with me. Perhaps there was something in my quietness that he felt wasn't appropriate for my development, so he would tell me about "my terrible intensity." As I would hold a microphone up to him, he would stare at me and say, "Now, I can use that terrible intensity at will and as I look at you . . . *there* . . . now I see you, I see the microphone, and I see nothing else." He was experiencing tunnel vision; he was giving me that ocular fixation that you have heard so much about. I was quivering a little bit trying to get it all recorded. Other times, he would say things like, "Manipulation is okay. We manipulate food when we put salt in it. After all, I am very gentle, yes, but there is an iron fist in my velvet glove."

The natural hypothesis is that he was very angry, very intense. He had learned to channel that intensity into his own therapeutic healing. In that sense, I feel, he is an example of the archetype of the wounded healer who, curing himself, learns to cure others. I marvel at that terrible intensity coming from a 17-year-old boy, that outrage against fate and anger at the doctor for *daring* to tell a mother—not his mother, but *a* mother—that her son would not live.

In my simplistic thinking, as I was discussing some of these things with Jay earlier today, I said, "I really think his creativity came out of his anger." Jay was not impressed, and a couple of moments later, he let drop, "Well, that is a very old theory, of course." I felt foolish, but that question is what I would like to throw open to Jay Haley and Carl Whitaker: "What *are* your ideas about Milton's creativity?" We are all unfinished people here. All of our concepts are unfinished. We are not going to come to the complete answer this afternoon, but I would like to act as *if* we were going to try to find the answer. I would like all of us to have the courage to share some of our personal experiences that may have bearing, to see just where we are on this issue of creativity and the making of a human existence. *(Applause.)*

*Carl A. Whitaker:*

I suppose that Jay Haley having done such a great job yesterday, I really need to start out and make sure that I am here. *(Whitaker pinches himself.) (Laughter.)* As he was finishing his discussion—he was talking about creativity—I suddenly remembered my childhood. I, too, was brought up on a dairy farm, except mine was up near Lake Placid, instead of northern Wisconsin. I remember being out in the fields about three-quarters of a mile from the house when we broke a whiffletree, that piece of wood that connects the two horses. Then there was an easy decision. Could I make it back to the barn, a half-hour back, and find some wood and come back and fix it, or could I find something nearby that I could make it work with? I finally found an old tree that was uprooted and broke off one end. I tied it up with a piece of strap off the reins and made my way back home with the team so that I didn't have to take that extra walk.

So part of my sense of creativity is that it comes out of necessity. You get in a corner. Let me give you another example. For 15 years, I have gone to the psychiatric ward in our university hospital at Madison once a week to see the family of an inpatient. I have one hour with each family, and that is all that I will ever have. By the next week there will be another family, and the first one will be gone, so it's either now or never. These interviews have been unique experiences, and some of the things that have come to me in them have been the strange ways in which I trick myself. I think I hypnotize myself in the occupational sense as well as in the personal sense. I have experienced a gradually increasing willingness to share my pain and my horror and my anger at the family scenes that I run into. I recall one week the residents hadn't scheduled any family, and they didn't call to tell me. I went up to the ward and was irritated that I had to tramp all the way back downstairs. They had set me up to feel like a dope again. So, the next week, I scheduled two families in my office—one from one to two, which was the interview hour, and one from two to three, which was the discussion hour—and then the residents called up and said, "We've got a family. You are supposed to be up here. They are already here." I said, "I've got two families scheduled. I forgot all about it. I double-scheduled myself in my little book." As I walked back toward the office, I was thinking, "What in the hell am I going to do?" I got on the telephone in my office and said, "You take a good history, and I will be up there in an hour." I saw my first family; I told them what a mess I was in. The second family came in, and I said, "I have got a problem. I've agreed to do a consultation up on the ward with a new family who have come from Illinois or Iowa. Would you guys come up and help me?" So we took the five members of that family up on the ward to those 20 people in the other family and *that* family did a consultation on the new family. That is an example, at least in my world, in which anger produced creativity—but it was a funny flip because I had to corner myself first. *(Applause.)*

*Jay Haley:*

This is a time for free associating, I think. (*Laughter.*) I think there has always been a problem in investigating creativity, and I don't know of a single research project that has attempted it and has come out with anything. I remember one at the University of California; they gave a vast number of psychological tests to creative people, and the creative people that I knew wouldn't have put up with those tests. The people that they tested weren't the most appropriate ones. It's a difficult problem.

About the idea that anger causes creativity—I think that it causes action in many situations, but it can also obstruct creativity. There are different kinds of creativity. There's the kind that lays down something new, and once that is laid down all kinds of things can be done with it. The man who invented the wheel did something rather extraordinary, but the person who applied wheels in new ways had the advantage that somebody else had already invented the wheel. I think that Erickson was in many ways the one who did that original invention.

Let me give a small example. I had a woman patient who had a lot of problems; one relatively minor problem was that if she took a shower or a bath she couldn't do it with the bathroom door closed because she was afraid that the bathroom would flood and she would drown. She was a swimming teacher so she felt that this was a problem. While I was dealing with other issues, I hypnotized her and said that during the week she would realize that she had taken a shower with the bathroom door closed. She came in the next week and said, "A funny thing happened this week. I took a shower, and after I finished I noticed that I had closed the bathroom door. So the next day, I did the same thing. I closed the door and took a shower. I don't seem to have that problem anymore." I said, "That's nice. We can go to more important problems," and we went on. I didn't devise the simple principle that I applied. Erickson created the idea that if you give a post-hypnotic suggestion for something to happen after a particular act, the person has to do the particular act in order to carry out the post-hypnotic suggestion.

I think that that is an extraordinary idea, really, but once somebody has produced that idea, anyone can think of an infinite number of ways of using it. I think the problem for all of us is how to achieve a way of thinking in that basic way rather than only developing the ideas that are already present. *(Applause.)*

*Ernest Rossi:*

I want to share one personal experience about the way I work when I am writing, something about the role of negativity in my creative process. Then I want to say something about Milton and how we relate to his work.

Over the years, I developed a habit of writing for a few hours in the morning; this has been a pattern I have had for about 15 years now. About five or six years ago I discovered one of the ways that some of my better ideas come. Usually a better idea comes along when I am writing away and thinking usually two or three paragraphs ahead of what I am actually writing. That's the way I work. I will come to a point where I think, "Say, this is important. What am I going to do with that? Is that it? No, no . . . definitely, that's not it." I thus reject the new idea and continue writing without it. What I suddenly discovered one day is that when I get to saying, "No, no . . . that's not it," *that* is usually it, the new idea, the new way of saying something, the new question to ask. Usually my mind rejects it first. Is that just one of my quirks or is this a general aspect of negativity? There are lots of stories about the devil, Lucifer, the light bringer, the negative, that initiates the new. I am currently exploring the idea that the creative and new tends to come in the negative form. Does that idea have implications for psychopathology—that all symptoms are forms of communication, new insights that our cortex cannot express verbally because of our learned limitations, so our body tries to express these new insights, these new patterns, in body language. The body is really not suited to expressing what is cognitively new, however, and does such a poor job of it that we recognize that something is wrong and thus say the body language is a symptom or bad habit. Hiding behind these symptoms, the odd and idiosyncratic within ourselves, is the new, the creative, struggling for recognition within our consciousness.

The thing that I want to say about our relationship to Milton's work comes from what has happened to me personally since he died. My mind has gone on sabbatical. It's like mush. I can't think. I can't do any intellectual work. Partly, I know, there is a struggle going on in me. I know that for the eight years I'd known him, I've dedicated myself to his work.

However, after all, there was an Ernest Rossi before Milton H. Erickson came along. When I wrote my first book on dreams and the growth of personality, before I met Milton, I was tuned in to my own creativity. I thought I was doing interesting work on the phenomenology of dreams and how new consciousness evolves in psychotherapy, and then I ran into the accident that was Milton H. Erickson, and I felt that there was something more important that I had to learn. For eight long years you might say that I really sacrificed some of Ernie Rossi. I put me, whatever I am, on hold for a little while, because there was a sense of urgency about trying to learn something about Milton's work. As much as possible, I tried to keep Ernie Rossi out of it although, as Jay said yesterday, there is probably a lot of evidence in my work of how Milton used the metaphors of my own mind to communicate his message. For that I am sorry, because I really tried to communicate Milton H. Erickson's story and creativity as much as possible.

What is the struggle going on in me now? Is this just mourning, grief? I'm sure that's part of it, but there is a part of me that is rebellious and angry. I want to say, "To hell with it. I am going to drop all of the

Erickson work and go back to where I was and pick up my consciousness stuff." There's a great struggle going on in me to find Ernie Rossi again and differentiate from Milton H. Erickson, just as earlier there was a struggle to differentiate myself from Franz Alexander, who was one of my teachers, and from Spurgeon English, who is at this Congress, who was also one of my early teachers.

One of the problems with this conference is that we hear all the wonderful things about Milton H. Erickson, all the marvelous cures, all the fantastic powers, and compared to all that, what am I? People come to me with great expectation. They think that if I am an Ericksonian hypnotherapist I am going to be able to help them experience all those marvelous classical hypnotic phenomena. I'm going to be able to use double binds and indirect suggestion. I can do hardly any of that. I am just a raw beginner, just learning how to do some of that, and part of me doesn't *want* to know how to do even that much. I've got my own consciousness. I've got other things that I'm more interested in when I work with people. Besides, I will never be Milton H. Erickson, and if I try too hard to be Milton H. Erickson, I will always be a nothing because, dammit, I will never be able to do it his way.

People keep whispering to me, "Didn't Milton ever have failures?" (*Laughter.*) Yes, I think he had failures. At one time, I wanted to do a paper about some of his failures, but the thinking became so clouded and complex that I gave up because I couldn't follow Milton's thinking. (*Laughter.*) Milton would say, "Now see this, this is black," and I would say, "Yes, it's black." Then Milton would present an argument, "Now you see how, in effect, from this point of view it is really white. You are really talking about a patient's symptom, and that is why you think it is a failure, but it is really not a failure." I would say, "What? Oh, I see. I see, if you look at it that way. Yeah, I guess." Now, were these rationalizations or was Erickson really on meta-levels that I've never been able to achieve? (*Laughter.*) For years, every time I'd come to his home—and for a while it was every week or a week a month—he would always greet me with a new puzzle. I guess he was trying to train me to use my mind, but I never succeeded in solving his puzzles. *(Laughter.)* Because I was such a poor student, I would have to ask a lot of questions, and he would be tempted sometimes to answer some of them. (*Laughter.*)

I really suspect Milton failed a lot in every session as well as succeeded a lot in every session. At least that's the way I work, and I'm going to hang onto that ideology, that view of myself. Every session I fail some and every session I succeed some, and I want to be able to see both sides. That is the only way I can remain a human being; that is the only way I can remain Ernie Rossi, in the face of having been with Milton H. Erickson. *(Applause.)*

*Carl A. Whitaker:*

I guess they want you to be Ernie Rossi. *(Applause.)*

I'd like to pick up on something you said about creativity because I have a funny experience of becoming creative when I have acknowledged my defeat. The first time that happened was in Austin, Texas. I was put in a funny booth with a videotape and two or three cameras. The booth was a room within a room, a weird looking place. The family that I was given to interview included the patient's brother and the brother's girlfriend and the girlfriend's mother. (*Laughter.*) I thought to myself, "This is ridiculous. To hell with them," and it turned out to be a great interview. I don't know what it had to with anything, but it was as though they had completely defeated me, so then I could be there.

I had another experience like that in Lyman Wynne's clinic in Rochester. I was seeing the family of a psychotic patient who thought he was Christ. I was doing a regular, routine family evaluation. I got about halfway through, and it was boring me, and I thought, "This is ridiculous." Here I am in front of all these students, and I'd like to make it worthwhile, and I'm goofing again, at which point I suddenly had an idea. Looking back on it, metaphorically, it feels as though my manipulative left brain gave up. All of a sudden I said, "You know, I think I know what is the trouble. You weren't baptized. (*Laughter.*) If Daddy will be John the Baptist and Mother will be Virgin Mary—she looks like she would do it all right—and if you three sisters-in-law will be Martha, Mary and Mary Magdalene—which one would like to be Mary Magdalene? One of them said, 'Oh, I'd love to be Mary Magdalene.' " *(Laughter.)* All of a sudden the patient got up from across the room and walked over to me and said, "Look, Doc, cut it out, will you? I'm not really Christ. That's all ridiculous!" *(Laughter.)*

The problem is I don't know how to do it to myself. I have to get to some point where I give up being Superman. *(To Haley)* Could you give up being Superman?

*Jay Haley:*

Nope. (*Laughter.*) I've tried though. It takes a lot of effort even to try.

When Dr. Rossi spoke of people trying to be like Erickson, I had a vision of 2000 people here in purple shirts . . . (*Laughter.*) . . . all trying to talk his way and behave his way. It isn't really what Erickson had in mind. *(Whitaker touches Rossi's purple tie. Laughter. Rossi takes off his tie and jacket. The audience laughs and applauds. Whitaker gets up and picks one of the mums that decorated the stage and places it on the table in front of Rossi. Rossi picks a mum himself and puts it in his shirt pocket. Applause. Rossi puts the flower Whitaker gave him onto Whitaker's lapel. Whitaker pounds his chest, Tarzan fashion. Laughter.)*

Well, as I was saying . . . I think that one of the things that Erickson most emphasized is managing to find your own way of working that fits your own particular style. You notice that problem most if you do live supervision behind a one-way mirror. I watch a trainee in a room with a family, and I have an idea what might be good for that family. My problem is that I know that trainee doesn't work that way, so I have to think of something else for him to do. What I have begun to recognize is that it isn't a matter so much of limitations as just different ways that people are. Everyone has to find his own particular way, I think, and Erickson certainly emphasized that.

An interesting similarity between Carl and Erickson is that both of them emphasize that in a session you should follow your impulses. Erickson did a lot of strategic planning and careful arranging of things, but often he would just follow an impulse and assume that it was the correct impulse that came up in the interview. It is inevitable any one person here will have a different impulse from any other person here. Those differences are in the nature of the very complex situation each person is in personally, as well as the position he is in during the therapeutic encounter. It wouldn't be possible to duplicate what Milton did in the way that Milton did it, and I think it would be strange if anybody really set out to want to do that.

The gentleman who formerly had the purple tie on will now speak.

*Ernest Rossi:*

I think that it is time to allow the audience to speak. Are there any statements or questions you would like to share with us?

*Carl A. Whitaker:*

Let me interrupt you because I had a thought a few minutes ago. *(Laughter.)* Milton was always defeated by his body, and it may well be that massive, continual, repeated defeat was what gave him guts enough to move like he really was rather than the way that most of us move—the way that we ought to be, or wish we could be, or somebody else thinks we ought to be, or Mother said we should have been.

Back in 1948 I was consultant to Warm Springs, and I was only invited down once in something like four years and only because one of the polio victims had a delusion that her teeth were turning green because of the atomic energy that was coming out of Oak Ridge. One of the things that was tremendously impressive there was the euphoria of these 75, 100, 120 polio victims. It was as though they were so glad to be alive that it made the rest of us feel depressed as hell just wandering through the place. I don't know what that has to do with Milton, *(to Rossi)* but that hit me very powerfully with what you were saying a minute ago.

*Ernest Rossi:*

A continual encounter with death or pain may make us thankful for whatever we have. One of Erickson's real gifts was that, in the face of continual defeat, he continually made an effort to make something creative out of it. Someone told me the story that at one point he was having visual problems. There were circles forming in front of his eyes. He was trying to go to sleep, and he looked through those circles and imagined himself going into a deep trance. Again, he used his symptoms, his physical disabilities in a creative way. This is the process the modern holistic people call "channeling." Erickson found ways of turning disabilities into positive things, out of sheer desperation, I am sure, with anger, but also with more and more love as he progressed in his life.

PART XVI

# *Keynote Address*

*Carl Whitaker, M.D., did not have much personal contact with Milton Erickson. In fact, they had met on only one occasion. Because he was not directly familiar with Erickson, Whitaker was not a member of the original Congress faculty. After Bateson's death, we searched for someone to present one of the keynote addresses. We looked for an expert outside the field of hypnosis. Part of Bateson's effectiveness had been derived from the fact that he was an anthropologist and, therefore, could comment on psychiatry from a unique perspective. Whitaker could comment on Ericksonian approaches from the vantage point of a family therapist.*

*After he was invited to speak at the Congress, we found out that Whitaker had a special fondness for Gregory Bateson. Whitaker explained that he had sought Bateson out as a mentor during his early years in psychiatry. Perhaps it was partially due to his special feeling for Bateson that Whitaker accepted the invitation to present one of the keynote addresses.*

*Whitaker was also invited to the Congress because of the many characteristics that he shared with Milton Erickson, including a strong emphasis on application rather than theory, remarkable flexibility in approach, and an emphasis on the positive strength of the human unconscious. Erickson is considered to be the father of modern hypnosis. Concomitantly, Whitaker is considered to be one of the fathers of family therapy. In regard to clinical applications, both would rather do it than talk about it; in some cases teaching can be best accomplished by modeling.*

*Carl Whitaker is a unique therapist and teacher. He has a wonderfully warm and humorous style of using symbolic processes to provoke growthful responses from the unconscious. He was invited to sit with us in our livingroom, but in his inimitable style, we wound up with him in the backyard.*

Chapter 43

# Hypnosis and Family Depth Therapy

*Carl A. Whitaker*

Since I am still alive to take poetic license and talk with you about myself and my professional living from that podium old men have fun with, I intend to take full advantage of this opportunity. I'm glad to share with Jay Haley who uses the podium of experience rather than old age. I tremble a bit to think of what will happen when he has both old age plus his massive perception to offer.

I must make it clear that I'm a lumper, not a shredder, and at times some people have reframed this as stupid. I'm interested in *my* depth, not the family's depth. I have no interest in individual symptoms, that is, in taking the family off the spot like the state hospital did in "treating" the identified patient. Once he was off the spot it cured the family like debtor prisons cured the debtors. I'm searching for my pathology, not yours and not the family's pathology. I share my pathology with patients, whether it's the somatic substitutes for my psychological stress, my parasympathetic attacks, my skin itching, or my asthma, which I think of as reciprocal with the psychosis of my high school days.

Furthermore, you must recognize that I'm not interested in being therapist to the culture and the pathology that it's induced. I make no effort to respond to the culture's demand that I play missionary to everyone who has been damaged and shows up at my door. This has to do with my discovery some time back that what happens to missionaries is that they get eaten up by cannibals.

Psychotherapy is an absurd, lifetime adventure. Like an abstract artist I'm looking for better expression of my life, not only in relation to significant others, but also in relation to myself. If I'm lucky, a creation may happen during therapy that bridges my inner self and the inner self of others, the family or even an audience. It may happen, but I don't work for that.

Since I was first called for this strange interlude in your hypnotic conference, I keep asking, "Lord, why me?" I really accepted as a way to share my grief at the loss of both Milton and Gregory Bateson, one of the greats in my beginning as a therapist.

I feel somewhat like a bastard at a family picnic of you hypnotists and hypnotic subjects, but am reminded of when I was a child and we had 100 persons at the Whitaker reunion. My mother was the only one on the Barnett side of the family. So I was trained for this.

I also suspect that my early work as a child on the dairy farm feeding 100 cows, 100 chickens, a dozen pigs and a half dozen horses and 23 cats made psychotherapy a natural process. I also spent many, many hours shoveling cow manure, which is very heavy—that gave me good training. I would never have guessed when I was a simple schizophrenic in high school that I would give up my OB-GYN training and become a psychiatrist just because I fell in love with schizophrenia. Now it is more and more clear that we're all schizophrenics in the middle of the night although we wake up and make believe nothing happened. Our highest integrity is limited to the sleep hours.

The opportunity to talk about family therapy within the framework of hypnosis left me quite frightened, but only after I'd accepted the challenge to come here. Having decided to try, it dawned on me that hypnosis derives quite automatically from the experience each of us has in his infant years. Some mothering person defines and prescribes our character structure. That character structure is only mildly, if at all, changed by all these wonderful ponderous efforts we make to be helpful. We try to bring about a state I'd call "undue influence" on those who come complaining about this hypnosis their mother put upon them. I hasten to add, for political reasons, of course, that I'm not talking about mother as an individual but the culture expressed through the family and as further expressed through the mother. *I hereby define this hypnosis as original sin #2.* Like our closet homosexuality, we each hide the post-hypnotic sacred cow image she left us with very carefully. Or, as Schatzman, in his *Soul Murder,* adds very nicely, "They taught that you don't do this thing that I'm now telling you because I tell you to do it. You do it because you know inside yourself that it is the right thing to do."

Let me back up for a minute. We old men claim the right to tell fables about our childhood. Growing up on a Lake Placid area dairy farm, I was trained for the first 13 years to save the world and, of course, now in this venerated moment, I can be clear that my mother is looking down at her white knight and his Christ-like saving the world against all the evil pressures from the latest devil. In my early teens, she helped switch me from being Christ to being an M.D., which of course was merely a paradoxical ploy. It's taken me many years of being the patient and many more years of being a covert patient disguised as therapist to discover how carefully I was hypnotized. First of all, I was "told" I should grow up to be whatever I wanted to be. This made the fact of her veneration for the church, her respectful devotion to the minister and playing the organ for our country church so much more powerful. It helped me gain this cloistered podium, which is not unlike that one. In my teen years, I wanted the admiration she had for our local doc. She and I also stored away in my motivational brain cells the veneration she had for her high school chum who became superintendent of a New York State mental hospital. This family controlled post-hypnotic suggestion not only included modeling after my father as a dairy farmer workaholic but the more subtle hypnosis of my nonhuman environment. My garage looks like the tool shed on my childhood farm and I even make my two-hundred dollar suit look like overalls in loyalty to that father. So it's easy for me to say to the wife of a Wisconsin dairy farm family, "How long after you married did you find out your husband loved the cows more than he did you?" She says, "Oh, I always knew that." The significance of this kind of hypnosis and its overall power was delightfully apparent a few years ago when our six children were home for Christmas vacation with spouses and grandchildren. The dinner table was more crowded than in those young days when the children knew that the way to spark the old man into involvement was to spill milk, but now in one meal I arranged to spill milk three times, thus reactivating my hypnosis and theirs in a return to the "good old days."

## UNDUE INFLUENCE

To define the "undue influence" quality of psychotherapy, one needs to develop only a few components of the original infantile induction. The first of these is the quality of *isolation*. The fearsome world is outside. Mother and I are the real world. I once recorded, for 100 hours of therapy, the time from the beginning of the interview until the word mother was first used. It turned out to be approximately five minutes. Secondly, recapitulation of the childhood hypnosis is facilitated by the freedom to move close and to move away, that *flux* so characteristic of sexual intercourse, breast-feeding, family belongingness and independence. A third component in the evolution of undue influence or the reactivation of mother's hypnosis is the freedom to "talk about" or metacommunicate. There's nothing mother did easier than saying, "Yes, dear, that's nice. No, dear, don't do that. Tell me about school." It's also characteristic of psychotherapy that we move toward a meta-experience. In my office, this usually involves *playing* with puzzles, throwing Nerf balls or Nerf frisbees, playing murderous fun experiences with Bataca bats and the occurrence of endless deliberate, accidental or intuitive meta-signals. Or, even as we're doing now, metacommunicating about meta-patterns.

The fourth component is not generally accepted. The best recapitulation of the family scene includes two parents. We call it co-therapy. The mother's hypnotic effect is not induced by her but by the "they."

One of my schizophrenics, many years ago, in the process of her recovery, had a dream. She was backed up against the wall by her mother, who had both hands around my patient's neck. Mother then glanced down to the far end of the long state hospital hall where father was seated in a rocking chair and quietly rocking back and forth. As mother looked down the hall, father gently nodded his head. At this point the patient was clear in her dream that mother would go on and choke her to death. Hypnosis can be merely a dyadic event but I assume it is more powerful if there is a "they," that mysterious paranoid other that gives the child a group to belong to, an experience of triangulation and a training in how to live in aloneness.

Family psychotherapy also includes the formation of a *meta-family,* that suprafamily that includes, in my model, two therapists or more—I've used up to 12. In this process reactivating the hypnotic experience is much more covert and therefore perhaps much more invasive.

Assuming, as I do, that hypnosis is always bilateral, it starts out with one therapist being willing to be hypnotized by the patient, or by the family—that is, daring to be vulnerable. Haley, Bateson et al. called it a double bind. Daring to care is the way we usually verbalize it. Without the anesthesia of that caring I suspect the powerhouse system we call the family would not allow undue influence. In the family versus the therapy team contest it's very clear that after the first few interviews the family has the greater power.

## FAMILY HYPNOSIS

The hypnotic induction of a family begins most easily through the development of an emerging sense of the whole, a family nationalism: "The Campbells never quit fighting." Affect contributions come from the subsystems, whether it's each generation as an entity or sexually identified subgroups or collusive triangles. They are, of course, supported by the detailed contributions of individuals. These symbolic icons include the father (known in the good old days as the Heavenly Father) and the executive officer (known in the good old days as the Virgin Mother). Such a double bind!—the untouchable dreamer and the master of the soup kitchen!

We label Erickson's concept of gaining control "the battle for structure." It's more overt and direct in family therapy than in individual therapy. The successful battle for control is usually fought over the telephone before the first interview. Whatever the family expects is expanded to demand more time and more people, to deny overt requests for hospitalization, or medication, or long-term therapy plans. It has almost become a rule that if you can't be accepted as parent before the first interview it will be very difficult to take control during the first interview. Once control is established, the therapist must augment his own caring. Once the family has become part of the treatment suprasystem, it is easier to change the interactional system if you change the therapist and his orientation. Family therapy is also characterized by the indirectness that was Erickson's forte. The use of obtuse, circumventing, confusing invasions by the therapist is very useful. Direct educational approaches are ordinarily uesless. Family therapists have long been clear that direct exposure of the family's deeply hidden dynamics may resolve the crisis—or result in further protectiveness. In fact, it's probably wise to leave the identified patient completely on the sidelines for the entire therapy. Changing the family as a symptom context is like changing an alcoholic spouse. It's more useful than any effort to change the identified patient. It doesn't help to treat lobar pneumonia as though it were just a cough; it may even be fatal.

In psychotherapy we struggle endlessly with the fact that most people live fragmented lives. They are preoccupied with the horrors and the glories of the past or they are preoccupied with the horrors and the glories of the future. They don't live; they just use their left brain to endlessly think about living. This kind of meta-living is just like metacommunication—the disease that all psychotherapists are suffering from. We spend our lives talking about talking, and many times never say anything. Even worse, if we're not very careful, metacommunicating contaminates the rest of our living and the rest of our talking. Medical students who are learning psychotherapy say, "The problem with this racket is that whenever I go on a date, I end up being a psychotherapist instead of a boyfriend, and I don't know how I get there."

We even do it with each other. If I can't be your therapist, I flip the other side of the coin and become your patient. We not only have the disease ourselves, but we're carriers. We contaminate our patients, and that's bad by itself. But it's even worse because almost all marriages in America now are bilateral pseudo-therapy projects. She's just the girl for him as soon as she gets over her compulsiveness, and he's just the man for her as soon as she gets him over his alcoholism. And then they spend the first five years of their marriage (it used to be ten years) trying to be better psychotherapists and better patients until it becomes a therapeutic impasse, and then they come for help. So when you see a couple, it's really not psychotherapy, it's supervision. They are trying to learn how to be better psychotherapists or better patients or both.

What is the essential objective of psychotherapy? If it's really second-degree psychotherapy, and not counseling or adequacy training or psychological education or some other contaminant, maybe it's to get rid of the past (good and bad) and the future (good and bad) and just be. That is, develop your personhood or your capacity to be who you are, wherever you are, etc. Ehrenwahl called that the existential shift. And every once in a while I get a patient who has it happen. It is a very exciting thing to have happen. The language change is dramatic. One talks in the present.

A patient I saw yesterday, mother of two anorexia nervosa daughters and the wife of a systems analyst husband, said, "I called my daughter to talk about the appointment today, and then I called you and you were upset about it. So I called her back, knowing that if it was to be different, she would be there, and if it wasn't to be different she wouldn't be at her apartment." This was kind of a strange emersion in the present-tense world of her living process. It was all right with her, whichever way the world turned; she would be accepting of it even ahead of time. The thing that was strange is not that she did it, but that it's such a surprise. I never seem to expect it. The present tense isn't something that we live in.

Anybody who is really studying the few grown-up people in the world will say that the most dramatic part about them is their personhood; they are a presence. Barbara Betz says, "The dynamics of psychotherapy are in the person of the therapist." I have had personal contact with three or four people whom I think could say the ABC's and it would be a personally significant experience for the other guy. One was Alan Gregg, who was president of the Rockefeller Foundation. One is Isaac Bashevis Singer, the Nobel Prize winning Jewish writer. There are a couple more. One was a Welsh preacher I heard lecture when I was in college. I went up to talk to him about what to do about my life. We had a very interesting talk. When I got through I said good-bye. He shook hands and said, "Give my regards to your father." This was 50 years ago and I can't forget it. It was the strangest experience. It was out of nowhere. An eerie kind of validation of me. We had said nothing about my father. It was like his peculiar kind of perception, a peculiar kind of Ericksonian way of saying "I'm glad to have met you."

I had a similar experience with Gregory Bateson when I was a resident. I wrote to several people who were exciting to me and asked to meet them at the American Psychiatric Association convention. I did that two or three times with Gregory Bateson. He and I would go into a bar and sit down for a drink. You didn't have to say anything to Gregory; all you had to do was say, "Hello" and from then on he cooked. I think Gregory could have said the ABC's and I would have grown by the experience. I was learning from him how to focus myself—how to be all in one place—how to be all in one direction. That's the existential shift—how to narrow your world until you're in the present tense. I think the change of language has to do with the disappearance of the conditional tense, the disappearance of the mythological themes: "I wish it could be," "I think it should have been,"—the "shoulds," "woulds," or "coulds." All of those seem to fall away. It has some of the quality of the manic patient who within three minutes will name 250 things. He's not thinking, he's just seeing and putting it in words. He is letting his unconscious take over, only crossing the corpus callosum into the verbal analytic side for the sake of communication. There is no programming it through the computer to see whether it agrees with past conclusions, conceptual frameworks, parental orders or cultural demands. It's really very exciting. But I think it's like a sexual turn-on in that you can respond to it or not respond to it. I am amazed when I hear it. Often I may not have heard it.

In therapy, once the family has a firm attachment to its meta-family, the process becomes one of increasing communication freedom with the opening of new options and extensive experience in the back-and-forth traffic across the corpus callosum from right brain total gestalt and intuition, to left brain symbolic use of language in consciousness and operationalized by the organizational capacities of the whole person. It used to be said that the process was mostly an effort to develop communication. Now it feels to me as though much of the traffic is in the other direction. We use our hypnotic-like power to expand access to primary process by way of play, by way of metaphor, by way of precipitating behavioral interactions and by way of body contact. The most graphic and powerful educator in this evolution, of course, is the young child. Hypnotic induction by way of cuddling the one-year-old is like magic in family therapy. Further support for our therapeutic project may evolve from an invasion of the three-generational or four-generational family system and hopefully we cultural cryptologists can help them by means of a short course in family code-breaking.

When therapy is successful, there develops in the therapeutic system cues which enable the therapist and later the family itself to regress to an infantile mother-child role set. The family is thus prepared to regress in the service of the family ego and simultaneously gain freedom to help the individuals and subgroups regress in the service of their individual maturing. The basis for this process evolves from the initial freedom of the therapist or the therapeutic team to rehypnotize themselves. The therapists must learn to modify the covert hypnosis of childhood and its subliminal cue turn-ons to an increasing freedom for self-hypnosis, and thereby an increased freedom to move in and out of this self-hypnosis and thereby the gradual emergence of free-flowing creative impulses. This movement inevitably preciptates anxiety in the therapist. This is in direct contrast with the ancient dictum that psychotherapy is a process in which one of the dyad is anxious—and hopefully that one is not the therapist. I'm convinced that the hypnosis is bilateral and hopefully the therapist is self-hypnotized and does it first. Many times I fear that the family hypnotizes the therapist first and then he struggles to break out of his own hypnosis by trying to hypnotize the family. Many times he doesn't make it and then the therapeutic party is a flop.

Though I had read little of Erickson before being invited to this lecture, and although I've never done hypnosis in any deliberate way, I find, in reading Jay Haley and Erickson, many similarities to my methodology for working with the family on a growth model. This is based on an assumption that the family itself is the patient. One can take the family where it operationally exists, joining it not where it thinks it is but where you observe it to be. A family may ask for help with a delinquent teenager or a drug-abusing college student when it's very clear that this symptom of the family's pain is covering more serious problems. Every family presents with a face-saving symptom even if it is a schizophrenic family member. Behind that is father's loneliness or mother's obesity or father's drive toward a coronary out of his bitter war with mother or maybe her loss of self-esteem. The schizophrenic may also have thrust his holy spirit into the triangle of father/mother and one or both mothers-in-law. Precipitation of the family into being more seriously concerned with the early death of father or the suicidal impulses of mother may escalate the family into a kind of bewildered confusion and those multiple stress reverberations that Erickson so neatly responded to in his work.

Subsumed in the process of the family's pain and their inability to break out of their lifetime chaos and its crippling effect is the presence of culture-induced stress. This is injected under the name of such themes as religion, nationalism, societal roles or ethnic tensions. Samples of these pressures are widespread; e.g., "We can only think in words," "You must love the other and not yourself," "Self-worth is measured in dollars," "Life is for working," "Nations, like women, are in constant danger of rape," "Only women love children."

Time is the essential presence of mother in the now and the clock is itself our god. So the induction of a useful stage of undue influence which I call hypnosis allows that isolation which gives the family the courage to defy some of these cultural hypnotic tricks.

The first step, then, in good family therapy is the freedom of the therapist to allow himself to be hypnotized, that is, to conquer his own fear of being unduly influenced. This involves, as David Rioch once said, a kind of maturity that he defined as *the capacity to be immature.* Can the therapist accept his vulnerability and allow an identification with the family and the submersion of his personhood into the family?

The second step in inducing deliberate undue influence is to invade the family and then to back off from the family. It's like a repeated hypnosis and rupture of hypnosis. The therapist allows himself to be induced and repeatedly escapes again, thus modeling for the family its freedom to regress and to fight its way free of the hypnotic spell put on it by the therapist. The process patterns later freedom on the part of the family to regress without needing to be hypnotized by the therapist and he thus patterns for the family courage for joining and individuating by the individuals and the subgroups within it. They learn to move into and out of hypnosis without the need of an outside vector, either by induction from the therapist or by the culture.

Successful therapy may lead the family to expand its boundaries to include its neighbors and even the "family of man." Then we can define family maturity as a nonhypnotic state of enjoying the absurdity of hypnotizing each individual and each person hypnotizing the family.

One other way of describing psychotherapy is to say that the family is the person and the therapist is the context. Furthermore, every family is crazy, that is, each lives in a world of pathological, irrational components. The therapist is expected to replace the chaotic component that society represents. When the therapist dares to become crazy he double binds the patient and sets up an arrangement such that the patient is forced to take the opposite pole of their interactional system and fulfill the sane and phobic role. This shift (back and forth across the corpus callosum if you will) sets up a contract. The patient can be crazy or sane depending upon the pressure. In just such fashion, the family as a system can become crazy or sane, intimate, silly, ridiculous, fun-loving, or at another time, rational, systematized, organized, and socially corrective. When that takes place, the family becomes therapeutic to its individual members.

Let's return for a moment to my own particular hypnotic life pattern. I began in 1945 to have episodes of going to sleep when I was the therapist. For the first four or five years I was horribly embarrassed, struggled to keep myself awake, apologized, went for therapy to break it up, etc. Gradually, as I became more tolerant of the beingness that was me, I dared to bring my dreams back from the sleep. Time after time they proved relevant to the therapeutic component of the interview.

Hypnosis is undoubtedly possible without the awareness of either the therapist or the family in the same sense that a couple fall in love without either one of them knowing what each has done to the other or what has happened to them. Psychotherapy then can be an experiential microproject of parenting. It's my assumption that the pressure for biological healing is identical in a weak back or a weak spirit. The universal objective is growth, that is, increased integration and increased personhood. Living demands a better integration in the body of the individual as well as in the family system as a body. The chief complaint that the family fronts with is a face-saver, a test pattern in the family's drive for change and the effort to seduce the therapist into developing a suprafamily in which the therapist and the co-therapist will take over.

Hypnosis is a bilateral two-person event just like craziness and suicide. Craziness involves someone who's willing to be crazy and someone who's insistent upon being sane. In the family, it is usually the mother who has a phobia about craziness. In suicide the two-person event includes someone who wants to be dead and someone else who will benefit by or wants that person dead.

The uses of projection within the family are very similar to those the hypnotist utilizes, except that the family therapist becomes the hypnotist and stage director. One of the most obvious dreams is the pairing between a father and daughter, or mother and son. When a divorce action is imminent, we suggest that the family sell the house and buy two condominiums or rent two apartments and daughter could cook for dad and son could take out the garbage for mother. If worse came to worst, father and mother could get together while son and daughter went out to a movie. Similar systems imbedded in the multigeneration projections that are covert in every family can be exposed by a facetious, tongue-in-cheek process within the family pattern. For example, the parentified son can be teased into demanding an adult status with the therapist and then cut down to child size. The therapist may tease him about taking over mother's job—that if he's going to be mother's mother and he is going to tell her how to spend the money or handle the household, then mother will have to be his little girl and he will have to cook for her, and that would make him his own grandmother. If he became the mother then he would be married to his own father, and that would make him a homosexual. The post-hypnotic residuals of such right brain fun often echo through the livingroom, diningroom and into the backyard.

The induction system in family therapy is thus focused to change the family as a whole and carefully not change any individual member. This may include a kind of hypnotic assault on the scapegoat. The therapist begins in the first interview to disconfirm the scapegoat, refusing to talk about his problem and possibly refusing to talk to the scapegoat about anything. In a similar manner he disconfirms mother by insisting that the person farthest outside the family start the family history. Father is not permitted to talk about any individual, not even himself, but must talk about the family's style of living over time and its dynamics of operation, and even its daily schedule. Once the family has conceded to the therapist's role as a senior parent person and has accepted the offer to regress and be childlike, this can be reinforced by all sorts of childlike actions, usually instigated by the therapist. I potentiate this meta-living by playing with puzzles, throwing Nerf balls and Nerf frisbees, playing with teddy bears, offering children of any age a baby bottle or sitting on the floor at mother's or father's feet to play with the little children while talking with the grown-ups. In fact, the therapist's becoming childlike may be a model for instigating regression and a bilateral hypnosis. In my interaction with families I may also become their child inside myself. They may often represent in my inner transference experience my mother, my father, my sister, or my brother.

Part of the usefulness of family therapy as a discipline lies in the effort to break through a mythology in our culture about psychotherapy as helpfulness. The therapist may himself be deeply stained with this. Generations of religious servant monk models have left their mark. Most of us are typical do-gooders who carefully disguise our delusion that a Thanksgiving turkey is the best way to take care of welfare patients. If we can only learn to do the right thing, all psychological ills will pass away. Behind this are other multiple generation myths: We were conceived in sin, giving is more blessed than receiving, I am the sinful one and the least worthy of all God's children, and self-denial is the best way to get into heaven. Self-denial is the basis for being seen as a good person in our social structure.

One of the most powerful factors in establishing undue influence is the clarity with which the therapist accepts the fact that he is not up to *doing anything* for the family. He's there for his own growth, for his own enjoyment of himself and for his enjoyment of the family. This makes it possible for them to take the responsibility for their own expansion, their own struggle, and for changing their mythological rules.

One psychotic, after 17 years of treatment by various, sophisticated agents and spending two years in co-therapy with us, was asked what had made the difference between this two years and his previous episodes. (He was pretty well cured—well, not quite—he went to medical school.) He said, "Oh, it was one hour. One day you and Tom Malone and I were here for a whole hour and nobody was up to anything. I had never experienced that kind of beingness before nor have I since. It changed my entire world."

In trying to relate my family psychotherapy to the world of the hypnotist I need to be historical again. I recall the accidental discovery in 1945 that sucking up a baby bottle full of milk flipped one manic psychotic into health in less than two weeks. I decided that the bottle-feeding mother process was curative. For the next three years I fed everybody from a bottle, holding most patients in my lap while rocking and singing nursery rhymes to them. Then the technique lost its flavor. I have never been able to do it again. It was as though I was developing my own maternal, affective competence. I spent the next two years instigating a physical struggle with almost every patient, with arm-wrestling, hand-wrestling, etc. That too lost its value as I became more in charge of the therapy and needed less manipulation. I was by then less easily captured by the double bind of the patient or, if you will, not so easily hypnotized.

Success in family therapy seems to result from increasing the power of the family and then its generosity in the use and distribution of its power to the individuals and to the subgroups. With the increasing individuation thus created, there comes increasing homeostasis, that is, the family's increased freedom to expand its boundaries and contract them follows as the therapist expands himself within the interview and contracts himself as he returns to his personal and professional life after the family has terminated the interview.

The extended family conference may present the most graphic description of family system dynamics. Even if the conference seems to be unproductive in character, the results frequently reveal an increased integration within the family and its members and an openness to including neighbors and even "the family of man."

In the very beginning of family therapy one must expand the family's commitment to itself as a unit, a living, operating self-actualizing system. Unique to family therapy is our greater freedom for confrontation than in working with individual patients. I call this availability a transference phenomenon. Apparently Erickson called this "the establishment of trust." It may be facilitated by a complete denial of the identified patient and helping the father to define his parental power vector and to expose his isolation and loneliness. Help in developing group stress is aided by joining forces with the little children or the white-knight scapegoat. Behind this is our effort to participate in the anxiety-ridden unconscious of the family itself. Deliberately inducing paranoia about death, about divorce, about craziness, about suicidal impulses, murderous impulses and the time changes in the family tends to open parts of the unconscious that are carefully covered. I firmly believe the family's homeostasis is so powerful that the therapist need not fear that he will overwhelm the family. The only danger in family therapy is that the therapist may be impotent or be extruded by the family.

Mobilizing the family by inducing anxiety brings a better morale and increases its power to neutralize the family in-fighting and actuate an operational readiness for change in the family system.

Once a trusting relationship has been set up with the family, the therapist's own personal concerns with what the family is doing to damage itself or failing to do to correct its pain become a basic factor in defusing or detumescing the scapegoat and in establishing a readiness on the part of the family to struggle with the family pathology. There's considerable similarity in this to Erickson's system of finding a common enemy and joining the family in its war against the school system or physical illness or an existential impulse for suicide or craziness.

Inducing mystification in the family is further amplified by an irrational disruption of the interview when the therapist and the co-therapist suddenly move out of pattern. Diversional techniques—playing with Nerf balls, sitting on the floor to play with one of the children without explanation—relieve the family's tension. Involving three teenage children with three Nerf frisbees in a tossing game tends to leave the family quite defenseless and their fear about fear or anxiety about anxiety is often dissipated or at least disrupted. It's hard to play and still moan about craziness. It's amazing what happens, if, in the middle of an interview, you suddenly have the impulse to go to the bathroom, so you get up and go to the bathroom; or you suddenly have the impulse to go out and get your telephone messages, so you get up and go get your telephone messages. And, if you feel like it and one looks like an interesting telephone call, you make the call. You come back ten minutes later and they say, "Where were you?" You say, "What do you mean?" "Well, what did you go out for?" "I didn't want to be here." "Well, you didn't say anything about it." "I know." "Well, why didn't you say something?" "I didn't want to."

It's this strange process of being more yourself than they dare to be. For example, a father says something and I say, "You know, I think you are lying." He says, "I'm not lying." I say, "What does that have to do with it?" He replies, "Well, you shouldn't say I'm lying if I'm not." So I say, "I didn't say that you were lying. I just said that I thought you were lying." "Well, I'm not." "Well, it doesn't make any difference to me. I'm just telling you what I thought. And I'm very old and very stubborn and don't expect me to change my mind just because you disagree with me."

I'm through.

# Name Index

References for M.H. Erickson include only citations of specific works within the text.

# Subject Index

SKETCHES BY BOZ
AND OTHER EARLY PAPERS
1833–39

THE DENT UNIFORM EDITION OF

# DICKENS' JOURNALISM

## SKETCHES BY BOZ

AND OTHER EARLY PAPERS

1833–39

EDITED BY MICHAEL SLATER

*With illustrations by George Cruikshank*

Ohio State University Press

COLUMBUS

Published in the United States by the Ohio State University Press
Published simultaneously in Great Britain by J. M. Dent

*Sketches by Boz* first published in Everyman's Library in 1907
*Study Under Three Heads* first published in *Reprinted Pieces* in Everyman's Library in 1921

Chronology from *The Dickens Index* by Nicolas Bentley, Michael Slater, and Nina Burgis (1988); reprinted with permission from Oxford University Press

Library of Congress Cataloging-in-Publication Data
Dickens, Charles, 1812–1870.
Sketches by Boz and other early papers, 1833–39 / edited by Michael Slater; with illustrations by George Cruikshank.
p. cm. — (The Dent uniform edition of Dickens' journalism)
ISBN 0-8142-0629-8 (alk. paper)
I. Slater, Michael. II. Cruikshank, 1792–1878. III. Title.
IV. Title: Sketches by Boz. V. Series: Dickens, Charles, 1812–1870. Journalism.
PR4570.A2S57 1994
823'.8—dc20 93-36399
CIP

Filmset in Baskerville by Selwood Systems, Midsomer Norton.
Printed in Great Britain by Butler & Tanner Ltd., Frome and London,
for J. M. Dent, Orion Publishing Group, London.



The paper in this book meets the guidelines for permanence and durability of the Committee on Production Guidelines for Book Longevity of the Council on Library Resources.

9 8 7 6 5 4 3 2 1

# CONTENTS

*Characters*



*Tales*

OTHER EARLY PAPERS

# PREFACE

*The Dent Uniform Edition of Dickens' Journalism* presents, for the first time in annotated form, all the journalism that Dickens published in collected form during his lifetime, *Sketches by Boz*, *Reprinted Pieces* and *The Uncommercial Traveller*. It also includes an early pamphlet, *Sunday Under Three Heads*, and a substantial selection of the many essays and reviews that were never collected by Dickens himself yet contain much material of outstanding interest. The earliest of these papers, those contributed to *Bentley's Miscellany*, were first collected as *The Mudfog Papers* by G. Bentley in 1880 (reprinted 1984). The later essays and reviews were first gathered together by B.W. Matz, the first editor of *The Dickensian* in 1908, as part of the National Edition of Dickens's works. The *Miscellaneous Papers*, as they were called, were reprinted with additions and retitled *Collected Papers* by Matz's successor, Walter Dexter, in the luxurious limited Nonesuch Edition (1937). Since then there has been one reprint of *Miscellaneous Papers* (1983) but the great mass of all this vintage Dickens writing has remained largely unobtainable outside libraries.

The texts of *Sketches by Boz* and the other material in Vol. 1, and of *Reprinted Pieces* and *The Uncommercial Traveller*, are those of the Charles Dickens Edition (the last edition of his works to be published in Dickens's lifetime). Misprints have been corrected and hyphens omitted in accordance with modern usage (for example, 'to-day' becomes 'today').

In order to fully understand and appreciate Dickens's journalistic achievement the modern reader inevitably needs a certain amount of background information and explanatory annotation. This Uniform Edition supplies such help in the form of headnotes preceding each piece, supplemented at the end of the volume by an index that is also a glossary and a dictionary of proper names. It is hoped that this combination, will, while avoiding a proliferation of footnotes, provide readers with all necessary information.

M.S.

# INTRODUCTION

*Sketches by Boz*, Dickens's first book, which consists mainly of collected journalistic pieces written between December 1833 and December 1836, has a complicated publishing history. Its familiar divisions – 'Our Parish', 'Scenes', 'Characters' and 'Tales' – were not arrived at until late 1837 when Dickens was preparing a composite, serialised reissue of the two-volume *Sketches by Boz* of February 1836 and the one-volume *Sketches by Boz: Second Series* of December 1836. And he did not stop revising the text until 1850 when *Sketches* was included in the first collected edition of his works. This introduction traces the intricate story of the moulding of Dickens's earliest writings into *Sketches by Boz* as we know it, and I wish to acknowledge at the outset a general indebtedness to the pioneer work of Kathleen Tillotson in *Dickens at Work* (1957; jointly written with John Butt), and to Duane DeVries's detailed study of the genesis of *Sketches* in his *Dickens's Apprentice Years* (1976).

The summer of 1833 was a critical time for the 21-year-old Dickens. In May his passion for the pretty banker's daughter Maria Beadnell was finally, and painfully, quenched and the Parliamentary recess had left him temporarily jobless (he had been working as a reporter for *The Mirror of Parliament*, a rival of Hansard's, also reporting debates for the *True Sun*). At this juncture, Dickens, who was fiercely ambitious, even though now deprived of the spur of 'bettering himself' in the eyes of the Beadnells, decided the time had come to heat up one of the other irons he had in the fire as regards his future career. He had, 'for some time past', been noting down materials for a projected series of magazine articles to be entitled 'Our Parish' and had also had an idea for a novel – perhaps the one that became *Oliver Twist* three and a half years later (*Pilgrim*, Vol. 1, p. 34). Now he made his first attempt on the literary market with a comic tale about the miseries of a misanthropic middle-aged bachelor forced to venture into the outer suburbs to pay a Sunday visit to some vulgar relatives who hope he will make their horrible child his heir. Years later, in the Preface to the Cheap (1847) Edition of *Pickwick*, Dickens described how, 'stealthily one evening at twilight', he dropped this manuscript 'with fear and trembling into a dark letter box, in a dark office, up a dark court in Fleet Street'. The letter box belonged to a small circulation journal called the *Monthly Magazine*, recently bought by a former aide-de-camp to Simon Bolivar, one Captain Holland who hoped to use it to forward the cause of Radicalism.

Holland liked Dickens's offering and published it in the December number of the *Monthly* under the title 'A Dinner at Poplar Walk' (Dickens later retitled it 'Mr Minns and his Cousin'). He invited further contributions from its author whilst regretting that he could not offer payment. But Dickens was so happy to see his work 'in all the glory of print' that he was content over the next year to supply six more tales to the *Monthly* – 'Mrs Joseph Porter', 'Horatio Sparkins', 'The Bloomsbury Christening', 'The Boarding House', 'The Steam Excursion' and 'Mr Watkins Tottle'. These farcical stories, in which Dickens's literary skills can clearly be seen developing, have for their subject matter the social and material preoccupations of nineteenth-century middle and lower class life: legacy-hunting, gentility, getting daughters well married, keeping up with the Joneses, and so on. Kathryn Chittick has pointed out that the earlier ones are set in a higher social sphere than any the young Dickens was personally familiar with, but that with 'The Boarding House' (May and August 1834) he 'finally stakes out his peculiar caste and territory', that special field of interest which Forster defined as 'a sort of life between the middle class and the low which, having few attractions for bookish observers, was quite unhackneyed ground'. It is, interestingly, with the second instalment of 'The Boarding House' that Dickens first used the pen-name 'Boz', as though to announce his coming into his literary own, and to signal that he wished his scattered pieces now to be thought of as the work of one distinctive writer. 'Boz' became his trademark, having originated as a family joke: one of his younger brothers was nicknamed 'Moses' after Dr Primrose's son in Goldsmith's *Vicar of Wakefield*; the little boy pronounced it 'Boses', which became shortened to 'Boz' (whether the 'o' should be short or long is a recurrent matter of debate for Dickens devotees).

The *Monthly Magazine* stories attracted a certain amount of approving notice from contemporary reviewers but did not make a great mark, perhaps because they were not sufficiently distinct from other comic journalism and popular drama treating similar subjects. One of them, 'The Bloomsbury Christening', was in fact turned into 'an amusing interlude' at the Adelphi Theatre by the popular comic actor, J.B. Buckstone (and was reviewed with rueful humour by Dickens himself). Dickens's real originality emerged in the five 'Street Sketches' he contributed under his 'Boz' signature to the *Morning Chronicle* between late September and early November 1834, shortly after he had succeeded in being taken on to the permanent staff of this paper, the leading Liberal voice in the British press.

These five sketches, 'Omnibuses', 'Shops and their Tenants', 'The Old

Bailey' (later retitled 'Criminal Courts'), 'Shabby-genteel People' and 'Brokers' and Marine-store Shops', represented something completely new in descriptions of London. Essayists like Charles Lamb, Leigh Hunt and Washington Irving had written romantically about the city with a particular predilection for its quaint old corners and antiquarian associations (Dickens was later to attempt this vein himself in the guise of Master Humphrey), and Pierce Egan in his hugely popular *Life in London* (1820) had taken his readers on rowdy sprees into the night-houses, 'boozing kens' and other lowlife attractions of the metropolis. But it was left to Dickens, the trained reporter, with eyes that missed nothing, and ears that picked up the actual language of the streets rather than the stylised slang of Egan's work, to astonish the readers of the *Chronicle* and, later, the reading public in general with the 'startling fidelity' with which he rendered the sights and sounds of ordinary daily life in the streets of London – the cheery insolence of omnibus cads, for example, or the desperate attempts of 'shabby-genteel' men to keep up appearances. But 'Boz' is not simply an animated camera cum tape recorder. He has a heart and invokes our sympathy for the poor girl struggling vainly to make a living as a 'fancy stationer', or the impoverished mother whose young son has already become a criminal. Already in these sketches Dickens is experimenting, very effectively, with that blending of the wildly comic and the intensely pathetic that was to win and keep him such thousands of devoted readers in after years.

It was not customary for features like these sketches in a daily newspaper to be noticed in the contemporary press (unlike comic tales in a magazine). But they were well received – we know that the *Chronicle*'s editor John Black thought highly of them – and he was invited to contribute similar work to the new tri-weekly paper, the *Evening Chronicle*, established in January 1835 under the editorship of Dickens's future father-in-law, George Hogarth. Up to this point Dickens had earned nothing by his writings except possibly for the one tale, 'Sentiment', he had published not in the *Monthly* but in *Bell's Weekly Magazine* (7 June 1834). Now, however, he felt he had sufficiently established himself as a writer (as distinct from as a journalist) to ask for payment for his literary work over and above his weekly reporter's salary of five guineas. He proposed to Hogarth to write as 'Boz' a series of twenty 'Sketches of London', and asked for an increase of two guineas in his salary. It was promptly agreed.

The series began on 31 January 1835 with a comic essay on transport in London, 'Hackney Coach Stands', paralleling 'Omnibuses' which had been his first offering for the *Morning Chronicle*. This was followed a week later by 'Gin Shops', which strikes a grimmer note than any 'Boz' had yet sounded in its vivid description of the 'filth and squalid misery' of the area surrounding the opulent gin shops, a note heard again a few months later in 'The Pawnbroker's Shop' (Dickens places these two papers together in his final arrangement of *Sketches*). 'Gin Shops' also ends with some fierce polemic directed against Temperance Societies which condemn gin drinkers but can provide 'no antidote against hunger and disease'. The majority of these *Evening Chronicle* sketches, however, either belong to the 'Parish' series, predominantly comic with occasional passages of pathos, or focus on London at play (for example, 'Greenwich Fair', 'Astley's'). Apart from the harshly supercilious tone of 'Private Theatres', the dominant attitude of 'Boz' in these sketches is one of delighted and sympathetic observation of popular metropolitan diversions. Other sketches draw directly on Dickens's experiences as a Parliamentary reporter and, in 'Early Coaches', the unsocial hours travelling which was part of his job as a newspaperman.

The *Evening Chronicle* series ended with the last of the 'Parish' sketches, 'The Ladies' Societies', which seems to be reverting to the genre of the *Monthly Magazine* tales in that it is a comic story about social one-upmanship in the suburban middle classes. The Brown and Johnson Parker ladies with their competing charitable organisations clearly come from the same world as the rival Taunton and the Briggs families in 'The Steam Excursion', although they are less dramatised and there is less of farce and more of generalised social satire in the narrative. This sketch, together with the four other 'Parish' ones which cluster in the second half of the *Evening Chronicle* series, seems to indicate a desire in Dickens to return to stories about characters rather than confining himself to 'Scenes'. This is borne out by a new series entitled 'Scenes and Characters' that he began contributing to *Bell's Life in London* in September 1835, immediately following the end of the *Evening Chronicle* series. For *Bell's Life* he also used a different pen-name; he writes as 'Tibbs', a name humorously borrowed from one of his own *Monthly Magazine* stories, 'The Boarding House', the joke being that Mr Tibbs spends most of his time in that story trying to tell a story but never succeeds because his wife is always interrupting him ('He was a melancholy specimen of the story-teller. He was the Wandering Jew of Joe Millerism'). So Dickens, by now very much a writer conscious of having a public, both ensures the recognition of the common authorship of the *Monthly* tales and *Bell's Life* sketches, and shares a running joke about that authorship with his readers.

Like the *Chronicle*, *Bell's Life* was Liberal in its politics but was a weekly paper which carried sporting news and comic features as well as news, so was more recreational in character. Indeed, as Kathryn Chittick has noted, it was 'established in 1822 to take advantage of the fad for Egan's *Life in London*'. For it Dickens wrote twelve papers, five of which are comic tales about farcical mishaps in the social life of characters drawn from the 'Tibbs' class or just below it – 'Miss Evans and the Eagle', 'The Dancing Academy', 'Making a Night of It', 'Love and Oysters' (retitled 'The

Misplaced Attachment of Mr John Dounce' when collected) and 'The Vocal Dressmaker' (also later retitled 'The Mistaken Milliner'). They are much funnier because more sharply focussed than the *Monthly* tales. Dickens is absolutely sure of his ground and does not – except in 'Love and Oysters' – need to fall back on stock farce types and situations as he had done in the earlier stories. The Camden Town belle Miss Jemima Evans and her young man 'with his hair carefully twisted into the outer corner of each eye till it formed a variety of that description of semi-curls, usually known as "aggerewators" '; Miss Amelia Martin 'chirruping' at the fateful wedding party in a Somers Town front parlour; Mr Augustus Cooper preparing for his entry into society at Signor Billsmethi's dancing academy off Gray's Inn Lane; Mr Thomas Potter and his fellow clerk Mr Robert Smithers getting themselves ignominiously turned out of the City Theatre after over-indulging in mild Havannahs and strong liquor – Dickens makes us see, and hear, all these characters in their very precisely located settings. He also treated *Bell*'s readers to a full-length portrait and history of an omnibus cad, a wonderfully impudent species of humanity that he had shown himself fascinated by in the *Chronicle* sketches.

In addition, the *Bell*'s series includes four sketches which are continuous with the *Chronicle* ones, one indeed, 'The Streets at Night', directly complementing 'The Streets – Morning' (*Evening Chronicle*, 21 July 1835). The others, 'Seven Dials', 'The Prisoners' Van' and 'The Parlour' (which becomes 'The Parlour Orator' when collected), present London sights and scenes very much in the manner of sketching 'Boz' rather than of anecdotal 'Tibbs'. 'The Prisoners' Van' echoes 'The Pawnbroker's Shop' in its juxtaposing of hardened female degradation and a young girl not yet completely ruined but (no doubt with an eye to *Bell*'s more raffish readers, 'swells' and men about town) Dickens is here much more urgent and direct in his comments on the situation:

> These things pass before our eyes, day after day, and hour after hour – they have become such matters of course, that they are utterly disregarded. The progress of these girls in crime will be as rapid as the flight of a pestilence, resembling it too in its baneful influence and widespreading infection.

Two other *Bell*'s sketches, 'Christmas Festivities' (published 27 December 1835; retitled 'A Christmas Dinner' when collected) and 'The New Year' (published 3 January 1836), are seasonal pieces, probably written to round out the series to the dozen items contracted. The last *Bell*'s sketch to be published on 17 January was, in fact, 'The Streets – Night', the concluding words of which perhaps allude to the forthcoming collection of *Sketches by Boz* in volume form:

> Scenes like this are continued until three or four o'clock in the morning; and

> even when they close, fresh ones open to the inquisitive novice. But as a description of all of them, however slight, would require a volume, the contents of which, however instructive, would be by no means pleasing, we make our bow, and drop the curtain.

One might even suspect Dickens of a somewhat disingenuous come-on here, in that potential buyers of the volume edition of *Sketches by Boz* might well be led by this to expect the contents to include some exposés of metropolitan nightlife.

In fact, the two volumes published by John Macrone on 6 February 1836 contained only three new pieces: 'A Visit to Newgate', perhaps his most powerfully imaginative piece to date; a gruesomely melodramatic tale, 'The Black Veil'; and 'The Great Winglebury Duel'. The first two were written specifically for inclusion in this collection, but the third, apparently intended for the *Monthly Magazine* but perhaps kept back because Dickens had decided to dramatise it (see below, p. 389), may have been put in to boost the 'tales' element in the collection. The rest of the contents of the two volumes consisted of all the *Monthly Magazine* tales apart from the very first one, nearly all the *Morning* and *Evening Chronicle* sketches, and just four from the *Bell's* series. The collection had been planned by Macrone and Dickens at least since October 1835, when we find the first surviving reference to it in Dickens's letters (*Pilgrim*, Vol. 1, p. 81*f.*) and a very distinguished illustrator recruited in the person of George Cruikshank, proudly referred to by Dickens in his preface. To those who might not yet be heavily aware of 'Boz', the scope and interest of the little volumes was made clear by Dickens's full title – *Sketches by Boz, illustrative of Everyday Life, and Everyday People.*

That Dickens worked hard on revising the texts of the sketches and tales chosen for inclusion was first documented in detail by Kathleen Tillotson in *Dickens at Work* (1957). She shows that his revisions went a good deal beyond minor stylistic tinkering and the removal of topicalities, particularly in the introductory and concluding paragraphs. One of the most extreme instances was the cancellation (probably, as Tillotson suggests, for reasons of space at a late stage in the preparation of the volumes) of two substantial opening paragraphs in 'The Prisoners' Van'. The first of these, quoted by Tillotson, might well serve as an introduction to 'Boz's' sketches in general:

> We have a most extraordinary partiality for lounging about the streets. Whenever we have an hour or two to spare, there is nothing we enjoy more than a little amateur vagrancy – walking up one street and down another, and staring into shop windows, and gazing about as if, instead of being on intimate terms with every shop and house in Holborn, the Strand, Fleet Street and Cheapside, the whole were an unknown region to our wandering mind. We

> revel in a crowd of any kind – a street 'row' is our delight – even a woman in a fit is by no means to be despised, especially in a fourth-rate street, where all the female inhabitants run out of their houses, and discharge large jugs of cold water over the patient, as if she were dying of spontaneous combustion, and wanted putting out. Then a drunken man – what can be more charming than a regular drunken man, who sits in a doorway for half an hour, holding a dialogue with the crowd, of which his portion is generally limited to repeated inquiries of 'I say – I'm all right, an't I?' and then suddenly gets up, without any ostensible cause of inducement, and runs down the street with tremendous swiftness for a hundred yards or so, when he falls into another doorway, where the first feeble words he imperfectly articulates to the policeman who lifts him up are, 'Let's av-drop-somethin' to drink?' – we say again, can anything be more charming than this sort of thing? And what, we ask, can be expected but popular discontent, when Temperance Societies interfere with the amusements of people?

While it is clear that Dickens took great trouble over the texts of his collected tales and sketches he does not, on the other hand, seem to have been greatly exercised about their arrangement. The six 'Parish' sketches are grouped together at the beginning of the first volume. After that there seems to be no apparent order in the sequence in which the items are printed. It may well be that a sense of the variety of London life was the very effect aimed at.

The reception of the two volumes we now call *Sketches by Boz: First Series* was everything a young author might have hoped for. George Hogarth gave it what Dickens called a 'beautiful notice' in the *Morning Chronicle* on 11 February, calling its author 'a close and acute observer of character and manners, with a strong sense of the ridiculous and a graphic faculty of placing in the most whimsical and amusing lights the follies and absurdities of human nature'. He added, 'He has the power, too, of producing tears as well as laughter' through his pictures of 'the vices and wretchedness which abound in this vast city'. 'Two more amusing volumes have not appeared this season', declared the *Sun*. The *Athenaeum* praised the work's 'admirable truth'. Other journals extolled its 'racy humour an irresistible wit', the 'little touches of pathos scattered here and there' and the 'amazing reality' of the 'graphic descriptions'. Cruikshank's illustrations won very high praise too. The *Court Journal* (which called 'Boz' 'a kind of Boswell to society ... an old favourite of ours') thought that they might be considered the best things the great artist had ever done. In America, where the book appeared as *Watkins Tottle and Other Sketches*, Edgar Allan Poe praised it in the *Southern Literary Messenger* (June 1836); one of the pieces that he singled out, unsurprisingly, was 'The Black Veil', which he described as 'an act of stirring tragedy, and evincing lofty powers in the writer'.

Long before Poe's notice was published in Richmond, Virginia, however, Dickens had begun reaping the rewards of 'the great success of my book', as he called it, in a letter to his uncle Thomas Barrow (March 1836; *Pilgrim*, Vol. 1, p. 144). A second edition was called for and duly appeared (with further textual revisions) in August, and Macrone and Dickens began planning a two-volume sequel, *Sketches by Boz: Second Series*. Meanwhile, Dickens was approached by another firm of publishers. Chapman and Hall, impressed by the success of his *Sketches*, invited Dickens to write the letterpress for their new project, *Pickwick Papers*, to be published in twenty monthly numbers to accompany illustrations by another famous comic artist, Robert Seymour. The 'emolument' being as Dickens ebulliently put it, 'too tempting to resist' (*Pilgrim*, Vol. 1, p. 129), he 'thought of Mr Pickwick and began'. The first number appeared at the end of March and probably explains why no more 'Sketches by Boz. New Series' appeared in the *Morning Chronicle* following 'Our Next-door Neighbour' on 18 March. Dickens's energies were sufficiently occupied with *Pickwick*, contributing to Chapman and Hall's other new project *The Library of Fiction* (a comic tale, 'The Tuggses at Ramsgate', in April and, in June, 'A Little Talk about Spring, and the Sweeps', later retitled 'The First of May') and dashing off his fierce little pamphlet *Sunday Under Three Heads*, provoked by Sir Andrew Agnew's reintroduction in Parliament of his notorious 'Sunday Bill'.

Even before the 'rocket-like' ascent of *Pickwick*'s popularity began, with Sam Weller's appearance in the fourth (June) number, Dickens had clearly become hot property in the publishing world. 'He is courted and made up to by all the literary Gentleman (*sic*)', his adored young sister-in-law, Mary Hogarth, wrote to her cousin on 15 May 1836, 'and has more to do in that way than he can well manage' (*Pilgrim*, Vol. 1, p. 689). During the spring and summer of 1836 he made agreements to write a three-volume historical novel, *Gabriel Vardon, The Locksmith of London*, for Macrone, and a children's book for another publisher, Thomas Tegg, and two three-volume novels, one of them to be *Gabriel Vardon,* for yet a fourth publisher, Richard Bentley. He was also concerned with preparations for the staging of his dramatisation of 'The Great Winglebury Duel', working on the libretto of an operetta, *The Village Coquettes*, and was still full time on the *Morning Chronicle.*

Beyond all this, he had to bear in mind the need to write enough new sketches to fill the projected two-volume *Second Series.* He was offered very good terms for fortnightly contributions from the editor of the *Carlton Chronicle*, a journal which circulated, as Dickens told Macrone, 'all among the nobs' who would 'buy the book' (*Pilgrim*, Vol. 1, p. 160). So he decided to abandon the projected 'New Series' in the *Chronicle* and embark on one for the *Carlton* entitled 'Leaves from an Unpublished Volume. By "Boz", (which will be torn out once a fortnight)'. In fact, only two papers appeared in this series, 'The Hospital Patient' on 6 August, and 'Hackney Cabs, and Their Drivers' on 17 September, six weeks rather than a fortnight later. Presumably the terms turned out not to be quite as good as Dickens had expected, or he decided that the *Carlton* was not a very secure vehicle. He reverted, therefore, to the aborted *Chronicle* series and produced, in the month between 24 September and 26 October, four little masterpieces of the genre – 'Meditations in Monmouth Street', 'Scotland Yard', 'Doctors' Commons' and 'Vauxhall Gardens by Day'.

The signing of an agreement with Bentley on 4 November to edit a new monthly journal, *Bentley's Miscellany*, to appear in January, and the now assured success of *Pickwick*, enabled Dickens to resign from the *Chronicle*. He was eager to do so as a result of increasing difficulties with its owner, Easthope (or 'Blasthope' as Dickens called him). He did resign on 5 November and that was the end of the 'New Series'. The publication date for *Sketches by Boz: Second Series* was drawing near, but it had by now been agreed that there should be only one volume so that Dickens had enough material. The volume duly appeared, again illustrated by Cruikshank, on 17 December.

This *Second Series* volume contained all the tales and sketches so far uncollected apart (for some reason – perhaps objections on the part of Chapman and Hall?) from 'The Tuggses at Ramsgate'. 'To finish the volume with *éclat*', Dickens wrote a *grand guignol* piece, 'The Drunkard's Death', over which, he told the printer, he had 'taken great pains' (*Pilgrim*, Vol. 1, p. 208). As for the *First Series*, Dickens carefully revised the texts of nearly all the pieces he included, and in two cases amalgamated two existing sketches to form one long one. So 'The "House"' and 'Bellamy's' were united to form 'A Parliamentary Sketch: With a Few Portraits' and 'Some Account of an Omnibus Cad' was combined with 'Hackney Cabs, and Their Drivers' to form 'The Last Cab-driver, and the First Omnibus Cad'. His very first publication, 'A Dinner at Poplar Walk' also now found a place between hard covers with its new title, 'Mr Minns and his Cousin', and numerous textual revisions. The volume opens with 'The Streets – Morning' paired with 'The Streets – Night'. 'Making a Night of It' seems to be appropriately placed next, and 'Criminal Courts' might be considered a suitable sequel to the story of the nocturnal escapade of Mr Thomas Potter and his friend. After that, however, the order of contents appears to be as random as in the *First Series* – apart from the use of 'The Drunkard's Death' to give the book a striking conclusion.

Shortly after the publication of the *Second Series* Dickens began his somewhat turbulent period as the editor of *Bentley's*. He had contracted to supply one sheet – that is, about sixteen pages – of his own writing to each number of the magazine, a condition that became a meaty bone of contention between himself and Bentley as the months went by. He intended to begin a serial in the first (January) number but was pressed with other work. He dashed off a comic tale instead. This was 'The Public Life of Mr Tulrumble, once Mayor of Mudfog', about the farcical humiliations undergone by the vainglorious Tulrumble as a result of his determination to have a mayoral show to rival the Lord Mayor of London's. It is very like the *Monthly Magazine* tales, differing only in its provincial setting and in being rather more spun-out. I have not included it in this edition as its place is in a collected edition of Dickens's shorter fiction rather than of his journalism (the tales in *Sketches* are rather different in that Dickens himself made them an integral part of his first volume of collected journalism).

In the last paragraph of 'Tulrumble' Dickens suggests that he may write some more Mudfog 'chronicles' – provincial variants on the 'Our Parish' papers, as it were – and indeed the next issue of *Bentley's* does carry a story mentioning Mudfog. This, however, proves to be the first two chapters of *Oliver Twist*, with Oliver being born in Mudfog workhouse, and it evidently transcends from the start any sort of occasional satire on parochial life. The name Mudfog appears only in the first sentence, and disappears even from that when the novel comes to be separately published. From the February issue onwards, the instalments of *Oliver* constitute Dickens's personal contribution to the *Miscellany* – eked out on two occasions by other material. In March he wrote 'The Pantomime of Life', which is unlike any of his earlier 'Boz' sketches but rather looks forward to some of the satirical essays he was later to write for *Household Words*. In May he contributed 'Some Particulars Concerning a Lion' which, by contrast, is very much in the 'Boz' vein, although lacking in the topographical precision so omnipresent in *Sketches*. Later on, in October 1836 and September 1837, when he was particularly hard pressed with *Oliver*, he was to fall back on the Mudfog idea and use the name in connection with two satirical pieces on the British Association for the Advancement of Science (see below, pp. 513–51).

Meanwhile, Macrone, smarting from a sense of injustice as he considered Dickens had reneged on his promise to write a novel for him, and realising that there would never now be a second volume to the *Second Series*, decided to profit from Dickens's now dazzling celebrity by reissuing *Sketches*, of which he held the copyright, in monthly numbers resembling those in which *Pickwick Papers* was appearing. Dickens was distressed, believing that he might appear to be flooding the literary market with his secondhand wares at a time when he already had two novels in progress. The difficulty was eventually resolved by Chapman and Hall's buying the copyright from Macrone and Dickens's agreeing to their issuing the work in monthly numbers (with pink covers, however, to distinguish it clearly from *Pickwick* in its green ones). Chapman and Hall used the wonderful cover that Cruikshank had designed for Macrone, and Cruikshank, who was illustrating *Oliver Twist* and other material in *Bentley's*, agreed to provide some new illustrations to *Sketches* so that each of the twenty monthly numbers should have its full quota of two illustrations.

For this serialised reissue Dickens added one hitherto uncollected item, 'The Tuggses at Ramsgate', and once again made extensive textual revisions throughout. He was particularly careful, apparently, to remove anything that might expose him to charges of vulgarity or being too 'broad' (see *Dickens at Work*, p. 57: 'the aphrodisiac effect of the oysters upon Mr John Dounce is toned down by two cautious alterations', etc.). He was now, Professor Tillotson comments, 'established as a popular "family" author, and also as the editor of a periodical himself; he had a keener sense of his audience and of his responsibilities towards it'. It was also in this edition, later published in volume form, that he first grouped the tales and sketches into the four divisions which have been preserved in all editions ever since. The group entitled 'Our Parish' had already been brought together in the *First Series* and now a seventh sketch, 'Our Next-door Neighbour', was added, no doubt because like them it presented 'Boz' as living in a particular locality and, to some extent, interacting with people in it rather than ranging London as a detached spectator. 'The Tuggses at Ramsgate' and the two melodramatic stories, 'The Black Veil' and 'The Drunkard's Death', group themselves with the *Monthly Magazine* tales, and all the *Chronicle* and *Bell's Life* sketches fall naturally into two groups, one predominantly concerned with places and the other with people (only 'The Last Cab-driver, and the First Omnibus Cad' might be thought to have got into the wrong category).

'The Drunkard's Death' retained its prominent position as the last item in the book. One of the two other pieces Dickens had specially written for volume publication, 'A Visit to Newgate', is also given a prominent position as the last in the 'Scenes' series. These three pieces, incidentally ('The Black Veil' being the third), are the only wholly non-comic pieces in the entire book. It seems as though the young Dickens made a distinction between material intended for serial publication and material to be published only in volume form. The former might happily mingle comedy and satire with pathos, but the latter demanded 'high seriousness' (which in the 1830s meant melodrama).

The next edition of *Sketches* was for the first collected edition of Dickens's works called the Cheap Edition. This began to appear in 1850 and *Sketches* was one of the first volumes in the series to be published. Dickens made a number of interesting textual revisions (see *Dickens at Work*, pp. 59–61), and he wrote a new preface, very deprecatory in tone, which has tended to be the only one reproduced in modern editions. This preface, with its references to 'imperfections' and 'obvious marks of haste and inexperience' has probably been responsible to a considerable degree for the comparative neglect of *Sketches* in the history of Dickens criticism. Dickens let the Preface stand in the last edition of the work to be published in his lifetime, the 1868 Charles Dickens Edition (which reprinted the text established in the Cheap Edition). It was no doubt what Forster primarily had in mind when he wrote in 1872 in *The Life of Dickens* (1872–74) that Dickens 'decidedly underrated' the achievement of the *Sketches*. Forster went on to give them high praise:

> ... the first sprightly runnings of his genius are undoubtedly here ... The observation shown throughout is nothing short of wonderful. Things are painted literally as they are; and whatever the picture, whether of everyday vulgar, shabby-genteel, or downright low, with neither the condescending air which is affectation, nor the too familiar one that is slang ...

Well before 1850, however, in fact by the time the 1839 edition of *Sketches* appeared in volume form after the conclusion of its publication in monthly parts Dickens had, as he put it, 'burst the Bentleian bonds' (*Pilgrim*, Vol. 1, p. 504), in other words resigned from the irksome editing of *Bentley's Miscellany* (see below, p. 500). The monthly serialisation of *Nicholas Nickleby* was proceeding triumphantly and for the next decade he was to be primarily occupied with an astonishing series of extraordinary novels, culminating in *David Copperfield* (1849–50). But the journalist in him also needed an outlet and a congenial one was at hand in the distinguished Radical weekly *The Examiner*, now edited by Forster, until in 1850 Dickens became 'conductor' of his own weekly journal, *Household Words*. It was in the pages of this periodical and in those of its successor, *All The Year Round*, that virtually all his later journalism was to appear.

MICHAEL SLATER

*Birkbeck College, University of London, 1994*

Note:

A paper entitled 'Mr Robert Bolton, the "Gentleman connected with the Press"' published in the August 1838 number of *Bentley's Miscellany* has been traditionally ascribed to Dickens and included in the so-called '*Mudfog Papers*'. As W. J. Carlton showed in his 'Who Wrote "Mr Robert Bolton"?' in *The Dickensian* (Vol. 44 [1958], 178–81), however, this was certainly not Dickens's work. It has, therefore, been omitted from this edition.

# THE FIRST PUBLICATION OF DICKENS'S SKETCHES IN SERIAL AND VOLUME FORM

A *Monthly Magazine* 'Tales'

| | | | |
|---|---|---|---|
| 1833 | Dec. | | A Dinner At Poplar Walk |
| 1834 | Jan. | | Mrs Joseph Porter 'Over the Way' |
| | Feb. | | Horatio Sparkins |
| | Apr. | | The Bloomsbury Christening |
| | May | | The Boarding House |
| | June | 7 | Sentiment! [unsigned, in *Bell's Weekly Magazine*] [All the above were unsigned] |
| | Aug. | | The Boarding House – No. 2 [This was the first sketch signed 'Boz'] |
| | Oct. | | The Steam Excursion |
| 1835 | Jan. | | A Passage in the Life of Mr Watkins Tottle, Chapter the First |
| | Feb. | | A Passage in the Life of Mr Watkins Tottle, Chapter the Second |

B *Morning Chronicle* 'Street Sketches'

| | | | |
|---|---|---|---|
| 1834 | Sept. | 26 | Omnibuses |
| | Oct. | 10 | Shops and their Tenants |
| | | 23 | The Old Bailey |
| | Nov. | 5 | Shabby-genteel People |
| | Dec. | 15 | Brokers' and Marine Store Shops |

C *Evening Chronicle* 'Sketches of London'

| | | | |
|---|---|---|---|
| 1835 | Jan. | 31 | Hackney Coach Stands |
| | Feb. | 7 | Gin Shops |
| | | 19 | Early Coaches |
| | | 28 | The Parish (The Beadle – The Parish Engine – The Schoolmaster) |

| | | |
|---|---|---|
| Mar. | 7 | The 'House' |
| | 17 | London Recreations |
| Apr. | 7 | Public Dinners |
| | 11 | Bellamy's |
| | 16 | Greenwich Fair |
| | 23 | Thoughts about People |
| May | 9 | Astley's |
| | 19 | Our Parish (The Curate – The Old Lady – The Half Pay Captain) |
| June | 6 | The River |
| | 18 | Our Parish (The Four Sisters) |
| | 30 | The Pawnbroker's Shop |
| July | 14 | Our Parish (The Election for Beadle) |
| | 21 | The Streets – Morning |
| | 28 | Our Parish (The Broker's Man) |
| Aug. | 11 | Private Theatres |
| | 20 | Our Parish (The Ladies' Societies) |

D *Bell's Life in London* 'Scenes and Characters' (by 'Tibbs')

| | | | |
|---|---|---|---|
| 1835 | Sept. | 27 | Seven Dials |
| | Oct. | 4 | Miss Evans and 'The Eagle' |
| | | 11 | The Dancing Academy |
| | | 18 | Making a Night of It |
| | | 25 | Love and Oysters |
| | Nov. | 1 | Some Account of an Omnibus Cad |
| | | 22 | The Vocal Dressmaker |
| | | 29 | The Prisoners' Van |
| | Dec. | 13 | The Parlour |
| | | 27 | Christmas Festivities |
| 1836 | Jan. | 3 | The New Year |
| | | 17 | The Streets at Night |

E *Sketches by Boz* (February 1836)

Vol. 1

The Parish (6 chapters)
Miss Evans and 'The Eagle'
Shops and their Tenants
Thoughts about People
A Visit to Newgate
London Recreations
The Boarding-House (2 chapters)
Hackney-Coach Stands

Vol. 2

Passage in the Life of Mr Watkins Tottle (2 chapters)
The Black Veil
Shabby-genteel People
Horatio Sparkins
The Pawnbroker's Shop
The Dancing Academy
Early Coaches

Vol. 1 (*cont.*)

Brokers and Marine-store Shops
The Bloomsbury Christening
Gin Shops
Public Dinners
Astley's
Greenwich Fair
The Prisoners' Van
A Christmas Dinner

Vol. 2 (*cont.*)

The River
Private Theatres
The Great Winglebury Duel
Omnibuses
Mrs Joseph Porter
The Steam Excursion
Sentiment

F Sketches and tales published in various places during 1836

| | |
|---|---|
| Mar. 18 | Our Next-door Neighbours (*Morning Chronicle*) |
| Apr. | The Tuggs's at Ramsgate (*The Library of Fiction*, Vol. 1, No. 1) |
| June | A Little Talk about Spring and the Sweeps (*The Library of Fiction*, Vol. 1, No. 3) |
| Aug. 6 | The Hospital Patient (*Carlton Chronicle*) |
| Sept. 17 | Hackney Cabs, and Their Drivers (*Carlton Chronicle*) |
| Sept. 24 | Meditations in Monmouth Street (*Morning Chronicle*) |
| Oct. 4 | Scotland Yard (*Morning Chronicle*) |
| Oct. 11 | Doctors' Commons (*Morning Chronicle*) |
| Oct. 26 | Vauxhall – Gardens by Day (*Morning Chronicle*) |

[The last four of the above were published under the heading *Sketches by Boz, New Series*]

G *Sketches by Boz: Second Series* (December 1836)

The Streets by Morning
The Streets by Night
Making a Night of It
Criminal Courts
Scotland-Yard
The New Year
Meditations in Monmouth-Street
Our Next-door Neighbours
The Hospital Patient
Seven Dials
The Mistaken Milliner
Doctors' Commons
Misplaced Attachment of Mr John Dounce
Vauxhall Gardens by Day

A Parliamentary Sketch – with a few Portraits
Mr Minns and his Cousin
The last Cab-driver, and the First Omnibus Cad
The Parlour Orator
The First of May
The Drunkard's Death

H *Sketches by Boz:* 20 monthly parts, 1 Nov. 1837–1 June 1839 – Complete in one volume, 1839. [Contents definitively arranged in four sections: 'Seven Sketches From Our Parish'; 'Scenes'; 'Characters'; 'Tales']

Note:
Macrone reprinted his second edition of *Sketches*, First Series, in 1837 without Dickens's agreement as a 'Third Edition'.

# SELECT BIBLIOGRAPHY

Ackroyd, Peter, *Dickens*, Sinclair-Stevenson, 1990. The best modern biography (though difficult to use for reference purposes) – an astonishing combination of exhaustive research and insight into the workings of Dickens's imagination. Excellent discussion of *Sketches* in ch. 7.

Axton, William F., *Circle of Fire: Dickens' Vision and Style and the Popular Victorian Theatre*, University of Kentucky Press, 1966. Argues for 'The Pantomime of Life' as a key text for understanding Dickens's '*theatrum mundi*' approach to sketch- and fiction-writing; also relates the *Bentley* 'Mudfog' papers to the serialisation of *Oliver Twist.*

Butt, J., and Tillotson, K., *Dickens at Work*, Methuen University Paperback edn, 1968 (first pub. 1957). Detailed and illuminating account of Dickens's revisions of the texts of *Sketches.* Cited in headnotes as Butt and Tillotson.

Chittick, Kathryn, *The Critical Reception of Charles Dickens, 1833–41*, Garland Publishing, New York, 1989. Exhaustive listing of contemporary reviews and notices of *Sketches by Boz* and of Dickens's other early works.

Chittick, Kathryn, *Dickens and the 1830s*, Cambridge University Press, 1990. Sets Dickens's early journalism and fiction in its historical and biographical context with impeccable scholarship and highly illuminating results.

Costigan, Edward, 'Drama and Everyday Life in *Sketches by Boz*', *Review of English Studies*, n.s., Vol. 27 (1976), pp. 401–21. Demonstrates the close relationship between the style and the structure of *Sketches* and the contemporary stage.

DeVries, Duane, *Dickens' Apprentice Years. The Making of a Novelist*, The Harvester Press, 1976. Detailed study of the textual and publishing history of *Sketches*, which reprints several interesting passages that Dickens omitted when preparing items for volume publication. Cited in headnotes as DeVries.

Easson, Angus, 'Who is Boz? Dickens and his Sketches', *The Dickensian*, Vol. 81 (1985), pp. 13–22. Examines the nature and function of the persona of 'Boz' in *Sketches.*

Forster, John, *The Life of Dickens*, ed. A.J. Hoppé for the Everyman's Library, 1969 (2 vols). The best modern edition of the classic Dickens biography by his lifelong friend (first published 1872–4).

HILL, T.W. 'Notes on *Sketches by Boz*', *The Dickensian*, Vols 46 (pp. 206–13), 47 (pp. 41–8, 102–7, 154–8, 210–18), and 48 (pp. 32–7, 90–4), 1950–2. Pioneering work of annotation. Cited in headnotes as Hill.

HOUSE, M., and STOREY, G. (eds), *The Letters of Charles Dickens* (The Pilgrim Edition), Vol. 1, 1820–39, Oxford University Press, 1965. Cited in headnotes as *Pilgrim*.

MILLER, J. Hillis, 'The Fiction of Realism: *Sketches by Boz*, *Oliver Twist*, and Cruikshank's Illustrations', in *Charles Dickens and George Cruikshank*, William Andrews Clark Memorial Library, University of California, 1971. Fascinating study of metonymy as 'a structuring principle' in *Sketches* (Boz's work is analogous to that of a detective or archaeologist ...').

SCHWARZBACH, F.S., *Dickens and the City*, University of London, the Athlone Press, 1979. Ch. 1, 'Fiction for the Metropolis', calls attention to the essentially metropolitan spirit and outlook of *Sketches*.

# DICKENS'S LIFE AND TIMES – TO 1839

## EARLY LIFE

| | *Dickens's Family Life* | *Historical and Literary Background* |
|---|---|---|
| 1809 | John Dickens, a clerk in the Royal Navy Pay Office, marries Elizabeth Barrow (13 June) at St Mary-le-Strand, London. | |
| 1810 | Frances ('Fanny') Dickens born (28 Oct.; died 1848). | |
| 1811 | | Prince of Wales becomes Prince Regent owing to madness of George III. Shelley expelled from Oxford. |
| 1812 | CD born (7 Feb.) Mile End Terrace, Portsmouth. Family moves to 16 Hawk Street (June). | Napoleon invades Russia. War between UK and USA. Luddite riots. Byron's *Childe Harold*, Cantos i and ii published. |
| 1813 | Family moves to 39 Wish Street, Southsea (Dec.). | Battle of Leipzig between the Allies and Napoleon's forces. Jane Austen's *Pride and Prejudice* published. |
| 1814 | Alfred Dickens born (Mar.; died Sept.). | Allies capture Paris. Napoleon abdicates. Jane Austen's *Mansfield Park*, Scott's *Waverley*, and Wordsworth's *The Excursion* published. |
| 1815 | John Dickens posted back to London (Jan.). Family move to Norfolk Street, St Pancras. | Battle of Waterloo. Byron's *Hebrew Melodies*, Scott's *Guy Mannering*, and Wordsworth's *White Doe of Rylstone* published. |
| 1816 | Letitia Dickens born (died 1893). | Coleridge settles at Highgate, publishes 'Christabel' and 'Kubla Khan'. Scott's *The Antiquary* and *Tales of My Landlord* and Jane Austen's *Emma* published. |
| 1817 | John Dickens posted first to Sheerness, then (Apr.) to Chatham Dockyard. Family settles at 2 Ordnance Terrace, Chatham (Dec.). | Death of Princess Charlotte, daughter of the Prince Regent. Keats's *Poems*, Byron's *Manfred*, and Coleridge's *Biographia Literaria* published. Jane Austen dies. |
| 1818 | | Keats's *Endymion*, Scott's *Heart of Midlothian*, Mary Shelley's *Frankenstein*, and Jane Austen's *Northanger Abbey* and *Persuasion* published. |

| | | |
|---|---|---|
| 1819 | Harriet Dickens born (died 1822). | Peterloo Massacre. Scott's *Ivanhoe*, Shelley's *The Cenci*, Byron's *Don Juan* (first two cantos) published. |
| 1820 | Frederick Dickens born (died 1868). | Death of George III, accession of George IV. Shelley's *Prometheus Unbound*, Keats's *Hyperion*, and Washington Irving's *Sketch-Book* published. |
| 1821 | Family moves to St Mary's Place. CD begins education at William Giles's school, writes a tragedy, *Misnar, the Sultan of India.* | Greek War of Independence. Keats dies. De Quincey's *Confessions of an Opium Eater*, Scott's *Kenilworth*, and Shelley's *Adonais* published. |
| 1822 | Alfred Dickens born (died 1860). John Dickens recalled to London (summer), settles at 16 Bayham Street, Camden Town. CD follows family to London, his schooling broken off. | Shelley dies. Byron's *Vision of Judgement* and Scott's *Fortunes of Nigel* and *Peveril of the Peak* published. |
| 1823 | Fanny Dickens becomes boarder at Royal Academy of Music (Apr.). Family moves to 4 Gower Street North (26 Dec.) where Mrs Dickens attempts to start a school but without success. | Death penalty abolished in Britain for over 100 crimes. Construction of present British Museum building begun. Mechanics' Institutes founded in London and Glasgow. Scott's *Quentin Durward* and Lamb's *Essays of Elia* published. |
| 1824 | CD sent to work at Warren's Blacking Factory (late Jan./early Feb.). John Dickens arrested for debt (20 Feb.) and sent to Marshalsea Prison where Elizabeth and the younger children join him after some weeks. CD placed in lodgings with a family friend in Camden Town, subsequently in other lodgings in Lant Street, Southwark. John Dickens obtains release from the Marshalsea under the Insolvent Debtors Act (28 May). Family moves to 29 Johnson Street, Somers Town. | Death of Byron. Beethoven's Ninth Symphony performed (Vienna). British workers allowed to unionize. W.S. Landor's *Imaginary Conversations* and Mary Russell Mitford's *Our Village* published. |
| 1825 | John Dickens retires on pension from Navy Pay Office (9 Mar.). CD removed from Blacking Factory and sent to Wellington House Academy, Hampstead Road (? late Mar./early Apr.). | First passenger railway in UK (Stockton–Darlington) opened (Stephenson's 'Rocket'). Manzoni's *I promessi sposi* and Hazlitt's *Spirit of the Age* published. |
| 1826 | John Dickens working as Parliamentary correspondent for the *British Press.* | University College, London, founded, also Royal Zoological Society. Mendelssohn's Overture to *A Midsummer Night's Dream*, |

| | | |
|---|---|---|
| | | Fenimore Cooper's *Last of the Mohicans*, and Disraeli's *Vivian Grey* published. |
| 1827 | Family evicted for non-payment of rates (Mar.). CD leaves school, becomes clerk at Ellis & Blackmore, solicitors, and then at Charles Molloy's, solicitor. Augustus Dickens born (died 1858). | Battle of Navarino, Turkish fleet destroyed by British, French, and Russian fleets. Deaths of Blake and Beethoven. Schubert's *Winterreise* performed. Constable paints *The Cornfield.* Heine's *Buch der Lieder* published, also the first Baedeker travel guide. |
| 1828 | John Dickens working as reporter for the *Morning Herald.* | Greek independence declared. Wellington becomes Prime Minister and Andrew Jackson President of the USA. Constable paints *Salisbury Cathedral.* Death of Goya. Dumas *père's Les Trois Mousquetaires*, Scott's *Tales of a Grandfather*, and Bulwer-Lytton's *Pelham* published. |
| 1829 | Family move to 10 Norfolk Street, Fitzroy Square. CD, having learned shorthand, works as freelance reporter at Doctors' Commons. | Peel establishes Metropolitan Police in London. Catholic Emancipation Act. Horse-drawn omnibuses in London. Daguerre and Niepce form partnership to develop their photographic inventions. Delacroix paints *Sardanapalus* and Turner *Ulysses Deriding Polyphemus*. Balzac's *Les Chouans* published. |

## CAREER

| | *CD's Personal Life* | *Writing Career* | *Historical and Literary Background* |
|---|---|---|---|
| 1830 | Admitted as a reader at the British Museum (Feb.). Falls in love with banker's daughter Maria Beadnell (May). | | Death of George IV, accession of William IV. 'July Revolution' in France, accession of Louis Philippe. Lyell's *Principles of Geology* begins publication. Tennyson's *Poems, chiefly lyrical* published. |
| 1831 | Begins work as reporter for *The Mirror of Parliament* edited by his uncle, J.M. Barrow. | | Reform Bill passed by House of Commons, vetoed by the Lords. Peacock's *Crotchet Castle* and Hugo's *Notre Dame de Paris* published. |
| 1832 | Parliamentary reporter on the *True Sun*. Granted audition at Covent | | Reform Bill passed. Darwin begins publishing *Narrative of the Surveying Voyages of H.M.S. Adventure and Beagle* |

| | | | |
|---|---|---|---|
| | Garden Theatre but illness prevents his attendance. | | and Harriet Martineau begins publishing *Illustrations of Political Economy.* Bulwer-Lytton's *Eugene Aram*, Tennyson's *Poems*, and Mrs Trollope's *Domestic Manners of the Americans* published. |
| 1833 | Produces private theatricals at his parents' home in Bentinck St. Ends affair with Maria Beadnell. | CD's first story 'A Dinner at Poplar Walk' (later titled 'Mr Minns and his Cousin', *SB*) published in the *Monthly Magazine.* | First steamship crossing of the Atlantic. Slavery abolished throughout British Empire. Carlyle's *Sartor Resartus* and Lamb's *Last Essays of Elia* published. Newman, Pusey, Keble, and others begin issuing *Tracts for the Times* (beginning of the Oxford Movement in the Church of England). |
| 1834 | Becomes reporter on the *Morning Chronicle* and meets Catherine Hogarth (Aug.). Takes chambers at 13 Furnival's Inn, Holborn (Dec.). | Six more stories published in the *Monthly Magazine*, also one in *Bell's Weekly Magazine*; five 'Street Sketches' published in the *Morning Chronicle.* | Poor Law Amendment Act (the New Poor Law). Transportation of 'Tolpuddle Martyrs'. Destruction by fire of old Houses of Parliament. Ainsworth's *Rookwood*, Balzac's *Père Goriot*, Lady Blessington's *Conversations with Lord Byron*, Bulwer-Lytton's *Last Days of Pompeii* and Marryat's *Peter Simple* published. Deaths of Coleridge and Lamb. |
| 1835 | Becomes engaged to Catherine Hogarth (?May). | Two more stories in the *Monthly Magazine*, twenty 'Sketches of London' in the *Evening Chronicle*, ten 'Scenes and Characters' in *Bell's Life in London.* | Municipal Reform Act. Browning's *Paracelsus*, Clare's *The Rural Muse*, and Wordsworth's *Yarrow Revisited, and Other Poems* published. |
| 1836 | Moves into larger chambers at 15 Furnival's Inn (Feb.). Marries Catherine Hogarth at St Luke's, Chelsea (2 Apr.). Honey-moon at Chalk (Kent). Leaves staff | Two more 'Scenes and Characters' in *Bell's Life*, two contributions to *The Library of Fiction* and one to *Carlton Chronicle*, four 'Sketches by Boz: New Series' in *The Morning Chronicle. Sketches by Boz: First Series* published (8 Feb.). | Chartist Movement begins. Forster's *Lives of the Statesmen of the Commonwealth*, and Lockhart's *Life of Scott* begin publication; Marryat's *Mr Midshipman Easy* published. |

| | | | |
|---|---|---|---|
| | of the *Morning Chronicle* (?Nov.). First meeting with John Forster (Dec.). | *Pickwick Papers* begins serialization in 20 monthly numbers (31 Mar.), *Sunday Under Three Heads* (June). *The Strange Gentleman* produced at the St James's Theatre (29 Sept.) followed by *The Village Coquettes* (22 Dec.). *Sketches by Boz: Second Series* published (17 Dec.). | |
| 1837 | First child (Charles) born (6 Jan.). Move to 48 Doughty Street (Apr.). Death of Mary Hogarth, CD's sister-in-law (7 May). First visit to Europe (France and Belgium – July) and first family holiday at Broadstairs (Sept.). | First number of *Bentley's Miscellany* (ed. by CD) appears (1 Jan.). First of the 'Mudfog Papers' appears in it. *Oliver Twist* serialized in *Bentley's* in 24 monthly instalments from the 2nd number. *Is She His Wife?* produced at the St James's (3 Mar.). *Pickwick Papers* published in one volume (17 Nov.). | Death of William IV, accession of Victoria. Carlyle's *French Revolution* published. Death of Grimaldi, the clown. |
| 1838 | Expedition to Yorkshire schools with H.K. Browne (Jan./Feb.), second child (Mary) born. | *Sketches of Young Gentlemen* (10 Feb.) and *Memoirs of Joseph Grimaldi* (26 Feb.). *Nicholas Nickleby* begins serialization in 20 monthly numbers (31 Mar.). *Oliver Twist* published (9 Nov.). | Anti-Corn Law League founded in Manchester. First Afghan war breaks out. Daguerre–Niepce method of photography presented to the Académies des Sciences et des Beaux Arts, Paris. |
| 1839 | Resigns editorship of *Bentley's Miscellany* (31 Jan.). Third child (Kate) born. Moves to 1 Devonshire Place, Regent's Park. | *The Loving Ballad of Lord Bateman* published (June). *Nicholas Nickleby* published in volume form (23 Oct.). | First Opium Wars between Britain and China. Turner paints *The Fighting Téméraire*. Ainsworth's *Jack Sheppard* published. |

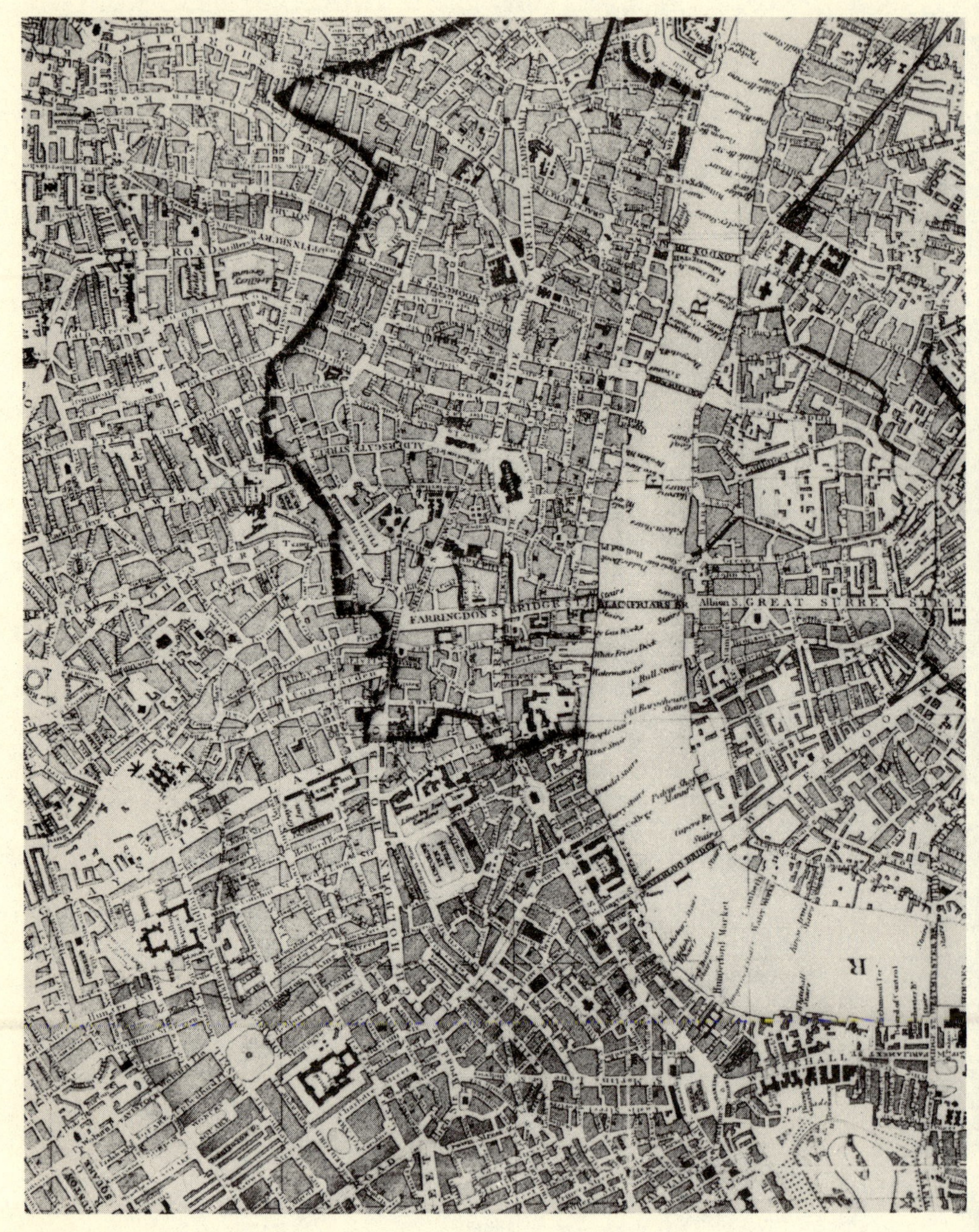


*Part of map from Joseph Cross's* London Guide *(1837).*
*By permission of the British Library*

# ILLUSTRATIONS

*By George Cruikshank*

Note: where titles differ from the original ones the latter are given in brackets.

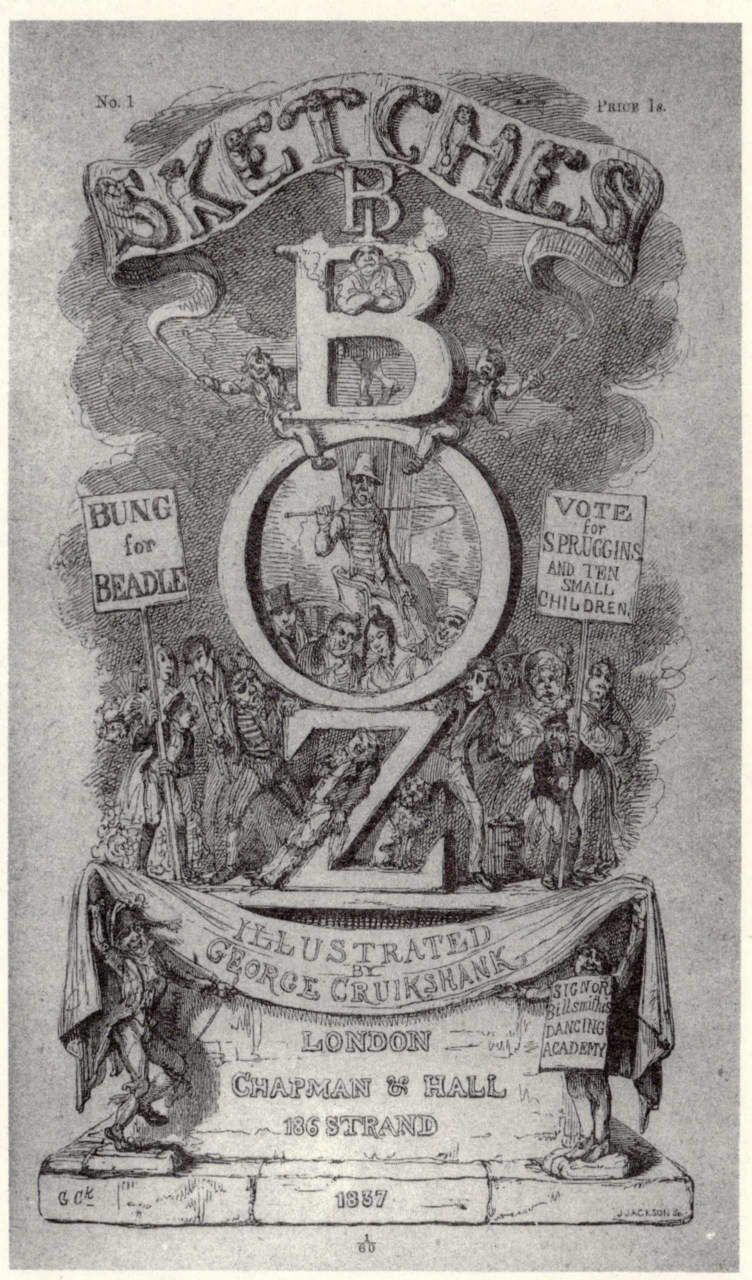
No. 1
Price 1s.
SKETCHES
BY
BOZ
BUNG for BEADLE
VOTE for SPRUGGINS AND TEN SMALL CHILDREN!
ILLUSTRATED BY GEORGE CRUIKSHANK
SIGNOR Billsmith's DANCING ACADEMY
LONDON
CHAPMAN & HALL
186 STRAND
1837

# DICKENS'S PREFACES TO *SKETCHES BY BOZ*

## Preface to the First Edition of the First Series

In humble imitation of a prudent course, universally adopted by aeronauts, the Author of these volumes throws them up as his pilot balloon, trusting it may catch some favourable current, and devoutly and earnestly hoping it may *go off well* – a sentiment in which his Publisher cordially concurs.

Unlike the generality of pilot balloons which carry no car, in this one it is very possible for a man to embark, not only himself, but all his hopes of future fame, and all his chances of future success. Entertaining no inconsiderable feeling of trepidation, at the idea of making so perilous a voyage in so frail a machine, alone and unaccompanied, the author was naturally desirous to secure the assistance and companionship of some well-known individual, who had frequently contributed to the success, though his well-earned reputation rendered it impossible for him ever to have shared the hazard, of similar undertakings. To whom, as possessing the requisite in an eminent degree, could he apply but to George Cruikshank? The application was readily heard, and at once acceded to: this is their first voyage in company, but it may not be the last.

If any further excuse be wanted for adding this book to the hundreds which every season produces, the Author may be permitted to plead the very favourable reception, which several of the following sketches received, on their original appearance in different periodicals. In behalf of the remainder, he can only entreat the kindness and favour of the public: his object has been to present little pictures of life and manners as they really are; and should they be approved of, he hopes to repeat his experiment with increased confidence, and on a more extensive scale.

Furnival's Inn, February 1836

## Preface to the Second Edition of the First Series

The Second Edition of a work, while it affords its author an opportunity of returning his warmest thanks to the Public, for their favourable reception of the first impression, furnishes in itself the best of all possible apologies for his again intruding upon their notice, with a few words in his individual capacity.

The words which the Author feels it necessary to say, in the present instance, are few indeed. He has to vindicate himself from no censure – to notice no illiberality – to complain of no attack. He has only in one single sentence, to acknowledge, with feelings of the deepest gratitude, the kindness and indulgence with which these volumes have been universally received, and the unlooked-for success with which his efforts have been crowned.

If the pen that designed these little outlines, should present its labours frequently to the Public hereafter; if it should produce fresh sketches, and even connected works of fiction of a higher grade, they have only themselves to blame. They have encouraged a young and unknown writer, by their patronage and approval, they have stimulated him to fresh efforts, by their liberality and praise; and if they *will* be guilty of such actions, they must be content to bear the consequences which naturally result from them.

Furnival's Inn, 1 August 1836

## Preface to the Second Series

If brevity be the soul of wit, anywhere, it is most especially so, in a preface; firstly, because those who do read such things as prefaces, prefer them, like grace before meat, in an epigrammatic form; and, secondly, because nine hundred and ninety-nine people out of every thousand, never read a preface at all.

Some of these sketches were written before the appearance of the former series, and the remainder have been added at different periods since that time. The author ventures to hope that they may experience as favourable a reception as the first productions of his pen; and that the present volume will not be considered an unwelcome, or inappropriate sequel, to the two which preceded it.

With these few words, he gives a modest tap at the door of the public with his Christmas Piece, when, perhaps, he may imagine the following dialogue to ensue, founded on the well-known precedent of the charity boys and the housemaid.

*Publisher* (to author) – *You* knock.

*Author* (to publisher) – No – you. (Here the Publisher seizes the knocker, and gives a loud rap at the door.)

*Public* (suspiciously, and with the door ajar) – Well; what do *you* want?

*Publisher* – Please, will you look at this Christmas Piece; me and the other boy goes partners in it.

*Public* – Go away; we have so many knocks of the same kind, at this time of year, that we are tired of answering the door. Go away.

*Publisher* (pushing it) – No; but do look at it, please. It's all his own doing, except the pictures; and they're capital, let alone the writing. [Here the public gradually softens, and takes the Christmas Piece in; upon which the Publisher makes a bow, and retires] – while the author lingers behind, for one instant, to repeat an old form with much sincerity; and to express his hearty wish that his best friend, the Public, may enjoy 'a merry Christmas, and a happy new year.'

Furnival's Inn, 17 December 1836

## Advertisement to the First Collected Edition

The following pages contain the earliest productions of their Author, written from time to time to meet the exigencies of a Newspaper or a Magazine. They were originally published in two series; the first in two volumes, and the second in one. Several editions having been exhausted, both are now published together in one volume, uniform with the *Pickwick Papers* and *Nicholas Nickleby.*

London, 15 May 1839

## Preface to the First Cheap Edition

The whole of these Sketches were written and published, one by one, when I was a very young man. They were collected and re-published while I was still a very young man; and sent into the world with all their imperfections (a good many) on their heads.

They comprise my first attempts at authorship – with the exception of certain tragedies achieved at the mature age of eight or ten, and represented with great applause to overflowing nurseries. I am conscious of their often being extremely crude and ill-considered, and bearing obvious marks of haste and inexperience; particularly in that section of the present volume which is comprised under the general head of Tales.

But as this collection is not originated now, and was very leniently and favourably received when it was first made, I have not felt it right either to remodel or expunge, beyond a few words and phrases here and there.

London, October 1850

The above preface was reprinted without any alteration or addition in the Charles Dickens Edition of *Sketches by Boz* (1868).

# Sketches by Boz

## Illustrative of Everyday Life, and Everyday People

# OUR PARISH

*A Bibliographical Note:*

The first six sketches grouped under this title originally appeared in the series of 'Sketches of London' (twenty sketches in all) published in the *Evening Chronicle* between January and August 1835; they all carried the sub-title 'Our Parish'. For publication dates see headnote to each individual sketch below. They were brought together and placed at the beginning of Vol. 1 of *Sketches by Boz* (2 vols, 1836) under the general title of 'The Parish', each sketch being designated a chapter and given the title found here.

For the 1839 edition of *Sketches*, 'complete in one volume', the general title reverted to being 'Our Parish'. A sixth chapter, 'Our Next-door Neighbour', was also added; it had originally appeared in the *Morning Chronicle*, 18 March 1836, and been included in *Sketches by Boz: Second Series* (1837) as 'Our Next-door Neighbours'.

*Historical Note:*

The parish was, until the Local Government Act of 1894, the basic administrative division of the country. At the centre (not necessarily the geographical centre) of each parish stands the parish church which belongs of course, to the established state church, the Church of England, and it was in the vestry of the church that the parishioners originally met for purposes of making bye-laws, dealing with rates (local taxes) and to discuss all matters concerned with the welfare of the local community. More spacious meeting places had to be found as the population increased but the name vestry continued to be used to denote the assembly. The parishioners who were legally responsible for parochial administration were called churchwardens (their number and method of appointment varied greatly from parish to parish) and by the early nineteenth century each parish had a salaried vestry clerk, usually a professional lawyer, who acted as secretary to the vestry and registrar of its proceedings. The parish was responsible for relieving the poor within its area, provided that they belonged to the parish by birth or 'settlement', and overseers of the poor were appointed by local justices of the peace to administer the Poor Laws. Until the New Poor Law of 1834, satirised by Dickens in *Oliver Twist* (1837–8), paupers could either be given 'outdoor relief' – food, fuel etc. – in their own homes, or be placed in the 'House' (the workhouse). The parish was responsible for maintaining the workhouse, appointing its master and seeing to the day-to-day running of the place. The parish would also maintain a school for pauper children with a very poorly paid schoolmaster (these masters were, Philip Collins notes in *Dickens and Education* [1963] p. 121, 'elderly men who turned to teaching when other work failed'). A cut above him would be the master of the national school, maintained not by the parish but by the Church of England.

One parish official figures prominently in Dickens's work – the beadle (notably Bumble in *Oliver Twist*). His elaborate traditional costume of cocked hat, gold-laced coat and 'large-headed staff' contrasted with the very menial nature of the duties that this paid official carried out at the behest of the churchwardens and overseers. His duties included clearing the streets of vagrants, helping to collect the Poor Rate, keeping order in the church during services and 'crying' the notices of Vestry meetings – 'in short,' observe the Webbs, 'to be on hand whenever any superior officer of the parish required an assistant, a messenger, or a porter' (Sidney and Beatrice Webb, *English Local Government* [1906], Vol. 1, pp. 126–7; quoted by P. Schlicke in his 'Bumble and the Poor Law Satire of *Oliver Twist*', *The Dickensian*, Vol. 71 [1975], pp. 149–56). See this article for further details about the role and status of parish beadles.

For later satire on vestries by Dickens see the essay 'Our Vestry' (1852) in *Reprinted Pieces* (Vol. III of this edition of the journalism).

## Chapter One

### *The Beadle – The Parish Engine – The Schoolmaster*

First published in the *Evening Chronicle*, 28 February 1835 ('Sketches of London No. 4').

How much is conveyed in those two short words – 'The Parish'! And with how many tales of distress and misery, of broken fortune and ruined hope, too often of unrelieved wretchedness and successful knavery, are they associated! A poor man, with small earnings, and a large family, just manages to live on from hand to mouth, and to procure food from day to day; he has barely sufficient to satisfy the present cravings of nature, and can take no heed of the future. His taxes are in arrear, quarter-day passes by, another quarter-day arrives: he can procure no more quarter for himself, and is summoned by – the parish. His goods are distrained, his children are crying with cold and hunger, and the very bed on which his sick wife is lying, is dragged from beneath her. What can he do? To whom is he to apply for relief? To private charity? To benevolent individuals? Certainly not – there is his parish. There are the parish vestry, the parish infirmary, the parish surgeon, the parish officers, the parish beadle. Excellent institutions, and gentle, kind-hearted men. The woman dies – she is buried by the parish. The children have no protector – they are taken care of by the parish. The man first neglects, and afterwards cannot obtain, work – he is relieved by the parish; and when distress and drunkenness have done their work upon him, he is maintained, a harmless babbling idiot, in the parish asylum.

The parish beadle is one of the most, perhaps *the* most, important member of the local administration. He is not so well off as the churchwardens, certainly, nor is he so learned as the vestry clerk, nor does he order things quite so much his own way as either of them. But his power is very great, notwithstanding; and the dignity of his office is never impaired by the absence of efforts on his part to maintain it. The beadle of our parish is a splendid fellow. It is quite delightful to hear him, as he explains the state of the existing poor laws to the deaf old woman in the board room passage on business nights; and to hear what he said to the senior churchwarden, and what the senior churchwarden said to him; and

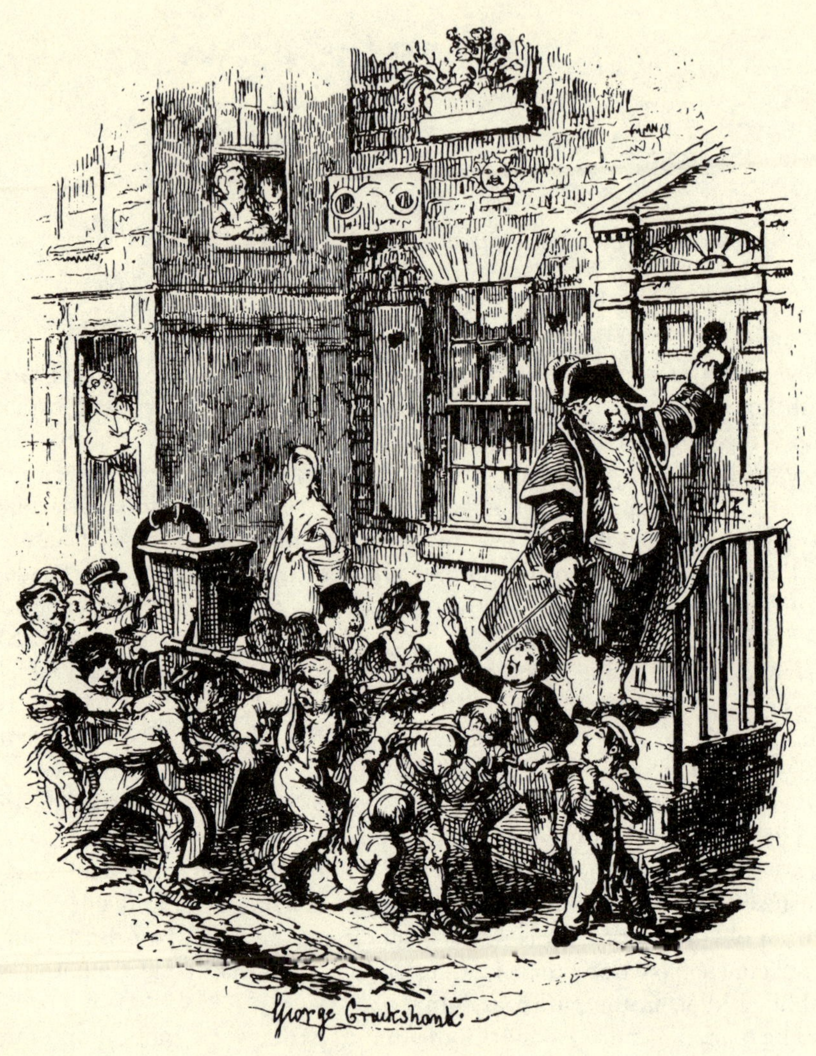


*The Parish Engine*

what 'we' (the beadle and the other gentlemen) came to the determination of doing. A miserable-looking woman is called into the board room, and represents a case of extreme destitution, affecting herself – a widow, with six small children. 'Where do you live?' inquires one of the overseers. 'I rents a two-pair back, gentlemen, at Mrs Brown's, Number 3, Little King William's Alley, which has lived there this fifteen year, and knows me to be very hard-working and industrious, and when my poor husband was alive, gentlemen, as died in the hospital,' – 'Well, well,' interrupts the overseer, taking a note of the address, 'I'll send Simmons, the beadle, tomorrow morning, to ascertain whether your story is correct; and if so, I suppose you must have an order into the House – Simmons, go to this woman's the first thing tomorrow morning, will you?' Simmons bows assent, and ushers the woman out. Her previous admiration of 'the board' (who all sit behind great books, and with their hats on) fades into nothing before her respect for her lace-trimmed conductor; and her account of what has passed inside, increases – if that be possible – the marks of respect, shown by the assembled crowd, to that solemn functionary. As to taking out a summons, it's quite a hopeless case if Simmons attends it, on behalf of the parish. He knows all the titles of the Lord Mayor by heart; states the case without a single stammer: and it is even reported that on one occasion he ventured to make a joke, which the Lord Mayor's head footman (who happened to be present) afterwards told an intimate friend, confidentially, was almost equal to one of Mr Hobler's.

See him again on Sunday in his state coat and cocked hat, with a large-headed staff for show in his left hand, and a small cane for use in his right. How pompously he marshals the children into their places! and how demurely the little urchins look at him askance as he surveys them when they are all seated, with a glare of the eye peculiar to beadles! The churchwardens and overseers being duly installed in their curtained pews, he seats himself on a mahogany bracket, erected expressly for him at the top of the aisle, and divides his attention between his prayer book and the boys. Suddenly, just at the commencement of the communion service, when the whole congregation is hushed into a profound silence, broken only by the voice of the officiating clergyman, a penny is heard to ring on the stone floor of the aisle with astounding clearness. Observe the generalship of the beadle. His involuntary look of horror is instantly changed into one of perfect indifference, as if he were the only person present who had not heard the noise. The artifice succeeds. After putting forth his right leg now and then, as a feeler, the victim who dropped the money ventures to make one or two distinct dives after it; and the beadle, gliding softly round, salutes his little round head, when it again appears above the seats, with divers double knocks, administered with the cane before noticed, to the intense delight of three young men in an adjacent pew, who cough violently at intervals until the conclusion of the sermon.

Such are a few traits of the importance and gravity of a parish beadle – a gravity which has never been disturbed in any case that has come under our observation, except when the services of that particularly useful machine, a parish fire engine, are required: then indeed all is bustle. Two little boys run to the beadle as fast as their legs will carry them, and report from their own personal observation that some neighbouring chimney is on fire; the engine is hastily got out, and a plentiful supply of boys being obtained, and harnessed to it with ropes, away they rattle over the pavement, the beadle, running – we do not exaggerate – running at the side, until they arrive at some house, smelling strongly of soot, at the door of which the beadle knocks with considerable gravity for half an hour. No attention being paid to these manual applications, and the turn-cock having turned on the water, the engine turns off amidst the shouts of the boys; it pulls up once more at the workhouse, and the beadle 'pulls up' the unfortunate householder next day, for the amount of his legal reward. We never saw a parish engine at a regular fire but once. It came up in gallant style – three miles and a half an hour, at least; there was a capital supply of water, and it was first on the spot. Bang went the pumps – the people cheered – the beadle perspired profusely; but it was unfortunately discovered, just as they were going to put the fire out, that nobody understood the process by which the engine was filled with water; and that eighteen boys, and a man, had exhausted themselves in pumping for twenty minutes, without producing the slightest effect!

The personages next in importance to the beadle, are the master of the workhouse and the parish schoolmaster. The vestry-clerk, as everybody knows, is a short, pudgy little man, in black, with a thick gold watch-chain of considerable length, terminating in two large seals and a key. He is an attorney, and generally in a bustle; at no time more so, than when he is hurrying to some parochial meeting, with his gloves crumpled up in one hand, and a large red book under the other arm. As to the churchwardens and overseers, we exclude them altogether, because all we know of them is, that they are usually respectable tradesmen, who wear hats with brims inclined to flatness, and who occasionally testify in gilt letters on a blue ground, in some conspicuous part of the church, to the important fact of a gallery having been enlarged and beautified, or an organ rebuilt.

The master of the workhouse is not, in our parish – nor is he usually in any other – one of that class of men the better part of whose existence has passed away, and who drag out the remainder in some inferior situation, with just enough thought of the past, to feel degraded by, and discontented with, the present. We are unable to guess precisely to our own satisfaction what station the man can have occupied before; we should think he had been an inferior sort of attorney's clerk, or else the master of a national school – whatever he was, it is clear his present position is a change for the better. His income is small certainly, as the rusty black coat and threadbare velvet collar demonstrate: but then he lives free of house-rent, has a limited allowance of coals and candles, and an almost unlimited allowance of authority in his petty kingdom. He is a tall, thin, bony man; always wears shoes and black cotton stockings with his surtout; and eyes you, as you pass his parlour window, as if he wished you were a pauper, just to give you a specimen of his power. He is an admirable specimen of a small tyrant: morose, brutish, and ill-tempered; bullying to his inferiors, cringing to his superiors, and jealous of the influence and authority of the beadle.

Our schoolmaster is just the very reverse of this amiable official. He has been one of those men one occasionally hears of, on whom misfortune seems to have set her mark; nothing he ever did, or was concerned in, appears to have prospered. A rich old relation who had brought him up, and openly announced his intention of providing for him, left him 10,000*l.* in his will, and revoked the bequest in a codicil. Thus unexpectedly reduced to the necessity of providing for himself, he procured a situation in a public office. The young clerks below him, died off as if there were a plague among them; but the old fellows over his head, for the reversion of whose places he was anxiously waiting, lived on and on, as if they were immortal. He speculated and lost. He speculated again and won – but never got his money. His talents were great; his disposition easy, generous and liberal. His friends profited by the one, and abused the other. Loss succeeded loss; misfortune crowded on misfortune; each successive day brought him nearer the verge of hopeless penury, and the quondam friends who had been warmest in their professions, grew strangely cold and indifferent. He had children whom he loved, and a wife on whom he doted. The former turned their backs on him; the latter died broken-hearted. He went with the stream – it had ever been his failing, and he had not courage sufficient to bear up against so many shocks – he had never cared for himself, and the only being who had cared for him, in his poverty and distress, was spared to him no longer. It was at this period that he applied for parochial relief. Some kind-hearted man who had known him in happier times, chanced to be churchwarden that year, and through his interest he was appointed to his present situation.

He is an old man now. Of the many who once crowded round him in all the hollow friendship of boon-companionship, some have died, some have fallen like himself, some have prospered – all have forgotten him. Time and misfortune have mercifully been permitted to impair his memory, and use has habituated him to his present condition. Meek, uncomplaining, and zealous in the discharge of his duties, he has been allowed to hold his situation long beyond the usual period; and he will no doubt continue to hold it, until infirmity renders him incapable, or death releases him. As the grey-headed old man feebly paces up and down the sunny side of the little courtyard between school hours, it would be difficult, indeed, for the most intimate of his former friends to recognise their once gay and happy associate, in the person of the Pauper Schoolmaster.

## Chapter Two

*The Curate – The Old Lady – The Half Pay Captain*

First published in the *Evening Chronicle* 19 May 1835 ('Sketches of London No. 12'). In the Church of England a curate is a priest, usually young, appointed to assist the parish priest. For the probable original of 'the Old Lady' (Mrs Mary Newnham, a neighbour of the Dickens family in Ordnance Terrace, Chatham, when Dickens was a child) see W.J. Carlton's article in *The Dickensian*, Vol. 49 (1953), pp. 149–52. Naval or military officers who were retired or not on active service were placed on half pay.

We commenced our last chapter with the beadle of our parish, because we are deeply sensible of the importance and dignity of his office. We will begin the present, with the clergyman. Our curate is a young gentleman of such prepossessing appearance, and fascinating manners, that within one month after his first appearance in the parish, half the young-lady inhabitants were melancholy with religion, and the other half desponding with love. Never were so many young ladies seen in our parish church on Sunday before; and never had the little round angels' faces on Mr Tomkins's monument in the side aisle, beheld such devotion on earth as they all exhibited. He was about five-and-twenty when he first came to astonish the parishioners. He parted his hair on the centre of his forehead in the form of a Norman arch, wore a brilliant of the first water on the fourth finger on his left hand (which he always applied to his left cheek when he read prayers), and had a deep sepulchral voice of unusual solemnity. Innumerable were the calls made by prudent mammas on our new curate, and innumerable the invitations with which he was assailed, and which, to do him justice, he readily accepted. If his manner in the pulpit had created an impression in his favour, the sensation was increased tenfold, by his appearance in private circles. Pews in the immediate vicinity of the pulpit or reading desk rose in value; sittings in the centre aisle were at a premium: an inch of room in the front row of the gallery could not be procured for love or money; and some people even went so far as to assert that the three Miss Browns, who had an obscure family pew just behind the churchwardens', were detected, one Sunday, in the free seats by the communion table, actually lying in wait for the curate as he passed to the vestry! He began to preach extempore sermons, and even grave papas caught the infection. He got out of bed at half past twelve o'clock one winter's night, to half-baptise a washerwoman's child in a slop basin, and the gratitude of the parishioners knew no bounds – the very churchwardens grew generous, and insisted on the parish defraying the expense of the watch-box on wheels, which the new curate had ordered for himself, to perform the funeral service in, in wet weather. He sent three pints of gruel and a quarter of a pound of tea to a poor woman who had been brought to bed of four small children, all at once – the parish were charmed. He got up a subscription for her – the woman's fortune was made. He spoke for one hour and twenty-five minutes, at an anti-slavery meeting at the Goat and Boots – the enthusiasm was at its height. A proposal was set on foot for presenting the curate with a piece of plate, as a mark of esteem for his valuable services rendered to the parish. The list of subscriptions was filled up in no time; the contest was, not who should escape the contribution, but who should be the foremost to subscribe. A splendid silver inkstand was made, and engraved with an appropriate inscription; the curate was invited to a public breakfast, at the before-mentioned Goat and Boots; the inkstand was presented in a neat speech by Mr Gubbins, the ex-churchwarden, and acknowledged by the curate in terms which drew tears into the eyes of all present – the very waiters were melted.

One could have supposed that, by this time, the theme of universal admiration was lifted to the very pinnacle of popularity. No such thing. The curate began to cough; four fits of coughing one morning between the Litany and the Epistle, and five in the afternoon service. Here was a discovery – the curate was consumptive. How interestingly melancholy! If the young ladies were energetic before, their sympathy and solicitude now knew no bounds. Such a man as the curate – such a dear – such a perfect love – to be consumptive! It was too much. Anonymous presents of blackcurrant jam, and lozenges, elastic waistcoats, bosom friends, and warm stockings, poured in upon the curate until he was as completely fitted out, with winter clothing, as if he were on the verge of an expedition to the North Pole: verbal bulletins of the state of his health were circulated throughout the parish half-a-dozen times a day; and the curate was in the very zenith of his popularity.

About this period a change came over the spirit of the parish. A very quiet, respectable, dozing old gentleman, who had officiated in our chapel of ease for twelve years previously, died one fine morning, without having given any notice whatever of his intention. This circumstance gave rise to counter-sensation the first; and the arrival of his successor occasioned counter-sensation the second. He was a pale, thin, cadaverous man, with large black eyes, and long straggling black hair: his dress was slovenly in the extreme, his manner ungainly, his doctrines startling; in short, he was in every respect the antipodes of the curate. Crowds of our female parishioners flocked to hear him; at first, because he was *so* odd-looking, then because his face was *so* expressive, then because he preached *so* well; and at last, because they really thought that, after all, there was something about him which it was quite impossible to describe. As to the curate, he was all very well; but certainly, after all, there was no denying that – that – in short, the curate wasn't a novelty, and the other clergyman was. The inconstancy of public opinion is proverbial: the congregation migrated one by one. The curate coughed till he was black in the face – it was in vain. He respired with difficulty – it was equally ineffectual in awakening sympathy. Seats are once again to be had in any part of our parish church, and the chapel of ease is going to be enlarged, as it is crowded to suffocation every Sunday!

The best known and most respected among our parishioners, is an old lady, who resided in our parish long before our name was registered in the list of baptisms. Our parish is a suburban one, and the old lady lives in a neat row of houses in the most airy and pleasant part of it. The house is her own; and it, and everything about it, except the old lady herself, who looks a little older than she did ten years ago, is in just the same state as when the old gentleman was living. The little front parlour, which is the old lady's ordinary sitting room, is a perfect picture of quiet neatness; the carpet is covered with brown Holland, the glass and picture frames are carefully enveloped in yellow muslin; the table covers are never taken off, except when the leaves are turpentined and bees'-waxed, an operation which is regularly commenced every other morning at half past nine o'clock – and the little nicknacks are always arranged in precisely the same manner. The greater part of these are presents from little girls whose parents live in the same row; but some of them, such as the two old-fashioned watches (which never keep the same time, one being always a quarter of an hour too slow, and the other a quarter of an hour too fast), the little picture of the Princess Charlotte and Prince Leopold as they appeared in the Royal Box at Drury Lane Theatre, and others of the same class, have been in the old lady's possession for many years. Here the old lady sits with her spectacles on, busily engaged in needlework – near the window in summertime; and if she sees you coming up the steps, and you happen to be a favourite, she trots out to open the street door for you before you knock, and as you must be fatigued after that hot walk, insists on your swallowing two glasses of sherry before you exert yourself by talking. If you call in the evening you will find her cheerful, but rather more serious than usual, with an open Bible on the table before her, of which 'Sarah', who is just as neat and methodical as her mistress, regularly reads two or three chapters in the parlour aloud.

The old lady sees scarcely any company, except the little girls before noticed, each of whom has always a regular fixed day for a periodical tea-drinking with her, to which the child looks forward as the greatest treat of its existence. She seldom visits at a greater distance than the next door but one on either side; and when she drinks tea here, Sarah runs out first and knocks a double knock, to prevent the possibility of her 'Missis's' catching cold by having to wait at the door. She is very scrupulous in returning these little invitations, and when she asks Mr and Mrs So-and-so, to meet Mr and Mrs Somebody-else, Sarah and she dust the urn, and the best china tea-service, and the Pope Joan board; and the visitors are received in the drawing room in great state. She has but few relations, and they are scattered about in different parts of the country, and she seldom sees them. She has a son in India, whom she always describes to you as a fine, handsome fellow – so like the profile of his poor dear father over the sideboard, but the old lady adds, with a mournful shake of the head, that he has always been one of her greatest trials; and that indeed he once almost broke her heart; but it pleased God to enable her to get the better of it, and she would prefer your never mentioning the subject to her again. She has a great number of pensioners: and on Saturday, after she comes back from market, there is a regular levee of old men and women in the passage, waiting for their weekly gratuity. Her name always heads the list of any benevolent subscriptions, and hers are always the most liberal donations to the Winter Coal and Soup Distribution Society. She subscribed twenty pounds towards the erection of an organ in our parish church, and was so overcome the first Sunday the children sang to it, that she was obliged to be carried out by the pew opener. Her entrance into church on Sunday is always the signal for a little bustle in the side aisle, occasioned by a general rise among the poor people, who bow and curtsey until the pew opener has ushered the old lady into her accustomed seat, dropped a respectful curtsey and shut the door: and the same ceremony is repeated on her leaving church, when she walks home with the family next door but one, and talks about the sermon all the way, invariably opening the conversation by asking the youngest boy where the text was.

Thus, with the annual variation of a trip to some quiet place on the sea coast, passes the old lady's life. It has rolled on in the same unvarying and benevolent course for many years now, and must at no distant period be brought to its final close. She looks forward to its termination, with calmness and without apprehension. She has everything to hope and nothing to fear.

A very different personage, but one who has rendered himself very conspicuous in our parish, is one of the old lady's next-door neighbours. He is an old naval officer on half pay, and his bluff and unceremonious behaviour disturbs the old lady's domestic economy, not a little. In the first place, he *will* smoke cigars in the front court, and when he wants something to drink with them – which is by no means an uncommon circumstance – he lifts up the old lady's knocker with his walking stick, and demands to have a glass of table ale, handed over the rails. In addition to this cool proceeding, he is a bit of a Jack of all trades, or to use his own words, 'a regular Robinson Crusoe'; and nothing delights him better than to experimentalise on the old lady's property. One morning he got up early, and planted three or four roots of full-grown marigolds in every bed of her front garden, to the inconceivable astonishment of the old lady, who actually thought when she got up and looked out of the window, that it was some strange eruption which had come out in the night. Another time he took to pieces the eight-day clock on the front landing, under pretence of cleaning the works, which he put together again, by some undiscovered process, in so wonderful a manner, that the large hand has done nothing but trip up the little one ever since. Then he took to breeding silk worms, which he *would* bring in two or three times a day, in little paper boxes, to show the old lady, generally dropping a worm or two at every visit. The consequence was, that one morning a very stout silk worm was discovered in the act of walking upstairs – probably with the view of inquiring after his friends, for, on further inspection, it appeared that some of his companions had already found their way to every room in the house. The old lady went to the seaside in despair, and during her absence he completely effaced the name from her brass door plate, in his attempts to polish it with aqua-fortis.

But all this is nothing to his seditious conduct in public life. He attends every vestry meeting that is held; always opposes the constituted authorities of the parish, denounces the profligacy of the churchwardens, contests legal points against the vestry clerk, *will* make the tax gatherer call for his money till he won't call any longer, and then he sends it: finds fault with the sermon every Sunday, says that the organist ought to be ashamed of himself, offers to back himself for any amount to sing the psalms better than all the children put together, male and female; and, in short, conducts himself in the most turbulent and uproarious manner. The worst of it is, that having a high regard for the old lady, he wants to make her a convert to his views, and therefore walks into her little parlour with his newspaper in his hand, and talks violent politics by the hour. He is a charitable, open-hearted old fellow at bottom, after all; so, although he puts the old lady a little out occasionally, they agree very well in the main, and she laughs as much at each feat of his handiwork when it is all over, as anybody else.

## Chapter Three

### *The Four Sisters*

First published in the *Evening Chronicle*, 18 June 1835 ('Sketches of London No. 14').

The row of houses in which the old lady and her troublesome neighbour reside, comprises, beyond all doubt, a greater number of characters within its circumscribed limits, than all the rest of the parish put together. As we cannot, consistently with our present plan, however, extend the number of our parochial sketches beyond six, it will be better, perhaps, to select the most peculiar, and to introduce them at once without further preface.

The four Miss Willises, then, settled in our parish thirteen years ago. It is a melancholy reflection that the old adage, 'time and tide wait for no man', applies with equal force to the fairer portion of the creation; and willingly would we conceal the fact, that even thirteen years ago the Miss Willises were far from juvenile. Our duty as faithful parochial chroniclers, however, is paramount to every other consideration, and we are bound to state, that thirteen years since, the authorities in matrimonial cases considered the youngest Miss Willis in a very precarious state, while the eldest sister was positively given over, as being far beyond all human hope. Well, the Miss Willises took a lease of the house; it was fresh painted and papered from top to bottom: the paint inside was all wainscoted, the marble all cleaned, the old grates taken down, and register-stoves, you could see to dress by, put up; four trees were planted in the back garden, several small baskets of gravel sprinkled over the front one, vans of elegant furniture arrived, spring blinds were fitted to the windows, carpenters who had been employed in the various preparations, alterations, and repairs, made confidential statements to the different maidservants in the row, relative to the magnificent scale on which the Miss Willises were commencing; the maidservants told their 'Missises', the Missises told their friends, and vague rumours were circulated throughout the parish, that No. 25, in Gordon Place, had been taken by four maiden ladies of immense property.

At last, the Miss Willises moved in; and then the 'calling' began. The house was the perfection of neatness – so were the four Miss Willises.

Everything was formal, stiff, and cold – so were the four Miss Willises. Not a single chair of the whole set was ever seen out of its place – not a single Miss Willis of the whole four was ever seen out of hers. There they always sat, in the same places, doing precisely the same things at the same hour. The eldest Miss Willis used to knit, the second to draw, the two others to play duets on the piano. They seemed to have no separate existence, but to have made up their minds just to winter through life together. They were three long graces in drapery, with the addition, like a school dinner, of another long grace afterwards – the three fates with another sister – the Siamese twins multiplied by two. The eldest Miss Willis grew bilious – the four Miss Willises grew bilious immediately. The eldest Miss Willis grew ill-tempered and religious – the four Miss Willises were ill-tempered and religious directly. Whatever the eldest did, the others did, and whatever anybody else did, they all disapproved of; and thus they vegetated – living in Polar harmony among themselves, and, as they sometimes went out, or saw company 'in a quiet way' at home, occasionally iceing the neighbours. Three years passed over in this way, when an unlooked-for and extraordinary phenomenon occurred. The Miss Willises showed symptoms of summer, the frost gradually broke up; a complete thaw took place. Was it possible? one of the four Miss Willises was going to be married!

Now, where on earth the husband came from, by what feelings the poor man could have been actuated, or by what process of reasoning the four Miss Willises succeeded in persuading themselves that it was possible for a man to marry one of them, without marrying all them, are questions too profound for us to resolve: certain it is, however, that the visits of Mr Robinson (a gentleman in a public office, with a good salary and a little property of his own, beside) were received – that the four Miss Willises were courted in due form by the said Mr Robinson – that the neighbours were perfectly frantic in their anxiety to discover which of the four Miss Willises was the fortunate fair, and that the difficulty they experienced in solving the problem was not at all lessened by the announcement of the eldest Miss Willis, – '*We* are going to marry Mr Robinson.'

It was very extraordinary. They were so completely identified, the one with the other, that the curiosity of the whole row – even of the old lady herself – was roused almost beyond endurance. The subject was discussed at every little card table and tea-drinking. The old gentleman of silk worm notoriety did not hesitate to express his decided opinion that Mr Robinson was of Eastern descent, and contemplated marrying the whole family at once; and the row, generally, shook their heads with considerable gravity, and declared the business to be very mysterious. They hoped it might all end well; it certainly had a very singular appearance, but still it would be uncharitable to express any opinion without good grounds to go upon, and certainly the Miss Willises were *quite* old enough to judge for themselves, and to be sure people ought to know their own business best, and so forth.

At last, one fine morning, at a quarter before eight o'clock AM, two glass coaches drove up to the Miss Willises' door, at which Mr Robinson had arrived in a cab ten minutes before, dressed in a light blue coat and double-milled kersey pantaloons, white neckerchief, pumps, and dress gloves, his manner denoting, as appeared from the evidence of the housemaid at No. 23, who was sweeping the doorsteps at the time, a considerable degree of nervous excitement. It was also hastily reported on the same testimony, that the cook who opened the door, wore a large white bow of unusual dimensions, in a much smarter head-dress than the regulation cap to which the Miss Willises invariably restricted the somewhat excursive tastes of female servants in general.

The intelligence spread rapidly from house to house. It was quite clear that the eventful morning had at length arrived; the whole row stationed themselves behind their first and second floor blinds, and waited the result in breathless expectation.

At last the Miss Willises' door opened; the door of the first glass coach did the same. Two gentlemen, and a pair of ladies to correspond – friends of the family, no doubt; up went the steps, bang went the door, off went the first glass coach, and up came the second.

The street door opened again; the excitement of the whole row increased – Mr Robinson and the eldest Miss Willis. 'I thought so,' said the lady at No. 19; 'I always said it was *Miss* Willis!' – 'Well, I never!' ejaculated the young lady at No. 18 to the young lady at No. 17. – 'Did you ever, dear!' responded the young lady at No. 17 to the young lady at No. 18. 'It's too ridiculous!' exclaimed a spinster of an *un*certain age, at No. 16, joining in the conversation. But who shall portray the astonishment of Gordon Place, when Mr Robinson handed in *all* the Miss Willises, one after the other, and then squeezed himself into an acute angle of the glass coach, which forthwith proceeded at a brisk pace, after the other glass coach, which other glass coach had itself proceeded, at a brisk pace, in the direction of the parish church! Who shall depict the perplexity of the clergyman, when *all* the Miss Willises knelt down at the communion table, and repeated the responses incidental to the marriage service in an audible voice – or who shall describe the confusion which prevailed, when – even after the difficulties thus occasioned had been adjusted – *all* the Miss Willises went into hysterics at the conclusion of the ceremony, until the sacred edifice resounded with their united wailings!

As the four sisters and Mr Robinson continued to occupy the same house after this memorable occasion, and as the married sister, whoever she was, never appeared in public without the other three, we are not quite clear that the neighbours ever would have discovered the real Mrs Robinson, but for a circumstance of the most gratifying description, which *will* happen occasionally in the best regulated families. Three quarter-days elapsed, and the row, on whom a new light appeared to have been bursting for some time, began to speak with a sort of implied confidence on the subject, and to wonder how Mrs Robinson – the youngest Miss Willis that was – got on; and servants might be seen running up the steps, about nine or ten o'clock every morning, with 'Missis's compliments, and wishes to know how Mrs Robinson finds herself this morning?' And the answer always was, 'Mrs Robinson's compliments, and she's in very good spirits, and doesn't find herself any worse.' The piano was heard no longer, the knitting needles were laid aside, drawing was neglected, and mantua-making and millinery, on the smallest scale imaginable, appeared to have become the favourite amusement of the whole family. The parlour wasn't quite as tidy as it used to be, and if you called in the morning, you would see lying on a table, with old newspaper carelessly thrown over them, two or three particularly small caps, rather larger than if they had been made for a moderate sized doll, with a small piece of lace, in the shape of a horseshoe, let in behind: or perhaps a white robe, not very large in circumference, but very much out of proportion in point of length, with a little tucker round the top, and a frill round the bottom; and once when we called, we saw a long white roller, with a kind of blue margin down each side, the probable use of which, we were at a loss to conjecture. Then we fancied that Mr Dawson, the surgeon, &c., who displays a large lamp with a different colour in every pane of glass, at the corner of the row, began to be knocked up at night oftener than he used to be; and once we were very much alarmed by hearing a hackney coach stop at Mrs Robinson's door, at half past two o'clock in the morning, out of which there emerged a fat old woman, in a cloak and nightcap, with a bundle in one hand, and a pair of pattens in the other, who looked as if she had been suddenly knocked up out of bed for some very special purpose.

When we got up in the morning, we saw that the knocker was tied up in an old white kid glove; and we, in our innocence (we were in a state of bachelorship then), wondered what on earth it all meant, until we heard the eldest Miss Willis, *in propriâ personâ*, say, with great dignity, in answer to the next inquiry, '*My* compliments, and Mrs Robinson's doing as well as can be expected, and the little girl thrives wonderfully.' And then, in common with the rest of the row, our curiosity was satisfied, and we began to wonder it had never occurred to us what the matter was, before.

## Chapter Four

### *The Election for Beadle*

First published in the *Evening Chronicle*, 14 July 1835 ('Sketches of London No. 16')

A great event has recently occurred in our parish. A contest of paramount interest has just terminated; a parochial convulsion has taken place. It has been succeeded by a glorious triumph, which the country – or at least the parish – it is all the same – will long remember. We have had an election; an election for beadle. The supporters of the old beadle system have been defeated in their stronghold, and the advocates of the great new beadle principles have achieved a proud victory.

Our parish, which, like all other parishes, is a little world of its own, has long been divided into two parties, whose contentions, slumbering for a while, have never failed to burst forth with unabated vigour, on any occasion on which they could by possibility be renewed. Watching rates, lighting rates, paving rates, sewer's rates, church rates, poor's rates – all sorts of rates, have been in their turn the subjects of a grand struggle; and as to questions of patronage, the asperity and determination with which they have been contested is scarcely credible.

The leader of the official party – the steady advocate of the church-wardens, and the unflinching supporter of the overseers – is an old gentleman who lives in our row. He owns some half a dozen houses in it, and always walks on the opposite side of the way, so that he may be able to take in a view of the whole of his property at once. He is a tall, thin, bony man, with an interrogative nose, and little restless perking eyes, which appear to have been given him for the sole purpose of peeping into other people's affairs with. He is deeply impressed with the importance of our parish business, and prides himself, not a little, on his style of addressing the parishioners in vestry assembled. His views are rather confined than extensive; his principles more narrow than liberal. He has been heard to declaim very loudly in favour of the liberty of the press, and advocates the repeal of the stamp duty on newspapers, because the daily journals who now have a monopoly of the public, never give *verbatim* reports of vestry meetings. He would not appear egotistical for the world,

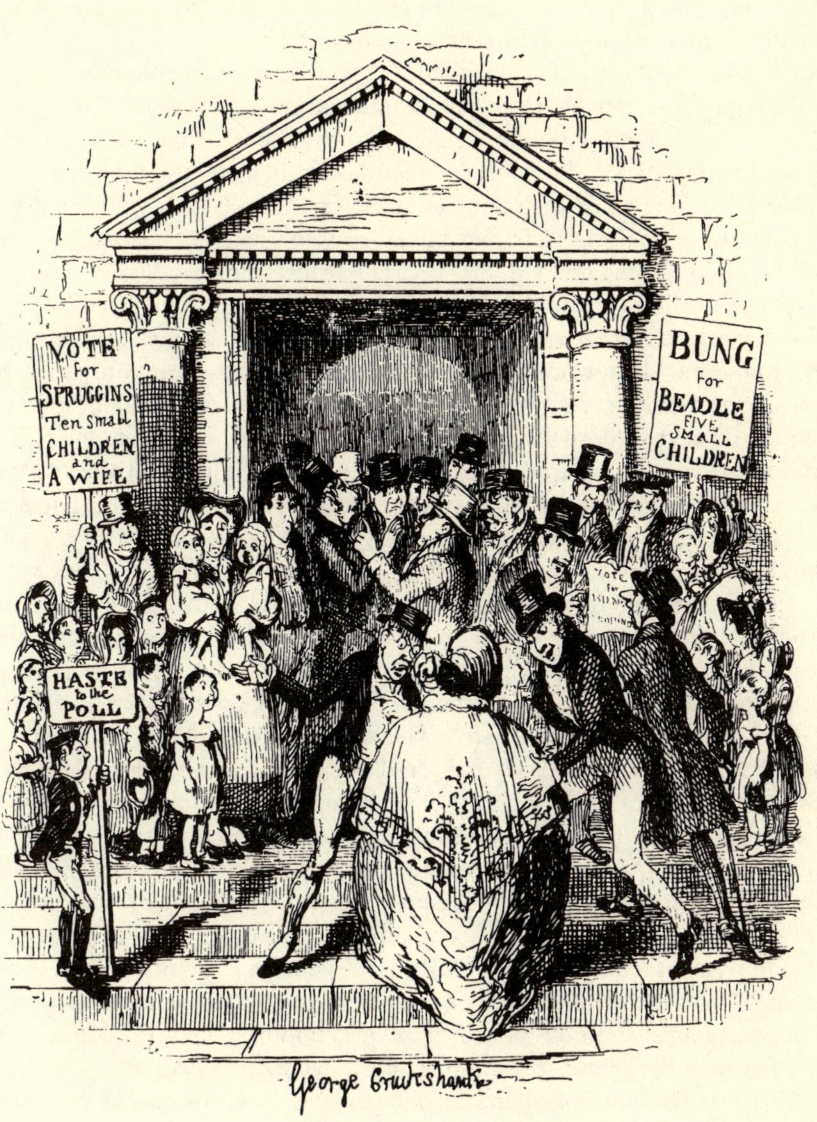


*The Election for Beadle*

but at the same time he must say, that there *are* speeches – that celebrated speech of his own, on the emoluments of the sexton, and the duties of the office, for instance – which might be communicated to the public, greatly to their improvement and advantage.

His great opponent in public life is Captain Purday, the old naval officer on half pay, to whom we have already introduced our readers. The captain being a determined opponent of the constituted authorities, whoever they may chance to be, and our other friend being their steady supporter, with an equal disregard of their individual merits, it will readily be supposed that occasions for their coming into direct collision are neither few nor far between. They divided the vestry fourteen times on a motion for heating the church with warm water instead of coals: and made speeches about liberty and expenditure, and prodigality and hot water, which threw the whole parish into a state of excitement. Then the captain, when he was on the visiting committee, and his opponent overseer, brought forward certain distinct and specific charges relative to the management of the workhouse, boldly expressed his total want of confidence in the existing authorities, and moved for 'a copy of the recipe by which the paupers' soup was prepared, together with any documents relating thereto'. This the overseer steadily resisted; he fortified himself by precedent, appealed to the established usage, and declined to produce the papers, on the ground of the injury that would be done to the public service, if documents of a strictly private nature, passing between the master of the workhouse and the cook, were to be thus dragged to light on the motion of any individual member of the vestry. The motion was lost by a majority of two; and then the captain, who never allows himself to be defeated, moved for a committee of inquiry into the whole subject. The affair grew serious: the question was discussed at meeting after meeting, and vestry after vestry; speeches were made, attacks repudiated, personal defiances exchanged, explanations received, and the greatest excitement prevailed, until at last, just as the question was going to be finally decided, the vestry found that somehow or other, they had become entangled in a point of form, from which it was impossible to escape with propriety. So the motion was dropped, and everybody looked extremely important, and seemed quite satisfied with the meritorious nature of the whole proceeding.

This was the state of affairs in our parish a week or two since, when Simmons, the beadle, suddenly died. The lamented deceased had over-exerted himself, a day or two previously, in conveying an aged female, highly intoxicated, to the strong room of the workhouse. The excitement thus occasioned, added to a severe cold, which this indefatigable officer had caught in his capacity of director of the parish engine, by inadvertently playing over himself instead of a fire, proved too much for a constitution already enfeebled by age; and the intelligence was conveyed to the Board one evening that Simmons had died, and left his respects.

The breath was scarcely out of the body of the deceased functionary, when the field was filled with competitors for the vacant office, each of whom rested his claims to public support, entirely on the number and extent of his family, as if the office of beadle were originally instituted as an encouragement for the propagation of the human species. 'Bung for Beadle. Five small children!' – 'Hopkins for Beadle. Seven small children!!' – 'Timkins for Beadle. Nine small children!!!' Such were the placards in large black letters on a white ground, which were plentifully pasted on the walls, and posted in the windows of the principal shops. Timkins's success was considered certain: several mothers of families half promised their votes, and the nine small children would have run over the course, but for the production of another placard, announcing the appearance of a still more meritorious candidate. 'Spruggins for Beadle. Ten small children (two of them twins), and a wife!!!' There was no resisting this; ten small children would have been almost irresistible in themselves, without the twins, but the touching parenthesis about that interesting production of nature, and the still more touching allusion to Mrs Spruggins, must ensure success. Spruggins was the favourite at once, and the appearance of his lady, as she went about to solicit votes (which encouraged confident hopes of a still further addition to the house of Spruggins at no remote period), increased the general prepossession in his favour. The other candidates, Bung alone excepted, resigned in despair. The day of election was fixed; and the canvass proceeded with briskness and perseverance on both sides.

The members of the vestry could not be supposed to escape the contagious excitement inseparable from the occasion. The majority of the lady inhabitants of the parish declared at once for Spruggins; and the *quondam* overseer took the same side, on the ground that men with large families always had been elected to the office, and that although he must admit that, in other respects, Spruggins was the least qualified candidate of the two, still it was an old practice, and he saw no reason why an old practice should be departed from. This was enough for the captain. He immediately sided with Bung, canvassed for him personally in all directions, wrote squibs on Spruggins, and got his butcher to skewer them up on conspicuous joints in his shop-front; frightened his neighbour, the old lady, into a palpitation of the heart, by the awful denunciations of Spruggins's party; and bounced in and out, and up and down, and backwards and forwards, until all the sober inhabitants of the parish thought it inevitable that he must die of a brain fever, long before the election began.

The day of the election arrived. It was no longer an individual struggle, but a party contest between the ins and outs. The question was, whether the withering influence of the overseers, the domination of the churchwardens, and the blighting despotism of the vestry clerk, should be allowed to render the election of beadle a form – a nullity: whether they should impose a vestry-elected beadle on the parish, to do their bidding and forward their views, or whether the parishioners, fearlessly asserting their undoubted rights, should elect an independent beadle of their own.

The nomination was fixed to take place in the vestry, but so great was the throng of anxious spectators, that it was found necessary to adjourn to the church, where the ceremony commenced with due solemnity. The appearance of the churchwardens and overseers, and the ex-churchwardens and ex-overseers, with Spruggins in the rear, excited general attention. Spruggins was a little thin man, in rusty black, with a long pale face, and a countenance expressive of care and fatigue, which might either be attributed to the extent of his family or the anxiety of his feelings. His opponent appeared in a cast-off coat of the captain's – a blue coat with bright buttons: white trousers, and that description of shoes familiarly known by the appellation of 'high-lows'. There was a serenity in the open countenance of Bung – a kind of moral dignity in his confident air – an 'I wish you may get it' sort of expression in his eye – which infused animation into his supporters, and evidently dispirited his opponents.

The ex-churchwarden rose to propose Thomas Spruggins for beadle. He had known him long. He had had his eye upon him closely for years; he had watched him with twofold vigilance for months. (A parishioner here suggested that this might be termed 'taking a double sight,' but the observation was drowned in loud cries of 'Order!') He would repeat that he had had his eye upon him for years, and this he would say, that a more well-conducted, a more well behaved, a more sober, a more quiet man, with a more well regulated mind, he had never met with. A man with a larger family he had never known (cheers). The parish required a man who could be depended on ('Hear!' from the Spruggins side, answered by ironical cheers from the Bung party). Such a man he now proposed ('No', 'Yes'). He would not allude to individuals (the ex-churchwarden continued, in the celebrated negative style adopted by great speakers). He would not advert to a gentleman who had once held a high rank in the service of his majesty; he would not say, that that gentleman was no gentleman; he would not assert, that that man was no man; he would not say, that he was a turbulent parishioner; he would not say, that he had grossly misbehaved himself, not only on this, but on all former occasions; he would not say, that he was one of those discontented and treasonable spirits; who carried confusion and disorder wherever they went; he would not say, that he harboured in his heart envy, and hatred, and malice, and all uncharitableness. No! He wished to have everything comfortable and pleasant, and, therefore, he would say – nothing about him (cheers).

The captain replied in a similar parliamentary style. He would not say, he was astonished at the speech they had just heard; he would not say, he was disgusted (cheers). He would not retort the epithets which had been hurled against him (renewed cheering); he would not allude to men once in office, but now happily out of it, who had mismanaged the workhouse, ground the paupers, diluted the beer, slack-baked the bread, boned the meat, heightened the work, and lowered the soup (tremendous cheers). He would not ask what such men deserved (a voice, 'Nothing a-day, and find themselves!'). He would not say, that one burst of general indignation should drive them from the parish they polluted with their presence ('Give it him!'). He would not allude to the unfortunate man who had been proposed – he would not say, as the vestry's tool, but as Beadle. He would not advert to that individual's family; he would not say, that nine children, twins, and a wife, were very bad examples for pauper imitation (loud cheers). He would not advert in detail to the qualifications of Bung. The man stood before him, and he would not say in his presence, what he might be disposed to say of him if he were absent. (Here Mr Bung telegraphed to a friend near him, under cover of his hat, by contracting his left eye, and applying his right thumb to the tip of his nose). It had been objected to Bung that he had only five children ('Hear, hear!' from the opposition). Well; he had yet to learn that the legislature had affixed any precise amount of infantine qualification to the office of beadle; but taking it for granted that an extensive family were a great requisite, he entreated them to look to facts, and compare *data*, about which there could be no mistake. Bung was 35 years of age. Spruggins – of whom he wished to speak with all possible respect – was 50. Was it not more than possible – was it not very probable – that by the time Bung attained the latter age, he might see around him a family, even exceeding in number and extent that to which Spruggins at present laid claim? (deafening cheers and waving of handkerchiefs). The captain concluded, amidst loud applause, by calling upon the parishioners to sound the tocsin, rush to the poll, free themselves from dictation, or be slaves for ever.

On the following day the polling began, and we never have had such a bustle in our parish since we got up our famous anti-slavery petition, which was such an important one that the House of Commons ordered it to be printed, on the motion of the member for the district. The captain engaged two hackney coaches and a cab for Bung's people – the cab for the drunken voters, and the two coaches for the old ladies, the greater portion of whom, owing to the captain's impetuosity, were driven up to the poll and home again, before they recovered from their flurry sufficiently to know, with any degree of clearness, what they had been doing. The opposite party wholly neglected these precautions, and the consequence was, that a great many ladies who were walking leisurely up to the church – for it was a very hot day – to vote for Spruggins, were artfully decoyed into the coaches, and voted for Bung. The captain's arguments, too, had produced considerable effect: the attempted influence of the vestry produced a greater. A threat of exclusive dealing was clearly established against the vestry clerk – a case of heartless and profligate atrocity. It appeared that the delinquent had been in the habit of purchasing six penn'orth of muffins, weekly, from an old woman who rents a small house in the parish, and resides among the original settlers; on her last weekly visit, a message was conveyed to her through the medium of the cook, couched in mysterious terms, but indicating with sufficient clearness, that the vestry clerk's appetite for muffins, in future, depended entirely on her vote on the beadleship. This was sufficient: the stream had been turning previously, and the impulse thus administered directed its final course. The Bung party ordered one shilling's-worth of muffins weekly for the remainder of the old woman's natural life; the parishioners were loud in their exclamations; and the fate of Spruggins was sealed.

It was in vain that the twins were exhibited in dresses of the same pattern, and nightcap to match, at the church door: the boy in Mrs Spruggins's right arm, and the girl in her left – even Mrs Spruggins herself failed to be an object of sympathy any longer. The majority attained by Bung on the gross poll was four hundred and twenty-eight, and the cause of the parishioners triumphed.

## Chapter Five

### *The Broker's Man*

First published in the *Evening Chronicle*, 28 July 1835 ('Sketches of London No. 18'). Brokers (dealers in second-hand furniture) were employed by the courts to value debtors' household effects that might be distrained for non-payment of rent or other debts. They would place a man in the debtor's house to ensure that no goods were removed during the time allowed for their owner to try to raise the money to settle the debt.

The excitement of the late election has subsided, and our parish being once again restored to a state of comparative tranquillity, we are enabled to devote our attention to those parishioners who take little share in our party contests or in the turmoil and bustle of public life. And we feel sincere pleasure in acknowledging here, that in collecting materials for this task we have been greatly assisted by Mr Bung himself, who has imposed on us a debt of obligation which we fear we can never repay. The life of this gentleman has been one of a very chequered description: he has undergone transitions – not from grave to gay, for he never was grave – not from lively to severe, for severity forms no part of his disposition; his fluctuations have been between poverty in the extreme, and poverty modified, or, to use his own emphatic language, 'between nothing to eat and just half enough'. He is not, as he forcibly remarks, 'one of those fortunate men who, if they were to dive under one side of a barge stark-naked, would come up on the other, with a new suit of clothes on, and a ticket for soup in the waistcoat pocket': neither is he one of those whose spirit has been broken beyond redemption by misfortune and want. He is just one of the careless, good-for-nothing, happy fellows, who float, cork-like, on the surface, for the world to play at hockey with: knocked here, and there, and everywhere: now to the right, then to the left, again up in the air, and anon to the bottom, but always reappearing and bounding with the stream buoyantly and merrily along. Some few months before he was prevailed upon to stand a contested election for the office of beadle, necessity attached him to the service of a broker; and on the opportunities he here acquired of ascertaining the condition of most of the poor inhabitants of the parish, his patron, the captain, first

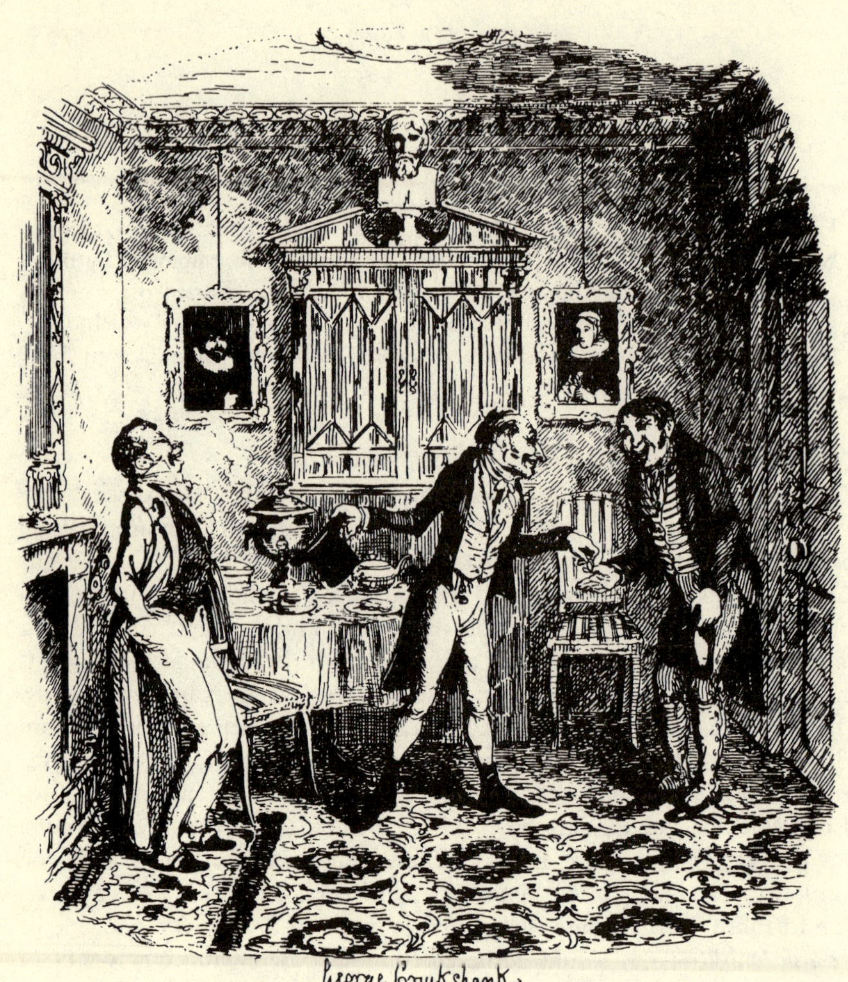


*The Broker's Men*

grounded his claims to public support. Chance threw the man in our way a short time since. We were, in the first instance, attracted by his prepossessing impudence at the election; we were not surprised, on further acquaintance, to find him a shrewd, knowing fellow, with no inconsiderable power of observation; and, after conversing with him a little, were somewhat struck (as we dare say our readers have frequently been in other cases) with the power some men seem to have, not only of sympathising with, but to all appearance of understanding feelings to which they themselves are entire strangers. We had been expressing to the new functionary our surprise that he should ever have served in the capacity to which we have just adverted, when we gradually led him into one or two professional anecdotes. As we are induced to think, on reflection, that they will tell better in nearly his own words than with any attempted embellishments of ours, we will at once entitle them

### *Mr Bung's Narrative*

'It's very true, as you say, sir,' Mr Bung commenced, 'that a broker's man's is not a life to be envied; and in course you know as well as I do, though you don't say it, that people hate and scout 'em because they're the ministers of wretchedness, like, to poor people. But what could I do, sir? The thing was no worse because I did it, instead of somebody else; and if putting me in possession of a house would put me in possession of three and sixpence a day, and levying a distress on another man's goods would relieve my distress and that of my family, it can't be expected but what I'd take the job and go through with it. I never liked it, God knows; I always looked out for something else, and the moment I got other work to do, I left it. If there is anything wrong in being the agent in such matters – not the principal, mind you – I'm sure the business, to a beginner like I was, at all events, carries its own punishment along with it. I wished again and again that the people would only blow me up, or pitch into me – that I wouldn't have minded, it's all in my way; but it's the being shut up by yourself in one room for five days, without so much as an old newspaper to look at, or anything to see out o' the winder but the roofs and chimneys at the back of the house, or anything to listen to but the ticking, perhaps, of an old Dutch clock, the sobbing of the missis now and then, the low talking of friends in the next room, who speak in whispers, lest 'the man' should overhear them, or perhaps the occasional opening of the door, as a child peeps in to look at you, and then runs half-frightened away – it's all this, that makes you feel sneaking somehow, and ashamed of yourself; and then, if it's winter time, they just give you fire enough to make you think you'd like more, and bring in your grub as if they wished it 'ud choke you – as I dare say they do, for the matter of that, most heartily. If they're very civil, they make you up a bed in the room at night, and if they don't, your master sends one in for you; but there you are, without being washed or shaved all the time, shunned by everybody, and spoken to by no one, unless someone comes in at dinner time, and asks you whether you want any more, in a tone as much as to say, 'I hope you don't', or, in the evening, to inquire whether you wouldn't rather have a candle, after you've been sitting in the dark half the night. When I was left in this way, I used to sit, think, think, thinking, till I felt as lonesome as a kitten in a wash-house copper with the lid on; but I believe the old brokers' men who are regularly trained to it, never think at all. I have heard some on 'em say, indeed, that they don't know how!

'I put in a good many distresses in my time (continued Mr Bung), and in course I wasn't long in finding, that some people are not as much to be pitied as others are, and that people with good incomes who get into difficulties, which they keep patching up day after day, and week after week, get so used to these sort of things in time, that at last they come scarcely to feel them at all. I remember the very first place I was put in possession of, was a gentleman's house in this parish here, that everybody would suppose couldn't help having money if he tried. I went with old Fixem, my old master, 'bout half arter eight in the morning; rang the area-bell; servant in livery opened the door: "Governor at home?" – "Yes, he is," says the man; "but he's breakfasting just now." "Never mind," says Fixem, "just you tell him there's a gentleman here, as wants to speak to him partickler." So the servant he opens his eyes, and stares about him all ways – looking for the gentleman, as it struck me, for I don't think anybody but a man as was stone-blind would mistake Fixem for one; and as for me, I was as seedy as a cheap cowcumber. Hows'ever, he turns round, and goes to the breakfast parlour, which was a little snug sort of room at the end of the passage, and Fixem (as we always did in that profession), without waiting to be announced, walks in arter him, and before the servant could get out, "Please, sir, here's a man as wants to speak to you," looks in at the door as familiar and pleasant as may be. "Who the devil are you, and how dare you walk into a gentleman's house without leave?" says the master, as fierce as a bull in fits. "My name", says Fixem, winking to the master to send the servant away, and putting the warrant into his hands folded up like a note, "My name's Smith," says he, "and I called from Johnson's about that business of Thompson's." – "Oh," says the other, quite down on him directly, "How *is* Thompson?" says he. "Pray sit down, Mr Smith: John, leave the room." Out went the servant; and the gentleman and Fixem looked at one another till they couldn't look any longer, and then they varied the amusements by looking at me, who had been standing on the mat all this time. "Hundred and fifty pounds, I see," said the gentleman at last. "Hundred and fifty pound," said Fixem, "besides cost of levy, sheriff's poundage, and all other incidental expenses." – "Um," says the gentleman, "I shan't be able to settle this before tomorrow afternoon." – "Very sorry; but I shall be obliged to leave my man here till then," replies Fixem, pretending to look very miserable over it. "That's very unfort'nate," says the gentleman, "for I have got a large party here tonight, and I'm ruined if those fellows of mine get an inkling of the matter – just step here, Mr Smith," says he, after a short pause. So Fixem walks with him up to the window, and after a good deal of whispering, and a little chinking of suverins, and looking at me, he comes back and says, "Bung, you're a handy fellow, and very honest, I know. This gentleman wants an assistant to clean the plate and wait at table today, and if you're not particularly engaged," says old Fixem, grinning like mad, and shoving a couple of suverins into my hand, "he'll be very glad to avail himself of your services." Well, I laughed: and the gentleman laughed, and we all laughed; and I went home and cleaned myself, leaving Fixem there, and when I went back, Fixem went away, and I polished up the plate, and waited at table, and gammoned the servants, and nobody had the least idea I was in possession, though it very nearly came out after all; for one of the last gentlemen who remained, came downstairs into the hall where I was sitting pretty late at night, and putting half-a-crown into my hand, says, "Here, my man," says he, "run and get me a coach, will you?" I thought it was a do, to get me out of the house, and was just going to say so, sulkily enough, when the gentleman (who was up to everything) came running downstairs, as if he was in great anxiety. "Bung," says he, pretending to be in a consuming passion. "Sir," says I. "Why the devil an't you looking after that plate?" – "I was just going to send him for a coach for me," says the other gentleman. "And I was just a-going to say," says I – "Anybody else, my dear fellow," interrupts the master of the house, pushing me down the passage to get me out of the way – "anybody else; but I have put this man in possession of all the plate and valuables, and I cannot allow him, on any consideration whatever, to leave the house. Bung, you scoundrel, go and count those forks in the breakfast parlour instantly." You may be sure I went laughing pretty hearty when I found it was all right. The money was paid next day, with the addition of something else for myself, and that was the best job that I (and I suspect old Fixem too) ever got in that line.

'But this is the bright side of the picture, sir, after all,' resumed Mr Bung, laying aside the knowing look, and flash air, with which he had repeated the previous anecdote – 'and I'm sorry to say, it's the side one sees very, very seldom, in comparison with the dark one. The civility which money will purchase, is rarely extended to those who have none; and there's a consolation even in being able to patch up one difficulty, to make way for another, to which very poor people are strangers. I was once put into a house down George's Yard – that little dirty court at the back of the gas works; and I never shall forget the misery of them people, dear me! It was a distress for half a year's rent – two pound ten, I think. There was only two rooms in the house, and as there was no passage, the lodgers upstairs always went through the room of the people of the house, as they passed in and out; and every time they did so – which, on the average, was about four times every quarter of an hour – they blowed up quite frightful: for their things had been seized too, and included in the inventory. There was a little piece of enclosed dust in front of the house, with a cinder path leading up to the door, and an open rainwater butt on one side. A dirty striped curtain, on a very slack string, hung in the window, and a little triangular bit of broken looking glass rested on the sill inside. I suppose it was meant for the people's use, but their appearance was so wretched, and so miserable, that I'm certain they never could have plucked up courage to look themselves in the face a second time, if they survived the fright of doing so once. There was two or three chairs, that might have been worth, in their best days, from eightpence to a shilling apiece; a small deal table, an old corner cupboard with nothing in it, and one of those bedsteads which turn up half way, and leave the bottom legs sticking out for you to knock your head against, or hang your hat upon; no bed, no bedding. There was an old sack, by way of rug, before the fireplace, and four or five children were grovelling about, among the sand on the floor. The execution was only put in, to get 'em out of the house, for there was nothing to take to pay the expenses; and here I stopped for three days, though that was a mere form too: for, in course, I knew, and we all knew, they could never pay the money. In one of the chairs, by the side of the place where the fire ought to have been, was an old 'ooman – the ugliest and dirtiest I ever see – who sat rocking herself backwards and forwards, backwards and forwards, without once stopping, except for an instant now and then, to clasp together the withered hands which, with these exceptions, she kept constantly rubbing upon her knees, just raising and depressing her fingers convulsively, in time to the rocking of the chair. On the other side sat the mother with an infant in her arms, which cried till it cried itself to sleep, and when it 'woke, cried till it cried itself off again. The old 'ooman's voice I never heard: she seemed completely stupefied; and as to the mother's, it would have been better if she had been so too, for misery had changed her to a devil. If you had heard how she cursed the little naked children as was rolling on the floor, and seen how savagely she struck the infant when it cried with hunger, you'd have shuddered as much as I did. There they remained all the time: the children ate a morsel of bread once or twice, and I gave 'em best part of the dinners my missis brought me, but the woman ate nothing; they never even laid on the bedstead, nor was the room swept or cleaned all the time. The neighbours were all too poor themselves to take any notice of 'em, but from what I could make out from the abuse of the woman upstairs, it seemed the husband had been transported a few weeks before. When the time was up, the landlord and old Fixem too, got rather frightened about the family, and so they made a stir about it, and had 'em taken to the workhouse. They sent the sick couch for the old 'ooman, and Simmons took the children away at night. The old 'ooman went into the infirmary, and very soon died. The children are all in the house to this day, and very comfortable they are in comparison. As to the mother, there was no taming her at all. She had been a quiet, hard-working woman, I believe, but her misery had actually drove her wild; so after she had been sent to the house of correction half-a-dozen times, for throwing inkstands at the overseers, blaspheming the churchwardens, and smashing everybody as come near her, she burst a blood vessel one mornin', and died too; and a happy release it was, both for herself and the old paupers, male and female, which she used to tip over in all directions, as if they were so many skittles and she the ball.

'Now this was bad enough,' resumed Mr Bung, taking a half-step towards the door, as if to intimate that he had nearly concluded. 'This was bad enough, but there was a sort of quiet misery – if you understand what I mean by that, sir – about a lady at one house I was put into, as touched me a good deal more. It doesn't matter where it was exactly: indeed, I'd rather not say, but it was the same sort o' job. I went with Fixem in the usual way – there was a year's rent in arrear; a very small servant girl opened the door, and three or four fine-looking little children was in the front parlour we were shown into, which was very clean, but very scantily furnished, much like the children themselves. "Bung," says Fixem to me, in a low voice, when we were left alone for a minute, "I know something about this here family, and my opinion is, it's no go." "Do you think they can't settle?" says I, quite anxiously; for I liked the looks of them children. Fixem shook his head, and was just about to reply, when the door opened, and in come a lady, as white as ever I see any one in my days, except about the eyes, which were red with crying. She walked in, as firm as I could have done; shut the door carefully after her, and sat herself down with a face as composed as if it was made of stone. "What is the matter, gentlemen?" says she, in a surprisin' steady voice. "*Is* this an execution?" "It is, mum," says Fixem. The lady looked at him as steady as ever: she didn't seem to have understood him. "It is, mum," says Fixem again; "this is my warrant of distress, mum," says he, handing it over as polite as if it was a newspaper which had been bespoke arter the next gentleman.

'The lady's lip trembled as she took the printed paper. She cast her eye over it, and old Fixem began to explain the form, but I saw she wasn't reading it, plain enough, poor thing. "Oh, my God!" says she, suddenly a-bursting out crying, letting the warrant fall, and hiding her face in her hands. "Oh, my God! what will become of us!" The noise she made, brought in a young lady of about nineteen or twenty, who, I suppose, had been a-listening at the door, and who had got a little boy in her arms: she sat him down in the lady's lap, without speaking, and she hugged the poor little fellow to her bosom, and cried over him, till even old Fixem put on his blue spectacles to hide the two tears, that was a-trickling down, one on each side of his dirty face. "Now, dear ma," says the young lady, "you know how much you have borne. For all our sakes – for pa's sake," says she, "don't give way to this!" – "No, no, I won't!" says the lady, gathering herself up hastily, and drying her eyes; "I am very foolish, but I'm better now – much better." And then she roused herself up, went with us into every room while we took the inventory, opened all the drawers of her own accord, sorted the children's little clothes to make the work easier; and, except doing everything in a strange sort of hurry, seemed as calm and composed as if nothing had happened. When we came downstairs again, she hesitated a minute or two, and at last says, "Gentlemen," says she, "I am afraid I have done wrong, and perhaps it may bring you into trouble. I secreted just now", she says, "the only trinket I have left in the world – here it is." So she lays down on the table a little miniature mounted in gold. "It's a miniature", she says, "of my poor dear father! I little thought once, that I should ever thank God for depriving me of the original, but I do, and have done for years back, most fervently. Take it away, sir," she says, "it's a face that never turned from me in sickness or distress, and I can hardly bear to turn from it now, when, God knows, I suffer both in no ordinary degree." I couldn't say nothing, but I raised my head from the inventory which I was filling up, and looked at Fixem; the old fellow nodded to me significantly, so I ran my pen through the "*Mini*" I had just written, and left the miniature on the table.

'Well, sir, to make short of a long story, I was left in possession, and in possession I remained; and though I was an ignorant man, and the master of the house a clever one, I saw what he never did, but what he would give worlds now (if he had 'em) to have seen in time. I saw, sir, that his wife was wasting away, beneath cares of which she never complained, and griefs she never told. I saw that she was dying before his eyes; I knew that one exertion from him might have saved her, but he never made it. I don't blame him: I don't think he *could* rouse himself. She had so long anticipated all his wishes, and acted for him, that he was a lost man when left to himself. I used to think when I caught sight of her, in the clothes she used to wear, which looked shabby even upon her, and would have been scarcely decent on anyone else, that if I was a gentleman it would wring my very heart to see the woman that was a smart and merry girl when I courted her, so altered through her love for me. Bitter cold and damp weather it was, yet, though her dress was thin, and her shoes none of the best, during the whole three days, from morning to night, she was out of doors running about to try and raise the money. The money *was* raised and the execution was paid out. The whole family crowded into the room where I was, when the money arrived. The father was quite happy as the inconvenience was removed – I dare say he didn't know how; the children looked merry and cheerful again; the eldest girl was bustling about, making preparations for the first comfortable meal they had had since the distress was put in; and the mother looked pleased to see them all so. But if ever I saw death in a woman's face, I saw it in hers that night.

'I was right, sir,' continued Mr Bung, hurriedly passing his coat sleeve over his face; 'the family grew more prosperous, and good fortune arrived. But it was too late. Those children are motherless now, and their father would give up all he has since gained – house, home, goods, money: all that he has, or ever can have, to restore the wife he has lost.'

## Chapter Six

### *The Ladies' Societies*

First published in the *Evening Chronicle*, 20 August 1835 ('Sketches of London No. 20'). The Irish orator mentioned in the last paragraph was in the original *Chronicle* version of this sketch called 'Mr Somebody O'Something, a celebrated Catholic renegade and Protestant bigot'. This was changed in the 1836 volume edition to 'Mr Mortimer O'Silly-one' and further modified before the version here was arrived at. Butt and Tillotson (p. 47) identify the target of Dickens's lampooning as the Rev. Mortimer O'Sullivan who addressed meetings at Exeter Hall describing the condition of the Irish Protestant clergy in June and July 1835; they quote the *Morning Chronicle*'s condemnation of his 'bombastic, frothy, nonsensical style' of speaking.

Our parish is very prolific in ladies' charitable institutions. In winter, when wet feet are common, and colds not scarce, we have the ladies' soup distribution society, the ladies' coal distribution society, and the ladies' blanket distribution society; in summer, when stone fruits flourish and stomach aches prevail, we have the ladies' dispensary, and the ladies' sick visitation committee; and all the year round we have the ladies' child's examination society, the ladies' bible and prayer book circulation society, and the ladies' childbed linen monthly loan society. The two latter are decidedly the most important; whether they are productive of more benefit than the rest, it is not for us to say, but we can take upon ourselves to affirm, with the utmost solemnity, that they create a greater stir and more bustle, than all the others put together.

We should be disposed to affirm, on the first blush of the matter, that the bible and prayer book society is not so popular as the childbedlinen society; the bible and prayer book society has, however, considerably increased in importance within the last year or two, having derived some adventitious aid from the factious opposition of the child's examination society; which factious opposition originated in manner following: – When the young curate was popular, and all the unmarried ladies in the parish took a serious turn, the charity children all at once became objects of peculiar and especial interest. The three Miss Browns (enthusiastic admirers of the curate) taught, and exercised, and examined, and re-examined the unfortunate children, until the boys grew pale, and the girls consumptive, with study and fatigue. The three Miss Browns stood it out very well, because they relieved each other; but the children, having no relief at all, exhibited decided symptoms of weariness and care. The unthinking part of the parishioners laughed at all this, but the more reflective portion of the inhabitants abstained from expressing any opinion on the subject until that of the curate had been clearly ascertained.

The opportunity was not long wanting. The curate preached a charity sermon on behalf of the charity school, and in the charity sermon aforesaid, expatiated in glowing terms on the praiseworthy and indefatigable exertions of certain estimable individuals. Sobs were heard to issue from the three Miss Browns' pew; the pew opener of the division was seen to hurry down the centre aisle to the vestry door, and to return immediately, bearing a glass of water in her hand. A low moaning ensued; two more pew openers rushed to the spot, and the three Miss Browns, each supported by a pew opener, were led out of the church, and led in again after the lapse of five minutes with white pocket handkerchiefs to their eyes, as if they had been attending a funeral in the churchyard adjoining. If any doubt had for a moment existed, as to whom the allusion was intended to apply, it was at once removed. The wish to enlighten the charity children became universal, and the three Miss Browns were unanimously besought to divide the school into classes, and to assign each class to the superintendence of two young ladies.

A little learning is a dangerous thing, but a little patronage is more so; the three Miss Browns appointed all the old maids, and carefully excluded the young ones. Maiden aunts triumphed, mammas were reduced to the lowest depths of despair, and there is no telling in what act of violence the general indignation against the three Miss Browns might have vented itself, had not a perfectly providential occurrence changed the tide of public feeling. Mrs Johnson Parker, the mother of seven extremely fine girls – all unmarried – hastily reported to several other mammas of several other unmarried families, that five old men, six old women, and children innumerable, in the free seats near her pew, were in the habit of coming to church every Sunday, without either bible or prayer book. Was this to be borne in a civilised country? Could such things be tolerated in a Christian land? Never! A ladies' bible and prayer book distribution society was instantly formed: president, Mrs Johnson Parker; treasurers, auditors, and secretary, the Misses Johnson Parker: subscriptions were entered into, books were bought, all the free-seat people provided therewith, and when the first lesson was given out, on the first Sunday succeeding these events, there was such a dropping of books, and rustling of leaves, that it was morally impossible to hear one word of the service for five minutes afterwards.

The three Miss Browns, and their party, saw the approaching danger, and endeavoured to avert it by ridicule and sarcasm. Neither the old men nor the old women could read their books, now they had got them, said the three Miss Browns. Never mind; they could learn, replied Mrs Johnson Parker. The children couldn't read either, suggested the three Miss Browns. No matter; they could be taught, retorted Mrs Johnson Parker. A balance of parties took place. The Miss Browns publicly examined – popular feeling inclined to the child's examination society. The Miss Johnson Parkers publicly distributed – a reaction took place in favour of the prayer book distribution. A feather would have turned the scale, and a feather did turn it. A missionary returned from the West Indies; he was to be presented to the Dissenters' Missionary Society on his marriage with a wealthy widow. Overtures were made to the Dissenters by the Johnson Parkers. Their object was the same, and why not have a joint meeting of the two societies? The proposition was accepted. The meeting was duly heralded by public announcement, and the room was crowded to suffocation. The missionary appeared on the platform; he was hailed with enthusiasm. He repeated a dialogue he had heard between two negroes, behind a hedge, on the subject of distribution societies; the approbation was tumultuous. He gave an imitation of the two negroes in broken English; the roof was rent with applause. From that period we date (with one trifling exception) a daily increase in the popularity of the distribution society, and an increase of popularity, which the feeble and impotent opposition of the examination party has only tended to augment.

Now, the great points about the childbedlinen monthly loan society are, that it is less dependent on the fluctuations of public opinion than either the distribution or the child's examination; and that, come what may, there is never any lack of objects on which to exercise its benevolence. Our parish is a very populous one, and, if anything, contributes, we should be disposed to say, rather more than its due share to the aggregate amount of births in the metropolis and its environs. The consequence is, that the monthly loan society flourishes, and invests its members with a most enviable amount of bustling patronage. The society (whose only notion of dividing time would appear to be its allotment into months) holds monthly tea-drinkings, at which the monthly report is received, a secretary elected for the month ensuing, and such of the monthly boxes as may not happen to be out on loan for the month, carefully examined.

We were never present at one of these meetings, from all of which it is scarcely necessary to say, gentlemen are carefully excluded; but Mr Bung has been called before the board once or twice, and we have his authority for stating that its proceedings are conducted with great order and regularity: not more than four members being allowed to speak at one time on any pretence whatever. The regular committee is composed exclusively of married ladies, but a vast number of young unmarried ladies of from eighteen to twenty-five years of age, respectively, are admitted as honorary members, partly because they are very useful in replenishing the boxes, and visiting the confined; partly because it is highly desirable that they should be initiated, at an early period, into the more serious and matronly duties of after-life; and partly because prudent mammas have not unfrequently been known to turn this circumstance to wonderfully good account in matrimonial speculations.

In addition to the loan of the monthly boxes (which are always painted blue, with the name of the society in large white letters on the lid), the society dispense occasional grants of beef tea, and a composition of warm beer, spice, eggs, and sugar, commonly known by the name of 'caudle', to its patients. And here again the services of the honorary members are called into requisition, and most cheerfully conceded. Deputations of twos or threes are sent out to visit the patients, and on these occasions there is such a tasting of caudle and beef tea, such a stirring about of little messes in tiny saucepans on the hob, such a dressing and undressing of infants, such a tying, and folding, and pinning; such a nursing and warming of little legs and feet before the fire, such a delightful confusion of talking and cooking, bustle, importance and officiousness, as never can be enjoyed in its full extent but on similar occasions.

In rivalry of these two institutions, and as a last expiring effort to acquire parochial popularity, the child's examination people determined, the other day, on having a grand public examination of the pupils; and the large school room of the national seminary was, by and with the consent of the parish authorities, devoted to the purpose. Invitation circulars were forwarded to all the principal parishioners, including, of course, the heads of the other two societies, for whose especial behoof and edification the display was intended; and a large audience was confidently anticipated on the occasion. The floor was carefully scrubbed the day before, under the immediate superintendence of the three Miss Browns; forms were placed across the room for the accommodation of the visitors, specimens in writing were carefully selected, and as carefully patched and touched up, until they astonished the children who had written them, rather more than the company who read them; sums in compound addition were rehearsed and re-rehearsed until all the children had the totals by heart; and the preparations altogether were on the most laborious and most comprehensive scale. The morning arrived: the children were yellow-soaped and flannelled, and towelled, till their faces shone again; every pupil's hair was carefully combed into his or her eyes, as the case might be; the girls were adorned with snow-white tippets, and caps bound round the head by a single purple ribbon: the necks of the elder boys were fixed into collars of startling dimensions.

The doors were thrown open, and the Misses Brown and Co. were discovered in plain white muslin dresses, and caps of the same – the child's examination uniform. The room filled: the greetings of the company were loud and cordial. The distributionists trembled for their popularity was at stake. The eldest boy fell forward, and delivered a propitiatory address from behind his collar. It was from the pen of Mr Henry Brown; the applause was universal, and the Johnson Parkers were aghast. The examination proceeded with success, and terminated in triumph. The child's examination society gained a momentary victory, and the Johnson Parkers retreated in despair.

A secret council of the distributionists was held that night, with Mrs Johnson Parker in the chair, to consider of the best means of recovering the ground they had lost in the favour of the parish. What could be done? Another meeting! Alas! who was to attend it? The Missionary would not do twice; and the slaves were emancipated. A bold step must be taken. The parish must be astonished in some way or other; but no one was able to suggest what the step should be. At length, a very old lady was heard to mumble, in indistinct tones, 'Exeter Hall'. A sudden light broke in upon the meeting. It was unanimously resolved, that a deputation of old ladies should wait upon a celebrated orator, imploring his assistance, and the favour of a speech; and the deputation should also wait on two or three other imbecile old women, not resident in the parish, and entreat their attendance. The application was successful, the meeting was held; the orator (an Irishman) came. He talked of green isles – other shores – vast Atlantic – bosom of the deep – Christian charity – blood and extermination – mercy in hearts – arms in hands – altars and homes – household gods. He wiped his eyes, he blew his nose, and he quoted Latin. The effect was tremendous – the Latin was a decided hit. Nobody knew exactly what it was about, but everybody knew it must be affecting, because even the orator was overcome. The popularity of the distribution society among the ladies of our parish is unprecedented; and the child's examination is going fast to decay.

## Chapter Seven

### *Our Next-door Neighbour*

First published in both the *Morning Chronicle* and the *Evening Chronicle*, 18 March 1836, under the heading 'Sketches by Boz – New Series' (see Graham Mott's article in *The Dickensian*, Vol. 80 [1984], pp. 114–16). See bibliographical note above (p. 3) for details of volume publication.

We are very fond of speculating as we walk through a street, on the character and pursuits of the people who inhabit it; and nothing so materially assists us in these speculations as the appearance of the house doors. The various expressions of the human countenance afford a beautiful and interesting study; but there is something in the physiognomy of street door knockers, almost as characteristic, and nearly as infallible. Whenever we visit a man for the first time, we contemplate the features of his knocker with the greatest curiosity, for we well know, that between the man and his knocker, there will inevitably be a greater or less degree of resemblance and sympathy.

For instance, there is one description of knocker that used to be common enough, but which is fast passing away – a large round one, with the jolly face of a convivial lion smiling blandly at you, as you twist the sides of your hair into a curl, or pull up your shirt collar while you are waiting for the door to be opened; we never saw that knocker on the door of a churlish man – so far as our experience is concerned, it invariably bespoke hospitality and another bottle.

No man ever saw this knocker on the door of a small attorney or bill-broker; they always patronise the other lion; a heavy ferocious-looking fellow, with a countenance expressive of savage stupidity – a sort of grand master among the knockers, and a great favourite with the selfish and brutal.

Then there is a little pert Egyptian knocker, with a long thin face, a pinched-up nose, and a very sharp chin; he is most in vogue with your government office people, in light drabs and starched cravats; little spare priggish men, who are perfectly satisfied with their own opinions, and consider themselves of paramount importance.

We were greatly troubled a few years ago, by the innovation of a new

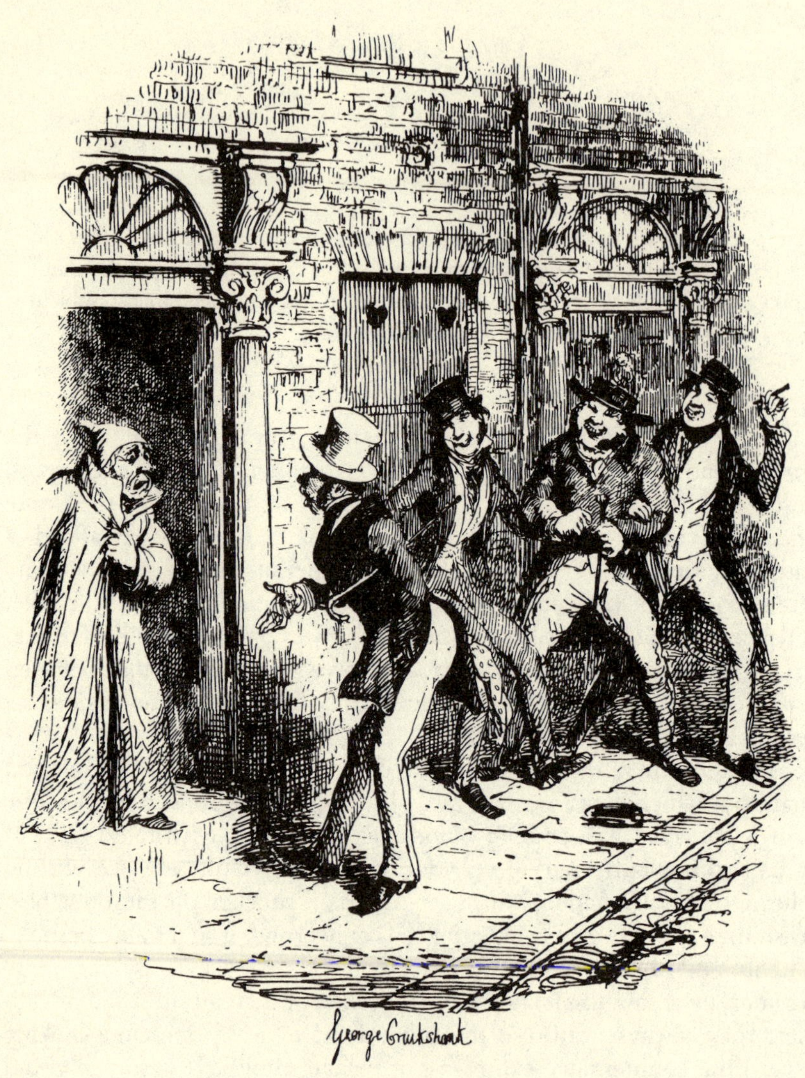


*Our Next-door Neighbours*

kind of knocker, without any face at all, composed of a wreath, depending from a hand or small truncheon. A little trouble and attention, however, enabled us to overcome this difficulty, and to reconcile the new system to our favourite theory. You will invariably find this knocker on the doors of cold and formal people, who always ask you why you *don't* come, and never say *do*.

Everybody knows the brass knocker is common to suburban villas, and extensive boarding schools; and having noticed this genus we have recapitulated all the most prominent and strongly defined species.

Some phrenologists affirm, that the agitation of a man's brain by different passions, produces corresponding developments in the form of his skull. Do not let us be understood as pushing our theory to the full length of asserting, that any alteration in a man's disposition would produce a visible effect on the feature of his knocker. Our position merely is, that in such a case, the magnetism which must exist between a man and his knocker, would induce the man to remove, and seek some knocker more congenial to his altered feelings. If you ever find a man changing his habitation without any reasonable pretext, depend on it, that, although he may not be aware of the fact himself, it is because he and his knocker are at variance. This is a new theory, but we venture to launch it, nevertheless, as being quite as ingenious and infallible as many thousands of the learned speculations which are daily broached for public good and private fortune making.

Entertaining these feelings on the subject of knockers, it will be readily imagined with what consternation we viewed the entire removal of the knocker from the door of the next house to the one we lived in, some time ago, and the substitution of a bell. This was a calamity we had never anticipated. The bare idea of anybody being able to exist without a knocker, appeared so wild and visionary, that it had never for one instant entered our imagination.

We sauntered moodily from the spot, and bent our steps towards Eaton Square, then just building. What was our astonishment and indignation to find that bells were fast becoming the rule, and knockers the exception! Our theory trembled beneath the shock. We hastened home; and fancying we foresaw in the swift progress of events, its entire abolition, resolved from that day forward to vent our speculations on our next-door neighbours in person. The house adjoining ours on the left hand was uninhabited, and we had, therefore, plenty of leisure to observe our next-door neighbours on the other side.

The house without the knocker was in the occupation of a city clerk, and there was a neatly written bill in the parlour window intimating that lodgings for a single gentleman were to be let within.

It was a neat, dull little house, on the shady side of the way, with new, narrow floorcloth in the passage, and new, narrow stair carpets up to the first floor. The paper was new, and the paint was new, and the furniture was new; and all three, paper, paint, and furniture, bespoke the limited means of the tenant. There was a little red and black carpet in the drawing room, with a border of flooring all the way round; a few stained chairs and a Pembroke table. A pink shell was displayed on each of the little sideboards, which, with the addition of a tea-tray and caddy, a few more shells on the mantlepiece, and three peacock's feathers tastefully arranged above them, completed the decorative furniture of the apartment.

This was the room destined for the reception of the single gentleman during the day, and a little back room on the same floor was assigned as his sleeping apartment by night.

The bill had not been long in the window, when a stout, good-humoured looking gentleman, of about five-and-thirty, appeared as a candidate for the tenancy. Terms were soon arranged, for the bill was taken down immediately after his first visit. In a day or two the single gentleman came in, and shortly afterwards his real character came out.

First of all, he displayed a most extraordinary partiality for sitting up till three or four o'clock in the morning, drinking whiskey and water, and smoking cigars; then he invited friends home, who used to come at ten o'clock, and begin to get happy about the small hours, when they evinced their perfect contentment by singing songs with half a dozen verses of two lines each, and a chorus of ten, which chorus used to be shouted forth by the whole strength of the company, in the most enthusiastic and vociferous manner, to the great annoyance of the neighbours, and the special discomfort of another single gentleman overhead.

Now, this was bad enough, occurring as it did three times a week on the average, but this was not all; for when the company *did* go away, instead of walking quietly down the street, as anybody else's company would have done, they amused themselves by making alarming and frightful noises, and counterfeiting the shrieks of females in distress; and one night, a red-faced gentleman in a white hat knocked in the most urgent manner at the door of the powdered-headed old gentleman at No. 3, and when the powdered-headed old gentleman, who thought one of his married daughters must have been taken ill prematurely, had groped downstairs, and after a great deal of unbolting and key-turning, opened the street door, the red-faced man in the white hat said he hoped he'd excuse his giving him so much trouble, but he'd feel obliged if he'd favour him with a glass of cold spring water, and the loan of a shilling for a cab to take him home, on which the old gentleman slammed the door and went upstairs, and threw the contents of his water jug out of the window – very straight, only it went over the wrong man; and the whole street was involved in confusion.

A joke's a joke; and even practical jests are very capital in their way, if you can only get the other party to see the fun of them; but the population of our street were so dull of apprehension, as to be quite lost to a sense of the drollery of this proceeding: and the consequence was, that our next-door neighbour was obliged to tell the single gentleman, that unless he gave up entertaining his friends at home, he really must be compelled to part with him. The single gentleman received the remonstrance with great good humour, and promised from that time forward, to spend his evenings at a coffee house – a determination which afforded general and unmixed satisfaction.

The next night passed off very well, everybody being delighted with the change; but on the next, the noises were renewed with greater spirit than ever. The single gentleman's friends being unable to see him in his own house every alternate night, had come to the determination of seeing him home every night; and what with the discordant greetings of the friends at parting, and the noise created by the single gentleman in his passage upstairs, and his subsequent struggles to get his boots off, the evil was not to be borne. So our next-door neighbour gave the single gentleman, who was a very good lodger in other respects, notice to quit; and the single gentleman went away, and entertained his friends in other lodgings.

The next applicant for the vacant first floor was of a very different character from the troublesome single gentleman who had just quitted it. He was a tall, thin gentleman, with a profusion of brown hair, reddish whiskers, and very slightly developed moustaches. He wore a braided surtout, with frogs behind, light grey trousers, and wash leather gloves, and had altogether rather a military appearance. So unlike the roystering single gentleman. Such insinuating manners, and such a delightful address! So seriously disposed, too! When he first came to look at the lodgings, he inquired most particularly whether he was sure to be able to get a seat in the parish church; and when he had agreed to take them, he requested to have a list of the different local charities, as he intended to subscribe his mite to the most deserving among them.

Our next-door neighbour was now perfectly happy. He had got a lodger at last, of just his own way of thinking – a serious, well-disposed man, who abhorred gaiety, and loved retirement. He took down the bill with a light heart, and pictured in imagination a long series of quiet Sundays, on which he and his lodger would exchange mutual civilities and Sunday papers.

The serious man arrived, and his luggage was to arrive from the country next morning. He borrowed a clean shirt, and a prayer book, from our next-door neighbour, and retired to rest at an early hour, requesting that he might be called punctually at ten o'clock next morning – not before, as he was much fatigued.

He *was* called, and did not answer: he was called again, but there was no reply. Our next-door neighbour became alarmed, and burst the door open. The serious man had left the house mysteriously; carrying with him the shirt, the prayer book, a teaspoon, and the bedclothes.

Whether this occurrence, coupled with the irregularities of his former lodger, gave our next-door neighbour an aversion to single gentlemen, we know not; we only know that the next bill which made its appearance in the parlour window intimated generally, that there were furnished apartments to let on the first floor. The bill was soon removed. The new lodgers at first attracted our curiosity, and afterwards excited our interest.

They were a young lad of eighteen or nineteen, and his mother, a lady of about fifty, or it might be less. The mother wore a widow's weeds, and the boy was also clothed in deep mourning. They were poor – very poor; for their only means of support arose from the pittance the boy earned, by copying writings, and translating for booksellers.

They had removed from some country place and settled in London; partly because it afforded better chances of employment for the boy, and partly, perhaps, with the natural desire to leave a place where they had been in better circumstances, and where their poverty was known. They were proud under their reverses, and above revealing their wants and privations to strangers. How bitter those privations were, and how hard the boy worked to remove them, no one ever knew but themselves. Night after night, two, three, four hours after midnight, could we hear the occasional raking up of the scanty fire, or the hollow and half stifled cough, which indicated his being still at work; and day after day, could we see more plainly that nature had set that unearthly light in his plaintive face, which is the beacon of her worst disease.

Actuated, we hope, by a higher feeling than mere curiosity, we contrived to establish, first an acquaintance, and then a close intimacy, with the poor strangers. Our worst fears were realised; the boy was sinking fast. Through a part of the winter, and the whole of the following spring and summer, his labours were unceasingly prolonged: and the mother attempted to procure needlework, embroidery – anything for bread.

A few shillings now and then, were all she could earn. The boy worked steadily on; dying by minutes, but never once giving utterance to complaint or murmur.

One beautiful autumn evening we went to pay our customary visit to the invalid. His little remaining strength had been decreasing rapidly for two or three days preceding, and he was lying on the sofa at the open window, gazing at the setting sun. His mother had been reading the Bible to him, for she closed the book as we entered, and advanced to meet us.

'I was telling William,' she said, 'that we must manage to take him into the country somewhere, so that he may get quite well. He is not ill, you know, but he is not very strong, and has exerted himself too much lately.' Poor thing! The tears that streamed through her fingers, as she turned aside, as if to adjust her close widow's cap, too plainly showed how fruitless was the attempt to deceive herself.

We sat down by the head of the sofa, but said nothing, for we saw the breath of life was passing gently but rapidly from the young form before us. At every respiration, his heart beat more slowly.

The boy placed one hand in ours, grasped his mother's arm with the other, drew her hastily towards him, and fervently kissed her cheek. There was a pause. He sunk back upon his pillow, and looked long and earnestly in his mother's face.

'William, William!' murmured the mother, after a long interval, 'don't look at me so – speak to me, dear!'

The boy smiled languidly, but an instant afterwards his features resolved into the same cold, solemn gaze.

'William, dear William! rouse yourself; don't look at me so, love – pray don't! Oh, my God! what shall I do!' cried the widow, clasping her hands in agony – 'my dear boy! he is dying!'

The boy raised himself by a violent effort, and folded his hands together – 'Mother! dear, dear mother, bury me in the open fields – anywhere but in these dreadful streets. I should like to be where you can see my grave, but not in these close crowded streets; they have killed me; kiss me again, mother; put your arm round my neck—'

He fell back, and a strange expression stole upon his features; not of pain or suffering, but an indescribable fixing of every line and muscle.

The boy was dead.

# SCENES

## Chapter One

### *The Streets – Morning*

First published in the *Evening Chronicle*, 21 July 1835 ('Sketches of London No. 17') and collected in the *Second Series* as 'The Streets by Morning'. The detail about the office boys being tempted by stale tarts outside pastry cooks' shops derives from Dickens's own boyhood experience when he was working at the blacking factory and walking daily to the Strand from Camden Town. See *David Copperfield* ch. 11: 'I could not resist the stale pastry put out at half price on trays at the confectioners' doors in Tottenham Court Road; and I often spent in that the money I should have kept for my dinner'.

The appearance presented by the streets of London an hour before sunrise, on a summer's morning, is most striking even to the few whose unfortunate pursuits of pleasure, or scarcely less unfortunate pursuits of business, cause them to be well acquainted with the scene. There is an air of cold, solitary desolation about the noiseless streets which we are accustomed to see thronged at other times by a busy, eager crowd, and over the quiet, closely shut buildings, which throughout the day are swarming with life and bustle, that is very impressive.

The last drunken man, who shall find his way home before sunlight, has just staggered heavily along, roaring out the burden of the drinking song of the previous night: the last houseless vagrant whom penury and police have left in the streets, has coiled up his chilly limbs in some paved corner, to dream of food and warmth. The drunken, the dissipated, and the wretched have disappeared; the more sober and orderly part of the population have not yet awakened to the labours of the day, and the stillness of death is over the streets; its very hue seems to be imparted to them, cold and lifeless as they look in the grey, sombre light of daybreak. The coach stands in the larger thoroughfares are deserted; the night houses are closed; and the chosen promenades of profligate misery are empty.

An occasional policeman may alone be seen at the street corners,

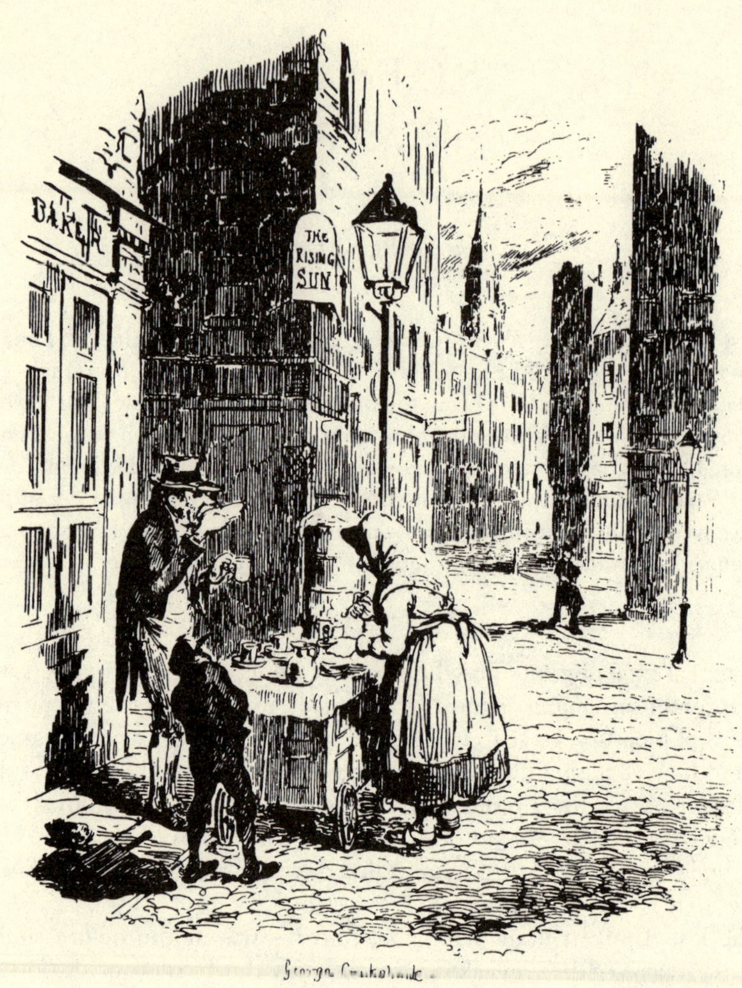


*The Streets. Morning*

listlessly gazing on the deserted prospect before him; and now and then a rakish-looking cat runs stealthily across the road and descends his own area with as much caution and slyness – bounding first on the water butt, then on the dust hole, and then alighting on the flagstones – as if he were conscious that his character depended on his gallantry of the preceding night escaping public observation. A partially opened bedroom window here and there, bespeaks the heat of the weather, and the uneasy slumbers of its occupant; and the dim scanty flicker of the rushlight, through the window blind, denotes the chamber of watching or sickness. With these few exceptions, the streets present no signs of life, nor the houses of habitation.

An hour wears away; the spires of the churches and roofs of the principal buildings are faintly tinged with the light of the rising sun; and the streets, by almost imperceptible degrees, begin to resume their bustle and animation. Market carts roll slowly along: the sleepy waggoner impatiently urging on his tired horses, or vainly endeavouring to awaken the boy, who, luxuriously stretched on the top of the fruit baskets, forgets, in happy oblivion, his long cherished curiosity to behold the wonders of London.

Rough, sleepy-looking animals of strange appearance, something between ostlers and hackney coachmen, begin to take down the shutters of early public houses; and little deal tables, with the ordinary preparations for a street breakfast, make their appearance at the customary stations. Numbers of men and women (principally the latter), carrying upon their heads heavy baskets of fruit, toil down the park side of Piccadilly, on their way to Covent Garden, and, following each other in rapid succession, form a long straggling line from thence to the turn of the road at Knightsbridge.

Here and there, a bricklayer's labourer, with the day's dinner tied up in a handkerchief, walks briskly to his work, and occasionally a little knot of three or four schoolboys on a stolen bathing expedition rattle merrily over the pavement, their boisterous mirth contrasting forcibly with the demeanour of the little sweep, who, having knocked and rung till his arm aches, and being interdicted by a merciful legislature from endangering his lungs by calling out, sits patiently down on the doorstep, until the housemaid may happen to awake.

Covent Garden market, and the avenues leading to it, are thronged with carts of all sorts, sizes, and descriptions, from the heavy lumbering waggon, with its four stout horses, to the jingling costermonger's cart, with its consumptive donkey. The pavement is already strewed with decayed cabbage leaves, broken hay bands, and all the indescribable litter of a vegetable market; men are shouting, carts backing, horses neighing, boys fighting, basket-women talking, piemen expatiating on the excellence of their pastry, and donkeys braying. These and a hundred other sounds form a compound discordant enough to a Londoner's ears, and remarkably disagreeable to those of country gentlemen who are sleeping at the Hummums for the first time.

Another hour passes away, and the day begins in good earnest. The servant of all work, who, under the plea of sleeping very soundly, has utterly disregarded 'Missis's' ringing for half an hour previously, is warned by Master (whom Missis has sent up in his drapery to the landing place for that purpose), that it's half past six, whereupon she awakes all of a sudden, with well feigned astonishment, and goes downstairs very sulkily, wishing, while she strikes a light, that the principle of spontaneous combustion would extend itself to coals and kitchen range. When the fire is lighted, she opens the street door to take in the milk, when, by the most singular coincidence in the world, she discovers that the servant next door has just taken in her milk too, and that Mr Todd's young man over the way is, by an equally extraordinary chance, taking down his master's shutters. The inevitable consequence is, that she just steps, milk jug in hand, as far as next door, just to say 'good morning' to Betsy Clark, and that Mr Todd's young man just steps over the way to say 'good morning' to both of 'em; and as the aforesaid Mr Todd's young man is almost as good-looking and fascinating as the baker himself, the conversation quickly becomes very interesting, and probably would become more so, if Betsy Clark's Missis, who always will be a-followin' her about, didn't give an angry tap at her bedroom window, on which Mr Todd's young man tries to whistle coolly, as he goes back to his shop much faster than he came from it; and the two girls run back to their respective places, and shut their street doors with surprising softness, each of them poking their heads out of the front parlour window, a minute afterwards, however, ostensibly with the view of looking at the mail which just then passes by, but really for the purpose of catching another glimpse of Mr Todd's young man, who being fond of mails, but more of females, takes a short look at the mails, and a long look at the girls, much to the satisfaction of all parties concerned.

The mail itself goes on to the coach office in due course, and the passengers who are going out by the early coach, stare with astonishment at the passengers who are coming in by the early coach, who look blue and dismal, and are evidently under the influence of that odd feeling produced by travelling, which makes the events of yesterday morning seem as if they had happened at least six months ago, and induces people to wonder with considerable gravity whether the friends and relations they took leave of a fortnight before, have altered much since they have left them. The coach office is all alive, and the coaches which are just going out, are surrounded by the usual crowd of Jews and nondescripts, who seem to consider, Heaven knows why, that it is quite impossible any man can mount a coach without requiring at least sixpennyworth of oranges, a penknife, a pocket book, a last year's annual, a pencil case, a piece of sponge, and a small series of caricatures.

Half an hour more, and the sun darts his bright rays cheerfully down the still half-empty streets, and shines with sufficient force to rouse the dismal laziness of the apprentice, who pauses every other minute from his task of sweeping out the shop and watering the pavement in front of it, to tell another apprentice similarly employed, how hot it will be today, or to stand with his right hand shading his eyes, and his left resting on the broom, gazing at the 'Wonder', or the 'Tally-ho', or the 'Nimrod', or some other fast coach, till it is out of sight, when he re-enters the shop, envying the passengers on the outside of the fast coach, and thinking of the old red brick house 'down in the country', where he went to school: the miseries of the milk and water, and thick bread and scrapings, fading into nothing before the pleasant recollection of the green field the boys used to play in, and the green pond he was caned for presuming to fall into, and other schoolboy associations.

Cabs, with trunks and band boxes between the drivers' legs and outside the apron, rattle briskly up and down the streets on their way to the coach office or steam packet wharfs; and the cab drivers and hackney coachmen who are on the stand polish up the ornamental part of their dingy vehicles – the former wondering how people can prefer 'them wild beast cariwans of homnibuses, to a riglar cab with a fast trotter', and the latter admiring how people can trust their necks into one of 'them crazy cabs, when they can have a 'spectable 'ackney cotche with a pair of 'orses as von't run away with no vun'; a consolation unquestionably founded on fact, seeing that a hackney coach horse never was known to run at all, 'except,' as the smart cabman in front of the rank observes, 'except one, and *he* run back'ards'.

The shops are now completely opened, and apprentices and shopmen are busily engaged in cleaning and decking the windows for the day. The bakers' shops in town are filled with servants and children waiting for the drawing of the first batch of rolls – an operation which was performed a full hour ago in the suburbs: for the early clerk population of Somers and Camden Towns, Islington, and Pentonville, are fast pouring into the city, or directing their steps towards Chancery Lane and the Inns of Court. Middle-aged men, whose salaries have by no means increased in the same proportion as their families, plod steadily along, apparently with no object in view but the counting house; knowing by sight almost everybody they meet or overtake, for they have seen them every morning (Sundays excepted) during the last twenty years, but speaking to no one. If they do happen to overtake a personal acquaintance, they just exchange a hurried salutation, and keep walking on, either by his side or in front of him, as his rate of walking may chance to be. As to stopping to shake hands, or to take the friend's arm, they seem to think that as it is not included in their salary, they have no right to do it. Small office lads in large hats, who are made men before they are boys, hurry along in pairs, with their first coat carefully brushed, and the white trousers of last Sunday plentifully besmeared with dust and ink. It evidently requires a considerable mental struggle to avoid investing part of the day's dinner money in the purchase of the stale tarts so temptingly exposed in dusty tins at the pastry cooks' doors; but a consciousness of their own importance and the receipt of seven shillings a week, with the prospect of an early rise to eight, comes to their aid, and they accordingly put their hats a little more on one side, and look under the bonnets of all the milliners' and staymakers' apprentices they meet – poor girls! – the hardest worked, the worst paid, and too often, the worst used class of the community.

Eleven o'clock, and a new set of people fill the streets. The goods in the shop window are invitingly arranged; the shopmen in their white neckerchiefs and spruce coats, look as if they couldn't clean a window if their lives depended on it; the carts have disappeared from Covent Garden; the waggoners have returned, and the costermongers repaired to their ordinary 'beats' in the suburbs; clerks are at their offices, and gigs, cabs, omnibuses, and saddle horses, are conveying their masters to the same destination. The streets are thronged with a vast concourse of people, gay and shabby, rich and poor, idle and industrious; and we come to the heat, bustle, and activity of NOON.

## Chapter Two

### *The Streets – Night*

First published in *Bell's Life in London*, 17 January 1836 ('Scenes and Characters No. 12') and collected in the *Second Series* as 'The Streets at Night'. *Bell's Life* was a popular weekly paper which carried sports reports and comic features as well as news. At this date, theatre programmes would consist of several pieces (melodramas, farces, etc.) lasting from 6 p.m. until around midnight with patrons being admitted at half price after the main piece (usually around 8.30 p.m.). The 'harmonic meeting' described at the end of this sketch was a very popular early nineteenth-century institution. It would take place in a special large room, usually upstairs, in a public house with an MC, some professional singers, and patrons joining in the choruses and glees; a forerunner of the music-hall. See the descriptions of the vocalist Little Swills at the Sol's Arms in *Bleak House*, chs 11, 19, 32, 33, 39.

But the streets of London, to be beheld in the very height of their glory, should be seen on a dark, dull, murky winter's night, when there is just enough damp gently stealing down to make the pavement greasy, without cleansing it of any of its impurities; and when the heavy lazy mist, which hangs over every object, makes the gas lamps look brighter, and the brilliantly-lighted shops more splendid, from the contrast they present to the darkness around. All the people who are at home on such a night as this, seem disposed to make themselves as snug and comfortable as possible; and the passengers in the streets have excellent reason to envy the fortunate individuals who are seated by their own firesides.

In the larger and better kind of streets, dining parlour curtains are closely drawn, kitchen fires blaze brightly up, and savoury steams of hot dinners salute the nostrils of the hungry wayfarer, as he plods wearily by the area railings. In the suburbs, the muffin boy rings his way down the little street, much more slowly than he is wont to do; for Mrs Macklin, of No 4, has no sooner opened her little street door, and screamed out 'Muffins!' with all her might, than Mrs Walker, at No 5, puts her head out of the parlour window, and screams 'Muffins!' too; and Mrs Walker has scarcely got the words out of her lips, than Mrs Peplow, over the way, lets loose Master Peplow, who darts down the street, with a velocity which

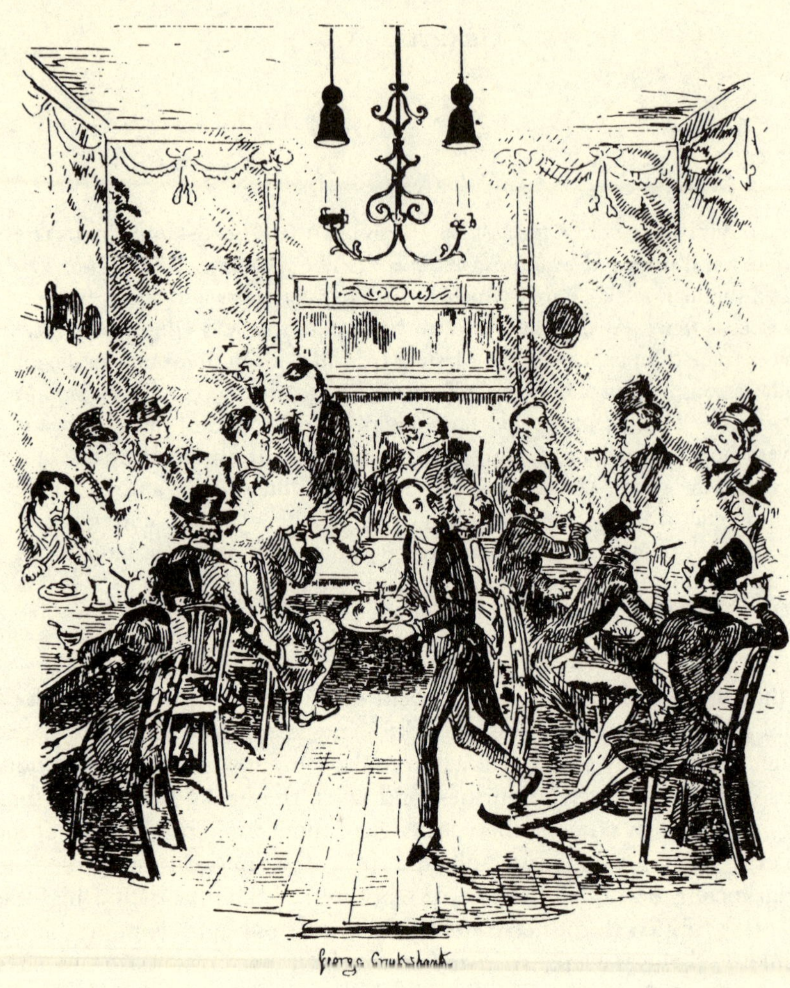


*A Harmonic Meeting*

nothing but buttered muffins in perspective could possibly inspire, and drags the boy back by main force, whereupon Mrs Macklin and Mrs Walker, just to save the boy trouble, and to say a few neighbourly words to Mrs Peplow at the same time, run over the way and buy their muffins at Mrs Peplow's door, when it appears from the voluntary statement of Mrs Walker, that her 'kittle's jist a-biling, and the cups and sarsers ready laid', and that, as it was such a wretched night out o' doors, she'd made up her mind to have a nice hot comfortable cup o' tea – a determination at which, by the most singular coincidence, the other two ladies had simultaneously arrived.

After a little conversation about the wretchedness of the weather and the merits of tea, with a digression relative to the viciousness of boys as a rule, and the amiability of Master Peplow as an exception, Mrs Walker sees her husband coming down the street; and as he must want his tea, poor man, after his dirty walk from the Docks, she instantly runs across, muffins in hand, and Mrs Macklin does the same, and after a few words to Mrs Walker, they all pop into their little houses, and slam their little street doors, which are not opened again for the remainder of the evening, except to the nine o'clock 'beer', who comes round with a lantern in front of his tray, and says, as he lends Mrs Walker 'Yesterday's 'Tiser', that he's blessed if he can hardly hold the pot, much less feel the paper, for it's one of the bitterest nights he ever felt, 'cept the night when the man was frozen to death in the Brickfield.

After a little prophetic conversation with the policeman at the street corner, touching a probable change in the weather, and the setting in of a hard frost, the nine o'clock beer returns to his master's house, and employs himself for the remainder of the evening, in assiduously stirring the tap room fire, and deferentially taking part in the conversation of the worthies assembled round it.

The streets in the vicinity of the Marsh Gate and Victoria Theatre present an appearance of dirt and discomfort on such a night, which the groups who lounge about them in no degree tend to diminish. Even the little block tin temple sacred to baked potatoes, surmounted by a splendid design in variegated lamps, looks less gay than usual; and as to the kidney pie stand, its glory has quite departed. The candle in the transparent lamp, manufactured of oil paper, embellished with 'characters', has been blown out fifty times, so the kidney pie merchant, tired with running backwards and forwards to the next wine vaults, to get a light, has given up the idea of illumination in despair, and the only signs of his 'whereabout', are the bright sparks, of which a long irregular train is whirled down the street every time he opens his portable oven to hand a hot kidney pie to a customer.

Flatfish, oyster, and fish vendors linger hopelessly in the kennel, in vain endeavouring to attract customers; and the ragged boys who usually disport themselves about the streets, stand crouched in little knots in some projecting doorway, or under the canvas blind of a cheesemonger's, where great flaring gaslights, unshaded by any glass, display huge piles of bright red and pale yellow cheeses, mingled with little fivepenny dabs of dingy bacon, various tubs of weekly Dorset, and cloudy rolls of 'best fresh'.

Here they amuse themselves with theatrical converse, arising out of their last half-price visit to the Victoria gallery, admire the terrific combat, which is nightly encored, and expatiate on the inimitable manner in which Bill Thompson can 'come the double monkey', or go through the mysterious involutions of a sailor's hornpipe.

It is nearly eleven o'clock, and the cold thin rain which has been drizzling so long, is beginning to pour down in good earnest; the baked potato man has departed – the kidney pie man has just walked away with his warehouse on his arm – the cheesemonger has drawn in his blind, and the boys have dispersed. The constant clicking of pattens on the slippy and uneven pavement, and the rustling of umbrellas, as the wind blows against the shop windows, bear testimony to the inclemency of the night; and the policeman, with his oilskin cape buttoned closely round him, seems as he holds his hat on his head, and turns round to avoid the gust of wind and rain which drives against him at the street corner, to be very far from congratulating himself on the prospect before him.

The little chandler's shop with the cracked bell behind the door, whose melancholy tinkling has been regulated by the demand for quarterns of sugar and half ounces of coffee, is shutting up. The crowds which have been passing to and fro during the whole day, are rapidly dwindling away; and the noise of shouting and quarrelling which issues from the public houses, is almost the only sound that breaks the melancholy stillness of the night.

There was another, but it has ceased. That wretched woman with the infant in her arms, round whose meagre form the remnant of her own scanty shawl is carefully wrapped, has been attempting to sing some popular ballad, in the hope of wringing a few pence from the compassionate passer-by. A brutal laugh at her weak voice is all she has gained. The tears fall thick and fast down her own pale face; the child is cold and hungry, and its low half stifled wailing adds to the misery of its wretched mother, as she moans aloud, and sinks despairingly down on a cold damp doorstep.

Singing! How few of those who pass such a miserable creature as this, think of the anguish of heart, the sinking of soul and spirit, which the very effort of singing produces. Bitter mockery! Disease, neglect, and starvation, faintly articulating the words of the joyous ditty, that has enlivened your hours of feasting and merriment, God knows how often!

It is no subject of jeering. The weak tremulous voice tells a fearful tale of want and famishing; and the feeble singer of this roaring song may turn away, only to die of cold and hunger.

One o'clock! Parties returning from the different theatres foot it through the muddy streets; cabs, hackney coaches, carriages, and theatre omnibuses, roll swiftly by; watermen with dim dirty lanterns in their hands, and large brass plates upon their breasts, who have been shouting and rushing about for the last two hours, retire to their watering houses, to solace themselves with the creature comforts of pipes and purl; the half price pit and box frequenters of the theatre throng to the different houses of refreshment; and chops, kidneys, rabbits, oysters, stout, cigars, and 'goes' innumerable, are served up amidst a noise and confusion of smoking, running, knife clattering, and waiter chattering, perfectly indescribable.

The more musical portion of the play-going community betake themselves to some harmonic meeting. As a matter of curiosity let us follow them thither for a few moments.

In a lofty room of spacious dimensions, are seated some eighty or a hundred guests knocking little pewter measures on the tables, and hammering away, with the handles of their knives, as if they were so many trunk makers. They are applauding a glee, which has just been executed by the three 'professional gentlemen' at the top of the centre table, one of whom is in the chair – the little pompous man with the bald head just emerging from the collar of his green coat. The others are seated on either side of him – the stout man with the small voice, and the thin-faced dark man in black. The little man in the chair is a most amusing personage, – *such* condescending grandeur, and *such* a voice!

'Bass!' as the young gentleman near us with the blue stock forcibly remarks to his companion, 'bass! I b'lieve you; he can go down lower than any man: so low sometimes that you can't hear him.' And so he does. To hear him growling away, gradually lower and lower down, till he can't get back again, is the most delightful thing in the world, and it is quite impossible to witness unmoved the impressive solemnity with which he pours forth his soul in 'My 'art's in the 'ighlands', or 'The brave old Hoak'. The stout man is also addicted to sentimentality, and warbles, 'Fly, fly from the world, my Bessy, with me,' or some such song, with ladylike sweetness, and in the most seductive tones imaginable.

'Pray give your orders, gen'l'm'n – pray give your orders,' – says the pale-faced man with the red head; and demands for 'goes' of gin and 'goes' of brandy, and pints of stout, and cigars of peculiar mildness, are vociferously made from all parts of the room. The 'professional gentlemen' are in the very height of their glory, and bestow condescending nods, or even a word or two of recognition, on the better-known frequenters of the room, in the most bland and patronising manner possible.

That little round-faced man, with the small brown surtout, white stockings and shoes, is in the comic line; the mixed air of self-denial, and mental consciousness of his own powers, with which he acknowledges the call of the chair, is particularly gratifying. 'Gen'l'men,' says the little pompous man, accompanying the word with a knock of the president's hammer on the table – 'Gen'l'men, allow me to claim your attention – our friend, Mr Smuggins, will oblige.' – 'Bravo!' shout the company; and Smuggins, after a considerable quantity of coughing by way of symphony, and a most facetious sniff or two, which afford general delight, sings a comic song, with a fal-de-ral – tol-de-ral chorus at the end of every verse, much longer than the verse itself. It is received with unbounded applause, and after some aspiring genius has volunteered a recitation, and failed dismally therein, the little pompous man gives another knock, and says, 'Gen'l'men, we will attempt a glee, if you please.' This announcement calls forth tumultuous applause, and the more energetic spirits express the unqualified approbation it affords them, by knocking one or two stout glasses off their legs – a humorous device; but one which frequently occasions some slight altercation when the form of paying the damage is proposed to be gone through by the waiter.

Scenes like these are continued until three or four o'clock in the morning; and even when they close, fresh ones open to the inquisitive novice. But as a description of all of them, however slight, would require a volume, the contents of which, however instructive, would be by no means pleasing, we make our bow, and drop the curtain.

## Chapter Three

### *Shops and Their Tenants*

First published in the *Morning Chronicle*, 10 October 1834 ('Street Sketches No. 2'). The appearance on the house of a brass plate inscribed 'Ladies' School' as a 'sign of poverty' would have had a personal resonance for Dickens, remembering his mother's vain efforts to ward off the family's economic collapse by starting a school.

What inexhaustible food for speculation do the streets of London afford! We never were able to agree with Sterne in pitying the man who could travel from Dan to Beersheba, and say that all was barren; we have not the slightest commiseration for the man who can take up his hat and stick, and walk from Covent Garden to St Paul's Churchyard, and back into the bargain, without deriving some amusement – we had almost said instruction – from his perambulation. And yet there are such beings: we meet them every day. Large black stocks and light waistcoats, jet canes and discontented countenances, are the characteristics of the race; other people brush quickly by you, steadily plodding on to business, or cheerfully running after pleasure. These men linger listlessly past, looking as happy and animated as a policeman on duty. Nothing seems to make an impression on their minds: nothing short of being knocked down by a porter, or run over by a cab, will disturb their equanimity. You will meet them on a fine day in any of the leading thoroughfares: peep through the window of a west end cigar shop in the evening, if you can manage to get a glimpse between the blue curtains which intercept the vulgar gaze, and you see them in their only enjoyment of existence. There they are lounging about, on round tubs and pipe boxes, in all the dignity of whiskers and gilt watchguards; whispering soft nothings to the young lady in amber, with the large earrings, who, as she sits behind the counter in a blaze of adoration and gaslight, is the admiration of all the female servants in the neighbourhood, and the envy of each milliner's apprentice within two miles around.

One of our principal amusements is to watch the gradual progress – the rise or fall – of particular shops. We have formed an intimate acquaintance with several, in different parts of town, and are perfectly acquainted with their whole history. We could name offhand, twenty at least, which we are quite sure have paid no taxes for the last six years. They are never inhabited for more than two months consecutively, and, we verily believe, have witnessed every retail trade in the directory.

There is one, whose history is a sample of the rest, in whose fate we have taken especial interest, having had the pleasure of knowing it ever since it has been a shop. It is on the Surrey side of the water – a little distance beyond the Marsh Gate. It was originally a substantial, good-looking private house enough; the landlord got into difficulties, the house got into Chancery, the tenant went away, and the house went to ruin. At this period our acquaintance with it commenced; the paint was all worn off; the windows were broken, the area was green with neglect and the overflowings of the water butt; the butt itself was without a lid, and the street door was the very picture of misery. The chief pastime of the children in the vicinity had been to assemble in a body on the steps, and take it in turn to knock loud double knocks at the door, to the great satisfaction of the neighbours generally, and especially of the nervous old lady next door but one. Numerous complaints were made, and several small basins of water discharged over the offenders, but without effect. In this state of things, the marine store dealer at the corner of the street, in the most obliging manner took the knocker off, and sold it: and the unfortunate house looked more wretched than ever.

We deserted our friend for a few weeks. What was our surprise, on our return, to find no trace of its existence! In its place was a handsome shop, fast approaching to a state of completion, and on the shutters were large bills, informing the public that it would shortly be opened with 'an extensive stock of linen drapery and haberdashery'. It opened in due course; there was the name of the proprietor 'and Co.' in gilt letters, almost too dazzling to look at. Such ribbons and shawls! and two such elegant young men behind the counter, each in a clean collar and white neckcloth, like the lover in a farce. As to the proprietor, he did nothing but walk up and down the shop, and hand seats to the ladies, and hold important conversations with the handsomest of the young men, who was shrewdly suspected by the neighbours to be the 'Co.'. We saw all this with sorrow; we felt a fatal presentiment that the shop was doomed – and so it was. Its decay was slow, but sure. Tickets gradually appeared in the windows; then rolls of flannel, with labels on them, were stuck outside the door; then a bill was pasted on the street door, intimating that the first floor was to let *un*furnished; then one of the young men disappeared altogether, and the other took to a black neckerchief, and the proprietor took to drinking. The shop became dirty, broken panes of glass remained unmended, and the stock disappeared piecemeal. At last the company's man came to cut off the water, and then the linen draper cut off himself, leaving the landlord his compliments and the key.

The next occupant was a fancy stationer. The shop was more modestly painted than before, still it was neat; but somehow we always thought, as we passed, that it looked like a poor and struggling concern. We wished the man well, but we trembled for his success. He was a widower evidently, and had employment elsewhere, for he passed us every morning on his road to the city. The business was carried on by his eldest daughter. Poor girl! she needed no assistance. We occasionally caught a glimpse of two or three children, in mourning like herself, as they sat in the little parlour behind the shop; and we never passed at night without seeing the eldest girl at work, either for them, or in making some elegant little trifle for sale. We often thought, as her pale face looked more sad and pensive in the dim candlelight, that if those thoughtless females who interfere with the miserable market of poor creatures such as these knew but one half of the misery they suffer, and the bitter privations they endure, in their honourable attempts to earn a scanty subsistence, they would, perhaps, resign even opportunities for the gratification of vanity, and an immodest love of self-display, rather than drive them to a last dreadful resource, which it would shock the delicate feelings of these *charitable* ladies to hear named.

But we are forgetting the shop. Well, we continued to watch it, and every day showed too clearly, the increasing poverty of its inmates. The children were clean, it is true, but their clothes were threadbare and shabby; no tenant had been procured for the upper part of the house, from the letting of which, a portion of the means of paying the rent was to have been derived, and a slow, wasting consumption prevented the eldest girl from continuing her exertions. Quarter-day arrived. The landlord had suffered from the extravagance of his last tenant, and he had no compassion for the struggles of his successor; he put in an execution. As we passed one morning, the broker's men were removing the little furniture there was in the house, and a newly posted bill informed us it was again 'To Let'. What became of the last tenant we never could learn; we believe the girl is past all suffering, and beyond all sorrow. Gold help her! We hope she is.

We were somewhat curious to ascertain what would be the next stage – for that the place had no chance of succeeding now, was perfectly clear. The bill was soon taken down, and some alterations were being made in the interior of the shop. We were in a fever of expectation; we exhausted conjecture – we imagined all possible trades, none of which were perfectly reconcilable with our idea of the gradual decay of the tenement. It opened, and we wondered why we had not guessed at the real state of the case before. The shop – not a large one at the best of times – had been converted into two: one was a bonnet-shape maker's, the other was opened by a tobacconist, who also dealt in walking sticks and Sunday newspapers; the two were separated by a thin partition, covered with tawdry striped paper.

The tobacconist remained in possession longer than any tenant within our recollection. He was a red-faced, impudent, good-for-nothing dog, evidently accustomed to take things as they came, and to make the best of a bad job. He sold as many cigars as he could, and smoked the rest. He occupied the shop as long as he could make peace with the landlord, and when he could no longer live in quiet, he very coolly locked the door, and bolted himself. From this period, the two little dens have undergone innumerable changes. The tobacconist was succeeded by a theatrical hairdresser, who ornamented the windows with a great variety of 'characters', and terrific combats. The bonnet-shape maker gave place to a greengrocer, and the histrionic barber was succeeded, in his turn, by a tailor. So numerous have been the changes, that we have of late done little more than mark the peculiar but certain indications of a house being poorly inhabited. It has been progressing by almost imperceptible degrees. The occupiers of the shops have gradually given up room after room, until they have only reserved the little parlour for themselves. First there appeared a brass plate on the private door, with 'Ladies' School' legibly engraved thereon; shortly afterwards we observed a second brass plate, then a bell, and then another bell.

When we paused in front of our old friend, and observed these signs of poverty, which are not to be mistaken, we thought as we turned away, that the house had attained its lowest pitch of degradation. We were wrong. When we last passed it, a 'dairy' was established in the area, and a party of melancholy-looking fowls were amusing themselves by running in at the front door, and out at the back one.

## Chapter Four

### *Scotland Yard*

First published in the *Morning Chronicle*, 4 October 1836 ('Sketches by Boz New Series No. 2'). Scotland Yard took its name from the palace of the kings of Scotland which stood there until 1701. In 1829 Peel located the headquarters of his newly formed Metropolitan Police in Whitehall Place where it remained until 1890; it soon came to be known as 'Scotland Yard' then simply 'the Yard'. In 1890 the Yard moved to a site in Cannon Row, near Westminster Bridge, which was then called New Scotland Yard (now the Norman Shaw Building); and in 1967 moved again, to its present location in Victoria Street.

Scotland Yard is a small – a very small – tract of land, bounded on one side by the river Thames, on the other by the gardens of Northumberland House: abutting at one end on the bottom of Northumberland Street, at the other on the back of Whitehall Place. When this territory was first accidentally discovered by a country gentleman who lost his way in the Strand, some years ago, the original settlers were found to be a tailor, a publican, two eating-house keepers, and a fruit pie maker; and it was also found to contain a race of strong and bulky men, who repaired to the wharfs in Scotland Yard regularly each morning, about five or six o'clock, to fill heavy waggons with coal, with which they proceeded to distant places up the country, and supplied the inhabitants with fuel. When they had emptied their waggons, they again returned for a fresh supply; and this trade was continued throughout the year.

As the settlers derived their subsistence from ministering to the wants of these primitive traders, the articles exposed for sale, and the places where they were sold, bore strong outward marks of being expressly adapted to their tastes and wishes. The tailor displayed in his window a Lilliputian pair of leather gaiters, and a diminutive round frock, while each doorpost was appropriately garnished with a model of a coal sack. The two eating-house keepers exhibited joints of a magnitude, and puddings of a solidity, which coalheavers alone could appreciate; and the fruit pie maker displayed on his well scrubbed window board large white compositions of flour and dripping, ornamented with pink stains, giving rich promise of the fruit within, which made their huge mouths water, as they lingered past.

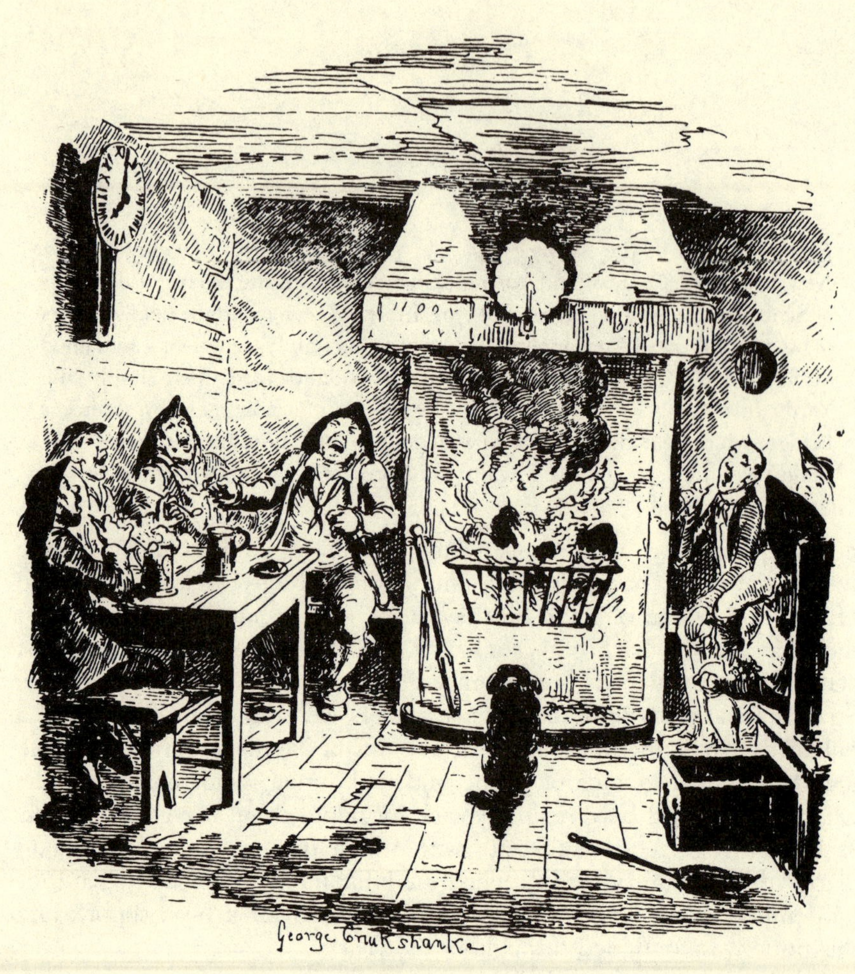


*Scotland Yard*

But the choicest spot in all Scotland Yard was the old public house in the corner. Here, in a dark wainscoted room of ancient appearance, cheered by the glow of a mighty fire, and decorated with an enormous clock, whereof the face was white, and the figures black, sat the lusty coalheavers, quaffing large draughts of Barclay's best, and puffing forth volumes of smoke, which wreathed heavily above their heads, and involved the room in a thick dark cloud. From this apartment might their voices be heard on a winter's night, penetrating to the very bank of the river, as they shouted out some sturdy chorus, or roared forth the burden of a popular song; dwelling upon the last few words with a strength and length of emphasis which made the very roof tremble above them.

Here, too, would they tell old legends of what the Thames was in ancient times, when the Patent Shot Manufactory wasn't built, and Waterloo Bridge had never been thought of; and then they would shake their heads with portentous looks, to the deep edification of the rising generation of heavers, who crowded round them, and wondered where all this would end; whereat the tailor would take his pipe solemnly from his mouth, and say, how that he hoped it might end well, but he very much doubted whether it would or not, and couldn't rightly tell what to make of it – a mysterious expression of opinion, delivered with a semi-prophetic air, which never failed to elicit the fullest concurrence of the assembled company; and so they would go on drinking and wondering till ten o'clock came, and with it the tailor's wife to fetch him home, when the little party broke up, to meet again in the same room, and say and do precisely the same things, on the following evening at the same hour.

About this time the barges that came up the river began to bring vague rumours to Scotland Yard of somebody in the city having been heard to say, that the Lord Mayor had threatened in so many words to pull down the old London Bridge, and build up a new one. At first these rumours were disregarded as idle tales, wholly destitute of foundation, for nobody in Scotland Yard doubted that if the Lord Mayor contemplated any such dark design, he would just be clapped up in the Tower for a week or two, and then killed off for high treason.

By degrees, however, the reports grew stronger, and more frequent, and at last a barge, laden with numerous chaldrons of the best Wallsend, brought up the positive intelligence that several of the arches of the old bridge were stopped, and that preparations were actually in progress for constructing the new one. What an excitement was visible in the old tap room on that memorable night! Each man looked into his neighbour's face, pale with alarm and astonishment, and read therein an echo of the sentiments which filled his own breast. The oldest heaver present proved to demonstration, that the moment the piers were removed, all the water in the Thames would run clean off, and leave a dry gulley in its place.

What was to become of the coal barges – of the trade of Scotland Yard – of the very existence of its population? The tailor shook his head more sagely than usual, and grimly pointing to a knife on the table, bid them wait and see what happened. He said nothing – not he; but if the Lord Mayor didn't fall a victim to popular indignation, why he would be rather astonished; that was all.

They did wait; barge after barge arrived, and still no tidings of the assassination of the Lord Mayor. The first stone was laid; it was done by a Duke – the King's brother. Years passed away, and the bridge was opened by the King himself. In course of time the piers were removed; and when the people in Scotland Yard got up next morning in the confident expectation of being able to step over to Pedlar's Acre without wetting the soles of their feet, they found to their unspeakable astonishment that the water was just where it used to be.

A result so different from that which they had anticipated from this first improvement, produced its full effect upon the inhabitants of Scotland Yard. One of the eating house keepers began to court public opinion, and to look for customers among a new class of people. He covered his little dining tables with white cloths, and got a painter's apprentice to inscribe something about hot joints from twelve to two, in one of the little panes of his shop window. Improvement began to march with rapid strides up the very threshold of Scotland Yard. A new market sprung up at Hungerford, and the Police Commissioners established their office in Whitehall Place. The traffic in Scotland Yard increased; fresh Members were added to the House of Commons, Metropolitan Representatives found it a near cut, and many other foot passengers followed their example.

We marked the advance of civilisation, and beheld it with a sigh. The eating-house keeper who manfully resisted the innovation of tablecloths, was losing ground every day, as his opponent gained it, and a deadly feud sprung up between them. The genteel one no longer took his evening's pint in Scotland Yard, but drank gin and water at a 'parlour' in Parliament Street. The fruit pie maker still continued to visit the old room, but he took to smoking cigars, and began to call himself a pastry cook, and to read the papers. The old heavers still assembled round the ancient fireplace, but their talk was mournful: and the loud song and the joyous shout were heard no more.

And what is Scotland Yard now? How have its old customs changed; and how has the ancient simplicity of its inhabitants faded away! The old tottering public house is converted into a spacious and lofty 'wine vaults'; gold leaf has been used in the construction of the letters which emblazon its exterior, and the poet's art has been called into requisition, to intimate that if you drink a certain description of ale, you must hold fast by the rail. The tailor exhibits in his window the pattern of a foreign-looking brown surtout, with silk buttons, a fur collar, and fur cuffs. He wears a stripe down the outside of each leg of his trousers: and we have detected his assistants (for he has assistants now) in the act of sitting on the shop board in the same uniform.

At the other end of the little row of houses a bootmaker has established himself in a brick box, with the additional innovation of a first floor; and here he exposes for sale, boots – real Wellington boots – an article which a few years ago, none of the original inhabitants had ever seen or heard of. It was but the other day, that a dressmaker opened another little box in the middle of the row; and when we thought that the spirit of change could produce no alteration beyond that, a jeweller appeared, and not content with exposing gilt rings and copper bracelets out of number, put up an announcement, which still sticks in his window, that 'ladies' ears may be pierced within'. The dressmaker employs a young lady who wears pockets in her apron; and the tailor informs the public that gentlemen may have their own materials made up.

Amidst all this change, and restlessness, and innovation, there remains but one old man, who seems to mourn the downfall of this ancient place. He holds no converse with human kind, but, seated on a wooden bench at the angle of the wall which fronts the crossing from Whitehall Place, watches in silence the gambols of his sleek and well-fed dogs. He is the presiding genius of Scotland Yard. Years and years have rolled over his head; but in fine weather or in foul, hot or cold, wet or dry, hail, rain, or snow, he is still in his accustomed spot. Misery and want are depicted in his countenance; his form is bent by age, his head is grey with length of trial, but there he sits from day to day, brooding over the past; and thither he will continue to drag his feeble limbs, until his eyes have closed upon Scotland Yard, and upon the world together.

A few years hence, and the antiquary of another generation looking into some mouldy record of the strife and passions that agitated the world in these times, may glance his eye over the pages we have just filled: and not all his knowledge of the history of the past, not all his black-letter lore, or his skill in book collecting, not all the dry studies of a long life, or the dusty volumes that have cost him a fortune, may help him to the whereabouts, either of Scotland Yard or of any one of the landmarks we have mentioned in describing it.

## CHAPTER FIVE

### *Seven Dials*

First published in *Bell's Life in London*, 27 September 1837 ('Scenes and Characters No. 1'). The area known as Seven Dials formed part of the parish of St Giles-in-the-Fields in west-central London. It was laid out as a speculative venture in the late seventeenth century by Thomas Neale, Master of the Royal Mint. Seven streets converged on a central space in the middle of which was a Doric column surmounted by a hexagonal stone, each face of which bore a sundial facing the opening of one of the streets (or, in one case, two streets which opened into the same angle of this central area). The column was removed in 1773, but has recently been replaced by a replica. By the early nineteenth century the whole area of St Giles had become a notorious 'rookery' or densely populated slum containing a large criminal element. In his fragment of autobiography, printed by Forster in *Life of Dickens*, Dickens recalls his childhood fascination with St Giles: 'what wild visions of prodigies of wickedness, want, and beggary, arose in my mind out of that place!' In referring to Warren's Blacking Warehouse and its proprietor's famous rhymed advertisements Dickens is also touching on his own memories of the time when he was a 'little labouring hind' in a rival warehouse established by Warren's brother and bought by James Lamert, a family acquaintance of the Dickenses.

We have always been of opinion that if Tom King and the Frenchman had not immortalised Seven Dials, Seven Dials would have immortalised itself. Seven Dials! the region of song and poetry – first effusions, and last dying speeches: hallowed by the names of Catnach and of Pitts – names that will entwine themselves with costermongers and barrel organs, when penny magazines shall have superseded penny yards of song, and capital punishment be unknown!

Look at the construction of the place. The gordian knot was all very well in its way: so was the maze of Hampton Court: so is the maze at the Beulah Spa: so were the ties of stiff white neckcloths, when the difficulty of getting one on was only to be equalled by the apparent impossibility of ever getting it off again. But what involutions can compare with those of Seven Dials? Where is there such another maze of streets,

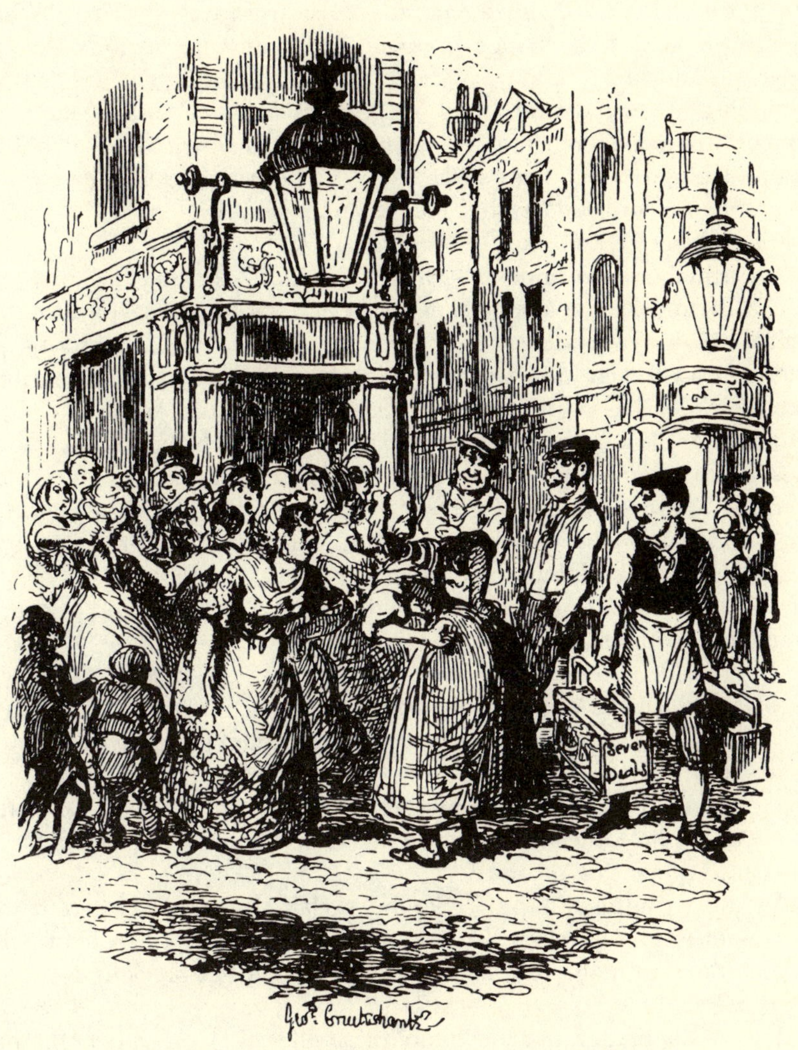


*Seven Dials*

courts, lanes, and alleys? Where such a pure mixture of Englishmen and Irishmen, as in this complicated part of London? We boldly aver that we doubt the veracity of the legend to which we have adverted. We *can* suppose a man rash enough to inquire at random – at a house with lodgers too for a Mr Thompson, with all but the certainty before his eyes of finding at least two or three Thompsons in any house of moderate dimensions; but a Frenchman – a Frenchman in Seven Dials! Pooh! He was an Irishman. Tom King's education had been neglected in his infancy, and as he couldn't understand half the man said, he took it for granted he was talking French.

The stranger who finds himself in 'The Dials' for the first time, and stands Belzoni like, at the entrance of seven obscure passages, uncertain which to take, will see enough around him to keep his curiosity and attention awake for no inconsiderable time. From the irregular square into which he has plunged, the streets and courts dart in all directions, until they are lost in the unwholesome vapour which hangs over the house tops, and renders the dirty perspective uncertain and confined; and lounging at every corner, as if they came there to take a few gasps of such air as has found its way so far, but is too much exhausted already, to be enabled to force itself into the narrow alleys around, are groups of people, whose appearance and dwellings would fill any mind but a regular Londoner's with astonishment.

On one side, a little crowd has collected round a couple of ladies, who having imbibed the contents of various 'three-outs' of gin and bitters in the course of the morning, have at length differed on some point of domestic arrangement, and are on the eve of settling the quarrel satisfactorily, by an appeal to blows, greatly to the interest of other ladies who live in the same house, and tenements adjoining, and who are all partisans on one side or other.

'Vy don't you pitch into her, Sarah?' exclaims one half dressed matron by way of encouragement. 'Vy don't you? if *my* 'usband had treated her with a drain last night, unbeknown to me, I'd tear her precious eyes out – a wixen!'

'What's the matter, ma'am?' inquires another old woman, who has just bustled up to the spot.

'Matter!' replies the first speaker, talking *at* the obnoxious combatant, 'matter! Here's poor dear Mrs Sulliwin, as has five blessed children of her own, can't go out a-charing for one arternoon, but what hussies must be a-comin', and 'ticing avay her oun' 'usband, as she's been married to twelve year come next Easter Monday, for I see the certificate ven I vas a-drinkin' a cup o' tea vith her, only the werry last blessed Ven'sday as ever vas sent. I 'appen'd to say promiscuously, "Mrs Sulliwin," says I——'

'What do you mean by hussies?' interrupts a champion of the other party, who has evinced a strong inclination throughout to get up a branch fight on her own account ('Hooroar,' ejaculates a pot-boy in parenthesis, 'put the kye-bosk on her, Mary!'). 'What do you mean by hussies?' reiterates the champion.

'Niver mind,' replies the opposition expressively, 'niver mind; *you* go home, and, ven you're quite sober, mend your stockings.'

This somewhat personal allusion, not only to the lady's habits of intemperance, but also to the state of her wardrobe, rouses her utmost ire, and she accordingly complies with the urgent request of the bystanders to 'pitch in', with considerable alacrity. The scuffle became general, and terminates, in minor play bill phraseology, with 'arrival of the policeman, interior of the station house, and impressive *dénouement*.'

In addition to the numerous groups who are idling about the gin shops and squabbling in the centre of the road, every post in the open space has its occupant, who leans against it for hours, with listless perseverance. It is odd enough that one class of men in London appear to have no enjoyment beyond leaning against posts. We never saw a regular bricklayer's labourer take any other recreation, fighting excepted. Pass through St Giles's in the evening of a week day, there they are in their fustian dresses, spotted with brick dust and whitewash, leaning against posts. Walk through Seven Dials on Sunday morning: there they are again, drab or light corduroy trousers, Blucher boots, blue coats, and great yellow waistcoats, leaning against posts. The idea of a man dressing himself in his best clothes, to lean against a post all day!

The peculiar character of these streets, and the close resemblance each one bears to its neighbour, by no means tends to decrease the bewilderment in which the unexperienced wayfarer through 'the Dials' finds himself involved. He traverses streets of dirty, straggling houses, with now and then an unexpected court composed of buildings as ill proportioned and deformed as the half naked children that wallow in the kennels. Here and there, a little dark chandler's shop, with a cracked bell hung up behind the door to announce the entrance of a customer, or betray the presence of some young gentleman in whom a passion for shop tills has developed itself at an early age: others, as if for support, against some handsome lofty building, which usurps the place of a low dingy public house; long rows of broken and patched windows expose plants that may have flourished when 'the Dials' were built, in vessels as dirty as 'the Dials' themselves; and shops for the purchase of rags, bones, old iron, and kitchen stuff, vie in cleanliness with the bird fanciers' and rabbit dealers', which one might fancy so many arks, but for the irresistible conviction that no bird in its proper senses, who was permitted to leave one of them, would ever come back again. Brokers' shops, which would seem to have been established by humane individuals, as refuges for destitute bugs, interspersed with announcements of day-schools, penny theatres, petition writers, mangles, and music for balls or routs, complete the 'still life' of the subject; and dirty men, filthy women, squalid children, fluttering shuttlecocks, noisy battledores, reeking pipes, bad fruit, more than doubtful oysters, attenuated cats, depressed dogs, and anatomical fowls, are its cheerful accompaniments.

If the external appearance of the houses, or a glance at their inhabitants, presents but few attractions, a closer acquaintance with either is little calculated to alter one's first impression. Every room has its separate tenant, and every tenant is, by the same mysterious dispensation which causes a country curate to 'increase and multiply' most marvellously, generally the head of a numerous family.

The man in the shop, perhaps, is in the baked 'jemmy' line, or the firewood and hearthstone line, or any other line which requires a floating capital of eighteen pence or thereabouts: and he and his family live in the shop, and the small back parlour behind it. Then there is an Irish labourer and *his* family in the back kitchen, and a jobbing man – carpet beater and so forth – with *his* family in the front one. In the front one-pair, there's another man with another wife and family, and in the back one-pair, there's 'a young 'oman as takes in tambour work, and dresses quite genteel', who talks a good deal about 'my friend', and can't 'a-bear anything low'. The second floor front, and the rest of the lodgers, are just a second edition of the people below, except a shabby-genteel man in the back attic, who has his half pint of coffee every morning from the coffee shop next door but one, which boasts a little front den called a coffee room, with a fireplace, over which is an inscription, politely requesting that, 'to prevent mistakes', customers will 'please to pay on delivery'. The shabby-genteel man is an object of some mystery, but as he leads a life of seclusion, and never was known to buy anything beyond an occasional pen, except half pints of coffee, penny loaves, and ha'porths of ink, his fellow-lodgers very naturally suppose him to be an author; and rumours are current in the Dials, that he writes poems for Mr Warren.

Now anybody who passed through the Dials on a hot summer's evening, and saw the different women of the house gossiping on the steps, would be apt to think that all was harmony among them, and that a more primitive set of people than the native Diallers could not be imagined. Alas! the man in the shop ill treats his family; the carpet beater extends his professional pursuits to his wife; the one-pair front has an undying feud with the two-pair front, in consequence of the two-pair front persisting in dancing over his (the one-pair front's) head, when he and his family have retired for the night; the two-pair back *will* interfere with the front kitchen's children; the Irishman comes home drunk every other night, and attacks everybody; and the one-pair back screams at everything. Animosities spring up between floor and floor; the very cellar asserts his equality. Mrs A. 'smacks' Mrs B.'s child, for 'making faces'. Mrs B. forthwith throws cold water over Mrs A.'s child for 'calling names'. The husbands are embroiled – the quarrel becomes general – an assault is the consequence, and a police officer the result.

## Chapter Six

### *Meditations in Monmouth Street*

First published in the *Morning Chronicle*, 11 October 1836 ('Sketches by Boz, New Series No. 1'). Monmouth Street formed the boundary of Seven Dials on the northwest, now the eastern section of Shaftesbury Avenue.

We have always entertained a particular attachment towards Monmouth Street, as the only true and real emporium for second hand wearing apparel. Monmouth Street is venerable from its antiquity, and respectable from its usefulness. Holywell Street we despise; the red-headed and red-whiskered Jews who forcibly haul you into their squalid houses, and thrust you into a suit of clothes, whether you will or not, we detest.

The inhabitants of Monmouth Street are a distinct class; a peaceable and retiring race, who immure themselves for the most part in deep cellars, or small back parlours, and who seldom come forth into the world, except in the dusk and coolness of the evening, when they may be seen seated, in chairs on the pavement, smoking their pipes, or watching the gambols of their engaging children as they revel in the gutter, a happy troop of infantine scavengers. Their countenances bear a thoughtful and a dirty cast, certain indications of their love of traffic; and their habitations are distinguished by that disregard of outward appearance and neglect of personal comfort, so common among people who are constantly immersed in profound speculations, and deeply engaged in sedentary pursuits.

We have hinted at the antiquity of our favourite spot. 'A Monmouth Street laced coat' was a byword a century ago; and still we find Monmouth Street the same. Pilot greatcoats with wooden buttons have usurped the place of the ponderous laced coats with full skirts; embroidered waistcoats with large flaps have yielded to double-breasted checks with roll collars; and three-cornered hats of quaint appearance have given place to the low crowns and broad brims of the coachman school; but it is the times that have changed, not Monmouth Street. Through every alteration and every change, Monmouth Street has still remained the burial place of the fashions; and such, to judge from all present appearances, it will remain until there are no more fashions to bury.

We love to walk among these extensive groves of the illustrious dead,

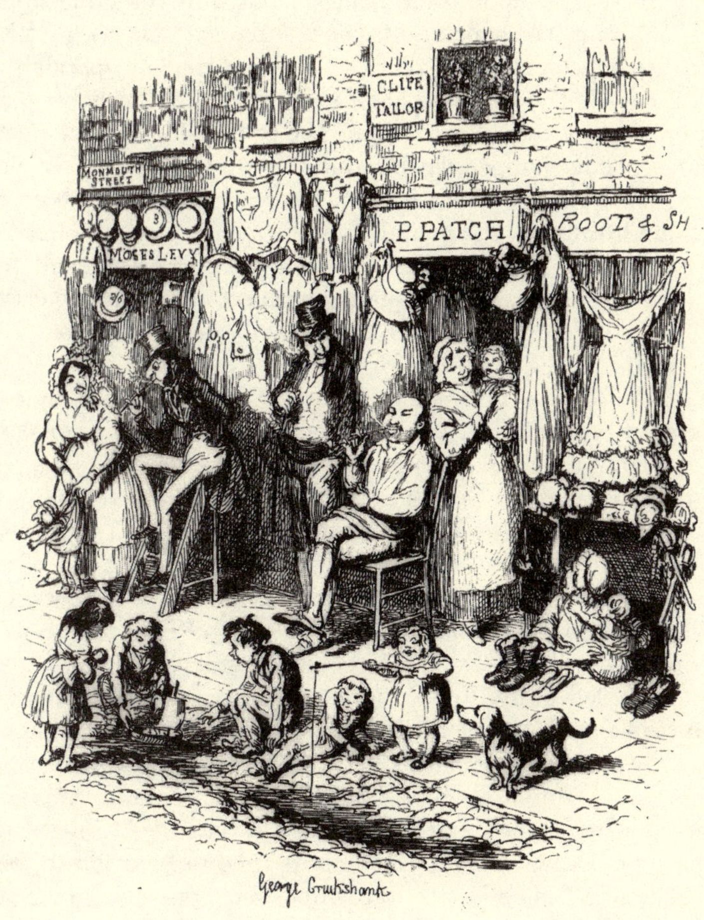


*Monmouth Street*

and to indulge in the speculations to which they give rise; now fitting a deceased coat, then a dead pair of trousers, and anon the mortal remains of a gaudy waistcoast, upon some being of our own conjuring up, and endeavouring, from the shape and fashion of the garment itself, to bring its former owner before our mind's eye. We have gone on speculating in this way, until whole rows of coats have started from their pegs, and buttoned up, of their own accord, round the waists of imaginary wearers; lines of trousers have jumped down to meet them; waistcoats have almost burst with anxiety to put themselves on; and half an acre of shoes have suddenly found feet to fit them, and gone stumping down the street with a noise which has fairly awakened us from our pleasant reverie, and driven us slowly away, with a bewildered stare, an object of astonishment to the good people of Monmouth Street, and of no slight suspicion to the policemen at the opposite street corner.

We were occupied in this manner the other day, endeavouring to fit a pair of lace-up half-boots on an ideal personage, for whom, to say the truth, they were full a couple of sizes too small, when our eyes happened to alight on a few suits of clothes ranged outside a shop window, which it immediately struck us, must at different periods have all belonged to, and been worn by, the same individual, and had now, by one of those strange conjunctions of circumstances which will occur sometimes, come to be exposed together for sale in the same shop. The idea seemed a fantastic one, and we looked at the clothes again with a firm determination not to be easily led away. No, we were right; the more we looked, the more we were convinced of the accuracy of our previous impression. There was the man's whole life written as legibly on those clothes, as if we had his autobiography engrossed on parchment before us.

The first was a patched and much soiled skeleton suit; one of those straight blue cloth cases in which small boys used to be confined, before belts and tunics had come in, and old notions had gone out: an ingenious contrivance for displaying the full symmetry of a boy's figure, by fastening him into a very tight jacket, with an ornamental row of buttons over each shoulder, and then buttoning his trousers over it, so as to give his legs the appearance of being hooked on, just under the armpits. This was the boy's dress. It had belonged to a town boy, we could see; there was a shortness about the legs and arms of the suit; and a bagging at the knees, peculiar to the rising youth of London streets. A small day school he had been at, evidently. If it had been a regular boys' school they wouldn't have let him play on the floor so much, and rub his knees so white. He had an indulgent mother too, and plenty of halfpence, as the numerous smears of some sticky substance about the pockets, and just below the chin, which even the salesman's skill could not succeed in disguising, sufficiently betokened. They were decent people, but not overburdened with riches, or he would not have so far outgrown the suit when he passed into those corduroys with the round jacket; in which he went to a boys' school, however, and learnt to write – and in ink of pretty tolerable blackness, too, if the place where he used to wipe his pen might be taken as evidence.

A black suit and the jacket changed into a diminutive coat. His father had died, and the mother had got the boy a message lad's place in some office. A long worn suit that one; rusty and threadbare before it was laid aside, but clean and free from soil to the last. Poor woman! We could imagine her assumed cheerfulness over the scanty meal, and the refusal of her own small portion, that her hungry boy might have enough. Her constant anxiety for his welfare, her pride in his growth mingled sometimes with the thought, almost too acute to bear, that as he grew to be a man his old affection might cool, old kindnesses fade from his mind, and old promises be forgotten – the sharp pain that even then a careless word or a cold look would give her – all crowded on our thoughts as vividly as if the very scene were passing before us.

These things happen every hour, and we all know it; and yet we felt as much sorrow when we saw, or fancied we saw – it makes no difference which – the change that began to take place now, as if we had just conceived the bare possibility of such a thing for the first time. The next suit, smart but slovenly; meant to be gay, and yet not half so decent as the threadbare apparel; redolent of the idle lounge, and the blackguard companions, told us, we thought, that the widow's comfort had rapidly faded away. We could imagine that coat – imagine! we could see it; we *had* seen it a hundred times – sauntering in company with three or four other coats of the same cut, about some place of profligate resort at night.

We dressed, from the same shop window in an instant, half a dozen boys of from fifteen to twenty; and putting cigars into their mouths, and their hands into their pockets, watched them as they sauntered down the street, and lingered at the corner, with the obscene jest, and the oft repeated oath. We never lost sight of them, till they had cocked their hats a little more on one side, and swaggered into the public house; and then we entered the desolate home, where the mother sat late in the night, alone; we watched her, as she paced the room in feverish anxiety, and every now and then opened the door, looked wistfully into the dark and empty street, and again returned, to be again and again disappointed. We beheld the look of patience with which she bore the brutish threat, nay, even the drunken blow; and we heard the agony of tears that gushed from her very heart, as she sank upon her knees in her solitary and wretched apartment.

A long period had elapsed, and a greater change had taken place, by the time of casting off the suit that hung above. It was that of a stout, broad-shouldered, sturdy-chested man; and we knew at once, as anybody would, who glanced at that broad-skirted green coat, with the large metal buttons, that its wearer seldom walked forth without a dog at his heels, and some idle ruffian, the very counterpart of himself, at his side. The vices of the boy had grown with the man, and we fancied his home then – if such a place deserve the name.

We saw the bare and miserable room, destitute of furniture, crowded with his wife and children, pale, hungry, and emaciated; the man cursing their lamentations, staggering to the tap room, from whence he had just returned, followed by his wife and a sickly infant, clamouring for bread; and heard the street wrangle and noisy recrimination that his striking her occasioned. And then imagination led us to some metropolitan workhouse, situated in the midst of crowded streets and alleys, filled with noxious vapours, and ringing with boisterous cries, where an old and feeble woman, imploring pardon for her son, lay dying in a close dark room, with no child to clasp her hand, and no pure air from heaven to fan her brow. A stranger closed the eyes that settled into a cold unmeaning glare, and strange ears received the words that murmured from the white and half closed lips.

A coarse round frock, with a worn cotton neckerchief, and other articles of clothing of the commonest description, completed the history. A prison, and the sentence – banishment or the gallows. What would the man have given then, to be once again the contented humble drudge of his boyish years; to have been restored to life, but for a week, a day, an hour, a minute, only for so long a time as would enable him to say one word of passionate regret to, and hear one sound of heartfelt forgiveness from, the cold and ghastly form that lay rotting in the pauper's grave! The children wild in the streets, the mother a destitute widow; both deeply tainted with the deep disgrace of the husband and father's name, and impelled by sheer necessity, down the precipice that had led him to a lingering death, possibly of many years' duration, thousands of miles away. We had no clue to the end of the tale; but it was easy to guess its termination.

We took a step or two further on, and by way of restoring the naturally cheerful tone of our thoughts, began fitting visionary feet and legs into a cellar board full of boots and shoes, with a speed and accuracy that would have astonished the most expert artist in leather, living. There was one pair of boots in particular – a jolly, good-tempered, hearty-looking, pair of tops, that excited our warmest regard; and we had got a fine, red-faced, jovial fellow of a market gardener into them, before we had made their acquaintance half a minute. They were just the very thing for him. There were his huge fat legs bulging over the tops, and fitting them too tight to admit of his tucking in the loops he had pulled them on by; and his knee cords with an interval of stocking; and his blue apron tucked up round his waist; and his red neckerchief and blue coat, and a white hat stuck on one side of his head; and there he stood with a broad grin on that great red face whistling away, as if any other idea but that of being happy and comfortable had never entered his brain.

This was the very man after our own heart; we knew all about him; we had seen him coming up to Covent Garden in his green chaise cart, with the fat tubby little horse, half a thousand times; and even while we cast an affectionate look upon his boots, at that instant, the form of a coquettish servant maid suddenly sprung into a pair of Denmark satin shoes that stood beside them, and we at once recognised the very girl who accepted his offer of a ride, just on this side the Hammersmith suspension bridge, the very last Tuesday morning we rode into town from Richmond.

A very smart female, in a showy bonnet, stepped into a pair of grey cloth boots, with black fringe and binding, that were studiously pointing out their toes on the other side of the top-boots, and seemed very anxious to engage his attention, but we didn't observe that our friend the market gardener appeared at all captivated with these blandishments; for beyond giving a knowing wink when they first began, as if to imply that he quite understood their end and object, he took no further notice of them. His indifference, however, was amply recommended by the excessive gallantry of a very old gentleman with a silver headed stick, who tottered into a pair of large list shoes, that were standing in one corner of the board, and indulged in a variety of gestures expressive of his admiration of the lady in the cloth boots, to the immeasurable amusement of a young fellow we put into a pair of long quartered pumps, who we thought would have split the coat that slid down to meet him, with laughing.

We had been looking on at this little pantomime with great satisfaction for some time, when, to our unspeakable astonishment, we perceived that the whole of the characters, including a numerous *corps de ballet* of boots and shoes in the background, into which we had been hastily thrusting as many feet as we could press into the service, were arranging themselves in order for dancing; and some music striking up at the moment, to it they went without delay. It was perfectly delightful to witness the agility of the market gardener. Out went the boots, first on one side, then on the other, then cutting, then shuffling, then setting to the Denmark satins, then advancing, then retreating, then going round, and then repeating the whole of the evolutions again, without appearing to suffer in the least from the violence of the exercise.

Nor were the Denmark satins a bit behindhand, for they jumped and bounded about in all directions; and though they were neither so regular, nor so true to the time as the cloth boots, still, as they seemed to do it from the heart, and to enjoy it more, we candidly confess that we preferred their style of dancing to the other. But the old gentleman in the list shoes was the most amusing object in the whole party; for, besides his grotesque attempts to appear youthful, and amorous, which were sufficiently entertaining in themselves, the young fellow in the pumps managed so artfully that every time the old gentleman advanced to salute the lady in the cloth boots, he trod with his whole weight on the old fellow's toes, which made him roar with anguish, and rendered all the others like to die of laughing.

We were in the full enjoyment of these festivities when we heard a shrill, and by no means musical voice, exclaim, 'Hope you'll know me agin, imperence!' and on looking intently forward to see from whence the sound came, we found that it proceeded, not from the young lady in the cloth boots, as we had at first been inclined to suppose, but from a bulky lady of elderly appearance who was seated in a chair at the head of the cellar steps, apparently for the purpose of superintending the sale of the articles arranged there.

A barrel organ, which had been in full force close behind us, ceased playing; the people we had been fitting into the shoes and boots took to flight at the interruption; and as we were conscious that in the depth of our meditations we might have been rudely staring at the old lady for half an hour without knowing it, we took to flight too, and were soon immersed in the deepest obscurity of the adjacent 'Dials'.

## Chapter Seven

### *Hackney Coach Stands*

First published in the *Evening Chronicle*, 31 January 1835 ('Sketches of London No. 1'). Hackney coaches had plied for hire in London since Stuart times and were often the former private coaches of noble families, hence Dickens's reference to 'a faded coat of arms'. The London Hackney Carriage Act of 1831 fixed coach fares. Drivers could charge by either distance or time. Fares were fixed at one shilling for up to a mile, and then sixpence for every half mile beyond that, or one shilling for up to thirty minutes, increasing by sixpence every fifteen minutes after that. Cabs cost eightpence a mile. The increasing popularity of cabs (particularly the light and speedy Hansom cab, patented in 1834), and omnibuses (first introduced in 1829) gradually drove the old hackney coaches out of business. See below p. 142.

We maintain that hackney coaches, properly so called, belong solely to the metropolis. We may be told, that there are hackney coach stands in Edinburgh; and not to go quite so far for a contradiction to our position, we may be reminded that Liverpool, Manchester, 'and other large towns' (as the Parliamentary phrase goes), have *their* hackney coach stands. We readily concede to these places, the possession of certain vehicles, which may look almost as dirty; and even go almost as slowly, as London hackney coaches; but that they have the slightest claim to compete with the metropolis, either in point of stands, drivers, or cattle, we indignantly deny.

Take a regular, ponderous, rickety, London hackney coach of the old school, and let any man have the boldness to assert, if he can, that he ever beheld any object on the face of the earth which at all resembles it, unless, indeed, it were another hackney coach of the same date. We have recently observed on certain stands, and we say it with deep regret, rather dapper green chariots, and coaches of polished yellow, with four wheels of the same colour as the coach, whereas it is perfectly notorious to every one who has studied the subject, that every wheel ought to be of a different colour, and a different size. These are innovations, and, like other miscalled improvements, awful signs of the restlessness of the public mind, and the little respect paid to our time-honoured institutions. Why should hackney

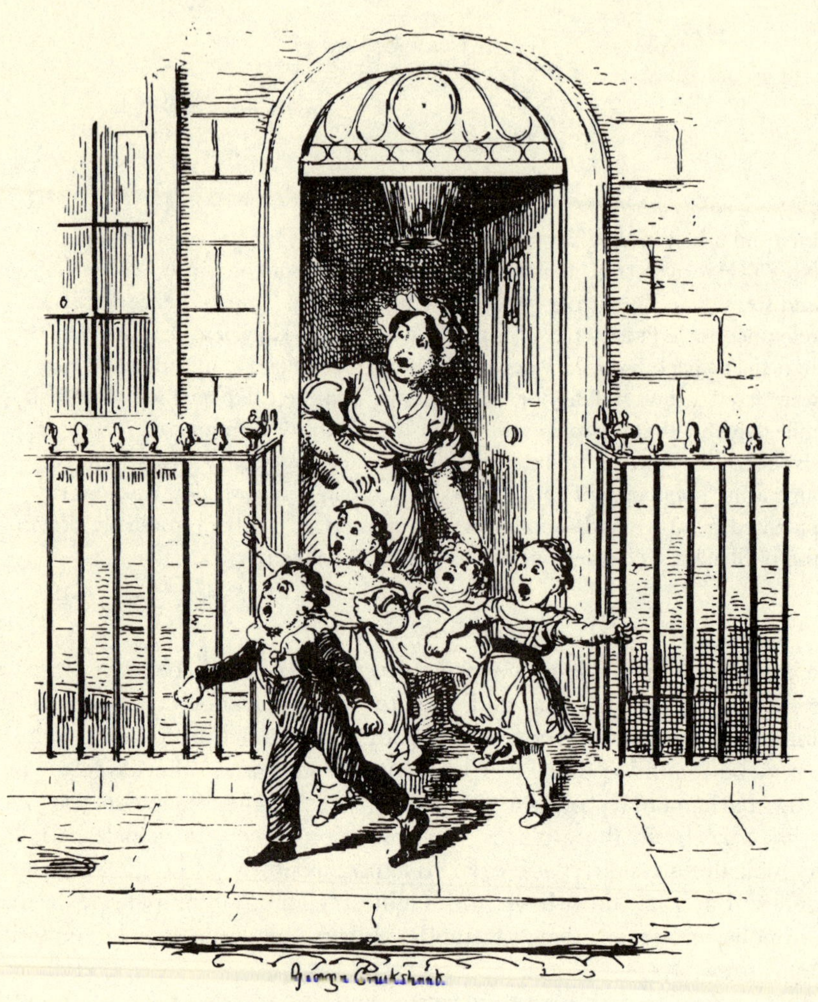

*Hackney Coach Stands*

coaches be clean? Our ancestors found them dirty, and left them so. Why should we, with a feverish wish to 'keep moving', desire to roll along at the rate of six miles an hour, while they were content to rumble over the stones at four? These are solemn considerations. Hackney coaches are part and parcel of the law of the land; they were settled by the Legislature; plated and numbered by the wisdom of Parliament.

Then why have they been swamped by cabs and omnibuses? Or why should people be allowed to ride quickly for eightpence a mile, after Parliament had come to the solemn decision that they should pay a shilling a mile for riding slowly? We pause for a reply; – and, having no chance of getting one, begin a fresh paragraph.

Our acquaintance with hackney coach stands is of long standing. We are a walking book of fares, feeling ourselves half bound, as it were, to be always in the right on contested points. We know all the regular watermen within three miles of Covent Garden by sight, and should be almost tempted to believe that all the hackney coach horses in that district knew us by sight too, if one half of them were not blind. We take great interest in hackney coaches, but we seldom drive, having a knack of turning ourselves over when we attempt to do so. We are as great friends to horses, hackney coach and otherwise, as the renowned Mr Martin, of costermonger notoriety, and yet we never ride. We keep no horse, but a clothes horse; enjoy no saddle so much as a saddle of mutton; and, following our own inclinations, have never followed the hounds. Leaving these fleeter means of getting over the ground, or of depositing oneself upon it, to those who like them, by hackney coach stands we take our stand.

There is a hackney coach stand under the very window at which we are writing; there is only one coach on it now, but it is a fair specimen of the class of vehicles to which we have alluded – a great, lumbering, square concern of a dingy yellow colour (like a bilious brunette), with very small glasses, but very large frames; the panels are ornamented with a faded coat of arms, in shape something like a dissected bat, the axletree is red, and the majority of the wheels are green. The box is partially covered by an old greatcoat, with a multiplicity of capes, and some extraordinary looking clothes; and the straw, with which the canvas cushion is stuffed, is sticking up in several places, as if in rivalry of the hay, which is peeping through the chinks in the boot. The horses, with drooping heads, and each with a mane and tail as scanty and straggling as those of a worn out rocking horse, are standing patiently on some damp straw, occasionally wincing, and rattling the harness; and now and then one of them lifts his mouth to the ear of his companion as if he were saying, in a whisper, that he should like to assassinate the coachman. The coachman himself is in the watering house; and the waterman, with his hands forced into his pockets as far as they can possibly go, is dancing the 'double shuffle', in front of the pump, to keep his feet warm.

The servant girl, with the pink ribbons, at No 5, opposite, suddenly opens the street door, and four small children forthwith rush out, and scream 'Coach!' with all their might and main. The waterman darts from the pump, seizes the horses by their respective bridles, and drags them, and the coach too, round to the house, shouting all the time for the coachman at the very top, or rather very bottom of his voice, for it is a deep bass growl. A response is heard from the tap room; the coachman, in his wooden-soled shoes, makes the street echo again as he runs across it; and then there is such a struggling, and backing, and grating of the kennel, to get the coach door opposite the house door, that the children are in perfect ecstasies of delight. What a commotion! The old lady, who has been stopping there for the last month, is going back to the country. Out comes box after box, and one side of the vehicle is filled with luggage in no time; the children get into everybody's way, and the youngest, who has upset himself in his attempts to carry an umbrella, is borne off wounded and kicking. The youngsters disappear, and a short pause ensues, during which the old lady is, no doubt, kissing them all round in the back parlour. She appears at last, followed by her married daughter, all the children, and both the servants, who, with the joint assistance of the coachman and waterman, manage to get her safely into the coach. A cloak is handed in, and a little basket, which we could almost swear contains a small black bottle, and a paper of sandwiches. Up go the steps, bang goes the door, 'Golden Cross, Charing Cross, Tom,' says the waterman; 'Goodbye, grandma,' cry the children, off jingles the coach at the rate of three miles an hour, and the mamma and children retire into the house, with the exception of one little villain, who runs up the street at the top of his speed, pursued by the servant; not ill pleased to have such an opportunity of displaying her attractions. She brings him back, and, after casting two or three gracious glances across the way, which are either intended for us or the potboy (we are not quite certain which), shuts the door, and the hackney coach stand is again at a standstill.

We have been frequently amused, with the intense delight with which a 'servant of all work', who is sent for a coach, deposits herself inside; and the unspeakable gratification which boys, who have been despatched on a similar errand, appear to derive from mounting the box. But we never recollect to have been more amused with a hackney coach party, than one we saw early the other morning in Tottenham Court Road. It was a wedding party, and emerged from one of the inferior streets near Fitzroy Square. There were the bride, with a thin white dress, and a great red face; and the bridesmaid, a little, dumpy, good-humoured young woman, dressed, of course, in the same appropriate costume; and the bridegroom and his chosen friend, in blue coats, yellow waistcoats, white trousers, and Berlin gloves to match. They stopped at the corner of the street, and called a coach with an air of indescribable dignity. The moment they were in, the bridesmaid threw a red shawl, which she had, no doubt, brought on purpose, negligently over the number on the door, evidently to delude pedestrians into the belief that the hackney coach was a private carriage; and away they went, perfectly satisfied that the imposition was successful, and quite unconscious that there was a great staring number stuck up behind, on a plate as large as a schoolboy's slate. A shilling a mile! – the ride was worth five, at least, to them.

What an interesting book a hackney coach might produce, if it could carry as much in its head as it does in its body! The autobiography of a broken-down hackney coach would surely be as amusing as the autobiography of a broken down hackneyed dramatist; and it might tell as much of its travels *with* the pole, as others have of their expeditions *to* it. How many stories might be related of the different people it had conveyed on matters of business or profit – pleasure or pain! And how many melancholy tales of the same people at different periods! The country girl – the showy, over dressed woman – the drunken prostitute! The raw apprentice – the dissipated spendthrift – the thief!

Talk of cabs! Cabs are all very well in cases of expedition, when it's a matter of neck or nothing, life or death, your temporary home or your long one. But, besides a cab's lacking that gravity of deportment which so peculiarly distinguishes a hackney coach, let it never be forgotten that a cab is a thing of yesterday, and that he never was anything better. A hackney cab has always been a hackney cab, from his first entry into life; whereas a hackney coach is a remnant of past gentility, a victim to fashion, a hanger on of an old English family, wearing their arms, and, in days of yore, escorted by men wearing their livery, stripped of his finery, and thrown upon the world, like a once smart footman when he is no longer sufficiently juvenile for his office, progressing lower and lower in the scale of four-wheeled degradation, until at last it comes to – *a stand!*

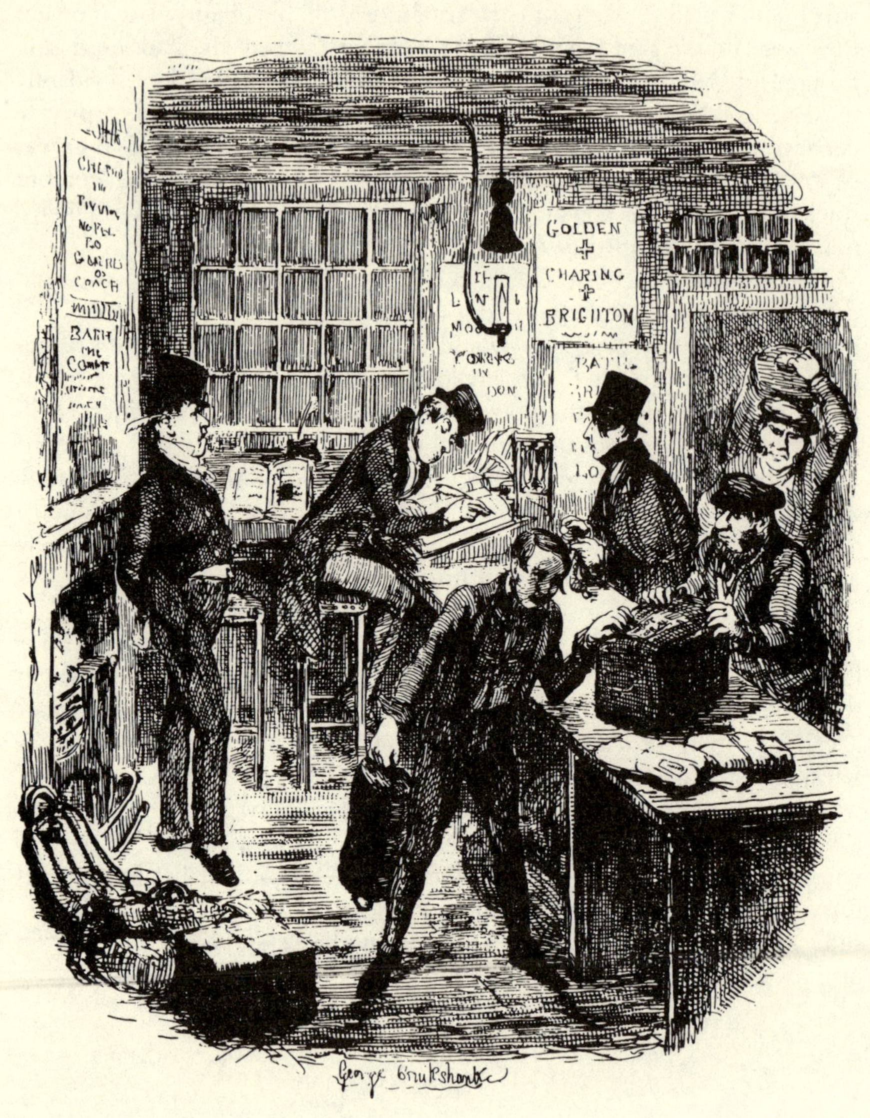


*Early Coaches (see p. 134)*

## Chapter Eight

### *Doctors' Commons*

First published in the *Morning Chronicle*, 11 October 1836 ('Sketches by Boz, New Series No. 3'). Doctors' Commons was a college of lawyers situated close to St Paul's Cathedral where a series of courts was convened in the same hall. One of these was the Court of Arches, the consistory court of the Province of Canterbury in the organisation of the Church of England. It dealt with divorce cases as well as the kind of petty squabbles connected with a church or vestry that Dickens ridicules here. Other courts dealt with probate of wills and with Admiralty cases. Only lawyers holding the degree of Doctor of Law from either Oxford or Cambridge University had the right to appear in these courts; attached to them were proctors who did the work of solicitors. As a young man Dickens worked (1829–31) as a shorthand reporter in Doctors' Commons, an experience which left him with a lasting contempt for its antiquated, self-serving rituals. In *David Copperfield* David is articled to Mr Spenlow, a proctor in Doctors' Commons, and this gives Dickens further scope to satirise the institution as both farcical and corrupt, 'a very pleasant profitable little affair of private theatricals' – see *David Copperfield* chs 23, 33, 39. For the original of the case of Bumple *v.* Sludberry here, a case that Dickens reported, 18 November 1830, see William J. Carlton, *Charles Dickens Shorthand Writer* (1926) pp. 57–67. Doctors' Commons ceased to exist in 1867 when its functions were transferred to the High Court (with the Arches Court becoming the Archbishop of Canterbury's Court of Appeal) and the buildings were demolished soon afterwards.

Walking without any definite object through St Paul's Churchyard, a little while ago, we happened to turn down a street entitled 'Paul's Chain', and keeping straight forward for a few hundred yards, found ourself, as a natural consequence, in Doctors' Commons. Now Doctors' Commons being familiar by name to everybody, as the place where they grant marriage licenses to love-sick couples, and divorces to unfaithful ones; register the wills of people who have any property to leave, and punish hasty gentlemen who call ladies by unpleasant names, we no sooner discovered that we were really within its precincts, than we felt a laudable desire to become better acquainted therewith; and as the first object of our curiosity was the Court, whose decrees can even unloose the bonds of matrimony, we procured a direction to it; and bent our steps thither without delay.

Crossing a quiet and shady courtyard, paved with stone, and frowned upon by old red brick houses, on the doors of which were painted the names of sundry learned civilians, we paused before a small, green-baized, brass-headed-nailed door, which yielding to our gentle push, at once admitted us into an old quaint-looking apartment, with sunken windows, and black carved wainscoting, at the upper end of which, seated on a raised platform, of semicircular shape, were about a dozen solemn-looking gentlemen, in crimson gowns and wigs.

At a more elevated desk in the centre, sat a very fat and red-faced gentleman, in tortoiseshell spectacles, whose dignified appearance announced the judge; and round a long green-baized table below, something like a billiard table without the cushions and pockets, were a number of very self-important-looking personages, in stiff neckcloths, and black gowns with white fur collars, whom we at once set down as proctors. At the lower end of the billiard table was an individual in an armchair, and a wig, whom we afterwards discovered to be the registrar; and seated behind a little desk, near the door, were a respectable-looking man in black, of about twenty-stone weight or thereabouts, and a fat-faced, smirking, civil-looking body, in a black gown, black kid gloves, knee shorts, and silks, with a shirt frill in his bosom, curls on his head, and a silver staff in his hand, whom we had no difficulty in recognising as the officer of the Court. The latter, indeed, speedily set our mind at rest upon this point, for, advancing to our elbow, and opening a conversation forthwith, he had communicated to us, in less than five minutes, that he was the apparitor, and the other the court keeper; that this was the Arches Court, and therefore the counsel wore red gowns, and the proctors fur collars; and that when the other Courts sat there, they didn't wear red gowns or fur collars either; with many other scraps of intelligence equally interesting. Besides these two officers, there was a little thin old man, with long grizzly hair, crouched in a remote corner, whose duty, our communicative friend informed us, was to ring a large hand bell when the Court opened in the morning, and who, for aught his appearance betokened to the contrary, might have been similarly employed for the last two centuries at least.

The red-faced gentleman in the tortoiseshell spectacles had got all the talk to himself just then, and very well he was doing it, too, only he spoke very fast, but that was habit; and rather thick, but that was good living. So we had plenty of time to look about us. There was one individual who amused us mightily. This was one of the bewigged gentlemen in the red robes, who was straddling before the fire in the centre of the Court, in the attitude of the brazen Colossus, to the complete exclusion of everybody else. He had gathered up his robe behind, in much the same manner as a slovenly woman would her petticoats on a very dirty day, in order that he might feel the full warmth of the fire. His wig was put on all awry, with the tail straggling about his neck; his scanty grey trousers and short black gaiters, made in the worst possible style, imparted an additional inelegant appearance to his uncouth person; and his limp, badly-starched shirt collar almost obscured his eyes. We shall never be able to claim any credit as a physiognomist again, for, after a careful scrutiny of this gentleman's countenance, we had come to the conclusion that it bespoke nothing but conceit and silliness, when our friend with the silver staff whispered in our ear that he was no other than a doctor of civil law, and heaven knows what besides. So of course we were mistaken, and he must be a very talented man. He conceals it so well though – perhaps with the merciful view of not astonishing ordinary people too much – that you would suppose him to be one of the stupidest dogs alive.

The gentleman in the spectacles having concluded his judgment, and a few minutes having been allowed to elapse, to afford time for the buzz in the Court to subside, the registrar called on the next cause, which was 'the office of the Judge promoted by Bumple against Sludberry'. A general movement was visible in the Court at this announcement, and the obliging functionary with silver staff whispered us that 'there would be some fun now, for this was a brawling case'.

We were not rendered much the wiser by this piece of information, till we found by the opening speech of the counsel for the promoter, that, under a half obsolete statute of one of the Edwards, the Court was empowered to visit with the penalty of excommunication, any person who should be proved guilty of the crime of 'brawling', or 'smiting', in any church, or vestry adjoining thereto; and it appeared, by some eight-and-twenty affidavits, which were duly referred to, that on a certain night, at a certain vestry meeting, in a certain parish particularly set forth, Thomas Sludberry, the party appeared against in that suit, had made use of, and applied to Michael Bumple, the promoter, the words 'You be blowed'; and that, on the said Michael Bumple and others remonstrating with the said Thomas Sludberry, on the impropriety of his conduct, the said Thomas Sludberry repeated the aforesaid expression, 'You be blowed'; and furthermore desired and requested to know, whether the said Michael Bumple 'wanted anything for himself'; adding 'that if the said Michael Bumple did want anything for himself, he, the said Thomas Sludberry, was the man to give it him'; at the same time making use of other heinous and sinful expressions, all of which, Bumple submitted, came within the intent and meaning of the Act; and therefore he, for the soul's health and chastening of Sludberry, prayed for sentence of excommunication against him accordingly.

Upon these facts a long argument was entered into, on both sides, to the great edification of a number of persons interested in the parochial squabbles, who crowded the Court; and when some very long and grave speeches had been made *pro* and *con*, the red-faced gentleman in the tortoiseshell spectacles took a review of the case, which occupied half an hour more, and then pronounced upon Sludberry the awful sentence of excommunication for a fortnight, and payment of the costs of the suit. Upon this, Sludberry, who was a little, red-faced, sly-looking, ginger beer seller, addressed the Court, and said, if they'd be good enough to take off the costs, and excommunicate him for the term of his natural life instead, it would be much more convenient to him, for he never went to church at all. To this appeal the gentleman in the spectacles made no other reply than a look of virtuous indignation; and Sludberry and his friends retired. As the man with the silver staff informed us that the Court was on the point of rising, we retired too – pondering, as we walked away, upon the beautiful spirit of these ancient ecclesiastical laws, the kind and neighbourly feelings they are calculated to awaken, and the strong attachment to religious institutions which they cannot fail to engender.

We were so lost in these meditations, that we had turned into the street, and run up against a door post, before we recollected where we were walking. On looking upwards to see what house we had stumbled upon, the words 'Prerogative Office', written in large characters, met our eye; and as we were in a sightseeing humour and the place was a public one, we walked in.

The room into which we walked was a long, busy-looking place, partitioned off, on either side, into a variety of little boxes, in which a few clerks were engaged in copying or examining deeds. Down the centre of the room were several desks, nearly breast high, at each of which, three or four people were standing, poring over large volumes. As we knew that they were searching for wills, they attracted our attention at once.

It was curious to contrast the lazy indifference of the attorneys' clerks who were making a search for some legal purpose, with the air of earnestness and interest which distinguished the strangers to the place, who were looking up the will of some deceased relative; the former pausing every now and then with an impatient yawn, or raising their heads to look at the people who passed up and down the room; the latter stooping over the book, and running down column after column of names in the deepest abstraction.

There was one little dirty-faced man in a blue apron, who after a whole morning's search, extending some fifty years back, had just found the will to which he wished to refer, which one of the officials was reading to him in a low hurried voice from a thick vellum book with large clasps. It was perfectly evident that the more the clerk read, the less the man with the blue apron understood about the matter. When the volume was first brought down, he took off his hat, smoothed down his hair, smiled with great self-satisfaction, and looked up in the reader's face with the air of a man who had made up his mind to recollect every word he heard. The first two or three lines were intelligible enough; but then the technicalities began, and the little man began to look rather dubious. Then came a whole string of complicated trusts, and he was regularly at sea. As the reader proceeded, it was quite apparent that it was a hopeless case, and the little man, with his mouth open and his eyes fixed upon his face, looked on with an expression of bewilderment and perplexity irresistibly ludicrous.

A little further on, a hard-featured old man with a deeply wrinkled face, was intently perusing a lengthy will with the aid of a pair of horn spectacles: occasionally pausing from his task, and slily noting down some brief memorandum of the bequests contained in it. Every wrinkle about his toothless mouth, and sharp keen eyes, told of avarice and cunning. His clothes were nearly threadbare, but it was easy to see that he wore them from choice and not from necessity; all his looks and gestures down to the very small pinches of snuff which he every now and then took from a little tin canister, told of wealth, and penury, and avarice.

As he leisurely closed the register, put up his spectacles, and folded his scraps of paper in a large leathern pocket book, we thought what a nice hard bargain he was driving with some poverty-stricken legatee, who, tired of waiting year after year, until some life-interest should fall in, was selling his chance, just as it began to grow most valuable, for a twelfth part of its worth. It was a good speculation – a very safe one. The old man stowed his pocket book carefully in the breast of his greatcoat, and hobbled away with a leer of triumph. That will had made him ten years younger at the lowest computation.

Having commenced our observations, we should certainly have extended them to another dozen of people at least, had not a sudden shutting up and putting away of the worm-eaten old books, warned us that the time for closing the office had arrived; and thus deprived us of a pleasure, and spared our readers an infliction.

We naturally fell into a train of reflection as we walked homewards, upon the curious old records of likings and dislikings; of jealousies and revenges; of affection defying the power of death, and hatred pursued beyond the grave, which these depositories contain; silent but striking tokens, some of them, of excellence of heart, and nobleness of soul; melancholy examples, others, of the worst passions of human nature. How many men as they lay speechless and helpless on the bed of death, would have given worlds but for the strength and power to blot out the silent evidence of animosity and bitterness, which now stands registered against them in Doctors' Commons!

## Chapter Nine

### *London Recreations*

First published in the *Evening Chronicle*, 17 March 1835 ('Sketches of London No. 6') with a concluding paragraph that was omitted when the sketch was collected for publication in *Sketches: First Series* and never restored. See DeVries, p. 78.

The wish of persons in the humbler classes of life, to ape the manners and customs of those whom fortune has placed above them, is often the subject of remark, and not unfrequently of complaint. The inclination may, and no doubt does, exist to a great extent, among the small gentility – the would-be aristocrats – of the middle classes. Tradesmen and clerks, with fashionable novel-reading families, and circulating-library-subscribing daughters, get up small assemblies in humble imitation of Almack's, and promenade the dingy 'large room' of some second-rate hotel with as much complacency as the enviable few who are privileged to exhibit their magnificence in that exclusive haunt of fashion and foolery. Aspiring young ladies, who read flaming accounts of some 'fancy fair in high life', suddenly grow desperately charitable; visions of admiration and matrimony float before their eyes; some wonderfully meritorious institution, which, by the strangest accident in the world, has never been heard of before, is discovered to be in a languishing condition: Thomson's great room, or Johnson's nursery ground, is forthwith engaged, and the aforesaid young ladies, from mere charity, exhibit themselves for three days, from twelve to four, for the small charge of one shilling per head! With the exception of these classes of society, however, and a few weak and insignificant persons, we do not think the attempt at imitation to which we have alluded, prevails in any great degree. The different character of the recreations of different classes, has often afforded us amusement; and we have chosen it for the subject of our present sketch, in the hope that it may possess some amusement for our readers.

If the regular City man, who leaves Lloyd's at five o'clock and drives home to Hackney, Clapton, Stamford Hill, or elsewhere, can be said to have any daily recreation beyond his dinner, it is his garden. He never does anything to it with his own hands; but he takes great pride in it

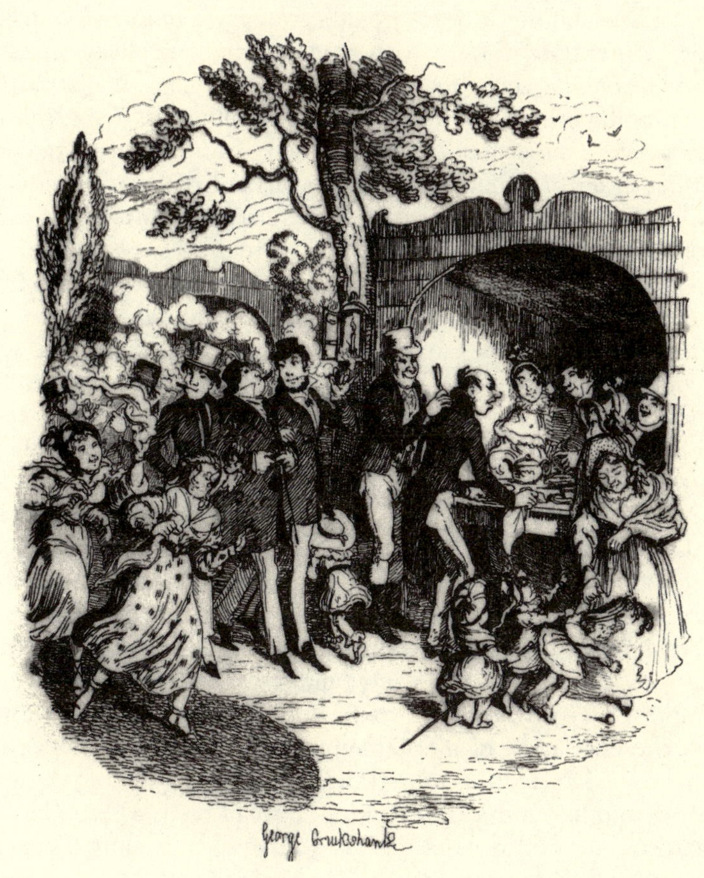


*London Recreations*

notwithstanding; and if you are desirous of paying your addresses to the youngest daughter, be sure to be in raptures with every flower and shrub it contains. If your poverty of expression compel you to make any distinction between the two, we would certainly recommend your bestowing more admiration on his garden than his wine. He always takes a walk round it, before he starts for town in the morning, and is particularly anxious that the fishpond should be kept specially neat. If you call on him on Sunday in summertime, about an hour before dinner, you will find him sitting in an armchair, on the lawn behind the house, with a straw hat on, reading a Sunday paper. A short distance from him you will most likely observe a handsome paroquet in a large brass-wire cage; ten to one but the two eldest girls are loitering in one of the side walks accompanied by a couple of young gentlemen, who are holding parasols over them – of course only to keep the sun off – while the younger children, with the under nursery-maid, are strolling listlessly about in the shade. Beyond these occasions, his delight in his garden appears to arise more from the consciousness of possession than actual enjoyment of it. When he drives you down to dinner on a weekday, he is rather fatigued with the occupations of the morning, and tolerably cross into the bargain; but when the cloth is removed, and he has drunk three or four glasses of his favourite port, he orders the French windows of his dining room (which of course look into the garden) to be opened, and throwing a silk handkerchief over his head, and leaning back in his armchair, descants at considerable length upon its beauty, and the cost of maintaining it. This is to impress you – who are a young friend of the family – with a due sense of the excellence of the garden, and the wealth of its owner; and when he has exhausted the subject, he goes to sleep.

There is another and a very different class of men, whose recreation is their garden. An individual of this class resides some short distance from town – say in the Hampstead Road, or the Kilburn Road, or any other road where the houses are small and neat, and have little slips of back garden. He and his wife – who is as clean and compact a little body as himself – have occupied the same house ever since he retired from business twenty years ago. They have no family. They once had a son, who died at about five years old. The child's portrait hangs over the mantelpiece in the best sitting room, and a little cart he used to draw about is carefully preserved as a relic.

In fine weather the old gentleman is almost constantly in the garden; and when it is too wet to go into it, he will look out of the window at it, by the hour together. He has always something to do there, and you will see him digging and sweeping, and cutting, and planting, with manifest delight. In springtime, there is no end to the sowing of seeds, and sticking little bits of wood over them, with labels, which look like epitaphs to their memory; and in the evening, when the sun has gone down, the perseverance with which he lugs a great watering pot about is perfectly astonishing. The only other recreation he has is the newspaper, which he peruses every day, from beginning to end, generally reading the most interesting pieces of intelligence to his wife during breakfast. The old lady is very fond of flowers, as the hyacinth glasses in the parlour window, and geranium pots in the little front court, testify. She takes great pride in the garden too: and when one of the four fruit trees produces rather a larger gooseberry than usual, it is carefully preserved under a wine glass on the sideboard, for the edification of visitors, who are duly informed that Mr So-and-so planted the tree which produced it, with his own hands. On a summer's evening, when the large watering pot has been filled and emptied some fourteen times, and the old couple have quite exhausted themselves by trotting about, you will see them sitting happily together in the little summer house, enjoying the calm and peace of the twilight, and watching the shadows as they fall upon the garden, and gradually growing thicker and more sombre, obscure the tints of their gayest flowers – no bad emblem of the years that have silently rolled over their heads, deadening in their course the brightest hues of early hopes and feelings which have long since faded away. These are their only recreations, and they require no more. They have within themselves the materials of comfort and content; and the only anxiety of each, is to die before the other.

This is no ideal sketch. There *used* to be many old people of this description; their numbers may have diminished, and may decrease still more. Whether the course female education has taken of late days – whether the pursuit of giddy frivolities, and empty nothings, has tended to unfit women for that quiet domestic life, in which they show far more beautifully than in the most crowded assembly, is a question we should feel little gratification in discussing: we hope not.

Let us turn now to another portion of the London population, whose recreations present about as strong a contrast as can well be conceived – we mean the Sunday pleasurers; and let us beg our readers to imagine themselves stationed by our side in some well known rural 'Tea gardens'.

The heat is intense this afternoon, and the people, of whom there are additional parties arriving every moment, look as warm as the tables which have been recently painted, and have the appearance of being red hot. What a dust and noise! Men and women – boys and girls – sweethearts and married people – babies in arms, and children in chaises – pipes and shrimps – cigars and periwinkles – tea and tobacco. Gentlemen in alarming waistcoats, and steel watchguards, promenading about, three abreast, with surprising dignity (or as the gentleman in the next box facetiously observes, 'cutting it uncommon fat!') – ladies, with great, long, white pocket handkerchiefs like small table cloths in their hands, chasing one another on the grass in the most playful and interesting manner, with the view of attracting the attention of the aforesaid gentlemen – husbands in perspective ordering bottles of ginger beer for the objects of their affections, with a lavish disregard of expense; and the said objects washing down huge quantities of 'shrimps' and 'winkles', with an equal disregard of their own bodily health and subsequent comfort – boys, with great silk hats just balanced on the top of their heads, smoking cigars, and trying to look as if they liked them – gentlemen in pink shirts and blue waistcoats, occasionally upsetting either themselves, or somebody else, with their own canes.

Some of the finery of these people provokes a smile, but they are all clean, and happy, and disposed to be good natured and sociable. Those two motherly-looking women in the smart pelisses, who are chatting so confidentially, inserting a 'ma'am', at every fourth word, scraped an acquaintance about a quarter of an hour ago: it originated in admiration of the little boy who belongs to one of them – that diminutive specimen of mortality in the three-cornered pink satin hat with black feathers. The two men in the blue coats and drab trousers, who are walking up and down, smoking their pipes, are their husbands. The party in the opposite box are a pretty fair specimen of the generality of the visitors. These are the father and mother, and old grandmother: a young man and woman, and an individual addressed by the euphonious title of 'Uncle Bill', who is evidently the wit of the party. They have some half-dozen children with them, but it is scarcely necessary to notice the fact, for that is a matter of course here. Every woman in 'the gardens', who has been married for any length of time, must have had twins on two or three occasions; it is impossible to account for the extent of juvenile population in any other way.

Observe the inexpressible delight of the old grandmother, at Uncle Bill's splendid joke of 'tea for four: bread and butter for forty'; and the loud explosion of mirth which follows his wafering a paper 'pigtail' on the waiter's collar. The young man is evidently 'keeping company' with Uncle Bill's niece: and Uncle Bill's hints – such as 'Don't forget me at the dinner, you know', 'I shall look out for the cake, Sally', 'I'll be godfather to your first – wager it's a boy', and so forth, are equally embarrassing to the young people, and delightful to the elder ones. As to the old grandmother, she is in perfect ecstasies, and does nothing but laugh herself into fits of coughing, until they have finished the 'gin and water warm with', of which Uncle Bill ordered 'glasses round' after tea, 'just to keep the night air out, and do it up comfortable and riglar arter sitch an astonishing hot day!'

It is getting dark, and the people begin to move. The field leading to town is quite full of them; the little hand-chaises are dragged wearily along, the children are tired, and amuse themselves and the company generally by crying, or resort to the much more pleasant expedient of going to sleep – the mothers begin to wish they were at home again – sweethearts grow more sentimental than ever, as the time for parting arrives – the gardens look mournful enough, by the light of the two lanterns which hang against the trees for the convenience of smokers – and the waiters who have been running about incessantly for the last six hours, think they feel a little tired, as they count their glasses and their gains.

## Chapter Ten

### *The River*

First published in the *Evening Chronicle*, 6 June 1835 ('Sketches of London No. 13').

'Are you fond of the water?' is a question very frequently asked, in hot summer weather, by amphibious-looking young men. 'Very', is the general reply. 'An't you?' – 'Hardly ever off it', is the response, accompanied by sundry adjectives, expressive of the speaker's heartfelt admiration of that element. Now, with all respect for the opinion of society in general, and cutter clubs in particular, we humbly suggest that some of the most painful reminiscences in the mind of every individual who has occasionally disported himself on the Thames, must be connected with his aquatic recreations. Who ever heard of a successful water party? – or to put the question in a still more intelligible form, who ever saw one? We have been on water excursions out of number, but we solemnly declare that we cannot call to mind one single occasion of the kind, which was not marked by more miseries than any one would suppose could be reasonably crowded into the space of some eight or nine hours. Something has always gone wrong. Either the cork of the salad dressing has come out, or the most anxiously expected member of the party has not come out, or the most disagreeable man in company would come out, or a child or two have fallen into the water, or the gentleman who undertook to steer has endangered everybody's life all the way, or the gentlemen who volunteered to row have been 'out of practice', and performed very alarming evolutions, putting their oars down into the water and not being able to get them up again, or taking terrific pulls without putting them in at all; in either case, pitching over on the backs of their heads with startling violence, and exhibiting the soles of their pumps to the 'sitters' in the boat, in a very humiliating manner.

We grant that the banks of the Thames are very beautiful at Richmond and Twickenham, and other distant havens, often sought though seldom reached; but from the 'Red-us' back to Blackfriars Bridge, the scene is wonderfully changed. The Penitentiary is a noble building, no doubt, and the sportive youths who 'go in' at that particular part of the river, on a summer's evening, may be all very well in perspective; but young ladies will colour up, and look perseveringly the other way, while the married dittoes cough slightly, and stare very hard at the water, you feel awkward – especially if you happen to have been attempting the most distant approach to sentimentality, for an hour or two previously.

Although experience and suffering have produced in our minds the result we have just stated, we are by no means blind to a proper sense of the fun which a looker on may extract from the amateurs of boating. What can be more amusing than Searle's yard on a fine Sunday morning? It's a Richmond tide, and some dozen boats are preparing for the reception of the parties who have engaged them. Two or three fellows in great trousers and Guernsey shirts, are getting them ready by easy stages; now coming down the yard with a pair of sculls and a cushion – then having a chat with the 'jack', who, like all his tribe, seems to be wholly incapable of doing anything but lounging about – then going back again, and returning with a rudder line and a stretcher – then solacing themselves with another chat – and then wondering, with their hands in their capacious pockets, 'where them gentlemen's got to as ordered the six'. One of these, the head man, with the legs of his trousers carefully tucked up at the bottom, to admit the water, we presume – for it is an element in which he is infinitely more at home than on land – is quite a character, and shares with the defunct oyster-swallower the celebrated name of 'Dando'. Watch him, as taking a few minutes' respite from his toils, he negligently seats himself on the edge of a boat, and fans his broad bushy chest with a cap scarcely half so furry. Look at his magnificent, though reddish whiskers, and mark the somewhat native humour with which he 'chaffs' the boys and 'prentices, or cunningly gammons the gen'lm'n into the gift of a glass of gin, of which we verily believe he swallows in one day as much as any six ordinary men, without ever being one atom the worse for it.

But the party arrives, and Dando, relieved from his state of uncertainty, starts up into activity. They approach in full aquatic costume, with round blue jackets, striped shirts, and caps of all sizes and patterns, from the velvet skull cap of French manufacture, to the easy head dress familiar to the students of the old spelling books, as having, on the authority of the portrait, formed part of the costume of the Reverend Mr Dilworth.

This is the most amusing time to observe a regular Sunday water party. There has evidently been up to this period no inconsiderable degree of boasting on everybody's part relative to his knowledge of navigation; the sight of the water rapidly cools their courage, and the air of self-denial with which each of them insists on somebody else's taking an oar, is perfectly delightful. At length, after a great deal of changing and fidgeting, consequent upon the election of a stroke oar: the inability of one gentleman to pull on this side, of another to pull on that, and of a third to pull at all, the boat's crew are seated. 'Shove her off!' cries the coxswain, who looks as easy and comfortable as if he were steering in the Bay of Biscay. The order is obeyed; the boat is immediately turned completely round, and proceeds towards Westminster Bridge, amidst such a splashing and struggling as never was seen before, except when the Royal George went down. 'Back wa'ater, sir,' shouts Dando, 'Back wa'ater, you sir, aft'; upon which everybody thinking he must be the individual referred to, they all back water, and back comes the boat, stern first, to the spot whence it started. 'Back water, you sir, aft; pull round, you sir, for'ad, can't you?' shouts Dando, in a frenzy of excitement. 'Pull round, Tom, can't you?' re-echoes one of the party. 'Tom an't for'ad,' replies another. 'Yes, he is,' cries a third; and the unfortunate young man, at the imminent risk of breaking a blood vessel, pulls and pulls, until the head of the boat fairly lies in the direction of Vauxhall Bridge. 'That's right – now pull all on you!' shouts Dando again, adding, in an undertone, to somebody by him, 'Blowed if hever I see sich a set of muffs!' and away jogs the boat in a zigzag direction, every one of the six oars dipping into the water at a different time; and the yard is once more clear, until the arrival of the next party.

A well-contested rowing match on the Thames is a very lively and interesting scene. The water is studded with boats of all sorts, kinds, and descriptions; places in the coal barges at the different wharfs are let to crowds of spectators, beer and tobacco flow freely about; men, women, and children wait for the start in breathless expectation; cutters of six and eight oars glide gently up and down, waiting to accompany their *protégés* during the race; bands of music add to the animation, if not to the harmony of the scene; groups of watermen are assembled at the different stairs, discussing the merits of the respective candidates; and the prize wherry, which is rowed slowly about by a pair of sculls, is an object of general interest.

Two o'clock strikes, and everybody looks anxiously in the direction of the bridge through which the candidates for the prize will come – half-past two, and the general attention which has been preserved so long begins to flag, when suddenly a gun is heard, and a noise of distant hurra'ing along each bank of the river – every head is bent forward – the noise draws nearer and nearer – the boats which have been waiting at the bridge start briskly up the river, and a well-manned galley shoots through the arch, the sitters cheering on the boats behind them, which are not yet visible.

'Here they are,' is the general cry – and through darts the first boat, the men in her, stripped to the skin, and exerting every muscle to preserve the advantage they have gained – four other boats follow close astern;

there are not two boats' length between them – the shouting is tremendous, and the interest intense. 'Go on, Pink' – 'Give it her, Red' – 'Sulliwin for ever'– 'Bravo! George' – 'Now, Tom, now – now – now – why don't your partner stretch out?' – 'Two pots to a pint on Yellow,' &c., &c. Every little public house fires its gun, and hoists its flag; and the men who win the heat, come in, amidst a splashing and shouting, and banging and confusion, which no one can imagine who has not witnessed it, and of which any description would convey a very faint idea.

One of the most amusing places we know, is the steam wharf of the London Bridge, or St Katharine's Dock Company, on a Saturday morning in summer, when the Gravesend and Margate steamers are usually crowded to excess; and as we have just taken a glance at the river above bridge, we hope our readers will not object to accompany us on board a Gravesend packet.

Coaches are every moment setting down at the entrance to the wharf, and the stare of bewildered astonishment with which the 'fares' resign themselves and their luggage into the hands of the porters, who seize all the packages at once as a matter of course, and run away with them, heaven knows where, is laughable in the extreme. A Margate boat lies alongside the wharf, the Gravesend boat (which starts first) lies alongside that again; and as a temporary communication is formed between the two, by means of a plank and handrail, the natural confusion of the scene is by no means diminished.

'Gravesend?' inquires a stout father of a stout family, who follow him, under the guidance of their mother, and a servant, at the no small risk of two or three of them being left behind in the confusion. 'Gravesend?'

'Pass on, if you please, sir,' replies the attendant – 'other boat, sir.'

Hereupon the stout father, being rather mystified, and the stout mother rather distracted by maternal anxiety, the whole party deposit themselves in the Margate boat, and after having congratulated himself on having secured very comfortable seats, the stout father sallies to the chimney to look for his luggage, which he has a faint recollection of having given some man, something, to take somewhere. No luggage, however, bearing the most remote resemblance to his own, in shape or form, is to be discovered; on which the stout father calls very loudly for an officer, to whom he states the case, in the presence of another father of another family – a little thin man – who entirely concurs with him (the stout father) in thinking that it's high time something was done with these steam companies, and that as the Corporation Bill failed to do it, something else must; for really people's property is not to be sacrificed in this way; and that if the luggage isn't restored without delay, he will take care it shall be put in the papers, for the public is not to be the victim of these great monopolies. To this, the officer, in his turn, replies, that that company, ever since it has been St Kat'rine's Dock Company, has protected life and property; that if it had been the London Bridge Wharf Company, indeed, he shouldn't have wondered, seeing that the morality of that company (they being the opposition) can't be answered for, by no one; but as it is, he's convinced there must be some mistake, and he wouldn't mind making a solemn oath afore a magistrate that the gentleman'll find his luggage afore he gets to Margate.

Here the stout father, thinking he is making a capital point, replies, that as it happens, he is not going to Margate at all, and that 'Passenger to Gravesend' was on the luggage, in letters of full two inches long; on which the officer rapidly explains the mistake, and the stout mother, and the stout children, and the servant, are hurried with all possible despatch on board the Gravesend boat, which they reach just in time to discover that their luggage is there, and that their comfortable seats are not. Then the bell, which is the signal for the Gravesend boat starting, begins to ring most furiously: and people keep time to the bell, by running in and out of our boat at a double-quick pace. The bell stops; the boat starts: people who have been taking leave of their friends on board, are carried away against their will; and people who have been taking leave of their friends on shore, find that they have performed a very needless ceremony, in consequence of their not being carried away at all. The regular passengers, who have season tickets, go below to breakfast; people who have purchased morning papers, compose themselves to read them; and people who have not been down the river before, think that both the shipping and the water look a great deal better at a distance.

When we get down about as far as Blackwall, and begin to move at a quicker rate, the spirits of the passengers appear to rise in proportion. Old women who have brought large wicker hand baskets with them, set seriously to work at the demolition of heavy sandwiches, and pass round a wine glass, which is frequently replenished from a flat bottle like a stomach warmer, with considerable glee: handing it first to the gentleman in the foraging cap, who plays the harp – partly as an expression of satisfaction with his previous exertions, and partly to induce him to play 'Dumbledumb-deary', for 'Alick' to dance to; which being done, Alick, who is a damp earthy child in red worsted socks, takes certain small jumps upon the deck, to the unspeakable satisfaction of his family circle. Girls who have brought the first volume of some new novel in their reticule, become extremely plaintive, and expatiate to Mr Brown, or young Mr O'Brien, who has been looking over them, on the blueness of the sky, and brightness of the water; on which Mr Brown or Mr O'Brien, as the case may be, remarks in a low voice that he has been quite insensible of late to the beauties of nature – that his whole thoughts and wishes have centred in one object alone – whereupon the young lady looks up, and failing in her attempt to appear unconscious, looks down again; and turns over the next leaf with great difficulty, in order to afford opportunity for a lengthened pressure of the hand.

Telescopes, sandwiches, and glasses of brandy and water cold without, begin to be in great requisition; and bashful men who have been looking down the hatchway at the engine, find, to their great relief, a subject on which they can converse with one another – and a copious one too – Steam.

'Wonderful thing steam, sir.' 'Ah! (a deep drawn sigh) it is indeed, sir.' 'Great power, sir.' 'Immense – immense!' 'Great deal done by steam, sir.' 'Ah! (another sigh at the immensity of the subject and a knowing shake of the head) you may say that, sir.' 'Still in its infancy, they say, sir.' Novel remarks of this kind, are generally the commencement of a conversation which is prolonged until the conclusion of the trip, and, perhaps, lays the foundation of a speaking acquaintance between half a dozen gentlemen, who, having their families at Gravesend, take season tickets for the boat, and dine on board regularly every afternoon.

## Chapter Eleven

### *Astley's*

First published in the *Evening Chronicle*, 9 May 1835 ('Sketches of London, No. 11'). Philip Astley, a former cavalry sergeant-major, opened a riding school and exhibition of horsemanship in Lambeth, near Westminster Bridge, in 1770. It subsequently became a circus, and then a combination of theatre and circus with a stage and 'the circle' in front of it, called Astley's (later Royal Astley's) Amphitheatre. It was finally demolished in 1893. Dickens makes several references to it and its delights in his later work and it is visited by characters in two of his novels, the Nubbles family in *The Old Curiosity Shop* ch. 39, and Mr George in *Bleak House* ch. 21. The delighted observation towards the end of this sketch of contemporary 'Minor Theatre' acting conventions and the absurdities of melodrama plots looks forward to the glorious Crummles episodes in *Nicholas Nickleby.*

We never see any very large, staring, black Roman capitals, in a book, or shop window, or placarded on a wall, without their immediately recalling to our mind an indistinct and confused recollection of the time when we were first initiated in the mysteries of the alphabet. We almost fancy we see the pin's point following the letter, to impress its form more strongly on our bewildered imagination; and wince involuntarily, as we remember the hard knuckles with which the reverend old lady who instilled into our mind the first principles of education for ninepence per week, or ten and sixpence per quarter, was wont to poke our juvenile head occasionally, by way of adjusting the confusion of ideas in which we were generally involved. The same kind of feeling pursues us in many other instances, but there is no place which recalls so strongly our recollections of childhood as Astley's. It was not a 'Royal Amphitheatre' in those days, nor had Ducrow arisen to shed the light of classic taste and portable gas over the sawdust of the circus; but the whole character of the place was the same, the pieces were the same, the clown's jokes were the same, the riding masters were equally grand, the comic performers equally witty, the tragedians equally hoarse, and the 'highly trained chargers' equally spirited. Astley's has altered for the better – we have changed for the worse. Our histrionic taste is gone, and with shame we must confess, that we are far more delighted and amused with the audience, than with the pageantry we once so highly appreciated.

We like to watch a regular Astley's party in the Easter or Midsummer holidays – pa and ma, and nine or ten children, varying from five foot six to two foot eleven: from fourteen years of age to four. We had just taken our seat in one of the boxes, in the centre of the house, the other night, when the next was occupied by just such a party as we should have attempted to describe, had we depicted our *beau idéal* of a group of Astley's visitors.

First of all, there came three little boys and a little girl, who, in pursuance of pa's directions, issued in a very audible voice from the box door, occupied the front row; then two more little girls were ushered in by a young lady, evidently the governess. Then came three more little boys, dressed like the first, in blue jackets and trousers, with lay down shirt collars: then a child in a braided frock, and high state of astonishment, with very large round eyes, opened to their utmost width, was lifted over the seats – a process which occasioned a considerable display of little pink legs – then came ma and pa, and then the eldest son, a boy of fourteen years old, who was evidently trying to look as if he did not belong to the family.

The first five minutes were occupied in taking the shawls off the little girls, and adjusting the bows which ornamented their hair; then it was providentially discovered that one of the little boys was seated behind a pillar and could not see, so the governess was stuck behind the pillar, and the boy lifted into her place. Then pa drilled the boys, and directed the stowing away of their pocket handkerchiefs, and ma having first nodded and winked to the governess to pull the girls' frocks a little more off their shoulders, stood up to review the little troop – an inspection which appeared to terminate much to her own satisfaction, for she looked with a complacent air at pa, who was standing up at the further end of his seat. Pa returned the glance, and blew his nose very emphatically; and the poor governess peeped out from behind the pillar, and timidly tried to catch ma's eye, with a look expressive of her high admiration of the whole family. Then two of the little boys who had been discussing the point whether Astley's was more than twice as large as Drury Lane, agreed to refer it to 'George' for his decision; at which 'George', who was no other than the young gentleman before noticed, waxed indignant, and remonstrated in no very gentle terms on the gross impropriety of having his name repeated in so loud a voice at a public place, on which all the children laughed very heartily, and one of the little boys wound up by expressing his opinion, that 'George began to think himself quite a man now', whereupon both pa and ma laughed too; and George (who carried a dress cane and was cultivating whiskers) muttered that 'William always was encouraged in his impertinence'; and assumed a look of profound contempt, which lasted the whole evening.

The play began, and the interest of the little boys knew no bounds. Pa was clearly interested too, although he very unsuccessfully endeavoured to look as if he wasn't. As for ma, she was perfectly overcome by the drollery of the principal comedian, and laughed till every one of the immense bows on her ample cap trembled, at which the governess peeped out from behind the pillar again, and whenever she could catch ma's eye, put her handkerchief to her mouth, and appeared, as in duty bound, to be in convulsions of laughter also. Then when the man in the splendid armour vowed to rescue the lady or perish in the attempt, the little boys applauded vehemently, especially one little fellow who was apparently on a visit to the family, and had been carrying on a child's flirtation, the whole evening, with a small coquette of twelve years old, who looked like a model of her mamma on a reduced scale; and who, in common with the other little girls (who, generally speaking, have even more coquettishness about them than much older ones), looked very properly shocked, when the knight's squire kissed the princess's confidential chambermaid.

When the scenes in the circle commenced, the children were more delighted than ever; and the wish to see what was going forward, completely conquering pa's dignity, he stood up in the box, and applauded as loudly as any of them. Between each feat of horsemanship, the governess leant across to ma, and retailed the clever remarks of the children on that which had preceded: and ma, in the openness of her heart, offered the governess an acidulated drop, and the governess, gratified to be taken notice of, retired behind her pillar again with a brighter countenance: and the whole party seemed quite happy except the exquisite in the back of the box, who, being too grand to take any interest in the children, and too insignificant to be taken notice of by anybody else, occupied himself, from time to time, in rubbing the place where the whiskers ought to be, and was completely alone in his glory.

We defy anyone who has been to Astley's two or three times, and is consequently capable of appreciating the perseverance with which precisely the same jokes are repeated night after night, and season after season, not to be amused with one part of the performance at least – we mean the scenes in the circle. For ourself, we know that when the hoop, composed of jets of gas, is let down, the curtain drawn up for the convenience of the half-price on their ejectment from the ring, the orange peel cleared away, and the sawdust shaken, with mathematical precision, into a complete circle, we feel as much enlivened as the youngest child present; and actually join in the laugh which follows the clown's shrill shout of 'Here we are!' just for old acquaintance' sake. Nor can we quite divest ourself of our old feeling of reverence for the riding-master, who follows the clown with a long whip in his hand, and bows to the audience with graceful dignity. He is none of your second-rate riding-masters in nankeen dressing-gowns, with brown frogs, but the regular gentleman attendant on the principal riders, who always wear a military uniform with a tablecloth inside the breast of the coat, in which costume he forcibly reminds one of a fowl trussed for roasting. He is – but why should we attempt to describe that of which no description can convey an adequate idea? Everybody knows the man, and everybody remembers his polished boots, his graceful demeanour, stiff, as some misjudging persons have in their jealousy considered it, and the splendid head of black hair, parted high on the forehead, to impart to the countenance an appearance of deep thought and poetic melancholy. His soft and pleasing voice, too, is in perfect unison with his noble bearing, as he humours the clown by indulging in a little badinage; and the striking recollection of his own dignity, with which he exclaims, 'Now sir, if you please, inquire for Miss Woolford, sir', can never be forgotten. The graceful air, too, with which he introduces Miss Woolford into the arena, and, after assisting her to the saddle, follows her fairy courser round the circle, can never fail to create a deep impression in the bosom of every female servant present.

When Miss Woolford, and the horse, and the orchestra, all stop together to take breath, he urbanely takes part in some such dialogue as the following (commenced by the clown): ' I say, sir!' – 'Well, sir?' (it's always conducted in the politest manner). – 'Did you ever happen to hear I was in the army, sir?' – 'No, sir.' – 'Oh, yes, sir – I can go through my exercise, sir.' – 'Indeed, sir!' – 'Shall I do it now, sir?' – 'If you please, sir; come, sir – make haste' (a cut with the long whip, and 'Ha' done now – I don't like it,' from the clown). Here the clown throws himself to the ground, and goes through a variety of gymnastic convulsions, doubling himself up, and untying himself again, and making himself look very like a man in the most hopeless extreme of human agony, to the vociferous delight of the gallery, until he is interrupted by a second cut from the long whip, and a request to see 'what Miss Woolford's stopping for?' On which, to the inexpressible mirth of the gallery, he exclaims, 'Now, Miss Woolford, what can I come for to go, for to fetch, for to bring, for to carry, for to do for you, ma'am?' On the lady's announcing with a sweet smile that she wants the two flags, they are, with sundry grimaces, procured and handed up; the clown facetiously observing after the performance of the latter ceremony – 'He he, oh! I say, sir, Miss Woolford knows me; she smiled at me.' Another cut from the whip, a burst from the orchestra, a start from the horse, and round goes Miss Woolford again on her graceful performance, to the delight of every member of the audience, young or old. The next pause affords an opportunity for similar witticisms, the only additional fun being that of the clown making ludicrous grimaces at the riding-master every time his back is turned; and finally quitting the circle by jumping over his head, having previously directed his attention another way.

Did any of our readers ever notice the class of people, who hang about the stage doors of our minor theatres in the daytime? You will rarely pass one of these entrances without seeing a group of three or four men conversing on the pavement, with an indescribable public-house-parlour swagger, and a kind of conscious air, peculiar to people of this description. They always seem to think they are exhibiting; the lamps are ever before them. That young fellow in the faded brown coat, and very full light green trousers, pulls down the wristbands of his check shirt, as ostentatiously as if it were of the finest linen, and cocks the white hat of the summer-before-last as knowingly over his right eye, as if it were a purchase of yesterday. Look at the dirty white Berlin gloves, and the cheap silk handkerchief stuck in the bosom of his threadbare coat. Is it possible to see him for an instant, and not come to the conclusion that he is the walking gentleman who wears a blue surtout, clean collar, and white trousers, for half an hour, and then shrinks into his worn-out scanty clothes: who has to boast night after night of his splendid fortune, with the painful consciousness of a pound a week and his boots to find; to talk of his father's mansion in the country, with a dreary recollection of his own two-pair back, in the New Cut; and to be envied and flattered as the favoured lover of a rich heiress, remembering all the while that the ex-dancer at home is in the family way and out of an engagement?

Next to him, perhaps, you will see a thin pale man, with a very long face, in a suit of shining black, thoughtfully knocking that part of his boot which once had a heel, with an ash stick. He is the man who does the heavy business, such as prosy fathers, virtuous servants, curates, landlords, and so forth.

By the way, talking of fathers, we should very much like to see some piece in which all the dramatis personæ were orphans. Fathers are invariably great nuisances on the stage, and always have to give the hero or heroine a long explanation of what was done before the curtain rose, usually commencing with 'It is now nineteen years, my dear child, since your blessed mother (here the old villain's voice falters) confided you to my charge. You were then an infant,' &c., &c. Or else they have to discover, all of a sudden, that somebody whom they have been in constant communication with, during three long acts, without the slightest suspicion, is their own child: in which case they exclaim, 'Ah! what do I see? This bracelet! That smile! These documents! Those eyes! Can I believe my senses? – It must be! – Yes – it is, it is my child! – 'My father!' exclaims the child; and they fall into each other's arms, and look over each other's shoulders, and the audience give three rounds of applause.

To return from this digression, we were about to say that these are the sort of people whom you see talking, and attitudinising, outside the stage doors of our minor theatres. At Astley's they are always more numerous than at any other place. There is generally a groom or two, sitting on the windowsill, and two or three dirty shabby-genteel men in checked neckerchiefs, and sallow linen, lounging about, and carrying, perhaps, under one arm, a pair of stage shoes badly wrapped up in a piece of old newspaper. Some years ago we used to stand looking, open-mouthed, at these men, with a feeling of mysterious curiosity, the very recollection of which provokes a smile at the moment we are writing. We could not believe that the beings of light and elegance, in milk-white tunics, salmon-coloured legs, and blue scarfs, who flitted on sleek cream-coloured horses before our eyes at night, with all the aid of lights, music, and artificial flowers, could be the pale, dissipated-looking creatures we beheld by day.

We can hardly believe it now. Of the lower class of actors we have seen something, and it requires no great exercise of imagination to identify the walking gentleman with the 'dirty swell', the comic singer with the public house chairman, or the leading tragedian with drunkenness and distress; but these other men are mysterious beings, never seen out of the ring, never beheld but in the costume of gods and sylphs. With the exception of Ducrow, who can scarcely be classed among them, who ever knew a rider at Astley's, or saw him but on horseback? Can our friend in the military uniform, ever appear in threadbare attire, or descend to the comparatively un-wadded costume of everyday life? Impossible! We cannot – we will not – believe it.

## Chapter Twelve

### *Greenwich Fair*

First published in the *Evening Chronicle*, 16 April 1835 ('Sketches of London No. 9'). Easter Monday fell on 20 April in 1835 so this sketch was very timely: fairs were held at Greenwich twice a year, at Easter and at Whitsun, until 1857. Stalls and sideshows of all kinds stretched from the gates of Greenwich Park to Deptford Creek, one of the most famous being Richardson's, the booth of the itinerant showman John Richardson (1761–1837) where pantomimes were performed and severely truncated melodramas such as the one Dickens describes here. For more about Richardson and his shows, see P. Schlicke, *Dickens and Popular Entertainment* (1985). The 'majestic building' referred to in this sketch is Greenwich Hospital, now the Royal Naval College, built by Wren in the late seventeenth century as an asylum for the aged or disabled seamen, the 'pensioners' mentioned in this sketch; the 'voices of the boys' refers to the choir in the College chapel. Greenwich Park is laid out on a steep hill at the top of which stands the Royal Observatory (built 1675–6).

If the Parks be 'the lungs of London', we wonder what Greenwich Fair is – a periodical breaking out, we suppose, a sort of spring-rash: a three days' fever, which cools the blood for six months afterwards, and at the expiration of which London is restored to its old habits of plodding industry, as suddenly and completely as if nothing had ever happened to disturb them.

In our earlier days, we were a constant frequenter of Greenwich Fair, for years. We have proceeded to, and returned from it, in almost every description of vehicle. We cannot conscientiously deny the charge of having once made the passage in a spring van, accompanied by thirteen gentlemen, fourteen ladies, an unlimited number of children, and a barrel of beer; and we have a vague recollection of having, in later days, found ourself the eighth outside, on the top of a hackney coach, at something past four o'clock in the morning, with a rather confused idea of our own name, or place of residence. We have grown older since then, and quiet, and steady: liking nothing better than to spend our Easter, and all our other holidays, in some quiet nook, with people of whom we shall never

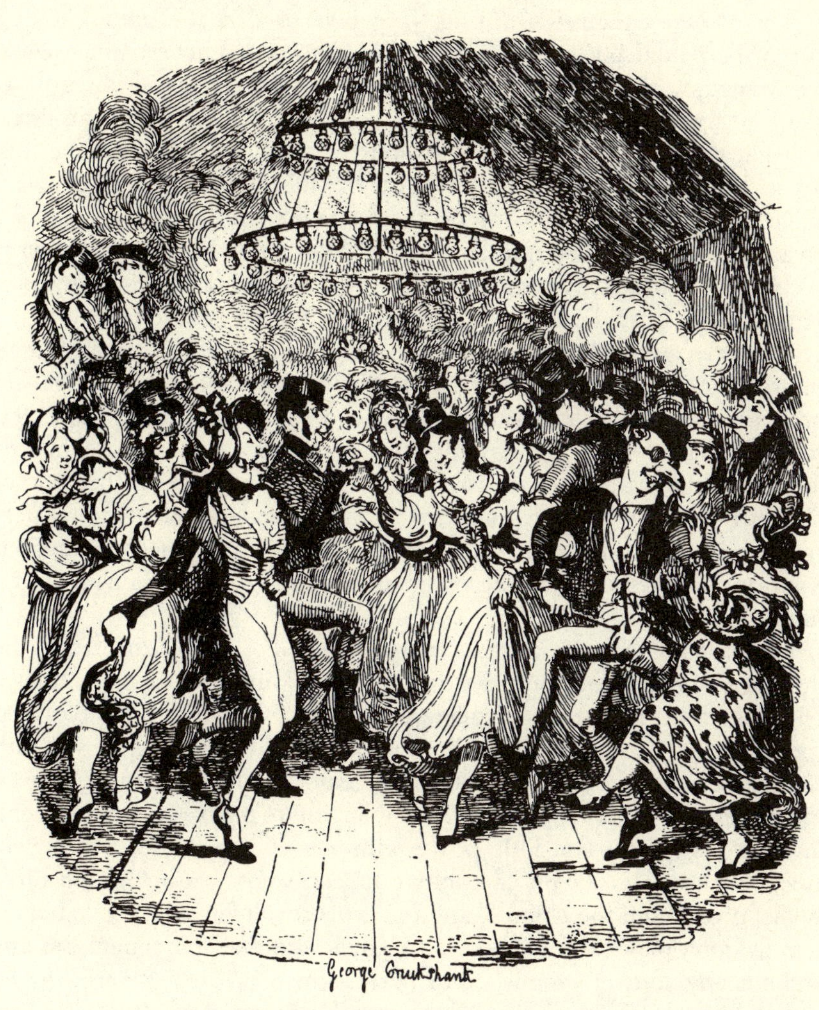

*Greenwich Fair*

tire; but we think we still remember something of Greenwich Fair, and of those who resort to it. At all events we will try.

The road to Greenwich during the whole of Easter Monday, is in a state of perpetual bustle and noise. Cabs, hackney coaches, 'shay' carts, coal waggons, stages, omnibuses, sociables, gigs, donkey chaises – all crammed with people (for the question never is, what the horse can draw, but what the vehicle will hold), roll along at their utmost speed; the dust flies in clouds, ginger beer corks go off in volleys, the balcony of every public house is crowded with people, smoking and drinking, half the private houses are turned into tea shops, fiddles are in great request, every little fruit shop displays its stall of gilt gingerbread and penny toys; turnpike men are in despair; horses won't go on, and wheels will come off; ladies in 'carawans' scream with fright at every fresh concussion, and their admirers find it necessary to sit remarkably close to them, by way of encouragement; servants-of-all-work, who are not allowed to have followers, and have got a holiday for the day, make the most of their time with the faithful admirer who waits for a stolen interview at the corner of the street every night, when they go to fetch the beer – apprentices grow sentimental, and straw bonnet makers kind. Everybody is anxious to get on, and actuated by the common wish to be at the fair, or in the park, as soon as possible.

Pedestrians linger in groups at the roadside, unable to resist the allurements of the stout proprietress of the 'Jack-in-the-box, three shies a penny', or the more splendid offers of the man with three thimbles and a pea on a little round board, who astonishes the bewildered crowd with some such address as, 'Here's the sort o' game to make you laugh seven years arter you're dead, and turn ev'ry air on your ed grey vith delight! Three thimbles and vun little pea – with a vun, two, three, and a two, three, vun: catch him who can, look on, keep your eyes open, and niver say die! niver mind the change, and the expense: all fair and above board: them as don't play can't vin, and luck attend the ryal sportsman! Bet any gen'lm'n any sum of money, from harf-a-crown up to a suverin, as he doesn't name the thimble as kivers the pea!' Here some greenhorn whispers his friend that he distinctly saw the pea roll under the middle thimble – an impression which is immediately confirmed by a gentleman in top boots, who is standing by, and who, in a low tone, regrets his own inability to bet, in consequence of having unfortunately left his purse at home, but strongly urges the stranger not to neglect such a golden opportunity. The 'plant' is successful, the bet is made, the stranger of course loses: and the gentleman with the thimble consoles him, as he pockets the money, with an assurance that it's 'all the fortin of war! this time I vin, next time you vin: niver mind the loss of two bob and a bender! Do it up in a small parcel, and break out in a fresh place. Here's the sort o' game,' &c. –

and the eloquent harangue, with such variations as the speaker's exuberant fancy suggests, is again repeated to the gaping crowd, reinforced by the accession of several newcomers.

The chief place of resort in the daytime, after the public houses, is the park, in which the principal amusement is to drag young ladies up the steep hill which leads to the Observatory, and then drag them down again, at the very top of their speed, greatly to the derangement of their curls and bonnet caps, and much to the edification of lookers on from below. 'Kiss in the Ring', and 'Threading my Grandmother's Needle', too, are sports which receive their full share of patronage. Love-sick swains, under the influence of gin and water, and the tender passion, become violently affectionate: and the fair objects of their regard enhance the value of stolen kisses, by a vast deal of struggling, and holding down of heads, and cries of 'Oh! Ha' done, then, George – Oh, do tickle him for me, Mary – Well, I never!' and similar Lucretian ejaculations. Little old men and women, with a small basket under one arm, and a wine glass, without a foot, in the other hand, tender 'a drop o' the right sort' to the different groups; and young ladies, who are persuaded to indulge in a drop of the aforesaid right sort, display a pleasing degree of reluctance to taste it, and cough afterwards with great propriety.

The old pensioners, who, for the moderate charge of a penny, exhibit the masthouse, the Thames and shipping, the place where the men used to hang in chains, and other interesting sights, through a telescope, are asked questions about objects within the range of glass, which it would puzzle a Solomon to answer; and requested to find out particular houses in particular streets, which it would have been a task of some difficulty for Mr Horner (not the young gentleman who ate mince pies with his thumb, but the man of Colosseum notoriety) to discover. Here and there, where some three or four couple are sitting on the grass together, you will see a sunburnt woman in a red cloak 'telling fortunes' and prophesying husbands, which it requires no extraordinary observation to describe, for the originals are before her. Thereupon, the lady concerned laughs and blushes, and ultimately buries her face in an imitation cambric handkerchief, and the gentleman described looks extremely foolish, and squeezes her hand, and fees the gipsy liberally; and the gipsy goes away, perfectly satisfied also: and the prophecy, like many other prophecies of greater importance fulfils itself in time.

But it grows dark: the crowd has gradually dispersed, and only a few stragglers are left behind. The light in the direction of the church shows that the fair is illuminated; and the distant noise proves it to be filling fast. The spot, which half an hour ago was ringing with the shouts of boisterous mirth, is as calm and quiet as if nothing could disturb its serenity; the fine old trees, the majestic building at their feet, with the noble river beyond, glistening in the moonlight, appear in all their beauty, and under their most favourable aspect; the voices of the boys, singing their evening hymn, are borne gently on the air; and the humblest mechanic who has been lingering on the grass so pleasant to the feet that beat the same dull round from week to week in the paved streets of London, feels proud to think as he surveys the scene before him, that he belongs to the country which has selected such a spot as a retreat for its oldest and best defenders in the decline of their lives.

Five minutes' walking brings you to the fair; a scene calculated to awaken very different feelings. The entrance is occupied on either side by the vendors of gingerbread and toys: the stalls are gaily lighted up, the most attractive goods profusely disposed, and unbonneted young ladies in their zeal for the interest of their employers, seize you by the coat, and use all the blandishments of 'Do, dear' – 'There's a love' – 'Don't be cross, now,' &c., to induce you to purchase half a pound of the real spice nuts, of which the majority of the regular fair-goers carry a pound or two as a present supply, tied up in a cotton pocket handkerchief. Occasionally you pass a deal table, on which are exposed pen'orths of pickled salmon (fennel included), in little white saucers: oysters, with shells as large as cheeseplates, and divers specimens of a species of snail (*wilks,* we think they are called), floating in a somewhat bilious-looking green liquid. Cigars, too, are in great demand; gentlemen must smoke, of course, and here they are, two a penny, in a regular authentic cigar-box, with a lighted tallow candle in the centre.

Imagine yourself in an extremely dense crowd, which swings you to and fro, and in and out, and every way but the right one; add to this the screams of women, the shouts of boys, the clanging of gongs, the firing of pistols, the ringing of bells the bellowings of speaking trumpets, the squeaking of penny dittoes, the noise of a dozen bands, with three drums in each, all playing different tunes at the same time, the hallooing of showmen, and an occasional roar from the wild beast shows; and you are in the very centre and heart of the fair.

This immense booth, with the large stage in front, so brightly illuminated with variegated lamps, and pots of burning fat, is 'Richardson's', where you have a melodrama (with three murders and a ghost), a pantomime, a comic song, an overture, and some incidental music, all done in five and twenty minutes.

The company are now promenading outside in all the dignity of wigs, spangles, red ochre, and whitening. See with what a ferocious air the gentleman who personates the Mexican chief, paces up and down, and with what an eye of calm dignity the principal tragedian gazes on the crowd below, or converses confidentially with the harlequin! The four clowns, who are engaged in a mock broadsword combat, may be all very well for the low-minded holidaymakers; but these are the people for the reflective portion of the community. They look so noble in those Roman dresses, with their yellow legs and arms, long black curly heads, bushy eyebrows, and scowl expressive of assassination, and vengeance, and everything else that is grand and solemn. Then, the ladies – were there ever such innocent and awful-looking beings; as they walk up and down the platform in twos and threes, with their arms round each other's waists, or leaning for support on one of those majestic men! Their spangled muslin dresses and blue satin shoes and sandals (a *leetle* the worse for wear) are the admiration of all beholders; and the playful manner in which they check the advances of the clown, is perfectly enchanting.

'Just a-going to begin! Pray come for'erd, come for'erd', exclaims the man in the countryman's dress, for the seventieth time: and people force their way up the steps in crowds. The band suddenly strikes up, the harlequin and columbine set the example, reels are formed in less than no time, the Roman heroes place their arms akimbo, and dance with considerable agility; and the leading tragic actress, and the gentleman who enacts the 'swell' in the pantomime, foot it to perfection. 'All in to begin', shouts the manager, when no more people can be induced to 'come for'erd', and away rush the leading members of the company to do the dreadful in the first piece.

A change of performance takes place every day during the fair, but the story of the tragedy is always pretty much the same. There is a rightful heir, who loves a young lady, and is beloved by her; and a wrongful heir, who loves her too, and isn't beloved by her; and the wrongful heir gets hold of the rightful heir, and throws him into a dungeon, just to kill him off when convenient, for which purpose he hires a couple of assassins – a good one and a bad one – who, the moment they are left alone, get up a little murder on their own account, the good one killing the bad one, and the bad one wounding the good one. Then the rightful heir is discovered in prison, carefully holding a long chain in his hands, and seated despondingly in a large armchair; and the young lady comes in to two bars of soft music, and embraces the rightful heir; and then the wrongful heir comes in to two bars of quick music (technically called 'a hurry'), and goes on in the most shocking manner, throwing the young lady about as if she was nobody, and calling the rightful heir 'Ar-recreant – ar-wretch!' in a very loud voice, which answers the double purpose of displaying his passion, and preventing the sound being deadened by the sawdust. The interest becomes intense; the wrongful heir draws his sword, and rushes on the rightful heir; a blue smoke is seen, a gong is heard, and a tall white figure (who has been all the time, behind the armchair, covered over with a tablecloth), slowly rises to the tune of 'Oft in the stilly night'. This is no other than the ghost of the rightful heir's father, who was killed by the wrongful heir's father, at sight of which the wrongful heir becomes apoplectic, and is literally 'struck all of a heap', the stage not being large enough to admit of his falling down at full length. Then the good assassin staggers in, and says he was hired in conjunction with the bad assassin, by the wrongful heir, to kill the rightful heir; and he's killed a good many people in his time, but he's very sorry for it, and won't do so any more – a promise which he immediately redeems, by dying off hand without any nonsense about it. Then the rightful heir throws down his chain; and then two men, a sailor and a young woman (the tenantry of the rightful heir) come in, and the ghost makes dumb motions to them, which they, by supernatural interference, understand – for no one else can; and the ghost (who can't do anything without blue fire) blesses the rightful heir and the young lady, by half suffocating them with smoke: and then a muffin bell rings, and the curtain drops.

The exhibitions next in popularity to these itinerant theatres are the travelling menageries, or, to speak more intelligibly, the 'Wild beast shows', where a military band in beefeater's costume, with leopard-skin caps, play incessantly; and where large highly coloured representations of tigers tearing men's heads open, and a lion being burnt with red-hot irons to induce him to drop his victim, are hung outside, by way of attracting visitors.

The principal officer at these places is generally a very tall, hoarse man, in a scarlet coat, with a cane in his hand, with which he occasionally raps the pictures we have just noticed, by way of illustrating his description – something in this way. 'Here, here, here; the lion, the lion (tap), exactly as he is represented on the canvas outside (three taps): no waiting, remember; no deception. The fe-ro-cious lion (tap, tap) who bit off the gentleman's head last Cambervel vos a twelvemonth, and has killed on average three keepers a year ever since he arrived at matoority. No extra charge on this account recollect; the price of admission is only sixpence.' This address never fails to produce a considerable sensation, and sixpences flow into the treasury with wonderful rapidity.

The dwarfs are also objects of great curiosity, and as a dwarf, a giantess, a living skeleton, a wild Indian, 'a young lady of singular beauty, with perfectly white hair and pink eyes', and two or three other natural curiosities, are usually exhibited together for the small charge of a penny, they attract very numerous audiences. The best thing about a dwarf is, that he has always a little box, about two feet six inches high, into which, by long practice, he can just manage to get, by doubling himself up like a boot-jack; this box is painted outside like a six-roomed house, and as the crowd see him ring a bell, or fire a pistol out of the first-floor window, they verily believe that it is his ordinary town residence, divided like other mansions into drawing rooms, dining parlour, and bedchambers. Shut up in this case, the unfortunate little object is brought out to delight the throng by holding a facetious dialogue with the proprietor: in the course of which, the dwarf (who is always particularly drunk) pledges himself to sing a comic song inside, and pays various compliments to the ladies to induce them to 'come for'erd' with great alacrity. As a giant is not so easily moved, a pair of indescribables of most capacious dimensions, and a huge shoe, are usually brought out, into which two or three stout men get all at once, to the enthusiastic delight of the crowd, who are quite satisfied with the solemn assurance that these habiliments form part of the giant's everyday costume.

The grandest and most numerously frequented booth in the whole fair, however, is 'The Crown and Anchor' – a temporary ballroom – we forget how many hundred feet long, the price of admission to which is one shilling. Immediately on your right hand as you enter, after paying your money, is a refreshment place, at which cold beef, roast and boiled, French rolls, stout, wine, tongue, ham, even fowls, if we recollect right, are displayed in tempting array. There is a raised orchestra, and the place is boarded all the way down, in patches, just wide enough for a country dance.

There is no master of the ceremonies in this artificial Eden – all is primitive, unreserved, and unstudied. The dust is blinding, the heat insupportable, the company somewhat noisy, and in the highest spirits possible: the ladies, in the height of their innocent animation, dancing in the gentlemen's hats, and the gentlemen promenading 'the gay and festive scene' in the ladies' bonnets, or with the more expensive ornaments of false noses, and low-crowned, tinder-box-looking-hats: playing children's drums, and accompanied by ladies on the penny trumpet.

The noise of these various instruments, the orchestra, the shouting, the 'scratchers', and the dancing, is perfectly bewildering. The dancing itself beggars description – every figure lasts about an hour, and the ladies bounce up and down the middle, with a degree of spirit which is quite indescribable. As to the gentlemen, they stamp their feet against the ground, every time 'hands four round' begins, go down the middle and up again, with cigars in their mouths, and silk handkerchiefs in their hands, and whirl their partners round, nothing loth, scrambling and falling, and embracing, and knocking up against the other couples, until they are fairly tired out, and can move no longer. The same scene is repeated again and again (slightly varied by an occasional 'row') until a late hour at night: and a great many clerks and 'prentices find themselves next morning with aching heads, empty pockets, damaged hats, and a very imperfect recollection of how it was they did *not* get home.

## Chapter Thirteen

### *Private Theatres*

First published in the *Evening Chronicle*, 11 August 1835 ('Sketches of London No. 19'). As Dickens records, there were many little private theatres scattered throughout early nineteenth-century London. They were run by speculators trading on the readiness of stage-struck youngsters to pay for the privilege of performing classic roles. They attracted much official disapproval. In July 1829, for example, the Mansion House magistrates' court heard from a policeman, who had witnessed 'romping ... and very indecent conduct' among the young patrons of the Catherine Street Theatre that Dickens mentions here, that 'the mischiefs produced in society by places of this kind were incalculable'. Dickens's harsh and scornful tone may result from a determination to distance himself from a less than reputable aspect of his own recent past: according to the reminiscences of George Lear, who had been young Dickens's fellow solicitor's clerk in 1827, Dickens may have acted in private theatres. Even if he did not act himself, however, he certainly went with Lear to see another clerk from their office, Thomas Potter (see headnote to 'Making a Night of It', p. 265 below), perform at such places. Lear's reminiscences appear in F.G. Kitton's *Charles Dickens by Pen and Pencil* (1890).

'Richard the Third. – Duke of Glo'ster, 2*l.*; Earl of Richmond, 1*l.*; Duke of Buckingham, 15*s.*; Catesby, 12*s.*; Tressel, 10*s.* 6*d.*; Lord Stanley, 5*s.*; Lord Mayor of London, 2*s.* 6*d.*'

Such are the written placards wafered up in the gentlemen's dressing room, or the green room (where there is any), at a private theatre; and such are the sums extracted from the shop till, or overcharged in the office expenditure, by the donkeys who are prevailed upon to pay for permission to exhibit their lamentable ignorance and boobyism on the stage of a private theatre. This they do, in proportion to the scope afforded by the character for the display of their imbecility. For instance, the Duke of Glo'ster is well worth two pounds, because he has it all to himself; he must wear a real sword, and what is better still, he must draw it several times in the course of the piece. The soliloquies alone are well worth fifteen shillings; then there is the stabbing King Henry – decidedly cheap

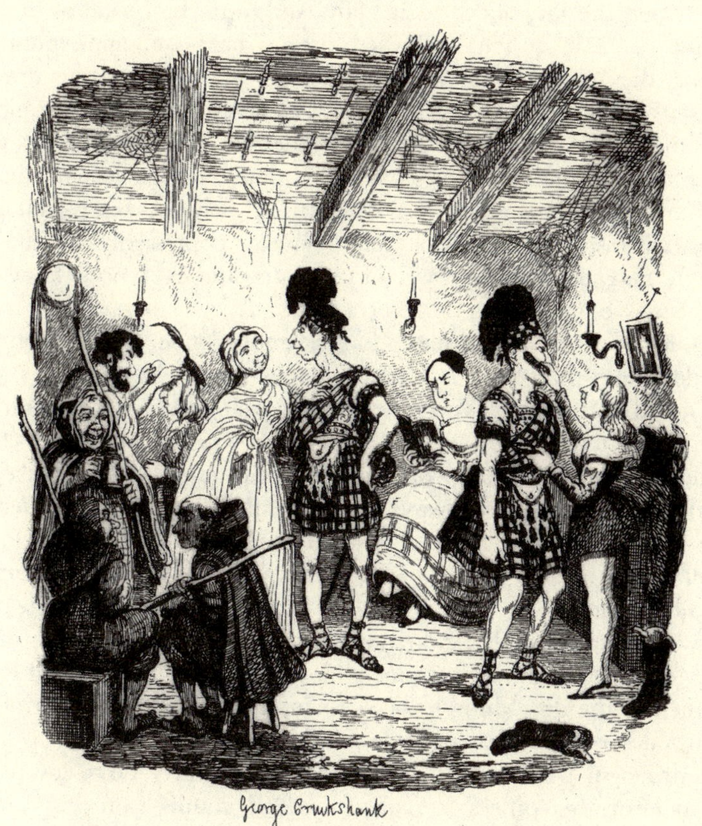

*Private Theatres*

at three-and-sixpence, that's eighteen-and-sixpence; bullying the coffin bearers – say eighteen-pence, though it's worth much more – that's a pound. Then the love scene with Lady Ann, and the bustle of the fourth act can't be dear at ten shillings more – that's only one pound ten, including the 'off with his head!' – which is sure to bring down the applause, and it is very easy to do – 'Orf with his ed' (very quick and loud; – then slow and sneeringly) – 'So much for Bu-u-u-uckingham!' Lay the emphasis on the 'uck'; get yourself gradually into a corner, and work with your right hand, while you're saying it, as if you were feeling your way, and it's sure to do. The tent scene is confessedly worth half-a-sovereign, and so you have the fight in, gratis, and everybody knows what an effect may be produced by a good combat. One – two – three – four – over; then, one – two – three – four – under; then thrust; then dodge and slide about; then fall down on one knee; then fight upon it, and then get up again and stagger. You may keep on doing this, as long as it seems to take – say ten minutes – and then fall down (backwards, if you can manage it without hurting yourself), and die game: nothing like it for producing an effect. They always do it at Astley's and Sadler's Wells, and if they don't know how to do this sort of thing, who in the world does? A small child, or a female in white, increases the interest of a combat materially – indeed, we are not aware that a regular legitimate terrific broadsword combat could be done without; but it would be rather difficult, and somewhat unusual, to introduce this effect in the last scene of Richard the Third, so the only thing to be done is, just to make the best of a bad bargain, and be as long as possible fighting it out.

The principal patrons of private theatres are dirty boys, low copying clerks in attorneys' offices, capacious-headed youths from city counting houses, Jews whose business, as lenders of fancy dresses, is a sure passport to the amateur stage, shopboys who now and then mistake their masters' money for their own; and a choice miscellany of idle vagabonds. The proprietor of a private theatre may be an ex-scene-painter, a low coffee house keeper, a disappointed eighth-rate actor, a retired smuggler, or uncertificated bankrupt. The theatre itself may be in Catherine Street, Strand, the purlieus of the city, the neighbourhood of Gray's Inn Lane, or the vicinity of Sadler's Wells; or it may, perhaps, form the chief nuisance of some shabby street, on the Surrey side of Waterloo Bridge.

The lady performers pay nothing for their characters, and it is needless to add, are usually selected from one class of society; the audiences are necessarily of much the same character as the performers, who receive, in return for their contributions to the management, tickets to the amount of the money they pay.

All the minor theatres in London, especially the lowest, constitute the centre of a little stage-struck neighbourhood. Each of them has an audience exclusively its own; and at any you will see dropping into the pit at half price, or swaggering into the back of a box, if the price of admission be a reduced one, divers boys of from fifteen to twenty-one years of age, who throw back their coat and turn up their wristbands, after the portraits of Count D'Orsay, hum tunes and whistle when the curtain is down, by way of persuading the people near them, that they are not at all anxious to have it up again, and speak familiarly of the inferior performers as Bill Such-a-one, and Ned So-and-so, or tell each other how a new piece called *The Unknown Bandit of the Invisible Cavern*, is in rehearsal; how Mister Palmer is to play *The Unknown Bandit*; how Charley Scarton is to take the part of an English sailor, and fight a broadsword combat with six unknown bandits, at one and the same time (one theatrical sailor is always equal to half a dozen men at least); how Mister Palmer and Charley Scarton are to go through a double hornpipe in fetters in the second act; how the interior of the invisible cavern is to occupy the whole extent of the stage; and other town-surprising theatrical announcements. These gentlemen are the amateurs – the *Richards*, *Shylocks*, *Beverleys*, and *Othellos* – the *Young Dorntons*, *Rovers*, *Captain Absolutes*, and *Charles Surfaces* – of a private theatre.

See them at the neighbouring public house or the theatrical coffee shop! They are the kings of the place, supposing no real performers to be present; and roll about, hats on one side, and arms akimbo, as if they had actually come into possession of eighteen shillings a week, and a share of a ticket night. If one of them does but know an Astley's supernumerary he is a happy fellow. The mingled air of envy and admiration with which his companions will regard him, as he converses familiarly with some mouldy-looking man in a fancy neckerchief, whose partially corked eyebrows, and half-rouged face, testify to the fact of his having just left the stage or the circle, sufficiently shows in what high admiration these public characters are held.

With the double view of guarding against the discovery of friends or employers, and enhancing the interest of an assumed character, by attaching a high-sounding name to its representative, these geniuses assume fictitious names, which are not the least amusing part of the play-bill of a private theatre. Belville, Melville, Treville, Berkeley, Randolph, Byron, St Clair, and so forth, are among the humblest; and the less imposing titles of Jenkins, Walker, Thomson, Barker, Solomons, &c., are completely laid aside. There is something imposing in this, and it is an excellent apology for shabbiness into the bargain. A shrunken, faded coat, a decayed hat, a patched and soiled pair of trousers – nay, even a very dirty shirt (and none of these appearances are very uncommon among the members of the *corps dramatique*), may be worn for the purpose of disguise, and to prevent any troublesome inquiries or explanations about employment and pursuits; everybody is a gentleman at large, for the occasion, and there are none of those unpleasant and unnecessary distinctions to which even genius must occasionally succumb elsewhere. As to the ladies (God bless them), they are quite above any formal absurdities; the mere circumstance of your being behind the scenes is a sufficient introduction to their society – for of course they know that none but strictly respectable persons would be admitted into that close fellowship with them, which acting engenders. They place implicit reliance on the manager, no doubt; and as to the manager, he is all affability when he knows you well, – or, in other words, when he has pocketed your money once, and entertains confident hopes of doing so again.

A quarter before eight – there will be a full house tonight – six parties in the boxes, already; four little boys and a woman in the pit; and two fiddles and a flute in the orchestra, who have got through five overtures since seven o'clock (the hour fixed for the commencement of the performances), and have just begun the sixth. There will be plenty of it, though, when it does begin, for there is enough in the bill to last six hours at least.

That gentleman in the white hat and checked shirt, brown coat and brass buttons, lounging behind the stage box on the O. P. side, is Mr Horatio St Julien, alias Jem Larkins. His line is genteel comedy – his father's, coal and potato. He *does* Alfred Highflier in the last piece, and very well he'll do it – at the price. The party of gentlemen in the opposite box, to whom he has just nodded, are friends and supporters of Mr Beverley (otherwise Loggins), the *Macbeth* of the night. You observe their attempts to appear easy and gentlemanly, each member of the party, with his feet cocked upon the cushion in front of the box! They let them do these things here, upon the same humane principle which permits poor people's children to knock double knocks at the door of an empty house – because they can't do it anywhere else. The two stout men in the centre box, with an opera glass ostentatiously placed before them, are friends of the proprietor – opulent country managers, as he confidentially informs every individual among the crew behind the curtain – opulent country managers looking out for recruits; a representation which Mr Nathan, the dresser, who is in the manager's interest, and has just arrived with the costumes, offers to confirm upon oath if required – corroborative evidence, however, is quite unnecessary, for the gulls believe it at once.

The stout Jewess who has just entered is the mother of the pale bony little girl, with the necklace of blue glass beads, sitting by her; she is being brought up to 'the profession'. Pantomime is to be her line, and she is coming out tonight, in a hornpipe after the tragedy. The short thin man beside Mr St Julien, whose white face is so deeply seared with the smallpox, and whose dirty shirt-front is inlaid with open-work, and embossed with coral studs like ladybirds, is the low comedian and comic singer of the establishment. The remainder of the audience – a tolerably numerous one by this time – are a motley group of dupes and blackguards.

The footlights have just made their appearance: the wicks of the six little oil lamps round the only tier of boxes are being turned up, and the additional light thus afforded serves to show the presence of dirt, and absence of paint, which forms a prominent feature in the audience part of the house. As these preparations, however, announce the speedy commencement of the play, let us take a peep 'behind', previous to the ringing up.

The little narrow passages beneath the stage are neither especially clean nor too brilliantly lighted; and the absence of any flooring, together with the damp mildewy smell which pervades the place, does not conduce in any great degree to their comfortable appearance. Don't fall over this plate basket – it's one of the 'properties' – the caldron for the witches' cave; and the three uncouth-looking figures, with broken clothes-props in their hands, who are drinking gin and water out of a pint pot, are the weird sisters. This miserable room, lighted by candles in sconces placed at lengthened intervals round the wall, is the dressing room, common to the gentlemen performers, and the square hole in the ceiling is *the* trap door of the stage above. You will observe that the ceiling is ornamented with the beams that support the boards, and tastefully hung with cobwebs.

The characters in the tragedy are all dressed, and their own clothes are scattered in hurried confusion over the wooden dresser which surrounds the room. That snuff-shop-looking figure, in front of the glass, is *Banquo*: and the young lady with the liberal display of legs, who is kindly painting his face with a hare's foot, is dressed for *Fleance*. The large woman, who is consulting the stage directions in Cumberland's edition of *Macbeth*, is the *Lady Macbeth* of the night; she is always selected to play the part, because she is tall and stout, and *looks* a little like Mrs Siddons – at a considerable distance. That stupid-looking milksop, with light hair and bow legs – a kind of man whom you can warrant town-made – is fresh caught; he plays *Malcolm* tonight, just to accustom himself to an audience. He will get on better by degrees; he will play *Othello* in a month, and in a month more, will very probably be apprehended on a charge of embezzlement. The black-eyed female with whom he is talking so earnestly, is dressed for the 'gentlewoman'. It is *her* first appearance, too – in that character. The boy of fourteen who is having his eyebrows smeared with soap and whitening, is *Duncan*, King of Scotland; and the two dirty men with the corked countenances, in very old green tunics, and dirty drab boots, are the 'army'.

'Look sharp below there, gents,' exclaims the dresser, a red-headed and red-whiskered Jew, calling through the trap, 'they're a-going to ring up. The flute says he'll be blowed if he plays any more, and they're getting precious noisy in front.' A general rush immediately takes place to the half dozen little steep steps leading to the stage, and the heterogeneous group are soon assembled at the side scenes, in breathless anxiety and motley confusion.

'Now,' cries the manager, consulting the written list which hangs behind the first P. S. wing, 'Scene 1, open country – lamps down – thunder and lightning – all ready, White?' [This is addressed to one of the army.] 'All ready.' – 'Very well. Scene 2, front chamber. Is the front chamber down?' – 'Yes.' – 'Very well.' – 'Jones' [to the other army who is up in the flies]. 'Hallo!' – 'Wind up the open country when we ring up.' – 'I'll take care.' – 'Scene 3, back perspective with practical bridge. Bridge ready, White? Got the tressels there?' – 'All right.'

'Very well. Clear the stage,' cries the manager, hastily packing every member of the company into the little space there is between the wings and the wall, and one wing and another. 'Places, places. Now then, Witches – Duncan – Malcolm – bleeding officer – where's the bleeding officer?' – 'Here!' replies the officer, who has been rose pinking for the character. 'Get ready, then; now, White, ring the second music bell.' The actors who are to be discovered, are hastily arranged, and the actors who are not to be discovered place themselves, in their anxiety to peep at the house, just where the audience can see them. The bell rings, and the orchestra, in acknowledgment of the call, play three distinct chords. The bell rings –the tragedy (!) opens – and our description closes.

## Chapter Fourteen

### *Vauxhall Gardens by Day*

First published in the *Morning Chronicle*, 26 October 1836 ('Sketches by Boz, New Series No. 4'). Vauxhall Gardens was a public pleasure ground situated to the northeast of the Lambeth end of Vauxhall Bridge. Originally called the New Spring Garden when the place was opened in 1660, the name was changed to Vauxhall Gardens in 1728. The Gardens were famous for their musical entertainment, brilliant illuminations and fireworks, and were popular among all classes during the eighteenth and early nineteenth centuries. For a vivid description of a pleasure party visiting the Gardens see Thackeray's *Vanity Fair*, ch. 6. By 1836, however, Vauxhall's popularity had waned, especially among the more respectable classes, and, in an effort to boost profits, the proprietors tried the experiment of opening the Gardens during the day. They were finally closed in 1859. The comic singer bearing 'the name of one of the English counties' referred to by Dickens was the well known Paul Bedford (?1792–1871).

There was a time when if a man ventured to wonder how Vauxhall Gardens would look by day, he was hailed with a shout of derision at the absurdity of the idea. Vauxhall by daylight! A porter pot without porter, the House of Commons without the Speaker, a gas lamp without the gas – pooh, nonsense, the thing was not to be thought of. It was rumoured, too, in those times, that Vauxhall Gardens by day were the scene of secret and hidden experiments; that there, carvers were exercised in the mystic art of cutting a moderate-sized ham into slices thin enough to pave the whole of the grounds; that beneath the shade of the tall trees, studious men were constantly engaged in chemical experiments, with the view of discovering how much water a bowl of negus could possibly bear; and that in some retired nooks, appropriated to the study of ornithology, other sage and learned men were, by a process known only to themselves, incessantly employed in reducing fowls to a mere combination of skin and bone.

Vague rumours of this kind, together with many others of a similar nature, cast over Vauxhall Gardens an air of deep mystery; and as there is a great deal in the mysterious, there is no doubt that to a good many

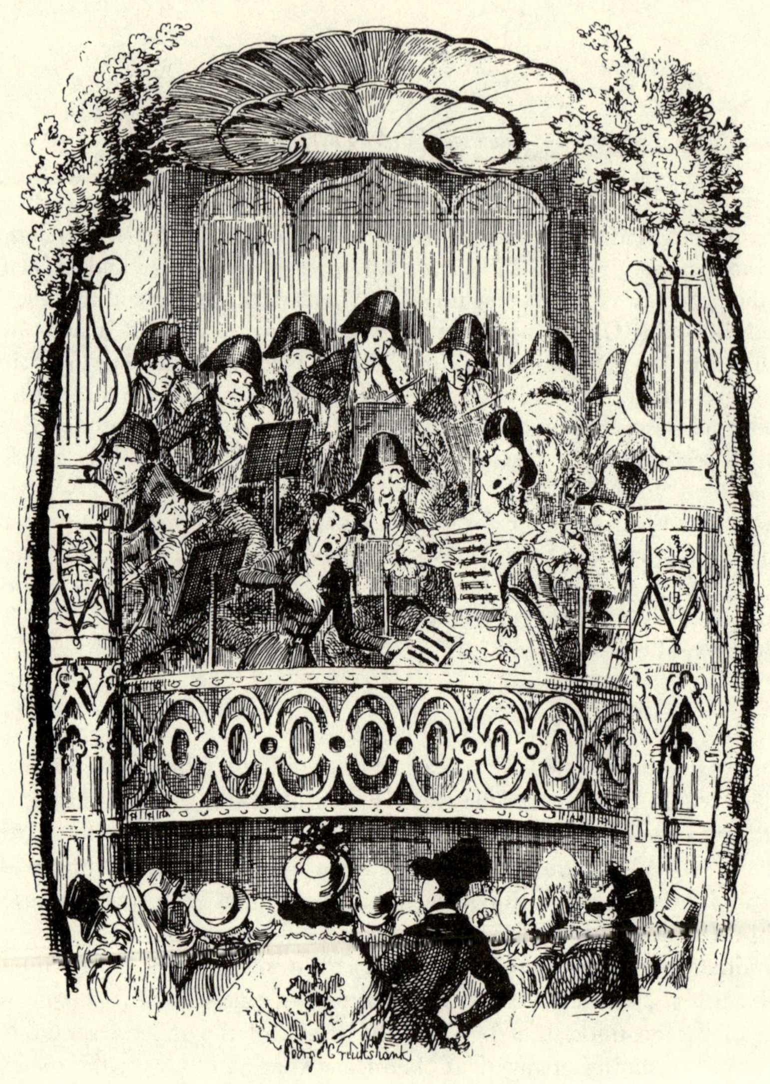


*Vauxhall Gardens by Day*

people, at all events, the pleasure they afforded was not a little enhanced by this very circumstance.

Of this class of people we confess to having made one. We loved to wander among these illuminated groves, thinking of the patient and laborious researches which had been carried on there during the day, and witnessing their results in the suppers which were served up beneath the light of lamps and to the sound of music at night. The temples and saloons and cosmoramas and fountains glittered and sparkled before our eyes; the beauty of the lady singers and the elegant deportment of the gentlemen, captivated our hearts; a few hundred thousand of additional lamps dazzled our senses; a bowl or two of punch bewildered our brains; and we were happy.

In an evil hour, the proprietors of Vauxhall Gardens took to opening them by day. We regretted this, as rudely and harshly disturbing that veil of mystery which had hung about the property for many years, and which none but the noonday sun, and the late Mr Simpson, had ever penetrated. We shrunk from going; at this moment we scarcely know why. Perhaps a morbid consciousness of approaching disappointment – perhaps a fatal presentiment – perhaps the weather; whatever it was, we did *not* go until the second or third announcement of a race between two balloons tempted us, and we went.

We paid our shilling at the gate, and then we saw for the first time, that the entrance, if there had been any magic about it at all, was now decidedly disenchanted, being, in fact, nothing more nor less than a combination of very roughly painted boards and sawdust. We glanced at the orchestra and supper room as we hurried past – we just recognised them, and that was all. We bent our steps to the firework ground; there, at least, we should not be disappointed. We reached it, and stood rooted to the spot with mortification and astonishment. *That* the Moorish tower – that wooden shed with a door in the centre, and daubs of crimson and yellow all round, like a gigantic watch case! *That* the place where night after night we had beheld the undaunted Mr Blackmore make his terrific ascent, surrounded by flames of fire, and peals of artillery, and where the white garments of Madame Somebody (we forget even her name now), who nobly devoted her life to the manufacture of fireworks, had so often been seen fluttering in the wind, as she called up a red, blue, or parti-coloured light to illumine her temple! *That* the – but at this moment the bell rang; the people scampered away, pell-mell, to the spot from whence the sound proceeded; and we, from the mere force of habit, found ourself running among the first, as if for very life.

It was for the concert in the orchestra. A small party of dismal men in cocked hats were 'executing' the overture to *Tancredi*, and a numerous assemblage of ladies and gentlemen, with their families, had rushed from their half emptied stout mugs in the supper boxes, and crowded to the spot. Intense was the low murmur of admiration when a particularly small gentleman, in a dress coat, led on a particularly tall lady in a blue sarcenet pelisse and bonnet of the same, ornamented with large white feathers, and forthwith commenced a plaintive duet.

We knew the small gentleman well; we had seen a lithographed semblance of him, on many a piece of music, with his mouth wide open as if in the act of singing; a wine glass in his hand; and a table with two decanters and four pineapples on it in the background. The tall lady, too, we had gazed on, lost in raptures of admiration, many and many a time – how different people *do* look by daylight, and without punch, to be sure! It was a beautiful duet: first the small gentleman asked a question, and then the tall lady answered it; then the small gentleman and the tall lady sang together most melodiously; then the small gentleman went through a little piece of vehemence by himself, and got very tenor indeed, in the excitement of his feelings, to which the tall lady responded in a similar manner; then the small gentleman had a shake or two, after which the tall lady had the same, and then they both merged imperceptibly into the original air: and the band wound themselves up to a pitch of fury, and the small gentleman handed the tall lady out, and the applause was rapturous.

The comic singer, however, was the especial favourite; we really thought that a gentleman, with his dinner in a pocket handkerchief, who stood near us, would have fainted with excess of joy. A marvellously facetious gentleman that comic singer is; his distinguishing characteristics are, a wig approaching to the flaxen, and an aged countenance, and he bears the name of one of the English counties, if we recollect right. He sang a very good song about the seven ages, the first half hour of which afforded the assembly the purest delight; of the rest we can make no report, as we did not stay to hear any more.

We walked about, and met with a disappointment at every turn; our favourite views were mere patches of paint; the fountain that had sparkled so showily by lamplight, presented very much the appearance of a waterpipe that had burst; all the ornaments were dingy, and all the walks gloomy. There was a spectral attempt at rope-dancing in the little open theatre. The sun shone upon the spangled dresses of the performers, and their evolutions were about as inspiring and appropriate as a country dance in a family vault. So we retraced our steps to the firework ground, and mingled with the little crowd of people who were contemplating Mr Green.

Some half dozen men were restraining the impetuosity of one of the balloons, which was completely filled, and had the car already attached; and as rumours had gone abroad that a Lord was 'going up', the crowd were more than usually anxious and talkative. There was one little man in faded black, with a dirty face and a rusty black neckerchief with a red border, tied in a narrow wisp round his neck, who entered into conversation with everybody, and had something to say upon every remark that was made within his hearing. He was standing with his arms folded, staring up at the balloon, and every now and then vented his feelings of reverence for the aëronaut, by saying, as he looked round to catch somebody's eye, 'He's a rum 'un is Green; think o' this here being up'ards of his two hundredth ascent; ecod, the man as is ekal to Green never had the toothache yet, nor won't have within this hundred year, and that's all about it. When you meets with real talent, and native, too, encourage it, that's what I say'; and when he had delivered himself to this effect, he would fold his arms with more determination than ever, and stare at the balloon with a sort of admiring defiance of any other man alive, beyond himself and Green, that impressed the crowd with the opinion that he was an oracle.

'Ah, you're very right, sir,' said another gentleman, with his wife, and children, and mother, and wife's sister, and a host of female friends, in all the gentility of white pocket handkerchiefs, frills, and spencers, 'Mr Green is a steady man, sir, and there's no fear about him.'

'Fear!' said the little man: 'isn't it a lovely thing to see him and his wife a-going up in one balloon, and his own son and *his* wife a-jostling up against them in another, and all of them going twenty or thirty miles in three hours or so, and then coming back in pochayses? I don't know where this here science is to stop, mind you; that's what bothers me.'

Here there was a considerable talking among the females in the spencers.

'What's the ladies a-laughing at, sir?' inquired the little man, condescendingly.

'It's only my sister Mary,' said one of the girls, 'as says she hopes his lordship won't be frightened when he's in the car, and want to come out again.'

'Make yourself easy about that there, my dear,' replied the little man. 'If he was so much as to move a inch without leave, Green would jist fetch him a crack over the head with the telescope, as would send him into the bottom of the basket in no time, and stun him till they come down again.'

'Would he, though?' inquired the other man.

'Yes, would he,' replied the little one, 'and think nothing of it, neither, if he was the king himself. Green's presence of mind is wonderful.'

Just at this moment all eyes were directed to the preparations which were being made for starting. The car was attached to the second balloon, the two were brought pretty close together, and a military band commenced playing, with a zeal and fervour which would render the most timid man in existence but too happy to accept any means of quitting that particular spot of earth on which they were stationed. Then Mr Green, sr, and his noble companion entered one car, and Mr Green, jr, and *his* companion the other; and then the balloons went up, and the aërial travellers stood up, and the crowd outside roared with delight, and the two gentlemen who had never ascended before, tried to wave their flags, as if they were not nervous, but held on very fast all the while; and the balloons were wafted gently away, our little friend solemnly protesting, long after they were reduced to mere specks in the air, that he could still distinguish the white hat of Mr Green. The gardens disgorged their multitudes, boys ran up and down screaming 'bal-loon'; and in all the crowded thoroughfares people rushed out of their shops into the middle of the road, and having stared up in the air at two little black objects till they almost dislocated their necks, walked slowly in again, perfectly satisfied.

The next day there was a grand account of the ascent in the morning papers, and the public were informed how it was the finest day but four in Mr Green's remembrance; how they retained sight of the earth till they lost it behind the clouds; and how the reflection of the balloon on the undulating masses of vapour was gorgeously picturesque; together with a little science about the refraction of the sun's rays, and some mysterious hints respecting atmospheric heat and eddying currents of air.

There was also an interesting account how a man in a boat was distinctly heard by Mr Green, jun., to exclaim, 'My eye!' which Mr Green, jun., attributed to his voice rising to the balloon, and the sound being thrown back from its surface into the car; and the whole concluded with a slight allusion to another ascent next Wednesday, all of which was very instructive and very amusing, as our readers will see if they look to the papers. If we have forgotten to mention the date, they have only to wait till next summer, and take the account of the first ascent, and it will answer the purpose equally well.

## Chapter Fifteen

### *Early Coaches*

First published in the *Evening Chronicle*, 19 February 1835 ('Sketches of London No. 3'). In this sketch Dickens was evidently drawing on his own experiences as a reporter for the *Morning Chronicle* which frequently involved cross-country travelling at all hours of the day and night, and Cruikshank's illustration for this sketch (see p. 88 above) shows Dickens at the coach office. His box, labelled 'Mr Boz London', is being handed across the counter.

We have often wondered how many months' incessant travelling in a post-chaise it would take to kill a man; and wondering by analogy, we should very much like to know how many months of constant travelling in a succession of early coaches, an unfortunate mortal could endure. Breaking a man alive upon the wheel, would be nothing to breaking his rest, his peace, his heart – everything but his fast – upon four; and the punishment of Ixion (the only practical person, by-the-bye, who has discovered the secret of the perpetual motion) would sink into utter insignificance before the one we have suggested. If we had been a powerful churchman in those good times when blood was shed as freely as water, and men were mowed down like grass, in the sacred cause of religion, we would have lain by very quietly till we got hold of some especially obstinate miscreant, who positively refused to be converted to our faith, and then we would have booked him for an inside place in a small coach, which travelled day and night: and securing the remainder of the places for stout men with a slight tendency to coughing and spitting, we would have started him forth on his last travels; leaving him mercilessly to all the tortures which the waiters, landlords, coachmen, guards, boots, chambermaids, and other familiars on his line of road, might think proper to inflict.

Who has not experienced the miseries inevitably consequent upon a summons to undertake a hasty journey? You receive an intimation from your place of business – wherever that may be, or whatever you may be – that it will be necessary to leave town without delay. You and your family are forthwith thrown into a state of tremendous excitement; an express is immediately dispatched to the washerwoman's; everybody is in a bustle; and you, yourself, with a feeling of dignity which you cannot altogether conceal, sally forth to the booking office to secure your place. Here a painful consciousness of your own unimportance first rushes on your mind – the people are as cool and collected as if nobody were going out of town, or as if a journey of a hundred odd miles were a mere nothing. You enter a mouldy-looking room, ornamented with large posting bills; the greater part of the place enclosed behind a huge lumbering rough counter, and fitted up with recesses that look like the dens of the smaller animals in a travelling menagerie, without the bars. Some half dozen people are 'booking' brown-paper parcels, which one of the clerks flings into the aforesaid recesses with an air of recklessness which you, remembering the new carpet bag you bought in the morning, feel considerably annoyed at; porters, looking like so many Atlases, keep rushing in and out, with large packages on their shoulders; and while you are waiting to make the necessary inquiries, you wonder what on earth the booking office clerks can have been before they were booking office clerks; one of them with his pen behind his ear, and his hands behind him, is standing in front of the fire, like a full-length portrait of Napoleon; the other with his hat half off his head, enters the passengers' names in the books with a coolness which is inexpressibly provoking; and the villain whistles – actually whistles – while a man asks him what the fare is outside, all the way to Holyhead! – in frosty weather, too! They are clearly an isolated race, evidently possessing no sympathies or feelings in common with the rest of mankind. Your turn comes at last, and having paid the fare, you tremblingly inquire – 'What time will it be necessary for me to be here in the morning?' – 'Six o'clock', replies the whistler, carelessly pitching the sovereign you have just parted with, into a wooden bowl on the desk. 'Rather before than arter', adds the man with the semi-roasted unmentionables, with just as much ease and complacency as if the whole world got out of bed at five. You turn into the street, ruminating as you bend your steps homewards on the extent to which men become hardened in cruelty by custom.

If there be one thing in existence more miserable than another, it most unquestionably is the being compelled to rise by candlelight. If you ever doubted the fact, you are painfully convinced of your error, on the morning of your departure. You left strict orders, overnight, to be called at half-past four, and you have done nothing all night but doze for five minutes at a time, and start up suddenly from a terrific dream of a large church clock with the small hand running round, with astonishing rapidity, to every figure on the dial plate. At last, completely exhausted, you fall gradually into a refreshing sleep – your thoughts grow confused – the stage coaches, which have been 'going off' before your eyes all night, become less and less distinct, until they go off altogether; one moment you are driving with all the skill and smartness of an experienced whip –

the next you are exhibiting *à la* Ducrow, on the off-leader; anon you are closely muffled up, inside, and have just recognised in the person of the guard an old schoolfellow, whose funeral, even in your dream, you remember to have attended eighteen years ago. At last you fall into a state of complete oblivion, from which you are aroused, as if into a new state of existence, by a singular illusion. You are apprenticed to a trunk maker; how, or why, or when, or wherefore, you don't take the trouble to inquire; but there you are, pasting the lining in the lid of a portmanteau. Confound that other apprentice in the back shop, how he is hammering! – rap, rap, rap – what an industrious fellow he must be! you have heard him at work for half an hour past, and he has been hammering incessantly the whole time. Rap, rap, rap, again – he's talking now – what's that he said? Five o'clock! You make a violent exertion, and start up in bed. The vision is at once dispelled; the trunk maker's shop is your own bedroom, and the other apprentice your shivering servant, who has been vainly endeavouring to wake you for the last quarter of an hour, at the imminent risk of breaking either his own knuckles or the panels of the door.

You proceed to dress yourself, with all possible dispatch. The flaring flat candle with the long snuff gives light enough to show that the things you want are not where they ought to be, and you undergo a trifling delay in consequence of having carefully packed up one of your boots in your over-anxiety of the preceding night. You soon complete your toilet, however, for you are not particular on such an occasion, and you shaved yesterday evening; so mounting your Petersham greatcoat, and green travelling shawl, and grasping your carpet bag in your right hand, you walk lightly downstairs, lest you should awaken any of the family, and after pausing in the common sitting room for one moment, just to have a cup of coffee (the said common sitting room looking remarkably comfortable, with everything out of its place, and strewed with the crumbs of last night's supper), you undo the chain and bolts of the street door, and find yourself fairly in the street.

A thaw, by all that is miserable! The frost is completely broken up. You look down the long perspective of Oxford Street, the gaslights mournfully reflected on the wet pavement, and can discern no speck in the road to encourage the belief that there is a cab or a coach to be had – the very coachmen have gone home in despair. The cold sleet is drizzling down with that gentle regularity, which betokens a duration of four-and-twenty hours at least; the damp hangs upon the house tops and lamp posts and clings to you like an invisible cloak. The water is 'coming in' in every area, the pipes have burst, the water butts are running over; the kennels seem to be doing matches against time, pump handles descend of their own accord, horses in market carts fall down, and there's no one to help them up again, policemen look as if they had been carefully sprinkled with powdered glass; here and there a milkwoman trudges slowly along, with a bit of list round each foot to keep her from slipping; boys who 'don't sleep in the house', and are not allowed much sleep out of it, can't wake their masters by thundering at the shop door, and cry with the cold – the compound of ice, snow, and water on the pavement, is a couple of inches thick – nobody ventures to walk fast to keep himself warm, and nobody could succeed in keeping himself warm if he did.

It strikes a quarter past five as you trudge down Waterloo Place on your way to the Golden Cross, and you discover, for the first time, that you were called about an hour too early. You have not time to go back; there is no place open to go into, and you have, therefore, no resource but to go forward, which you do, feeling remarkably satisfied with yourself, and everything about you. You arrive at the office, and look wistfully up the yard for the Birmingham High-flier, which, for aught you can see, may have flown away altogether, for no preparations appear to be on foot for the departure of any vehicle in the shape of a coach. You wander into the booking office, which with the gaslights and blazing fire, looks quite comfortable by contrast – that is to say, if any place *can* look comfortable at half-past five on a winter's morning. There stands the identical book keeper in the same position as if he had not moved since you saw him yesterday. As he informs you, that the coach is up the yard, and will be brought round in about a quarter of an hour, you leave your bag, and repair to 'The Tap' – not with any absurd idea of warming yourself, because you feel such a result to be utterly hopeless, but for the purpose of procuring some hot brandy and water, which you do, – when the kettle boils! an event which occurs exactly two minutes and a half before the time fixed for the starting of the coach.

The first stroke of six peals from St Martin's church steeple just as you take the first sip of the boiling liquid. You find yourself at the booking office in two seconds, and the tap waiter finds himself much comforted by your brandy and water, in about the same period. The coach is out; the horses are in, and the guard and two or three porters are stowing the luggage away, and running up the steps of the booking office, and down the steps of the booking office, with breathless rapidity. The place, which a few minutes ago was so still and quiet, is now all bustle; the early vendors of the morning papers have arrived, and you are assailed on all sides with shouts of '*Times*, gen'lm'n, *Times*', 'Here's *Chron – Chron – Chron*', '*Herald*, ma'am', 'Highly interesting murder, gen'lm'n', 'Curious case o' breach o' promise, ladies'. The inside passengers are already in their dens, and the outsides, with the exception of yourself warm; they consist of two young men with very long hair, to which the sleet has communicated the appearance of crystallised rats' tails; one thin young woman cold and peevish, one old gentleman ditto ditto, and something in a cloak and cap, intended to represent a military officer; every member of the party, with a large stiff shawl over his chin, looking exactly as if he were playing a set of Pan's pipes.

'Take off the cloths, Bob,' says the coachman, who now appears for the first time, in a rough blue greatcoat, of which the buttons behind are so far apart, that you can't see them both at the same time. 'Now, gen'lm'n', cries the guard, with the waybill in his hand. 'Five minutes behind time already!' Up jump the passengers – the two young men smoking like lime kilns, and the old gentleman grumbling audibly. The thin young woman is got upon the roof, by dint of a great deal of pulling, and pushing, and helping and trouble, and she repays it by expressing her solemn conviction that she will never be able to get down again.

'All right,' sings out the guard at last, jumping up as the coach starts, and blowing his horn directly afterwards, in proof of the soundness of his wind. 'Let 'em go, Harry, give 'em their heads,' cried the coachman – and off we start as briskly as if the morning were 'all right', as well as the coach: and looking forward as anxiously to the termination of our journey, as we fear our readers will have done, long since, to the conclusion of our paper.

## Chapter Sixteen

### *Omnibuses*

First published in the *Morning Chronicle*, 26 September 1834 ('Street Sketches No. 1'). Omnibuses were first introduced in London by George Shillibeer in 1829 and soon competing firms were running them over the same routes. Passengers sat on two long rows of facing benches.

It is very generally allowed that public conveyances afford an extensive field for amusement and observation. Of all the public conveyances that have been constructed since the days of the Ark – we think that is the earliest on record – to the present time, commend us to an omnibus. A long stage is not to be despised, but there you have only six insides, and the chances are, that the same people go all the way with you – there is no change, no variety. Besides, after the first twelve hours or so, people get cross and sleepy, and when you have seen a man in his nightcap, you lose all respect for him; at least, that is the case with us. Then on smooth roads people frequently get prosy, and tell long stories, and even those who don't talk, may have very unpleasant predilections. We once travelled four hundred miles, inside a stagecoach, with a stout man, who had a glass of rum and water, warm, handed in at the window at every place where we changed horses. This was decidedly unpleasant. We have also travelled occasionally, with a small boy, of a pale aspect, with light hair, and no perceptible neck, coming up to town from school under the protection of the guard, and directed to be left at the Cross Keys till called for. This is, perhaps, even worse than rum and water in a close atmosphere. Then there is the whole train of evils consequent on the change of the coachman; and the misery of the discovery – which the guard is sure to make the moment you begin to doze – that he wants a brown paper parcel, which he distinctly remembers to have deposited under the seat on which you are reposing. A great deal of bustle and groping takes place, and when you are thoroughly awakened, and severely cramped, by holding your legs up by an almost supernatural exertion, while he is looking behind them, it suddenly occurs to him that he put it in the fore-boot. Bang goes the door; the parcel is immediately found; off starts the coach again; and the guard plays the key-bugle as loud as he can play it, as if in mockery of your wretchedness.

Now, you meet with none of these afflictions in an omnibus; sameness there can never be. The passengers change as often in the course of one journey as the figures in a kaleidoscope, and though not so glittering, are far more amusing. We believe there is no instance on record, of a man's having gone to sleep in one of these vehicles. As to long stories, would any man venture to tell a long story in an omnibus? and even if he did, where would be the harm? nobody could possibly hear what he was talking about. Again; children, though occasionally, are not often to be found in an omnibus; and even when they are, if the vehicle be full, as is generally the case, somebody sits upon them, and we are unconscious of their presence. Yes, after mature reflection, and considerable experience, we are decidedly of opinion that of all known vehicles, from the glass coach in which we were taken to be christened, to that sombre caravan in which we must one day make our last earthly journey, there is nothing like an omnibus.

We will back the machine in which we make our daily peregrination from the top of Oxford Street to the city, against any 'buss' on the road, whether it be for the gaudiness of its exterior, the perfect simplicity of its interior, or the native coolness of its cad. This young gentleman is a singular instance of self-devotion; his somewhat intemperate zeal on behalf of his employers is constantly getting him into trouble, and occasionally into the house of correction. He is no sooner emancipated, however, than he resumes the duties of his profession with unabated ardour. His principal distinction is his activity. His great boast is, 'that he can chuck an old gen'lm'n into the buss, shut him in, and rattle off, afore he knows where it's a-going to' – a feat which he frequently performs, to the infinite amusement of everyone but the old gentleman concerned, who, somehow or other, never can see the joke of the thing.

We are not aware that it has ever been precisely ascertained, how many passengers our omnibus will contain. The impression on the cad's mind evidently is, that it is amply sufficient for the accommodation of any number of persons that can be enticed into it. 'Any room?' cries a very hot pedestrian. 'Plenty o' room, sir', replies the conductor, gradually opening the door, and not disclosing the real state of the case until the wretched man is on the steps. 'Where?' inquires the entrapped individual, with an attempt to back out again. 'Either side, sir', rejoins the cad, shoving him in, and slamming the door. 'All right, Bill.' Retreat is impossible; the newcomer rolls about, till he falls down somewhere, and there he stops.

As we get into the city a little before ten, four or five of our party are regular passengers. We always take them up at the same places, and they generally occupy the same seats; they are always dressed in the same manner, and invariably discuss the same topics – the increasing rapidity of cabs, and the disregard of moral obligations evinced by omnibus men. There is a little testy old man, with a powdered head, who always sits on the right-hand side of the door as you enter, with his hands folded on the top of his umbrella. He is extremely impatient, and sits there for the purpose of keeping a sharp eye on the cad, with whom he generally holds a running dialogue. He is very officious in helping people in and out, and always volunteers to give the cad a poke with his umbrella, when anyone wants to alight. He usually recommends ladies to have sixpence ready, to prevent delay; and if anybody puts a window down, that he can reach, he immediately puts it up again.

'Now, what are you stopping for?' says the little man every morning, the moment there is the slightest indication of 'pulling up' at the corner of Regent Street, when some such dialogue as the following takes place between him and the cad:

'What are you stopping for?'

Here the cad whistles, and affects not to hear the question.

'I say [a poke], what are you stopping for?'

'For passengers, sir. Ba–nk. – Ty.'

'I know you're stopping for passengers; but you've no business to do so. *Why* are you stopping?'

'Vy sir, that's a difficult question. I think it is because we perfer stopping here to going on.'

'Now mind,' exclaims the little old man, with great vehemence, 'I'll pull you up tomorrow; I've often threatened to do it; now I will.'

'Thankee, sir,' replies the cad, touching his hat with a mock expression of gratitude; – 'werry much obliged to you indeed, sir.' Here the young men in the omnibus laugh very heartily, and the old gentleman gets very red in the face, and seems highly exasperated.

The stout gentleman in the white neckcloth, at the other end of the vehicle, looks very prophetic, and says that something must shortly be done with these fellows, or there's no saying where all this will end; and the shabby-genteel man with the green bag, expresses his entire concurrence in the opinion, as he has done regularly every morning for the last six months.

A second omnibus now comes up, and stops immediately behind us. Another old gentleman elevates his cane in the air, and runs with all his might towards our omnibus; we watch his progress with great interest; the door is opened to receive him, he suddenly disappears – he has been spirited away by the opposition. Hereupon the driver of the opposition taunts our people with his having 'regularly done 'em out of that old swell,' and the voice of the 'old swell' is heard, vainly protesting against this unlawful detention. We rattle off, the other omnibus rattles after us, and every time we stop to take up a passenger, they stop to take him too;

sometimes we get him; sometimes they get him; but whoever don't get him, say they ought to have had him, and the cads of the respective vehicles abuse one another accordingly.

As we arrive in the vicinity of Lincoln's Inn Fields, Bedford Row, and other legal haunts, we drop a great many of our original passengers, and take up fresh ones, who meet with a very sulky reception. It is rather remarkable, that the people already in an omnibus always look at new-comers, as if they entertained some undefined idea that they have no business to come in at all. We are quite persuaded the little old man has some notion of this kind, and that he considers their entry as a sort of negative impertinence.

Conversation is now entirely dropped; each person gazes vacantly through the window in front of him, and everybody thinks that his opposite neighbour is staring at him. If one man gets out at Shoe Lane, and another at the corner of Farringdon Street, the little old gentleman grumbles, and suggests to the latter, that if he had got out at Shoe Lane too, he would have saved them the delay of another stoppage; whereupon the young men laugh again, and the old gentleman looks very solemn, and says nothing more till he gets to the Bank, when he trots off as fast as he can, leaving us to do the same, and to wish, as we walk away, that we could impart to others any portion of the amusement we have gained for ourselves.

## Chapter Seventeen

### *The Last Cab Driver, and the First Omnibus Cad*

First published in this form in the *Second Series* (December 1836). The first part is an extensively revised version of 'Hackney Cabs and Their Drivers', originally published in a shortlived weekly, the *Carlton Chronicle*, 17 September 1836. The second, a similarly-revised version of 'Some Account of an Omnibus Cad', was first published in *Bell's Life in London*, 1 November 1835 ('Scenes and Characters No. 6'). For details of the revisions and the full text of the *Carlton* sketch see DeVries, pp. 158–66. The legal fare for cabs was eightpence a mile (see headnote to 'Hackney Coach Stands', p. 83 above); that this would leave fourpence change out of a shilling coin, which cab drivers seemed to have expected as their rightful tip. The reference to William Barker's 'quitting his ungrateful country' for 'a distant shore' is an allusion to the punishment of transportation to Australia for a set term of years.

Of all the cabriolet drivers whom we have ever had the honour and gratification of knowing by sight – and our acquaintance in this way has been most extensive – there is one who made an impression on our mind which can never be effaced, and who awakened in our bosom a feeling of admiration and respect, which we entertain a fatal presentiment will never be called forth again by any human being. He was a man of most simple and prepossessing appearance. He was a brown-whiskered, white-hatted, no-coated cabman; his nose was generally red, and his bright blue eye not unfrequently stood out in bold relief against a black border of artificial workmanship; his boots were of the Wellington form, pulled up to meet his corduroy knee-smalls, or at least to approach as near them as their dimensions would admit of; and his neck was usually garnished with a bright yellow handkerchief. In summer he carried in his mouth a flower; in winter, a straw – slight, but, to a contemplative mind, certain indications of a love of nature, and a taste for botany.

His cabriolet was gorgeously painted – a bright red; and wherever we went, City or West End, Paddington or Holloway, North, East, West, or South, there was the red cab, bumping up against the posts at the street corners, and turning in and out, among hackney coaches, and drays, and

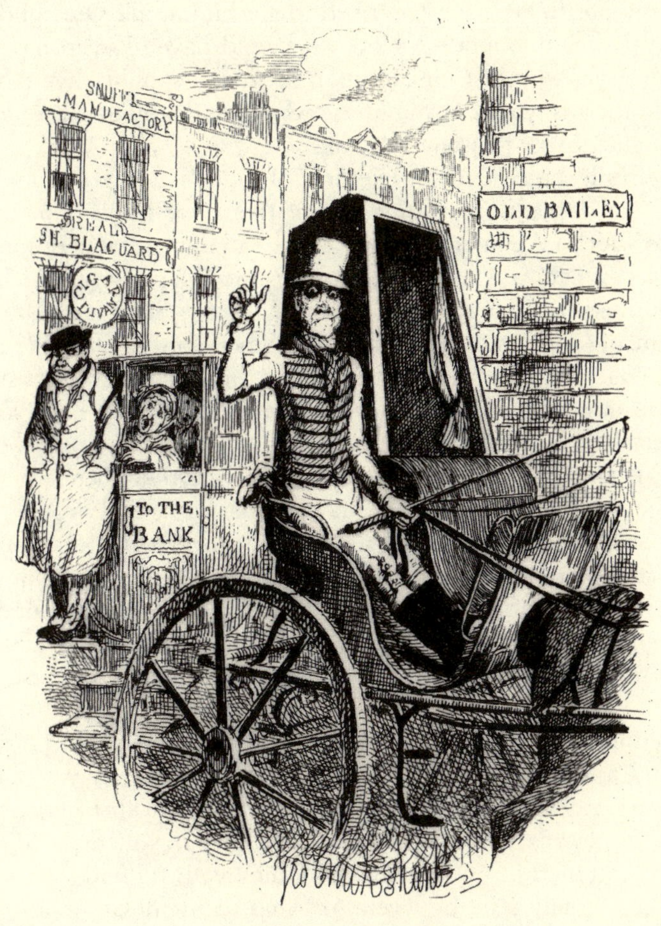


*The Last Cab Driver*

Note: Cruikshank depicts an 'outrigger'-style cab; these were rapidly replaced after the mid-1830s by the safer Hansom cabs with the driver in a seat behind his passengers.

carts, and waggons, and omnibuses, and contriving by some strange means or other, to get out of places which no other vehicle but the red cab could ever by any possibility have contrived to get into at all. Our fondness for that red cab was unbounded. How we should have liked to have seen it in the circle at Astley's! Our life upon it, that it should have performed such evolutions as would have put the whole company to shame – Indian chiefs, knights, Swiss peasants, and all.

Some people object to the exertion of getting into cabs, and others object to the difficulty of getting out of them; we think both these are objections which take their rise in perverse and ill-conditioned minds. The getting into a cab is a very pretty and graceful process, which, when well performed, is essentially melodramatic. First, there is the expressive pantomime of every one of the eighteen cabmen on the stand, the moment you raise your eyes from the ground. Then there is your own pantomime in reply – quite a little ballet. Four cabs immediately leave the stand, for your especial accommodation; and the evolutions of the animals who draw them are beautiful in the extreme, as they grate the wheels of the cabs against the curbstones, and sport playfully in the kennel. You single out a particular cab, and dart swiftly towards it. One bound, and you are on the first step; turn your body lightly round to the right, and you are on the second; bend gracefully beneath the reins, working round to the left at the same time, and you are in the cab. There is no difficulty in finding a seat: the apron knocks you comfortably into it at once, and off you go.

The getting out of a cab is, perhaps, rather more complicated in its theory, and a shade more difficult in its execution. We have studied the subject a great deal, and we think the best way is, to throw yourself out, and trust to chance for alighting on your feet. If you make the driver alight first, and then throw yourself upon him, you will find that he breaks your fall materially. In the event of your contemplating an offer of eightpence, on no account make the tender, or show the money, until you are safely on the pavement. It is very bad policy attempting to save the fourpence. You are very much in the power of a cabman, and he considers it a kind of fee not to do you any wilful damage. Any instruction, however, in the art of getting out of a cab, is wholly unnecessary if you are going any distance, because the probability is that you will be shot lightly out before you have completed the third mile.

We are not aware of any instance on record in which a cab-horse has performed three consecutive miles without going down once. What of that? It is all excitement. And in these days of derangement of the nervous system and universal lassitude, people are content to pay handsomely for excitement; where can it be procured at a cheaper rate?

But to return to the red cab; it was omnipresent. You had but to walk down Holborn, or Fleet Street, or any of the principal thoroughfares in which there is a great deal of traffic, and judge for yourself. You had hardly turned into the street, when you saw a trunk or two, lying on the ground: an uprooted post, a hatbox, a portmanteau, and a carpet-bag, strewed about in a very picturesque manner; a horse in a cab standing by, looking about him with great unconcern; and a crowd, shouting and screaming with delight, cooling their flushed faces against the glass windows of a chemist's shop. – 'What's the matter here, can you tell me?' – 'O'ny a cab, sir.' – 'Anybody hurt, do you know?' – 'O'ny the fare, sir. I see him a-turnin' the corner, and I ses to another gen'lm'n "That's a reg'lar little oss that, and he's a-comin' along raything sweet, an't he?" – "He just is," ses the other gen'lm'n, ven bump they cums agin the post, and out flies the fare like bricks.' Need we say it was the red cab; or that the gentleman with the straw in his mouth, who emerged so coolly from the chemist's shop and philosophically climbing into the little dickey, started off at full gallop, was the red cab's licensed driver?

The ubiquity of this red cab, and the influence it exercised over the risible muscles of justice itself, was perfectly astonishing. You walked into the justice-room of the Mansion House; the whole court resounded with merriment. The Lord Mayor threw himself back in his chair, in a state of frantic delight at his own joke; every vein in Mr Hobler's countenance was swollen with laughter, partly at the Lord Mayor's facetiousness, but more at his own; the constables and police officers were (as in duty bound) in ecstasies at Mr Hobler and the Lord Mayor combined; and the very paupers, glancing respectfully at the beadle's countenance, tried to smile, as even he relaxed. A tall, weazen-faced man, with an impediment in his speech, would be endeavouring to state a case of imposition against the red cab's driver; and the red cab's driver, and the Lord Mayor, and Mr Hobler, would be having a little fun among themselves, to the inordinate delight of everybody but the complainant. In the end, justice would be so tickled with the red cab driver's native humour, that the fine would be mitigated, and he would go away full gallop, in the red cab, to impose on somebody else without loss of time.

The driver of the red cab, confident in the strength of his own moral principles, like many other philosophers, was wont to set the feelings and opinions of society at complete defiance. Generally speaking, perhaps, he would as soon carry a fare safely to his destination, as he would upset him – sooner, perhaps, because in that case he not only got the money, but had the additional amusement of running a longer heat against some smart rival. But society made war upon him in the shape of penalties, and he must make war upon society in his own way. This was the reasoning of the red cab driver. So he bestowed a searching look upon the fare, as he put his hand in his waistcoat pocket, when he had gone half the mile, to get the money ready; and if he brought forth eightpence, out he went.

The last time we saw our friend was one wet evening in Tottenham Court Road, when he was engaged in a very warm and somewhat personal altercation with a loquacious little gentleman in a green coat. Poor fellow! there were great excuses to be made for him: he had not received above eighteenpence more than his fare, and consequently laboured under a great deal of very natural indignation. The dispute had attained a pretty considerable height, when at last the loquacious little gentleman, making a mental calculation of the distance, and finding that he had already paid more than he ought, avowed his unalterable determination to 'pull up' the cabman in the morning.

'Now, just mark this, young man,' said the little gentleman, 'I'll pull you up tomorrow morning.'

'No! will you though?' said our friend, with a sneer.

'I will,' replied the little gentleman, 'mark my words, that's all. If I live till tomorrow morning, you shall repent this.'

There was a steadiness of purpose, and indignation of speech, about this little gentleman, as he took an angry pinch of snuff, after this last declaration, which made a visible impression on the mind of the red cab driver. He appeared to hesitate for an instant. It was only for an instant; his resolve was soon taken.

'You'll pull me up, will you?' said our friend.

'I will,' rejoined the little gentleman, with even greater vehemence than before.

'Wery well,' said our friend, tucking up his shirt sleeves very calmly. 'There'll be three veeks for that. Wery good; that'll bring me up to the middle o' next month. Three veeks more would carry me on to my birthday, and then I've got ten pound to draw. I may as well get board, lodgin', and washin', till then, out of the county, as pay for it myself; consequently here goes!'

So, without more ado, the red cab driver knocked the little gentleman down, and then called the police to take himself into custody, with all the civility in the world.

A story is nothing without the sequel; and therefore we may state, that to our certain knowledge, the board, lodging, and washing, were all provided in due course. We happen to know the fact, for it came to our knowledge thus: we went over the House of Correction for the county of Middlesex shortly after, to witness the operation of the silent system; and looked on all the 'wheels' with the greatest anxiety, in search of our long lost friend. He was nowhere to be seen, however, and we began to think that the little gentleman in the green coat must have relented, when, as we were traversing the kitchen garden, which lies in a sequestered part of the prison, we were startled by hearing a voice, which apparently proceeded, from the wall, pouring forth its soul in the plaintive air of 'All round my hat', which was then just beginning to form a recognised portion of our national music.

We started – 'What voice is that?' said we.

The Governor shook his head.

'Sad fellow,' he replied, 'very sad. He positively refused to work on the wheel; so, after many trials, I was compelled to order him into solitary confinement. He says he likes it very much though, and I am afraid he does, for he lies on his back on the floor, and sings comic songs all day!'

Shall we add, that our heart had not deceived us; and that the comic singer was no other than our eagerly-sought friend, the red cab driver?

We have never seen him since, but we have strong reason to suspect that this noble individual was a distant relative of a waterman of our acquaintance, who, on one occasion, when we were passing the coach stand over which he presides, after standing very quietly to see a tall man struggle into a cab, ran up very briskly when it was all over (as his brethren invariably do), and, touching his hat, asked, as a matter of course, for 'a copper for the waterman'. Now, the fare was by no means a handsome man; and, waxing very indignant at the demand, he replied – 'Money! What for? Coming up and looking at me, I suppose!' – 'Vell , sir,' rejoined the waterman, with a smile of immovable complacency, '*that's* worth twopence.'

This identical waterman afterwards attained a very prominent station in society; and as we know something of his life, and have often thought of telling what we *do* know, perhaps we shall never have a better opportunity than the present.

Mr William Barker, then, for that was the gentleman's name, Mr William Barker was born — but why need we relate where Mr William Barker was born, or when? Why scrutinise the entries in parochial ledgers, or seek to penetrate the Lucinian mysteries of lying-in hospitals? Mr William Barker *was* born, or he had never been. There is a son – there was a father. There is an effect – there was a cause. Surely this is sufficient information for the most Fatima-like curiosity; and, if it be not, we regret our inability to supply any further evidence on the point. Can there be a more satisfactory, or more strictly parliamentary course? Impossible.

We at once avow a similar ability to record at what precise period, or by what particular process, this gentleman's patronymic, of William Barker, became corrupted into 'Bill Boorker'. Mr Barker acquired a high standing, and no inconsiderable reputation, among the members of that profession to which he more peculiarly devoted his energies; and to them he was generally known, either by the familiar appellation of 'Bill Boorker', or the flattering designation of 'Aggerawatin Bill,' the latter being a playful and expressive *sobriquet*, illustrative of Mr Barker's great talent in 'aggerawatin' and rendering wild such subjects of her Majesty as are conveyed from place to place, through the instrumentality of omnibuses. Of the early life of Mr Barker little is known, and even that little is involved in a considerable doubt and obscurity. A want of application, a restlessness of purpose, a thirsting after porter, a love of all that is roving and cadger-like in nature, shared in common with many other great geniuses, appear to have been his leading characteristics. The busy hum of a parochial free school, and the shady repose of a county gaol, were alike inefficacious in producing the slightest alteration in Mr Barker's disposition. His feverish attachment to change and variety nothing could repress; his native daring no punishment could subdue.

If Mr Barker can be fairly said to have had any weakness in his earlier years, it was an amiable one – love; love in its most comprehensive form – a love of ladies, liquids and pocket handkerchiefs. It was no selfish feeling; it was not confined to his own possessions, which but too many men regard with exclusive complacency. No; it was a nobler love – a general principle. It extended itself with equal force to the property of other people.

There is something very affecting in this. It is still more affecting to know, that such philanthropy is but imperfectly rewarded. Bow Street, Newgate, and Millbank, are a poor return for general benevolence, evincing itself in an irrepressible love for all created objects. Mr Barker felt it so. After a lengthened interview with the highest legal authorities, he quitted his ungrateful country with the consent, and at the expense, of its Government; proceeded to a distant shore; and there employed himself, like another Cincinnatus, in clearing and cultivating the soil – a peaceful pursuit, in which a term of seven years glided almost imperceptibly away.

Whether, at the expiration of the period we have just mentioned, the British Government required Mr Barker's presence here, or did not require his residence abroad, we have no distinct means of ascertaining. We should be inclined, however, to favour the latter position, inasmuch as we do not find that he was advanced to any other public post on his return, than the post at the corner of the Haymarket, where he officiated as assistant waterman to the hackney coach stand. Seated, in this capacity, on a couple of tubs near the curbstone, with a brass plate and number suspended round his neck by a massive chain, and his ankles curiously enveloped in haybands, he is supposed to have made those observations on human nature which exercised so material an influence over all his proceedings in later life.

Mr Barker had not officiated for many months in this capacity, when the appearance of the first omnibus caused the public mind to go in a new direction, and prevented a great many hackney coaches from going in any direction at all. The genius of Mr Barker at once perceived the whole extent of the injury that would be eventually inflicted on cab and coach stands, and, by consequence, on watermen also, by the progress of the system of which the first omnibus was a part. He saw, too, the necessity of adopting some more profitable profession; and his active mind at once perceived how much might be done in the way of enticing the youthful and unwary, and shoving the old and helpless, into the wrong bus, and carrying them off, until, reduced to despair, they ransomed themselves by the payment of sixpence a head, or, to adopt his own figurative expression in all its native beauty, 'till they was rig'larly done over, and forked out the stumpy'.

An opportunity for realising his fondest anticipations soon presented itself. Rumours were rife on the hackney coach stands, that a bus was building, to run from Lisson Grove to the Bank, down Oxford Street and Holborn; and the rapid increase of busses on the Paddington Road, encouraged the idea. Mr Barker secretly and cautiously inquired in the proper quarters. The report was correct; the 'Royal William' was to make its first journey on the following Monday. It was a crack affair altogether. An enterprising young cabman, of established reputation as a dashing whip – for he had compromised with the parents of three scrunched children, and just 'worked out' his fine, for knocking down an old lady – was the driver; and the spirited proprietor, knowing Mr Barker's qualifications, appointed him to the vacant office of cad on the very first application. The bus began to run, and Mr Barker entered into a new suit of clothes, and on a new sphere of action.

To recapitulate all the improvements introduced by this extraordinary man, into the omnibus system – gradually, indeed, but surely – would occupy a far greater space than we are enabled to devote to this imperfect memoir. To him is universally assigned the original suggestion of the practice which afterwards became so general – of the driver of a second bus keeping constantly behind the first one, and driving the pole of his vehicle either into the door of the other, every time it was opened, or through the body of any lady or gentleman who might make an attempt to get into it; a humorous and pleasant invention, exhibiting all that originality of idea, and fine bold flow of spirits, so conspicuous in every action of this great man.

Mr Barker had opponents of course; what man in public life has not? But even his worst enemies cannot deny that he has taken more old ladies and gentlemen to Paddington who wanted to go to the Bank, and more old ladies and gentlemen to the Bank who wanted to go to Paddington, than any six men on the road; and however much malevolent spirits may pretend to doubt the accuracy of the statement, they well know it to be an established fact, that he has forcibly conveyed a variety of ancient persons of either sex, to both places, who had not the slightest or most distant intention of going anywhere at all.

Mr Barker was the identical cad who nobly distinguished himself, some time since, by keeping a tradesman on the step – the omnibus going at full speed all the time – till he had thrashed him to his entire satisfaction, and finally throwing him away, when he had quite done with him. Mr Barker it *ought* to have been, who honestly indignant at being ignominiously ejected from a house of public entertainment, kicked the landlord in the knee, and thereby caused his death. We say it *ought* to have been Mr Barker, because the action was not a common one, and could have emanated from no ordinary mind.

It has now become matter of history; it is recorded in the Newgate Calendar; and we wish we could attribute this piece of daring heroism to Mr Barker. We regret being compelled to state that it was not performed by him. Would, for the family credit we could add, that it was achieved by his brother!

It was in the exercise of the nicer details of his profession, that Mr Barker's knowledge of human nature was beautifully displayed. He could tell at a glance where a passenger wanted to go to, and would shout the name of the place accordingly, without the slightest reference to the real destination of the vehicle. He knew exactly the kind of old lady that would be too much flurried by the process of pushing in and pulling out of the caravan, to discover where she had been put down, until too late; had an intuitive perception of what was passing in a passenger's mind when he inwardly resolved to 'pull that cad up tomorrow morning'; and never failed to make himself agreeable to female servants, whom he would place next the door, and talk to all the way.

Human judgment is never infallible, and it would occasionally happen that Mr Barker experimentalised with the timidity or forbearance of the wrong person, in which case a summons to a Police office was, on more than one occasion, followed by a committal to prison. It was not in the power of trifles such as these, however, to subdue the freedom of his spirit. As soon as they passed away, he resumed the duties of his profession with unabated ardour.

We have spoken of Mr Barker and of the red cab driver, in the past tense. Alas! Mr Barker has again become an absentee; and the class of men to which they both belonged are fast disappearing. Improvement has peered beneath the aprons of our cabs, and penetrated to the very innermost recesses of our omnibuses. Dirt and fustian will vanish before cleanliness and livery. Slang will be forgotten when civility becomes general: and that enlightened, eloquent, sage, and profound body, the Magistracy of London, will be deprived of half their amusement, and half their occupation.

## Chapter Eighteen

### *A Parliamentary Sketch*

First published in this form in the *Second Series* (December 1836). This sketch represents a combination of two earlier, extensively revised pieces. The first, 'The House', had appeared in the *Evening Chronicle*, 7 March 1835 ('Sketches of London No. 5'), and the second, 'Bellamy's', had appeared in the *Evening Chronicle*, 11 April 1835 ('Sketches of London No. 8'). For a discussion of the original sketches and how Dickens revised them, see W.J. Carlton, 'Portraits in "A Parliamentary Sketch"', *The Dickensian*, Vol. 50 (1954), pp. 100–109. See also Butt and Tillotson, pp. 52–3.

Dickens began work as a Parliamentary reporter for the *True Sun* in 1832 and from 1834 to 1836 worked in this capacity for the *Morning Chronicle*; he worked, therefore, both in the old Houses of Parliament before they were destroyed by fire in October 1834, and in the temporary building erected pending the completion of the present Houses of Parliament. His experience left him with a profound contempt for most MPs (satirised in Cornelius Brook Dingwall in 'Sentiment' – see below, p. 318) and for the standard of debate and general conduct in the House of Commons. In an autobiographical passage in *David Copperfield* he has David remark of his time as a Parliamentary reporter, 'I am sufficiently behind the scenes to know the worth of political life. I am quite an infidel about it and shall never be converted.'

The MPs described in this sketch were all identifiable (see 'Portraits in "A Parliamentary Sketch"'). The 'ferocious-looking gentleman' with a 'large black moustache' was Colonel Sibthorp, the highly eccentric ultra-Tory who represented Lincoln 1826–33 and 1834–55. 'Honest Tom' was the Radical Thomas Slingsby Duncombe (1796–1861) who became MP for the newly created borough of Finsbury in 1834; he had a reputation for being a dandy. The other member for Finsbury – his colleague – was Thomas Wakely (1795–1862) who founded the *Lancet* in 1823. The 'quiet, gentlemanly-looking man' was John Gully, a former prizefighter, MP for Pontefract 1832–7, while the 'old hard featured man' was George Byng, Liberal MP for Middlesex 1790–1847 (the phrase about the 'memory of man' alludes to a formula in Blackstone's *Commentaries on the Laws of England* – 'The memory of man runneth not to the contrary', i.e., from time immemorial). The phrase 'hereditary bondsman' applied to the Irish journalist derives from Byron's *Childe Harold* canto 2, stanza 76, referring to the Greeks under Turkish rule.

Bellamy's Kitchen was a coffee and chop house next door to the old House of Commons very popular among MPs both because of the good food and because the division bell rang on the premises. When the new Houses of Parliament were opened in 1847 Bellamy's closed down, since MPs had their own dining room in the new building.

The 'Lord's Day Bill Baronet' is Sir Andrew Agnew (1793–1849) who unsuccessfully introduced a Bill for the Better Observance of Sunday in 1833. See headnote to *Sunday Under Three Heads* below, p. 475 ff.

We hope our readers will not be alarmed at this rather ominous title. We assure them that we are not about to become political, neither have we the slightest intention of being more prosy than usual – if we can help it. It has occurred to us that a slight sketch of the general aspect of 'the House', and the crowds that resort to it on the night of an important debate, would be productive of some amusement: and as we have made some few calls at the aforesaid house in our time – have visited it quite often enough for our purpose, and a great deal too often for our personal peace and comfort – we have determined to attempt the description. Dismissing from our minds, therefore, all that feeling of awe, which vague ideas of breaches of privilege, Serjeant-at-Arms, heavy denunciations, and still heavier fees, are calculated to awaken, we enter at once into the building, and upon our subject.

Half-past four o'clock – and at five the mover of the Address will be 'on his legs', as the newspapers announce sometimes by way of novelty, as if speakers were occasionally in the habit of standing on their heads. The members are pouring in, one after the other, in shoals. The few spectators who can obtain standing room in the passages, scrutinise them as they pass, with the utmost interest, and the man who can identify a member occasionally, becomes a person of great importance. Every now and then you hear earnest whispers of 'That's Sir John Thomson.' 'Which? him with the gilt order round his neck?' 'No, no; that's one of the messengers – that other with the yellow gloves, is Sir John Thomson.' 'Here's Mr Smith.' 'Lor!' 'Yes, how d'ye do, sir? – (He is our new member) – How do you do, sir?' Mr Smith stops: turns round with an air of enchanting urbanity (for the rumour of an intended dissolution has been very extensively circulated this morning); seizes both the hands of his gratified constituent, and, after greeting him with the most enthusiastic warmth, darts into the lobby with an extraordinary display of ardour in the public cause, leaving an immense impression in his favour on the mind of his 'fellow-townsman'.

The arrivals increase in number, and the heat and noise increase in very unpleasant proportion. The livery servants form a complete lane on either side of the passage, and you reduce yourself into the smallest possible space to avoid being turned out. You see that stout man with the hoarse voice, in the blue coat, queer-crowned, broad-brimmed hat, white corduroy breeches, and great boots, who has been talking incessantly for half an hour past, and whose importance has occasioned no small quantity of mirth among the strangers. That is the great conservator of the peace of Westminster. You cannot fail to have remarked the grace with which he saluted the noble Lord who passed just now, or the excessive dignity of his air, as he expostulates with the crowd. He is rather out of temper now, in consequence of the very irreverent behaviour of those two young fellows behind him, who have done nothing but laugh all the time they have been here.

'Will they divide tonight, do you think, Mr —?' timidly inquires a little thin man in the crowd, hoping to conciliate the man of office.

'How *can* you ask such questions, sir?' replies the functionary, in an incredibly loud key, and pettishly grasping the thick stick he carries in his right hand. 'Pray do not, sir. I beg of you; pray do not, sir.' The little man looks remarkably out of his element, and the uninitiated part of the throng are in positive convulsions of laughter.

Just at this moment some unfortunate individual appears, with a very smirking air, at the bottom of the long passage. He has managed to elude the vigilance of the special constable downstairs, and is evidently congratulating himself on having made his way so far.

'Go back, sir – you must *not* come here', shouts the hoarse one, with tremendous emphasis of voice and gesture, the moment the offender catches his eye.

The stranger pauses.

'Do you hear, sir – will you go back?' continues the official dignitary, gently pushing the intruder some half dozen yards.

'Come, don't push me,' replies the stranger, turning angrily round.

'I will, sir.'

'You won't, sir.'

'Go out, sir.'

'Take your hands off me, sir.'

'Go out of the passage, sir.'

'You're a Jack-in-office, sir.'

'A what?' ejaculates he of the boots.

'A Jack-in-office, sir, and a very insolent fellow,' reiterates the stranger, now completely in a passion.

'Pray do not force me to put you out, sir!' retorts the other – 'pray do not – my instructions are to keep this passage clear – it's the Speaker's orders, sir.'

'D–n the Speaker, sir!' shouts the intruder.

'Here, Wilson! – Collins!' gasps the officer, actually paralysed at this insulting expression, which in his mind is all but high treason; 'take this man out – take him out, I say! How dare you, sir?' and down goes the unfortunate man five stairs at a time, turning round at every stoppage, to come back again, and denouncing bitter vengeance against the commander-in-chief, and all his supernumeraries.

'Make way, gentlemen, – pray make way for the Members, I beg of you!' shouts the zealous officer, turning back, and preceding a whole string of the liberal and independent.

You see this ferocious-looking gentleman, with a complexion almost as sallow as his linen, and whose large black moustache would give him the appearance of a figure in a hairdresser's window, if his countenance possessed the thought which is communicated to those waxen caricatures of the human face divine. He is a militia officer, and the most amusing person in the House. Can anything be more exquisitely absurd than the burlesque grandeur of his air, as he strides up to the lobby, his eyes rolling like those of a Turk's head in a cheap Dutch clock? He never appears without that bundle of dirty papers which he carries under his left arm, and which are generally supposed to be the miscellaneous estimates for 1804, or some equally important documents. He is very punctual in his attendance at the House, and his self-satisfied 'He-ar-He-ar', is not unfrequently the signal for a general titter.

This is the gentleman who once actually sent a messenger up to the Stranger's gallery in the old House of Commons, to inquire the name of an individual who was using an eye-glass, in order that he might complain to the Speaker that the person in question was quizzing him! On another occasion, he is reported to have repaired to Bellamy's kitchen – a refreshment room, where persons who are not Members are admitted on sufferance, as it were – and perceiving two or three gentlemen, at supper, who he was aware were not Members, and could not, in that place, very well resent his behaviour, he indulged in the pleasantry of sitting with his booted leg on the table at which they were supping! He is generally harmless, though, and always amusing.

By dint of patience, and some little interest with our friend the constable, we have contrived to make our way to the Lobby, and you can just manage to catch an occasional glimpse of the House, as the door is opened for the admission of Members. It is tolerably full already, and little groups of Members are congregated together here, discussing the interesting topics of the day.

That smart-looking fellow in the black coat with velvet facings and cuffs, who wears his *D'Orsay* hat so rakishly, is 'Honest Tom', a metropolitan representative; and the large man in the cloak with the white lining – not the man by the pillar; the other with the light hair hanging over his coat collar behind – is his colleague. The quiet gentlemanly-looking man in the blue surtout, grey trousers, white neckerchief, and gloves, whose closely-buttoned coat displays his manly figure and broad chest to great advantage, is a very well known character. He has fought a great many battles in his time, and conquered like the heroes of old, with no other arms than those the gods gave him. The old hard-featured man who is standing near him, is really a good specimen of a class of men now nearly extinct. He is a county Member, and has been from time whereof the memory of man is not to the contrary. Look at his loose, wide, brown coat, with capacious pockets on each side; the knee breeches and boots, the immensely long waistcoat, and silver watch chain dangling below it, the wide-brimmed brown hat, and the white handkerchief tied in a great bow, with straggling ends sticking out beyond his shirt frill. It is a costume one seldom sees nowadays, and when the few who wear it have died off, it will be quite extinct. He can tell you long stories of Fox, Pitt, Sheridan, and Canning, and how much better the House was managed in those times, when they used to get up at eight or nine o'clock, except on regular field-days, of which everybody was apprised beforehand. He has a great contempt for all young Members of Parliament, and thinks it quite impossible that a man can say anything worth hearing, unless he has sat in the House for fifteen years at least, without saying anything at all. He is of opinion that 'that young Macaulay' was a regular impostor; he allows that Lord Stanley may do something one of these days, but 'he's too young, sir – too young'. He is an excellent authority on points of precedent, and when he grows talkative, after his wine, will tell you how Sir Somebody Something, when he was whipper-in for the Government, brought four men out of their beds to vote in the majority, three of whom died on their way home again; how the House once divided on the question, that fresh candles be now brought in; how the Speaker was once upon a time left in the chair by accident, at the conclusion of business, and was obliged to sit in the House by himself for three hours, till some Member could be knocked up and brought back again, to move the adjournment; and a great many other anecdotes of a similar description.

There he stands, leaning on his stick; looking at the throng of Exquisites around him with most profound contempt; and conjuring up, before his mind's eye, the scenes he beheld in the old House, in days gone by, when his own feelings were fresher and brighter, and when, as he imagines, wit, talent, and patriotism flourished more brightly too.

You are curious to know who that young man in the rough greatcoat is, who has accosted every Member who has entered the House since we have been standing here. He is not a Member; he is only an 'hereditary bondsman', or, in other words, an Irish correspondent of an Irish newspaper, who has just procured his forty-second frank from a Member whom he never saw in his life before. There he goes again – another! Bless the man, he has his hat and pockets full already.

We will try our fortune at the Strangers' gallery, though the nature of the debate encourages very little hope of success. What on earth are you about? Holding up your order as if it were a talisman at whose command the wicket would fly open? Nonsense. Just preserve the order for an autograph, if it be worth keeping at all, and make your appearance at the door with your thumb and forefinger expressively inserted in you waistcoat pocket. This tall stout man in black is the doorkeeper. 'Any room?' 'Not an inch – two or three dozen gentlemen, waiting downstairs on the chance of somebody's going out.' Pull out your purse – 'Are you *quite* sure there's no room?' – 'I'll go and look,' replies the doorkeeper, with a wistful glance at your purse, 'but I'm afraid there's not.' He returns, and with real feeling assures you that it is morally impossible to get near the gallery. It is of no use waiting. When you are refused admission into the Strangers' gallery at the House of Commons, under such circumstances, you may return home thoroughly satisfied that the place must be remarkably full indeed.[1]

Retracing our steps through the long passage, descending the stairs and crossing Palace Yard, we halt at a small temporary doorway adjoining the King's entrance to the House of Lords. The order of the serjeant-at-arms will admit you into the Reporters' gallery, from whence you can obtain a tolerably good view of the House. Take care of the stairs, they are none of the best; through this little wicket – there. As soon as your eyes become a little used to the mist of the place, and the glare of the chandeliers below you, you will see that some unimportant personage on the Ministerial side of the House (to your right hand) is speaking, amidst a hum of voices and confusion which would rival Babel, but for the circumstance of its being all in one language.

The 'hear, hear', which occasioned that laugh, proceeded from our warlike friend with the moustache; he is sitting on the back seat against the wall, behind the Member who is speaking, looking as ferocious and intellectual as usual. Take one look around you, and retire! The body of the House and the side galleries are full of Members; some, with their legs on the back of the opposite seat; some, with theirs stretched out to their utmost length on the floor; some going out, others coming in; all talking, laughing, lounging, coughing, oh-ing, questioning, or groaning; presenting a conglomeration of noise and confusion, to be met with in no other place in existence, not even excepting Smithfield on a market day, or a cockpit in its glory.

[1] This paper was written before the practice of exhibiting Members of Parliament, like other curiosities, for the small charge of half-a-crown, was abolished.

But let us not omit to notice Bellamy's kitchen, or, in other words, the refreshment room, common to both Houses of Parliament, where Ministerialists and Oppositionists, Whigs and Tories, Radicals, Peers and Destructives, strangers from the gallery, and the more favoured strangers from below the bar, are alike at liberty to resort; where divers honourable members prove their perfect independence by remaining during the whole of a heavy debate, solacing themselves with the creature comforts; and whence they are summoned by whippers-in, when the House is on the point of dividing; either to give their 'conscientious votes' on questions of which they are conscientiously innocent of knowing anything whatever, or to find a vent for the playful exuberance of their wine-inspired fancies, in boisterous shouts of 'Divide', occasionally varied with a little howling, barking, crowing, or other ebullitions of senatorial pleasantry.

When you have ascended the narrow staircase which, in the present temporary House of Commons, leads to the place we are describing, you will probably observe a couple of rooms on your right hand, with tables spread for dining. Neither of these is the kitchen, although they are both devoted to the same purpose; the kitchen is further on to our left, up these half dozen stairs. Before we ascend the staircase, however, we must request you to pause in front of this little bar place with the sash windows; and beg your particular attention to the steady honest-looking old fellow in black, who is its sole occupant. Nicholas (we do not mind mentioning the old fellow's name, for if Nicholas be not a public man, who is? – and public men's names are public property) – Nicholas is the butler of Bellamy's, and has held the same place, dressed exactly in the same manner, and said precisely the same things, ever since the oldest of its present visitors can remember. An excellent servant Nicholas is – an unrivalled compounder of salad dressing – an admirable preparer of soda water and lemon – a special mixer of cold grog and punch – and, above all, an unequalled judge of cheese. If the old man have such a thing as vanity in his composition, this is certainly his pride; and if it be possible to imagine that anything in this world could disturb his impenetrable calmness, we should say it would be the doubting his judgment on this important point.

We needn't tell you all this, however, for if you have an atom of observation, one glance at his sleek, knowing-looking head and face – his prim white neckerchief, with the wooden tie into which it has been regularly folded for twenty years past, merging by imperceptible degrees into a small plaited shirt frill – and his comfortable-looking form encased in a well-brushed suit of black – would give you a better idea of his real character than a column of our poor description could convey.

Nicholas is rather out of his element now; he cannot see the kitchen as he used to in the old House; there, one window of his glass-case opened into the room, and then, for the edification and behoof of more juvenile questioners, he would stand for an hour together, answering deferential questions about Sheridan, and Perceval, and Castlereagh, and Heaven knows who beside, with manifest delight, always inserting a 'Mister' before every commoner's name.

Nicholas, like all men of his age and standing, has a great idea of the degeneracy of the times. He seldom expresses any political opinions, but we managed to ascertain, just before the passing of the Reform Bill, that Nicholas was a thorough Reformer. What was our astonishment to discover shortly after the meeting of the first reformed Parliament, that he was a most inveterate and decided Tory! It was very odd: some men change their opinions from necessity, others from expediency, others from inspiration; but that Nicholas should undergo any change in any respect, was an event we had never contemplated, and should have considered impossible. His strong opinion against the clause which empowered the metropolitan districts to return Members to Parliament, too, was perfectly unaccountable.

We discovered the secret at last; the metropolitan Members always dined at home. The rascals! As for giving additional Members to Ireland, it was even worse – decidedly unconstitutional. Why, sir, an Irish Member would go up there, and eat more dinner than three English Members put together. He took no wine; drank table-beer by the half-gallon; and went home to Manchester Buildings, or Millbank Street, for his whiskey and water. And what was the consequence? Why, the concern lost – actually lost, sir – by his patronage. A queer old fellow is Nicholas, and as completely a part of the building as the house itself. We wonder he ever left the old place, and fully expected to see in the papers, the morning after the fire, a pathetic account of an old gentleman in black, of decent appearance, who was seen at one of the upper windows when the flames were at their height, and declared his resolute intention of falling with the floor. He must have been got out by force. However, he was got out – here he is again, looking as he always does, as if he had been in a bandbox ever since the last session. There he is, at his old post every night, just as we have described him: and, as characters are scarce, and faithful servants scarcer, long may he be there, say we!

Now, when you have taken your seat in the kitchen, and duly noticed the large fire and roasting jack at one end of the room – the little table for washing glasses and draining jugs at the other – the clock over the window opposite St Margaret's Church – the deal tables and wax candles – the damask tablecloths and bare floor – the plate and china on the tables, and the gridiron on the fire; and a few other anomalies peculiar to the place – we will point out to your notice two or three of the people present, whose station or absurdities render them the most worthy of remark.

It is half-past twelve o'clock, and as the division is not expected for an hour or two, a few Members are lounging away the time here in preference to standing at the bar of the House, or sleeping in one of the side galleries. That singularly awkward and ungainly-looking man, in the brownish-white hat, with the straggling black trousers which reach about halfway down the legs of his boots, who is leaning against the meat screen, apparently deluding himself into the belief that he is thinking about something, is a splendid sample of a Member of the House of Commons concentrating in his own person the wisdom of a constituency. Observe the wig, of a dark hue but indescribable colour, for if it be naturally brown, it has acquired a black tint by long service, and if it be naturally black, the same cause has imparted to it a tinge of rusty brown; and remark how very materially the great blinker-like spectacles assist the expression of that most intelligent face. Seriously speaking, did you ever see a countenance so expressive of the most hopeless extreme of heavy dulness, or behold a form so strangely put together? He is no great speaker: but when he *does* address the House, the effect is absolutely irresistible.

The small gentleman with the sharp nose, who has just saluted him, is a Member of Parliament, an ex-Alderman, and a sort of amateur fireman. He, and the celebrated fireman's dog, were observed to be remarkably active at the conflagration of the two Houses of Parliament – they both ran up and down, and in and out, getting under people's feet, and into everybody's way, fully impressed with the belief that they were doing a great deal of good, and barking tremendously. The dog went quietly back to his kennel with the engine, but the gentleman kept up such an incessant noise for some weeks after the occurrence, that he became a positive nuisance. As no more Parliamentary fires have occurred, however, and as he has consequently had no more opportunities of writing to the newspapers to relate how, by way of preserving pictures he cut them out of their frames, and performed other great national services, he has gradually relapsed into his old state of calmness.

That female in black – not the one whom the Lord's Day Bill Baronet has just chucked under the chin; the shorter of the two – is 'Jane': the Hebe of Bellamy's. Jane is as great a character as Nicholas, in her way. Her leading features are a thorough contempt for the great majority of her visitors; her predominant quality, love of admiration, as you cannot fail to observe, if you mark the glee with which she listens to something the young Member near her mutters somewhat unintelligibly in her ear (for his speech is rather thick from some cause or other), and how playfully she digs the handle of a fork into the arm with which he detains her, by way of reply.

Jane is no bad hand at repartees, and showers them about, with a degree of liberality and total absence of reserve or constraint, which occasionally excites no small amazement in the minds of strangers. She cuts jokes with Nicholas, too, but looks up to him with a great deal of respect; the immovable stolidity with which Nicholas receives the aforesaid jokes, and looks on, at certain pastoral friskings and rompings (Jane's only recreations, and they are very innocent too) which occasionally take place in the passage, is not the least amusing part of his character.

The two persons who are seated at the table in the corner, at the farther end of the room, have been constant guests here, for many years past; and one of them has feasted within these walls many a time, with the most brilliant characters of a brilliant period. He has gone up to the other House since then; the greater part of his boon companions have shared Yorick's fate, and his visits to Bellamy's are comparatively few.

If he really be eating his supper now, at what hour can he possibly have dined! A second solid mass of rump steak has disappeared, and he eat the first in four minutes and three quarters, by the clock over the window. Was there ever such a personification of Falstaff! Mark the air with which he gloats over that Stilton, as he removes the napkin which has been placed beneath his chin to catch the superfluous gravy of the steak, and with what gusto he imbibes the porter which has been fetched, expressly for him, in the pewter pot. Listen to the hoarse sound of that voice, kept down as it is by layers of solids, and deep draughts of rich wine, and tell us if you ever saw such a perfect picture of a regular *gourmand*; and whether he is not exactly the man whom you would pitch upon as having been the partner of Sheridan's parliamentary carouses, the volunteer driver of the hackney coach that took him home, and the involuntary upsetter of the whole party?

What an amusing contrast between his voice and appearance, and that of the spare, squeaking old man, who sits at the same table, and who, elevating a little cracked bantam sort of voice to its highest pitch, invokes damnation upon his own eyes or somebody else's at the commencement of every sentence he utters. 'The Captain', as they call him, is a very old frequenter of Bellamy's; much addicted to stopping 'after the House is up' (an inexpiable crime in Jane's eyes), and a complete walking reservoir of spirits and water.

The old Peer – or rather, the old man – for his peerage is of comparatively recent date – has a huge tumbler of hot punch brought him; and the other damns and drinks, and drinks and damns, and smokes. Members arrive every moment in a great bustle to report that 'The Chancellor of the Exchequer's up', and to get glasses of brandy and water to sustain them during the division; people who have ordered supper, countermand it, and prepare to go downstairs, when suddenly a bell is heard to ring with tremendous violence, and a cry of 'Di-vi-sion!' is heard in the passage. This is enough; away rush the members pell-mell. The room is cleared is an instant; the noise rapidly dies away; you hear the creaking of the last boot on the last stair, and are left alone with the leviathan of rump steaks.

## Chapter Nineteen

### *Public Dinners*

First published in the *Evening Chronicle*, 7 April 1835 ('Sketches of London No.7'). Throughout the early and mid nineteenth century, public dinners were exclusively male affairs, ladies being admitted to a gallery overlooking the hall only after the actual eating was over, in time to hear the speeches. Dickens, who himself became a highly praised and much sought after speaker at such dinners, protested strongly against this segregation of the sexes at a Royal Society of Musicians Dinner, 8 March 1860 (see K.J. Fielding, *The Speeches of Charles Dickens*, [1960], p. 297).

All public dinners in London, from the Lord Mayor's annual banquet at Guildhall, to the Chimney sweepers' anniversary at White Conduit House; from the Goldsmiths' to the Butchers', from the Sheriffs' to the Licensed Victuallers'; are amusing scenes. Of all entertainments of this description, however, we think the annual dinner of some public charity is the most amusing. At a Company's dinner, the people are nearly all alike – regular old stagers, who make it a matter of business, and a thing not to be laughed at. At a political dinner, everybody is disagreeable, and inclined to speechify – much the same thing, by-the-bye; but at a charity dinner you see people of all sorts, kinds, and descriptions. The wine may not be remarkably special, to be sure, and we have heard some hard-hearted monsters grumble at the collection; but we really think the amusement to be derived from the occasion, sufficient to counterbalance even these disadvantages.

Let us suppose you are induced to attend a dinner of this description – 'Indigent Orphans' Friends' Benevolent Institution', we think it is. The name of the charity is a line or two longer, but never mind the rest. You have a distinct recollection, however, that you purchased a ticket at the solicitation of some charitable friend: and you deposit yourself in a hackney coach, the driver of which – no doubt that you may do the thing in style – turns a deaf ear to your earnest entreaties to be set down at the corner of Great Queen Street, and persists in carrying you to the very door of the Freemasons', round which a crowd of people are assembled to witness the entrance of the indigent orphans' friends. You hear great speculations

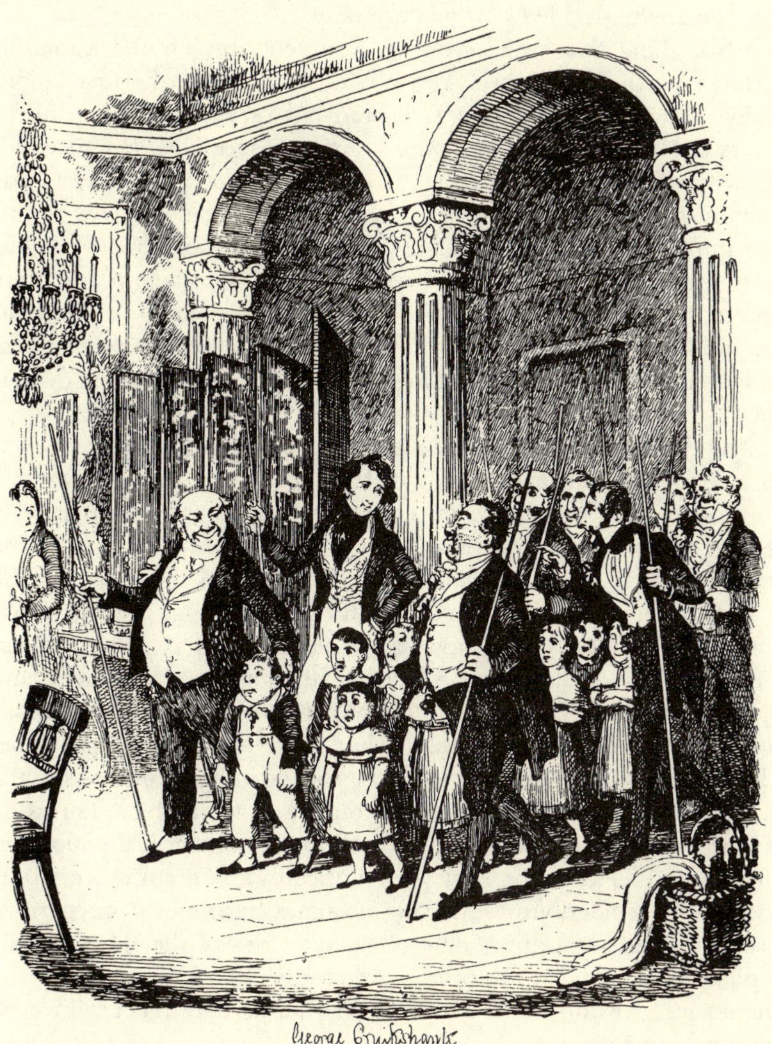


*Public Dinners*

Note: Cruikshank has depicted Dickens and himself (right) behind the leading stewards.

as you pay the fare, on the possibility of your being the noble Lord who is announced to fill the chair on the occasion, and are highly gratified to hear it eventually decided that you are only a 'wocalist'.

The first thing that strikes you, on your entrance, is the astonishing importance of the committee. You observe a door on the first landing, carefully guarded by two waiters, in and out of which stout gentlemen with very red faces keep running, with a degree of speed highly unbecoming the gravity of persons of their years and corpulency. You pause, quite alarmed at the bustle, and thinking, in your innocence, that two or three people must have been carried out of the dining room in fits, at least. You are immediately undeceived by the waiter – 'Upstairs, if you please, sir; this is the committee room.' Upstairs you go, accordingly; wondering, as you mount, what the duties of the committee can be, and whether they ever do anything beyond confusing each other, and running over the waiters.

Having deposited your hat and cloak, and received a remarkably small scrap of pasteboard in exchange (which, as a matter of course, you lose, before you require it again), you enter the hall, down which there are three long tables for the less distinguished guests, with a cross table on a raised platform at the upper end for the reception of the very particular friends of the indigent orphans. Being fortunate enough to find a plate without anybody's card in it, you wisely seat yourself at once, and have a little leisure to look about you. Waiters, with wine baskets in their hands, are placing decanters of sherry down the tables, at very respectable distances; melancholy-looking salt cellars, and decayed vinegar cruets, which might have belonged to the parents of the indigent orphans in their time, are scattered at distant intervals on the cloth; and the knives and forks look as if they had done duty at every public dinner in London since the accession of George the First. The musicians are scraping and grating and screwing tremendously – playing no notes but notes of preparation; and several gentlemen are gliding along the sides of the tables, looking into plate after plate with frantic eagerness, the expression of their countenances growing more and more dismal as they meet with everybody's card but their own.

You turn round to take a look at the table behind you, and – not being in the habit of attending public dinners – are somewhat struck by the appearance of the party on which your eyes rest. One of its principal members appears to be a little man, with a long and rather inflamed face, and grey hair brushed bolt upright in front; he wears a wisp of black silk round his neck, without any stiffener, as an apology for a neckerchief, and is addressed by his companions by the familiar appellation of 'Fitz', or some such monosyllable. Near him is a stout man in a white neckerchief and buff waistcoat, with shining dark hair, cut very short in front, and a great round healthy-looking face, on which he studiously preserves a half sentimental simper. Next him, again, is a large-headed man, with black hair and bushy whiskers; and opposite them are two or three others, one of whom is a little round-faced person in a dress-stock and blue under-waistcoat. There is something peculiar in their air and manner, though you could hardly describe what it is; you cannot divest yourself of the idea that they have come for some other purpose than mere eating and drinking. You have no time to debate the matter, however, for the waiters (who have been arranged in lines down the room, placing the dishes on table) retire to the lower end; the dark man in the blue coat and bright buttons, who has the direction of the music, looks up to the gallery, and calls out 'band' in a very loud voice; out burst the orchestra, up rise the visitors, in march fourteen stewards, each with a long wand in his hand, like the evil genius in a pantomime; then the chairman, then the titled visitors; they all make their way up the room, as fast as they can, bowing, and smiling, and smirking, and looking remarkably amiable. The applause ceases, grace is said, the clatter of plates and dishes begins; and everyone appears highly gratified, either with the presence of the distinguished visitors, or the commencement of the anxiously expected dinner.

As to the dinner itself – the mere dinner – it goes off much the same everywhere. Tureens of soup are emptied with awful rapidity – waiters take plates of turbot away, to get lobster sauce, and bring back plates of lobster sauce without turbot; people who can carve poultry, are great fools if they own it, and people who can't have no wish to learn. The knives and forks form a pleasing accompaniment to Auber's music, and Auber's music would form a pleasing accompaniment to the dinner, if you could hear anything besides the cymbals. The substantials disappear – moulds of jelly vanish like lightning – hearty eaters wipe their foreheads, and appear rather overcome by their recent exertions – people who have looked very cross hitherto, become remarkably bland, and ask you to take wine in the most friendly manner possible – old gentlemen direct your attention to the ladies' gallery, and take great pains to impress you with the fact that the charity is always peculiarly favoured in this respect – everyone appears disposed to become talkative – and the hum of conversation is loud and general.

'Pray, silence, gentlemen, if you please, for *Non nobis!*' shouts the toast-master with stentorian lungs – a toast master's shirt-front, waistcoat, and neckerchief, by-the-bye, always exhibit three distinct shades of cloudy white. – 'Pray, silence, gentlemen, for *Non nobis!*' The singers, whom you discover to be no other than the very party that excited your curiosity at first, after 'pitching' their voices immediately begin *too-too*ing most dismally, on which the regular old stagers burst into occasional cries of – 'Sh – Sh – waiters! – Silence, waiters – stand still, waiters – keep back, waiters,' and other exorcisms, delivered in a tone of indignant remonstrance. The grace is soon concluded, and the company resume their seats. The uninitiated portion of the guests applaud *Non nobis* as vehemently as if it were a capital comic song, greatly to the scandal and indignation of the regular diners, who immediately attempt to quell this sacrilegious approbation, by cries of 'Hush, hush!' whereupon the others, mistaking these sounds for hisses, applaud more tumultuously than before, and, by way of placing their approval beyond the possibility of doubt, shout '*Encore!*' most vociferously.

The moment the noise ceases, up starts the toast master: – 'Gentlemen, charge your glasses, if you please!' Decanters having been handed about, and glasses filled, the toast master proceeds, in a regular ascending scale: 'Gentlemen – *air* – you – all charged? Pray – silence – gentlemen – for – the cha–i–r!' The chairman rises, and after stating that he feels it quite unnecessary to preface the toast he is about to propose, with any observations whatever, wanders into a maze of sentences, and flounders about in the most extraordinary manner, presenting a lamentable spectacle of mystified humanity, until he arrives at the words, 'constitutional sovereign of these realms', at which elderly gentlemen exclaim 'Bravo!' and hammer the table tremendously with their knife handles. 'Under any circumstances, it would give him the greatest pride, it would give him the greatest pleasure – he might almost say, it would afford him satisfaction [cheers] to propose that toast. What must be his feelings, then, when he has the gratification of announcing, that he has received her Majesty's commands to apply to the Treasurer of her Majesty's Household, for her Majesty's annual donation of 25*l.* in aid of the funds of this charity!' This announcement (which has been regularly made by every chairman, since the first foundation of the charity, forty-two years ago) calls forth the most vociferous applause; the toast is drunk with a great deal of cheering and knocking; and 'God save the Queen' is sung by the 'professional gentlemen'; the unprofessional gentlemen joining in the chorus, and giving the national anthem an effect which the newspapers, with great justice, describe as 'perfectly electrical'.

The other 'loyal' and 'patriotic' toasts having been drunk with all due enthusiasm, a comic song having been well sung by the gentleman with the small neckerchief, and a sentimental one by the second of the party, we come to the most important toast of the evening – 'Prosperity to the charity'. Here again we are compelled to adopt newspaper phraseology, and to express our regret at being 'precluded from giving even the substance of the noble lord's observations'. Suffice it to say, that the speech, which is somewhat of the longest, is rapturously received; and the toast having been drunk, the stewards (looking more important than ever) leave the room, and presently return, heading a procession of indigent orphans, boys and girls, who walk round the room, curtseying and bowing, and treading on each other's heels, and looking very much as if they would like a glass of wine apiece, to the high gratification of the company generally, and especially of the lady patronesses in the gallery. *Exeunt* children, and re-enter stewards, each with a blue plate in his hand. The band plays a lively air; the majority of the company put their hands into their pockets and look rather serious; and the noise of sovereigns, rattling on crockery, is heard from all parts of the room.

After a short interval, occupied in singing and toasting, the secretary puts on his spectacles, and proceeds to read the report and list of subscriptions, the latter being listened to with great attention. 'Mr Smith, one guinea – Mr Tompkins, one guinea – Mr Wilson, one guinea – Mr Hickson, one guinea – Mr Nixon, one guinea – Mr Charles Nixon, one guinea – [hear, hear!] – Mr James Nixon, one guinea – Mr Thomas Nixon, one pound one [tremendous applause]. Lord Fitz Binkle, the chairman of the day, in addition to an annual donation of fifteen pounds – thirty guineas [prolonged knocking: several gentlemen knock the stems off their wine glasses, in the vehemence of their approbation]. Lady Fitz Binkle, in addition to an annual donation of ten pound – twenty pound,' [protracted knocking and shouts of 'Bravo!']. The list being at length concluded, the chairman rises, and proposes the health of the secretary, than whom he knows no more zealous or estimable individual. The secretary, in returning thanks, observes that *he* knows no more excellent individual than the chairman – except the senior officer of the charity, whose health *he* begs to propose. The senior officer, in returning thanks, observes that *he* knows no more worthy man than the secretary – except Mr Walker, the auditor, whose health *he* begs to propose. Mr Walker, in returning thanks, discovers some other estimable individual, to whom alone the senior officer is inferior – and so they go on toasting and lauding and thanking: the only other toast of importance being 'The Lady Patronesses now present!' on which all the gentlemen turn their faces towards the ladies' gallery, shouting tremendously; and little priggish men, who have imbibed more wine than usual, kiss their hands and exhibit distressing contortions of visage.

We have protracted our dinner to so great a length, that we have hardly time to add one word by way of grace. We can only entreat our readers not to imagine, because we have attempted to extract some amusement from a charity dinner, that we are at all disposed to underrate, either the excellence of the benevolent institutions with which London abounds, or the estimable motives of those who support them.

## Chapter Twenty

### *The First of May*

First published as 'A Little Talk about Spring and the Sweeps' in Chapman and Hall; new monthly publication, *The Library of Fiction; or Family Story-teller; Consisting of Original Tales, Essays and Sketches of Character*, No. 3, 31 May 1836 (For Dickens's only other publication in this series see below, p. 327 ['The Tuggses at Ramsgate']). May Day was a traditional holiday for sweeps as for other workers. Groups of sweeps would parade the streets in fancy dress while one of them called 'Jack-in-the-Green' would be hidden in a portable framework of leaves and branches. Money would be solicited from passers by by a woman carrying a brass ladle using some such formula as that used by Dickens for the first of his epigraphs; the second epigraph refers to the recent legislation prohibiting sweeps from advertising their presence by calling out in the streets (see Dickens's ironic reference to this in 'The Streets – Morning', p. 51, above; see also his allusion to the Jack-in-the-Green and lady with the brass ladle in 'The Bloomsbury Christening', below, p. 453). For a detailed discussion of this sketch see G.C. Phillips, 'Dickens and the Chimney-Sweepers', *The Dickensian*, Vol. 59 (1963), pp. 28–44.

'Now ladies, up in the sky-parlour: only once a year, if you please!'
Young Lady with Brass Ladle.

'Sweep – sweep – sw-e-ep!'
Illegal Watchword.

The first of May! There is a merry freshness in the sound, calling to our minds a thousand thoughts of all that is pleasant in nature and beautiful in her most delightful form. What man is there, over whose mind a bright spring morning does not exercise a magic influence – carrying him back to the days of his childish sports, and conjuring up before him the old green field with its gently waving trees, where the birds sang as he has never heard them since – where the butterfly fluttered far more gaily than he ever sees him now, in all his ramblings – where the sky seemed bluer, and the sun shone more brightly – where the air blew more freshly over greener grass, and sweeter-smelling flowers – where everything wore a richer and more brilliant hue than it is ever dressed in now! Such are the

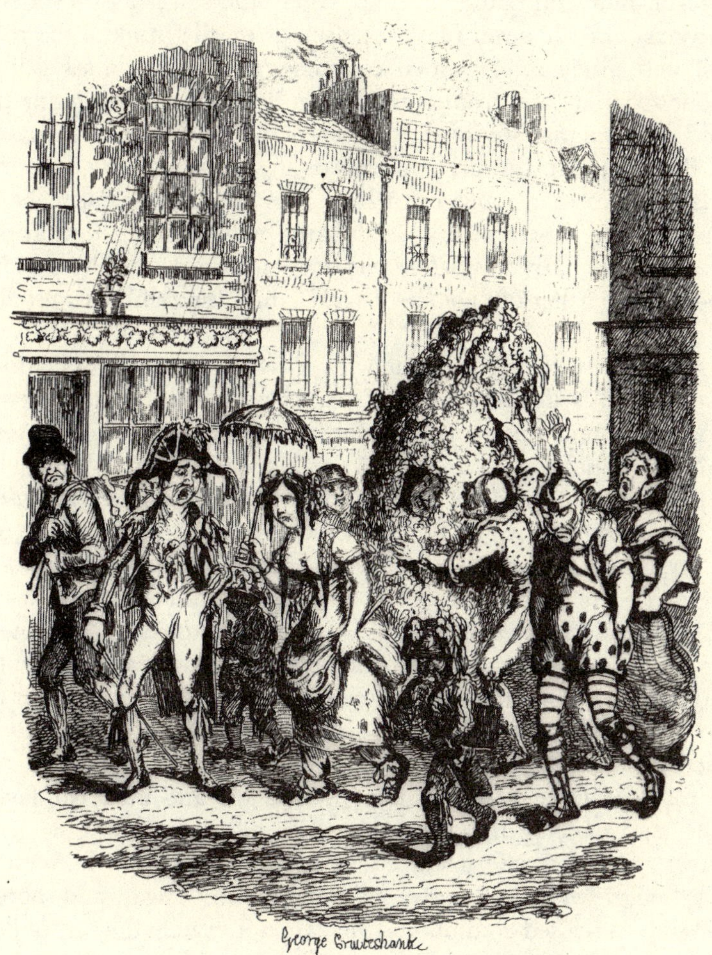


*The First of May*

deep feelings of childhood, and such are the impressions which every lovely object stamps upon its heart! The hardy traveller wanders through the maze of thick and pathless woods, where the sun's rays never shone, and heaven's pure air never played; he stands on the brink of the roaring waterfall, and, giddy and bewildered, watches the foaming mass as it leaps from stone to stone, and from crag to crag; he lingers in the fertile plains of a land of perpetual sunshine, and revels in the luxury of their balmy breath. But what are the deep forests, or the thundering waters, or the richest landscapes that bounteous nature ever spread, to charm the eyes, and captivate the senses of man, compared with the recollection of the old scenes of his early youth? Magic scenes indeed; for the fancies of childhood dressed them in colours brighter than the rainbow, and almost as fleeting!

In former times, spring brought with it not only such associations as these, connected with the past, but sports and games for the present – merry dances round rustic pillars, adorned with emblems of the season, and reared in honour of its coming. Where are they now? Pillars we have, but they are no longer rustic ones; and as to dancers, they are used to rooms, and lights, and would not show well in the open air. Think of the immorality, too! What would your sabbath enthusiasts say, to an aristocratic ring encircling the Duke of York's column in Carlton Terrace – a grand *poussette* of the middle classes, round Alderman Waithman's monument in Fleet Street, – or a general hands-four-round of ten-pound householders, at the foot of the Obelisk in St George's Fields? Alas! romance can make no head against the riot act; and pastoral simplicity is not understood by the police.

Well; many years ago we began to be a steady and matter-of-fact sort of people, and dancing in spring being beneath our dignity, we gave it up, and in course of time it descended to the sweeps – a fall certainly, because, though sweeps are very good fellows in their way, and moreover very useful in a civilised community, they are not exactly the sort of people to give the tone to the little elegances of society. The sweeps, however, got the dancing to themselves, and they kept it up, and handed it down. This was a severe blow to the romance of springtime, but it did not entirely destroy it either; for a portion of it descended to the sweeps with the dancing, and rendered them objects of great interest. A mystery hung over the sweeps in those days. Legends were in existence of wealthy gentlemen who had lost children, and who, after many years of sorrow and suffering, had found them in the character of sweeps. Stories were related of a young boy who, having been stolen from his parents in his infancy, and devoted to the occupation of chimney sweeping, was sent, in the course of his professional career, to sweep the chimney of his mother's bedroom; and how, being hot and tired when he came out of the chimney, he got into the bed he had so often slept in as an infant, and was discovered and recognised therein by his mother, who once every year of her life, thereafter, requested the pleasure of the company of every London sweep, at half-past one o'clock, to roast beef, plum pudding, porter, and sixpence.

Such stories as these, and there were many such, threw an air of mystery round the sweeps, and produced for them some of those good effects which animals derive from the doctrine of the transmigration of souls. No one (except the masters) thought of ill-treating a sweep, because no one knew who he might be, or what nobleman's or gentleman's son he might turn out. Chimney sweeping was, by many believers in the marvellous, considered as a sort of probationary term, at an earlier or later period of which, divers young noblemen were to come into possession of their rank and title: and the profession was held by them in great respect accordingly.

We remember, in our young days, a little sweep about our own age, with curly hair and white teeth, whom we so devoutly and sincerely believed to be the lost son and heir of some illustrious personage – an impression which was resolved into an unchangeable conviction on our infant mind, by the subject of our speculations informing us, one day, in reply to our question, propounded a few moments before his ascent to the summit of the kitchen chimney, 'that he believed he'd been born in the vurkis, but he'd never know'd his father.' We felt certain, from that time forth, that he would one day be owned by a lord; and we never heard the church bells ring, or saw a flag hoisted in the neighbourhood, without thinking that the happy event had at last occurred, and that his long-lost parent had arrived in a coach and six, to take him home to Grosvenor Square. He never came, however; and, at the present moment, the young gentleman in question is settled down as a master sweep in the neighbourhood of Battle Bridge, his distinguishing characteristics being a decided antipathy to washing himself, and the possession of a pair of legs very inadequate to the support of his unwieldy and corpulent body.

The romance of spring having gone out before our time, we were fain to console ourselves as we best could with the uncertainty that enveloped the birth and parentage of its attendant dancers, the sweeps; and we *did* console ourselves with it, for many years. But even this wretched source of comfort received a shock from which it has never recovered – a shock which has been in reality its death blow. We could not disguise from ourselves the fact that whole families of sweeps were regularly born of sweeps, in the rural districts of Somers Town and Camden Town – that the eldest son succeeded to the father's business, that the other branches assisted him therein, and commenced on their own account; that their children again, were educated to the profession; and that about their identity there could be no mistake whatever. We could not be blind, we say, to this melancholy truth, but we could not bring ourselves to admit it, nevertheless, and we lived on for some years in a state of voluntary ignorance. We were roused from our pleasant slumber by certain dark insinuations thrown out by a friend of ours, to the effect that children in the lower ranks of life were beginning to *choose* chimney sweeping as their particular walk; that applications had been made by various boys to the constituted authorities, to allow them to pursue the object of their ambition with the full concurrence and sanction of the law; that the affair, in short, was becoming one of mere legal contract. We turned a deaf ear to these rumours at first, but slowly and surely they stole upon us. Month after month, week after week, nay, day after day, at last, did we meet with accounts of similar applications. The veil was removed, all mystery was at an end, and chimney sweeping had become a favourite and chosen pursuit. There is no longer any occasion to steal boys; for boys flock in crowds to bind themselves. The romance of the trade has fled, and the chimney sweeper of the present day is no more like unto him of thirty years ago, than is a Fleet Street pickpocket to a Spanish brigand, or Paul Pry to Caleb Williams.

This gradual decay and disuse of the practice of leading noble youths into captivity, and compelling them to ascend chimneys, was a severe blow, if we may so speak, to the romance of chimney sweeping, and to the romance of spring at the same time. But even this was not all, for some few years ago the dancing on May-day began to decline; small sweeps were observed to congregate in twos or threes, unsupported by a 'green', with no 'My Lord' to act as master of the ceremonies, and no 'My Lady' to preside over the exchequer. Even in companies where there was a 'green' it was an absolute nothing – a mere sprout – and the instrumental accompaniments rarely extended beyond the shovels and a set of Pan pipes, better known to the many, as a 'mouth organ'.

These were signs of the times, portentous omens of a coming change; and what was the result which they shadowed forth? Why, the master sweeps, influenced by a restless spirit of innovation, actually interposed their authority, in opposition to the dancing, and substituted a dinner – an anniversary dinner at White Conduit House – where clean faces appeared in lieu of black ones smeared with rose pink; and knee cords and tops superseded nankeen drawers and rosetted shoes.

Gentlemen who were in the habit of riding shy horses; and steady going people who have no vagrancy in their souls, lauded this alteration to the skies, and the conduct of the master sweeps was described as beyond the reach of praise. But how stands the real fact? Let any man deny, if he can, that when the cloth had been removed, fresh pots and pipes laid upon the table, and the customary loyal and patriotic toasts proposed, the celebrated Mr Sluffen, of Adam and Eve Court, whose authority not the most malignant of our opponents can call in question, expressed himself in a manner following: 'That now he'd cotcht the cheerman's hi, he vished he might be jolly vell blessed, if he worn't a goin' to have his innings, vich he vould say these here obserwashuns – that how some mischeevus coves as know'd nuffin about the consarn, had tried to sit people agin the mas'r swips, and take the shine out o' their bis'nes, and the bread out o' the traps o' their preshus kids, by a makin' o' this here remark, as chimblies could be as vell svept by 'sheenery as by boys; and that the makin' use o' boys for that there purpuss vos barbareous; veras, he 'ad been a chummy – he begged the cheerman's parding for usin' such a wulgar hexpression – more nor thirty year – he might say he'd been born in a chimbley – and he know'd uncommon vell as 'sheenery vos vus nor o' no use; and as to kerhewelty to the boys, everybody in the chimbley line know'd as vell as he did, that they liked the climbin' better nor nuffin as vos.' From this day, we date the total fall of the last lingering remnant of May-day dancing, among the *élite* of the profession: and from this period we commence a new era in that portion of our spring associations which relates to the 1st of May.

We are aware that the unthinking part of the population will meet us here, with the assertion that dancing on May-day still continues – that 'greens' are annually seen to roll along the streets – that youths in the garb of clowns precede them, giving vent to the ebullitions of their sportive fancies; and that lords and ladies follow in their wake.

Granted. We are ready to acknowledge that in outward show, these processions have greatly improved: we do not deny the introduction of solos on the drum; we will even go so far as to admit an occasional fantasia on the triangle, but here our admissions end. We positively deny that the sweeps have art or part in these proceedings. We distinctly charge the dustmen with throwing what they ought to clear away, into the eyes of the public. We accuse scavengers, brickmakers, and gentlemen who devote their energies to the costermongering line, with obtaining money once a year, under false pretences. We cling with peculiar fondness to the custom of days gone by, and have shut out conviction as long as we could, but it has forced itself upon us; and we now proclaim to a deluded public, that the May-day dancers are *not* sweeps. The size of them, alone, is sufficient to repudiate the idea. It is a notorious fact that the widely spread taste for register stoves has materially increased the demand for small boys; whereas the men who, under a fictitious character, dance about the streets on the first of May nowadays, would be a tight fit in a kitchen flue, to say nothing of the parlour. This is strong presumptive evidence, but we have positive proof – the evidence of our own senses. And here is our testimony.

Upon the morning of the second of the merry month of May, in the year of our Lord one thousand eight hundred and thirty-six, we went out for a stroll, with a kind of forlorn hope of seeing something or other which might induce us to believe that it was really spring, and not Christmas. After wandering as far as Copenhagen House, without meeting anything calculated to dispel our impression that there was a mistake in the almanacks, we turned back down Maiden Lane, with the intention of passing through the extensive colony lying between it and Battle Bridge, which is inhabited by proprietors of donkey carts, boilers of horse flesh, makers of tiles, and sifters of cinders; through which colony we should have passed, without stoppage or interruption, if a little crowd gathered round a shed had not attracted our attention, and induced us to pause.

When we say a 'shed', we do not mean the conservatory sort of building which, according to the old song, Love tenanted when he was a young man, but a wooden house with windows stuffed with rags and paper, and a small yard at the side, with one dust-cart, two baskets, a few shovels, and little heaps of cinders, and fragments of china and tiles, scattered about it. Before this inviting spot we paused; and the longer we looked, the more we wondered what exciting circumstance it could be, that induced, the foremost members of the crowd to flatten their noses against the parlour window, in the vain hope of catching a glimpse of what was going on inside. After staring vacantly about us for some minutes, we appealed, touching the cause of this assemblage, to a gentleman in a suit of tarpaulin, who was smoking his pipe on our right hand; but as the only answer we obtained was a playful inquiry whether our mother had disposed of her mangle, we determined to await the issue in silence.

Judge of our virtuous indignation, when the street door of the shed opened, and a party emerged therefrom, clad in the costume and emulating the appearance, of May-day sweeps!

The first person who appeared was 'my lord', habited in a blue coat and bright buttons, with gilt paper tacked over the seams, yellow knee breeches, pink cotton stockings, and shoes; a cocked hat, ornamented with shreds of various coloured paper, on his head, a *bouquet* the size of a prize cauliflower in his button hole, a long Belcher handkerchief in his right hand, and a thin cane in his left. A murmur of applause ran through the crowd (which was chiefly composed of his lordship's personal friends), when this graceful figure made his appearance, which swelled into a burst of applause as his fair partner in the dance bounded forth to join him. Her ladyship was attired in pink crape over bed furniture, with a low body and short sleeves. The symmetry of her ankles was partially concealed by a very perceptible pair of frilled trousers; and the inconvenience which might have resulted from the circumstance of her white satin shoes being a few sizes too large, was obviated by their being firmly attached to her legs with strong tape sandals.

Her head was ornamented with a profusion of artificial flowers; and in her hand she bore a large brass ladle, wherein to receive what she figuratively denominated 'the tin'. The other characters were a young gentleman in girl's clothes and a widow's cap; two clowns who walked upon their hands in the mud, to the immeasurable delight of all the spectators; a man with a drum; another man with a flageolet; a dirty woman in a large shawl, with a box under her arm for the money, – and last, though not least, the 'green', animated by no less a personage than our identical friend in the tarpaulin suit.

The man hammered away at the drum, the flageolet squeaked, the shovels rattled, the 'green' rolled about, pitching first on one side and then on the other; my lady threw her right foot over her left ankle, and her left foot over her right ankle, alternately; my lord ran a few paces forward, and butted at the 'green', and then a few paces backward upon the toes of the crowd, and then went to the right, and then to the left, and then dodged my lady round the 'green'; and finally drew her arm through his, and called upon the boys to shout, which they did lustily – for this was the dancing.

We passed the same group, accidentally, in the evening. We never saw a 'green' so drunk, a lord so quarrelsome (no: not even in the house of peers after dinner), a pair of clowns so melancholy, a lady so muddy, or a party so miserable.

How has May-day decayed!

## Chapter Twenty-one

### *Brokers' and Marine-store Shops*

First published in the *Morning Chronicle*, 15 December 1834 ('Street Sketches No. 5'). An example of the black doll trade sign that Dickens mentions can be seen in the illustration by 'Phiz' (H.K. Browne) 'Tom-All-Alone's' in *Bleak House*, where it embellishes Krook's rag and bone shop. The term 'Marine-store' originally applied to shops in seaport towns selling miscellaneous items that might be needed on board ship; it was gradually extended to mean shops anywhere that dealt in second-hand items.

When we affirm that brokers' shops are strange places, and that if an authentic history of their contents could be procured, it would furnish many a page of amusement, and many a melancholy tale, it is necessary to explain the class of shops to which we allude. Perhaps when we make use of the term 'Brokers' Shop', the minds of our readers will at once picture large, handsome warehouses, exhibiting a long perspective of French-polished dining tables, rosewood chiffoniers, and mahogany wash-hand-stands, with an occasional vista of a four-post bedstead and hangings, and an appropriate foreground of dining room chairs. Perhaps they will imagine that we mean an humble class of second-hand furniture repositories. Their imagination will then naturally lead them to that street at the back of Long Acre, which is composed almost entirely of brokers' shops; where you walk through groves of deceitful, showy-looking furniture, and where the prospect is occasionally enlivened by a bright red, blue, and yellow hearth rug, embellished with the pleasing device of a mail coach at full speed, or a strange animal, supposed to have been originally intended for a dog, with a mass of worsted work in his mouth, which conjecture has likened to a basket of flowers.

This, by-the-bye, is a tempting article to young wives in the humbler ranks of life, who have a first-floor front to furnish – they are lost in admiration, and hardly know which to admire most. The dog is very beautiful, but they have a dog already on the best tea tray, and two more on the mantelpiece. Then, there is something so genteel about that mail coach; and the passengers outside (who are all hat) give it such an air of reality!

The goods here are adapted to the taste, or rather to the means, of cheap purchasers. There are some of the most beautiful *looking* Pembroke tables that were ever beheld: the wood as green as the trees in the Park, and the leaves almost as certain to fall off in the course of a year. There is also a most extensive assortment of tent and turn up bedsteads, made of stained wood, and innumerable specimens of that base imposition on society – a sofa bedstead.

A turn up bedstead is a blunt, honest piece of furniture; it may be slightly disguised with a sham drawer; and sometimes a mad attempt is even made to pass it off for a bookcase; ornament it as you will, however, the turn up bedstead seems to defy disguise, and to insist on having it distinctly understood that he is a turn up bedstead, and nothing else – that he is indispensably necessary, and that being so useful, he disdains to be ornamental.

How different is the demeanour of a sofa bedstead! Ashamed of its real use, it strives to appear an article of luxury and gentility – an attempt in which it miserably fails. It has neither the respectability of a sofa, nor the virtues of a bed; every man who keeps a sofa bedstead in his house, becomes a party to a wilful and designing fraud – we question whether you could insult him more, than by insinuating that you entertain the least suspicion of its real use.

To return from this digression, we beg to say, that neither of these classes of brokers' shops forms the subject of this sketch. The shops to which we advert, are immeasurably inferior to those on whose outward appearance we have slightly touched. Our readers must often have observed in some by street, in a poor neighbourhood, a small dirty shop, exposing for sale the most extraordinary and confused jumble of old, worn-out, wretched articles, that can well be imagined. Our wonder at their ever having been bought, is only to be equalled by our astonishment at the idea of their ever being sold again. On a board, at the side of the door, are placed about twenty books – all odd volumes; and as many wine glasses – all different patterns; several locks, an old earthenware pan, full of rusty keys; two or three gaudy chimney ornaments – cracked, of course; the remains of a lustre, without any drops; a round frame like a capital O, which has once held a mirror; a flute, complete with the exception of the middle joint; a pair of curling irons; and a tinder box. In front of the shop window are ranged some half dozen high backed chairs, with spinal complaints and wasted legs; a corner cupboard; two or three very dark mahogany tables with flaps like mathematical problems; some pickle jars, some surgeons' ditto, with gilt labels and without stoppers; an unframed portrait of some lady who flourished about the beginning of the thirteenth century, by an artist who never flourished at all; an incalculable host of miscellanies of every description, including bottles and cabinets, rags and bones, fenders and street door knockers, fire irons, wearing apparel and bedding, a hall lamp, and a room door. Imagine, in addition to this incongruous mass, a black doll in a white frock, with two faces – one looking up the street, and the other looking down, swinging over the door; a board with the squeezed up inscription 'Dealer in marine stores', in lanky white letters, whose height is strangely out of proportion to their width; and you have before you precisely the kind of shop to which we wish to direct your attention.

Although the same heterogeneous mixture of things will be found at all these places, it is curious to observe how truly and accurately some of the minor articles which are exposed for sale – articles of wearing apparel, for instance – mark the character of the neighbourhood. Take Drury Lane and Covent Garden for example.

This is essentially a theatrical neighbourhood. There is not a potboy in the vicinity who is not, to a greater or lesser extent, a dramatic character. The errand boys and chandler's shopkeepers' sons are all stage-struck: they 'gets up' plays in back kitchens hired for the purpose, and will stand before a shop window for hours, contemplating a great staring portrait of Mr Somebody or other, of the Royal Coburg Theatre, 'as he appeared in the character of Tongo the Denounced'. The consequence is, that there is not a marine-store shop in the neighbourhood, which does not exhibit for sale some faded articles of dramatic finery, such as three or four pairs of soiled buff boots with turnover red tops, heretofore worn by a 'fourth robber', or 'fifth mob'; a pair of rusty broadswords, a few gauntlets, and certain resplendent ornaments, which, if they were yellow instead of white, might be taken for insurance plates of the Sun Fire Office. There are several of these shops in the narrow streets and dirty courts, of which there are so many near the national theatres, and they all have tempting goods of this description, with the addition, perhaps, of a lady's pink dress covered with spangles; white wreaths, stage shoes, and a tiara like a tin lamp reflector. They have been purchased of some wretched supernumeraries, or sixth-rate actors, and are now offered for the benefit of the rising generation, who, on condition of making certain weekly payments, amounting in the whole to about ten times their value, may avail themselves of such desirable bargains.

Let us take a very different quarter, and apply it to the same test. Look at a marine-store dealer's, in that reservoir of dirt, drunkenness, and drabs: thieves, oysters, baked potatoes, and pickled salmon – Ratcliff Highway. Here, the wearing apparel is all nautical. Rough blue jackets, with mother-of-pearl buttons, oil skin hats, coarse checked shirts, and large canvas trousers that look as if they were made for a pair of bodies instead of a pair of legs, are the staple commodities. Then, there are large bunches of cotton pocket handkerchiefs, in colour and pattern unlike any one ever saw before, with the exception of those on the backs of the three young ladies without bonnets who passed just now. The furniture is much the same as elsewhere, with the addition of one or two models of ships, and some old prints of naval engagements in still older frames. In the window are a few compasses, a small tray containing silver watches in clumsy thick cases; and tobacco boxes, the lid of each ornamented with a ship, or an anchor, or some such trophy. A sailor generally pawns or sells all he has before he has been long ashore, and if he does not, some favoured companion kindly saves him the trouble. In either case, it is an even chance that he afterwards unconsciously repurchases the same things at a higher price than he gave for them at first.

Again: pay a visit with a similar object, to a part of London, as unlike both of these as they are to each other. Cross over to the Surrey side, and look at such shops of this description as are to be found near the King's Bench prison, and in 'the Rules.' How different, and how strikingly illustrative of the decay of some of the unfortunate residents of this part of the metropolis! Imprisonment and neglect have done their work. There is contamination in the profligate denizens of a debtor's prison; old friends have fallen off; the recollection of former prosperity has passed away; and with it all thoughts for the past, all care for the future. First, watches and rings, then cloaks, coats, and all the more expensive articles of dress, have found their way to the pawnbroker's. That miserable resource has failed at last, and the sale of some trifling article at one of these shops has been the only mode left of raising a shilling or two, to meet the urgent demands of the moment. Dressing cases and writing desks, too old to pawn but too good to keep; guns, fishing rods, musical instruments, all in the same condition; have first been sold, and the sacrifice has been but slightly felt. But hunger must be allayed, and what has already become a habit is easily resorted to, when an emergency arises. Light articles of clothing, first of the ruined man, then of his wife, at last of their children, even of the youngest, have been parted with, piecemeal. There they are, thrown carelessly together until a purchaser presents himself, old, and patched and repaired, it is true; but the make and materials tell of better days; and the older they are, the greater the misery and destitution of those whom they once adorned.

## Chapter Twenty-Two

### *Gin Shops*

First published in the *Evening Chronicle*, 7 February 1835.

It is a remarkable circumstance, that different trades appear to partake of the disease to which elephants and dogs are especially liable, and to run stark, staring, raving mad, periodically. The great distinction between the animals and the trades is, that the former run mad with a certain degree of propriety – they are very regular in their irregularities. We know the period at which the emergency will arise, and provide against it accordingly. If an elephant run mad, we are all ready for him – kill or cure – pills or bullets, calomel in conserve of roses, or lead in a musket barrel. If a dog happen to look unpleasantly warm in the summer months, and to trot about the shady side of the streets with a quarter of a yard of tongue hanging out of his mouth, a thick leather muzzle, which has been previously prepared in compliance with the thoughtful injunctions of the Legislature, is instantly clapped over his head, by way of making him cooler, and he either looks remarkably unhappy for the next six weeks, or becomes legally insane, and goes mad, as it were, by Act of Parliament. But these trades are as eccentric as comets; nay, worse, for no one can calculate on the recurrence of the strange appearances which betoken the disease. Moreover, the contagion is general, and the quickness with which it diffuses itself, almost incredible.

We will cite two or three cases in illustration of our meaning. Six or eight years ago, the epidemic began to display itself among the linen drapers and haberdashers. The primary symptoms were an inordinate love of plate glass, and a passion for gaslights and gilding. The disease gradually progressed, and at last attained a fearful height. Quiet dusty old shops in different parts of town, were pulled down; spacious premises with stuccoed fronts and gold letters, were erected instead; floors were covered with Turkey carpets; roofs supported by massive pillars; doors knocked into windows, a dozen squares of glass into one; one shopman into a dozen; and there is no knowing what would have been done, if it had not been fortunately discovered, just in time, that the Commissioners in Bankruptcy were as competent to decide such cases as the Commissioners

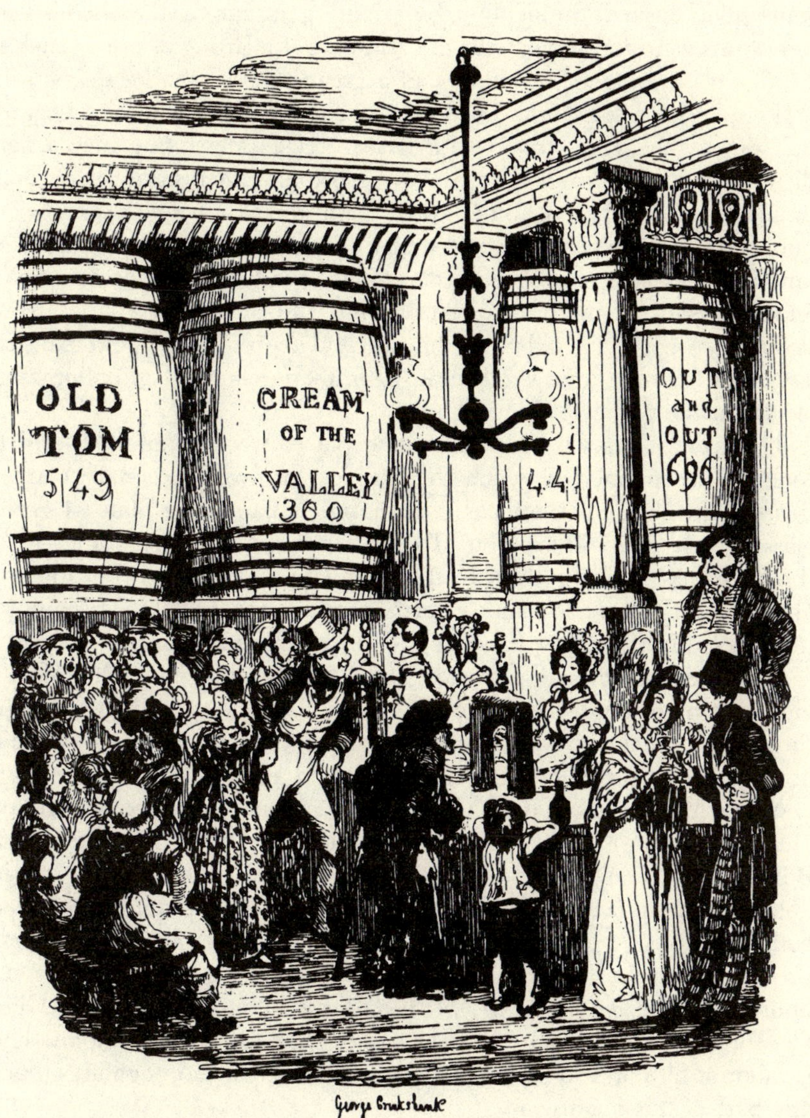
OLD
TOM
5|49
CREAM
OF THE
VALLEY
360
44
OUT
and
OUT
696
George Cruikshank

*The Gin Shop*

of Lunacy, and that a little confinement and gentle examination did wonders. The disease abated. It died away. A year or two of comparative tranquillity ensued. Suddenly it burst out again among the chemists; the symptoms were the same, with the addition of a strong desire to stick the royal arms over the shop door, and a great rage for mahogany, varnish, and expensive floor cloth. Then the hosiers were infected, and began to pull down their shop fronts with frantic recklessness. The mania again died away, and the public began to congratulate themselves on its entire disappearance, when it burst forth with tenfold violence among the publicans, and keepers of 'wine vaults'. From that moment it has spread among them with unprecedented rapidity, exhibiting a concatenation of all the previous symptoms; onward it has rushed to every part of town, knocking down all the old public houses, and depositing splendid mansions, stone balustrades, rosewood fittings, immense lamps, and illuminated clocks, at the corner of every street.

The extensive scale on which these places were established, and the ostentatious manner in which the business of even the smallest among them is divided into branches is amusing. A handsome plate of ground glass in one door directs you 'To the Counting house', another to the 'Bottle Department'; a third to the 'Wholesale Department'; a fourth to 'The Wine Promenade'; and so forth, until we are in daily expectation of meeting with a 'Brandy Bell', or a 'Whiskey Entrance'. Then, ingenuity is exhausted in devising attractive titles for the different descriptions of gin; and the dram-drinking portion of the community as they gaze upon the gigantic black and white announcements, which are only to be equalled in size by the figures beneath them, are left in a state of pleasing hesitation between 'The Cream of the Valley', 'The Out and Out', 'The No Mistake', 'The Good for Mixing', 'The Real Knock-me-down', 'The celebrated Butter Gin', 'The regular Flare-up', and a dozen other, equally inviting, and wholesome *liqueurs*. Although places of this description are to be met with in every second street, they are invariably numerous and splendid in precise proportion to the dirt and poverty of the surrounding neighbourhood. The gin shops in and near Drury Lane, Holborn, St Giles's, Covent Garden, and Clare Market, are the handsomest in London. There is more of filth and squalid misery near those great thoroughfares than in any part of this mighty city.

We will endeavour to sketch the bar of a large gin shop, and its ordinary customers, for the edification of such of our readers as may not have had opportunities of observing such scenes; and on the chance of finding one well suited to our purpose, we will make for Drury Lane, through the narrow streets and dirty courts which divide it from Oxford Street, and that classical spot adjoining the brewery at the bottom of Tottenham Court Road, best known to the initiated as the 'Rookery'.

The filthy and miserable appearance of this part of London can hardly be imagined by those (and there are many such) who have not witnessed it. Wretched houses with broken windows patched with rags and paper: every room let out to a different family, and in many instances to two or even three – fruit and 'sweet-stuff' manufacturers in the cellars, barbers and red herring vendors in the front parlours, cobblers in the back; a bird fancier in the first floor, three families on the second, starvation in the attics, Irishmen in the passage, a 'musician' in the front kitchen, and a charwoman and five hungry children in the back one – filth everywhere – a gutter before the houses and a drain behind – clothes drying and slops emptying, from the windows; girls of fourteen or fifteen, with matted hair, walking about barefoot, and in white greatcoats, almost their only covering; boys of all ages, in coats of all sizes and no coats at all; men and women, in every variety of scanty and dirty apparel, lounging, scolding, drinking, smoking, squabbling, fighting, and swearing.

You turn the corner. What a change! All is light and brilliancy. The hum of many voices issues from that splendid gin shop which forms the commencement of the two streets opposite; and the gay building with the fantastically ornamented parapet, the illuminated clock, the plate glass windows surrounded by stucco rosettes, and its profusion of gaslights in richly gilt burners, is perfectly dazzling when contrasted with the darkness and dirt we have just left. The interior is even gayer than the exterior. A bar of French-polished mahogany, elegantly carved, extends the whole width of the place; and there are two side aisles of great casks, painted green and gold, enclosed within a light brass rail, and bearing such inscriptions as 'Old Tom, 549'; 'Young Tom, 360'; 'Samson, 1421' – the figures agreeing, we presume, with 'gallons', understood. Beyond the bar is a lofty and spacious saloon, full of the same enticing vessels, with a gallery running round it, equally well furnished. On the counter, in addition to the usual spirit apparatus, are two or three little baskets of cakes and biscuits, which are carefully secured at the top with wickerwork, to prevent their contents being unlawfully abstracted. Behind it are two showily dressed damsels with large necklaces, dispensing the spirits and 'compounds'. They are assisted by the ostensible proprietor of the concern, a stout coarse fellow in a fur cap, put on very much on one side to give him a knowing air, and to display his sandy whiskers to the best advantage.

The two old washerwomen, who are seated on the little bench to the left of the bar, are rather overcome by the head dresses and haughty demeanour of the young ladies who officiate. They receive their half-quartern of gin and peppermint, with considerable deference, prefacing a request for 'one of them soft biscuits', with a 'Jist be good enough, ma'am'. They are quite astonished at the impudent air of the young fellow in a brown coat and bright buttons, who, ushering in his two companions, and walking up to the bar in as careless a manner as if he had been used to green and gold ornaments all his life, winks at one of the young ladies with singular coolness, and calls for a 'kervorten and a three-out-glass', just as if the place were his own. 'Gin for you, sir?' says the young lady when she has drawn it: carefully looking every way but the right one, to show that the wink had no effect upon her. 'For me, Mary, my dear,' replies the gentleman in brown. 'My name an't Mary as it happens,' says the young girl, rather relaxing as she delivers the change. 'Well, if it an't, it ought to be,' responds the irresistible one; 'all the Marys as ever *I* see, was handsome gals'. Here the young lady, not precisely remembering how blushes are managed in such cases, abruptly ends the flirtation by addressing the female in the faded feathers who has just entered, and who, after stating explicitly, to prevent any subsequent misunderstanding, that 'this gentleman pays', calls for 'a glass of port wine and a bit of sugar'.

Those two old men who came in 'just to have a drain', finished their third quartern a few seconds ago; they have made themselves crying drunk; and the fat comfortable-looking elderly women, who had 'a glass of rum-srub' each, having chimed in with their complaints on the hardness of the times, one of the women has agreed to stand a glass round, jocularly observing that 'grief never mended no broken bones, and as good people's wery scarce, what I says is, make the most on 'em, and that's all about it!' a sentiment which appears to afford unlimited satisfaction to those who have nothing to pay.

It is growing late, and the throng of men, women, and children, who have been constantly going in and out, dwindles down to two or three occasional stragglers – cold, wretched-looking creatures, in the last stage of emaciation and disease. The knot of Irish labourers at the lower end of the place, who have been alternately shaking hands with, and threatening the life of each other, for the last hour, become furious in their disputes, and finding it impossible to silence one man, who is particularly anxious to adjust the difference, they resort to the expedient of knocking him down and jumping on him afterwards. The man in the fur cap, and the potboy rush out: a scene of riot and confusion ensues; half the Irishmen get shut out, and the other half get shut in; the potboy is knocked among the tubs in no time; the landlord hits everybody, and everybody hits the landlord; the barmaids scream; the police come in; the rest is a confused mixture of arms, legs, staves, torn coats, shouting, and struggling. Some of the party are borne off to the station house, and the remainder slink home to beat their wives for complaining, and kick the children for daring to be hungry.

We have sketched this subject very slightly, not only because our limits compel us to do so, but because, if it were pursued farther, it would be painful and repulsive. Well disposed gentlemen, and charitable ladies, would alike turn with coldness and disgust from a description of the drunken besotted men, and wretched broken down miserable women, who form no inconsiderable portion of the frequenters of these haunts; forgetting, in the pleasant consciousness of their own rectitude, the poverty of the one, and the temptation of the other. Gin drinking is a great vice in England, but wretchedness and dirt are a greater; and until you improve the homes of the poor, or persuade a half famished wretch not to seek relief in the temporary oblivion of his own misery, with the pittance which, divided among his family, would furnish a morsel of bread for each, gin shops will increase in number and splendour. If Temperance Societies would suggest an antidote against hunger, filth, and foul air, or could establish dispensaries for the gratuitous distribution of bottles of Lethe water, gin palaces would be numbered among the things that were.

## Chapter Twenty-three

### *The Pawnbroker's Shop*

First published in the *Evening Chronicle*, 30 June 1835 ('Sketches of London No. 16'). For another illustration of the kind of shop that Dickens describes here, with private booths for the more fastidious customer, see Phiz's illustration, 'Martin meets an Acquaintance at the House of a Mutual Relation' in *Martin Chuzzlewit*.

Of the numerous receptacles for misery and distress with which the streets of London unhappily abound, there are, perhaps, none which present such striking scenes as the pawnbrokers' shops. The very nature and description of these places occasions their being but little known, except to the unfortunate beings whose profligacy or misfortune drives them to seek the temporary relief they offer. The subject may appear, at first sight, to be anything but an inviting one, but we venture on it nevertheless, in the hope that, as far as the limits of our present paper are concerned, it will present nothing to disgust even the most fastidious reader.

There are some pawnbrokers' shops of a very superior description. There are grades in pawning as in everything else, and distinctions must be observed even in poverty. The aristocratic Spanish cloak and the plebeian calico shirt, the silver fork and the flat iron, the muslin cravat and the Belcher neckerchief, would but ill assort together; so the better sort of pawnbroker calls himself a silversmith, and decorates his shop with handsome trinkets and expensive jewellery, while the more humble money lender boldly advertises his calling, and invites observation. It is with pawnbrokers' shops of the latter class, that we have to do. We have selected one for our purpose, and will endeavour to describe it.

The pawnbroker's shop is situated near Drury Lane, at the corner of a court, which affords a side entrance for the accommodation of such customers as may be desirous of avoiding the observation of the passers by, or the chance of recognition in a public street. It is a low, dirty-looking, dusty shop, the door of which stands always doubtfully a little way open: half inviting, half repelling the hesitating visitor, who, if he be as yet uninitiated, examines one of the old garnet brooches in the window for a minute or two with affected eagerness, as if he contemplated making

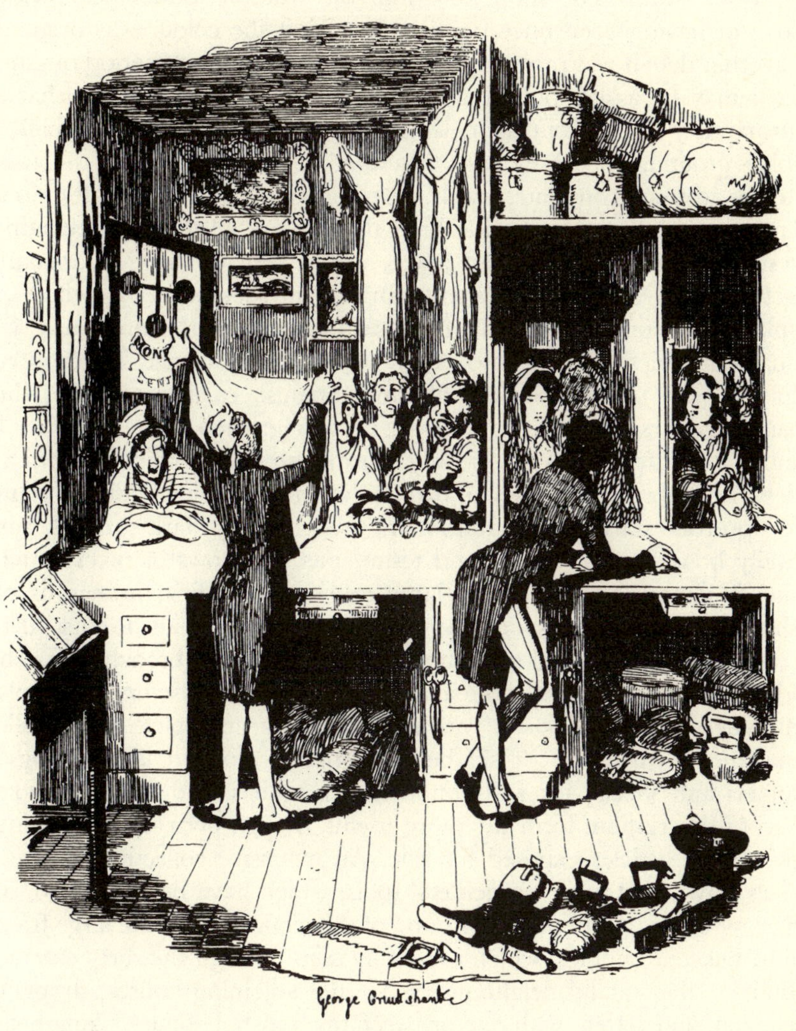


*The Pawnbroker's Shop*

a purchase; and then looking cautiously round to ascertain that no one watches him, hastily slinks in: the door closing of itself after him, to just its former width. The shop front and the window frames bear evident marks of having been once painted; but what the colour was originally, or at what date it was probably laid on, are at this remote period questions which may be asked, but cannot be answered. Tradition states that the transparency in the front door, which displays at night three red balls on a blue ground, once bore also, inscribed in graceful waves, the words 'Money advanced on plate, jewels, wearing apparel, and every description of property,' but a few illegible hieroglyphics are all that now remain to attest the fact. The plate and jewels would seem to have disappeared, together with the announcement, for the articles of stock, which are displayed in some profusion in the window, do not include any very valuable luxuries of either kind. A few old china cups; some modern vases, adorned with paltry paintings of three Spanish cavaliers playing three Spanish guitars; or a party of boors carousing: each boor with one leg painfully elevated in the air, by way of expressing his perfect freedom and gaiety; several sets of chessmen, two or three flutes, a few fiddles, a round-eyed portrait staring in astonishment from a very dark ground; some gaudily bound prayer books and testaments, two rows of silver watches quite as clumsy and almost as large as Ferguson's first; numerous old-fashioned table and teaspoons, displayed, fan-like, in half dozens; strings of coral with great broad gilt snaps; cards of rings and brooches, fastened and labelled separately, like the insects in the British Museum; cheap silver penholders and snuff boxes, with a masonic star, complete the jewellery department; while five or six beds in smeary clouded ticks, strings of blankets and sheets, silk and cotton handkerchiefs, and wearing apparel of every description, form the more useful, though even less ornamental, part, of the articles exposed for sale. An extensive collection of planes, chisels, saws, and other carpenters' tools, which have been pledged, and never redeemed, form the foreground of the picture; while the large frames full of ticketed bundles, which are dimly seen through the dirty casement upstairs – the squalid neighbourhood – the adjoining houses, straggling, shrunken, and rotten, with one or two filthy, unwholesome-looking heads, thrust out of every window, and old red pans and stunted plants exposed on the tottering parapets, to the manifest hazard of the heads of the passers by – the noisy men loitering under the archway at the corner of the court, or about the gin shop next door – and their wives patiently standing on the curbstone, with large baskets of cheap vegetables slung round them for sale, are its immediate auxiliaries.

If the outside of the pawnbroker's shop be calculated to attract the attention, or excite the interest, of the speculative pedestrian, its interior cannot fail to produce the same effect in an increased degree. The front door, which we have before noticed, opens into the common shop, which is the resort of all those customers whose habitual acquaintance with such scenes renders them indifferent to the observation of their companions in poverty. The side door opens into a small passage from which some half dozen doors (which may be secured on the inside by bolts) open into a corresponding number of little dens, or closets, which face the counter. Here, the more timid or respectable portion of the crowd shroud themselves from the notice of the remainder, and patiently wait until the gentleman behind the counter, with the curly black hair, diamond ring, and double silver watchguard, shall feel disposed to favour them with his notice – a consummation which depends considerably on the temper of the aforesaid gentleman for the time being.

At the present moment, this elegantly attired individual is in the act of entering the duplicate he has just made out, in a thick book: a process from which he is diverted occasionally, by a conversation he is carrying on with another young man similarly employed at a little distance from him, whose allusions to 'that last bottle of soda water last night', and 'how regularly round my hat he felt himself when the young 'ooman gave 'em in charge', would appear to refer to the consequences of some stolen joviality of the preceding evening. The customers generally, however, seem unable to participate in the amusement derivable from this source, for an old sallow-looking woman, who has been leaning with both arms on the counter with a small bundle before her, for half an hour previously, suddenly interrupts the conversation by addressing the jewelled shopman – 'Now, Mr Henry, do make haste, there's a good soul, for my two grandchildren's locked up at home, and I'm afeer'd of the fire.' The shopman slightly raises his head with an air of deep abstraction, and resumes his entry with as much deliberation as if he were engraving. 'You're in a hurry, Mrs Tatham, this ev'nin', an't you?' is the only notice he deigns to take, after the lapse of five minutes or so. 'Yes, I am indeed, Mr Henry; now, do serve me next, there's a good creetur. I wouldn't worry you, only it's all along o' them botherin' children.' 'What have you got here?' inquires the shopman, unpinning the bundle – 'old concern, I suppose – pair o' stays and a petticut. You must look up somethin' else, old 'ooman; I can't lend you anything more upon them; they're completely worn out by this time, if it's only by putting in, and taking out again, three times a week.' 'Oh! you're a rum un, you are,' replies the old woman, laughing extremely, as in duty bound; 'I wish I'd got the gift of the gab like you; see if I'd be up the spout so often then! No, no; it an't the petticut; it's a child's frock and a beautiful silk ankecher, as belongs to my husband. He gave four shillin' for it, the werry same blessed day as he broke his arm.' – 'What do you want upon these?' inquires Mr Henry, slightly glancing at the articles, which in all probability are old acquaintances. 'What do you want upon these?' – 'Eighteenpence.' – 'Lend you ninepence.' – 'Oh, make it a shillin; there's a dear – do now?' – 'Not another farden.' – 'Well, I suppose I must take it.' The duplicate is made out, one ticket pinned on the parcel, the other given to the old woman; the parcel is flung carelessly down into a corner, and some other customer prefers his claim to be served without further delay.

The choice falls on an unshaven, dirty, sottish-looking fellow, whose tarnished paper cap, stuck negligently over one eye, communicates an additionally repulsive expression to his very uninviting countenance. He was enjoying a little relaxation from his sedentary pursuits a quarter of an hour ago, in kicking his wife up the court. He has come to redeem some tools: – probably to complete a job with, an account of which he has already received some money, if his inflamed countenance and drunken stagger may be taken as evidence of the fact. Having waited some little time, he makes his presence known by venting his ill humour on a ragged urchin, who, being unable to bring his face on a level with the counter by any other process, has employed himself in climbing up, and then hooking himself on with his elbows – an uneasy perch, from which he has fallen at intervals, generally alighting on the toes of the person in his immediate vicinity. In the present case, the unfortunate little wretch has received a cuff which sends him reeling to the door; and the donor of the blow is immediately the object of general indignation.

'What do you strike the boy for, you brute?' exclaims a slipshod woman, with two flat irons in a little basket. 'Do you think he's your wife, you willin?' 'Go and hang yourself!' replies the gentleman addressed, with a drunken look of savage stupidity, aiming at the same time a blow at the woman which fortunately misses its object. 'Go and hang yourself; and wait till I come and cut you down.' – 'Cut you down,' rejoins the woman, 'I wish I had the cutting of you up, you wagabond! (loud). Oh! you precious wagabond! (rather louder). Where's your wife, you willin? (louder still; women of this class are always sympathetic, and work themselves into a tremendous passion on the shortest notice). Your poor dear wife as you uses worser nor a dog – strike a woman – you a man! (very shrill); I wish I had you – I'd murder you, I would, if I died for it!' – 'Now be civil,' retorts the man fiercely. 'Be civil, you wiper!' ejaculates the woman contemptuously. 'An't it shocking?' she continues, turning round, and appealing to an old woman who is peeping out of one of the little closets we have before described, and who has not the slightest objection to join in the attack, possessing, as she does, the comfortable conviction that she is bolted in. 'An't it shocking, ma'am? (Dreadful! says the old woman in a parenthesis, not exactly knowing what the question refers to.) He's got a wife, ma'am, as takes in mangling, and is as 'dustrious and hard working a young 'ooman as can be, (very fast) as lives in the back parlour of our 'ous, which my husband and me lives in the front one (with great rapidity) – and we hears him a beaten' on her sometimes when he comes home drunk, the whole night through, and not only a beaten' her, but beaten' his own child, too, to make her more miserable – ugh, you beast! and she, poor creater, won't swear the peace agin him, nor do nothin', because she likes the wretch arter all – worse luck!' Here, as the woman has completely run herself out of breath, the pawnbroker himself, who has just appeared behind the counter in a gay dressing gown, embraces the favourable opportunity of putting in a word: – 'Now I won't have none of this sort of thing on my premises!' he interposes with an air of authority. 'Mrs Mackin, keep yourself to yourself, or you don't get fourpence for a flat iron here; and Jinkins, you leave your ticket here till you're sober, and send your wife for them two planes, for I won't have you in my shop at no price; so make yourself scarce, before I make you scarcer.'

This eloquent address produces anything but the effect desired; the women rail in concert; the man hits about him in all directions, and is in the act of establishing an indisputable claim to gratuitous lodgings for the night, when the entrance of his wife, a wretched worn-out woman, apparently in the last stage of consumption, whose face bears evident marks of recent ill usage, and whose strength seems hardly equal to the burden – light enough, God knows! – of the thin, sickly child she carries in her arms, turns his cowardly rage in a safer direction. 'Come home, dear,' cries the miserable creature, in an imploring tone; '*do* come home, there's a good fellow, and go to bed.' – 'Go home yourself,' rejoins the furious ruffian. 'Do come home quietly,' repeats the wife, bursting into tears. 'Go home yourself,' retorts the husband again, enforcing his argument by a blow which sends the poor creature flying out of the shop. Her 'natural protector' follows her up the court, alternately venting his rage in accelerating her progress, and in knocking the little scanty blue bonnet of the unfortunate child over its still more scanty and faded-looking face.

In the last box, which is situated in the darkest and most obscure corner of the shop, considerably removed from either of the gaslights, are a young delicate girl of about twenty, and an elderly female, evidently her mother from the resemblance between them, who stand at some distance back, as if to avoid the observation even of the shopman. It is not their first visit to a pawnbroker's shop, for they answer without a moment's hesitation the usual questions, put in a rather respectful manner, and in a much lower tone than usual, of 'What name shall I say? – Your own property, of course? – Where do you live? – Housekeeper or lodger?' They bargain, too, for a higher loan than the shopman is at first inclined to offer, which a perfect stranger would be little disposed to do; and the elder female urges her daughter on, in scarcely audible whispers, to exert her utmost powers of persuasion to obtain an advance of the sum, and expatiate on the value of the articles they have brought to raise a present supply upon. They are a small gold chain and a 'Forget-me-not' ring: the girl's property, for they are both too small for the mother; given her in better times; prized, perhaps, once, for the giver's sake, but parted with now without a struggle; for want has hardened the mother, and her example has hardened the girl, and the prospect of receiving money, coupled with a recollection of the misery they have both endured from the want of it – the coldness of old friends – the stern refusal of some, and the still more galling compassion of others – appears to have obliterated the consciousness of self-humiliation, which the idea of their present situation would once have aroused.

In the next box is a young female, whose attire, miserably poor but extremely gaudy, wretchedly cold but extravagantly fine, too plainly bespeaks her station. The rich satin gown with its faded trimmings, the worn out thin shoes, and pink silk stockings, the summer bonnet in winter, and the sunken face, where a daub of rouge only serves as an index to the ravages of squandered health never to be regained, and lost happiness never to be restored, and where the practised smile is a wretched mockery of the misery of the heart, cannot be mistaken. There is something in the glimpse she has just caught of her young neighbour, and in the sight of the little trinkets she has offered in pawn, that seems to have awakened in this woman's mind some slumbering recollection, and to have changed, for an instant, her whole demeanour. Her first hasty impulse was to bend forward as if to scan more minutely the appearance of her half-concealed companions; her next, on seeing them involuntarily shrink from her, to retreat to the back of the box, cover her face with her hands, and burst into tears.

There are strange chords in the human heart, which will lie dormant through years of depravity and wickedness, but which will vibrate at last to some slight circumstance apparently trivial in itself, but connected by some undefined and indistinct association with past days that can never be recalled, and with bitter recollections from which the most degraded creature in existence cannot escape.

There has been another spectator, in the person of a woman in the common shop; the lowest of the low; dirty, unbonneted, flaunting, and slovenly. Her curiosity was at first attracted by the little she could see of the group; then her attention. The half-intoxicated leer changed to an expression of something like interest, and a feeling similar to that we have described, appeared for a moment, and only a moment, to extend itself even to her bosom.

Who shall say how soon these women may change places? The last has but two more stages – the hospital and the grave. How many females situated as her two companions are, and as she may have been once, have terminated the same wretched course, in the same wretched manner! One is already tracing her footsteps with frightful rapidity. How soon may the other follow her example! How many have done the same!

## Chapter Twenty-four

### *Criminal Courts*

First published with the title 'The Old Bailey' in the *Morning Chronicle*, 23 October 1834 ('Street Sketches No. 3') and retitled for inclusion in the *Second Series*, 1837. The scene at the end of this sketch looks forward to two notable scenes in *Oliver Twist*, Fagin in the dock (ch. 52) and the Artful Dodger in court (ch. 43). The undignified custom of allowing Newgate gaolers to take money from sightseers wishing to get into the courts is mentioned by Dickens again in *Great Expectations*, ch. 20, when Pip, in London for the first time, finds himself at Newgate where 'an exceedingly dirty and partially drunk minister of justice asked me if I would like to step in and hear a trial or two: informing me that he could give me a front place for half a crown, whence I should command a full view of the Lord Chief Justice in his wig and robes – mentioning that awful personage like waxwork, and presently offering him at the reduced price of eighteenpence'. In the same passage in the novel appear all the other details mentioned at the beginning of this sketch – the whipping place, the 'dark building on one side of the yard, in which is kept the gibbet', and the Debtors' Door 'out of which culprits came to be hanged'. The fetters over the door (not mentioned in the *Great Expectations* passage) were architectural embellishments, many times larger than actual fetters; they disappeared with the rest of the prison when it was demolished in 1902 (the main gateway, however, may still be seen in the London Museum).

We shall never forget the mingled feelings of awe and respect with which we used to gaze on the exterior of Newgate in our schoolboy days. How dreadful its rough heavy walls, and low massive doors, appeared to us – the latter looking as if they were made for the express purpose of letting people in, and never letting them out again. Then the fetters over the debtors' door, which we used to think were a *bonâ fide* set of irons, just hung up there for convenience sake, ready to be taken down at a moment's notice, and riveted on the limbs of some refractory felon! We were never tired of wondering how the hackney coachmen on the opposite stand could cut jokes in the presence of such horrors, and drink pots of half-and-half so near the last drop.

Often have we strayed here, in sessions time, to catch a glimpse of the whipping place, and that dark building on one side of the yard, in which is kept the gibbet with all its dreadful apparatus, and on the side of which we half expected to see a brass plate, with the inscription 'Mr Ketch'; for we never imagined that the distinguished functionary could by possibility live anywhere else! The days of these childish dreams have passed away, and with them many other boyish ideas of a gayer nature. But we still retain so much of our original feeling, that to this hour we never pass the building without something like a shudder.

What London pedestrian is there who has not, at some time or other, cast a hurried glance through the wicket at which prisoners are admitted into this gloomy mansion, and surveyed the few objects he could discern, with an indescribable feeling of curiosity? The thick door, plated with iron and mounted with spikes, just low enough to enable you to see, leaning over them, an ill-looking fellow in a broad-brimmed hat, Belcher handkerchief and top boots: with a brown coat, something between a greatcoat and a 'sporting' jacket, on his back, and an immense key in his left hand. Perhaps you are lucky enough to pass, just as the gate is being opened; then, you see on the other side of the lodge, another gate, the image of its predecessor, and two or three more turnkeys, who look like multiplications of the first one, seated round a fire which just lights up the whitewashed apartment sufficiently to enable you to catch a hasty glimpse of these different objects. We have a great respect for Mrs Fry, but she certainly ought to have written more romances than Mrs Radcliffe.

We were walking leisurely down the Old Bailey, some time ago, when, as we passed this identical gate, it was opened by the officiating turnkey. We turned quickly round, as a matter of course, and saw two persons descending the steps. We could not help stopping and observing them.

They were an elderly woman, of decent appearance, though evidently poor, and a boy of about fourteen or fifteen. The woman was crying bitterly; she carried a small bundle in her hand, and the boy followed at a short distance behind her. Their little history was obvious. The boy was her son, to whose early comfort she had perhaps sacrificed her own – for whose sake she had borne misery without repining, and poverty without a murmur – looking steadily forward to the time when he who had so long witnessed her struggles for himself might be enabled to make some exertions for their joint support. He had formed dissolute connexions; idleness had led to crime; and he had been committed to take his trial for some petty theft. He had been long in prison, and, after receiving some trifling additional punishment, had been ordered to be discharged that morning. It was his first offence, and his poor old mother, still hoping to reclaim him, had been waiting at the gate to implore him to return home.

We cannot forget the boy; he descended the steps with a dogged look, shaking his head with an air of bravado and obstinate determination. They walked a few paces, and paused. The woman put her hand upon his shoulder in an agony of entreaty, and the boy sullenly raised his head as if in refusal. It was a brilliant morning, and every object looked fresh and happy in the broad, gay sunlight; he gazed round him for a few moments, bewildered with the brightness of the scene, for it was long since he had beheld anything save the gloomy walls of a prison. Perhaps the wretchedness of his mother made some impression on the boy's heart; perhaps some undefined recollection of the time when he was a happy child, and she his only friend and best companion, crowded on him – he burst into tears; and covering his face with one hand, and hurriedly placing the other in his mother's, walked away with her.

Curiosity has occasionally led us into both Courts at the Old Bailey. Nothing is so likely to strike the person who enters them for the first time, as the calm indifference with which the proceedings are conducted; every trial seems a mere matter of business. There is a great deal of form, but no compassion; considerable interest, but no sympathy. Take the Old Court for example. There sit the Judges, with whose great dignity everybody is acquainted, and of whom therefore we need say more. Then, there is the Lord Mayor in the centre, looking as cool as a Lord Mayor *can* look, with an immense *bouquet* before him, and habited in all the splendour of his office. Then, there are the Sheriffs, who are almost as dignified as the Lord Mayor himself; and the Barristers, who are quite dignified enough in their own opinion; and the spectators, who having paid for their admission, look upon the whole scene as if it were got up especially for their amusement. Look upon the whole group in the body of the Court – some wholly engrossed in the morning papers, others carelessly conversing in low whispers, and others, again, quietly dozing away an hour – and you can scarcely believe that the result of the trial is a matter of life or death to one wretched being present. But turn your eyes to the dock; watch the prisoner attentively for a few moments; and the fact is before you, in all its painful reality. Mark how restlessly he has been engaged for the last ten minutes, in forming all sorts of fantastic figures with the herbs which are strewed upon the ledge before him; observe the ashy paleness of his face when a particular witness appears, and how he changes his position and wipes his clammy forehead and feverish hands, when the case for the prosecution is closed, as if it were a relief to him to feel that the jury knew the worst.

The defence is concluded; the judge proceeds to sum up the evidence; and the prisoner watches the countenances of the jury, as a dying man, clinging to life to the very last, vainly looks in the face of his physician for a slight ray of hope. They turn round to consult; you can almost hear the man's heart beat, as he bites the stalk of rosemary, with a desperate effort to appear composed. They resume their places – a dead silence prevails as the foreman delivers in the verdict – 'Guilty!' A shriek bursts from a female in the gallery; the prisoner casts one look at the quarter from whence the noise proceeded; and is immediately hurried from the dock by the gaoler. The clerk directs one of the officers of the Court to 'take the woman out', and fresh business is proceeded with, as if nothing had occurred.

No imaginary contrast to a case like this, could be as complete as that which is constantly presented in the New Court, the gravity of which is frequently disturbed in no small degree, by the cunning and pertinacity of juvenile offenders. A boy of thirteen is tried, say for picking the pocket of some subject of her Majesty, and the offence is about as clearly proved as an offence can be. He is called upon for his defence, and contents himself with a little declamation about the jurymen and his country – asserts that all the witnesses have committed perjury, and hints that the police force generally have entered into a conspiracy 'again' him. However probable this statement may be, it fails to convince the Court, and some such scene as the following then takes place:

*Court:* Have you any witnesses to speak to your character, boy?

*Boy:* Yes, my lord; fifteen gen'lm'n is a vaten outside, and vos a vaten all day yesterday, vich they told me the night afore my trial vos a comin' on.

*Court:* Inquire for these witnesses.

Here, a stout beadle runs out, and vociferates for the witnesses at the very top of his voice; for you hear his cry grow fainter and fainter as he descends the steps into the courtyard below. After an absence of five minutes, he returns, very warm and hoarse, and informs the Court of what it knew perfectly well before – namely, that there are no such witnesses in attendance. Hereupon, the boy sets up a most awful howling; screws the lower parts of the palms of his hands into the corners of his eyes; and endeavours to look the picture of injured innocence. The jury at once find him 'guilty', and his endeavours to squeeze out a tear or two are redoubled. The governor of the gaol then states, in reply to an inquiry from the bench, that the prisoner has been under his care twice before. This the urchin resolutely denies in some such terms as – 'S'elp me, gen'lm'n, I never vos in trouble afore – indeed, my Lord, I never vos. It's all a howen to my having a twin brother, vich has wrongfully got into trouble, and vich is so exactly like me, that no vun ever knows the difference atween us.'

This representation, like the defence, fails in producing the desired effect, and the boy is sentenced, perhaps, to seven years' transportation. Finding it impossible to excite compassion, he gives vent to his feelings in an imprecation bearing reference to the eyes of 'old big vig!' and as he declines to take the trouble of walking from the dock, is forthwith carried out, congratulating himself on having succeeded in giving everybody as much trouble as possible.

## Chapter Twenty-five

### *A Visit to Newgate*

Specially written for the first collection of *Sketches* in volume form (the *First Series*), 1836. Dickens added the footnote (p. 195) in the 1837–9 monthly parts issue of *Sketches* (the last sentence was not added until the Charles Dickens Edition, 1868, however). Newgate prison had been built to replace the prison destroyed by the Gordon Rioters in 1780 (an event that Dickens was to describe in vivid detail in *Barnaby Rudge*, 1841); it stood until 1902 when it was demolished to make way for the Central Criminal Court (the Old Bailey). Dickens visited Newgate, as well as the House of Correction at Coldbath Fields, Clerkenwell, on 5 November 1835, accompanied by his publisher, Macrone, and an American journalist, N. P. Willis. The three condemned men described by Dickens were identified by W. J. Carlton ('The Third Man at Newgate', *Review of English Studies*, n.s., Vol. VIII [1957], pp. 402–7) as Robert Swan, a guardsman convicted of robbery with menaces; John Smith, and John Pratt, convicted of a homosexual offence. Swan was reprieved by the King, as Dickens's footnote states; Smith and Pratt were hanged outside Newgate on 27 November.

'The force of habit' is a trite phrase in everybody's mouth; and it is not a little remarkable that those who use it most as applied to others, unconsciously afford in their own persons singular examples of the power which habit and custom exercise over the minds of men, and of the little reflection they are apt to bestow on subjects with which every day's experience has rendered them familiar. If Bedlam could be suddenly removed like another Aladdin's palace, and set down on the space now occupied by Newgate, scarcely one man out of a hundred, whose road to business every morning lies through Newgate Street, or the Old Bailey, would pass the building without bestowing a hasty glance on its small, grated windows, and a transient thought upon the condition of the unhappy beings immured in its dismal cells; and yet these same men, day by day, and hour by hour, pass and repass this gloomy depository of the guilt and misery of London, in one perpetual stream of life and bustle, utterly unmindful of the throng of wretched creatures pent up within it – nay, not even knowing, or if they do, not heeding, the fact, that as they pass one particular angle of the massive wall with a light laugh or a merry whistle, they stand within one yard of a fellow creature, bound and helpless, whose hours are numbered, from whom the last feeble ray of hope has fled for ever, and whose miserable career will shortly terminate in a violent and shameful death. Contact with death, even in its least terrible shape, is solemn and appalling. How much more awful is it to reflect on this near vicinity to the dying – to men in full health and vigour, in the flower of youth or the prime of life, with all their faculties, and perceptions as acute and perfect as your own; but dying, nevertheless – dying as surely – with the hand of death imprinted upon them as indelibly – as if mortal disease had wasted their frames to shadows, and corruption had already begun!

It was with some such thoughts as these that we determined, not many weeks since, to visit the interior of Newgate – in an amateur capacity, of course; and, having carried our intention into effect, we proceed to lay its results before our readers, in the hope – founded more upon the nature of the subject, than on any presumptuous confidence in our own descriptive powers – that this paper may not be found wholly devoid of interest. We have only to premise, that we do not intend to fatigue the reader with any statistical accounts of the prison; they will be found at length in numerous reports of numerous committees, and a variety of authorities of equal weight. We took no notes, made no memoranda, measured none of the yards, ascertained the exact number of inches in no particular room: are unable even to report of how many apartments the gaol is composed.

We saw the prison, and saw the prisoners; and what we did see, and what we thought, we will tell at once in our own way.

Having delivered our credentials to the servant who answered our knock at the door of the governor's house, we were ushered into the 'office'; a little room, on the right-hand side as you enter, with two windows looking into the Old Bailey: fitted up like an ordinary attorney's office, or merchant's counting house, with the usual fixtures – a wainscoted partition, a shelf or two, a desk, a couple of stools, a pair of clerks, an almanack, a clock, and a few maps. After a little delay, occasioned by sending into the interior of the prison for the officer whose duty it was to conduct us, that functionary arrived; a respectable-looking man of about two or three and fifty, in a broad-brimmed hat, and full suit of black, who, but for his keys, would have looked quite as much like a clergyman as a turnkey. We were disappointed; he had not even top boots on. Following our conductor by a door opposite to that at which we had entered, we arrived at a small room, without any other furniture than a little desk, with a book for visitors' autographs, and a shelf, on which were a few boxes for papers, and casts of the heads and faces of the two notorious murderers, Bishop and Williams; the former, in particular, exhibiting a style of head and set of features, which might have afforded sufficient moral grounds for his instant execution at any time, even had there been no other evidence against him. Leaving this room also, by an opposite door, we found ourself in the lodge which opens on the Old Bailey; one side of which is plentifully garnished with a choice collection of heavy sets of irons, including those worn by the redoubtable Jack Sheppard – genuine; and those *said* to have been graced by the sturdy limbs of the no less celebrated Dick Turpin – doubtful. From this lodge, a heavy oaken gate, bound with iron, studded with nails of the same material, and guarded by another turnkey, opens on a few steps, if we remember right, which terminate in a narrow and dismal stone passage, running parallel with the Old Bailey, and leading to the different yards, through a number of tortuous and intricate windings, guarded in their turn by huge gates and gratings, whose appearance is sufficient to dispel at once the slightest hope of escape that any newcomer may have entertained; and the very recollection of which, on eventually traversing the place again, involves one in a maze of confusion.

It is necessary to explain here, that the buildings in the prison, or in other words the different wards – form a square, of which the four sides abut respectively on the Old Bailey, the old College of Physicians (now forming a part of Newgate Market), the Sessions House, and Newgate Street. The intermediate space is divided into several paved yards, in which the prisoners take such air and exercise as can be had in such a place. These yards, with the exception of that in which prisoners under sentence of death are confined (of which we shall presently give a more detailed description), run parallel with Newgate Street, and consequently from the Old Bailey, as it were, to Newgate Market. The women's side is in the right wing of the prison nearest the Sessions House. As we were introduced into this part of the building first, we will adopt the same order, and introduce our readers to it also.

Turning to the right, then, down the passage to which we just now adverted, omitting any mention of intervening gates – for if we noticed every gate that was unlocked for us to pass through, and locked again as soon as we had passed, we should require a gate at every comma – we came to a door composed of thick bars of wood, through which were discernible, passing to and fro in a narrow yard, some twenty women: the majority of whom, however, as soon as they were aware of the presence of strangers, retreated to their wards. One side of this yard is railed off at a considerable distance, and formed into a kind of iron cage, about five feet ten inches in height, roofed at the top, and defended in front by iron bars, from which the friends of the female prisoners communicate with them. In one corner of this singular looking den, was a yellow, haggard, decrepit old woman, in a tattered gown that had once been black, and the remains of an old straw bonnet, with faded ribbon of the same hue, in earnest conversation with a young girl – a prisoner, of course – of about two-and-twenty. It is impossible to imagine a more poverty-stricken object, or a creature so borne down in soul and body, by excess of misery and destitution, as the old woman. The girl was a good-looking robust female, with a profusion of hair streaming about in the wind – for she had no bonnet on – and a man's silk pocket handkerchief loosely thrown over a most ample pair of shoulders. The old woman was talking in that low, stifled tone of voice which tells so forcibly of mental anguish; and every now and then burst into an irrepressible sharp, abrupt cry of grief, the most distressing sound that ears can hear. The girl was perfectly unmoved. Hardened beyond all hope of redemption, she listened doggedly to her mother's entreaties, whatever they were: and, beyond inquiring after 'Jem', and eagerly catching at the few halfpence her miserable parent had brought her, took no more apparent interest in the conversation than the most unconcerned spectators. Heaven knows there were enough of them, in the persons of the other prisoners in the yard, who were no more concerned by what was passing before their eyes, and within their hearing, than if they were blind and deaf. Why should they be? Inside the prison, and out, such scenes were too familiar to them, to excite even a passing thought, unless of ridicule or contempt for feelings which they had long since forgotten.

A little farther on, a squalid-looking woman in a slovenly, thick-bordered cap, with her arms muffled in a large red shawl, the fringed ends of which straggled nearly to the bottom of a dirty white apron, was communicating some instructions to *her* visitor – her daughter evidently. The girl was thinly clad, and shaking with the cold. Some ordinary word of recognition passed between her and her mother when she appeared at the grating, but neither hope, condolence, regret, nor affection was expressed on either side. The mother whispered her instructions, and the girl received them with her pinched-up half-starved features twisted into an expression of careful cunning. It was some scheme for the woman's defence that she was disclosing, perhaps; and a sullen smile came over the girl's face for an instant, as if she were pleased: not so much at the probability of her mother's liberation, as at the chance of her 'getting off' in spite of her prosecutors. The dialogue was soon concluded; and with the same careless indifference with which they had approached each other, the mother turned towards the inner end of the yard, and the girl to the gate at which she had entered.

The girl belonged to a class – unhappily but too extensive – the very existence of which should make men's hearts bleed. Barely past her childhood, it required but a glance to discover that she was one of those children, born and bred in neglect and vice, who have never known what childhood is: who have never been taught to love and court a parent's smile, or to dread a parent's frown. The thousand nameless endearments of childhood, its gaiety and its innocence, are unlike unknown to them. They have entered at once upon the stern realities and miseries of life, and to their better nature it is almost hopeless to appeal in aftertimes, by any of the references which will awaken, if it be only for a moment, some good feeling in ordinary bosoms, however corrupt they may have become. Talk to *them* of parental solicitude, the happy days of childhood, and the merry games of infancy! Tell them of hunger and the streets, beggary and stripes, the gin shop, the station house, and the pawnbroker's, and they will understand you.

Two or three women were standing at different parts of the grating, conversing with their friends, but a very large proportion of the prisoners appeared to have no friends at all, beyond such of their old companions as might happen to be within the walls. So, passing hastily down the yard, and pausing only for an instant to notice the little incidents we have just recorded, we were conducted up a clean and well-lighted flight of stone stairs to one of the wards. There are several in this part of the building, but a description of one is a description of the whole.

It was a spacious, bare, whitewashed apartment, lighted, of course, by windows looking into the interior of the prison, but far more light and airy than one could reasonably expect to find in such a situation. There was a large fire with a deal table before it, round which ten or a dozen women were seated on wooden forms at dinner. Along both sides of the room ran a shelf; below it, at regular intervals, a row of large hooks were fixed in the wall, on each of which was hung the sleeping mat of a prisoner: her rug and blanket being folded up, and placed on the shelf above. At night, these mats are placed on the floor, each beneath the hook on which it hangs during the day; and the ward is thus made to answer the purposes both of a day-room and sleeping apartment. Over the fireplace was a large sheet of pasteboard, on which were displayed a variety of texts from Scripture, which were also scattered about the room in scraps about the size and shape of the copy slips which are used in schools. On the table was a sufficient provision of a kind of stewed beef and brown bread, in pewter dishes, which are kept perfectly bright, and displayed on shelves in great order and regularity when they are not in use.

The women rose hastily, on our entrance, and retired in a hurried manner to either side of the fireplace. They were all cleanly – many of them decently – attired, and there was nothing peculiar, either in their appearance or demeanour. One or two resumed the needlework which they had probably laid aside at the commencement of their meal; others gazed at the visitors with listless curiosity; and a few retired behind their companions to the very end of the room, as if desirous to avoid even the casual observation of the strangers. Some old Irish women, both in this and other wards, to whom the thing was no novelty, appeared perfectly indifferent to our presence, and remained standing close to the seats from which they had just risen; but the general feeling among the females seemed to be one of uneasiness during the period of our stay among them: which was very brief. Not a word was uttered during the time of our remaining, unless, indeed, by the wardswoman in reply to some question which we put to the turnkey who accompanied us. In every ward on the female side, a wardswoman is appointed to preserve order, and a similar regulation is adopted among the males. The wardsmen and wardswomen are all prisoners, selected for good conduct. They alone are allowed the privilege of sleeping on bedsteads; a small stump bedstead being placed in every ward for that purpose. On both sides of the gaol is a small receiving room, to which prisoners are conducted on their first reception, and whence they cannot be removed until they have been examined by the surgeon of the prison[1].

Retracing our steps to the dismal passage in which we found ourselves at first (and which, by-the-bye, contains three or four dark cells for the accommodation of refractory prisoners), we were led through a narrow yard to the 'school' – a portion of the prison set apart for boys under fourteen years of age. In a tolerable-sized room, in which were writing materials and some copy books, was the schoolmaster, with a couple of his pupils; the remainder having been fetched from an adjoining apartment, the whole were drawn up in line for our inspection. There were fourteen of them in all, some with shoes, some without; some in pinafores without jackets, others in jackets without pinafores, and one in scarce anything at all. The whole number, without an exception we believe, had been committed for trial on charges of pocket-picking; and fourteen such terrible little faces we never beheld. – There was not one redeeming feature among them – not a glance of honesty – not a wink expressive of anything but the gallows and the hulks, in the whole collection. As to anything like shame or contrition, that was entirely out of the question. They were evidently quite gratified at being thought worth the trouble of looking at; their idea appeared to be, that we had come to see Newgate as a grand affair, and that they were an indispensable part of the show; and every boy as he 'fell in' to the line, actually seemed as pleased and important as if he had done something excessively meritorious in getting there at

[1] The regulations of the prison relative to the confinement of prisoners during the day, their sleeping at night, their taking their meals, and other matters of gaol economy, have all been altered – greatly for the better – since this sketch was first published. Even the construction of the prison itself has been changed.

all. We never looked upon a more disagreeable sight, because we never saw fourteen such hopeless creatures of neglect, before.

On either side of the schoolyard is a yard for men, in one of which – that towards Newgate Street – prisoners of the more respectable class are confined. On the other, we have little description to offer, as the different wards necessarily partake of the same character. They are provided, like the wards on the women's side, with mats and rugs, which are disposed of in the same manner during the day; the only very striking difference between their appearance and that of the wards inhabited by the females, is the utter absence of any employment. Huddled together on two opposite forms, by the fireside, sit twenty men perhaps; here, a boy in livery; there, a man in a rough greatcoat and top boots; farther on, a desperate-looking fellow in his shirt sleeves, with an old Scotch cap upon his shaggy head; near him again, a tall ruffian, in a smock frock; next to him, a miserable being of distressed appearance, with his head resting on his hand; – all alike in one respect, all idle and listless. When they do leave the fire, sauntering moodily about, lounging in the window, or leaning against the wall, vacantly swinging their bodies to and fro. With the exception of a man reading an old newspaper, in two or three instances, this was the case in every ward we entered.

The only communication these men have with their friends, is through two close iron gratings, with an intermediate space of about a yard in width between the two, so that nothing can be handed across, nor can the prisoner have any communication by touch with the person who visits him. The married men have a separate grating, at which to see their wives, but its construction is the same.

The prison chapel is situated at the back of the governor's house: the latter having no windows looking into the interior of the prison. Whether the associations connected with the place – the knowledge that here a portion of the burial service is, on some dreadful occasions, performed over the quick and not upon the dead – cast over it a still more gloomy and sombre air than art has imparted to it, we know not, but its appearance is very striking. There is something in a silent and deserted place of worship, solemn and impressive at any time; and the very dissimilarity of this one from any we have been accustomed to, only enhances the impression. The meanness of its appointments – the bare and scanty pulpit, with the paltry painted pillars on either side – the women's gallery with its great heavy curtain – the men's with its unpainted benches and dingy front – the tottering little table at the altar, with the commandments on the wall above it, scarcely legible through lack of paint, and dust and damp – so unlike the velvet and gilding, the marble and wood, of a modern church – are strange and striking. There is one object, too, which rivets the attention and fascinates the gaze, and from which we may turn horror stricken in vain, for the recollections of it will haunt us, waking and sleeping, for a long time afterwards. Immediately below the reading desk, on the floor of the chapel, and forming the most conspicuous object in its little area, is *the condemned pew*; a huge black pen, in which the wretched people, who are singled out for death, are placed on the Sunday preceding their execution, in sight of all their fellow prisoners, from many of whom they may have been separated but a week before, to hear prayers for their own souls, to join in the responses of their own burial service, and to listen to an address, warning their recent companions to take example by their fate, and urging themselves, while there is yet time – nearly four-and-twenty hours – to 'turn, and flee from the wrath to come!' Imagine what have been the feelings of the men whom that fearful pew has enclosed, and of whom, between the gallows and the knife, no mortal remnant may now remain! Think of the hopeless clinging to life to the last, and the wild despair, far exceeding in anguish the felon's death itself, by which they have heard the certainty of their speedy transmission to another world, with all their crimes upon their heads, rung into their ears by the officiating clergyman!

At one time – and at no distant period either – the coffins of the men about to be executed, were placed in that pew, upon the seat by their side, during the whole service. It may seem incredible, but it is true. Let us hope that the increased spirit of civilisation and humanity which abolished this frightful and degrading custom, may extend itself to other usages equally barbarous; usages which have not even the plea of utility in their defence, as every year's experience has shown them to be more and more inefficacious.

Leaving the chapel, descending to the passage so frequently alluded to, and crossing the yard before noticed as being allotted to prisoners of a more respectable description than the generality of men confined here, the visitor arrives at a thick iron gate of great size and strength. Having been admitted through it by the turnkey on duty, he turns sharp round to the left, and pauses before another gate; and, having passed this last barrier, he stands in the most terrible part of this gloomy building – the condemned ward.

The press yard, well known by name to newspaper readers, from its frequent mention in accounts of executions, is at the corner of the building, and next to the ordinary's house, in Newgate Street: running from Newgate Street, towards the centre of the prison, parallel with Newgate Market. It is a long, narrow court, of which a portion of the wall in Newgate Street forms one end, and the gate the other. At the upper end, on the left hand – that is, adjoining the wall in Newgate Street – is a cistern of water, and at the bottom a double grating (of which the gate itself forms a part) similar to that before described. Through these grates the prisoners are allowed to see their friends; a turnkey always remaining in the vacant space between, during the whole interview. Immediately on the right as you enter, is a building containing the press room, day room, and cells; the yard is on every side surrounded by lofty walls guarded by *chevaux de frise*; and the whole is under the constant inspection of vigilant and experienced turnkeys.

In the first apartment into which we were conducted – which was at the top of a staircase, and immediately over the press room – were five-and-twenty or thirty prisoners, all under sentence of death, awaiting the result of the recorder's report – men of all ages and appearances, from a hardened old offender with swarthy face and grizzly beard of three days' growth, to a handsome boy, not fourteen years old, and of singularly youthful appearance even for that age, who had been condemned for burglary. There was nothing remarkable in the appearance of these prisoners. One or two decently dressed men were brooding with a dejected air over the fire; several little groups of two or three had been engaged in conversation at the upper end of the room, or in the windows; and the remainder were crowded round a young man seated at a table, who appeared to be engaged in teaching the younger ones to write. The room was large, airy, and clean. There was very little anxiety or mental suffering depicted in the countenance of any of the men; – they had all been sentenced to death, it is true, and the recorder's report had not yet been made; but we question whether there was a man among them, notwithstanding, who did not *know* that although he had undergone the ceremony, it never was intended that his life should be sacrificed. On the table lay a Testament, but there were no tokens of its having been in recent use.

In the press room below were three men, the nature of whose offence rendered it necessary to separate them even from their companions in guilt. It is a long, sombre room, with two windows sunk into the stone wall, and here the wretched men are pinioned on the morning of their execution, before moving towards the scaffold. The fate of one of these prisoners was uncertain; some mitigatory circumstances having come to light since his trial, which had been humanely represented in the proper quarter. The other two had nothing to expect from the mercy of the crown; their doom was sealed; no plea could be urged in extenuation of their crime, and they well knew that for them there was no hope in this world. 'The two short ones,' the turnkey whispered, 'were dead men.'

The man to whom we have alluded as entertaining some hopes of escape, was lounging, at the greatest distance he could place between himself and his companions, in the window nearest to the door. He was probably aware of our approach, and had assumed an air of courageous indifference; his face was purposely averted towards the window, and he stirred not an inch while we were present. The other two men were at the upper end of the room. One of them, who was imperfectly seen in the dim light, had his back towards us, and was stooping over the fire, with his right arm on the mantelpiece, and his head sunk upon it. The other was leaning on the sill of the farthest window. The light fell full upon him, and communicated to his pale, haggard face, and disordered hair, an appearance which, at that distance, was ghastly. His cheek rested upon his hand; and, with his face a little raised, and his eyes wildly staring before him, he seemed to be unconsciously intent on counting the chinks in the opposite wall. We passed this room again afterwards. The first man was pacing up and down the court with a firm military step – he had been a soldier in the foot guards – and a cloth cap jauntily thrown on one side of his head. He bowed respectfully to our conductor, and the salute was returned. The other two still remained in the positions we have described, and were as motionless as statues[1].

A few paces up the yard, and forming a continuation of the building, in which are the two rooms we have just quitted, lie the condemned cells. The entrance is by a narrow and obscure staircase leading to a dark passage, in which a charcoal stove casts a lurid tint over the objects in its immediate vicinity, and diffuses something like warmth around. From the left-hand side of this passage, the massive door of every cell on the story opens; and from it alone can they be approached. There are three of these passages, and three of these ranges of cells, one above the other; but in size, furniture and appearance, they are all precisely alike. Prior to the recorder's report being made, all the prisoners under sentence of death are removed from the day room at five o'clock in the afternoon, and locked up in these cells, where they are allowed a candle until ten o'clock; and here they remain until seven next morning. When the warrant for a prisoner's execution arrives, he is removed to the cells and confined in one of them until he leaves it for the scaffold. He is at liberty to walk in the yard; but, both in his walks and in his cell, he is constantly attended by a turnkey who never leaves him on any pretence.

We entered the first cell. It was a stone dungeon, eight feet long by six wide, with a bench at the upper end, under which were a common rug, a Bible, and prayer book. An iron candlestick was fixed into the wall at the side; and a small high window in the back admitted as much air and light as could struggle in between a double row of heavy, crossed iron bars. It contained no other furniture of any description.

Conceive the situation of a man, spending his last night on earth in this cell. Buoyed up with some vague and undefined hope of reprieve, he

[1] These two men were executed shortly afterwards. The other was respited during his Majesty's pleasure.

knew not why – indulging in some wild and visionary idea of escaping, he knew not how – hour after hour of the three preceding days allowed him for preparation, has fled with a speed which no man living would deem possible, for none but this dying man can know. He has wearied his friends with entreaties, exhausted the attendants with importunities, neglected in his feverish restlessness the timely warnings of his spiritual consoler; and, now that the illusion is at last dispelled, now that eternity is before him and guilt behind, now that his fears of death amount almost to madness, and an overwhelming sense of his helpless, hopeless state rushes upon him, he is lost and stupefied, and has neither thoughts to turn to, nor power to call upon, the Almighty Being, from whom alone he can seek mercy and forgiveness, and before whom his repentance can alone avail.

Hours have glided by, and still he sits upon the same stone bench with folded arms, heedless alike of the fast decreasing time before him, and the urgent entreaties of the good man at his side. The feeble light is wasting gradually, and the deathlike stillness of the street without, broken only by the rumbling of some passing vehicle which echoes mournfully through the empty yards, warns him that the night is waning fast away. The deep bell of St Paul's strikes – one! He heard it; it has roused him. Seven hours left! He paces the narrow limits of his cell with rapid strides, cold drops of terror starting on his forehead, and every muscle of his frame quivering with agony. Seven hours! He suffers himself to be led to his seat, mechanically takes the Bible which is placed in his hand, and tries to read and listen. No: his thoughts will wander. The book is torn and soiled by use – and like the book he read his lessons in, at school, just forty years ago! He has never bestowed a thought upon it, perhaps, since he left it as a child: and yet the place, the time, the room – nay, the very boys he played with, crowd as vividly before him as if they were scenes of yesterday; and some forgotten phrase, some childish word, rings in his ears like the echo of one uttered but a minute since. The voice of the clergyman recalls him to himself. He is reading from the sacred book its solemn promises of pardon for repentance, and its awful denunciation of obdurate men. He falls upon his knees and clasps his hands to pray. Hush! what sound was that? He starts upon his feet. It cannot be two yet. Hark! Two quarters have struck; – the third – the fourth. It is! Six hours left. Tell him not of repentance! Six hours' repentance for eight times six years of guilt and sin! He buries his face in his hands, and throws himself on the bench.

Worn with watching and excitement, he sleeps, and the same unsettled state of mind pursues him in his dreams. An insupportable load is taken from his breast; he is walking with his wife in a pleasant field, with the bright sky above them, and a fresh and boundless prospect on every side – how different from the stone walls of Newgate! She is looking – not as she did when he saw her for the last time in that dreadful place, but as she used when he loved her – long, long ago, before misery and ill treatment had altered her looks, and vice had changed his nature, and she is leaning upon his arm, and looking up into his face with tenderness and affection – and he does *not* strike her now, nor rudely shake her from him. And oh! how glad he is to tell her all he had forgotten in that last hurried interview, and to fall on his knees before her and fervently beseech her pardon for all the unkindness and cruelty that wasted her form and broke her heart! The scene suddenly changes. He is on his trial again: there are the judge and jury, and prosecutors, and witnesses, just as they were before. How full the court is – what a sea of heads – with a gallows, too, and a scaffold – and how all those people stare at *him!* Verdict, 'Guilty'. No matter; he will escape.

The night is dark and cold, the gates have been left open, and in an instant he is in the street, flying from the scene of his imprisonment like the wind. The streets are cleared, the open fields are gained and the broad wide country lies before him. Onward he dashes in the midst of darkness, over hedge and ditch, through mud and pool, bounding from spot to spot with a speed and lightness, astonishing even to himself. At length he pauses; he must be safe from pursuit now; he will stretch himself on that bank and sleep till sunrise.

A period of unconsciousness succeeds. He wakes, cold and wretched. The dull grey light of morning is stealing into the cell, and falls upon the form of the attendant turnkey. Confused by his dreams, he starts from his uneasy bed in momentary uncertainty. It is but momentary. Every object in the narrow cell is too frightfully real to admit of doubt or mistake. He is the condemned felon again, guilty and despairing; and in two hours more will be dead.

# CHARACTERS

## Chapter One

### *Thoughts About People*

First published in the *Evening Chronicle,* 23 April 1835 ('Sketches of London No. 10').

It is strange with how little notice, good, bad, or indifferent, a man may live and die in London. He awakens no sympathy in the breast of any single person; his existence is a matter of interest to no one save himself; he cannot be said to be forgotten when he dies, for no one remembered him when he was alive. There is a numerous class of people in this great metropolis who seem not to possess a single friend, and whom nobody appears to care for. Urged by imperative necessity in the first instance, they have resorted to London in search of employment, and the means of subsistence. It is hard, we know, to break the ties which bind us to our homes and friends, and harder still to efface the thousand recollections of happy days and old times, which have been slumbering in our bosoms for years, and only rush upon the mind, to bring before it associations connected with the friends we have left, the scenes we have beheld too probably for the last time, and the hopes we once cherished, but may entertain no more. These men, however, happily for themselves, have long forgotten such thoughts. Old country friends have died or emigrated; former correspondents have become lost, like themselves, in the crowd and turmoil of some busy city; and they have gradually settled down into mere passive creatures of habit and endurance.

We were seated in the enclosure of St James's Park the other day, when our attention was attracted by a man whom we immediately put down in our own mind as one of this class. He was a tall, thin, pale person, in a black coat, scanty grey trousers, little pinched up gaiters, and brown beaver gloves. He had an umbrella in his hand – not for use, for the day was fine – but, evidently, because he always carried one to the office in the morning. He walked up and down before the little patch of grass on which the chairs are placed for hire, not as if he were doing it for pleasure

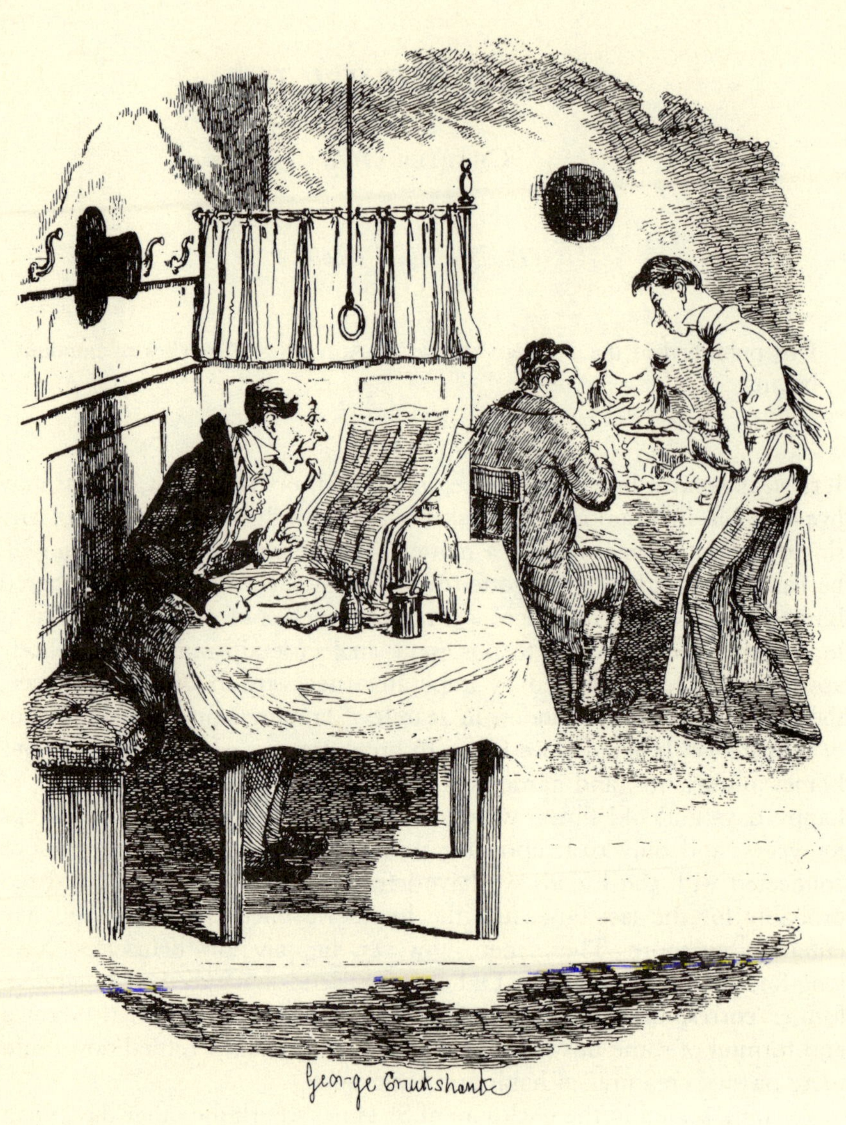

*The Poor Clerk*

or recreation, but as if it were a matter of compulsion, just as he would walk to the office every morning from the back settlements of Islington. It was Monday; he had escaped for four-and-twenty hours from the thraldom of the desk; and was walking here for exercise and amusement – perhaps for the first time in his life. We were inclined to think he had never had a holiday before, and that he did not know what to do with himself. Children were playing on the grass; groups of people were loitering about, chatting and laughing; but the man walked steadily up and down, unheeding and unheeded, his spare pale face looking as if it were incapable of bearing the expression of curiosity or interest.

There was something in the man's manner and appearance which told us, we fancied, his whole life, or rather his whole day, for a man of this sort has no variety of days. We thought we almost saw the dingy little back office into which he walks every morning, hanging his hat on the same peg, and placing his legs beneath the same desk: first, taking off that black coat which lasts the year through, and putting on the one which did duty last year, and which he keeps in his desk to save the other. There he sits till five o'clock, working on, all day, as regularly as the dial over the mantelpiece, whose loud ticking is as monotonous as his whole existence: only raising his head when someone enters the counting house, or when, in the midst of some difficult calculation, he looks up to the ceiling as if there were inspiration in the dusty skylight with a green knot in the centre of every pane of glass. About five, or half-past, he slowly dismounts from his accustomed stool, and again changing his coat, proceeds to his usual dining place, somewhere near Bucklersbury. The waiter recites the bill of fare in a rather confidential manner – for he is a regular customer – and after inquiring 'What's in the best cut?' and 'What was up last?' he orders a small plate of roast beef, with greens, and half a pint of porter. He has a small plate today, because greens are a penny more than potatoes, and he had 'two breads' yesterday, with the additional enormity of 'a cheese' the day before. This important point settled, he hangs up his hat – he took it off the moment he sat down – and bespeaks the paper after the next gentleman. If he can get it while he is at dinner, he eats with much greater zest; balancing it against the water bottle, and eating a bit of beef, and reading a line or two, alternately. Exactly at five minutes before the hour is up, he produces a shilling, pays the reckoning, carefully deposits the change in his waistcoat pocket (first deducting a penny for the waiter), and returns to the office, from which, if it is not foreign post night, he again sallies forth in about half an hour. He then walks home, at his usual pace, to his little back room at Islington, where he has his tea; perhaps solacing himself during the meal with the conversation of his landlady's little boy, whom he occasionally rewards with a penny, for solving problems in simple addition. Sometimes, there is a letter or two to take up to his employer's, in Russell Square; and then, the wealthy man of business, hearing his voice, calls out from the dining parlour, – 'Come in, Mr Smith'; and Mr Smith, putting his hat at the feet of one of the hall chairs, walks timidly in, and being condescendingly desired to sit down, carefully tucks his legs under his chair, and sits at a considerable distance from the table while he drinks the glass of sherry which is poured out for him by the eldest boy, and after drinking which, he backs and slides out of the room, in a state of nervous agitation from which he does not perfectly recover, until he finds himself once more in the Islington Road. Poor, harmless creatures such men are; contented but not happy; broken-spirited and humbled, they may feel no pain, but they never know pleasure.

Compare these men with another class of beings who, like them, have neither friend nor companion, but whose position in society is the result of their own choice. These are generally old fellows with white heads and red faces, addicted to port wine and Hessian boots, who from some cause, real or imaginary – generally the former, the excellent reason being that they are rich, and their relations poor – grow suspicious of everybody, and do the misanthropical in chambers, taking great delight in thinking themselves unhappy, and making everybody they come near, miserable. You may see such men as these anywhere; you will know them at coffee houses by their discontented exclamations and the luxury of their dinners; at theatres, by their always sitting in the same place and looking with a jaundiced eye on all the young people near them; at church, by the pomposity with which they enter, and the loud tone in which they repeat the responses; at parties, by their getting cross at whist and hating music. An old fellow of this kind will have his chambers splendidly furnished, and collect books, plate, and pictures about him in profusion; not so much for his own gratification, as to be superior to those who have the desire, but not the means, to compete with him. He belongs to two or three clubs, and is envied, and flattered, and hated by the members of them all. Sometimes he will be appealed to by a poor relation – a married nephew perhaps – for some little assistance: and then he will declaim with honest indignation on the improvidence of young married people, the worthlessness of a wife, the insolence of having a family, the atrocity of getting into debt with a hundred and twenty-five pounds a year, and other unpardonable crimes; winding up his exhortations with a complacent review of his own conduct, and a delicate allusion to parochial relief. He dies, some day after dinner, of apoplexy, having bequeathed his property to a Public Society, and the Institution erects a tablet to his memory, expressive of their admiration of his Christian conduct in this world, and their comfortable conviction of his happiness in the next.

But, next to our very particular friends, hackney coachmen, cabmen and cads, whom we admire in proportion to the extent of their cool impudence and perfect self-possession, there is no class of people who amuse us more than London apprentices. They are no longer an organised body, bound down by solemn compact to terrify his Majesty's subjects whenever it pleases them to take offence in their heads and staves in their hands. They are only bound, now, by indentures, and, as to their valour, it is easily restrained by the wholesome dread of the New Police, and a perspective view of a damp station house, terminating in a police office and a reprimand. They are still, however, a peculiar class, and not the less pleasant for being inoffensive. Can anyone fail to have noticed them in the streets on Sunday? And were there ever such harmless efforts at the grand and magnificent as the young fellows display! We walked down the Strand, a Sunday or two ago, behind a little group; and they furnished food for our amusement the whole way. They had come out of some part of the city; it was between three and four o'clock in the afternoon; and they were on their way to the Park. There were four of them, all arm-in-arm, with white kid gloves like so many bridegrooms, light trousers of unprecedented patterns, and coats for which the English language has yet no name – a kind of cross between a great coat and a surtout, with the collar of the one, the skirts of the other, and pockets peculiar to themselves.

Each of the gentlemen carried a thick stick, with a large tassel at the top, which he occasionally twirled gracefully round; and the whole four, by way of looking easy and unconcerned, were walking with a paralytic swagger irresistibly ludicrous. One of the party had a watch about the size and shape of a reasonable Ribstone pippin, jammed into his waistcoat pocket, which he carefully compared with the clocks at St Clement's and the New Church, the illuminated clock at Exeter 'Change, the clock of St Martin's Church, and the clock of the Horse Guards. When they at last arrived in St James's Park, the member of the party who had the best made boots on, hired a second chair expressly for his feet, and flung himself on this two-pennyworth of sylvan luxury with an air which levelled all distinctions between Brookes's and Snooks's, Crockford's and Bagnigge Wells.

We may smile at such people, but they can never excite our anger. They are usually on the best terms with themselves, and it follows almost as a matter of course, in good humour with everyone about them. Besides, they are always the faint reflection of higher lights; and, if they do display a little occasional foolery in their own proper persons, it is surely more tolerable than precocious puppyism in the Quadrant, whiskered dandyism in Regent Street and Pall Mall, or gallantry in its dotage anywhere.

## Chapter Two

### *A Christmas Dinner*

First published under the title 'Christmas Festivities' in *Bell's Life in London*, 27 December 1835 ('Scenes and Characters No. 10'). This, Dickens's first celebration in print of the season that is so strongly associated with him, looks forward, both in its general spirit and in many details, to the Christmas chapter of *Pickwick Papers* and the later Christmas Books and Stories.

Christmas time! That man must be a misanthrope indeed, in whose breast something like a jovial feeling is not roused – in whose mind some pleasant associations are not awakened – by the recurrence of Christmas. There are people who will tell you that Christmas is not to them what it used to be; that each succeeding Christmas has found some cherished hope, or happy prospect, of the year before, dimmed or passed away; that the present only serves to remind them of reduced circumstances and straitened incomes – of the feasts they once bestowed on hollow friends, and of the cold looks that meet them now, in adversity and misfortune. Never heed such dismal reminiscences. There are few men who have lived long enough in the world, who cannot call up such thoughts any day in the year. Then do not select the merriest of the three hundred and sixty-five, for your doleful recollections, but draw your chair nearer the blazing fire – fill the glass and send round the song – and if your room be smaller than it was a dozen years ago, or if your glass be filled with reeking punch, instead of sparkling wine, put a good face on the matter, and empty it off-hand, and fill another, and troll off the old ditty you used to sing, and thank God it's no worse. Look on the merry faces of your children (if you have any) as they sit round the fire. One little seat may be empty; one slight form that gladdened the father's heart, and roused the mother's pride to look upon, may not be there. Dwell not upon the past; think not that one short year ago, the fair child now resolving into dust, sat before you, with the bloom of health upon its cheek, and the gaiety of infancy in its joyous eye. Reflect upon your present blessings – of which every man has many – not on your past misfortunes, of which all men have some. Fill your glass again, with a merry face and contented heart. Our life on it, but your Christmas shall be merry, and your new year a happy one!

Who can be insensible to the outpourings of good feeling, and the honest interchange of affectionate attachment, which abound at this season of the year! A Christmas family party! We know nothing in nature more delightful! There seems a magic in the very name of Christmas. Petty jealousies and discords are forgotten; social feelings are awakened, in bosoms to which they have long been strangers; father and son, or brother and sister, who have met and passed with averted gaze, or a look of cold recognition, for months before, proffer and return the cordial embrace, and bury their past animosities in their present happiness. Kindly hearts that have yearned towards each other, but have been withheld by false notions of pride and self-dignity, are again reunited, and all is kindness and benevolence! Would that Christmas lasted the whole year through (as it ought), and that the prejudices and passions which deform our better nature, were never called into action among those to whom they should ever be strangers!

The Christmas family party that we mean, is not a mere assemblage of relations, got up at a week or two's notice, originating this year, having no family precedent in the last, and not likely to be repeated in the next. No. It is an annual gathering of all the accessible members of the family, young or old, rich or poor; and all the children look forward to it, for two months beforehand, in a fever of anticipation. Formerly, it was held at grandpapa's; but grandpapa getting old, and grandmamma getting old too, and rather infirm, they have given up housekeeping, and domesticated themselves with uncle George; so the party always takes place at uncle George's house, but grandmamma sends in most of the good things, and grandpapa always *will* toddle down, all the way to Newgate Market, to buy the turkey, which he engages a porter to bring home behind him in triumph, always insisting on the man's being rewarded with a glass of spirits, over and above his hire, to drink 'a merry Christmas and a happy new year' to aunt George. As to grandmamma, she is very secret and mysterious for two or three days beforehand, but not sufficiently so to prevent rumours getting afloat that she has purchased a beautiful new cap with pink ribbons for each of the servants, together with sundry books, and pen knives, and pencil cases, for the younger branches; to say nothing of divers secret additions to the order originally given by aunt George at the pastrycook's, such as another dozen of mince pies for the dinner, and a large plum cake for the children.

On Christmas Eve, grandmamma is always in excellent spirits, and after employing all the children, during the day, in stoning the plums, and all that, insists, regularly every year, on uncle George coming down into the kitchen, taking off his coat, and stirring the pudding for half an hour or so, which uncle George good-humouredly does, to the vociferous delight of the children and servants. The evening concludes with a glorious game of blind man's buff, in an early stage of which grandpapa takes great care to be caught, in order that he may have an opportunity of displaying his dexterity.

On the following morning, the old couple, with as many of the children as the pew will hold, go to church in great state: leaving aunt George at home dusting decanters and filling casters, and uncle George carrying bottles into the dining parlour, and calling for corkscrews, and getting into everybody's way.

When the church party return to lunch, grandpapa produces a small sprig of mistletoe from his pocket, and tempts the boys to kiss their little cousins under it – a proceeding which affords both the boys and the old gentleman unlimited satisfaction, but which rather outrages grandmamma's ideas of decorum, until grandpapa says that when he was just thirteen years and three months old, *he* kissed grandmamma under a mistletoe too, on which the children clap their hands, and laugh very heartily, as do aunt George and uncle George; and grandmamma looks pleased, and says, with a benevolent smile, that grandpapa was an impudent young dog, on which the children laugh very heartily again, and grandpapa more heartily than any of them.

But all these diversions are nothing to the subsequent excitement when grandmamma in a high cap, and slate-coloured silk gown; and grandpapa with a beautifully plaited shirt frill, and white neckerchief; seat themselves on one side of the drawing room fire, with uncle George's children and little cousins innumerable, seated in the front, waiting the arrival of the expected visitors. Suddenly a hackney coach is heard to stop, and uncle George, who has been looking out of the window, exclaims, 'Here's Jane!' on which the children rush to the door, and helter-skelter downstairs; and uncle Robert and aunt Jane, and the dear little baby, and the nurse, and the whole party, are ushered upstairs amidst tumultuous shouts of 'Oh, my!' from the children, and frequently repeated warnings not to hurt baby from the nurse. And grandpapa takes the child, and grandmamma kisses her daughter, and the confusion of the first entry has scarcely subsided, when some other aunts and uncles with more cousins arrive, and the grown up cousins flirt with each other, and so do the little cousins too, for that matter, and nothing is to be heard but a confused din of talking, laughing, and merriment.

A hesitating double knock at the street door, heard during a momentary pause in the conversation, excites a general inquiry of 'Who's that?' and two or three children, who have been standing at the window, announce in a low voice, that it's 'poor aunt Margaret'. Upon which, aunt George leaves the room to welcome the newcomer; and grandmamma draws herself up, rather stiff and stately; for Margaret married a poor man without her consent, and poverty not being a sufficiently weighty punishment for her offence, has been discarded by her friends, and debarred the society of her dearest relatives. But Christmas has come round, and the unkind feelings that have struggled against better dispositions during the year, have melted away before its genial influence, like half formed ice beneath the morning sun. It is not difficult in a moment of angry feeling for a parent to denounce a disobedient child; but to banish her at a period of general good will and hilarity, from the hearth round which she has sat on so many anniversaries of the same day, expanding by slow degrees from infancy to girlhood, and then bursting, almost imperceptibly, into a woman, is widely different. The air of conscious rectitude, and cold forgiveness, which the old lady has assumed, sits ill upon her; and when the poor girl is led in by her sister, pale in looks and broken in hope – not from poverty, for that she could bear, but from the consciousness of undeserved neglect, and unmerited unkindness – it is easy to see how much of it is assumed. A momentary pause succeeds; the girl breaks suddenly from her sister and throws herself, sobbing, on her mother's neck. The father steps hastily forward, and takes her husband's hand. Friends crowd round to offer their hearty congratulations, and happiness and harmony again prevail.

As to the dinner, it's perfectly delightful – nothing goes wrong, and everybody is in the very best of spirits, and disposed to please and be pleased. Grandpapa relates a circumstantial account of the purchase of the turkey, with a slight digression relative to the purchase of previous turkeys, on former Christmas-days, which grandmamma corroborates in the minutest particular. Uncle George tells stories, and carves poultry, and takes wine, and jokes with the children at the side table, and winks at the cousins that are making love, or being made love to, and exhilarates everybody with his good humour and hospitality; and when, at last, a stout servant staggers in with a gigantic pudding, with a sprig of holly in the top, there is such a laughing, and shouting, and clapping of little chubby hands, and kicking up of fat dumpy legs, as can only be equalled by the applause with which the astonishing feat of pouring lighted brandy into mince pies is received by the younger visitors. Then the dessert! – and the wine! – and the fun! Such beautiful speeches, and *such* songs, from aunt Margaret's husband, who turns out to be such a nice man, and *so* attentive to grandmamma! Even grandpapa not only sings his annual song with unprecedented vigour, but on being honoured with an unanimous *encore,* according to annual custom, actually comes out with a new one which nobody but grandmamma ever heard before; and a young scape-grace of a cousin, who has been in some disgrace with the old people, for certain heinous sins of omission and commission – neglecting to call, and persisting in drinking Burton Ale – astonishes everybody into convulsions of laughter by volunteering the most extraordinary comic songs that ever were heard. And thus the evening passes, in a strain of rational good will and cheerfulness, doing more to awaken the sympathies of every member of the party in behalf of his neighbour, and to perpetuate their good feeling during the ensuing year, than half the homilies that have ever been written, by half the Divines that have ever lived.

## Chapter Three

### *The New Year*

First published in *Bell's Life in London,* 3 January 1836 ('Scenes and Characters No. 11'). Dickens's 'thirty-six' in para. 3 is presumably an error for 'thirty-five'.

Next to Christmas day, the most pleasant annual epoch in existence is the advent of the New Year. There are a lachrymose set of people who usher in the New Year with watching and fasting, as if they were bound to attend as chief mourners at the obsequies of the old one. Now, we cannot but think it a great deal more complimentary, both to the old year that has rolled away, and to the New Year that is just beginning to dawn upon us, to see the old fellow out, and the new one in, with gaiety and glee.

There must have been some few occurrences in the past year to which we can look back, with a smile of cheerful recollection, if not with a feeling of heartfelt thankfulness. And we are bound by every rule of justice and equity to give the New Year credit for being a good one, until he proves himself unworthy the confidence we repose in him.

This is our view of the matter; and entertaining it, notwithstanding our respect for the old year, one of the few remaining moments of whose existence passes away with every word we write, here we are, seated by our fireside on this last night of the old year, one thousand eight hundred and thirty-six, penning this article with as jovial a face as if nothing extraordinary had happened, or was about to happen, to disturb our good humour.

Hackney coaches and carriages keep rattling up the street and down the street in rapid succession, conveying, doubtless, smartly dressed coachfuls to crowded parties; loud and repeated double knocks at the house with green blinds, opposite, announce to the whole neighbourhood that there's one large party in the street at all events; and we saw through the window, and through the fog too, till it grew so thick that we rung for candles, and drew our curtains, pastry cooks' men with green boxes on their heads, and rout-furniture-warehouse-carts, with cane seats and French lamps, hurrying to the numerous houses where an annual festival is held in honour of the occasion.

We can fancy one of these parties, we think, as well as if we were duly dress coated and pumped, and had just been announced at the drawing room door.

Take the house with the green blinds for instance. We know it is a quadrille party, because we saw some men taking up the front drawing room carpet while we sat at breakfast this morning, and if further evidence be required, and we must tell the truth, we just now saw one of the young ladies 'doing' another of the young ladies' hair, near one of the bedroom windows, in an unusual style of splendour, which nothing else but a quadrille party could possibly justify.

The master of the house with the green blinds is in a public office; we know the fact by the cut of his coat, the tie of his neckcloth, and the self-satisfaction of his gait – the very green blinds themselves have a Somerset House air about them.

Hark! – a cab! That's a junior clerk in the same office; a tidy sort of young man, with a tendency to cold and corns, who comes in a pair of boots with black cloth fronts, and brings his shoes in his coat pocket, which shoes he is at this very moment putting on in the hall. Now he is announced by the man in the passage to another man in a blue coat, who is a disguised messenger from the office.

The man on the first landing precedes him to the drawing room door. 'Mr Tupple!' shouts the messenger. 'How *are* you, Tupple?' says the master of the house, advancing from the fire, before which he has been talking politics and airing himself. 'My dear, this is Mr Tupple (a courteous salute from the lady of the house); Tupple my eldest daughter; Julia, my dear, Mr Tupple; Tupple, my other daughters; my son, sir'; Tupple rubs his hands very hard, and smiles as if it were all capital fun, and keeps constantly bowing and turning himself round, till the whole family have been introduced, when he glides into a chair at the corner of the sofa, and opens a miscellaneous conversation with the young ladies upon the weather, and the theatres, and the old year, and the last new murder, and the balloon, and the ladies' sleeves, and the festivities of the season, and a great many other topics of small talk.

More double knocks! what an extensive party! what an incessant hum of conversation and general sipping of coffee! We see Tupple now, in our mind's eye, in the height of his glory. He has just handed that stout old lady's cup to the servant; and now he dives among the crowd of young men by the door, to intercept the other servant, and secure the muffin plate for the old lady's daughter, before he leaves the room; and now, as he passes the sofa on his way back, he bestows a glance of recognition and patronage upon the young ladies, as condescending and familiar as if he had known them from infancy.

Charming person Mr Tupple – perfect ladies' man – such a delightful companion, too! Laugh! – nobody ever understood papa's jokes half so well as Mr Tupple, who laughs himself into convulsions at every fresh burst of facetiousness. Most delightful partner! talks through the whole set! and although he does seem at first rather gay and frivolous, so romantic and with so *much* feeling! Quite a love. No great favourite with the young men, certainly, who sneer at, and affect to despise him; but everybody knows that's only envy, and they needn't give themselves the trouble to depreciate his merits at any rate, for Ma says he shall be asked to every future dinner party, if it's only to talk to people between the courses, and distract their attention when there's any unexpected delay in the kitchen.

At supper, Mr Tupple shows to still greater advantage than he has done throughout the evening, and when Pa requests everyone to fill their glasses for the purpose of drinking happiness throughout the year, Mr Tupple is *so* droll: insisting on all the young ladies having their glasses filled, notwithstanding their repeated assurances that they never can, by any possibility, think of emptying them: and subsequently begging permission to say a few words on the sentiment which has just been uttered by Pa – when he makes one of the most brilliant and poetical speeches that can possibly be imagined, about the old year and the new one. After the toast has been drunk, and when the ladies have retired, Mr Tupple requests that every gentleman will do him the favour of filling his glass, for he has a toast to propose: on which all the gentlemen cry 'Hear! hear!' and pass the decanters accordingly: and Mr Tupple being informed by the master of the house that they are all charged, and waiting for his toast, rises, and begs to remind the gentlemen present, how much they have been delighted by the dazzling array of elegance and beauty which the drawing room has exhibited that night, and how their senses have been charmed, and their hearts captivated, by the bewitching concentration of female loveliness which that very room has so recently displayed. (Loud cries of 'Hear!') Much as he (Tupple) would be disposed to deplore the absence of the ladies, on other grounds, he cannot but derive some consolation from the reflection that the very circumstance of their not being present, enables him to propose a toast, which he would have otherwise been prevented from giving – that toast he begs to say is – 'The Ladies!' (Great applause.) The Ladies! among whom the fascinating daughters of their excellent host are alike conspicuous for their beauty, their accomplishments, and their elegance. He begs them to drain a bumper to 'The Ladies, and a happy new year to them!' (Prolonged approbation; above which the noise of the ladies dancing the Spanish dance among themselves, overhead, is distinctly audible.)

The applause consequent on this toast has scarcely subsided, when a young gentleman in a pink under-waistcoat, sitting towards the bottom of the table, is observed to grow very restless and fidgety, and to evince strong indications of some latent desire to give vent to his feelings in a speech, which the wary Tupple at once perceiving, determines to forestall by speaking himself. He, therefore, rises again, with an air of solemn importance, and trusts he may be permitted to propose another toast (unqualified approbation, and Mr Tupple proceeds). He is sure they must all be deeply impressed with the hospitality – he may say the splendour – with which they have been that night received by their worthy host and hostess. (Unbounded applause.) Although this is the first occasion on which he has had the pleasure and delight of sitting at that board, he has known his friend Dobble long and intimately; he has been connected with him in business – he wishes everybody present knew Dobble as well as he does. (A cough from the host.) He (Tupple) can lay his hand upon his (Tupple's) heart, and declare his confident belief that a better man, a better husband, a better father, a better brother, a better son, a better relation in any relation of life, than Dobble, never existed. (Loud cries of 'Hear!') They have seen him tonight in the peaceful bosom of his family; they should see him in the morning, in the trying duties of his office. Calm in the perusal of the morning papers, uncompromising in the signature of his name, dignified in his replies to the inquiries of stranger applicants, deferential in his behaviour to his superiors, majestic in his deportment to the messengers. (Cheers.) When he bears this merited testimony to the excellent qualities of his friend Dobble, what can he say in approaching such a subject as Mrs Dobble? Is it requisite for him to expatiate on the qualities of that amiable woman? No; he will spare his friend Dobble's feelings; he will spare the feelings of his friend – if he will allow him to have the honour of calling him so – Mr Dobble, junior. (Here Mr Dobble, junior, who has been previously distending his mouth to a considerable width, by thrusting a particularly fine orange into that feature, suspends operations, and assumes a proper appearance of intense melancholy.) He will simply say – and he is quite certain it is a sentiment in which all who hear him will readily concur – that his friend Dobble is as superior to any man he ever knew, as Mrs Dobble is far beyond any woman he ever saw (except her daughters); and he will conclude by proposing their worthy 'Host and Hostess, and may they live to enjoy many more new years!'

The toast is drunk with acclamation; Dobble returns thanks, and the whole party rejoin the ladies in the drawing room. Young men who were too bashful to dance before supper, find tongues and partners; the musicians exhibit unequivocal symptoms of having drunk the new year in, while the company were out; and dancing is kept up until far in the first morning of the new year.

We have scarcely written the last word of the previous sentence, when the first stroke of twelve peals from the neighbouring churches. There certainly – we must confess it now – is something awful in the sound. Strictly speaking, it may not be more impressive now than at any other time; for the hours steal as swiftly on at other periods, and their flight is little heeded. But we measure man's life by years, and it is a solemn knell that warns us we have passed another of the landmarks which stand between us and the grave. Disguise it as we may, the reflection will force itself on our minds, that when the next bell announces the arrival of a new year, we may be insensible alike of the timely warning we have so often neglected, and of all the warm feelings that glow within us now.

## Chapter Four

### *Miss Evans and the Eagle*

First published in *Bell's Life in London,* 4 October 1835 ('Scenes and Characters No. 2'). Green tea was luxury, as its price (seven shillings and sixpence) indicates. The Eagle was a tea garden in the City Road which became a kind of early music hall in 1825. Its large concert hall (the Rotunda) held over a thousand people and Hill suggests that the 'Miss Somebody in white satin' who sings Thomas Arne's 'The soldier tired' was Miss Fraser James whose portrait appears in Wroth's *Cremorne and the Later London Gardens* (1907). The aria, immensely popular with soprano singers, was written by Arne for his own translation of Metastasio's *Artaserse*: 'The soldier tired of war's alarms/Forswears the clang of hostile arms ...'

The Eagle later became the Grecian Theatre and in 1884 a Salvation Army Centre. In 1901 it was demolished and rebuilt as a public house, which still stands.

Mr Samuel Wilkins was a carpenter, a journeyman carpenter of small dimensions, decidedly below the middle size – bordering, perhaps, upon the dwarfish. His face was round and shining, and his hair carefully twisted into the outer corner of each eye, till it formed a variety of that description of semi-curls, usually known as 'aggerawators'. His earnings were all-sufficient for his wants, varying from eighteen shillings to one pound five, weekly – his manner undeniable – his sabbath waistcoats dazzling. No wonder that, with these qualifications, Samuel Wilkins found favour in the eyes of the other sex: many women have been captivated by far less substantial qualifications. But Samuel was proof against their blandishments, until at length his eyes rested on those of a Being for whom, from that time forth, he felt fate had destined him. He came, and conquered – proposed, and was accepted – loved, and was beloved. Mr Wilkins 'kept company' with Jemima Evans.

Miss Evans (or Ivins, to adopt the pronunciation most in vogue with her circle of acquaintance) had adopted in early life the useful pursuit of shoe-binding, to which she had afterwards superadded the occupation of a straw-bonnet maker. Herself, her maternal parent, and two sisters, formed an harmonious quartet in the most secluded portion of Camden

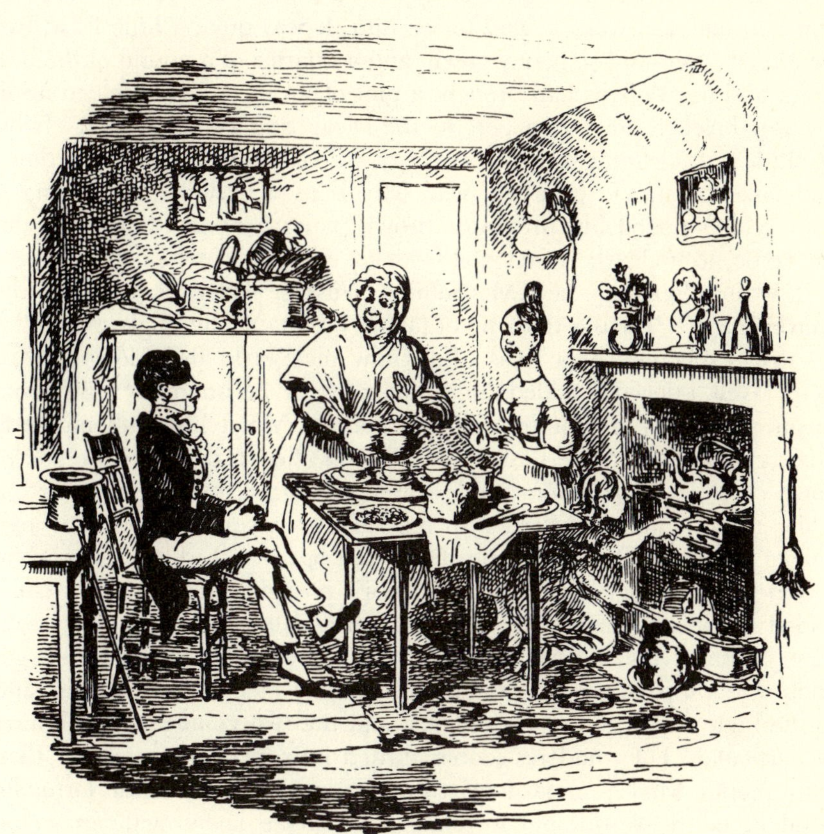

*Samuel Wilkins and the Evanses*

Town; and here it was that Mr Wilkins presented himself, one Monday afternoon, in his best attire, with his face more shining and his waistcoat more bright than either had ever appeared before. The family were just going to tea, and were *so* glad to see him. It was quite a little feast; two ounces of seven-and-sixpenny green, and a quarter of a pound of the best fresh; and Mr Wilkins had brought a pint of shrimps, neatly folded up in a clean belcher, to give a zest to the meal, and propitiate Mrs Ivins. Jemima was 'cleaning herself' upstairs; so Mr Samuel Wilkins sat down and talked domestic economy with Mrs Ivins, whilst the two youngest Miss Ivinses poked bits of lighted brown paper between the bars under the kettle, to make the water boil for tea.

'I wos a-thinking,' said Mr Samuel Wilkins, during a pause in the conversation – 'I wos a-thinking of taking J'mima to the Eagle tonight.' – 'O my!' exclaimed Mrs Ivins. 'Lor! how nice!' said the youngest Miss Ivins. 'Well, I declare!' added the youngest Miss Ivins but one. 'Tell J'mima to put on her white muslin, Tilly,' screamed Mrs Ivins, with motherly anxiety; and down came J'mima herself soon afterwards in a white muslin gown carefully hooked and eyed, a little red shawl, plentifully pinned, a white straw bonnet trimmed with red ribbons, a small necklace, a large pair of bracelets, Denmark satin shoes, and open-worked stockings; white cotton gloves on her fingers, and a cambric pocket handkerchief, carefully folded up, in her hand – all quite genteel and ladylike. And away went Miss J'mima Ivins and Mr Samuel Wilkins, and a dress cane with a gilt knob at the top, to the admiration and envy of the street in general, and to the high gratification of Mrs Ivins, and the two youngest Miss Ivinses in particular. They had no sooner turned into the Pancras Road, than who should Miss J'mima Ivins stumble upon, by the most fortunate accident in the world, but a young lady as she knew, with *her* young man! – And it is so strange how things do turn out sometimes – they were actually going to the Eagle too. So Mr Samuel Wilkins was introduced to Miss J'mima Ivins's friend's young man, and they all walked on together, talking, and laughing, and joking away like anything; and when they got as far as Pentonville, Miss Ivins's friend's young man *would* have the ladies go into the Crown to taste some shrub, which, after a great blushing and giggling, and hiding of faces in elaborate pocket handkerchiefs, they consented to do. Having tasted it once, they were easily prevailed upon to taste it again; and they sat out in the garden tasting shrub, and looking at the Busses alternately, till it was just the proper time to go to the Eagle; and then they resumed their journey, and walked very fast, for fear they should lose the beginning of the concert in the Rotunda.

'How ev'nly!' said Miss J'mima Ivins, and Miss J'mima Ivins's friend, both at once, when they had passed the gate and were fairly inside the gardens. There were the walks, beautifully gravelled and planted – and the refreshment boxes, painted and ornamented like so many snuff boxes – and the variegated lamps shedding their rich light upon the company's heads – and the place for dancing ready chalked for the company's feet – and a Moorish band playing at one end of the gardens – and an opposition military band playing away at the other. Then, the waiters were rushing to and fro with glasses of negus, and glasses of brandy and water, and bottles of ale, and bottles of stout; and ginger beer was going off in one place, and practical jokes were going on in another; and people were crowding to the door of the Rotunda; and in short the whole scene was, as Miss J'mima Ivins, inspired by the novelty, or the shrub, or both, observed – 'one of dazzling excitement'. As to the concert room, never was anything half so splendid. There was an orchestra for the singers, all paint, gilding, and plate glass; and such an organ! Miss J'mima Ivins's friend's young man whispered it had cost 'four hundred pound', which Mr Samuel Wilkins said was 'not dear neither'; an opinion in which the ladies perfectly coincided. The audience were seated on elevated benches round the room, and crowded into every part of it; and everybody was eating and drinking as comfortably as possible. Just before the concert commenced, Mr Samuel Wilkins ordered two glasses of rum and water 'warm with –' and two slices of lemon, for himself and the other young man, together with 'a pint o' sherry wine for the ladies, and some sweet carraway seed biscuits'; and they would have been quite comfortable and happy, only a strange gentleman with large whiskers *would* stare at Miss J'mima Ivins, and another gentleman in a plaid waistcoat *would* wink at Miss J'mima Ivins's friend; on which Miss J'mima Ivins's friend's young man exhibited symptoms of boiling over, and began to mutter about 'people's imperence', and 'swells out o' luck'; and to intimate, in oblique terms, a vague intention of knocking somebody's head off; which he was only prevented from announcing more emphatically, by both Miss J'mima Ivins and her friend threatening to faint away on the spot if he said another word.

The concert commenced – overture on the organ. 'How solemn!' exclaimed Miss J'mima Ivins, glancing, perhaps unconsciously, at the gentleman with the whiskers. Mr Samuel Wilkins, who had been muttering apart for some time past, as if he were holding a confidential conversation with the gilt knob of the dress cane, breathed hard – breathing vengeance, perhaps, – but said nothing. 'The soldier tired,' Miss Somebody in white satin. 'Ancore!' cried Miss J'mima Ivins's friend. 'Ancore!' shouted the gentleman in the plaid waistcoat immediately, hammering the table with a stout bottle. Miss J'mima Ivins's friend's young man eyed the man behind the waistcoat from head to foot, and cast a look of interrogative contempt towards Mr Samuel Wilkins. Comic song, accompanied on the organ. Miss J'mima Ivins was convulsed with laughter – so was the man with the whiskers. Everything the ladies did, the plaid waistcoat and whiskers did, by way of expressing unity of sentiment and congeniality of soul; and Miss J'mima Ivins, and Miss J'mima Ivins's friend, grew lively and talkative, as Mr Samuel Wilkins, and Miss J'mima Ivins's friend's young man, grew morose and surly in inverse proportion.

Now, if the matter had ended here, the little party might soon have recovered their former equanimity; but Mr Samuel Wilkins and his friend began to throw looks of defiance upon the waistcoat and whiskers. And the waistcoat and whiskers, by way of intimating the slight degree in which they were affected by the looks aforesaid, bestowed glances of increased admiration upon Miss J'mima Ivins and friend. The concert and vaudeville concluded, they promenaded the gardens. The waistcoat and whiskers did the same; and made divers remarks complimentary to the ankles of Miss J'mima Ivins and friend, in an audible tone. At length, not satisfied with these numerous atrocities, they actually came up and asked Miss J'mima Ivins, and Miss J'mima Ivins's friend, to dance without taking no more notice of Mr Samuel Wilkins, and Miss J'mima Ivins's friend's young man, than if they was nobody!

'What do you mean by that, scoundrel!' exclaimed Mr Samuel Wilkins, grasping the gilt-knobbed dress cane firmly in his right hand. 'What's the matter with *you,* you little humbug?' replied the whiskers. 'How dare you insult me and my friend?' inquired the friend's young man. 'You and your friend be hanged!' responded the waistcoat. 'Take that,' exclaimed Mr Samuel Wilkins. The ferrule of the gilt-knobbed dress cane was visible for an instant, and then the light of the variegated lamps shone brightly upon it as it whirled into the air, cane and all. 'Give it him,' said the waistcoat. 'Horficer!' screamed the ladies. Miss J'mima Ivins's beau, and the friend's young man, lay gasping on the gravel, and the waistcoat and whiskers were seen no more.

Miss J'mima Ivins and friend being conscious that the affray was in no slight degree attributable to themselves, of course went into hysterics forthwith; declared themselves the most injured of women; exclaimed, in incoherent ravings, that they had been suspected – wrongfully suspected – oh! that they should ever have lived to see the day – and so forth; suffered a relapse every time they opened their eyes and saw their unfortunate little admirers; and were carried to their respective abodes in a hackney coach, and a state of insensibility, compounded of shrub, sherry, and excitement.

## Chapter Five

### *The Parlour Orator*

First published under the title 'The Parlour' in *Bell's Life in London,* 13 December 1835 ('Scenes and Characters No. 9'). For the original opening paragraph of this sketch, describing different kinds of parlours, see DeVries, p. 169. Hill notes of the opening sentence that Dickens's 'lounge' represented a round trip of seven miles from Furnival's Inn where he was living at the time. The little greengrocer's reference to the 'twenty million that was paid for 'mancipation' alludes to the abolition of slavery throughout all British dominions. It had been decreed by Parliament in 1833 (the slave trade itself had been outlawed in 1807) at a cost to the nation of £20,000,000.

We had been lounging one evening, down Oxford Street, Holborn, Cheapside, Coleman Street, Finsbury Square, and so on, with the intention of returning westward, by Pentonville, and the New Road, where we began to feel rather thirsty, and disposed to rest for five or ten minutes. So we turned back towards an old, quiet, decent public house, which we remembered to have passed but a moment before (it was not far from the City Road), for the purpose of solacing ourself with a glass of ale. The house was none of your stuccoed, French-polished, illuminated palaces, but a modest public house of the old school, with a little old bar, and a little old landlord, who, with a wife and daughter of the same pattern, was comfortably seated in the bar aforesaid – a snug little room with a cheerful fire, protected by a large screen: from behind which the young lady emerged on our representing our inclination for a glass of ale.

'Won't you walk into the parlour, sir?' said the young lady, in seductive tones.

'You had better walk into the parlour, sir,' said the little old landlord, throwing his chair back, and looking round one side of the screen to survey our appearance.

'You had much better step into the parlour, sir,' said the little old lady, popping out her head on the other side of the screen.

We cast a slight glance around, as if to express our ignorance of the locality so much recommended. The little old landlord observed it; bustled out of the small door of the small bar; and forthwith ushered us into the parlour itself.

It was an ancient, dark-looking room, with oaken wainscoting, a sanded floor, and a high mantelpiece. The walls were ornamented with three or four old coloured prints in black frames, each print representing a naval engagement, with a couple of men-of-war banging away at each other most vigorously, while another vessel or two were blowing up in the distance, and the foreground presented a miscellaneous collection of broken masts and blue legs sticking up out of the water. Depending from the ceiling in the centre of the room, were a gaslight and bell pull; on each side were three or four long narrow tables, behind which was a thickly planted row of those slippery, shiny-looking wooden chairs, peculiar to hostelries of this description. The monotonous appearance of the sanded boards was relieved by an occasional spittoon; and a triangular pile of those useful articles adorned the two upper corners of the apartment.

At the furthest table, nearest the fire, with his face towards the door at the bottom of the room, sat a stoutish man of about forty, whose short, stiff, black hair curled closely round a broad high forehead, and a face to which something besides water and exercise had communicated a rather inflamed appearance. He was smoking a cigar, with his eyes fixed on the ceiling, and had that confident oracular air which marked him as the leading politician, general authority, and universal anecdote-relater, of the place. He had evidently just delivered himself of something very weighty; for the remainder of the company were puffing at their respective pipes and cigars in a kind of solemn abstraction, as if quite overwhelmed with the magnitude of the subject recently under discussion.

On his right hand sat an elderly gentleman with a white head, and broad-brimmed brown hat; on his left, a sharp-nosed, light-haired man in a brown surtout reaching nearly to his heels, who took a whiff at his pipe, and an admiring glance at the red-faced man, alternately.

'Very extraordinary!' said the light-haired man after a pause of five minutes. A murmur of assent ran through the company.

'Not at all extraordinary – not at all,' said the red-faced man, awakening suddenly from his reverie, and turning upon the light-haired man the moment he had spoken.

'Why should it be extraordinary? – why is it extraordinary? – prove it to be extraordinary!'

'Oh, if you come to that –' said the light-haired man, meekly.

'Come to that!' ejaculated the man with the red face; 'but we *must* come to that. We stand, in these times, upon a calm elevation of intellectual attainment, and not in the dark recess of mental deprivation. Proof is what I require – proof, and not assertions, in these stirring times. Every gen'lem'n that knows me, knows what was the nature and effect of my observations, when it was in the contemplation of the Old Street Suburban Representative Discovery Society, to recommend a candidate for that place in Cornwall there – I forget the name of it. 'Mr Snobee,' said Mr Wilson, 'is a fit and proper person to represent the borough in Parliament.' 'Prove it,' says I. 'He is a friend to Reform,' says Mr Wilson. 'Prove it,' says I. 'The abolitionist of the national debt, the unflinching opponent of pensions, the uncompromising advocate of the negro, the reducer of sinecures and the duration of Parliaments; the extender of nothing but the suffrages of the people,' says Mr Wilson. 'Prove it,' says I. 'His acts prove it,' says he. 'Prove *them*,' says I.

'And he could not prove them,' said the red-faced man, looking round triumphantly; 'and the borough didn't have him; and if you carried this principle to the full extent, you'd have no debt, no pensions, no sinecures, no negroes, no nothing. And then, standing upon an elevation of intellectual attainment, and having reached the summit of popular prosperity, you might bid defiance to the nations of the earth, and erect yourselves in the proud confidence of wisdom and superiority. This is my argument – this always has been my argument – and if I was a Member of the House of Commons tomorrow, I'd make 'em shake in their shoes with it.' And the red-faced man, having struck the table very hard with his clenched fist, to add weight to the declaration, smoked away like a brewery.

'Well!' said the sharp-nosed man, in a very slow and soft voice, addressing the company in general, 'I always do say, that of all the gentlemen I have the pleasure of meeting in this room, there is not one whose conversation I like to hear so much as Mr Rogers's, or who is such improving company.'

'Improving company!' said Mr Rogers, for that, it seemed, was the name of the red-faced man. 'You may say I am improving company, for I've improved you all to some purpose; though as to my conversation being as my friend Mr Ellis here describes it, that is not for me to say anything about. You, gentlemen, are the best judges on that point; but this I will say, when I came into this parish, and first used this room, ten years ago, I don't believe there was one man in it, who knew he was a slave – and now you all know it, and writhe under it. Inscribe that upon my tomb, and I am satisfied.'

'Why, as to inscribing it on your tomb,' said a little greengrocer with a chubby face, 'of course you can have anything chalked up, as you likes to pay for, so far as it relates to yourself and your affairs; but when you come to talk about slaves, and that there abuse, you'd better keep it in the family, 'cos I for one don't like to be called them names, night after night.'

'You *are* a slave,' said the red-faced man, 'and the most pitiable of all slaves.'

'Werry hard if I am,' interrupted the greengrocer, 'for I got no good out of the twenty million that was paid for 'mancipation, anyhow.'

'A willing slave,' ejaculated the red-faced man, getting more red with eloquence and contradiction – 'resigning the dearest birthright of your children – neglecting the sacred call of Liberty – who, standing imploringly before you, appeals to the warmest feelings of your heart, and points to your helpless infants, but in vain.'

'Prove it,' said the greengrocer.

'Prove it!' sneered the man with the red face. 'What! bending beneath the yoke of an insolent and factious oligarchy; bowed down by the domination of cruel laws; groaning beneath tyranny and oppression on every hand, at every side, and in every corner. Prove it! –' The red-faced man abruptly broke off, sneered melodramatically, and buried his countenance and his indignation together, in a quart pot.

'Ah, to be sure, Mr Rogers,' said a stout broker in a large waistcoat, who had kept his eyes fixed on this luminary all the time he was speaking. 'Ah, to be sure,' said the broker with a sigh, 'that's the point.'

'Of course, of course,' said divers members of the company, who understood almost as much about the matter as the broker himself.

'You had better let him alone, Tommy,' said the broker, by way of advice to the little greengrocer; 'he can tell what's o'clock by an eight day, without looking at the minute hand, he can. Try it on, on some other suit; it won't do with him, Tommy.'

'What is a man?' continued the red-faced specimen of the species, jerking his hat indignantly from its peg on the wall. 'What is an Englishman? Is he to be trampled upon by every oppressor? Is he to be knocked down at everybody's bidding? What's freedom? Not a standing army. What's a standing army? Not freedom. What's general happiness? Not universal misery. Liberty ain't the window tax, is it? The Lords ain't the Commons, are they?' And the red-faced man, gradually bursting into a radiating sentence, in which such adjectives as 'dastardly', 'oppressive', 'violent', and 'sanguinary', formed the most conspicuous words, knocked his hat indignantly over his eyes, left the room, and slammed the door after him.

'Wonderful man!' said he of the sharp nose.

'Splendid speaker!' added the broker.

'Great power!' said everybody but the greengrocer. And as they said it, the whole party shook their heads mysteriously, and one by one retired, leaving us alone in the old parlour.

If we had followed the established precedent in all such instances, we should have fallen into a fit of musing, without delay. The ancient appearance of the room – the old panelling of the wall – the chimney blackened with smoke and age – would have carried us back a hundred years at least, and we should have gone dreaming on, until the pewter pot on the table, or the little beer chiller on the fire, had started into life, and addressed to us a long story of days gone by. But, by some means or other, we were not in a romantic humour; and although we tried very hard to invest the furniture with vitality, it remained perfectly unmoved, obstinate, and sullen. Being thus reduced to the unpleasant necessity of musing about ordinary matters, our thoughts reverted to the red-faced man, and his oratorical display.

A numerous race are these red-faced men; there is not a parlour, or club room, or benefit society, or humble party of any kind, without its red-faced man. Weak-pated dolts they are, and a great deal of mischief they do to their cause, however good. So, just to hold a pattern one up, to know the others by, we took his likeness at once, and put him in here. And that is the reason why we have written this paper.

## Chapter Six

### *The Hospital Patient*

First published in the *Carlton Chronicle*, 6 August 1836. 'The Hospital Patient' was one of the pieces by Dickens contributed to this shortlived weekly paper which was launched on 11 June 1836 and survived only until 13 May 1837. In a number of ways, the piece looks forward to the character of Nancy in *Oliver Twist*.

In our rambles through the streets of London after evening has set in, we often pause beneath the windows of some public hospital, and picture to ourself the gloomy and mournful scenes that are passing within. The sudden moving of a taper as its feeble ray shoots from window to window, until its light gradually disappears, as if it were carried farther back into the room to the bedside of some suffering patient, is enough to awaken a whole crowd of reflections; the mere glimmering of the low-burning lamps, which, when all other habitations are wrapped in darkness and slumber, denote the chamber where so many forms are writhing with pain, or wasting with disease, is sufficient to check the most boisterous merriment.

Who can tell the anguish of those weary hours, when the only sound the sick man hears is the disjointed wanderings of some feverish slumberer near him, the low moan of pain, or perhaps the muttered, long-forgotten prayer of a dying man? Who, but they who have felt it, can imagine the sense of loneliness and desolation which must be the portion of those who in the hour of dangerous illness are left to be tended by strangers; for what hands, be they ever so gentle, can wipe the clammy brow, or smooth the restless bed, like those of mother, wife, or child?

Impressed with these thoughts, we have turned away through the nearly deserted streets; and the sight of the few miserable creatures still hovering about them has not tended to lessen the pain which such meditations awaken. The hospital is a refuge and resting place for hundreds, who but for such institutions must die in the streets and doorways; but what can be the feelings of some outcasts when they are stretched on the bed of sickness with scarcely a hope of recovery? The wretched woman who lingers about the pavement, hours after midnight, and the miserable

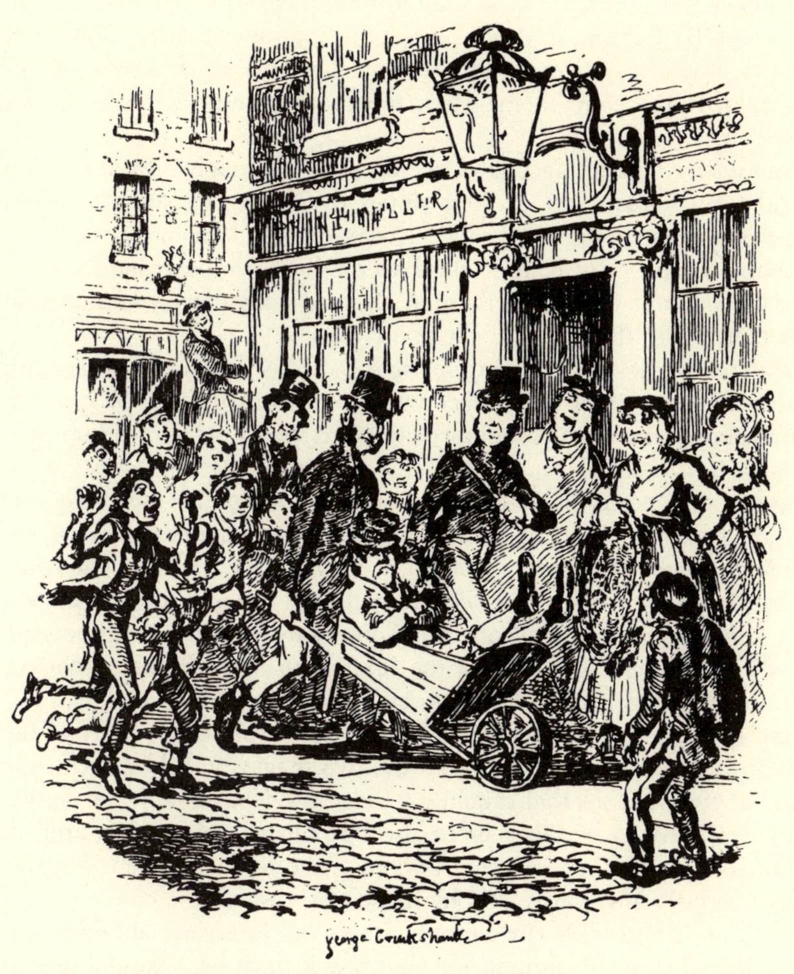


*A Pickpocket in Custody*

shadow of a man – the ghastly remnant that want and drunkenness have left – which crouches beneath a window ledge, to sleep where there is some shelter from the rain, have little to bind them to life, but what have they to look back upon, in death? What are the unwonted comforts of a roof and a bed to them, when the recollections of a whole life of debasement stalk before them; when repentance seems a mockery, and sorrow comes too late?

About a twelvemonth ago, as we were strolling through Covent Garden (we had been thinking about these things overnight), we were attracted by the very prepossessing appearance of a pickpocket, who having declined to take the trouble of walking to the Police Office, on the ground that he hadn't the slightest wish to go there at all, was being conveyed thither in a wheelbarrow, to the huge delight of a crowd.

Somehow, we never can resist joining a crowd, so we turned back with the mob, and entered the office, in company with our friend the pickpocket, a couple of policemen, and as many dirty-faced spectators as could squeeze their way in.

There was a powerful, ill-looking young fellow at the bar, who was undergoing an examination, on the very common charge of having, on the previous night, ill treated a woman, with whom he lived in some court hard by. Several witnesses bore testimony to acts of the grossest brutality; and a certificate was read from the house surgeon of a neighbouring hospital, describing the nature of the injuries the woman had received, and intimating that her recovery was extremely doubtful.

Some question appeared to have been raised about the identity of the prisoner; for when it was agreed that the two magistrates should visit the hospital at eight o'clock that evening, to take her deposition, it was settled that the man should be taken there also. He turned pale at this, and we saw him clench the bar very hard when the order was given. He was removed directly afterwards, and he spoke not a word.

We felt an irrepressible curiosity to witness this interview, although it is hard to tell why, at this instant, for we knew it must be a painful one. It was no very difficult matter for us to gain permission, and we obtained it.

The prisoner, and the officer who had him in custody, were already at the hospital when we reached it, and waiting the arrival of the magistrates in a small room below stairs. The man was handcuffed, and his hat was pulled forward over his eyes. It was easy to see, though, by the whiteness of his countenance, and the constant twitching of the muscles of his face, that he dreaded what was to come. After a short interval, the magistrates and clerk were bowed in by the house surgeon and a couple of young men who smelt very strong of tobacco smoke – they were introduced as 'dressers' – and after one magistrate had complained bitterly of the cold, and the other of the absence of any news in the evening paper, it was announced that the patient was prepared; and we were conducted to the 'casualty ward' in which she was lying.

The dim light which burnt in the spacious room, increased rather than diminished the ghastly appearance of the hapless creatures in the beds, which were ranged in two long rows on either side. In one bed lay a child enveloped in bandages, with its body half consumed by fire; in another, a female, rendered hideous by some dreadful accident, was wildly beating her clenched fists on the coverlet, in pain; on a third, there lay stretched a young girl, apparently in the heavy stupor often the immediate precursor of death: her face was stained with blood, and her breast and arms were bound up in folds of linen. Two or three of the beds were empty, and their recent occupants were sitting beside them, but with faces so wan, and eyes so bright and glassy, that it was fearful to meet their gaze. On every face was stamped the expression of anguish and suffering.

The object of the visit was lying at the upper end of the room. She was a fine young woman of about two or three and twenty. Her long black hair, which had been hastily cut from near the wounds on her head, streamed over the pillow in jagged and matted locks. Her face bore deep marks of the ill usage she had received; her hand was pressed upon her side, as if her chief pain were there; her breathing was short and heavy; and it was plain to see that she was dying fast. She murmured a few words in reply to the magistrate's inquiry whether she was in great pain; and, having been raised on the pillow by the nurse, looked vacantly upon the strange countenances that surrounded her bed. The magistrate nodded to the officer, to bring the man forward. He did so, and stationed him at the bedside. The girl looked on with a wild and troubled expression of face; but her sight was dim, and she did not know him.

'Take off his hat,' said the magistrate. The officer did as he was desired, and the man's features were disclosed.

The girl started up, with an energy quite preternatural; the fire gleamed in her heavy eyes, and the blood rushed to her pale and sunken cheeks. It was a convulsive effort. She fell back upon her pillow, and covering her scarred and bruised face with her hands, burst into tears. The man cast an anxious look towards her, but otherwise appeared wholly unmoved. After a brief pause the nature of the errand was explained, and the oath tendered.

'Oh, no, gentlemen,' said the girl, raising herself once more, and folding her hands together; 'no, gentlemen, for God's sake! I did it myself – it was nobody's fault – it was an accident. He didn't hurt me; he wouldn't for all the world. Jack, dear Jack, you know you wouldn't!'

Her sight was fast failing her, and her hand groped over the bedclothes in search of his. Brute as the man was, he was not prepared for this. He turned his face from the bed, and sobbed. The girl's colour changed, and her breathing grew more difficult. She was evidently dying.

'We respect the feelings which prompt you to this,' said the gentleman who had spoken first, 'but let me warn you not to persist in what you know to be untrue, until it is too late. It cannot save him.'

'Jack,' murmured the girl, laying her hand upon his arm, 'they shall not persuade me to swear your life away. He didn't do it, gentlemen. He never hurt me.' She grasped his arm tightly, and added, in a broken whisper, 'I hope God Almighty will forgive me all the wrong I have done, and the life I have led. God bless you, Jack. Some kind gentleman take my love to my poor old father. Five years ago, he said he wished I had died a child. Oh, I wish I had! I wish I had!'

The nurse bent over the girl for a few seconds, and then drew the sheet over her face. It covered a corpse.

## Chapter Seven

### *The Misplaced Attachment of Mr John Dounce*

First published under the title 'Love and Oysters' *Bell's Life in London,* 25 October 1835 ('Scenes and Characters No. 5'). Jones's jesting in the penultimate paragraph refers to the contemporary custom of supplying wedding guests with gloves.

If we had to make a classification of society, there are a particular kind of men whom we should immediately set down under the head of 'Old Boys'; and a column of most extensive dimensions the old boys would require. To what precise causes the rapid advance of old-boy population is to be traced, we are unable to determine. It would be an interesting and curious speculation, but, as we have not sufficient space to devote to it here, we simply state the fact that the numbers of the old boys have been gradually augmenting within the last few years, and that they are at this moment alarmingly on the increase.

Upon a general review of the subject, and without considering it minutely in detail, we should be disposed to sub-divide the old boys into two distinct classes – the gay old boys, and the steady old boys. The gay old boys are paunchy old men in the disguise of young ones, who frequent the Quadrant and Regent Street in the daytime: the theatres (especially theatres under lady management) at night; and who assume all the foppishness and levity of boys, without the excuse of youth or inexperience. The steady old boys are certain stout old gentlemen of clean appearance, who are always to be seen in the same taverns, at the same hours every evening, smoking and drinking in the same company.

There was once a fine collection of old boys to be seen round the circular table at Offley's every night, between the hours of half-past eight and half-past eleven. We have lost sight of them for some time. There were, and may be still, for aught we know, two splendid specimens in full blossom at the Rainbow Tavern in Fleet Street, who always used to sit in the box nearest the fireplace, and smoked long cherry stick pipes which went under the table, with the bowls resting on the floor. Grand old boys they were – fat, red-faced, white-headed old fellows – always there – one on one side the table, and the other opposite – puffing and drinking away

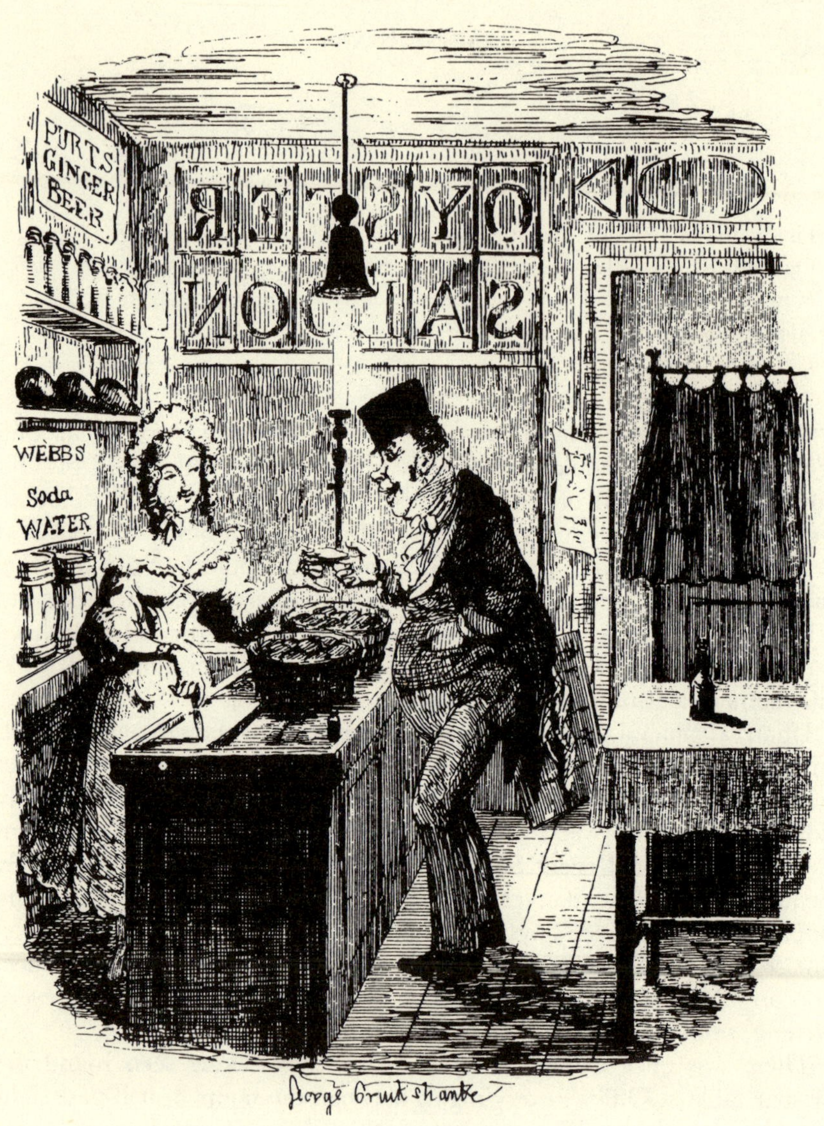


*Mr John Dounce*

in great state. Everybody knew them, and it was supposed by some people that they were both immortal.

Mr John Dounce was an old boy of the latter class (we don't mean immortal, but steady), a retired glove and braces maker, a widower, resident with three daughters – all grown up, and all unmarried – in Cursitor Street, Chancery Lane. He was a short, round, large-faced, tubbish sort of man, with a broad-brimmed hat, and a square coat; and had that grave, but confident, kind of roll, peculiar to old boys in general. Regular as clockwork – breakfast at nine – dress and tittivate a little – down to the Sir Somebody's Head – a glass of ale and the paper – come back again, and take daughters out for a walk – dinner at three – glass of grog and pipe – nap – tea – little walk – Sir Somebody's Head again – capital house – delightful evenings. There were Mr Harris, the law stationer, and Mr Jennings, the robe maker (two jolly young fellows like himself), and Jones, the barrister's clerk – rum fellow that Jones – capital company – full of anecdote! – and there they sat every night till just ten minutes before twelve, drinking their brandy and water, and smoking their pipes, and telling stories, and enjoying themselves with a kind of solemn joviality particularly edifying.

Sometimes Jones would propose a half price visit to Drury Lane or Covent Garden, to see two acts of a five-act play, and a new farce, perhaps, or a ballet, on which occasions the whole four of them went together: none of your hurrying and nonsense, but having their brandy and water first, comfortably, and ordering a steak and some oysters for their supper against they came back, and then walking coolly into the pit, when the 'rush' had gone in, as all sensible people do, and did when Mr Dounce was a young man, except when the celebrated Master Betty was at the height of his popularity, and then, sir, – then – Mr Dounce perfectly well remembered getting a holiday from business; and going to the pit doors at eleven o'clock in the forenoon, and waiting there till six in the afternoon, with some sandwiches in a pocket handkerchief and some wine in a phial; and fainting after all, with the heat and fatigue, before the play began; in which situation he was lifted out of the pit, into one of the dress boxes, sir, by five of the finest women of that day, sir, who compassionated his situation and administered restoratives, and sent a black servant, six foot high, in blue and silver livery, next morning with their compliments, and to know how he found himself, sir, by G—! Between the acts Mr Dounce, and Mr Harris, and Mr Jennings, used to stand up, and look round the house, and Jones – knowing fellow that Jones – knew everybody – pointed out the fashionable and celebrated Lady So-and-So in the boxes, at the mention of whose name Mr Dounce, after brushing up his hair, and adjusting his neckerchief, would inspect the aforesaid Lady So-and-So through an immense glass, and remark, either that she was a 'fine woman – very fine woman, indeed', or that 'there might be a little more of her, – eh, Jones?' just as the case might happen to be. When the dancing began, John Dounce and the other old boys were particularly anxious to see what was going forward on the stage, and Jones – wicked dog that Jones – whispered little critical remarks into the ears of John Dounce, which John Dounce retailed to Mr Harris, and Mr Harris to Mr Jennings; and then they all four laughed until the tears ran down out of their eyes.

When the curtain fell, they walked back together, two and two, to the steaks and oysters; and when they came to the second glass of brandy and water, Jones – hoaxing scamp, that Jones – used to recount how he had observed a lady in white feathers, in one of the pit boxes, gazing intently on Mr Dounce all the evening, and how he had caught Mr Dounce, whenever he thought no one was looking at him, bestowing ardent looks of intense devotion on the lady in return; on which Mr Harris and Mr Jennings used to laugh very heartily, and John Dounce more heartily than either of them, acknowledging, however, that the time *had* been when he *might* have done such things; upon which Mr Jones used to poke him in the ribs, and tell him he had been a sad dog in his time, which John Dounce with chuckles confessed. And after Mr Harris and Mr Jennings had preferred their claims to the character of having been sad dogs too, they separated harmoniously, and trotted home.

The decrees of Fate, and the means by which they are brought about, are mysterious and inscrutable. John Dounce had led this life for twenty years and upwards, without wish for change, or care for variety, when his whole social system was suddenly upset, and turned completely topsy-turvy – not by an earthquake, or some other dreadful convulsion of nature, as the reader would be inclined to suppose, but by the simple agency of an oyster; and thus it happened.

Mr John Dounce was returning one night from the Sir Somebody's Head, to his residence in Cursitor Street – not tipsy, but rather excited, for it was Mr Jennings's birthday, and they had had a brace of partridges for supper, and a brace of extra glasses afterwards, and Jones had been more than ordinarily amusing – when his eyes rested on a newly opened oyster shop, on a magnificent scale, with natives laid, one deep, in circular marble basins in the windows, together with little round barrels of oysters directed to Lords and Baronets, and Colonels and Captains, in every part of the habitable globe.

Behind the natives were the barrels, and behind the barrels was a young lady of about five-and-twenty, all in blue, and all alone – splendid creature, charming face and lovely figure! It is difficult to say whether Mr John Dounce's red countenance, illuminated as it was by the flickering gaslight in the window before which he paused, excited the lady's risibility, or whether a natural exuberance of animal spirits proved too much for that staidness of demeanour which the forms of society rather dictatorially prescribe. But certain it is, that the lady smiled; then put her finger upon her lip, with a striking recollection of what was due to herself; and finally retired, in oyster-like bashfulness, to the very back of the counter. The sad dog sort of feeling came strongly upon John Dounce: he lingered – the lady in blue made no sign. He coughed – still she came not. He entered the shop.

'Can you open me an oyster, my dear?' said Mr John Dounce.

'Dare say I can, sir,' replied the lady in blue, with playfulness. And Mr John Dounce eat one oyster, and then looked at the young lady, and then eat another, and then squeezed the young lady's hand as she was opening the third, and so forth, until he had devoured a dozen of those at eightpence in less than no time.

'Can you open me half-a-dozen more, my dear?' inquired Mr John Dounce.

'I'll see what I can do for you, sir,' replied the young lady in blue, even more bewitchingly than before; and Mr John Dounce eat half-a-dozen more of those at eightpence.

'You couldn't manage to get me a glass of brandy and water, my dear, I suppose?' said Mr John Dounce, when he had finished the oysters: in a tone which clearly implied his supposition that she could.

'I'll see, sir,' said the young lady: and away she ran out of the shop, and down the street, her long auburn ringlets shaking in the wind in the most enchanting manner; and back she came again, tripping over the coal cellar lids like a whipping top, with a tumbler of brandy and water, which Mr John Dounce insisted on her taking a share of, as it was regular ladies' grog – hot, strong, sweet, and plenty of it.

So the young lady sat down with Mr John Dounce, in a little red box with a green curtain, and took a small sip of the brandy and water, and a small look at Mr John Dounce, and then turned her head away, and went through various other serio-pantomimic fascinations, which forcibly reminded Mr John Dounce of the first time he courted his first wife, and which made him feel more affectionate than ever; in pursuance of which affection, and actuated by which feeling, Mr John Dounce sounded the young lady on her matrimonial engagements, when the young lady denied having formed any such engagements at all – she couldn't abear the men, they were such deceivers; thereupon Mr John Dounce inquired whether this sweeping condemnation was meant to include other than very young men; on which the young lady blushed deeply – at least she turned away her head, and said Mr John Dounce had made her blush, so of course she *did* blush – and Mr John Dounce was a long time drinking the brandy and water; and, at last, John Dounce went home to bed, and dreamed of his first wife, and his second wife, and the young lady, and partridges, and oysters, and brandy and water, and disinterested attachments.

The next morning, John Dounce was rather feverish with the extra brandy and water of the previous night; and, partly in the hope of cooling himself with an oyster, and partly with the view of ascertaining whether he owed the young lady anything or not, went back to the oyster shop. If the young lady had appeared beautiful by night, she was perfectly irresistible by day; and, from this time forward, a change came over the spirit of John Dounce's dream. He bought shirt pins; wore a ring on his third finger; read poetry; bribed a cheap miniature-painter to perpetrate a faint resemblance to a youthful face, with a curtain over his head, six large books in the background, and an open country in the distance (this he called his portrait); 'went on' altogether in such an uproarious manner, that the three Miss Dounces went off on small pensions, he having made the tenement in Cursitor Street too warm to contain them; and in short, comported and demeaned himself in every respect like an unmitigated old Saracen, as he was.

As to his ancient friends, the other old boys, at the Sir Somebody's Head, he dropped off from them by gradual degrees; for even when he did go there, Jones – vulgar fellow, that Jones – persisted in asking 'when it was to be?' and 'whether he was to have any gloves?' together with other inquiries of an equally offensive nature: at which not only Harris laughed, but Jennings also; so he cut the two altogether, and attached himself solely to the blue young lady at the smart oyster shop.

Now comes the moral of the story – for it has a moral after all. The last-mentioned young lady, having derived sufficient profit and emolument from John Dounce's attachment, not only refused, when matters came to a crisis, to take him for better for worse, but expressly declared, to use her own forcible words, that she 'wouldn't have him at no price'; and John Dounce, having lost his old friends, alienated his relations, and rendered himself ridiculous to everybody, made offers successively to a schoolmistress, a landlady, a feminine tobacconist, and a housekeeper; and, being directly rejected by each and every of them, was accepted by his cook, with whom he now lives, a henpecked husband, a melancholy monument of antiquated misery, and a living warning to all uxorious old boys.

## Chapter Eight

### *The Mistaken Milliner: A Tale of Ambition*

First published under the title 'The Vocal Dressmaker' in *Bell's Life in London,* 22 November 1835 ('Scenes and Characters No. 7'). The Jennings Rodolphs' duet, 'Red Ruffian, retire!', would seem to be an inspired invention on Dickens's part but the other songs mentioned are genuine. The lyrics of 'I am a Friar [of orders grey]' were written by John O'Keeffe, and the comic duet, 'The Time of Day', was, Hill notes, very popular at Vauxhall Gardens, the whole text being printed in *London Oddities* (1822). The first verse runs:

> I came up to town scarce six months ago,
> An awkward country clown, but now sir, quite a beau;
> I did but walk about to hear what folks should say
> And egad I soon found out what was the time of day.
> Too ral loo ral loo.

Miss Amelia Martin was pale, tallish, thin, and two-and-thirty – what ill natured people would call plain, and police reports interesting. She was a milliner and dressmaker, living on her business and not above it. If you had been a young lady in service, and had wanted Miss Martin, as a great many young ladies in service did, you would just have stepped up, in the evening, to number forty-seven, Drummond Street, George Street, Euston Square, and after casting your eye on a brass door plate, one foot ten by one and a half, ornamented with a great brass knob at each of the four corners, and bearing the inscription 'Miss Martin; millinery and dressmaking, in all its branches'; you'd just have knocked two loud knocks at the street door; and down would have come Miss Martin herself, in a merino gown of the newest fashion, black velvet bracelets on the genteelest principle, and other little elegancies of the most approved description.

If Miss Martin knew the young lady who called, or if the young lady who called had been recommended by any other young lady whom Miss Martin knew, Miss Martin would forthwith show her upstairs into the two-pair front, and chat she would – *so* kind, and *so* comfortable – it really wasn't like a matter of business, she was so friendly; and then Miss Martin, after contemplating the figure and general appearance of the young lady in service with great apparent admiration, would say how well she would look, to be sure, in a low dress with short sleeves; made very full in the skirts, with four tucks in the bottom; to which the young lady in service would reply in terms expressive of her entire concurrence in the notion, and of the virtuous indignation with which she reflected on the tyranny of 'Missis', who wouldn't allow a young girl to wear a short sleeve of an arternoon – no, nor nothing smart, not even a pair of ear-rings; let alone hiding people's heads of hair under them frightful caps. At the termination of this complaint, Miss Amelia Martin would distantly suggest certain dark suspicions that some people were jealous on account of their own daughters, and were obliged to keep their servants' charms under, for fear they should get married first, which was no uncommon circumstance – leastways she had known two or three young ladies in service, who had married a great deal better than their missises, and *they* were not very good looking either; and then the young lady would inform Miss Martin, in confidence, that how one of their young ladies was engaged to a young man and was a-going to be married, and Missis was so proud about it there was no bearing of her; but how she needn't hold her head quite so high neither, for, after all, he was only a clerk. And, after expressing due contempt for clerks in general, and the engaged clerk in particular, and the highest opinion possible of themselves and each other, Miss Martin and the young lady in service would bid each other goodnight, in a friendly but perfectly genteel manner: and the one went back to her 'place', and the other to her room on the second-floor front.

There is no saying how long Miss Amelia Martin might have continued this course of life; how extensive a connection she might have established among young ladies in service; or what amount her demands upon their quarterly receipts might have ultimately attained, had not an unforeseen train of circumstances directed her thoughts to a sphere of action very different from dressmaking or millinery.

A friend of Miss Martin's who had long been keeping company with an ornamental painter and decorator's journeyman, at last consented (on being at last asked to do so) to name the day which would make the aforesaid journeyman a happy husband. It was a Monday that was appointed for the celebration of the nuptials, and Miss Amelia Martin was invited, among others, to honour the wedding dinner with her presence. It was a charming party; Somers Town the locality, and a front parlour the apartment. The ornamental painter and decorator's journeyman had taken the house – no lodgings nor vulgarity of that kind, but a house – four beautiful rooms, and a delightful little washhouse at the end of the passage – which was the most convenient thing in the world, for the bridesmaids could sit in the front parlour and receive the company, and then run into the little washhouse and see how the pudding and boiled pork were getting on in the copper, and then pop back into the parlour again, as snug and comfortable as possible. And such a parlour as it was! Beautiful Kidderminster carpet – six brand-new cane-bottomed stained chairs – three wineglasses and a tumbler on each sideboard – farmer's girl and farmer's boy on the mantelpiece: girl tumbling over a stile, and boy spitting himself on the handle of a pitchfork – long white dimity curtains in the window – and, in short, everything on the most genteel scale imaginable.

Then, the dinner. There was baked leg of mutton at the top, boiled leg of mutton at the bottom, pair of fowls and leg of pork in the middle; porter pots at the corners; pepper, mustard, and vinegar in the centre; vegetables on the floor; and plum-pudding and apple-pie and tartlets without number: to say nothing of cheese, and celery, and watercresses, and all that sort of thing. As to the company! Miss Amelia Martin herself declared, on a subsequent occasion, that, much as she had heard of the ornamental painter's journeyman's connexion, she never could have supposed it was half so genteel. There was his father, such a funny old gentleman – and his mother, such a dear old lady – and his sister, such a charming girl – and his brother, such a manly-looking young man – with such a eye! But even all these were as nothing when compared with his musical friends, Mr and Mrs Jennings Rodolph, from White Conduit, with whom the ornamental painter's journeyman had been fortunate enough to contract an intimacy while engaged in decorating the concert room of that noble institution. To hear them sing separately was divine, but when they went through the tragic duet of 'Red Ruffian, retire!' it was, as Miss Martin afterwards remarked, 'thrilling'. And why (as Mr Jennings Rodolph observed) why were they not engaged at one of the patent theatres? If he was to be told that their voices were not powerful enough to fill the House, his only reply was, that he would back himself for any amount to fill Russell Square – a statement in which the company, after hearing the duet, expressed their full belief; so they all said it was shameful treatment; and both Mr and Mrs Jennings Rodolph said it was shameful too; and Mr Jennings Rodolph looked very serious, and said he knew who his malignant opponents were, but they had better take care how far they went, for if they irritated him too much he had not quite made up his mind whether he wouldn't bring the subject before Parliament; and they all agreed that it ''ud serve 'em quite right, and it was very proper that such people should be made an example of'. So Mr Jennings Rodolph said he'd think of it.

When the conversation resumed its former tone, Mr Jennings Rodolph claimed his right to call upon a lady, and the right being conceded, trusted Miss Martin would favour the company – a proposal which met with unanimous approbation, whereupon Miss Martin, after sundry hesitatings and coughings, with a preparatory choke or two, and an introductory declaration that she was frightened to death to attempt it before such great judges of the art, commenced a species of treble chirruping containing frequent allusions to some young gentleman of the name of Hen-e-ry, with an occasional reference to madness and broken hearts. Mr Jennings Rodolph frequently interrupted the progress of the song, by ejaculating 'Beautiful!' – 'Charming!' – 'Brilliant!' – 'Oh! splendid', &c.; and at its close the admiration of himself, and his lady, knew no bounds.

'Did you ever hear so sweet a voice, my dear?' inquired Mr Jennings Rodolph of Mrs Jennings Rodolph.

'Never; indeed I never did, love,' replied Mrs Jennings Rodolph.

'Don't you think Miss Martin, with a little cultivation, would be very like Signora Marra Boni, my dear?' asked Mr Jennings Rodolph.

'Just exactly the very thing that struck me, my love,' answered Mrs Jennings Rodolph.

And thus the time passed away; Mr Jennings Rodolph played tunes on a walking stick, and then went behind the parlour door and gave his celebrated imitations of actors, edge tools, and animals; Miss Martin sang several other songs with increased admiration every time; and even the funny old gentleman began singing. His song had properly seven verses, but as he couldn't recollect more than the first one, he sung that over seven times, apparently very much to his own personal gratification. And then all the company sang the national anthem with national independence – each for himself, without reference to the other – and finally separated: all declaring that they never had spent so pleasant an evening: and Miss Martin inwardly resolving to adopt the advice of Mr Jennings Rodolph, and to 'come out' without delay.

Now, 'coming out', either in acting, or singing, or society, or facetiousness, or anything else, is all very well, and remarkably pleasant to the individual principally concerned, if he or she can but manage to come out with a burst, and being out to keep out, and not go in again; but it does unfortunately happen that both consummations are extremely difficult to accomplish, and that the difficulties of getting out at all in the first instance, and if you surmount them, of keeping out in the second, are pretty much on a par, and no slight ones either – and so Miss Amelia Martin shortly discovered. It is a singular fact (there being ladies in the case) that Miss Amelia Martin's principal foible was vanity, and the leading characteristic of Mrs Jennings Rodolph an attachment to dress. Dismal wailings were heard to issue from the second-floor front of number forty-seven, Drummond Street, George Street, Euston Square; it was Miss Martin practising. Half suppressed murmurs disturbed the calm dignity of the White Conduit orchestra at the commencement of the season. It was the appearance of Mrs Jennings Rodolph in full dress, that occasioned them. Miss Martin studied incessantly – the practising was the consequence. Mrs Jennings Rodolph taught gratuitously now and then – the dresses were the result.

Weeks passed away; the White Conduit season had begun, and progressed, and was more than half over. The dress-making business had fallen off, from neglect; and its profits had dwindled away almost imperceptibly. A benefit night approached; Mr Jennings Rodolph yielded to the earnest solicitations of Miss Amelia Martin, and introduced her personally to the 'comic gentleman' whose benefit it was. The comic gentleman was all smiles and blandness – he had composed a duet expressly for the occasion, and Miss Martin should sing it with him. The night arrived; there was an immense room – ninety-seven sixpenn'orths of gin and water, thirty-two small glasses of brandy and water, five-and-twenty bottled ales, and forty-one neguses; and the ornamental painter's journeyman, with his wife and a select circle of acquaintance, were seated at one of the side tables near the orchestra. The concert began. Song – sentimental – by a light-haired young gentleman in a blue coat, and bright basket buttons – [applause]. Another song, doubtful, by another gentleman in another blue coat and more bright basket buttons – [increased applause]. Duet, Mr Jennings Rodolph, and Mrs Jennings Rodolph, 'Red Ruffian, retire!' – [great applause]. Solo, Miss Julia Montague (positively on this occasion only) – 'I am a Friar' – [enthusiasm]. Original duet, comic – Mr H. Taplin (the comic gentleman) and Miss Martin – 'The Time of Day'. 'Brayvo! – Brayvo!' cried the ornamental painter's journeyman's party, as Miss Martin was gracefully led in by the comic gentleman. 'Go to work, Harry,' cried the comic gentleman's personal friends. 'Tap—tap—tap,' went the leader's bow on the music desk. The symphony began, and was soon afterwards followed by a faint kind of ventriloquial chirping, proceeding apparently from the deepest recesses of the interior of Miss Amelia Martin. 'Sing out' – shouted one gentleman in a white greatcoat. 'Don't be afraid to put the steam on, old gal,' exclaimed another. 'S-s-s-s-s-s-s' – went the five-and-twenty bottled ales. 'Shame, shame!' remonstrated the ornamental painter's journeyman's party – 'S-s-s-s' went the bottled ales again, accompanied by all the gins, and a majority of the brandies.

'Turn them geese out,' cried the ornamental painter's journeyman's party, with great indignation.

'Sing out,' whispered Mr Jennings Rodolph.

'So I do,' responded Miss Amelia Martin.

'Sing louder,' said Mrs Jennings Rodolph.

'I can't,' replied Miss Amelia Martin.

'Off, off, off,' cried the rest of the audience.

'Bray-vo!' shouted the painter's party. It wouldn't do – Miss Amelia Martin left the orchestra, with much less ceremony than she had entered it; and, as she couldn't sing out, never came out. The general good humour was not restored until Mr Jennings Rodolph had become purple in the face, by imitating divers quadrupeds for half an hour, without being able to render himself audible; and, to this day, neither has Miss Amelia Martin's good humour been restored, nor the dresses made for and presented to Mrs Jennings Rodolph, nor the vocal abilities which Mr Jennings Rodolph once staked his professional reputation that Miss Martin possessed.

## CHAPTER NINE

### *The Dancing Academy*

First published in *Bell's Life in London,* 11 October 1835 ('Scenes and Characters No. 3'). All official and public advertisements were subject to a tax until 1833 and bore a stamp to show that the tax had been paid although the private placard advertisement carried by the boy would not have been liable for tax – hence the reference to the 'unstamped advertisement'. For a later description by Dickens of a private dancing academy (in Newman Street) see *Bleak House,* ch. 14.

Of all the dancing academies that ever were established, there never was one more popular in its immediate vicinity than Signor Billsmethi's, of the 'King's Theatre'. It was not in Spring Gardens, or Newman Street, or Berners Street, or Gower Street, or Charlotte Street, or Percy Street, or any other of the numerous streets which have been devoted time out of mind to professional people, dispensaries, and boarding houses; it was not in the West End at all – it rather approximated to the eastern portion of London, being situated in the populous and improving neighbourhood of Gray's Inn Lane. It was not a dear dancing academy – four-and-sixpence a quarter is decidedly cheap upon the whole. It was *very* select, the number of pupils being strictly limited to seventy-five, and a quarter's payment in advance being rigidly exacted. There was public tuition and private tuition – an assembly room and a parlour. Signor Billsmethi's family were always thrown in with the parlour, and included in parlour price; that is to say, a private pupil had Signor Billsmethi's parlour to dance *in,* and Signor Billsmethi's family to dance *with*; and when he had been sufficiently broken in in the parlour, he began to run in couples in the assembly room.

Such was the dancing academy of Signor Billsmethi, when Mr Augustus Cooper, of Fetter Lane, first saw an unstamped advertisement walking leisurely down Holborn Hill, announcing to the world that Signor Billsmethi, of the King's Theatre, intended opening for the season with a Grand Ball.

Now, Mr Augustus Cooper was in the oil and colour line – just of age, with a little money, a little business, and a little mother, who, having

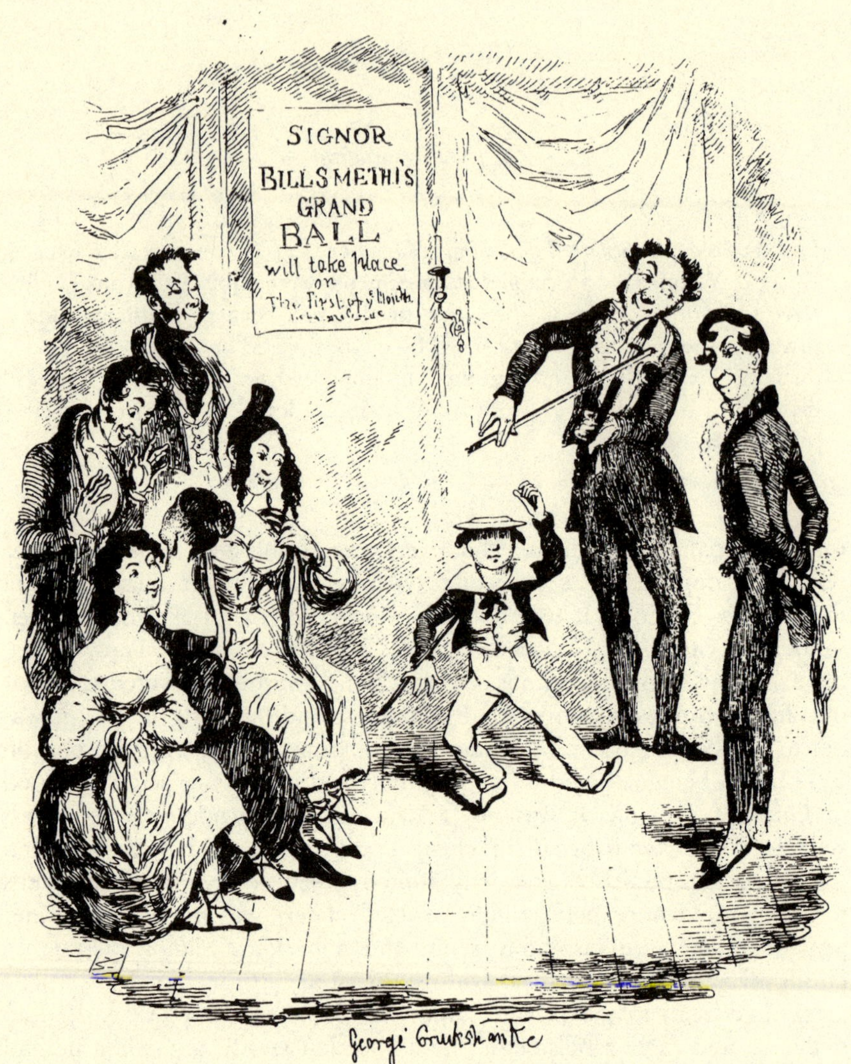
SIGNOR
BILLSMETHI'S
GRAND
BALL
will take place
on
The First of ye Month
George Cruikshank

*The Dancing Academy*

managed her husband and *his* business in his lifetime, took to managing her son and *his* business after his decease; and so, somehow or other, he had been cooped up in the little back parlour behind the shop on weekdays, and in a little deal box without a lid (called by courtesy a pew) at Bethel Chapel, on Sundays, and had seen no more of the world than if he had been an infant all his days; whereas Young White, at the gas-fitter's over the way, three years younger than him, had been flaring away like winkin' – going to the theatre – supping at harmonic meetings – eating oysters by the barrel – drinking stout by the gallon – even stopping out all night, and coming home as cool in the morning as if nothing had happened. So Mr Augustus Cooper made up his mind that he would not stand it any longer, and had that very morning expressed to his mother a firm determination to be 'blowed', in the event of his not being instantly provided with a street door key. And he was walking down Holborn Hill, thinking about all these things, and wondering how he could manage to get introduced into genteel society for the first time, when his eyes rested on Signor Billsmethi's announcement, which it immediately struck him was just the very thing he wanted; for he should not only be able to select a genteel circle of acquaintance at once, out of the five-and-seventy pupils at four-and-sixpence a quarter, but should qualify himself at the same time to go through a hornpipe in private society, with perfect ease to himself and great delight to his friends. So he stopped the unstamped advertisement – an animated sandwich, composed of a boy between two boards – and having procured a very small card with the Signor's address indented thereon, walked straight at once to the Signor's house – and very fast he walked too, for fear the list should be filled up, and the five-and-seventy completed, before he got there. The Signor was at home, and, what was still more gratifying, he was an Englishman! Such a nice man – and so polite! The list was not full, but it was a most extraordinary circumstance that there was only just one vacancy, and even that one would have been filled up, that very morning, only Signor Billsmethi was dissatisfied with the reference, and, being very much afraid that the lady wasn't select, wouldn't take her.

'And very much delighted I am, Mr Cooper,' said Signor Billsmethi, 'that I did *not* take her. I assure you, Mr Cooper – I don't say it to flatter you, for I know you're above it – that I consider myself extremely fortunate in having a gentleman of your manners and appearance, sir.'

'I am very glad of it too, sir,' said Augustus Cooper.

'And I hope we shall be better acquainted, sir,' said Signor Billsmethi.

'And I'm sure I hope we shall too, sir,' responded Augustus Cooper. Just then, the door opened, and in came a young lady, with her hair curled in a crop all over her head, and her shoes tied in sandals all over her ankles.

'Don't run away, my dear,' said Signor Billsmethi; for the young lady didn't know Mr Cooper was there when she ran in, and was going to run out again in her modesty, all in confusion, like. 'Don't run away, my dear,' said Signor Billsmethi, 'this is Mr Cooper – Mr Cooper, of Fetter Lane. Mr Cooper, my daughter, sir – Miss Billsmethi, sir, who I hope will have the pleasure of dancing many a quadrille, minuet, gavotte, country dance, fandango, double hornpipe, and farinagholkajingo with you, sir. She dances them all, sir; and so shall you, sir, before you're a quarter older, sir.'

And Signor Billsmethi slapped Mr Augustus Cooper on the back, as if he had known him a dozen years, – so friendly; – and Mr Cooper bowed to the young lady, and the young lady curtseyed to him, and Signor Billsmethi said they were as handsome a pair as ever he'd wish to see; upon which the young lady exclaimed, 'Lor, pa!' and blushed as red as Mr Cooper himself – you might have thought they were both standing under a red lamp at a chemist's shop; and before Mr Cooper went away it was settled that he should join the family circle that very night – taking them just as they were – no ceremony nor nonsense of that kind – and learn his positions in order that he might lose no time, and be able to come out at the forthcoming ball.

Well; Mr Augustus Cooper went away to one of the cheap shoemakers' shops in Holborn, where gentlemen's dress pumps are seven-and-sixpence, and men's strong walking just nothing at all, and bought a pair of the regular seven-and-sixpenny, long-quartered, town mades, in which he astonished himself quite as much as his mother, and sallied forth to Signor Billsmethi's. There were four other private pupils in the parlour: two ladies and two gentlemen. Such nice people! Not a bit of pride about them. One of the ladies in particular, who was in training for a Columbine, was remarkably affable; and she and Miss Billsmethi took such an interest in Mr Augustus Cooper, and joked, and smiled, and looked so bewitching, that he got quite at home, and learnt his steps in no time. After the practising was over, Signor Billsmethi, and Miss Billsmethi, and Master Billsmethi, and a young lady, and the two ladies, and the two gentlemen, danced a quadrille – none of your slipping and sliding about, but regular warm work, flying into corners, and diving among chairs, and shooting out at the door, – something like dancing! Signor Billsmethi in particular, notwithstanding his having a little fiddle to play all the time, was out on the landing every figure, and Master Billsmethi, when everybody else was breathless, danced a hornpipe, with a cane in his hand, and a cheese plate on his head, to the unqualified admiration of the whole company. Then, Signor Billsmethi insisted, as they were so happy, that they should all stay to supper, and proposed sending Master Billsmethi for the beer and spirits, whereupon the two gentlemen swore, 'strike 'em wulgar if they'd stand that'; and were just going to quarrel who should pay for it, when Mr Augustus Cooper said he would, if they'd have the kindness to allow him – and they *had* the kindness to allow him; and Master Billsmethi brought the beer in a can, and the rum in a quart pot. They had a regular night of it; and Miss Billsmethi squeezed Mr Augustus Cooper's hand under the table; and Mr Augustus Cooper returned the squeeze, and returned home too, at something to six o'clock in the morning, when he was put to bed by main force by the apprentice, after repeatedly expressing an uncontrollable desire to pitch his revered parent out of the second-floor window, and to throttle the apprentice with his own neck handkerchief.

Weeks had worn on, and the seven-and-six-penny town mades had nearly worn out, when the night arrived for the grand dress ball at which the whole of the five-and-seventy pupils were to meet together for the first time that season, and to take out some portion of their respective four-and-sixpences in lamp oil and fiddlers. Mr Augustus Cooper had ordered a new coat for the occasion – a two-pound-tenner from Turnstile. It was his first appearance in public; and, after a grand Sicilian shawl dance by fourteen young ladies in character, he was to open the quadrille department with Miss Billsmethi herself, with whom he had become quite intimate since his first introduction. It *was* a night! Everything was admirably arranged. The sandwich boy took the hats and bonnets at the street door; there was a turn up bedstead in the back parlour, on which Miss Billsmethi made tea and coffee for such of the gentlemen as chose to pay for it, and such of the ladies as the gentlemen treated; red port wine negus and lemonade were handed round at eighteenpence a head; and in pursuance of a previous engagement with the public house at the corner of the street, an extra potboy was laid on for the occasion. In short, nothing could exceed the arrangements, except the company. Such ladies! Such pink silk stockings! Such artificial flowers! Such a number of cabs! No sooner had one cab set down a couple of ladies, than another cab drove up and set down another couple of ladies, and they all knew: not only one another, but the majority of the gentlemen into the bargain, which made it all as pleasant and lively as could be. Signor Billsmethi, in black tights, with a large blue bow in his buttonhole, introduced the ladies to such of the gentlemen as were strangers: and the ladies talked away – and laughed they did – it was delightful to see them.

As to the shawl dance, it was the most exciting thing that ever was beheld; there was such a whisking, and rustling, and fanning, and getting ladies into a tangle with artificial flowers, and then disentangling them again! And as to Mr Augustus Cooper's share in the quadrille, he got through it admirably. He was missing from his partner, now and then, certainly, and discovered on such occasions to be either dancing with laudable perseverance in another set, or sliding about in perspective, without any definite object; but, generally speaking, they managed to shove him through the figure, until he turned up in the right place. Be this as it may, when he had finished, a great many ladies and gentlemen came up and complimented him very much, and said they had never seen a beginner do anything like it before; and Mr Augustus Cooper was perfectly satisfied with himself, and everybody else into the bargain; and 'stood' considerable quantities of spirits and water, negus, and compounds, for the use and behoof of two or three dozen very particular friends, selected from the select circle of five-and-seventy pupils.

Now, whether it was the strength of the compounds, or the beauty of the ladies, or what not, it did so happen that Mr Augustus Cooper encouraged, rather than repelled, the very flattering attentions of a young lady in brown gauze over white calico who had appeared particularly struck with him from the first; and when the encouragements had been prolonged for some time, Miss Billsmethi betrayed her spite and jealousy thereat by calling the young lady in brown gauze a 'creeter', which induced the young lady in brown gauze to retort, in certain sentences containing a taunt founded on the payment of four-and-sixpence a quarter, which reference Mr Augustus Cooper, being then and there in a state of considerable bewilderment, expressed his entire concurrence in. Miss Billsmethi, thus renounced, forthwith began screaming in the loudest key of her voice, at the rate of fourteen screams a minute; and being unsuccessful, in an onslaught on the eyes and face, first of the lady in gauze and then of Mr Augustus Cooper, called distractedly on the other three-and-seventy pupils to furnish her with oxalic acid for her own private drinking; and, the call not being honoured, made another rush at Mr Cooper, and then had her stay-lace cut, and was carried off to bed. Mr Augustus Cooper, not being remarkable for quickness of apprehension, was at a loss to understand what all this meant, until Signor Billsmethi explained it in a most satisfactory manner, by stating to the pupils, that Mr Augustus Cooper had made and confirmed divers promises of marriage to his daughter on divers occasions, and had now basely deserted her; on which the indignation of the pupils became universal; and as several chivalrous gentlemen inquired rather pressingly of Mr Augustus Cooper, whether he required anything for his own use, or, in other words, whether he 'wanted anything for himself', he deemed it prudent to make a precipitate retreat. And the upshot of the matter was, that a lawyer's letter came next day, and an action was commenced next week; and that Mr Augustus Cooper, after walking twice to the Serpentine for the purpose of drowning himself, and coming twice back without doing it, made a confidante of his mother, who compromised the matter with twenty pounds from the till: which made twenty pounds four shillings and sixpence paid to Signor Billsmethi, exclusive of treats and pumps. And Mr Augustus

Cooper went back and lived with his mother, and there he lives to this day; and as he has lost his ambition for society, and never goes into the world, he will never see this account of himself, and will never be any the wiser.

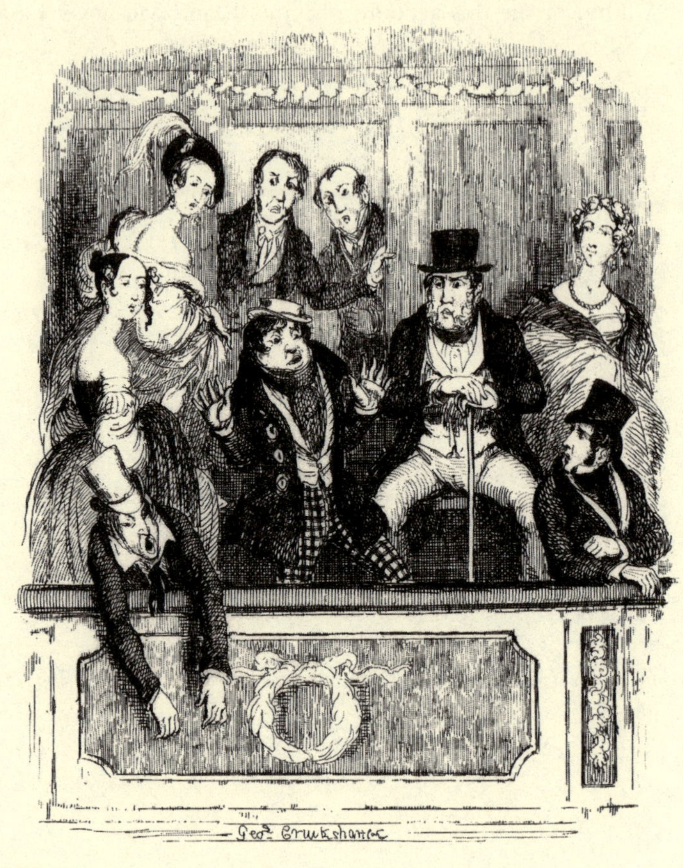


*Making a Night of It* *(see p. 267)*

## Chapter Ten

### *Shabby-genteel People*

First published in the *Morning Chronicle,* 5 November 1834 ('Street Sketches No. 4'). Scott's *Letters on Demonology and Witchcraft* appeared in the first volume in Murray's Family Library Series (1830) and the passage Dickens alludes to here describes the case of a man who was persecuted by visions during a period of sickness and depression; one of these visions was 'the apparition of a gentleman usher, dressed as if to wait on a Lord Lieutenant of Ireland ... arrayed in court dress, with bag and sword, tamboured waistcoat and chapeaubras who glided beside me like the ghost of Beau Nash'.

There are certain descriptions of people who, oddly enough, appear to appertain exclusively to the metropolis. You meet them, every day, in the streets of London, but no one ever encounters them elsewhere; they seem indigenous to the soil, and to belong as exclusively to London as its own smoke, or the dingy bricks and mortar. We could illustrate the remark by a variety of examples, but, in our present sketch, we will only advert to one class as a specimen – that class which is so aptly and expressively designated as 'shabby-genteel'.

Now, shabby people, God knows, may be found anywhere, and genteel people are not articles of greater scarcity out of London than in it; but this compound of the two – this shabby-gentility – is as purely local as the statue at Charing Cross, or the pump at Aldgate. It is worthy of remark, too, that only men are shabby-genteel; a woman is always either dirty and slovenly in the extreme, or neat and respectable, however poverty-stricken in appearance. A very poor man, 'who has seen better days', as the phrase goes, is a strange compound of dirty slovenliness and wretched attempts at faded smartness.

We will endeavour to explain our conception of the term which forms the title of this paper. If you meet a man, lounging up Drury Lane, or leaning with his back against a post in Long Acre, with his hands in the pockets of a pair of drab trousers plentifully besprinkled with grease spots: the trousers made very full over the boots, and ornamented with two cords down the outside of each leg – wearing, also, what has been a brown coat with bright buttons, and a hat very much pinched up at the side, cocked over his right eye – don't pity him. He is not shabby-genteel. The 'harmonic meetings' at some fourth-rate public house, or the purlieus of a private theatre, are his chosen haunts; he entertains a rooted antipathy to any kind of work, and is on familiar terms with several pantomime men at the large houses. But, if you see hurrying along a by-street, keeping as close as he can to the area railings, a man of about forty or fifty, clad in an old rusty suit of threadbare black cloth which shines with constant wear as if it had been beeswaxed – the trousers tightly strapped down, partly for the look of the thing and partly to keep his old shoes from slipping off at the heels, – if you observe, too, that his yellowish-white neckerchief is carefully pinned up, to conceal the tattered garment underneath, and that his hands are encased in the remains of an old pair of beaver gloves, you may set him down as a shabby-genteel man. A glance at that depressed face, and timorous air of conscious poverty, will make your heart ache – always supposing that you are neither a philosopher nor a political economist.

We were once haunted by a shabby-genteel man; he was bodily present to our senses all day, and he was in our mind's eye all night. The man of whom Sir Walter Scott speaks in his Demonology, did not suffer half the persecution from his imaginary gentleman usher in black velvet, that we sustained from our friend in quondam black cloth. He first attracted our notice, by sitting opposite to us in the reading room at the British Museum; and what made the man more remarkable was, that he always had before him a couple of shabby-genteel books – two old dog's-eared folios, in mouldy worm-eaten covers, which had once been smart. He was in his chair every morning, just as the clock struck ten; he was always the last to leave the room in the afternoon; and when he did, he quitted it with the air of a man who knew not where else to go for warmth and quiet. There he used to sit all day, as close to the table as possible, in order to conceal the lack of buttons on his coat: with his old hat carefully deposited at his feet, where he evidently flattered himself it escaped observation.

About two o'clock, you would see him munching a French roll or a penny loaf; not taking it boldly out of his pocket at once, like a man who knew he was only making a lunch; but breaking off little bits in his pocket, and eating them by stealth. He knew too well it was his dinner.

When we first saw this poor object, we thought it quite impossible that his attire could ever become worse. We even went so far as to speculate on the possibility of his shortly appearing in a decent second-hand suit. We knew nothing about the matter; he grew more and more shabby-genteel every day. The buttons dropped off his waistcoat one by one; then, he buttoned his coat; and when one side of the coat was reduced to the same condition as the waistcoat, he buttoned it over on the other side. He looked somewhat better at the beginning of the week than at the conclusion, because the neckerchief, though yellow, was not quite so dingy; and, in the midst of all this wretchedness, he never appeared without gloves and straps. He remained in this state for a week or two. At length, one of the buttons on the back of the coat fell off, and then the man himself disappeared, and we thought he was dead.

We were sitting at the same table about a week after his disappearance, and as our eyes rested on his vacant chair, we insensibly fell into a train of meditation on the subject of his retirement from public life. We were wondering whether he had hung himself, or thrown himself off a bridge – whether he really was dead or had only been arrested – when our conjectures were suddenly set at rest by the entry of the man himself. He had undergone some strange metamorphosis, and walked up the centre of the room with an air which showed he was fully conscious of the improvement in his appearance. It was very odd. His clothes were a fine, deep, glossy black; and yet they looked like the same suit; nay, there were the very darns with which old acquaintance had made us familiar. The hat, too – nobody could mistake the shape of that hat, with its high crown gradually increasing in circumference towards the top. Long service had imparted to it a reddish-brown tint; but now it was as black as the coat. The truth flashed suddenly upon us – they had been 'revived'. It is a deceitful liquid that black and blue reviver; we have watched its effects on many a shabby-genteel man. It betrays its victims into a temporary assumption of importance: possibly into the purchase of a new pair of gloves, or a cheap stock, or some other trifling article of dress. It elevates their spirits for a week, only to depress them, if possible, below their original level. It was so in this case; the transient dignity of the unhappy man decreased, in exact proportion as the 'reviver' wore off. The knees of the unmentionables, and the elbows of the coat, and the seams generally, soon began to get alarmingly white. The hat was once more deposited under the table, and its owner crept into his seat as quietly as ever.

There was a week of incessant small rain and mist. At its expiration the 'reviver' had entirely vanished, and the shabby-genteel man never afterwards attempted to effect any improvement in his outward appearance.

It would be difficult to name any particular part of town as the principal resort of shabby-genteel men. We have met a great many persons of this description in the neighbourhood of the Inns of Court. They may be met with in Holborn between eight and ten any morning; and whoever has the curiosity to enter the Insolvent Debtors' Court will observe, both among spectators and practitioners, a great variety of them. We never went on 'Change, by any chance, without seeing some shabby-genteel men, and we have often wondered what earthly business they can have there. They will sit there, for hours, leaning on great, dropsical, mildewed umbrellas, or eating Abernethy biscuits. Nobody speaks to them, nor they to anyone. On consideration, we remember to have occasionally seen two shabby-genteel men conversing together on 'Change, but our experience assures us that this is an uncommon circumstance, occasioned by the offer of a pinch of snuff, or some such civility.

It would be a task of equal difficulty, either to assign any particular spot for the residence of these beings, or to endeavour to enumerate their general occupations. We were never engaged in business with more than one shabby-genteel man; and he was a drunken engraver, and lived in a damp back parlour in a new row of houses at Camden Town, half street, half brick field, somewhere near the canal. A shabby-genteel man may have no occupation, or he may be a corn agent, or a coal agent, or a wine merchant, or a collector of debts, or a broker's assistant, or a broken down attorney. He may be a clerk of the lowest description, or a contributor to the press of the same grade. Whether our readers have noticed these men, in their walks, as often as we have, we know not; this we know – that the miserably poor man (no matter whether he owes his distresses to his own conduct, or that of others) who feels his poverty and vainly strives to conceal it, is one of the most pitiable objects in human nature. Such objects, with few exceptions, are shabby-genteel people.

## Chapter Eleven

### *Making a Night of It*

First published in *Bell's Life in London,* 18 October 1835 ('Scenes and Characters No. 4'). Damon and Pythias were ideal friends in classical legend. Pythias was condemned to death by Dionysius, Tyrant of Syracuse (405–367 BC), but given time to go home to settle his affairs. Damon pledged his own life as a guarantee of his friend's return, a gesture which so impressed Dionysius that when Pythias duly came back he spared his life. Hill notes that when Dickens was a junior clerk in the office of Ellis and Blackmore, solicitors, he had a colleague named Thomas Potter – see headnote to 'Private Theatres', above p. 120.

Damon and Pythias were undoubtedly very good fellows in their way: the former for his extreme readiness to put in special bail for a friend: and the latter for a certain trump-like punctuality in turning up just in the very nick of time, scarcely less remarkable. Many points in their character have, however, grown obsolete. Damons are rather hard to find, in these days of imprisonment for debt (except the sham ones, and they cost half-a-crown); and, as to the Pythiases, the few that have existed in these degenerate times, have had an unfortunate knack of making themselves scarce, at the very moment when their appearance would have been strictly classical. If the actions of these heroes, however, can find no parallel in modern times, their friendship can. We have Damon and Pythias on the one hand. We have Potter and Smithers on the other; and, lest the two last-mentioned names should never have reached the ears of our unenlightened readers, we can do no better than make them acquainted with the owners thereof.

Mr Thomas Potter, then, was a clerk in the city, and Mr Robert Smithers was a ditto in the same; their incomes were limited, but their friendship was unbounded. They lived in the same street, walked into town every morning at the same hour, dined at the same slap-bang every day, and revelled in each other's company every night. They were knit together by the closest ties of intimacy and friendship, or, as Mr Thomas Potter touchingly observed, they were 'thick-and-thin pals, and nothing but it'. There was a spice of romance in Mr Smithers's disposition, a ray of poetry, a gleam of misery, a sort of consciousness of he didn't exactly know what, coming across him he didn't precisely know why – which stood out in fine relief against the off hand, dashing, amateur pickpocket sort of manner, which distinguished Mr Potter in an eminent degree.

The peculiarity of their respective dispositions extended itself to their individual costume. Mr Smithers generally appeared in public in a surtout and shoes, with a narrow black neckerchief and a brown hat, very much turned up at the sides – peculiarities which Mr Potter wholly eschewed, for it was his ambition to do something in the celebrated 'kiddy' or stage coach way, and he had even gone so far as to invest capital in the purchase of a rough blue coat with wooden buttons, made upon the fireman's principle, in which, with the addition of a low-crowned, flowerpot-saucer-shaped hat, he had created no inconsiderable sensation at the Albion in Little Russell Street, and divers other places of public and fashionable resort.

Mr Potter and Mr Smithers had mutually agreed that, on the receipt of their quarter's salary, they would jointly and in company 'spend the evening' – an evident misnomer – the spending applying, as everybody knows, not to the evening itself but to all the money the individual may chance to be possessed of, on the occasion to which reference is made; and they had likewise agreed that, on the evening aforesaid, they would 'make a night of it' – an expressive term, implying the borrowing of several hours from tomorrow morning, adding them to the night before, and manufacturing a compound night of the whole.

The quarter-day arrived at last – we say at last, because quarter-days are as eccentric as comets: moving wonderfully quick when you have a good deal to pay, and marvellously slow when you have a little to receive. Mr Thomas Potter and Mr Robert Smithers met by appointment to begin the evening with a dinner; and a nice, snug, comfortable dinner they had, consisting of a little procession of four chops and four kidneys, following each other, supported on either side by a pot of the real draught stout, and attended by divers cushions of bread and wedges of cheese.

When the cloth was removed, Mr Thomas Potter ordered the waiter to bring in two goes of his best Scotch whiskey, with warm water and sugar, and a couple of his 'very mildest' Havannahs, which the waiter did. Mr Thomas Potter mixed his grog, and lighted his cigar; Mr Robert Smithers did the same; and then Mr Thomas Potter jocularly proposed as the first toast, 'the abolition of all offices whatever' (not sinecures, but counting houses), which was immediately drunk by Mr Robert Smithers, with enthusiastic applause. So they went on, talking politics, puffing cigars, and sipping whiskey and water, until the 'goes' – most appropriately so called – were both gone, which Mr Robert Smithers perceiving, immediately ordered in two more goes of the best Scotch whiskey, and two more of the very mildest Havannahs; and the goes kept coming in, and the mild Havannahs kept going out, until, what with the drinking, and lighting, and puffing, and the stale ashes on the table, and the tallow-grease on the cigars, Mr Robert Smithers began to doubt the mildness of the Havannahs, and to feel very much as if he had been sitting in a hackney coach with his back to the horses.

As to Mr Thomas Potter, he *would* keep laughing out loud, and volunteering inarticulate declarations that he was 'all right'; in proof of which he feebly bespoke the evening paper after the next gentleman, but finding it a matter of some difficulty to discover any news in its columns, or to ascertain distinctly whether it had any columns at all, walked slowly out to look for the moon, and, after coming back quite pale with looking up at the sky so long, and attempting to express mirth at Mr Robert Smithers having fallen asleep, by various galvanic chuckles, laid his head on his arm, and went to sleep also. When he awoke again, Mr Robert Smithers awoke too, and they both very gravely agreed that it was extremely unwise to eat so many pickled walnuts with the chops, as it was a notorious fact that they always made people queer and sleepy; indeed, if it had not been for the whiskey and cigars, there was no knowing what harm they mightn't have done 'em. So they took some coffee, and after paying the bill, – twelve and twopence the dinner, and the odd tenpence for the waiter – thirteen shillings in all – started out on their expedition to manufacture a night.

It was just half-past eight, so they thought they couldn't do better than go at half price to the slips at the City Theatre, which they did accordingly. Mr Robert Smithers, who had become extremely poetical after the settlement of the bill, enlivening the walk by informing Mr Thomas Potter in confidence that he felt an inward presentiment of approaching dissolution, and subsequently embellishing the theatre by falling asleep, with his head and both arms gracefully drooping over the front of the boxes.

Such was the quiet demeanour of the unassuming Smithers, and such were the happy effects of Scotch whiskey and Havannahs on that interesting person! But Mr Thomas Potter, whose great aim it was to be considered as a 'knowing card', a 'fastgoer', and so forth, conducted himself in a very different manner, and commenced going very fast indeed – rather too fast at last, for the patience of the audience to keep pace with him. On his first entry, he contented himself by earnestly calling upon the gentlemen in the gallery to 'flare up', accompanying the demand with another request, expressive of his wish that they would instantaneously 'form a union', both which requisitions were responded to, in the manner most in vogue on such occasions.

'Give that dog a bone!' cried one gentleman in his shirtsleeves.

'Where have you been a-having half a pint of intermediate beer?' cried a second. 'Tailor!' screamed a third. 'Barber's clerk!' shouted a fourth. 'Throw him O—VER!' roared a fifth; while numerous voices concurred in desiring Mr Thomas Potter to 'go home to his mother!' All these taunts Mr Thomas Potter received with supreme contempt, cocking the low-crowned hat a little more on one side, whenever any reference was made to his personal appearance, and, standing up with his arms a-kimbo, expressing defiance melodramatically.

The overture – to which these various sounds had been an *ad libitum* accompaniment – concluded, the second piece began, and Mr Thomas Potter, emboldened by impunity, proceeded to behave in a most unprecedented and outrageous manner. First of all, he imitated the shake of the principal female singer; then, groaned at the blue fire; then, affected to be frightened into convulsions of terror at the appearance of the ghost; and, lastly, not only made a running commentary, in an audible voice, upon the dialogue on the stage, but actually awoke Mr Robert Smithers, who, hearing his companion making a noise, and having a very indistinct notion where he was, or what was required of him, immediately, by way of imitating a good example, set up the most unearthly, unremitting, and appalling howling that ever audience heard. It was too much. 'Turn them out!' was the general cry. A noise, as of shuffling of feet, and men being knocked up with violence against wainscoting, was heard: a hurried dialogue of 'Come out!' – 'I won't!' – 'You shall!' – 'I shan't!' – 'Give me your card, Sir!' – 'You're a scoundrel, Sir!' and so forth, succeeded. A round of applause betokened the approbation of the audience, and Mr Robert Smithers and Mr Thomas Potter found themselves shot with astonishing swiftness into the road, without having had the trouble of once putting foot to ground during the whole progress of their rapid descent.

Mr Robert Smithers, being constitutionally one of the slowgoers, and having had quite enough of fastgoing, in the course of his recent expulsion, to last until the quarter-day then next ensuing at the very least, had no sooner emerged with his companion from the precincts of Milton Street, than he proceeded to indulge in circuitous references to the beauties of sleep, mingled with distant allusions to the propriety of returning to Islington, and testing the influence of their patent Bramahs over the street door locks to which they respectively belonged. Mr Thomas Potter, however, was valorous and peremptory. They had come out to make a night of it: and a night must be made. So Mr Robert Smithers, who was three parts dull, and the other dismal, despairingly assented; and they went into a wine vaults, to get materials for assisting them in making a night; where they found a good many young ladies, and various old gentlemen, and a plentiful sprinkling of hackney coachmen and cab drivers, all drinking and talking together; and Mr Thomas Potter and Mr

Robert Smithers drank small glasses of brandy, and large glasses of soda, until they began to have a very confused idea, either of things in general, or of anything in particular; and when they had done treating themselves they began to treat everybody else; and the rest of the entertainment was a confused mixture of heads and heels, black eyes and blue uniforms, mud and gaslights, thick doors, and stone paving.

Then, as standard novelists expressively inform us – 'all was a blank!' and in the morning the blank was filled up with the words 'STATION HOUSE', and the station house was filled up with Mr Thomas Potter, Mr Robert Smithers, and the major part of their wine vault companions of the preceding night, with a comparatively small portion of clothing of any kind. And it was disclosed at the Police Office, to the indignation of the Bench, and the astonishment of the spectators, how one Robert Smithers, aided and abetted by one Thomas Potter, had knocked down and beaten, in divers streets, at different times, five men, four boys, and three women; how the said Thomas Potter had feloniously obtained possession of five door knockers, two bell handles, and a bonnet; how Robert Smithers, his friend, had sworn at least forty pounds' worth of oaths, at the rate of five shillings apiece; terrified whole streets full of her Majesty's subjects with awful shrieks and alarms of fire; destroyed the uniforms of five policemen; and committed various other atrocities, too numerous to recapitulate. And the magistrate, after an appropriate reprimand, fined Mr Thomas Potter and Mr Robert Smithers five shillings each, for being what the law vulgarly terms drunk; and thirty-four pounds for seventeen assaults at forty shillings a-head, with liberty to speak to the prosecutors.

The prosecutors *were* spoken to, and Messrs Potter and Smithers lived on credit, for a quarter, as best they might; and, although the prosecutors expressed their readiness to be assaulted twice a week, on the same terms, they have never since been detected in 'making a night of it'.

## Chapter Twelve

### *The Prisoners' Van*

First published in *Bell's Life in London,* 29 November 1835 ('Scenes and Characters No. 9'). Cold Bath Fields was the Middlesex House of Correction where prisoners were punished with the 'mill', i.e., the treadmill. The girl in this sketch considers herself lucky that the magistrates have sentenced her to a short term in Cold Bath Fields rather than sending her for trial at the Quarter Sessions at the Old Bailey where she might have been sentenced to a longer term, to be served in 'the stone jug' (i.e., Newgate).

For the original opening paragraphs of the sketch, which began: 'We have a most extraordinary partiality for lounging about the streets . . .', see Introduction, p. xvi f. and DeVries, p. 169.

We were passing the corner of Bow Street, on our return from a lounging excursion the other afternoon, when a crowd, assembled round the door of the Police Office, attracted our attention. We turned up the street accordingly. There were thirty or forty people, standing on the pavement and half across the road; and a few stragglers were patiently stationed on the opposite side of the way – all evidently waiting in expectation of some arrival. We waited too, a few minutes, but nothing occurred; so we turned round to an unshorn, sallow-looking cobbler, who was standing next us with his hands under the bib of his apron, and put the usual question of 'What's the matter?' The cobbler eyed us from head to foot, with superlative contempt, and laconically replied 'Nuffin'.

Now, we were perfectly aware that if two men stop in the street to look at any given object, or even to gaze in the air, two hundred men will be assembled in no time; but as we knew very well that no crowd of people could by possibility remain in a street for five minutes without getting up a little amusement among themselves, unless they had some absorbing object in view, the natural inquiry next in order was, 'What are all these people waiting here for?' – 'Her Majesty's carriage,' replied the cobbler. This was still more extraordinary. We could not imagine what earthly business her Majesty's carriage could have at the Public Office, Bow Street. We were beginning to ruminate on the possible causes of such an uncommon appearance, when a general exclamation from all the boys in the crowd of 'Here's the wan!' caused us to raise our heads, and look up the street.

The covered vehicle, in which prisoners are conveyed from the police offices to the different prisons, was coming along at full speed. It then occurred to us, for the first time, that her Majesty's carriage was merely another name for the prisoners' van, conferred upon it, not only by reason of the superior gentility of the term, but because the aforesaid van is maintained at her Majesty's expense: having been originally started for the exclusive accommodation of ladies and gentlemen under the necessity of visiting the various houses of call known by the general denomination of 'Her Majesty's Gaols'.

The van drew up at the office door, and the people thronged round the steps, just leaving a little alley for the prisoners to pass through. Our friend the cobbler, and the other stragglers, crossed over, and we followed their example. The driver, and another man who had been seated by his side in front of the vehicle, dismounted, and were admitted into the office. The office door was closed after them, and the crowd were on the tiptoe of expectation.

After a few minutes' delay, the door again opened, and the two first prisoners appeared. They were a couple of girls, of whom the elder could not be more than sixteen, and the younger of whom had certainly not attained her fourteenth year. That they were sisters was evident from the resemblance which still subsisted between them, though two additional years of depravity had fixed their brand upon the elder girl's features, as legibly as if a red-hot iron had seared them. They were both gaudily dressed, the younger one especially; and, although there was a strong similarity between them in both respects, which was rendered the more obvious by their being handcuffed together, it is impossible to conceive a greater contrast than the demeanour of the two presented. The younger girl was weeping bitterly – not for display, or in the hope of producing effect, but for very shame; her face was buried in her handkerchief; and her whole manner was but too expressive of bitter and unavailing sorrow.

'How long are you for, Emily?' screamed a red-faced woman in the crowd. 'Six weeks and labour,' replied the elder girl with a flaunting laugh; 'and that's better than the stone jug anyhow; the mill's a deal better than the Sessions and here's Bella a-going too for the first time. Hold up your head, you chicken,' she continued, boisterously tearing the other girl's handkerchief away; 'Hold up your head, and show 'em your face. I an't jealous, but I'm blessed if I an't game!' – 'That's right, old gal,' exclaimed a man in a paper cap, who, in common with the greater part of the crowd, had been inexpressibly delighted with this little incident. – 'Right!' replied the girl; 'ah, to be sure; what's the odds, eh?' – 'Come! In with you,' interrupted the driver. 'Don't you be in a hurry, coachman,' replied the girl, 'and recollect I want to be set down in Cold Bath Fields – large house with a high garden wall in front; you can't mistake it. Hallo! Bella, where are you going to – you'll pull my precious arm off!' This was addressed to the younger girl, who, in her anxiety to hide herself in the caravan, had ascended the steps first, and forgotten the strain upon the handcuff. 'Come down, and let's show you the way.' And after jerking the miserable girl down with a force which made her stagger on the pavement, she got into the vehicle, and was followed by her wretched companion.

These two girls had been thrown upon London streets, their vices and debauchery, by a sordid and rapacious mother. What the younger girl was then, the elder had been once; and what the elder then was, the younger must soon become. A melancholy prospect, but how surely to be realised; a tragic drama, but how often acted! Turn to the prisons and police offices of London – nay, look into the very streets themselves. These things pass before our eyes, day after day, and hour after hour – they have become such matters of course, that they are utterly disregarded. The progress of these girls in crime will be as rapid as the flight of a pestilence, resembling it too in its baneful influence and wide-spreading infection. Step by step, how many wretched females, within the sphere of every man's observation, have become involved in a career of vice, frightful to contemplate; hopeless at its commencement, loathsome and repulsive in its course; friendless, forlorn, and unpitied, at its miserable conclusion!

There were other prisoners – boys of ten, as hardened in vice as men of fifty – a houseless vagrant, going joyfully to prison as a place of food and shelter, handcuffed to a man whose prospects were ruined, character lost, and family rendered destitute, by his first offence. Our curiosity, however, was satisfied. The first group had left an impression on our mind we would gladly have avoided, and would willingly have effaced.

The crowd dispersed; the vehicle rolled away with its load of guilt and misfortune; and we saw no more of the Prisoners' Van.

# TALES

## Chapter One

### *The Boarding House*

First published as 'The Boarding House' and 'The Boarding House No. 2' in the *Monthly Magazine,* May and August 1834. Dickens later adopted 'Tibbs' as his *nom-de-plume* for the twelve sketches collectively entitled 'Scenes and Characters' published in *Bell's Life in London,* 27 September 1835–17 January 1836.

#### *Chapter 1*

Mrs Tibbs was, beyond all dispute, the most tidy, fidgety, thrifty little personage that ever inhaled the smoke of London; and the house of Mrs Tibbs was, decidedly, the neatest in all Great Coram Street. The area and the area steps, and the street door and the street door steps, and the brass handle, and the door-plate, and the knocker, and the fan light, were all as clean and bright, as indefatigable whitewashing, and hearth-stoning, and scrubbing and rubbing, could make them. The wonder was, that the brass door plate, with the interesting inscription 'Mrs Tibbs', had never caught fire from constant friction, so perseveringly was it polished. There were meat-safe-looking blinds in the parlour windows, blue and gold curtains in the drawing room, and spring roller blinds, as Mrs Tibbs was wont in the pride of her heart to boast, 'all the way up'. The bell lamp in the passage looked as clear as a soap-bubble; you could see yourself in all the tables, and French polish yourself on any one of the chairs. The banisters were beeswaxed; and the very stair wires made your eyes wink, they were so glittering.

Mrs Tibbs was somewhat short of stature, and Mr Tibbs was by no means a large man. He had, moreover, very short legs, but, by way of indemnification, his face was peculiarly long. He was to his wife what the 0 is in 90 – he was of some importance *with* her – he was nothing without her. Mrs Tibbs was always talking. Mr Tibbs rarely spoke; but, if it were at any time possible to put in a word, when he should have said nothing

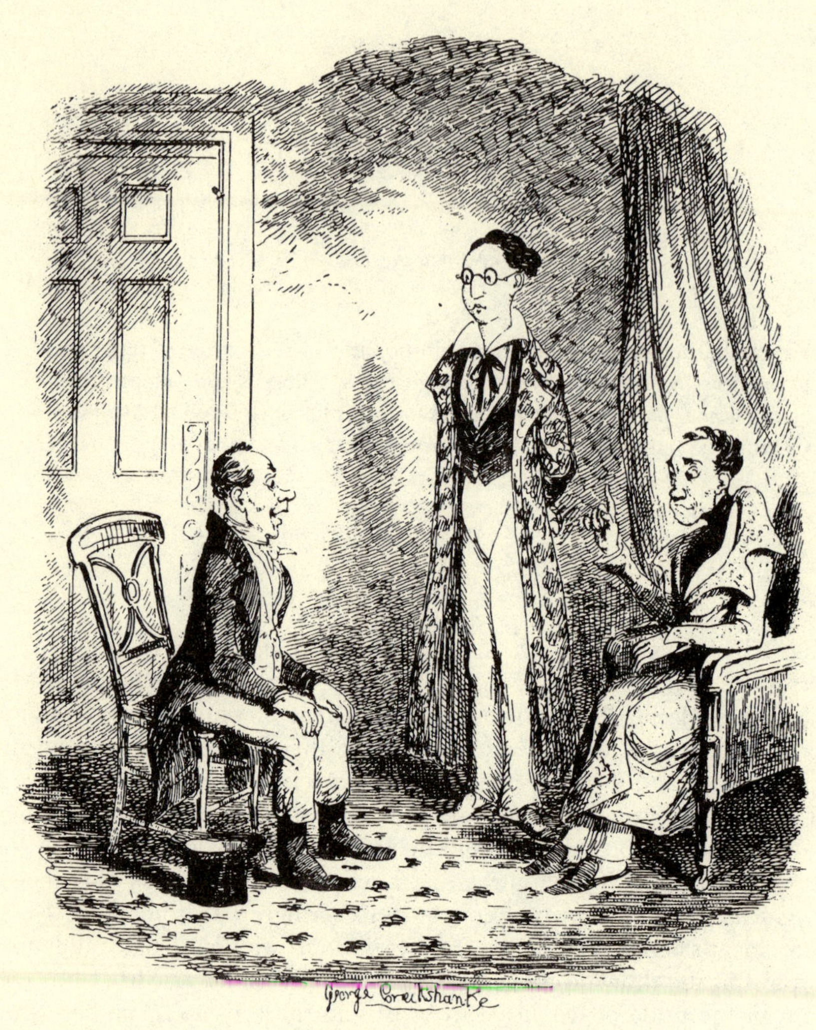


*The Boarding House (1)* *(see p. 284)*

at all, he had that talent. Mrs Tibbs detested long stories, and Mr Tibbs had one, the conclusion of which had never been heard by his most intimate friends. It always began, 'I recollect when I was in the volunteer corps, in eighteen hundred and six,' – but, as he spoke very slowly and softly, and his better half very quickly and loudly, he rarely got beyond the introductory sentence. He was a melancholy specimen of the storyteller. He was the wandering Jew of Joe Millerism.

Mr Tibbs enjoyed a small independence from the pension list – about 43*l.* 15*s.* 10*d.* a year. His father, mother, and five interesting scions from the same stock, drew a like sum from the revenue of a grateful country, though for what particular service was never known. But, as this said independence was not quite sufficient to furnish two people with *all* the luxuries of this life, it had occurred to the busy little spouse of Tibbs, that the best thing she could do with a legacy of 700*l.*, would be to take and furnish a tolerable house – somewhere in that partially explored tract of country which lies between the British Museum, and a remote village called Somers Town – for the reception of boarders. Great Coram Street was the spot pitched upon. The house had been furnished accordingly; two female servants and a boy engaged; and an advertisement inserted in the morning papers, informing the public that 'Six individuals would meet with all the comforts of a cheerful musical home in a select private family, residing within ten minutes' walk of' – everywhere. Answers out of number were received, with all sorts of initials; all the letters of the alphabet seemed to be seized with a sudden wish to go out boarding and lodging; voluminous was the correspondence between Mrs Tibbs and the applicants; and most profound was the secrecy observed. 'E.' didn't like this; 'I.' couldn't think of putting up with that; 'I.O.U.' didn't think the terms would suit him; and 'G.R.' had never slept in a French bed. The result, however, was that three gentlemen became inmates of Mrs Tibbs's house, on terms which were 'agreeable to all parties'. In went the advertisement again, and a lady with her two daughters proposed to increase – not their families, but Mrs Tibbs's.

'Charming woman, that Mrs Maplesone!' said Mrs Tibbs, as she and her spouse were sitting by the fire after breakfast; the gentlemen having gone out on their several avocations. 'Charming woman, indeed!' repeated little Mrs Tibbs, more by way of soliloquy than anything else, for she never thought of consulting her husband. 'And the two daughters are delightful. We must have some fish today; they'll join us at dinner for the first time.'

Mr Tibbs placed the poker at right angles with the fire shovel, and essayed to speak, but recollected he had nothing to say.

'The young ladies,' continued Mrs T, 'have kindly volunteered to bring their own piano.'

Tibbs thought of the volunteer story, but did not venture it. A bright thought struck him –

'It's very likely—' said he.

'Pray don't lean your head against the paper,' interrupted Mrs Tibbs; 'and don't put your feet on the steel fender; that's worse.'

Tibbs took his head from the paper, and his feet from the fender, and proceeded. 'It's very likely one of the young ladies may set her cap at young Mr Simpson, and you know a marriage—'

'A what!' shrieked Mrs Tibbs. Tibbs modestly repeated his former suggestion.

'I beg you won't mention such a thing,' said Mrs T. 'A marriage, indeed! – to rob me of my boarders – no, not for the world.'

Tibbs thought in his own mind that the event was by no means unlikely, but, as he never argued with his wife, he put a stop to the dialogue, by observing it was 'time to go to business'. He always went out at ten o'clock in the morning, and returned at five in the afternoon, with an exceedingly dirty face, and smelling mouldy. Nobody knew what he was, or where he went; but Mrs Tibbs used to say with an air of great importance, that he was engaged in the City.

The Miss Maplesones and their accomplished parent arrived in the course of the afternoon in a hackney coach, and accompanied by a most astonishing number of packages. Trunks, bonnet boxes, muff boxes and parasols, guitar cases, and parcels of all imaginable shapes, done up in brown paper, and fastened with pins, filled the passage. Then there was such a running up and down with the luggage, such scampering for warm water for the ladies to wash in, and such a bustle, and confusion, and heating of servants, and curling irons, as had never been known in Great Coram Street before. Little Mrs Tibbs was quite in her element, bustling about, talking incessantly, and distributing towels and soap, like a head nurse in a hospital. The house was not restored to its usual state of quiet repose, until the ladies were safely shut up in their respective bedrooms, engaged in the important occupation of dressing for dinner.

'Are these gals 'andsome?' inquired Mr Simpson of Mr Septimus Hicks, another of the boarders, as they were amusing themselves in the drawing room, before dinner, by lolling on sofas, and contemplating their pumps.

'Don't know,' replied Mr Septimus Hicks, who was a tallish, white-faced young man, with spectacles, and a black ribbon round his neck instead of a neckerchief – a most interesting person; a poetical walker of the hospitals, and a 'very talented young man'. He was fond of 'lugging' into conversation all sorts of quotations from Don Juan, without fettering himself by the propriety of their application; in which particular he was remarkably independent. The other, Mr Simpson, was one of those young men, who are in society what walking gentlemen are on the stage, only infinitely worse skilled in his vocation than the most indifferent artist. He was as empty-headed as the great bell of St Paul's; always dressed according to the caricatures published in the monthly fashions; and spelt Character with a K.

'I saw a devilish number of parcels in the passage when I came home,' simpered Mr Simpson.

'Materials for the toilet, no doubt,' rejoined the Don Juan reader.

> —Much linen, lace, and several pair
> Of stockings, slippers, brushes, combs, complete;
> With other articles of ladies fair,
> To keep them beautiful, or leave them neat.

'Is that from Milton?' inquired Mr Simpson.

'No – from Byron,' returned Mr Hicks, with a look of contempt. He was quite sure of his author, because he had never read any other. 'Hush! Here come the gals,' and they both commenced talking in a very loud key.

'Mrs Maplesone and the Miss Maplesones, Mr Hicks. Mr Hicks – Mrs Maplesone and the Miss Maplesones,' said Mrs Tibbs, with a very red face, for she had been superintending the cooking operations below stairs, and looked like a wax doll on a sunny day. 'Mr Simpson, I beg your pardon – Mr Simpson – Mrs Maplesone and the Miss Maplesones' – and *vice versa.* The gentlemen immediately began to slide about with much politeness, and to look as if they wished their arms had been legs, so little did they know what to do with them. The ladies smiled, curtseyed, and glided into chairs, and dived for dropped pocket-handkerchiefs: the gentlemen leant against two of the curtain pegs; Mrs Tibbs went through an admirable bit of serious pantomime with a servant who had come up to ask some question about the fish sauce; and then the two young ladies looked at each other; and everybody else appeared to discover something very attractive in the pattern of the fender.

'Julia, my love,' said Mrs Maplesone to her youngest daughter, in a tone loud enough for the remainder of the company to hear – 'Julia.'

'Yes, Ma.'

'Don't stoop.' – This was said for the purpose of directing general attention to Miss Julia's figure, which was undeniable. Everybody looked at her, accordingly, and there was another pause.

'We had the most uncivil hackney coachman today, you can imagine,' said Mrs Maplesone to Mrs Tibbs, in a confidential tone.

'Dear me!' replied the hostess, with an air of great commiseration. She couldn't say more, for the servant again appeared at the door, and commenced telegraphing most earnestly to her 'Missis'.

'I think hackney coachmen generally *are* uncivil,' said Mr Hicks, in his most insinuating tone.

'Positively I think they are,' replied Mrs Maplesone, as if the idea had never struck her before.

'And cabmen, too,' said Mr Simpson. This remark was a failure, for no one intimated, by word or sign, the slightest knowledge of the manners and customs of cabmen.

'Robinson, what *do* you want?' said Mrs Tibbs to the servant, who, by way of making her presence known to her mistress, had been giving sundry hems and sniffs outside the door during the preceding five minutes.

'Please ma'am, master wants his clean things,' replied the servant, taken off her guard. The two young men turned their faces to the window, and 'went off' like a couple of bottles of ginger beer; the ladies put their handkerchiefs to their mouths; and little Mrs Tibbs bustled out of the room to give Tibbs his clean linen, – and the servant warning.

Mr Calton, the remaining boarder, shortly afterwards made his appearance, and proved a surprising promoter of the conversation. Mr Calton was a superannuated beau – an old boy. He used to say of himself that although his features were not regularly handsome, they were striking. They certainly were. It was impossible to look at his face without being reminded of a chubby street door knocker, half lion half monkey; and the comparison might be extended to his whole character and conversation. He had stood still, while everything else had been moving. He never originated a conversation, or started an idea; but if any commonplace topic were broached, or, to pursue the comparison, if anybody *lifted him up,* he would hammer away with surprising rapidity. He had the tic douloureux occasionally, and then he might be said to be muffled, because he did not make quite as much noise as at other times, when he would go on prosing, rat-tat-tat the same thing over and over again. He had never been married; but he was still on the look-out for a wife with money. He had a life interest worth about 300*l.* a year – he was exceedingly vain, and inordinately selfish. He had acquired the reputation of being the very pink of politeness, and he walked round the park, and up Regent Street, every day.

This respectable personage had made up his mind to render himself exceedingly agreeable to Mrs Maplesone – indeed, the desire of being as amiable as possible extended itself to the whole party; Mrs Tibbs having considered it an admirable little bit of management to represent to the gentlemen that she had *some* reason to believe the ladies were fortunes, and to hint to the ladies, that all the gentlemen were 'eligible'. A little flirtation, she thought, might keep her house full, without leading to any other result.

Mrs Maplesone was an enterprising widow of about fifty: shrewd, scheming, and good-looking. She was amiably anxious on behalf of her daughters; in proof whereof she used to remark, that she would have no objection to marry again, if it would benefit her dear girls – she could have no other motive. The 'dear girls' themselves were not at all insensible to the merits of 'a good establishment'. One of them was twenty-five; the other, three years younger. They had been at different watering places, for four seasons; they had gambled at libraries, read books in balconies, sold at fancy fairs, danced at assemblies, talked sentiment – in short, they had done all that industrious girls could do – but, as yet, to no purpose.

'What a magnificent dresser Mr Simpson is!' whispered Matilda Maplesone to her sister Julia.

'Splendid!' returned the youngest. The magnificent individual alluded to wore a maroon-coloured dress coat, with a velvet collar and cuffs of the same tint – very like that which usually invests the form of the distinguished unknown who condescends to play the 'swell' in the pantomime at 'Richardson's Show.'

'What whiskers!' said Miss Julia.

'Charming!' responded her sister; 'and what hair!' His hair was like a wig, and distinguished by that insinuating wave which graces the shining locks of those *chef-d'œuvres* of art surmounting the waxen images in Bartellot's window in Regent Street; his whiskers meeting beneath his chin, seemed strings wherewith to tie it on, ere science had rendered them unnecessary by her patent invisible springs.

'Dinner's on the table, ma'am, if you please,' said the boy, who now appeared for the first time, in a revived black coat of his master's.

'Oh! Mr Calton, will you lead Mrs Maplesone? – Thank you.' Mr Simpson offered his arm to Miss Julia; Mr Septimus Hicks escorted the lovely Matilda; and the procession proceeded to the dining room. Mr Tibbs was introduced, and Mr Tibbs bobbed up and down to the three ladies like a figure in a Dutch clock, with a powerful spring in the middle of his body, and then dived rapidly into his seat at the bottom of the table, delighted to screen himself behind a soup tureen, which he could just see over, and that was all. The boarders were seated, a lady and gentleman alternately, like the layers of bread and meat in a plate of sandwiches; and then Mrs Tibbs directed James to take off the covers. Salmon, lobster sauce, giblet soup, and the usual accompaniments were *dis*-covered: potatoes like petrifactions, and bits of toasted bread, the shape and size of blank dice.

'Soup for Mrs Maplesone, my dear,' said the bustling Mrs Tibbs. She always called her husband 'my dear' before company. Tibbs, who had been eating his bread, and calculating how long it would be before he should get any fish, helped the soup in a hurry, made a small island on the tablecloth, and put his glass upon it to hide it from his wife.

'Miss Julia, shall I assist you to some fish?'

'If you please – very little – oh! plenty, thank you' (a bit about the size of a walnut put upon the plate).

'Julia is a *very* little eater,' said Mrs Maplesone to Mr Calton.

The knocker gave a single rap. He was busy eating the fish with his eyes: so he only ejaculated, 'Ah!'

'My dear,' said Mrs Tibbs to her spouse after everyone else had been helped, 'what do *you* take?' The inquiry was accompanied with a look intimating that he mustn't say fish, because there was not much left. Tibbs thought the frown referred to the island on the tablecloth; he therefore coolly replied, 'Why – I'll take a little – fish, I think.'

'Did you say fish, my dear?' (another frown).

'Yes, dear,' replied the villain, with an expression of acute hunger depicted in his countenance. The tears almost started to Mrs Tibbs's eyes, as she helped her 'wretch of a husband,' as she inwardly called him, to the last eatable bit of salmon on the dish.

'James, take this to your master, and take away your master's knife.' This was deliberate revenge, as Tibbs never could eat fish without one. He was, however, constrained to chase small particles of salmon round and round his plate with a piece of bread and a fork, the number of successful attempts being about one in seventeen.

'Take away, James,' said Mrs Tibbs, as Tibbs swallowed the fourth mouthful – and away went the plates like lightning.

'I'll take a bit of bread, James,' said the poor 'master of the house', more hungry than ever.

'Never mind your master now, James,' said Mrs Tibbs, 'see about the meat.' This was conveyed in the tone in which ladies usually give admonitions to servants in company, that is to say, a low one; but which, like a stage whisper, from its peculiar emphasis, is most distinctly heard by everybody present.

A pause ensued, before the table was replenished – a sort of parenthesis in which Mr Simpson, Mr Calton, and Mr Hicks, produced respectively a bottle of sauterne, bucellas, and sherry, and took wine with everybody – except Tibbs. No one ever thought of him.

Between the fish and an intimated sirloin, there was a prolonged interval.

Here was an opportunity for Mr Hicks. He could not resist the singularly appropriate quotation –

> But beef is rare within these oxless isles;
> Goats' flesh there is, no doubt, and kid, and mutton,
> And when a holiday upon them smiles,
> A joint upon their barbarous spits they put on.

'Very ungentlemanly behaviour,' thought little Mrs Tibbs, 'to talk in that way.'

'Ah,' said Mr Calton, filling his glass. 'Tom Moore is my poet.'

'And mine,' said Mrs Maplesone.

'And mine,' said Miss Julia.

'And mine,' added Mr Simpson.

'Look at his compositions,' resumed the knocker.

'To be sure,' said Simpson, with confidence.

'Look at Don Juan,' replied Mr Septimus Hicks.

'Julia's letter,' suggested Miss Matilda.

'Can anything be grander than the Fire Worshippers?' inquired Miss Julia.

'To be sure,' said Simpson.

'Or Paradise and the Peri,' said the old beau.

'Yes; or Paradise and the Peer,' repeated Simpson, who thought he was getting through it capitally.

'It's all very well,' replied Mr Septimus Hicks, who, as we have before hinted, never had read anything but Don Juan. 'Where will you find anything finer than the description of the siege, at the commencement of the seventh canto?'

'Talking of a siege,' said Tibbs, with a mouthful of bread – 'when I was in the volunteer corps, in eighteen hundred and six, our commanding officer was Sir Charles Rampart; and one day, when we were exercising on the ground on which the London University now stands, he says, says he, Tibbs (calling me from the ranks), Tibbs—'

'Tell your master, James,' interrupted Mrs Tibbs, in an awfully distinct tone, 'tell your master if he *won't* carve those fowls, to send them to me.' The discomfited volunteer instantly set to work, and carved the fowls almost as expeditiously as his wife operated on the haunch of mutton. Whether he ever finished the story is not known; but, if he did, nobody heard it.

As the ice was now broken, and the new inmates more at home, every member of the company felt more at ease. Tibbs himself most certainly did, because he went to sleep immediately after dinner. Mr Hicks and the ladies discoursed most eloquently about poetry, and the theatres, and Lord Chesterfield's Letters; and Mr Calton followed up what everybody said, with continuous double knocks. Mrs Tibbs highly approved of every observation that fell from Mrs Maplesone; and as Mr Simpson sat with a smile upon his face and said 'Yes,' or 'Certainly,' at intervals of about four minutes each, he received full credit for understanding what was going forward. The gentlemen rejoined the ladies in the drawing room very shortly after they had left the dining parlour. Mrs Maplesone and Mr Calton played cribbage, and the 'young people' amused themselves with music and conversation. The Miss Maplesones sang the most fascinating duets, and accompanied themselves on guitars, ornamented with bits of ethereal blue ribbon. Mr Simpson put on a pink waistcoat, and said he was in raptures; and Mr Hicks felt in the seventh heaven of poetry or the seventh canto of Don Juan – it was the same thing to him. Mrs Tibbs was quite charmed with the newcomers; and Mr Tibbs spent the evening in his usual way – he went to sleep, and woke up, and went to sleep again, and woke at suppertime.

We are not about to adopt the licence of novel-writers, and to let 'years roll on'; but we will take the liberty of requesting the reader to suppose that six months have elapsed, since the dinner we have described, and that Mrs Tibbs's boarders have, during that period, sang, and danced, and gone to theatres and exhibitions, together, as ladies and gentlemen, wherever they board, often do. And we will beg them, the period we have mentioned having elapsed, to imagine farther that Mr Septimus Hicks received, in his own bedroom (a front attic), at an early hour one morning, a note from Mr Calton, requesting the favour of seeing him, as soon as convenient to himself, in his (Calton's) dressing room, on the second floor back.

'Tell Mr Calton I'll come down directly,' said Mr Septimus to the boy. 'Stop – is Mr Calton unwell?' inquired this excited walker of hospitals, as he put on a bed-furniture-looking dressing-gown.

'Not as I knows on, sir,' replied the boy. 'Please, sir, he looked rather rum, as it might be.'

'Ah, that's no proof of his being ill,' returned Hicks, unconsciously. 'Very well: I'll be down directly.' Downstairs ran the boy with the message, and down went the excited Hicks himself, almost as soon as the message was delivered. 'Tap, tap.' 'Come in.' – Door opens, and discovers Mr Calton sitting in an easy chair. Mutual shakes of the hand exchanged, and Mr Septimus Hicks motioned to a seat. A short pause. Mr Hicks coughed, and Mr Calton took a pinch of snuff. It was one of those interviews where neither party knows what to say. Mr Septimus Hicks broke silence.

'I received a note – ' he said, very tremulously, in a voice like a Punch with a cold.

'Yes,' returned the other, 'you did.'

'Exactly.'

'Yes.'

Now, although this dialogue must have been satisfactory, both gentlemen felt there was something more important to be said; therefore they did as most men in such a situation would have done – they looked at the table with a determined aspect. The conversation had been opened, however, and Mr Calton had made up his mind to continue it with a regular double knock. He always spoke very pompously.

'Hicks,' said he, 'I have sent for you, in consequence of certain arrangements which are pending in this house, connected with a marriage.'

'With a marriage!' gasped Hicks, compared with whose expression of countenance, Hamlet's, when he sees his father's ghost, is pleasing and composed.

'With a marriage,' returned the knocker. 'I have sent for you to prove the great confidence I can repose in you.'

'And will you betray me?' eagerly inquired Hicks, who in his alarm had even forgotten to quote.

'*I* betray *you!* Won't *you* betray *me?*'

'Never; no one shall know, to my dying day, that you had a hand in the business,' responded the agitated Hicks, with an inflamed countenance, and his hair standing on end as if he were on the stool of an electrifying machine in full operation.

'People must know that, some time or other – within a year, I imagine,' said Mr Calton, with an air of great self-complacency. 'We *may* have a family.'

'*We!* – That won't affect you, surely?'

'The devil it won't!'

'No! how can it?' said the bewildered Hicks. Calton was too much inwrapped in the contemplation of his happiness to see the equivoque between Hicks and himself; and threw himself back in his chair. 'Oh, Matilda!' sighed the antique beau, in a lack-a-daisical voice, and applying his right hand a little to the left of the fourth button of his waistcoat, counting from the bottom. 'Oh, Matilda!'

'What Matilda?' inquired Hicks, starting up.

'Matilda Maplesone,' responded the other, doing the same.

'I marry her tomorrow morning,' said Hicks.

'It's false,' rejoined his companion: 'I marry her!'

'You marry her?'

'I marry her!'

'You marry Matilda Maplesone?'

'Matilda Maplesone.'

'*Miss* Maplesone marry *you*?'

'Miss Maplesone! No: Mrs Maplesone.'

'Good Heaven!' said Hicks, falling into his chair: 'You marry the mother, and I the daughter!'

'Most extraordinary circumstance!' replied Mr Calton, 'and rather inconvenient too; for the fact is, that owing to Matilda's wishing to keep her intention secret from her daughters until the ceremony had taken place, she doesn't like applying to any of her friends to give her away. I entertain an objection to making the affair known to my acquaintance just now; and the consequence is, that I sent to you to know whether you'd oblige me by acting as father.'

'I should have been most happy, I assure you,' said Hicks, in a tone of condolence; 'but, you see, I shall be acting as bridegroom. One character is frequently a consequence of the other; but it is not usual to act in both at the same time. There's Simpson – I have no doubt he'll do it for you.'

'I don't like to ask him,' replied Calton, 'he's such a donkey.'

Mr Septimus Hicks looked up at the ceiling, and down at the floor; at last an idea struck him. 'Let the man of the house, Tibbs, be the father,' he suggested; and then he quoted, as peculiarly applicable to Tibbs and the pair –

'Oh Powers of Heaven! what dark eyes meets she there?
'Tis – 'tis her father's – fixed upon the pair.'

'The idea has struck me already,' said Mr Calton: 'but, you see, Matilda, for what reason I know not, is very anxious that Mrs Tibbs should know nothing about it, till it's all over. It's a natural delicacy, after all, you know.'

'He's the best-natured little man in existence, if you manage him properly,' said Mr Septimus Hicks. 'Tell him not to mention it to his wife, and assure him she won't mind it, and he'll do it directly. My marriage is to be a secret one, on account of the mother and *my* father; therefore he must be enjoined to secrecy.'

A small double knock, like a presumptuous single one, was that instant heard at the street door. It was Tibbs; it could be no one else; for no one else occupied five minutes in rubbing his shoes. He had been out to pay the baker's bill.

'Mr Tibbs,' called Mr Calton in a very bland tone, looking over the banisters.

'Sir!' replied he of the dirty face.

'Will you have the kindness to step upstairs for a moment?'

'Certainly, sir,' said Tibbs, delighted to be taken notice of. The bedroom door was carefully closed, and Tibbs, having put his hat on the floor (as most timid men do), and been accommodated with a seat, looked as astounded as if he were suddenly summoned before the familiars of the Inquisition.

'A rather unpleasant occurrence, Mr Tibbs,' said Calton, in a very portentous manner, 'obliges me to consult you, and to beg you will not communicate what I am about to say, to your wife.'

Tibbs acquiesced, wondering in his own mind what the deuce the other could have done, and imagining that at least he must have broken the best decanters.

Mr Calton resumed; 'I am placed, Mr Tibbs, in rather an unpleasant situation.'

Tibbs looked at Mr Septimus Hicks, as if he thought Mr H.'s being in the immediate vicinity of his fellow-boarder might constitute the unpleasantness of his situation; but as he did not exactly know what to say, he merely ejaculated the monosyllable 'Lor!'

'Now,' continued the knocker, 'let me beg you will exhibit no manifestations of surprise, which may be overheard by the domestics, when I tell you – command your feelings of astonishment – that two inmates of this house intend to be married tomorrow morning.' And he drew back his chair several feet, to perceive the effect of the unlooked-for announcement.

If Tibbs had rushed from the room, staggered downstairs, and fainted in the passage – if he had instantaneously jumped out of the window into the mews behind the house, in an agony of surprise – his behaviour would have been much less inexplicable to Mr Calton than it was, when he put his hands into his inexpressible pockets, and said with a half chuckle, 'Just so.'

'You are not surprised, Mr Tibbs?' inquired Mr Calton.

'Bless you, no, sir,' returned Tibbs; 'after all, it's very natural. When two young people get together, you know—'

'Certainly, certainly,' said Calton, with an indescribable air of self-satisfaction.

'You don't think it's at all an out-of-the-way affair then?' asked Mr Septimus Hicks, who had watched the countenance of Tibbs in mute astonishment.

'No, sir,' replied Tibbs; 'I was just the same at his age.' He actually smiled when he said this.

'How devilish well I must carry my years!' thought the delighted old beau, knowing he was at least ten years older than Tibbs at that moment.

'Well, then, to come to the point at once,' he continued, 'I have to ask you whether you will object to act as father on the occasion?'

'Certainly not,' replied Tibbs; still without evincing an atom of surprise.

'You will not?'

'Decidedly not,' reiterated Tibbs, still as calm as a pot of porter with the head off.

Mr Calton seized the hand of the petticoat-governed little man, and vowed eternal friendship from that hour. Hicks, who was all admiration and surprise, did the same.

'Now, confess,' asked Mr Calton of Tibbs, as he picked up his hat, 'were you not a little surprised?'

'I b'lieve you!' replied that illustrious person, holding up one hand; 'I b'lieve you! When I first heard of it.'

'So sudden,' said Septimus Hicks.

'So strange to ask *me*, you know,' said Tibbs.

'So odd altogether!' said the superannuated love-maker; and then all three laughed.

'I say,' said Tibbs, shutting the door which he had previously opened, and giving full vent to a hitherto corked-up giggle, 'what bothers me is, what *will* his father say?'

Mr Septimus Hicks looked at Mr Calton.

'Yes; but the best of it is,' said the latter, giggling in his turn, 'I haven't got a father – he! he! he!'

'*You* haven't got a father. No; but *he* has,' said Tibbs.

'*Who* has?' inquired Septimus Hicks.

'Why *him*.'

'Him, who? Do you know my secret? Do you mean me?'

'You! No; you know who I mean,' returned Tibbs with a knowing wink.

'For Heaven's sake, whom *do* you mean?' inquired Mr Calton, who, like Septimus Hicks, was all but out of his senses at the strange confusion.

'Why, Mr Simpson, of course,' replied Tibbs; 'who else could I mean?'

'I see it all,' said the Byron-quoter; 'Simpson marries Julia Maplesone tomorrow morning!'

'Undoubtedly,' replied Tibbs, thoroughly satisfied, 'of course he does.'

It would require the pencil of Hogarth to illustrate – our feeble pen is inadequate to describe – the expression which the countenances of Mr Calton and Mr Septimus Hicks respectively assumed, at this unexpected announcement. Equally impossible is it to describe, although perhaps it is easier for our lady readers to imagine, what arts the three ladies could have used, so completely to entangle their separate partners. Whatever they were, however, they were successful. The mother was perfectly aware of the intended marriage of both daughters; and the young ladies were equally acquainted with the intention of their estimable parent. They agreed, however, that it would have a much better appearance if each feigned ignorance of the other's engagement; and it was equally desirable that all the marriages should take place on the same day, to prevent the discovery of one clandestine alliance, operating prejudicially on the others. Hence, the mystification of Mr Calton and Mr Septimus Hicks, and the pre-engagement of the unwary Tibbs.

On the following morning, Mr Septimus Hicks was united to Miss Matilda Maplesone. Mr Simpson also entered into a 'holy alliance' with Miss Julia; Tibbs acting as father, 'his first appearance in that character.' Mr Calton, not being quite so eager as the two young men, was rather struck by the double discovery; and as he had found some difficulty in getting any one to give the lady away, it occurred to him that the best mode of obviating the inconvenience would be not to take her at all. The lady, however, 'appealed', as her counsel said on the trial of the cause,

*Maplesone v. Calton,* for a breach of promise, 'with a broken heart, to the outraged laws of her country.' She recovered damages to the amount of 1,000*l.*, which the unfortunate knocker was compelled to pay. Mr Septimus Hicks having walked the hospitals, took it into his head to walk off altogether. His injured wife is at present residing with her mother at Boulogne. Mr Simpson, having the misfortune to lose his wife six weeks after marriage (by her eloping with an officer during his temporary sojourn in the Fleet Prison, in consequence of his inability to discharge her little mantua-maker's bill), and being disinherited by his father, who died soon afterwards, was fortunate enough to obtain a permanent engagement at a fashionable haircutter's; hairdressing being a science to which he had frequently directed his attention. In this situation he had necessarily many opportunities of making himself acquainted with the habits, and style of thinking, of the exclusive portion of the nobility of this kingdom. To this fortunate circumstance are we indebted for the production of those brilliant efforts of genius, his fashionable novels, which so long as good taste, unsullied by exaggeration, cant, and quackery, continues to exist, cannot fail to instruct and amuse the thinking portion of the community.

It only remains to add, that this complication of disorders completely deprived poor Mrs Tibbs of all her inmates, except the one whom she could have best spared – her husband. That wretched little man returned home, on the day of the wedding, in a state of partial intoxication; and, under the influence of wine, excitement, and despair, actually dared to brave the anger of his wife. Since that ill-fated hour he has constantly taken his meals in the kitchen, to which apartment, it is understood, his witticisms will be in future confined; a turn-up bedstead having been conveyed there by Mrs Tibbs's order for his exclusive accommodation. It is possible that he will be enabled to finish, in that seclusion, his story of the volunteers.

The advertisement has again appeared in the morning papers. Results must be reserved for another chapter.

## *Chapter the Second*

'Well!' said little Mrs Tibbs to herself, as she sat in the front parlour of the Coram Street mansion one morning, mending a piece of stair carpet off the first landing; – 'Things have not turned out so badly, either, and if I only get a favourable answer to the advertisement, we shall be full again.'

Mrs Tibbs resumed her occupation of making worsted lattice-work in the carpet, anxiously listening to the twopenny postman, who was hammering his way down the street at the rate of a penny a knock. The house

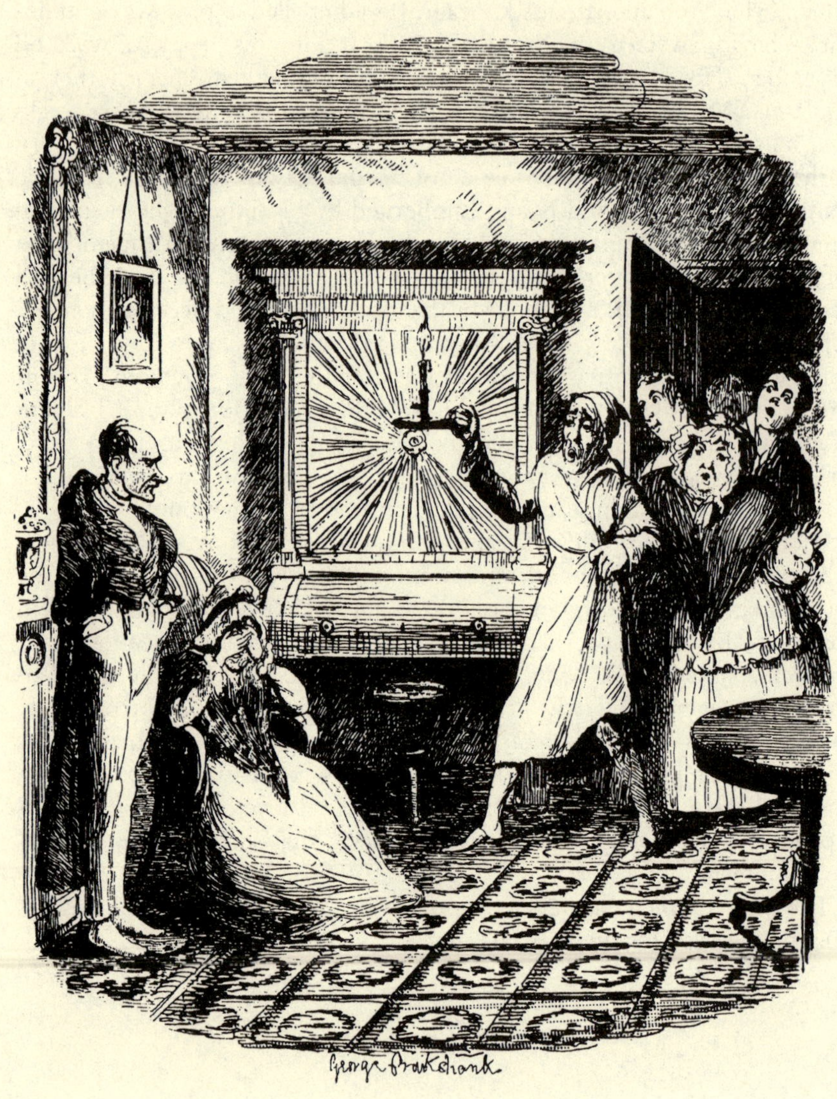


*The Boarding House (2)* *(see p. 304)*

was as quiet as possible. There was only one low sound to be heard – it was the unhappy Tibbs cleaning the gentlemen's boots in the back kitchen, and accompanying himself with a buzzing noise, in wretched mockery of humming a tune.

The postman drew near the house. He paused – so did Mrs Tibbs. A knock – a bustle – a letter – post-paid.

> T.I. presents compt. to I.T. and T.I. begs To say that i see the advertisement And she will Do Herself the pleasure of calling On you at 12 o'clock tomorrow morning.
>
> T.I. as To apologise to I.T. for the shortness Of the notice But i hope it will not unconvenience you.
>
> I remain yours Truly
> Wednesday evening.

Little Mrs Tibbs perused the document, over and over again; and the more she read it, the more was she confused by the mixture of the first and third person; the substitution of the 'i' for the 'T.I.'; and the transition from the 'I.T.' to the 'you'. The writing looked like a skein of thread in a tangle, and the note was ingeniously folded into a perfect square, with the direction squeezed up into the right-hand corner, as if it were ashamed of itself. The back of the epistle was pleasingly ornamented with a large red wafer, which, with the addition of divers ink stains, bore a marvellous resemblance to a black beetle trodden upon. One thing, however, was perfectly clear to the perplexed Mrs Tibbs. Somebody was to call at twelve. The drawing room was forthwith dusted for the third time that morning; three or four chairs were pulled out of their places, and a corresponding number of books carefully upset, in order that there might be a due absence of formality. Down went the piece of stair carpet before noticed, and up ran Mrs Tibbs 'to make herself tidy'.

The clock of New Saint Pancras Church struck twelve, and the Foundling, with laudable politeness, did the same ten minutes afterwards. Saint something else struck the quarter, and then there arrived a single lady with a double knock, in a pelisse the colour of the interior of a damson pie; a bonnet of the same, with a regular conservatory of artificial flowers; a white veil, and a green parasol, with a cobweb border.

The visitor (who was very fat and red-faced) was shown into the drawing room; Mrs Tibbs presented herself, and the negotiation commenced.

'I called in consequence of an advertisement,' said the stranger, in a voice as if she had been playing a set of Pan's pipes for a fortnight without leaving off.

'Yes!' said Mrs Tibbs, rubbing her hands very slowly, and looking the applicant full in the face – two things she always did on such occasions.

'Money isn't no object whatever to me,' said the lady, 'so much as living in a state of retirement and obtrusion.'

Mrs Tibbs, as a matter of course, acquiesced in such an exceedingly natural desire.

'I am constantly attended by a medical man,' resumed the pelisse wearer; 'I have been a shocking unitarian for some time – I, indeed, have had very little peace since the death of Mr Bloss.'

Mrs Tibbs looked at the relict of the departed Bloss, and thought he must have had very little peace in his time. Of course she could not say so; so she looked very sympathising.

'I shall be a good deal of trouble to you,' said Mrs Bloss; 'but for that trouble I am willing to pay. I am going through a course of treatment which renders attention necessary. I have one mutton chop in bed at half-past eight, and another at ten, every morning.'

Mrs Tibbs, as in duty bound, expressed the pity she felt for anybody placed in such a distressing situation; and the carnivorous Mrs Bloss proceeded to arrange the various preliminaries with wonderful despatch. 'Now mind,' said that lady, after terms were arranged; 'I am to have the second-floor front, for my bedroom?'

'Yes, ma'am.'

'And you'll find room for my little servant Agnes?'

'Oh! certainly.'

'And I can have one of the cellars in the area for my bottled porter.'

'With the greatest pleasure; – James shall get it ready for you by Saturday.'

'And I'll join the company at the breakfast table on Sunday morning,' said Mrs Bloss. 'I shall get up on purpose.'

'Very well,' returned Mrs Tibbs, in her most amiable tone; for satisfactory references had 'been given and required', and it was quite certain that the newcomer had plenty of money. 'It's rather singular,' continued Mrs Tibbs, with what was meant for a most bewitching smile, 'that we have a gentleman now with us, who is in a very delicate state of health – a Mr Gobler. – His apartment is the back drawing room.'

'The next room?' inquired Mrs Bloss.

'The next room,' repeated the hostess.

'How very promiscuous!' ejaculated the widow.

'He hardly ever gets up,' said Mrs Tibbs in a whisper.

'Lor!' cried Mrs Bloss, in an equally low tone.

'And when he is up,' said Mrs Tibbs, 'we never can persuade him to go to bed again.'

'Dear me!' said the astonished Mrs Bloss, drawing her chair nearer Mrs Tibbs. 'What is his complaint?'

'Why, the fact is,' replied Mrs Tibbs, with a most communicative air, 'he has no stomach whatever.'

'No what?' inquired Mrs Bloss, with a look of the most indescribable alarm.

'No stomach,' repeated Mrs Tibbs, with a shake of the head.

'Lord bless us! what an extraordinary case!' gasped Mrs Bloss, as if she understood the communication in its literal sense, and was astonished at a gentleman without a stomach finding it necessary to board anywhere.

'When I say he has no stomach,' explained the chatty little Mrs Tibbs, 'I mean that his digestion is so much impaired, and his interior so deranged, that his stomach is not of the least use to him; – in fact, it's an inconvenience.'

'Never heard such a case in my life!' exclaimed Mrs Bloss. 'Why, he's worse than I am.'

'Oh, yes!' replied Mrs Tibbs; – 'certainly.' She said this with great confidence, for the damson pelisse suggested that Mrs Bloss, at all events, was not suffering under Mr Gobler's complaint.

'You have quite incited my curiosity,' said Mrs Bloss, as she rose to depart. 'How I long to see him!'

'He generally comes down once a week,' replied Mrs Tibbs; 'I dare say you'll see him on Sunday.' With this consolatory promise Mrs Bloss was obliged to be contented. She accordingly walked slowly down the stairs, detailing her complaints all the way; and Mrs Tibbs followed her, uttering an exclamation of compassion at every step. James (who looked very gritty, for he was cleaning the knives) fell up the kitchen stairs, and opened the street door; and, after mutual farewells, Mrs Bloss slowly departed, down the shady side of the street.

It is almost superfluous to say, that the lady whom we have just shown out at the street door (and whom the two female servants are now inspecting from the second floor windows) was exceedingly vulgar, ignorant, and selfish. Her deceased better half had been an eminent cork cutter, in which capacity he had amassed a decent fortune. He had no relative but his nephew, and no friend but his cook. The former had the insolence one morning to ask for the loan of fifteen pounds; and, by way of retaliation, he married the latter next day; he made a will immediately afterwards, containing a burst of honest indignation against his nephew (who supported himself and two sisters on 100*l.* a year), and a bequest of his whole property to his wife. He felt ill after breakfast, and died after dinner. There is a mantelpiece-looking tablet in a civic parish church, setting forth his virtues, and deploring his loss. He never dishonoured a bill, or gave away a halfpenny.

The relict and sole executrix of this noble-minded man was an odd mixture of shrewdness and simplicity, liberality and meanness. Bred up as she had been, she knew no mode of living so agreeable as a boarding house; and having nothing to do, and nothing to wish for, she naturally imagined she must be very ill – an impression which was most assiduously promoted by her medical attendant, Dr Wosky, and her handmaid Agnes: both of whom, doubtless for good reasons, encouraged all her extravagant notions.

Since the catastrophe recorded in the last chapter, Mrs Tibbs had been very shy of young lady boarders. Her present inmates were all lords of the creation, and she availed herself of the opportunity of their assemblage at the dinner table, to announce the expected arrival of Mrs Bloss. The gentlemen received the communication with stoical indifference, and Mrs Tibbs devoted all her energies to prepare for the reception of the valetudinarian. The second-floor front was scrubbed, and washed, and flannelled, till the wet went through to the drawing room ceiling. Clean white counterpanes, and curtains, and napkins, water bottles as clear as crystal, blue jugs, and mahogany furniture, added to the splendour, and increased the comfort, of the apartment. The warming-pan was in constant requisition, and a fire lighted in the room every day. The chattels of Mrs Bloss were forwarded by instalments. First, there came a large hamper of Guinness's stout, and an umbrella; then, a train of trunks; then, a pair of clogs and a bandbox; then, an easy chair with an air-cushion; then, a variety of suspicious-looking packages; and – 'though last not least' – Mrs Bloss and Agnes: the latter in a cherry-coloured merino dress, open-work stockings, and shoes with sandals: like a disguised Columbine.

The installation of the Duke of Wellington as Chancellor of the University of Oxford was nothing, in point of bustle and turmoil, to the installation of Mrs Bloss in her new quarters. True, there was no bright doctor of civil law to deliver a classical address on the occasion; but there were several other old women present, who spoke quite as much to the purpose, and understood themselves equally well. The chop eater was so fatigued with the process of removal that she declined leaving her room until the following morning; so a mutton chop, pickle, a pill, a pint bottle of stout, and other medicines, were carried upstairs for her consumption.

'Why, what *do* you think, ma'am?' inquired the inquisitive Agnes of her mistress, after they had been in the house some three hours; 'what *do* you think, ma'am? the lady of the house is married.'

'Married!' said Mrs Bloss, taking the pill and a draught of Guinness – 'married! Unpossible!'

'She is indeed, ma'am,' returned the Columbine; 'and her husband, ma'am, lives – he – he – he – lives in the kitchen, ma'am.'

'In the kitchen!'

'Yes, ma'am: and he – he – he – the housemaid says, he never goes into the parlour except on Sundays; and that Mrs Tibbs makes him clean the gentlemen's boots; and that he cleans the windows, too, sometimes;

and that one morning early, when he was in the front balcony cleaning the drawing room windows, he called out to a gentleman on the opposite side of the way, who used to live here – "Ah! Mr Calton, sir, how are you?"' Here the attendant laughed till Mrs Bloss was in serious apprehension of her chuckling herself into a fit.

'Well, I never!' said Mrs Bloss.

'Yes. And please, ma'am, the servants give him gin and water sometimes; and then he cries, and says he hates his wife and the boarders, and wants to tickle them.'

'Tickle the boarders!' exclaimed Mrs Bloss, seriously alarmed.

'No, ma'am, not the boarders, the servants.'

'Oh, is that all!' said Mrs Bloss, quite satisfied.

'He wanted to kiss me as I came up the kitchen stairs, just now,' said Agnes, indignantly; 'but I gave it him – a little wretch!'

This intelligence was but too true. A long course of snubbing and neglect; his days spent in the kitchen, and his nights in the turn-up bedstead, had completely broken the little spirit that the unfortunate volunteer had ever possessed. He had no one to whom he could detail his injuries but the servants, and they were almost of necessity his chosen confidants. It is no less strange than true, however, that the little weaknesses which he had incurred, most probably during his military career, seemed to increase as his comforts diminished. He was actually a sort of journeyman Giovanni of the basement story.

The next morning, being Sunday, breakfast was laid in the front parlour at ten o'clock. Nine was the usual time, but the family always breakfasted an hour later on sabbath. Tibbs enrobed himself in his Sunday costume – a black coat, and exceedingly short, thin trousers; with a very large white waistcoat, white stockings and cravat, and Blucher boots – and mounted to the parlour aforesaid. Nobody had come down, and he amused himself by drinking the contents of the milkpot with a teaspoon.

A pair of slippers were heard descending the stairs. Tibbs flew to a chair; and a stern-looking man, of about fifty, with very little hair on his head, and a Sunday paper in his hand, entered the room.

'Good morning, Mr Evenson,' said Tibbs, very humbly, with something between a nod and a bow.

'How do you do, Mr Tibbs?' replied he of the slippers, as he sat himself down, and began to read his paper without saying another word.

'Is Mr Wisbottle in town today, do you know, sir?' inquired Tibbs, just for the sake of saying something.

'I should think he was,' replied the stern gentleman. 'He was whistling "The Light Guitar", in the next room to mine, at five o'clock this morning.'

'He's very fond of whistling,' said Tibbs, with a slight smirk.

'Yes – I ain't,' was the laconic reply.

Mr John Evenson was in the receipt of an independent income, arising chiefly from various houses he owned in the different suburbs. He was very morose and discontented. He was a thorough radical, and used to attend a great variety of public meetings, for the express purpose of finding fault with everything that was proposed. Mr Wisbottle, on the other hand, was a high Tory. He was clerk in the Woods and Forests Office, which he considered rather an aristocratic employment; he knew the peerage by heart, and could tell you, off-hand, where any illustrious personage lived. He had a good set of teeth, and a capital tailor. Mr Evenson looked on all these qualifications with profound contempt; and the consequence was that the two were always disputing, much to the edification of the rest of the house. It should be added, that, in addition to his partiality for whistling, Mr Wisbottle had a great idea of his singing powers. There were two other boarders, besides the gentleman in the back drawing room – Mr Alfred Tomkins and Mr Frederick O'Bleary. Mr Tomkins was a clerk in a wine house; he was a connoisseur in paintings, and had a wonderful eye for the picturesque. Mr O'Bleary was an Irishman, recently imported; he was in a perfectly wild state; and had come over to England to be an apothecary, a clerk in a government office, an actor, a reporter, or anything else that turned up – he was not particular. He was on familiar terms with two small Irish members, and got franks for everybody in the house. He felt convinced that his intrinsic merits must procure him a high destiny. He wore shepherd's plaid inexpressibles, and used to look under all the ladies' bonnets as he walked along the streets. His manners and appearance reminded one of Orson.

'Here comes Mr Wisbottle,' said Tibbs; and Mr Wisbottle forthwith appeared in blue slippers, and a shawl dressing gown, whistling *'Di piacer'*.

'Good morning, sir,' said Tibbs again. It was almost the only thing he ever said to anybody.

'How are you, Tibbs?' condescendingly replied the amateur; and he walked to the window, and whistled louder than ever.

'Pretty air, that!' said Evenson, with a snarl, and without taking his eyes off the paper.

'Glad you like it,' replied Wisbottle, highly gratified.

'Don't you think it would sound better, if you whistled it a little louder?' inquired the mastiff.

'No; I don't think it would,' rejoined the unconscious Wisbottle.

'I'll tell you what, Wisbottle,' said Evenson, who had been bottling up his anger for some hours – 'the next time you feel disposed to whistle "The Light Guitar" at five o'clock in the morning, I'll trouble you to whistle it with your head out o' window. If you don't, I'll learn the triangle – I will, by—'

The entrance of Mrs Tibbs (with the keys in a little basket) interrupted the threat, and prevented its conclusion.

Mrs Tibbs apologised for being down rather late; the bell was rung; James brought up the urn, and received an unlimited order for dry toast and bacon. Tibbs sat down at the bottom of the table, and began eating watercresses like a Nebuchadnezzar. Mr O'Bleary appeared, and Mr Alfred Tomkins. The compliments of the morning were exchanged, and the tea was made.

'God bless me!' exclaimed Tomkins, who had been looking out at the window. 'Here – Wisbottle – pray come here – make haste.'

Mr Wisbottle started from the table, and everyone looked up.

'Do you see,' said the connoisseur, placing Wisbottle in the right position – 'a little more this way: there – do you see how splendidly the light falls upon the left side of that broken chimney pot at No. 48?'

'Dear me! I see,' replied Wisbottle in a tone of admiration.

'I never saw an object stand out so beautifully against the clear sky in my life,' ejaculated Alfred. Everybody (except John Evenson) echoed the sentiment; for Mr Tomkins had a great character for finding out beauties which no one else could discover – he certainly deserved it.

'I have frequently observed a chimney pot in College Green, Dublin, which has a much better effect,' said the patriotic O'Bleary, who never allowed Ireland to be outdone on any point.

The assertion was received with obvious incredulity, for Mr Tomkins declared that no other chimney pot in the United Kingdom, broken or unbroken, could be so beautiful as the one at No. 48.

The room door was suddenly thrown open, and Agnes appeared, leading in Mrs Bloss, who was dressed in a geranium-coloured muslin gown, and displayed a gold watch of huge dimensions; a chain to match; and a splendid assortment of rings, with enormous stones. A general rush was made for a chair, and a regular introduction took place. Mr John Evenson made a slight inclination of the head; Mr Frederick O'Bleary, Mr Alfred Tomkins, and Mr Wisbottle, bowed like the mandarins in a grocer's shop; Tibbs rubbed hands, and went round in circles. He was observed to close one eye, and to assume a clockwork sort of expression with the other; this has been considered as a wink, and it has been reported that Agnes was its object. We repel the calumny, and challenge contradiction.

Mrs Tibbs inquired after Mrs Bloss's health in a low tone. Mrs Bloss, with a supreme contempt for the memory of Lindley Murray, answered the various questions in a most satisfactory manner; and a pause ensued, during which the eatables disappeared with awful rapidity.

'You must have been very much pleased with the appearance of the ladies going to the Drawing Room the other day, Mr O'Bleary?' said Mrs Tibbs, hoping to start a topic.

'Yes,' replied Orson, with a mouthful of toast.

'Never saw anything like it before, I suppose?' suggested Wisbottle.

'No – except the Lord Lieutenant's levees,' replied O'Bleary.

'Are they at all equal to our drawing rooms?'

'Oh, infinitely superior!'

'Gad! I don't know,' said the aristocratic Wisbottle, 'the Dowager Marchioness of Publiccash was most magnificently dressed, and so was the Baron Slappenbachenhausen.'

'What was he presented on?' inquired Evenson.

'On his arrival in England.'

'I thought so,' growled the radical; 'you never hear of these fellows being presented on their going away again. They know better than that.'

'Unless somebody pervades them with an apintment,' said Mrs Bloss, joining in the conversation in a faint voice.

'Well,' said Wisbottle, evading the point, 'it's a splendid sight.'

'And did it never occur to you,' inquired the radical, who never would be quiet; 'did it never occur to you, that you pay for these precious ornaments of society?'

'It certainly *has* occurred to me,' said Wisbottle, who thought this answer was a poser; 'it *has* occurred to me, and I am willing to pay for them.'

'Well, and it has occurred to me too,' replied John Evenson, 'and I ain't willing to pay for 'em. Then why should I? – I say, why should I?' continued the politician, laying down the paper, and knocking his knuckles on the table. 'There are two great principles – demand—'

'A cup of tea if you please, dear,' interrupted Tibbs.

'And supply—'

'May I trouble you to hand this tea to Mr Tibbs?' said Mrs Tibbs, interrupting the argument, and unconsciously illustrating it.

The thread of the orator's discourse was broken. He drank his tea and resumed the paper.

'If it's very fine,' said Mr Alfred Tomkins, addressing the company in general, 'I shall ride down to Richmond today, and come back by the steamer. There are some splendid effects of light and shade on the Thames; the contrast between the blueness of the sky and the yellow water is frequently exceedingly beautiful.' Mr Wisbottle hummed, 'Flow on, thou shining river.'

'We have some splendid steam-vessels in Ireland,' said O'Bleary.

'Certainly,' said Mrs Bloss, delighted to find a subject broached in which she could take part.

'The accommodations are extraordinary,' said O'Bleary.

'Extraordinary indeed,' returned Mrs Bloss. 'When Mr Bloss was alive, he was promiscuously obligated to go to Ireland on business. I went with him, and raly the manner in which the ladies and gentlemen were accommodated with berths, is not creditable.'

Tibbs, who had been listening to the dialogue, looked aghast, and evinced a strong inclination to ask a question, but was checked by a look from his wife. Mr Wisbottle laughed, and said Tomkins had made a pun; and Tomkins laughed too, and said he had not.

The remainder of the meal passed off as breakfasts usually do. Conversation flagged, and people played with their teaspoons. The gentlemen looked out at the window; walked about the room; and, when they got near the door, dropped off one by one. Tibbs retired to the back parlour by his wife's orders, to check the greengrocer's weekly account; and ultimately Mrs Tibbs and Mrs Bloss were left alone together.

'Oh dear!' said the latter, 'I feel alarmingly faint; it's very singular.' (It certainly was, for she had eaten four pounds of solids that morning.) 'By-the-bye,' said Mrs Bloss, 'I have not seen Mr What's-his-name yet.'

'Mr Gobler?' suggested Mrs Tibbs.

'Yes.'

'Oh!' said Mrs Tibbs, 'he is a most mysterious person. He has his meals regularly sent upstairs, and sometimes don't leave his room for weeks together.'

'I haven't seen or heard nothing of him,' repeated Mrs Bloss.

'I dare say you'll hear him tonight,' replied Mrs Tibbs; 'he generally groans a good deal on Sunday evenings.'

'I never felt such an interest in anyone in my life,' ejaculated Mrs Bloss. A little double-knock interrupted the conversation; Dr Wosky was announced, and duly shown in. He was a little man with a red face, – dressed of course in black, with a stiff white neckerchief. He had a very good practice, and plenty of money, which he had amassed by invariably humouring the worst fancies of all the females of all the families he had ever been introduced into. Mrs Tibbs offered to retire, but was entreated to stay.

'Well, my dear ma'am, and how are we?' inquired Wosky, in a soothing tone.

'Very ill, doctor – very ill.' said Mrs Bloss, in a whisper.

'Ah! we must take care of ourselves; – we must, indeed,' said the obsequious Wosky, as he felt the pulse of his interesting patient.

'How is your appetite?'

Mrs Bloss shook her head.

'Our friend requires great care,' said Wosky, appealing to Mrs Tibbs, who of course assented. 'I hope, however, with the blessing of Providence, that we shall be enabled to make her quite stout again.' Mrs Tibbs wondered in her own mind what the patient would be when she was made quite stout.

'We must take stimulants,' said the cunning Wosky – 'plenty of nourishment, and above all, we must keep our nerves quiet; we positively must not give way to our sensibilities. We must take all we can get,' concluded the doctor, as he pocketed his fee, 'and we must keep quiet.'

'Dear man!' exclaimed Mrs Bloss, as the doctor stepped into his carriage.

'Charming creature indeed – quite a lady's man!' said Mrs Tibbs, and Dr Wosky rattled away to make fresh gulls of delicate females, and pocket fresh fees.

As we had occasion, in a former paper, to describe a dinner at Mrs Tibbs's; and as one meal went off very like another on all ordinary occasions; we will not fatigue our readers by entering into any other detailed account of the domestic economy of the establishment. We will therefore proceed to events, merely premising that the mysterious tenant of the back drawing room was a lazy, selfish hypochondriac; always complaining and never ill. As his character in many respects closely assimilated to that of Mrs Bloss's, a very warm friendship soon sprung up between them. He was tall, thin, and pale; he always fancied he had a severe pain somewhere or other, and his face invariably wore a pinched, screwed-up expression; he looked, indeed, like a man who had got his feet in a tub of exceedingly hot water, against his will.

For two or three months after Mrs Bloss's first appearance in Coram Street, John Evenson was observed to become, every day, more sarcastic and more ill-natured; and there was a degree of additional importance in his manner, which clearly showed that he fancied he had discovered something, which he only wanted a proper opportunity of divulging. He found it at last.

One evening, the different inmates of the house were assembled in the drawing room engaged in their ordinary occupations. Mr Gobler and Mrs Bloss were sitting at a small card table near the centre window, playing cribbage; Mr Wisbottle was describing semicircles on the music stool, turning over the leaves of a book on the piano, and humming most melodiously; Alfred Tomkins was sitting at the round table, with his elbows duly squared, making a pencil sketch of a head considerably larger than his own; O'Bleary was reading Horace, and trying to look as if he understood it; and John Evenson had drawn his chair close to Mrs Tibbs's work table, and was talking to her very earnestly in a low tone.

'I can assure you, Mrs Tibbs,' said the radical, laying his forefinger on the muslin she was at work on; 'I can assure you, Mrs Tibbs, that nothing but the interest I take in your welfare would induce me to make this communication. I repeat, I fear Wisbottle is endeavouring to gain the affections of that young woman, Agnes, and that he is in the habit of meeting her in the store room on the first floor, over the leads. From my bedroom I distinctly heard voices there, last night. I opened my door immediately, and crept very softly on to the landing; there I saw Mr Tibbs, who it seems, had been disturbed also. – Bless me, Mrs Tibbs, you change colour!'

'No, no – it's nothing,' returned Mrs T. in a hurried manner; 'it's only the heat of the room.'

'A flush!' ejaculated Mrs Bloss from the card table; 'that's good for four.'

'If I thought it was Mr Wisbottle,' said Mrs Tibbs, after a pause, 'he should leave this house instantly.'

'Go!' said Mrs Bloss again.

'And if I thought,' continued the hostess with a most threatening air, 'if I thought he was assisted by Mr Tibbs – '

'One for his nob!' said Gobler.

'Oh,' said Evenson, in a most soothing tone – he liked to make mischief – 'I should hope Mr Tibbs was not in any way implicated. He always appeared to me very harmless.'

'I have generally found him so,' sobbed poor little Mrs Tibbs; crying like a watering pot.

'Hush! hush! pray – Mrs Tibbs – consider – we shall be observed – pray, don't!' said John Evenson, fearing his whole plan would be interrupted. 'We will set the matter at rest with the utmost care, and I shall be most happy to assist you in doing so.'

Mrs Tibbs murmured her thanks.

'When you think everyone has retired to rest tonight,' said Evenson very pompously, 'if you'll meet me without a light, just outside my bedroom door, by the staircase window, I think we can ascertain who the parties really are, and you will afterwards be enabled to proceed as you think proper.'

Mrs Tibbs was easily persuaded; her curiosity was excited, her jealousy was roused, and the arrangement was forthwith made. She resumed her work, and John Evenson walked up and down the room with his hands in his pockets, looking as if nothing had happened. The game of cribbage was over, and conversation began again.

'Well, Mr O'Bleary,' said the humming-top, turning round on his pivot, and facing the company, 'what did you think of Vauxhall the other night?'

'Oh, it's very fair,' replied Orson, who had been enthusiastically delighted with the whole exhibition.

'Never saw anything like that Captain Ross's set-out – eh?'

'No,' returned the patriot, with his usual reservation – 'except in Dublin.'

'I saw the Count de Canky and Captain Fitzthompson in the Gardens,' said Wisbottle; 'they appeared much delighted.'

'Then it *must* be beautiful,' snarled Evenson.

'I think the white bears is partickerlerly well done,' suggested Mrs Bloss. 'In their shaggy white coats, they look just like Polar bears – don't you think they do, Mr Evenson?'

'I think they look a great deal more like omnibus cads on all fours,' replied the discontented one.

'Upon the whole, I should have liked our evening very well,' gasped Gobler; 'only I caught a desperate cold which increased my pain dreadfully! I was obliged to have several shower-baths before I could leave my room.'

'Capital things those shower baths!' ejaculated Wisbottle.

'Excellent!' said Tomkins.

'Delightful!' chimed in O'Bleary. (He had once seen one, outside a tinman's.)

'Disgusting machines!' rejoined Evenson, who extended his dislike to almost every created object, masculine, feminine, or neuter.

'Disgusting, Mr Evenson!' said Gobler, in a tone of strong indignation – 'Disgusting! Look at their utility – consider how many lives they have saved by promoting perspiration.'

'Promoting perspiration, indeed,' growled John Evenson, stopping short in his walk across the large squares in the pattern of the carpet – 'I was ass enough to be persuaded some time ago to have one in my bedroom. 'Gad, I was in it once, and it effectually cured *me,* for the mere sight of it threw me into a profuse perspiration for six months afterwards.'

A titter followed this announcement, and before it had subsided James brought up 'the tray', containing the remains of a leg of lamb which had made its *début* at dinner; bread; cheese; an atom of butter in a forest of parsley; one pickled walnut and the third of another; and so forth. The boy disappeared, and returned again with another tray, containing glasses and jugs of hot and cold water. The gentlemen brought in their spirit bottles; the housemaid placed divers plated bedroom candlesticks under the card table; and the servants retired for the night.

Chairs were drawn round the table, and the conversation proceeded in the customary manner. John Evenson, who never ate supper, lolled on the sofa, and amused himself by contradicting everybody. O'Bleary ate as much as he could conveniently carry, and Mrs Tibbs felt a due degree of indignation thereat; Mr Gobler and Mrs Bloss conversed most affectionately on the subject of pill-taking, and other innocent amusements; and Tomkins and Wisbottle 'got into an argument'; that is to say, they both talked very loudly and vehemently, each flattering himself that he had got some advantage about something, and neither of them having more than a very indistinct idea of what they were talking about. An hour or two passed away; and the boarders and the brass candlesticks retired in pairs to their respective bedrooms. John Evenson pulled off his boots, locked his door, and determined to sit up until Mr Gobler had retired. He always sat in the drawing room an hour after everybody else had left it, taking medicine, and groaning.

Great Coram Street was hushed into a state of profound repose: it was nearly two o'clock. A hackney coach now and then rumbled slowly by; and occasionally some stray lawyer's clerk, on his way home to Somers Town, struck his iron heel on the top of the coal cellar with a noise resembling the click of a smoke jack. A low, monotonous, gushing sound was heard, which added considerably to the romantic dreariness of the scene. It was the water 'coming in' at number eleven.

'He must be asleep by this time,' said John Evenson to himself, after waiting with exemplary patience for nearly an hour after Mr Gobler had left the drawing room. He listened for a few moments; the house was perfectly quiet; he extinguished his rushlight, and opened his bedroom door. The staircase was so dark that it was impossible to see anything.

'S-s-s!' whispered the mischief-maker, making a noise like the first indication a catherine-wheel gives of the probability of its going off.

'Hush!' whispered somebody else.

'Is that you, Mrs Tibbs?'

'Yes, sir.'

'Where?'

'Here;' and the misty outline of Mrs Tibbs appeared at the staircase window, like the ghost of Queen Anne in the tent scene in Richard.

'This way, Mrs Tibbs,' whispered the delighted busybody: 'give me your hand – there! Whoever these people are, they are in the store room now, for I have been looking down from my window, and I could see that they accidentally upset their candlestick, and are now in darkness. You have no shoes on, have you?'

'No,' said little Mrs Tibbs, who could hardly speak for trembling.

'Well; I have taken my boots off, so we can go down, close to the store room door, and listen over the banisters'; and downstairs they both crept accordingly, every board creaking like a patent mangle on a Saturday afternoon.

'It's Wisbottle and somebody, I'll swear,' exclaimed the radical in an energetic whisper, when they had listened for a few moments.

'Hush – pray let's hear what they say!' exclaimed Mrs Tibbs, the gratification of whose curiosity was now paramount to every other consideration.

'Ah! if I could but believe you,' said a female voice coquettishly, 'I'd be bound to settle my missis for life.'

'What does she say?' inquired Mr Evenson, who was not quite so well situated as his companion.

'She says she'll settle her missis's life,' replied Mrs Tibbs. 'The wretch! they're plotting murder.'

'I know you want money,' continued the voice, which belonged to Agnes; 'and if you'd secure me the five hundred pound, I warrant she should take fire soon enough.'

'What's that?' inquired Evenson again. He could just hear enough to want to hear more.

'I think she says she'll set the house on fire,' replied the affrighted Mrs Tibbs. 'But, thank God, I'm insured in the Phœnix!'

'The moment I have secured your mistress, my dear,' said a man's voice in a strong Irish brogue, 'you may depend on having the money.'

'Bless my soul, it's Mr O'Bleary!' exclaimed Mrs Tibbs, in a parenthesis.

'The villain!' said the indignant Mr Evenson.

'The first thing to be done,' continued the Hibernian, 'is to poison Mr Gobler's mind.'

'Oh, certainly,' returned Agnes.

'What's that?' inquired Evenson again, in an agony of curiosity and a whisper.

'He says she's to mind and poison Mr Gobler,' replied Mrs Tibbs, aghast at this sacrifice of human life.

'And in regard of Mrs Tibbs,' continued O'Bleary. – Mrs Tibbs shuddered.

'Hush!' exclaimed Agnes, in a tone of the greatest alarm, just as Mrs Tibbs was on the extreme verge of a fainting fit. 'Hush!'

'Hush!' exclaimed Evenson, at the same moment, to Mrs Tibbs.

'There's somebody coming *up*stairs,' said Agnes to O'Bleary.

'There's somebody coming *down*stairs,' whispered Evenson to Mrs Tibbs.

'Go into the parlour, sir,' said Agnes to her companion. 'You will get there before whoever it is gets to the top of the kitchen stairs.'

'The drawing room, Mrs Tibbs!' whispered the astonished Evenson to his equally astonished companion; and for the drawing room they both made, plainly hearing the rustling of two persons, one coming downstairs, and one coming up.

'What can it be?' exclaimed Mrs Tibbs. 'It's like a dream. I wouldn't be found in this situation for the world!'

'Nor I,' returned Evenson, who could never bear a joke at his own expense. 'Hush! here they are at the door.'

'What fun!' whispered one of the newcomers. – It was Wisbottle.

'Glorious!' replied his companion, in an equally low tone. – This was Alfred Tomkins. 'Who would have thought it?'

'I told you so,' said Wisbottle, in a most knowing whisper. 'Lord bless you, he has paid her most extraordinary attention for the last two months. I saw 'em when I was sitting at the piano tonight.'

'Well, do you know I didn't notice it?' interrupted Tomkins.

'Not notice it!' continued Wisbottle. 'Bless you; I saw him whispering to her, and she crying; and then I'll swear I heard him say something about tonight when we were all in bed.'

'They're talking of *us*!' exclaimed the agonised Mrs Tibbs, as the painful suspicion, and a sense of their situation, flashed upon her mind.

'I know it – I know it,' replied Evenson, with a melancholy consciousness that there was no mode of escape.

'What's to be done? we cannot both stop here!' ejaculated Mrs Tibbs, in a state of partial derangement.

'I'll get up the chimney,' replied Evenson, who really meant what he said.

'You can't,' said Mrs Tibbs, in despair. 'You can't – it's a register stove.'

'Hush!' repeated John Evenson.

'Hush – hush!' cried somebody downstairs.

'What a d–d hushing!' said Alfred Tomkins, who began to get rather bewildered.

'There they are!' exclaimed the sapient Wisbottle, as a rustling noise was heard in the store room.

'Hark!' whispered both the young men.

'Hark!' repeated Mrs Tibbs and Evenson.

'Let me alone, sir,' said a female voice in the store room.

'Oh, Hagnes!' cried another voice, which clearly belonged to Tibbs, for nobody else ever owned one like it. 'Oh, Hagnes – lovely creature!'

'Be quiet, sir!' (A bounce.)

'Hag — '

'Be quiet, sir – I am ashamed of you. Think of your wife, Mr Tibbs. Be quiet, sir!'

'My wife!' exclaimed the valorous Tibbs, who was clearly under the influence of gin and water, and a misplaced attachment; 'I ate her! Oh, Hagnes! when I was in the volunteer corps, in eighteen hundred and—'

'I declare I'll scream. Be quiet, sir, will you?' (Another bounce and a scuffle.)

'What's that?' exclaimed Tibbs, with a start.

'What's what?' said Agnes, stopping short.

'Why, that!'

'Ah! you have done it nicely now, sir,' sobbed the frightened Agnes, as a tapping was heard at Mrs Tibbs's bedroom door, which would have beaten any dozen woodpeckers hollow.

'Mrs Tibbs! Mrs Tibbs!' called out Mrs Bloss. 'Mrs Tibbs, pray get up.' (Here the imitation of a woodpecker was resumed with tenfold violence.)

'Oh, dear – dear!' exclaimed the wretched partner of the depraved Tibbs. 'She's knocking at my door. We must be discovered! What will they think?'

'Mrs Tibbs! Mrs Tibbs!' screamed the woodpecker again.

'What's the matter?' shouted Gobler, bursting out of the back drawing room, like the dragon at Astley's.

'Oh, Mr Gobler!' cried Mrs Bloss, with a proper approximation to hysterics; 'I think the house is on fire, or else there's thieves in it. I have heard the most dreadful noises!'

'The devil you have!' shouted Gobler again, bouncing back into his den, in happy imitation of the aforesaid dragon, and returning immediately with a lighted candle. 'Why, what's this? Wisbottle! Tomkins! O'Bleary! Agnes! What the deuce! all up and dressed?'

'Astonishing!' said Mrs Bloss, who had run downstairs, and taken Mr Gobler's arm.

'Call Mrs Tibbs directly, somebody,' cried Gobler, turning into the front drawing room – 'What! Mrs Tibbs and Mr Evenson!!'

'Mrs Tibbs and Mr Evenson!' repeated everybody, as that unhappy pair were discovered: Mrs Tibbs seated in an armchair by the fireplace, and Mr Evenson standing by her side.

We must leave the scene that ensued to the reader's imagination. We could tell how Mrs Tibbs forthwith fainted away, and how it required the united strength of Mr Wisbottle and Mr Alfred Tomkins to hold her in her chair; how Mr Evenson explained, and how his explanation was evidently disbelieved; how Agnes repelled the accusations of Mrs Tibbs by proving that she was negotiating with Mr O'Bleary to influence her mistress's affections in his behalf; and how Mr Gobler threw a damp counterpane on the hopes of Mr O'Bleary by avowing that he (Gobler) had already proposed to, and been accepted by, Mrs Bloss; how Agnes was discharged from that lady's service; how Mr O'Bleary discharged himself from Mrs Tibbs's house, without going through the form of previously discharging his bill; and how that disappointed young gentleman rails against England and the English, and vows there is no virtue or fine feeling extant, 'except in Ireland'. We repeat that we *could* tell all this, but we love to exercise our self-denial, and we therefore prefer leaving it to be imagined.

The lady whom we have hitherto described as Mrs Bloss, is no more. Mrs Gobler exists: Mrs Bloss has left us for ever. In a secluded retreat in Newington Butts, far, far removed from the noisy strife of that great boarding house, the world, the enviable Gobler and his pleasing wife revel in retirement: happy in their complaints, their table, and their medicine; wafted through life by the grateful prayers of all the purveyors of animal food within three miles round.

We would willingly stop here, but we have a painful duty imposed upon us, which we must discharge. Mr and Mrs Tibbs have separated by mutual consent, Mrs Tibbs receiving one moiety of 43*l.* 15*s.* 10*d.*, which we before stated to be the amount of her husband's annual income, and Mr Tibbs the other. He is spending the evening of his days in retirement; and he is spending also, annually, that small but honourable independence. He resides among the original settlers at Walworth; and it has been stated, on unquestionable authority, that the conclusion of the volunteer story has been heard in a small tavern in that respectable neighbourhood.

The unfortunate Mrs Tibbs has determined to dispose of the whole of her furniture by public auction, and to retire from a residence in which she has suffered so much. Mr Robins has been applied to, to conduct the sale, and the transcendent abilities of the literary gentlemen connected with his establishment are now devoted to the task of drawing up the preliminary advertisement. It is to contain, among a variety of brilliant matter, seventy-eight words in large capitals, and six original quotations in inverted commas.

## Chapter Two

### *Mr Minns and his Cousin*

This was Dickens's first published work. It originally appeared under the title 'A Dinner at Poplar Walk' in the *Monthly Magazine*, December 1833, and was retitled and revised for inclusion in the *Second Series*. The original version was published in facsimile in *The Dickensian*, Vol. 30 (1934) pp. 3–10.

Mr Augustus Minns was a bachelor, of about forty as he said – of about eight-and-forty as his friends said. He was always exceedingly clean, precise, and tidy; perhaps somewhat priggish, and the most retiring man in the world. He usually wore a brown frock coat without a wrinkle, light inexplicables without a spot, a neat neckerchief with a remarkably neat tie, and boots without a fault; moveover, he always carried a brown silk umbrella with an ivory handle. He was a clerk in Somerset House, or, as he said himself, he held 'a responsible situation under Government.' He had a good and increasing salary, in addition to some 10,000*l.* of his own (invested in the funds), and he occupied a first floor in Tavistock Street, Covent Garden, where he had resided for twenty years, having been in the habit of quarrelling with his landlord the whole time: regularly giving notice of his intention to quit on the first day of every quarter, and as regularly countermanding it on the second. There were two classes of created objects which he held in the deepest and most unmingled horror; these were dogs, and children. He was not unamiable, but he could, at any time, have viewed the execution of a dog, or the assassination of an infant, with the liveliest satisfaction. Their habits were at variance with his love of order; and his love of order was as powerful as his love of life. Mr Augustus Minns had no relations in or near London, with the exception of his cousin, Mr Octavius Budden, to whose son, whom he had never seen (for he disliked the father), he had consented to become godfather by proxy. Mr Budden having realised a moderate fortune by exercising the trade or calling of a corn chandler, and having a great predilection for the country, had purchased a cottage in the vicinity of Stamford Hill, whither he retired with the wife of his bosom, and his only son, Master Alexander Augustus Budden. One evening as Mr and Mrs B. were admiring their son, discussing his various merits, talking over his education,

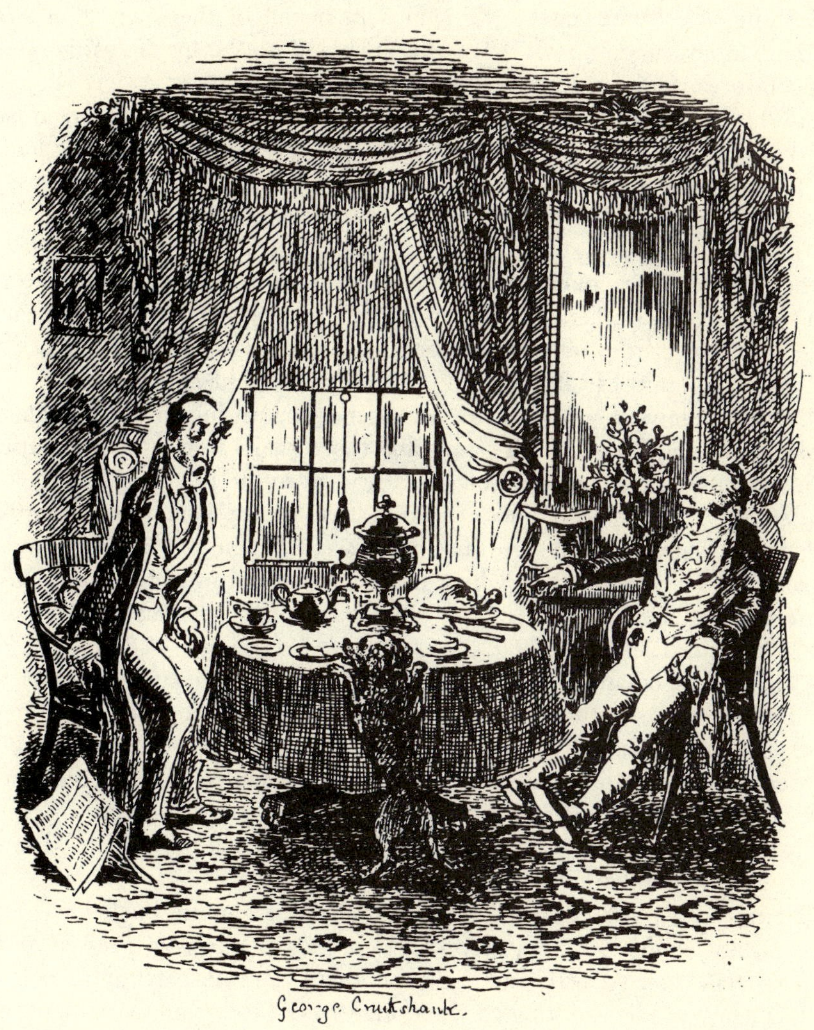


*Mr Minns and his Cousin*

and disputing whether the classics should be made an essential part thereof, the lady pressed so strongly upon her husband the propriety of cultivating the friendship of Mr Minns in behalf of their son, that Mr Budden at last made up his mind, that it should not be his fault if he and his cousin were not in future more intimate.

'I'll break the ice, my love,' said Mr Budden, stirring up the sugar at the bottom of his glass of brandy and water, and casting a sidelong look at his spouse to see the effect of the announcement of his determination, 'by asking Minns down to dine with us on Sunday.'

'Then pray, Budden, write to your cousin at once,' replied Mrs Budden. 'Who knows, if we could only get him down here, but he might take a fancy to our Alexander, and leave him his property? – Alick, my dear, take your legs off the rail of the chair!'

'Very true,' said Mr Budden, musing, 'very true indeed, my love!'

On the following morning, as Mr Minns was sitting at his breakfast table, alternately biting his dry toast and casting a look upon the columns of his morning paper, which he always read from the title to the printer's name, he heard a loud knock at the street door; which was shortly afterwards followed by the entrance of his servant, who put into his hands a particularly small card, on which was engraven in immense letters, 'Mr Octavius Budden, Amelia Cottage (Mrs B.'s name was Amelia), Poplar Walk, Stamford Hill.'

'Budden!' ejaculated Minns, 'what can bring that vulgar man here! – say I'm asleep – say I'm out, and shall never be home again – anything to keep him downstairs.'

'But please, sir, the gentleman's coming up,' replied the servant, and the fact was made evident by an appalling creaking of boots on the staircase accompanied by a pattering noise; the cause of which Minns could not, for the life of him, divine.

'Hem – show the gentleman in,' said the unfortunate bachelor. Exit servant, and enter Octavius preceded by a large white dog, dressed in a suit of fleecy hosiery, with pink eyes, large ears, and no perceptible tail.

The cause of the pattering on the stairs was but too plain. Mr Augustus Minns staggered beneath the shock of the dog's appearance.

'My dear fellow, how are you?' said Budden, as he entered.

He always spoke at the top of his voice, and always said the same thing half a dozen times.

'How are you, my hearty?'

'How do you do, Mr Budden? – pray take a chair!' politely stammered the discomfited Minns.

'Thank you – thank you – well – how are you, eh?'

'Uncommonly well, thank you,' said Minns, casting a diabolical look at the dog, who, with his hind legs on the floor, and his fore paws resting on the table, was dragging a bit of bread and butter out of a plate, preparatory to devouring it, with the buttered side next the carpet.

'Ah, you rogue!' said Budden to his dog; 'you see, Minns, he's like me, always at home, eh, my boy? – Egad, I'm precious hot and hungry! I've walked all the way from Stamford Hill this morning.'

'Have you breakfasted?' inquired Minns.

'Oh, no! – came to breakfast with you; so ring the bell, my dear fellow, will you? and let's have another cup and saucer, and the cold ham. – Make myself at home, you see!' continued Budden, dusting his boots with a table napkin. 'Ha! – ha! – ha! – 'pon my life, I'm hungry.'

Minns rang the bell, and tried to smile.

'I decidedly never was so hot in my life,' continued Octavius, wiping his forehead; 'well, but how are you, Minns? 'Pon my soul, you wear capitally!'

'D'ye think so?' said Minns; and he tried another smile.

''Pon my life, I do!'

'Mrs B. and – what's his name – quite well?'

'Alick – my son, you mean; never better – never better. But at such a place as we've got at Poplar Walk, you know, he couldn't be ill if he tried. When I first saw it, by Jove! it looked so knowing, with the front garden, and the green railings, and the brass knocker, and all that – I really thought it was a cut above me.'

'Don't you think you'd like the ham better,' interrupted Minns, 'if you cut it the other way?' He saw, with feelings which it is impossible to describe, that his visitor was cutting, or rather maiming, the ham, in utter violation of all established rules.

'No, thank ye,' returned Budden, with the most barbarous indifference to crime, 'I prefer it this way, it eats short. But I say, Minns, when will you come down and see us? You will be delighted with the place; I know you will. Amelia and I were talking about you the other night, and Amelia said – another lump of sugar, please; thank ye – she said, don't you think you could contrive, my dear, to say to Mr Minns, in a friendly way – come down, sir – damn the dog! he's spoiling your curtains, Minns – ha! – ha! – ha!' Minns leaped from his seat as though he had received the discharge from a galvanic battery.

'Come out, sir! – go out, hoo!' cried poor Augustus, keeping, nevertheless, at a very respectful distance from the dog; having read of a case of hydrophobia in the paper of that morning. By dint of great exertion, much shouting, and a marvellous deal of poking under the tables with a stick and umbrella, the dog was at last dislodged, and placed on the landing outside the door, where he immediately commenced a most appalling howling; at the same time vehemently scratching the paint off the two nicely varnished bottom panels, until they resembled the interior of a backgammon board.

'A good dog for the country that!' coolly observed Budden to the distracted Minns, 'but he's not much used to confinement. But now, Minns, when will you come down? I'll take no denial, positively. Let's see, today's Thursday. – Will you come on Sunday? We dine at five, don't say no – do.'

After a great deal of pressing, Mr Augustus Minns, driven to despair, accepted the invitation, and promised to be at Poplar walk on the ensuing Sunday, at a quarter before five to the minute.

'Now mind the direction,' said Budden: 'the coach goes from the Flower Pot, in Bishopsgate Street, every half-hour. When the coach stops at the Swan, you'll see, immediately opposite you, a white house.'

'Which is your house – I understand,' said Minns, wishing to cut short the visit, and the story, at the same time.

'No, no, that's not mine; that's Grogus's, the great ironmonger's. I was going to say – you turn down by the side of the white house till you can't go another step further – mind that! – and then you turn to your right, by some stables – well; close to you, you'll see a wall with "Beware of the Dog" written on it in large letters – (Minns shuddered) – go along by the side of that wall for about a quarter of a mile – and anybody will show you which is my place.'

'Very well – thank ye – goodbye.'

'Be punctual.'

'Certainly: good morning.'

'I say, Minns, you've got a card.'

'Yes, I have; thank ye.' And Mr Octavius Budden departed, leaving his cousin looking forward to his visit on the following Sunday, with the feelings of a penniless poet to the weekly visit of his Scotch landlady.

Sunday arrived; the sky was bright and clear; crowds of people were hurrying along the streets, intent on their different schemes of pleasure for the day; everything and everybody looked cheerful and happy except Mr Augustus Minns.

The day was fine, but the heat was considerable; when Mr Minns had fagged up the shady side of Fleet Street, Cheapside, and Threadneedle Street, he had become pretty warm, tolerably dusty, and it was getting late into the bargain. By the most extraordinary good fortune, however, a coach was waiting at the Flower Pot, into which Mr Augustus Minns got, on the solemn assurance of the cad that the vehicle would start in three minutes – that being the very utmost extremity of time it was allowed to wait by Act of Parliament. A quarter of an hour elapsed, and there were no signs of moving. Minns looked at his watch for the sixth time.

'Coachman, are you going or not?' bawled Mr Minns, with his head and half his body out of the coach window.

'Di–rectly, sir,' said the coachman, with his hands in his pockets, looking as much unlike a man in a hurry as possible.

'Bill, take them cloths off.' Five minutes more elapsed: at the end of which time the coachman mounted the box, from whence he looked down the street, and up the street, and hailed all the pedestrians for another five minutes.

'Coachman! if you don't go this moment, I shall get out,' said Mr Minns, rendered desperate by the lateness of the hour, and the impossibility of being in Poplar Walk at the appointed time.

'Going this minute, sir,' was the reply; – and, accordingly, the machine trundled on for a couple of hundred yards, and then stopped again. Minns doubled himself up in a corner of the coach, and abandoned himself to his fate, as a child, a mother, a bandbox and a parasol, became his fellow passengers.

The child was an affectionate and an amiable infant; the little dear mistook Minns for his other parent, and screamed to embrace him.

'Be quiet, dear,' said the mamma, restraining the impetuosity of the darling, whose little fat legs were kicking, and stamping, and twining themselves into the most complicated forms, in an ecstasy of impatience. 'Be quiet, dear, that's not your papa.'

'Thank Heaven I am not!' thought Minns, as the first gleam of pleasure he had experienced that morning shone like a meteor through his wretchedness.

Playfulness was agreeably mingled with affection in the disposition of the boy. When satisfied that Mr Minns was not his parent, he endeavoured to attract his notice by scraping his drab trousers with his dirty shoes, poking his chest with his mamma's parasol, and other nameless endearments peculiar to infancy, with which he beguiled the tediousness of the ride, apparently very much to his own satisfaction.

When the unfortunate gentleman arrived at the Swan, he found to his great dismay, that it was a quarter past five. The white house, the stables, the 'Beware of the Dog' – every landmark was passed, with a rapidity not unusual to a gentleman of a certain age when too late for dinner. After the lapse of a few minutes, Mr Minns found himself opposite a yellow brick house with a green door, brass knocker, and door plate, green window frames and ditto railings, with 'a garden' in front, that is to say, a small loose bit of gravelled ground, with one round and two scalene triangular beds, containing a fir tree, twenty or thirty bulbs, and an unlimited number of marigolds. The taste of Mr and Mrs Budden was further displayed by the appearance of a Cupid on each side of the door, perched upon a heap of large chalk flints, variegated with pink conch shells. His knock at the door was answered by a stumpy boy, in drab livery, cotton stockings and high-lows, who, after hanging his hat on one of the dozen brass pegs which ornamented the passage, denominated by courtesy 'The Hall', ushered him into a front drawing room commanding a very extensive view of the backs of the neighbouring houses. The usual ceremony of introduction, and so forth, over, Mr Minns took his seat: not a little agitated at finding that he was the last comer, and, somehow or other, the Lion of about a dozen people, sitting together in a small drawing room, getting rid of that most tedious of all time, the time preceding dinner.

'Well, Brogson,' said Budden, addressing an elderly gentleman in a black coat, drab knee breeches, and long gaiters, who, under pretence of inspecting the prints in an Annual, had been engaged in satisfying himself on the subject of Mr Minns's general appearance, by looking at him over the tops of the leaves – 'Well, Brogson, what do Ministers mean to do? Will they go out, or what?'

'Oh – why – really, you know, I'm the last person in the world to ask for news. Your cousin, from his situation, is the most likely person to answer the question.'

Mr Minns assured the last speaker, that although he was in Somerset House, he possessed no official communication relative to the projects of his Majesty's Ministers. But his remark was evidently received incredulously; and no further conjectures being hazarded on the subject, a long pause ensued, during which the company occupied themselves in coughing and blowing their noses, until the entrance of Mrs Budden caused a general rise.

The ceremony of introduction being over, dinner was announced, and downstairs the party proceeded accordingly – Mr Minns escorting Mrs Budden as far as the drawing room door, but being prevented, by the narrowness of the staircase, from extending his gallantry any farther. The dinner passed off as such dinners usually do. Ever and anon, amidst the clatter of knives and forks, and the hum of conversation, Mr B.'s voice might be heard, asking a friend to take wine, and assuring him he was glad to see him; and a great deal of by-play took place between Mrs B. and the servants, respecting the removal of the dishes, during which her countenance assumed all the variations of a weather glass, from 'stormy' to 'set fair'.

Upon the dessert and wine being placed on the table, the servant, in compliance with a significant look from Mrs B., brought down 'Master Alexander', habited in a sky-blue suit with silver buttons; and possessing hair of nearly the same colour as the metal. After sundry praises from his mother, and various admonitions as to his behaviour from his father, he was introduced to his godfather.

'Well, my little fellow – you are a fine boy, ain't you?' said Mr Minns, as happy as a tomtit on birdlime.

'Yes.'

'How old are you?'

'Eight next We'nsday. How old are *you*?'

'Alexander,' interrupted his mother, 'how dare you ask Mr Minns how old he is!'

'He asked me how old *I* was,' said the precocious child, to whom Minns had from that moment internally resolved that he never would bequeath one shilling. As soon as the titter occasioned by the observation had subsided, a little smirking man with red whiskers, sitting at the bottom of the table, who during the whole of dinner had been endeavouring to obtain a listener to some stories about Sheridan, called out, with a very patronising air, 'Alick, what part of speech is *be?*'

'A verb.'

'That's a good boy,' said Mrs Budden, with all a mother's pride. 'Now, you know what a verb is?'

'A verb is a word which signifies to be, to do, or to suffer; as, I am – I rule – I am ruled. Give me an apple, Ma.'

'I'll give you an apple,' replied the man with the red whiskers, who was an established friend of the family, or in other words was always invited by Mrs Budden, whether Mr Budden liked it or not, 'if you'll tell me what is the meaning of *be*.'

'Be?' said the prodigy, after a little hesitation – 'an insect that gathers honey.'

'No, dear,' frowned Mrs Budden; 'B double E is the substantive.'

'I don't think he knows much yet about *common* substantives,' said the smirking gentleman, who thought this an admirable opportunity for letting off a joke. 'It's clear he's not very well acquainted with *proper names*. He! he! he!'

'Gentlemen,' called out Mr Budden, from the end of the table, in a stentorian voice, and with a very important air, 'will you have the goodness to charge your glasses? I have a toast to propose.'

'Hear! hear!' cried the gentlemen, passing the decanters. After they had made the round of the table, Mr Budden proceeded – 'Gentlemen; there is an individual present—'

'Hear! hear!' said the little man with red whiskers.

'*Pray* be quiet, Jones,' remonstrated Budden.

'I say, gentlemen, there is an individual present,' resumed the host, 'in whose society I am sure we must take great delight – and – and – the conversation of that individual must have afforded to everyone present, the utmost pleasure.' ['Thank Heaven, he does not mean me!' thought Minns, conscious that his diffidence and exclusiveness had prevented his saying above a dozen words since he entered the house.] 'Gentlemen, I am but a humble individual myself, and I perhaps ought to apologise for allowing any individual feelings of friendship and affection for the person I allude to, to induce me to venture to rise, to propose the health of that person – a person that, I am sure – that is to say, a person whose virtues must endear him to those who know him – and those who have not the pleasure of knowing him, cannot dislike him.'

'Hear! hear!' said the company, in a tone of encouragement and approval.

'Gentlemen,' continued Budden, 'my cousin is a man who – who is a relation of my own.' (Hear! hear!) Minns groaned audibly. 'Who I am most happy to see here, and who, if he were not here, would certainly have deprived us of the great pleasure we all feel in seeing him. (Loud cries of hear!) Gentlemen, I feel that I have already trespassed on your attention for too long a time. With every feeling – of – with every sentiment of – of—'

'Gratification' – suggested the friend of the family.

'Of – gratification, I beg to propose the health of Mr Minns.'

'Standing, gentlemen!' shouted the indefatigable little man with the whiskers – 'and with the honours. Take your time from me, if you please. Hip! hip! hip! – Za! – Hip! hip! hip! – Za! – Hip! hip! – Za-a-a!'

All eyes were now fixed on the subject of the toast, who by gulping down port wine at the imminent hazard of suffocation, endeavoured to conceal his confusion. After as long a pause as decency would admit, he rose, but, as the newspapers sometimes say in their reports, 'we regret that we are quite unable to give even the substance of the honourable gentleman's observations'. The words 'present company – honour – present occasion', and 'great happiness' – heard occasionally, and repeated at intervals, with a countenance expressive of the utmost confusion and misery, convinced the company that he was making an excellent speech; and, accordingly, on his resuming his seat, they cried 'Bravo!' and manifested tumultuous applause. Jones who had been long watching his opportunity, then darted up.

'Budden,' said he, 'will you allow *me* to propose a toast?'

'Certainly,' replied Budden, adding in an undertone to Minns right across the table, 'Devilish sharp fellow that: you'll be very much pleased with his speech. He talks equally well on any subject.' Minns bowed, and Mr Jones proceeded:

'It has on several occasions, in various instances, under many circumstances, and in different companies, fallen to my lot to propose a toast to those by whom, at the time, I have had the honour to be surrounded. I have sometimes, I will cheerfully own – for why should I deny it? – felt the overwhelming nature of the task I have undertaken, and my own utter incapability to do justice to the subject. If such have been my feelings, however, on former occasions, what must they be now – now – under the extraordinary circumstances in which I am placed. (Hear! hear!) To describe my feelings accurately, would be impossible; but I cannot give you a better idea of them, gentlemen, than by referring to a circumstance which happens, oddly enough, to occur to my mind at the moment. On one occasion, when that truly great and illustrious man, Sheridan, was — '

Now, there is no knowing what new villainy in the form of a joke would have been heaped on the grave of that very ill-used man, Mr Sheridan, if the boy in drab had not at that moment entered the room in a breathless state, to report that, as it was a very wet night, the nine o'clock stage had come round, to know whether there was anybody going to town, as, in that case, he (the nine o'clock) had room for one inside.

Mr Minns started up; and, despite countless exclamations of surprise and entreaties to stay, persisted in his determination to accept the vacant place. But the brown silk umbrella was nowhere to be found; and as the coachman couldn't wait, he drove back to the Swan, leaving word for Mr Minns to 'run round' and catch him. However, as it did not occur to Mr Minns for some ten minutes or so, that he had left the brown silk umbrella with the ivory handle in the other coach, coming down; and, moreover, as he was by no means remarkable for speed, it is no matter of surprise that when he accomplished the feat of 'running round' to the Swan, the coach – the last coach – had gone without him.

It was somewhere about three o'clock in the morning, when Mr Augustus Minns knocked feebly at the street door of his lodgings in Tavistock Street, cold, wet, cross, and miserable. He made his will next morning, and his professional man informs us, in that strict confidence in which we inform the public, that neither the name of Mr Octavius Budden, nor of Mrs Amelia Budden, nor of Master Alexander Augustus Budden, appears therein.

## Chapter Three

*Sentiment*

First published in *Bell's Weekly Magazine,* 7 June 1834; Dickens's only contribution to this journal.

The Miss Crumptons, or to quote the authority of the inscription on the garden gate of Minerva House, Hammersmith, 'The Misses Crumpton', were two unusually tall, particularly thin, and exceedingly skinny personages: very upright, and very yellow. Miss Amelia Crumpton owned to thirty-eight, and Miss Maria Crumpton admitted she was forty; an admission which was rendered perfectly unnecessary by the self-evident fact of her being at least fifty. They dressed in the most interesting manner – like twins! and looked as happy and comfortable as a couple of marigolds run to seed. They were very precise, had the strictest possible ideas of propriety, wore false hair, and always smelt very strongly of lavender.

Minerva House, conducted under the auspices of the two sisters, was a 'finishing establishment for young ladies', where some twenty girls of the ages of from thirteen to nineteen inclusive, acquired a smattering of everything, and a knowledge of nothing; instruction in French and Italian, dancing lessons twice a week; and other necessaries of life. The house was a white one, a little removed from the roadside, with close palings in front. The bedroom windows were always left partly open, to afford a bird's-eye view of numerous little bedsteads with very white dimity furniture, and thereby impress the passer-by with a due sense of the luxuries of the establishment; and there was a front parlour hung round with highly varnished maps which nobody ever looked at, and filled with books which no one ever read, appropriated exclusively to the reception of parents, who, whenever they called, could not fail to be struck with the very deep appearance of the place.

'Amelia, my dear,' said Miss Maria Crumpton, entering the school room one morning, with her false hair in papers: as she occasionally did, in order to impress the young ladies with a conviction of its reality. 'Amelia, my dear, here is a most gratifying note I have just received. You needn't mind reading it aloud.'

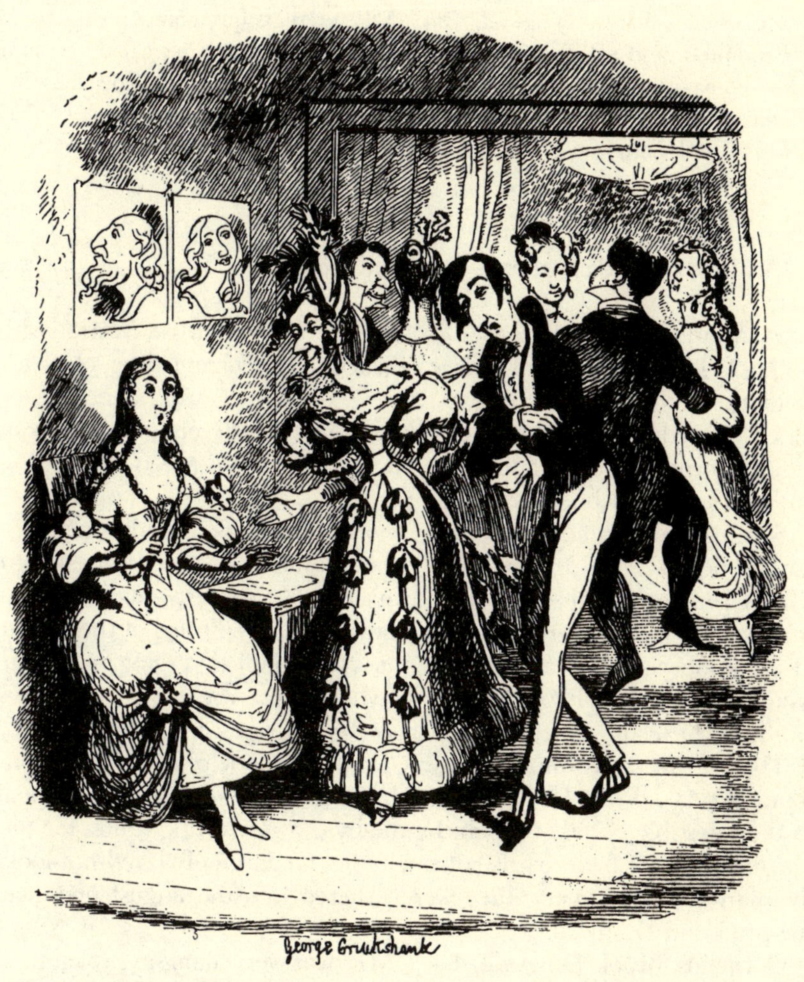


*Theodosius Introduced to the New Pupil* (see p. 323)

Miss Amelia, thus advised, proceeded to read the following note with an air of great triumph:

> Cornelius Brook Dingwall, Esq., MP, presents his compliments to Miss Crumpton, and will feel much obliged by Miss Crumpton's calling on him, if she conveniently can, tomorrow morning at one o'clock, as Cornelius Brook Dingwall, Esq., MP, is anxious to see Miss Crumpton on the subject of placing Miss Brook Dingwall under her charge.
>
> Adelphi.
> Monday morning.

'A Member of Parliament's daughter!' ejaculated Amelia, in an ecstatic tone.

'A Member of Parliament's daughter!' repeated Miss Maria, with a smile of delight, which, of course, elicited a concurrent titter of pleasure from all the young ladies.

'It's exceedingly delightful!' said Miss Amelia; whereupon all the young ladies murmured their admiration again. Courtiers are but schoolboys, and court ladies schoolgirls.

So important an announcement at once superseded the business of the day. A holiday was declared, in commemoration of the great event; the Miss Crumptons retired to their private apartment to talk it over; the smaller girls discussed the probable manners and customs of the daughter of a Member of Parliament; and the young ladies verging on eighteen wondered whether she was engaged, whether she was pretty, whether she wore much bustle, and many other *whethers* of equal importance.

The two Miss Crumptons proceeded to the Adelphi at the appointed time next day, dressed, of course, in their best style, and looking as amiable as they possibly could – which, by-the-bye, is not saying much for them. Having sent in their cards, through the medium of a red-hot-looking footman in bright livery, they were ushered into the august presence of the profound Dingwall.

Cornelius Brook Dingwall, Esq., MP, was very haughty, solemn, and portentous. He had, naturally, a somewhat spasmodic expression of countenance, which was not rendered the less remarkable by his wearing an extremely stiff cravat. He was wonderfully proud of the MP attached to his name, and never lost an opportunity of reminding people of his dignity. He had a great idea of his own abilities, which must have been a great comfort to him, as no one else had; and in diplomacy, on a small scale, in his own family arrangements, he considered himself unrivalled. He was a county magistrate, and discharged the duties of his station with all due justice and impartiality; frequently committing poachers, and occasionally committing himself. Miss Brook Dingwall was one of that numerous class of young ladies who, like adverbs, may be known by their answering to a commonplace question, and doing nothing else.

On the present occasion, this talented individual was seated in a small library at a table covered with papers, doing nothing, but trying to look busy, playing at shop. Acts of Parliament, and letters directed to 'Cornelius Brook Dingwall, Esq., MP', were ostentatiously scattered over the table; at a little distance from which, Mrs Brook Dingwall was seated at work. One of those public nuisances, a spoilt child, was playing about the room, dressed after the most approved fashion – in a blue tunic with a black belt a quarter of a yard wide, fastened with an immense buckle – looking like a robber in a melodrama, seen through a diminishing glass.

After a little pleasantry from the sweet child, who amused himself by running away with Miss Maria Crumpton's chair as fast as it was placed for her, the visitors were seated, and Cornelius Brook Dingwall, Esq., opened the conversation.

He had sent for Miss Crumpton, he said, in consequence of the high character he had received of her establishment from his friend, Sir Alfred Muggs.

Miss Crumpton murmured her acknowledgments to him (Muggs), and Cornelius proceeded.

'One of my principal reasons, Miss Crumpton, for parting with my daughter, is, that she has lately acquired some sentimental ideas, which it is most desirable to eradicate from her young mind.' (Here the little innocent before noticed, fell out of an armchair with an awful crash.)

'Naughty boy!' said his mamma, who appeared more surprised at his taking the liberty of falling down, than at anything else; 'I'll ring the bell for James to take him away.'

'Pray don't check him, my love,' said the diplomatist, as soon as he could make himself heard amidst the unearthly howling consequent upon the threat and the tumble. 'It all arises from his great flow of spirits.' This last explanation was addressed to Miss Crumpton.

'Certainly, sir,' replied the antique Maria: not exactly seeing, however, the connexion between a flow of animal spirits and a fall from an armchair.

Silence was restored, and the MP resumed: 'Now, I know nothing so likely to effect this object, Miss Crumpton, as her mixing constantly in the society of girls of her own age; and, as I know that in your establishment she will meet such as are not likely to contaminate her young mind, I propose to send her to you.'

The youngest Miss Crumpton expressed the acknowledgments of the establishment generally. Maria was rendered speechless by bodily pain. The dear little fellow, having recovered his animal spirits, was standing upon her most tender foot, by way of getting his face (which looked like a capital O in a red-lettered play bill) on a level with the writing table.

'Of course, Lavinia, will be a parlour boarder,' continued the enviable father; 'and on one point I wish my directions to be strictly observed. The fact is, that some ridiculous love affair, with a person much her inferior in life, has been the cause of her present state of mind. Knowing that of course, under your care, she can have no opportunity of meeting this person, I do not object to – indeed, I should rather prefer – her mixing with such society as you see yourself.'

This important statement was again interrupted by the high-spirited little creature, in the excess of his joyousness breaking a pane of glass, and nearly precipitating himself into an adjacent area. James was rung for; considerable confusion and screaming succeeded: two little blue legs were seen to kick violently in the air as the man left the room, and the child was gone.

'Mr Brook Dingwall would like Miss Brook Dingwall to learn everything,' said Mrs Brook Dingwall, who hardly ever said anything at all.

'Certainly,' said both the Miss Crumptons together.

'And as I trust the plan I have devised will be effectual in weaning my daughter from this absurd idea, Miss Crumpton,' continued the legislator, 'I hope you will have the goodness to comply, in all respects, with any request I may forward to you.'

The promise was of course made; and after a lengthened discussion, conducted on behalf of the Dingwalls with the most becoming diplomatic gravity, and on that of the Crumptons with profound respect, it was finally arranged that Miss Lavinia should be forwarded to Hammersmith on the next day but one, on which occasion the half yearly ball given at the establishment was to take place. It might divert the dear girl's mind. This, by the way, was another bit of diplomacy.

Miss Lavinia was introduced to her future governess, and both the Miss Crumptons pronounced her 'a most charming girl'; an opinion which, by a singular coincidence, they always entertained of any new pupil.

Courtesies were exchanged, acknowledgments expressed, condescension exhibited, and the interview terminated.

Preparations, to make use of theatrical phraseology, 'on a scale of magnitude never before attempted,' were incessantly made at Minerva House to give every effect to the forthcoming ball. The largest room in the house was pleasantly ornamented with blue calico roses, plaid tulips, and other equally natural-looking artificial flowers, the work of the young ladies themselves. The carpet was taken up, the folding doors were taken down, the furniture was taken out, and rout seats were taken in. The linen drapers of Hammersmith were astounded at the sudden demand for blue sarsenet ribbon, and long white gloves. Dozens of geraniums were purchased for bouquets, and a harp and two violins were bespoke from town, in addition to the grand piano already on the premises. The young ladies who were selected to show off on the occasion, and do credit to the establishment practised incessantly, much to their own satisfaction, and greatly to the annoyance of the lame old gentleman over the way; and a constant correspondence was kept up between the Misses Crumpton and the Hammersmith pastry cook.

The evening came; and then there was such a lacing of stays, and tying of sandals, and dressing of hair, as never can take place with a proper degree of bustle out of a boarding school. The smaller girls managed to be in everybody's way, and were pushed about accordingly; and the elder ones dressed, and tied, and flattered, and envied one another, as earnestly and sincerely as if they had actually *come out.*

'How do I look, dear?' inquired Miss Emily Smithers, the belle of the house, of Miss Caroline Wilson, who was her bosom friend, because she was the ugliest girl in Hammersmith, or out of it.

'Oh! charming, dear. How do I?'

'Delightful! you never looked so handsome,' returned the belle, adjusting her own dress, and not bestowing a glance on her poor companion.

'I hope young Hilton will come early,' said another young lady to Miss somebody else, in a fever of expectation.

'I'm sure he'd be highly flattered if he knew it,' returned the other, who was practising *l'été.*

'Oh! he's so handsome,' said the first.

'Such a charming person!' added a second.

'Such a *distingué* air!' said a third.

'Oh, what *do* you think?' said another girl, running into the room; 'Miss Crumpton says her cousin's coming.'

'What! Theodosius Butler?' said everybody in raptures.

'Is *he* handsome?' inquired a novice.

'No, not particularly handsome,' was the general reply; 'but, oh, so clever!'

Mr Theodosius Butler was one of those immortal geniuses who are to be met with in almost every circle. They have, usually, very deep, monotonous voices. They always persuade themselves that they are wonderful persons, and that they ought to be very miserable, though they don't precisely know why. They are very conceited, and usually possess half an idea; but, with enthusiastic young ladies, and silly young gentlemen, they are very wonderful persons. The individual in question, Mr Theodosius, had written a pamphlet containing some very weighty considerations on the expediency of doing something or other; and as every sentence contained a good many words of four syllables, his admirers took it for granted that he meant a good deal.

'Perhaps that's he,' exclaimed several young ladies, as the first pull of the evening threatened destruction to the bell of the gate.

An awful pause ensued. Some boxes arrived and a young lady – Miss Brook Dingwall, in full ball costume, with an immense gold chain round her neck, and her dress looped up with a single rose; an ivory fan in her hand, and a most interesting expression of despair in her face.

The Miss Crumptons inquired after the family, with the most excruciating anxiety, and Miss Brook Dingwall was formally introduced to her future companions. The Miss Crumptons conversed with the young ladies in the most mellifluous tones, in order that Miss Brook Dingwall might be properly impressed with their amiable treatment.

Another pull at the bell. Mr Dadson the writing master and his wife. The wife in green silk, with shoes and cap-trimmings to correspond: the writing master in a white waistcoat, black knee shorts, and ditto silk stockings, displaying a leg large enough for two writing masters. The young ladies whispered one another, and the writing master and his wife flattered the Miss Crumptons, who were dressed in amber, with long sashes, like dolls.

Repeated pulls at the bell, and arrivals too numerous to particularise: papas and mammas, and aunts and uncles, the owners and guardians of the different pupils; the singing master, Signor Lobskini, in a black wig; the piano-forte player and the violins; the harp, in a state of intoxication; and some twenty young men, who stood near the door, and talked to one another, occasionally bursting into a giggle. A general hum of conversation. Coffee handed round, and plentifully partaken of by fat mammas, who looked like the stout people who come on in pantomimes for the sole purpose of being knocked down.

The popular Mr Hilton was the next arrival; and he, having, at the request of the Miss Crumptons, undertaken the office of Master of the Ceremonies, the quadrilles commenced with considerable spirit. The young men by the door gradually advanced into the middle of the room, and in time became sufficiently at ease to consent to be introduced to partners. The writing master danced every set, springing about with the most fearful agility, and his wife played a rubber in the back parlour – a little room with five bookshelves, dignified by the name of the study. Setting her down to whist was a half-yearly piece of generalship on the part of the Miss Crumptons; it was necessary to hide her somewhere, on account of her being a fright.

The interesting Lavinia Brook Dingwall was the only girl present who appeared to take no interest in the proceedings of the evening. In vain was she solicited to dance; in vain was the universal homage paid to her as the daughter of a member of parliament. She was equally unmoved by the splendid tenor of the inimitable Lobskini, and the brilliant execution of Miss Lætitia Parsons, whose performance of 'The Recollections of Ireland' was universally declared to be almost equal to that of Moscheles himself. Not even the announcement of the arrival of Mr Theodosius Butler could induce her to leave the corner of the back drawing room in which she was seated.

'Now, Theodosius,' said Miss Maria Crumpton, after that enlightened pamphleteer had nearly run the gauntlet of the whole company, 'I must introduce you to our new pupil.'

Theodosius looked as if he cared for nothing earthly.

'She's the daughter of a member of parliament,' said Maria. – Theodosius started.

'And her name is—?' he inquired.

'Miss Brook Dingwall.'

'Great Heaven!' poetically exclaimed Theodosius, in a low tone.

Miss Crumpton commenced the introduction in due form. Miss Brook Dingwall languidly raised her head.

'Edward!' she exclaimed, with a half shriek, on seeing the well-known nankeen legs.

Fortunately, as Miss Maria Crumpton possessed no remarkable share of penetration, and as it was one of the diplomatic arrangements that no attention was to be paid to Miss Lavinia's incoherent exclamations, she was perfectly unconscious of the mutual agitation of the parties; and therefore, seeing that the offer of his hand for the next quadrille was accepted, she left him by the side of Miss Brook Dingwall.

'Oh, Edward!' exclaimed that most romantic of all romantic young ladies, as the light of science seated himself beside her, 'Oh, Edward, is it you?'

Mr Theodosius assured the dear creature, in the most impassioned manner, that he was not conscious of being anybody but himself.

'Then why – why – this disguise? Oh! Edward M'Neville Walter, what have I not suffered on your account?'

'Lavinia, hear me,' replied the hero, in his most poetic strain. 'Do not condemn me unheard. If anything that emanates from the soul of such a wretch as I, can occupy a place in your recollection – if any being, so vile, deserve your notice – you may remember that I once published a pamphlet (and paid for its publication) entitled "Considerations on the Policy of Removing the Duty on Beeswax." '

'I do – I do!' sobbed Lavinia.

'That,' continued the lover, 'was a subject to which your father was devoted, heart and soul.'

'He was – he was!' reiterated the sentimentalist.

'I knew it,' continued Theodosius, tragically; 'I knew it – I forwarded him a copy. He wished to know me. Could I disclose my real name? Never! No, I assumed that name which you have so often pronounced in tones of endearment. As M'Neville Walter, I devoted myself to the stirring cause; as M'Neville Walter, I gained your heart; in the same character I was ejected from your house by your father's domestics; and in no character at all have I since been enabled to see you. We now meet again, and I proudly own that I am – Theodosius Butler.'

The young lady appeared perfectly satisfied with this argumentative address, and bestowed a look of the most ardent affection on the immortal advocate of beeswax.

'May I hope,' said he, 'that the promise your father's violent behaviour interrupted, may be renewed?'

'Let us join this set,' replied Lavinia, coquettishly – for girls of nineteen *can* coquette.

'No,' ejaculated he of the nankeens; 'I stir not from this spot, writhing under this torture of suspense. May I – may I – hope?'

'You may.'

'The promise is renewed?'

'It is.'

'I have your permission?'

'You have.'

'To the fullest extent?'

'You know it,' returned the blushing Lavinia. The contortions of the interesting Butler's visage expressed his raptures.

We could dilate upon the occurrences that ensued. How Mr Theodosius and Miss Lavinia danced, and talked, and sighed for the remainder of the evening – how the Miss Crumptons were delighted thereat. How the writing master continued to frisk about with one-horse power, and how his wife, from some unaccountable freak, left the whist table in the little back parlour, and persisted in displaying her green head-dress in the most conspicuous part of the drawing room. How the supper consisted of small triangular sandwiches in trays, and a tart here and there by way of variety; and how the visitors consumed warm water disguised with lemon, and dotted with nutmeg, under the denomination of negus. These, and other matters of as much interest, however, we pass over, for the purpose of describing a scene of even more importance.

A fortnight after the date of the ball, Cornelius Brook Dingwall, Esq., MP, was seated at the same library table, and in the same room, as we have before described. He was alone, and his face bore an expression of deep thought and solemn gravity – he was drawing up 'A Bill for the better observance of Easter Monday.'

The footman tapped at the door – the legislator started from his reverie, and 'Miss Crumpton' was announced. Permission was given for Miss Crumpton to enter the *sanctum*; Maria came sliding in, and having taken her seat with a due portion of affectation, the footman retired, and the governess was left alone with the MP. Oh! how she longed for the presence of a third party! Even the facetious young gentleman would have been a relief.

Miss Crumpton began the duet. She hoped Mrs Brook Dingwall and the handsome little boy were in good health.

They were. Mrs Brook Dingwall and little Frederick were at Brighton.

'Much obliged to you, Miss Crumpton,' said Cornelius, in his most dignified manner, 'for your attention in calling this morning. I should have driven down to Hammersmith, to see Lavinia, but your account was so very satisfactory, and my duties in the House occupy me so much, that I determined to postpone it for a week. How has she gone on?'

'Very well indeed, sir,' returned Maria, dreading to inform the father that she had gone off.

'Ah, I thought the plan on which I proceeded would be a match for her.'

Here was a favourable opportunity to say that somebody else had been a match for her. But the unfortunate governess was unequal to the task.

'You have persevered strictly in the line of conduct I prescribed, Miss Crumpton?'

'Strictly, sir.'

'You tell me in your note that her spirits gradually improved.'

'Very much indeed, sir.'

'To be sure. I was convinced they would.'

'But I fear, sir,' said Miss Crumpton, with visible emotion, 'I fear the plan has not succeeded quite so well as we could have wished.'

'No!' exclaimed the prophet. 'Bless me! Miss Crumpton, you look alarmed. What has happened?'

'Miss Brook Dingwall, sir — '

'Yes, ma'am?'

'Has gone, sir' – said Maria, exhibiting a strong inclination to faint.

'Gone!'

'Eloped, sir.'

'Eloped! – Who with – when – where – how?' almost shrieked the agitated diplomatist.

The natural yellow of the unfortunate Maria's face changed to all the hues of the rainbow, as she laid a small packet on the Member's table.

He hurriedly opened it. A letter from his daughter, and another from Theodosius. He glanced over their contents – 'Ere this reaches you, far distant – appeal to feelings – love to distraction – beeswax – slavery,' &c., &c. He dashed his hand to his forehead, and paced the room with fearfully long strides, to the great alarm of the precise Maria.

'Now mind; from this time forward,' said Mr Brook Dingwall, suddenly stopping at the table, and beating time upon it with his hand; 'from this time forward, I never will, under any circumstances whatever, permit a man who writes pamphlets to enter any other room of this house but the kitchen. – I'll allow my daughter and her husband one hundred and fifty pounds a year, and never see their faces again: and, damme! ma'am, I'll bring in a bill for the abolition of finishing schools.'

Some time has elapsed since this passionate declaration. Mr and Mrs Butler are at present rusticating in a small cottage at Ball's Pond, pleasantly situated in the immediate vicinity of a brick field. They have no family. Mr Theodosius looks very important, and writes incessantly; but, in consequence of a gross combination on the part of publishers, none of his productions appear in print. His young wife begins to think that ideal misery is preferable to real unhappiness; and that a marriage contracted in haste, and repented at leisure, is the cause of more substantial wretchedness than she ever anticipated.

On cool reflection, Cornelius Brook Dingwall, Esq., MP, was reluctantly compelled to admit that the untoward result of his admirable arrangements was attributable, not to the Miss Crumptons, but his own diplomacy. He however consoles himself, like some other small diplomatists, by satisfactorily proving that if his plans did not succeed, they ought to have done so. Minerva House is *in statu quo*, and 'The Misses Crumpton' remain in the peaceable and undisturbed enjoyment of all the advantages resulting from their Finishing School.

## Chapter Four

### *The Tuggses at Ramsgate*

First published in the first number of Chapman and Hall's new monthly publication, *The Library of Fiction* ... , 31 March 1836. The first monthly number of *Pickwick Papers* was also issued by the same publishers on this day and *Pickwick*'s original illustrator Robert Seymour supplied two illustrations for this story also. Dickens's only other contribution to *The Library of Fiction* was 'A Little Talk about Spring and the Sweeps', published in the third number (see headnote to 'The First of May', p. 168, above).

Once upon a time there dwelt, in a narrow street on the Surrey side of the water, within three minutes' walk of old London Bridge. Mr Joseph Tuggs – a little dark-faced man, with shiny hair, twinkling eyes, short legs, and a body of very considerable thickness, measuring from the centre button of his waistcoat in front, to the ornamental buttons of his coat behind. The figure of the amiable Mrs Tuggs, if not perfectly symmetrical, was decidedly comfortable; and the form of her only daughter, the accomplished Miss Charlotte Tuggs, was fast ripening into that state of luxuriant plumpness which had enchanted the eyes, and captivated the heart, of Mr Joseph Tuggs in his earlier days. Mr Simon Tuggs, his only son, and Miss Charlotte Tuggs's only brother, was as differently formed in body, as he was differently constituted in mind, from the remainder of his family. There was that elongation in his thoughtful face, and that tendency to weakness in his interesting legs, which tell so forcibly of a great mind and romantic disposition. The slightest traits of character in such a being, possess no mean interest to speculative minds. He usually appeared in public, in capacious shoes with black cotton stockings; and was observed to be particularly attached to a black glazed stock, without a tie or ornament of any description.

There is perhaps no profession, however useful; no pursuit, however meritorious; which can escape the petty attacks of vulgar minds. Mr Joseph Tuggs was a grocer. It might be supposed that a grocer was beyond the breath of calumny; but no – the neighbours stigmatised him as a chandler; and the poisonous voice of envy distinctly asserted that he dispensed tea and coffee by the quartern, retailed sugar by the ounce, cheese by the

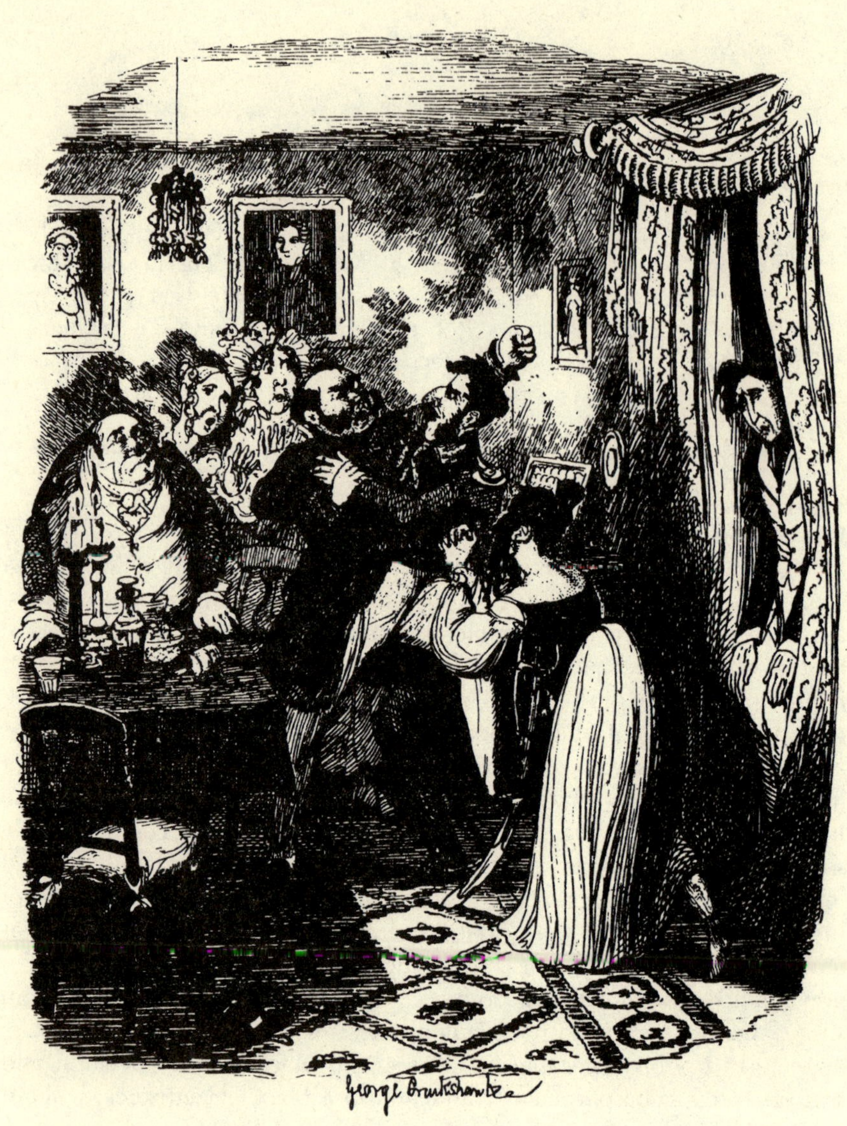

*The Tuggses at Ramsgate (see p. 344)*

slice, tobacco by the screw, and butter by the pat. These taunts, however, were lost upon the Tuggses. Mr Tuggs attended to the grocery department; Mrs Tuggs to the cheesemongery; and Miss Tuggs to her education. Mr Simon Tuggs kept his father's books, and his own counsel.

One fine spring afternoon, the latter gentleman was seated on a tub of weekly Dorset, behind the little red desk with a wooden rail, which ornamented a corner of the counter; when a stranger dismounted from a cab, and hastily entered the shop. He was habited in black cloth, and bore with him a green umbrella and a blue bag.

'Mr Tuggs?' said the stranger, inquiringly.

'*My* name is Tuggs,' replied Mr Simon.

'It's the other Mr Tuggs,' said the stranger, looking towards the glass door which led into the parlour behind the shop, and on the inside of which, the round face of Mr Tuggs, senior, was distinctly visible, peeping over the curtain.

Mr Simon gracefully waved his pen, as if in intimation of his wish that his father would advance. Mr Joseph Tuggs, with considerable celerity, removed his face from the curtain and placed it before the stranger.

'I come from the Temple,' said the man with the bag.

'From the Temple!' said Mrs Tuggs, flinging open the door of the little parlour and disclosing Miss Tuggs in perspective.

'From the Temple!' said Miss Tuggs and Mr Simon Tuggs at the same moment.

'From the Temple!' said Mr Joseph Tuggs, turning as pale as a Dutch cheese.

'From the Temple,' repeated the man with the bag; 'from Mr Cower's, the solicitor's. Mr Tuggs, I congratulate you, sir. Ladies, I wish you joy of your prosperity! We have been successful.' And the man with the bag leisurely divested himself of his umbrella and glove, as a preliminary to shaking hands with Mr Joseph Tuggs.

Now the words 'we have been successful,' had no sooner issued from the mouth of the man with the bag, than Mr Simon Tuggs rose from the tub of weekly Dorset, opened his eyes very wide, gasped for breath, made figures of eight in the air with his pen, and finally fell into the arms of his anxious mother, and fainted away without the slightest ostensible cause or pretence.

'Water!' screamed Mrs Tuggs.

'Look up, my son,' exclaimed Mr Tuggs.

'Simon! dear Simon!' shrieked Miss Tuggs.

'I'm better now,' said Mr Simon Tuggs. 'What! successful!' And then, as corroborative evidence of his being better, he fainted away again, and was borne into the little parlour by the united efforts of the remainder of the family, and the man with the bag.

To a casual spectator, or to any one unacquainted with the position of the family, this fainting would have been unaccountable. To those who understood the mission of the man with the bag, and were moreover acquainted with the excitability of the nerves of Mr Simon Tuggs, it was quite comprehensible. A long pending lawsuit respecting the validity of a will, had been unexpectedly decided; and Mr Joseph Tuggs was the possessor of twenty thousand pounds.

A prolonged consultation took place, that night, in the little parlour – a consultation that was to settle the future destinies of the Tuggses. The shop was shut up, at an unusually early hour; and many were the unavailing kicks bestowed upon the closed door by applicants for quarterns of sugar, or half-quarterns of bread, or penn'orths of pepper, which were to have been 'left till Saturday', but which fortune had decreed were to be left alone altogether.

'We must certainly give up business,' said Miss Tuggs.

'Oh, decidedly,' said Mrs Tuggs.

'Simon shall go to the bar,' said Mr Joseph Tuggs.

'And I shall always sign myself "Cymon" in future,' said his son.

'And I shall call myself Charlotta,' said Miss Tuggs.

'And you must always call *me* "Ma," and father "Pa," ' said Mrs Tuggs.

'Yes, and Pa must leave off all his vulgar habits,' interposed Miss Tuggs.

'I'll take care of all that,' responded Mr Joseph Tuggs, complacently. He was, at that very moment, eating pickled salmon with a pocket-knife.

'We must leave town immediately,' said Mr Cymon Tuggs.

Everybody concurred that this was an indispensable preliminary to being genteel. The question then arose. Where should they go?

'Gravesend?' mildly suggested Mr Joseph Tuggs. The idea was unanimously scouted. Gravesend was *low.*

'Margate?' insinuated Mrs Tuggs. Worse and worse – nobody there, but tradespeople.

'Brighton?' Mr Cymon Tuggs opposed an insurmountable objection. All the coaches had been upset, in turn, within the last three weeks; each coach had averaged two passengers killed, and six wounded; and, in every case, the newspapers had distinctly understood that 'no blame whatever was attributable to the coachman.'

'Ramsgate?' ejaculated Mr Cymon, thoughtfully. To be sure; how stupid they must have been, not to have thought of that before! Ramsgate was just the place of all others.

Two months after this conversation, the City of London Ramsgate steamer was running gaily down the river. Her flag was flying, her band was playing, her passengers were conversing; everything about her seemed gay and lively. – No wonder – the Tuggses were on board.

'Charming, ain't it?' said Mr Joseph Tuggs, in a bottle-green greatcoat, with a velvet collar of the same; and a blue travelling cap with a gold band.

'Soul inspiring,' replied Mr Cymon Tuggs – he was entered at the bar. 'Soul inspiring!'

'Delightful morning, sir!' said a stoutish, military-looking gentleman in a blue surtout buttoned up to his chin, and white trousers chained down to the soles of his boots.

Mr Cymon Tuggs took upon himself the responsibility of answering the observation. 'Heavenly!' he replied.

'You are an enthusiastic admirer of the beauties of Nature, sir?' said the military gentleman.

'I am, sir,' replied Mr Cymon Tuggs.

'Travelled much, sir?' inquired the military gentleman.

'Not much,' replied Mr Cymon Tuggs.

'You've been on the continent, of course?' inquired the military gentleman.

'Not exactly,' replied Mr Cymon Tuggs – in a qualified tone, as if he wished it to be implied that he had gone half way and come back again.

'You of course intend your son to make the grand tour, sir?' said the military gentleman, addressing Mr Joseph Tuggs.

As Mr Joseph Tuggs did not precisely understand what the grand tour was, or how such an article was manufactured, he replied. 'Of course.' Just as he said the word, there came tripping up, from her seat at the stern of the vessel, a young lady in a puce-coloured silk cloak, and boots of the same; with long black ringlets, large black eyes, brief petticoats, and unexceptionable ankles.

'Walter, my dear,' said the young lady to the military gentleman.

'Yes, Belinda, my love,' responded the military gentleman to the black-eyed young lady.

'What have you left me alone so long for?' said the young lady. 'I have been stared out of countenance by those rude young men.'

'What! stared at?' exclaimed the military gentleman, with an emphasis which made Mr Cymon Tuggs withdraw his eyes from the young lady's face with inconceivable rapidity. 'Which young men – where?' and the military gentleman clenched his fist, and glared fearfully on the cigar smokers around.

'Be calm, Walter, I entreat,' said the young lady.

'I won't,' said the military gentleman.

'Do, sir,' interposed Mr Cymon Tuggs. 'They ain't worth your notice.'

'No – no – they are not, indeed,' urged the young lady.

'I *will* be calm,' said the military gentleman. 'You speak truly, sir. I thank you for a timely remonstrance, which may have spared me the guilt of manslaughter.' Calming his wrath, the military gentleman wrung Mr Cymon Tuggs by the hand.

'My sister, sir!' said Mr Cymon Tuggs; seeing that the military gentleman was casting an admiring look towards Miss Charlotta.

'My wife, ma'am – Mrs Captain Waters,' said the military gentleman, presenting the black-eyed young lady.

'My mother, ma'am – Mrs Tuggs,' said Mr Cymon. The military gentleman and his wife murmured enchanting courtesies; and the Tuggses looked as unembarrassed as they could.

'Walter, my dear,' said the black-eyed young lady, after they had sat chatting with the Tuggses some half hour.

'Yes, my love,' said the military gentleman.

'Don't you think this gentleman (with an inclination of the head towards Mr Cymon Tuggs) is very much like the Marquis Carriwini?'

'Lord bless me, very!' said the military gentleman.

'It struck me the moment I saw him,' said the young lady, gazing intently, and with a melancholy air, on the scarlet countenance of Mr Cymon Tuggs. Mr Cymon Tuggs looked at everybody; and finding that everybody was looking at him, appeared to feel some temporary difficulty in disposing of his eyesight.

'So exactly the air of the marquis,' said the military gentleman.

'Quite extraordinary!' sighed the military gentleman's lady.

'You don't know the marquis, sir?' inquired the military gentleman.

Mr Cymon Tuggs stammered a negative.

'If you did,' continued Captain Walter Waters, 'you would feel how much reason you have to be proud of the resemblance – a most elegant man, with a most prepossessing appearance.'

'He is – he is indeed!' exclaimed Belinda Waters energetically. As her eye caught that of Mr Cymon Tuggs, she withdrew it from his features in bashful confusion.

All this was highly gratifying to the feelings of the Tuggses; and when, in the course of farther conversation, it was discovered that Miss Charlotta Tuggs was the *facsimile* of a titled relative of Mrs Belinda Waters, and that Mrs Tuggs herself was the very picture of the Dowager Duchess of Dobbleton, their delight in the acquisition of so genteel and friendly an acquaintance knew no bounds. Even the dignity of Captain Walter Waters relaxed to that degree, that he suffered himself to be prevailed upon by Mr Joseph Tuggs to partake of cold pigeon pie and sherry, on deck; and a most delightful conversation, aided by these agreeable stimulants, was prolonged until they ran alongside Ramsgate Pier.

'Good by'e, dear!' said Mrs Captain Waters to Miss Charlotta Tuggs, just before the bustle of landing commenced; 'we shall see you on the sands in the morning; and, as we are sure to have found lodgings before then, I hope we shall be inseparables for many weeks to come.'

'Oh! I hope so,' said Miss Charlotta Tuggs, emphatically.

'Tickets, ladies and gen'lm'n,' said the man on the paddle-box.

'Want a porter, sir?' inquired a dozen men in smock frocks.

'Now, my dear!' said Captain Waters.

'Good by'e!' said Mrs Captain Waters – 'good by'e, Mr Cymon!' and with a pressure of the hand which threw the amiable young man's nerves into a state of considerable derangement, Mrs Captain Waters disappeared among the crowd. A pair of puce-coloured boots were seen ascending the steps, a white handkerchief fluttered, a black eye gleamed. The Waterses were gone, and Mr Cymon Tuggs was alone in a heartless world.

Silently and abstractedly did that too sensitive youth follow his revered parents, and a train of smock frocks and wheelbarrows, along the pier, until the bustle of the scene around recalled him to himself. The sun was shining brightly; the sea, dancing to its own music, rolled merrily in; crowds of people promenaded to and fro; young ladies tittered; old ladies talked; nursemaids displayed their charms to the greatest possible advantage; and their little charges ran up and down, and to and fro, and in and out, under the feet, and between the legs, of the assembled concourse, in the most playful and exhilarating manner. There were old gentlemen, trying to make out objects through long telescopes; and young ones, making objects of themselves in open shirtcollars; ladies, carrying about portable chairs, and portable chairs carrying about invalids; parties, waiting on the pier for parties who had come by the steamboat; and nothing was to be heard but talking, laughing, welcoming, and merriment.

'Fly, sir?' exclaimed a chorus of fourteen men and six boys, the moment Mr Joseph Tuggs, at the head of his little party, set foot in the street.

'Here's the gen'lm'n at last!' said one, touching his hat with mock politeness. 'Werry glad to see you, sir, – been a-waitin' for you these six weeks. Jump in, if you please, sir!'

'Nice light fly and a fast trotter, sir,' said another: 'fourteen mile a hour, and surroundin' objects rendered inwisible by ex-treme welocity!'

'Large fly for your luggage, sir,' cried a third. 'Werry large fly here, sir – reg'lar bluebottle!'

'Here's *your* fly, sir!' shouted another aspiring charioteer, mounting the box, and inducing an old grey horse to indulge in some imperfect reminiscences of a canter. 'Look at him, sir! – temper of a lamb and haction of a steam-ingein!'

Resisting even the temptation of securing the services of so valuable a quadruped as the last named, Mr Joseph Tuggs beckoned to the proprietor of a dingy conveyance of a greenish hue, lined with faded striped calico; and, the luggage and the family having been deposited therein, the animal in the shafts, after describing circles in the road for a quarter of an hour, at last consented to depart in quest of lodgings.

'How many beds have you got?' screamed Mrs Tuggs out of the fly, to the woman who opened the door of the first house which displayed a bill intimating that apartments were to be let within.

'How many did you want, ma'am?' was, of course, the reply.

'Three.'

'Will you step in, ma'am?' Down got Mrs Tuggs. The family were delighted. Splendid view of the sea from the front windows – charming! A short pause. Back came Mrs Tuggs again. – One parlour and a mattress.

'Why the devil didn't they say so at first?' inquired Mr Joseph Tuggs, rather pettishly.

'Don't know,' said Mrs Tuggs.

'Wretches!' exclaimed the nervous Cymon. Another bill – another stoppage. Same question – same answer – similar result.

'What do they mean by this?' inquired Mr Joseph Tuggs, thoroughly out of temper.

'Don't know,' said the placid Mrs Tuggs.

'Orvis the vay here, sir,' said the driver, by way of accounting for the circumstance in a satisfactory manner; and off they went again, to make fresh inquiries, and encounter fresh disappointments.

It had grown dusk when the 'fly' – the rate of whose progress greatly belied its name – after climbing up four or five perpendicular hills, stopped before the door of a dusty house, with a bay window, from which you could obtain a beautiful glimpse of the sea – if you thrust half of your body out of it, at the imminent peril of falling into the area. Mrs Tuggs alighted. One ground floor sitting room, and three cells with beds in them upstairs. A double house. Family on the opposite side. Five children milk and watering in the parlour, and one little boy, expelled for bad behaviour, screaming on his back in the passage.

'What's the terms?' said Mrs Tuggs. The mistress of the house was considering the expediency of putting on an extra guinea; so she coughed slightly, and affected not to hear the question.

'What's the terms?' said Mrs Tuggs, in a louder key.

'Five guineas a week, ma'am, *with* attendance,' replied the lodging house keeper. (Attendance means the privilege of ringing the bell as often as you like, for your own amusement.)

'Rather dear,' said Mrs Tuggs.

'Oh dear, no, ma'am!' replied the mistress of the house, with a benign smile of pity at the ignorance of manners and customs with the observation betrayed, 'Very cheap!'

Such an authority was indisputable. Mrs Tuggs paid a week's rent in advance, and took the lodgings for a month. In an hour's time the family were seated at tea in their new abode.

'Capital srimps!' said Mr Joseph Tuggs.

Mr Cymon eyed his father with a rebellious scowl, as he emphatically said '*Shrimps.*'

'Well then, shrimps,' said Mr Joseph Tuggs. 'Srimps or shrimps, don't much matter.'

There was pity, blended with malignity, in Mr Cymon's eye, as he replied, 'Don't matter, father! What would Captain Waters say, if he heard such vulgarity?'

'Or what would dear Mrs Captain Waters say,' added Charlotta, 'if she saw mother – ma, I mean – eating them whole, heads and all!'

'It won't bear thinking of!' ejaculated Mr Cymon, with a shudder. 'How different,' he thought, 'from the Dowager Duchess of Dobbleton!'

'Very pretty woman, Mrs Captain Waters, is she not, Cymon?' inquired Miss Charlotta.

A glow of nervous excitement passed over the countenance of Mr Cymon Tuggs, as he replied, 'An angel of beauty!'

'Hallo!' said Mr Joseph Tuggs. 'Hallo, Cymon, my boy, take care. Married lady, you know'; and he winked one of his twinkling eyes knowingly.

'Why,' exclaimed Cymon, starting up with an ebullition of fury, as unexpected as alarming, 'why am I to be reminded of that blight of my happiness, and ruin of my hopes? Why am I to be taunted with the miseries which are heaped upon my head? Is it not enough to – to – to' and the orator paused; but whether for want of words, or lack of breath, was never distinctly ascertained.

There was an impressive solemnity in the tone of this address, and in the air with which the romantic Cymon, at its conclusion, rang the bell, and demanded a flat candlestick, which effectually forbade a reply. He stalked dramatically to bed, and the Tuggses went to bed too, half an hour afterwards, in a state of considerable mystification and perplexity.

If the pier had presented a scene of life and bustle to the Tuggses on their first landing at Ramsgate, it was far surpassed by the appearance of the sands on the morning after their arrival. It was a fine, bright, clear day, with a light breeze from the sea. There were the same ladies and gentlemen, the same children, the same nursemaids, the same telescopes, the same portable chairs. The ladies were employed in needlework, or watch guard making, or knitting, or reading novels; the gentlemen were reading newspapers and magazines; the children were digging holes in the sand with wooden spades, and collecting water therein; the nursemaids, with their youngest charges in their arms, were running in after the waves, and then running back with the waves after them; and, now and then, a little sailing boat either departed with a gay and talkative cargo of passengers, or returned with a very silent and particularly uncomfortable-looking one.

'Well, I never!' exclaimed Mrs Tuggs, as she and Mr Joseph Tuggs, and Miss Charlotta Tuggs, and Mr Cymon Tuggs, with their eight feet in a corresponding number of yellow shoes, seated themselves on four rush-bottomed chairs, which, being placed in a soft part of the sand, forthwith sunk down some two feet and a half – 'Well, I never!'

Mr Cymon, by an exertion of great personal strength, uprooted the chairs, and removed them further back.

'Why, I'm blessed if there ain't some ladies a-going in!' exclaimed Mr Joseph Tuggs, with intense astonishment.

'Lor, pa!' exclaimed Miss Charlotta.

'There *is,* my dear,' said Mr Joseph Tuggs. And, sure enough, four young ladies, each furnished with a towel, tripped up the steps of a bathing machine. In went the horse, floundering about in the water; round turned the machine; down sat the driver; and presently out burst the young ladies aforesaid, with four distinct splashes.

'Well, that's sing'ler, too!' ejaculated Mr Joseph Tuggs, after an awkward pause. Mr Cymon coughed slightly.

'Why, here's some gentlemen a-going in on this side!' exclaimed Mrs Tuggs, in a tone of horror.

Three machines – three horses – three flounderings – three turnings round – three splashes – three gentlemen, disporting themselves in the water like so many dolphins.

'Well, *that's* sing'ler!' said Mr Joseph Tuggs again. Miss Charlotta coughed this time, and another pause ensued. It was agreeably broken.

'How d'ye do, dear? We have been looking for you all the morning,' said a voice to Miss Charlotta Tuggs. Mrs Captain Waters was the owner of it.

'How d'ye do?' said Captain Walter Waters, all suavity; and a most cordial interchange of greetings ensued.

'Belinda, my love,' said Captain Walter Waters, applying his glass to his eye, and looking in the direction of the sea.

'Yes, my dear,' replied Mrs Captain Waters.

'There's Harry Thompson!'

'Where?' said Belinda, applying her glass to her eye.

'Bathing.'

'Lor, so it is! He don't see us, does he?'

'No, I don't think he does,' replied the captain. 'Bless my soul, how very singular!'

'What?' inquired Belinda.

'There's Mary Golding, too.'

'Lor! – where?' (Up went the glass again.)

'There!' said the captain, pointing to one of the young ladies before noticed, who, in her bathing costume, looked as if she was enveloped in a patent Mackintosh, of scanty dimensions.

'So it is, I declare!' exclaimed Mrs Captain Waters. 'How very curious we should see them both!'

'Very,' said the captain, with perfect coolness.

'It's the reg'lar thing here, you see,' whispered Mr Cymon Tuggs to his father.

'I see it is', whispered Mr Joseph Tuggs in reply. 'Queer though – ain't it?' Mr Cymon Tuggs nodded assent.

'What do you think of doing with yourself this morning?' inquired the captain. 'Shall we lunch at Pegwell?'

'I should like that very much indeed,' interposed Mrs Tuggs. She had never heard of Pegwell; but the word 'lunch' had reached her ears, and it sounded very agreeably.

'How shall we go?' inquired the captain; 'it's too warm to walk.'

'A shay?' suggested Mr Joseph Tuggs.

'Chaise,' whispered Mr Cymon.

'I should think one would be enough,' said Mr Joseph Tuggs aloud, quite unconscious of the meaning of the correction. 'However, two shays if you like.'

'I should like a donkey *so* much,' said Belinda.

'Oh, so should I!' echoed Charlotta Tuggs.

'Well, we can have a fly,' suggested the captain, 'and you can have a couple of donkeys.'

A fresh difficulty arose. Mrs Captain Waters declared it would be decidedly improper for two ladies to ride alone. The remedy was obvious. Perhaps young Mr Tuggs would be gallant enough to accompany them.

Mr Cymon Tuggs blushed, smiled, looked vacant, and faintly protested that he was no horseman. The objection was at once overruled. A fly was speedily found; and three donkeys – which the proprietor declared on his solemn asseveration to be 'three parts blood, and the other corn' – were engaged in the service.

'Kim up!' shouted one of the two boys who followed behind, to propel the donkeys, when Belinda Waters and Charlotta Tuggs had been hoisted, and pushed, and pulled, into their respective saddles.

'Hi – hi – hi!' groaned the other boy behind Mr Cymon Tuggs. Away went the donkey, with the stirrups jingling against the heels of Cymon's boots, and Cymon's boots nearly scraping the ground.

'Way – way! Wo–o–o–o–!' cried Mr Cymon Tuggs as well as he could, in the midst of the jolting.

'Don't make it gallop!' screamed Mrs Captain Waters, behind.

'My donkey *will* go into the public house!' shrieked Miss Tuggs in the rear.

'Hi – hi – hi!' groaned both the boys together; and on went the donkeys as if nothing would ever stop them.

Everything has an end, however; even the galloping of donkeys will cease in time. The animal which Mr Cymon Tuggs bestrode, feeling sundry uncomfortable tugs at the bit, the intent of which he could by no means divine, abruptly sidled against a brick wall, and expressed his uneasiness by grinding Mr Cymon Tuggs's leg on the rough surface. Mrs Captain Waters's donkey, apparently under the influence of some playfulness of spirit, rushed suddenly, head first, into a hedge, and declined to come out again: and the quadruped on which Miss Tuggs was mounted, expressed his delight at this humorous proceeding by firmly planting his forefeet against the ground, and kicking up his hind legs in a very agile, but somewhat alarming manner.

This abrupt termination to the rapidity of the ride naturally occasioned some confusion. Both the ladies indulged in vehement screaming for several minutes; and Mr Cymon Tuggs, besides sustaining intense bodily pain, had the additional mental anguish of witnessing their distressing situation, without having the power to rescue them, by reason of his leg being firmly screwed in between the animal and the wall. The efforts of the boys, however, assisted by the ingenious expedient of twisting the tail of the most rebellious donkey, restored order in a much shorter time than could have reasonably been expected, and the little party jogged slowly on together.

'Now let 'em walk,' said Mr Cymon Tuggs. 'It's cruel to overdrive 'em.'

'Werry well, sir,' replied the boy, with a grin at his companion, as if he understood Mr Cymon to mean that the cruelty applied less to the animals than to their riders.

'What a lovely day, dear!' said Charlotta.

'Charming; enchanting, dear!' responded Mrs Captain Waters. 'What a beautiful prospect, Mr Tuggs!'

Cymon looked full in Belinda's face, as he responded – 'Beautiful, indeed!' The lady cast down her eyes, and suffered the animal she was riding to fall a little back. Cymon Tuggs instinctively did the same.

There was a brief silence, broken only by a sigh from Mr Cymon Tuggs.

'Mr Cymon,' said the lady suddenly, in a low tone, 'Mr Cymon – I am another's.'

Mr Cymon expressed his perfect concurrence in a statement which it was impossible to controvert.

'If I had not been—' resumed Belinda; and there she stopped.

'What – what?' said Mr Cymon earnestly. 'Do not torture me. What would you say?'

'If I had not been' – continued Mrs Captain Waters – 'if, in earlier life, it had been my fate to have known, and been beloved by, a noble youth – a kindred soul – a congenial spirit – one capable of feeling and appreciating the sentiments which—'

'Heavens! what do I hear? exclaimed Mr Cymon Tuggs. 'Is it possible! can I believe my – Come up!' (This last unsentimental parenthesis was addressed to the donkey, who, with his head between his forelegs, appeared to be examining the state of his shoes with great anxiety.)

'Hi – hi – hi,' said the boys behind. 'Come up,' expostulated Cymon Tuggs again. 'Hi – hi – hi,' repeated the boys. And whether it was that the animal felt indignant at the tone of Mr Tuggs's command, or felt alarmed by the noise of the deputy proprietor's boots running behind him; or whether he burned with a noble emulation to outstrip the other donkeys; certain it is that he no sooner heard the second series of 'hi – hi's', than he started away, with a celerity of pace which jerked Mr Cymon's hat off instantaneously, and carried him to the Pegwell Bay hotel in no time, where he deposited his rider without giving him the trouble of dismounting, by sagaciously pitching him over his head into the very doorway of the tavern.

Great was the confusion of Mr Cymon Tuggs, when he was put right end uppermost by two waiters; considerable was the alarm of Mrs Tuggs in behalf of her son; agonizing were the apprehensions of Mrs Captain Waters on his account. It was speedily discovered, however, that he had not sustained much more injury than the donkey – he was grazed, and the animal was grazing – and then it *was* a delightful party to be sure! Mr and Mrs Tuggs, and the captain, had ordered lunch in the little garden behind: – small saucers of large shrimps, dabs of butter, crusty loaves, and bottled ale. The sky was without a cloud; there were flower pots and turf before them; the sea, from the foot of the cliff, stretching away as far as the eye could discern anything at all; vessels in the distance with sails as white, and as small, as nicely got up cambric handkerchiefs. The shrimps were delightful, the ale better, and the captain even more pleasant than either. Mrs Captain Waters was in *such* spirits after lunch! – chasing, first the captain across the turf, and among the flower pots; and then Mr Cymon Tuggs; and then Miss Tuggs; and laughing, too, quite boisterously. But as the captain said, it didn't matter; who knew what they were, there? For all the people of the house knew, they might be common people. To which Mr Joseph Tuggs responded, 'To be sure.' And then they went down the steep wooden steps a little further on, which led to the bottom of the cliff; and looked at the crabs, and the seaweed, and the eels, till it was more than fully time to go back to Ramsgate again. Finally, Mr

Cymon Tuggs ascended the steps last, and Mrs Captain Waters last but one; and Mr Cymon Tuggs discovered that the foot and ankle of Mrs Captain Waters were even more unexceptionable than he had at first supposed.

Taking a donkey towards his ordinary place of residence is a very different thing, and a feat much more easily to be accomplished, than taking him from it. It requires a great deal of foresight and presence of mind in the one case, to anticipate the numerous flights of his discursive imagination; whereas, in the other, all you have to do is to hold on, and place a blind confidence in the animal. Mr Cymon Tuggs adopted the latter expedient on his return, and his nerves were so little discomposed by the journey, that he distinctly understood they were all to meet again at the library in the evening.

The library was crowded. There were the same ladies, and the same gentlemen, who had been on the sands in the morning, and on the pier the day before. There were young ladies, in maroon-coloured gowns and black velvet bracelets, dispensing fancy articles in the shop, and presiding over games of chance in the concert room. There were marriageable daughters, and marriage-making mammas, gaming and promenading, and turning over music, and flirting. There were some male beaux doing the sentimental in whispers, and others doing the ferocious in moustache. There were Mrs Tuggs in amber, Miss Tuggs in sky-blue, Mrs Captain Waters in pink. There was Captain Waters in a braided surtout; there was Mr Cymon Tuggs in pumps and a gilt waistcoat; there was Mr Joseph Tuggs in a blue coat and a shirt frill.

'Numbers three, eight, and eleven!' cried one of the young ladies in the maroon-coloured gowns.

'Numbers three, eight, and eleven!' echoed another young lady in the same uniform.

'Number three's gone,' said the first young lady. 'Numbers eight and eleven!'

'Numbers eight and eleven!' echoed the second young lady.

'Number eight's gone, Mary Ann,' said the first young lady.

'Number eleven!' screamed the second.

'The numbers are all taken now, ladies, if you please,' said the first. The representatives of numbers three, eight, and eleven, and the rest of the numbers, crowded round the table.

'Will you throw, ma'am?' said the presiding goddess, handing the dice box to the eldest daughter of a stout lady, with four girls.

There was a profound silence among the lookers-on.

'Throw Jane, my dear,' said the stout lady. An interesting display of bashfulness – a little blushing in a cambric handkerchief – a whispering to a younger sister.

'Amelia, my dear, throw for your sister,' said the stout lady; and then she turned to a walking advertisement of Rowlands' Macassar Oil, who stood next her, and said, 'Jane is so *very* modest and retiring; but I can't be angry with her for it. An artless and unsophisticated girl is *so* truly amiable, that I often wish Amelia was more like her sister!'

The gentleman with the whiskers whispered his admiring approval.

'Now, my dear!' said the stout lady. Miss Amelia threw – eight for her sister, ten for herself.

'Nice figure, Amelia,' whispered the stout lady to a thin youth beside her.

'Beautiful!'

'And *such* a spirit! I am like you in that respect. I can *not* help admiring that life and vivacity. Ah! (a sigh) I wish I could make poor Jane a little more like my dear Amelia!'

The young gentleman cordially acquiesced in the sentiment; both he, and the individual first addressed, were perfectly contented.

'Who's this?' inquired Mr Cymon Tuggs of Mrs Captain Waters, as a short female, in a blue velvet hat and feathers, was led into the orchestra, by a fat man in black tights and cloudy Berlins.

'Mrs Tippin, of the London theatres,' replied Belinda, referring to the programme of the concert.

The talented Tippin having condescendingly acknowledged the clapping of hands and shouts of 'bravo!' which greeted her appearance, proceeded to sing the popular cavatina of 'Bid me discourse', accompanied on the piano by Mr Tippin; after which, Mr Tippin sang a comic song, accompanied on the piano by Mrs Tippin: the applause consequent upon which, was only to be exceeded by the enthusiastic approbation bestowed upon an air with variations on the guitar, by Miss Tippin, accompanied on the chin by Master Tippin.

Thus passed the evening; thus passed the days and evenings of the Tuggses, and the Waterses, for six weeks. Sands in the morning – donkeys at noon – pier in the afternoon – library at night – and the same people everywhere.

On that very night six weeks, the moon was shining brightly over the calm sea, which dashed against the feet of the tall gaunt cliffs, with just enough noise to lull the old fish to sleep, without disturbing the young ones, when two figures were discernible – or would have been, if anybody had looked for them – seated on one of the wooden benches which are stationed near the verge of the western cliff. The moon had climbed higher into the heavens, by two hours' journeying, since those figures first sat down – and yet they had moved not. The crowd of loungers had thinned and dispersed; the noise of itinerant musicians had died away; light after light had appeared in the windows of the different houses in the distance; blockade man after blockade man had passed the spot, wending his way towards his solitary post; and yet those figures had remained stationary. Some portions of the two forms were in deep shadow, but the light of the moon fell strongly on a puce-coloured boot and a glazed stock. Mr Cymon Tuggs and Mrs Captain Waters were seated on that bench. They spoke not, but were silently gazing on the sea.

'Walter will return tomorrow,' said Mrs Captain Waters, mournfully breaking silence.

Mr Cymon Tuggs sighed like a gust of wind through a forest of gooseberry bushes, as he replied 'Alas! he will.'

'Oh, Cymon!' resumed Belinda, 'the chaste delight, the calm happiness, of this one week of Platonic love, is too much for me!'

Cymon was about to suggest that it was too little for him, but he stopped himself, and murmured unintelligibly.

'And to think that even this gleam of happiness, innocent as it is,' exclaimed Belinda, 'is now to be lost for ever!'

'Oh, do not say for ever, Belinda,' exclaimed the excitable Cymon, as two strongly defied tears chased each other down his pale face – it was so long that there was plenty of room for a chase. 'Do not say for ever!'

'I must,' replied Belinda.

'Why?' urged Cymon, 'oh why? Such Platonic acquaintance as ours is so harmless, that even your husband can never object to it.'

'My husband!' exclaimed Belinda. 'You little know him. Jealous and revengeful; ferocious in his revenge – a maniac in his jealousy! Would you be assassinated before my eyes?' Mr Cymon Tuggs, in a voice broken by emotion, expressed his disinclination to undergo the process of assassination before the eyes of anybody.

'Then leave me,' said Mrs Captain Waters. 'Leave me, this night, for ever. It is late: let us return.'

Mr Cymon Tuggs sadly offered the lady his arm, and escorted her to her lodgings. He paused at the door – he felt a Platonic pressure of his hand. 'Goodnight,' he said, hesitating.

'Goodnight,' sobbed the lady. Mr Cymon Tuggs paused again.

'Won't you walk in, sir?' said the servant. Mr Tuggs hesitated. Oh, that hesitation! He *did* walk in.

'Goodnight!' said Mr Cymon Tuggs again, when he reached the drawing room.

'Goodnight!' replied Belinda; 'and, if at any period of my life, I – Hush!' The lady paused and stared, with a steady gaze of horror, on the ashy countenance of Mr Cymon Tuggs. There was a double knock at the street door.

'It is my husband!' said Belinda, as the captain's voice was heard below.

'And my family!' added Cymon Tuggs, as the voices of his relatives floated up the staircase.

'The curtain! The curtain!' gasped Mrs Captain Waters, pointing to the window, before which some chintz hangings were closely drawn.

'But I have done nothing wrong,' said the hesitating Cymon.

'The curtain!' reiterated the frantic lady: 'you will be murdered.' This last appeal to his feelings was irresistible. The dismayed Cymon concealed himself behind the curtain with pantomimic suddenness.

Enter the captain, Joseph Tuggs, Mrs Tuggs, and Charlotta.

'My dear,' said the captain, 'Lieutenant Slaughter.' Two iron-shod boots and one gruff voice was heard by Mr Cymon to advance, and acknowledge the honour of the introduction. The sabre of the lieutenant rattled heavily upon the floor, as he seated himself at the table. Mr Cymon's fears almost overcame his reason.

'The brandy, my dear!' said the captain. Here was a situation! They were going to make a night of it! And Mr Cymon Tuggs was pent up behind the curtain and afraid to breathe!

'Slaughter,' said the captain, 'a cigar?'

Now, Mr Cymon Tuggs never could smoke without feeling it indispensably necessary to retire immediately, and never could smell smoke without a strong disposition to cough. The cigars were introduced; the captain was a professed smoker; so was the lieutenant; so was Joseph Tuggs. The apartment was small, the door was closed, the smoke powerful: it hung in heavy wreaths over the room, and at length found its way behind the curtain. Cymon Tuggs held his nose, his mouth, his breath. It was all of no use – out came the cough.

'Bless my soul!' said the captain, 'I beg your pardon, Miss Tuggs. You dislike smoking?'

'Oh, no; I don't indeed,' said Charlotta.

'It makes you cough.'

'Oh dear no.'

'You coughed just now.'

'Me, Captain Waters! Lor! how can you say so?'

'Somebody coughed,' said the captain.

'I certainly thought so,' said Slaughter. No; everybody denied it.

'Fancy,' said the captain.

'Must be,' echoed Slaughter.

Cigars resumed – more smoke – another cough – smothered, but violent.

'Damned odd!' said the captain, staring about him.

'Sing'ler!' ejaculated the unconscious Mr Joseph Tuggs.

Lieutenant Slaughter looked first at one person mysteriously, then at another: then laid down his cigar, then approached the window on tiptoe, and pointed with his right thumb over his shoulder, in the direction of the curtain.

'Slaughter!' ejaculated the captain, rising from table, 'what do you mean?'

The lieutenant in reply, drew back the curtain and discovered Mr Cymon Tuggs behind it: pallid with apprehension, and blue with wanting to cough.

'Aha!' exclaimed the captain, furiously. 'What do I see? Slaughter, your sabre!'

'Cymon!' screamed the Tuggses.

'Mercy!' said Belinda.

'Platonic!' gasped Cymon.

'Your sabre!' roared the captain: 'Slaughter – unhand me – the villain's life!'

'Murder!' screamed the Tuggses.

'Hold him fast, sir!' faintly articulated Cymon.

'Water!' exclaimed Joseph Tuggs – and Mr Cymon Tuggs and all the ladies forthwith fainted away, and formed a tableau.

Most willingly would we conceal the disastrous termination of the six weeks' acquaintance. A troublesome form, and an arbitrary custom, however, prescribe that a story should have a conclusion, in addition to a commencement; we have therefore no alternative. Lieutenant Slaughter brought a message – the captain brought an action. Mr Joseph Tuggs interposed – the lieutenant negotiated. When Mr Cymon Tuggs recovered from the nervous disorder into which misplaced affection, and exciting circumstances, had plunged him, he found that his family had lost their pleasant acquaintance; that his father was minus fifteen hundred pounds; and the captain plus the precise sum. The money was paid to hush the matter up, but it got abroad notwithstanding; and there are not wanting some who affirm that three designing imposters never found more easy dupes, than did Captain Waters, Mrs Waters, and Lieutenant Slaughter, in the Tuggses at Ramsgate.

## Chapter Five

### *Horatio Sparkins*

First published in the *Monthly Magazine,* February 1834.

'Indeed, my love, he paid Teresa very great attention on the last assembly night,' said Mrs Malderton, addressing her spouse, who, after the fatigues of the day in the City, was sitting with a silk handkerchief over his head, and his feet on the fender, drinking his port; – 'very great attention; and I say again, every possible encouragement ought to be given him. He positively must be asked down here to dine.'

'Who must?' inquired Mr Malderton.

'Why, you know whom I mean, my dear – the young man with the black whiskers and the white cravat, who has just come out at our assembly, and whom all the girls are talking about. Young—dear me! what's his name? – Marianne, what *is* his name?' continued Mrs Malderton, addressing her youngest daughter, who was engaged in netting a purse, and looking sentimental.

'Mr Horatio Sparkins, ma,' replied Miss Marianne, with a sigh.

'Oh! yes, to be sure – Horatio Sparkins,' said Mrs Malderton. 'Decidedly the most gentleman-like young man I ever saw. I am sure in the beautifully made coat he wore the other night, he looked like – like—'

'Like Prince Leopold, ma – so noble, so full of sentiment!' suggested Marianne, in a tone of enthusiastic admiration.

'You should recollect, my dear,' resumed Mrs Malderton, 'that Teresa is now eight-and-twenty; and that it really is very important that something should be done.'

Miss Teresa Malderton was a very little girl, rather fat, with vermilion cheeks, but good-humoured, and still disengaged, although, to do her justice, the misfortune arose from no lack of perseverance on her part. In vain had she flirted for ten years; in vain had Mr and Mrs Malderton assiduously kept up an extensive acquaintance among the young eligible bachelors of Camberwell, and even of Wandsworth and Brixton; to say nothing of those who 'dropped in' from town. Miss Malderton was as well known as the lion on the top of Northumberland House, and had an equal chance of 'going off'.

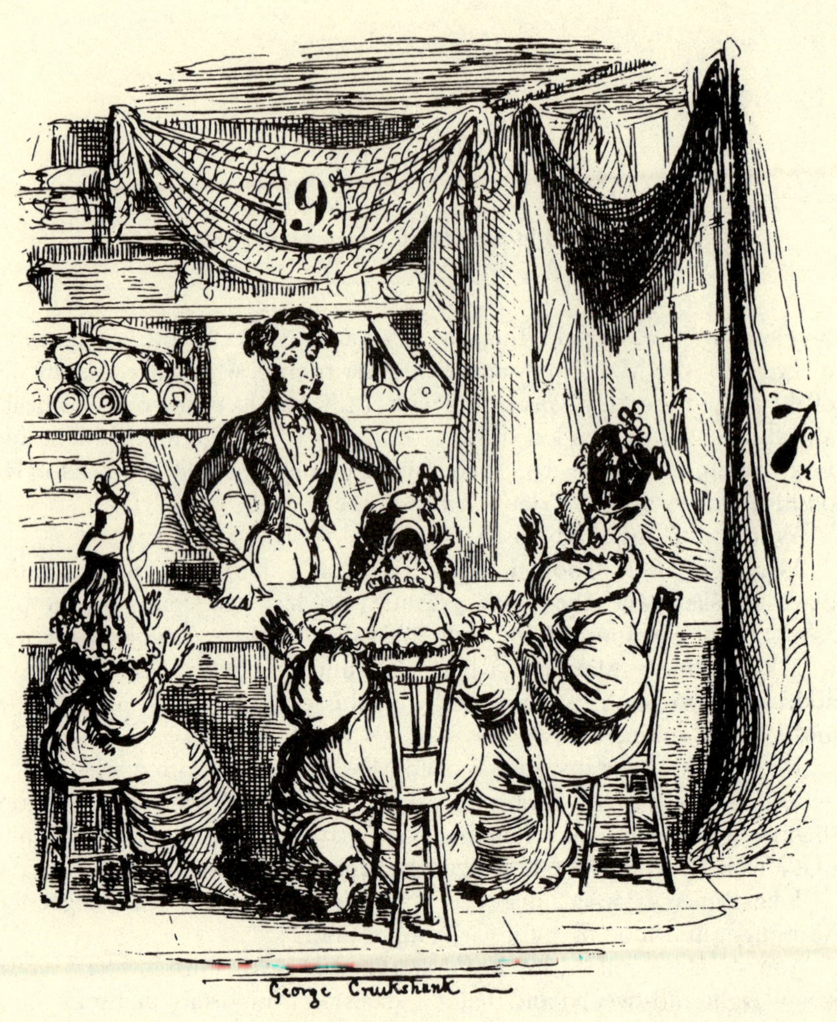


*Horatio Sparkins* *(see p. 358)*

'I am quite sure you'd like him,' continued Mrs Malderton, 'he is so gentlemanly!'

'So clever!' said Miss Marianne.

'And has such a flow of language!' added Miss Teresa.

'He has a great respect for you, my dear,' said Mrs Malderton to her husband. Mr Malderton coughed, and looked at the fire.

'Yes, I'm sure he's very much attached to pa's society,' said Miss Marianne.

'No doubt of it,' echoed Miss Teresa.

'Indeed, he said as much to me in confidence,' observed Mrs Malderton.

'Well, well,' returned Mr Malderton, somewhat flattered; 'if I see him at the assembly tomorrow, perhaps I'll ask him down. I hope he knows we live at Oak Lodge, Camberwell, my dear?'

'Of course – and that you keep a one-horse carriage.'

'I'll see about it,' said Mr Malderton, composing himself for a nap; 'I'll see about it.'

Mr Malderton was a man whose whole scope of ideas was limited to Lloyd's, the Exchange, the India House, and the Bank. A few successful speculations had raised him from a situation of obscurity and comparative poverty, to a state of affluence. As frequently happens in such cases, the ideas of himself and his family became elevated to an extraordinary pitch as their means increased; they affected fashion, taste, and many other fooleries, in imitation of their betters, and had a very decided and becoming horror of anything which could, by possibility, be considered *low.* He was hospitable from ostentation, illiberal from ignorance, and prejudiced from conceit. Egotism and the love of display induced him to keep an excellent table: convenience, and a love of good things of this life, ensured him plenty of guests. He liked to have clever men, or what he considered such, at his table, because it was a great thing to talk about; but he never could endure what he called 'sharp fellows'. Probably he cherished this feeling out of compliment to his two sons, who gave their respected parent no uneasiness in that particular. The family were ambitious of forming acquaintances and connexions in some sphere of society superior to that in which they themselves moved; and one of the necessary consequences of this desire, added to their utter ignorance of the world beyond their own small circle, was, that anyone who could lay claim to an acquaintance with people of rank and title, had a sure passport to the table at Oak Lodge, Camberwell.

The appearance of Mr Horatio Sparkins at the assembly had excited no small degree of surprise and curiosity among its regular frequenters. Who could he be? He was evidently reserved, and apparently melancholy. Was he a clergyman? – He danced too well. A barrister? – He said he was not called. He used very fine words, and talked a great deal. Could he be a distinguished foreigner, come to England for the purpose of describing the country, its manners and customs; and frequenting public balls and public dinners, with the view of becoming acquainted with high life, polished etiquette, and English refinement? – No, he had not a foreign accent. Was he a surgeon, a contributor to the magazines, a writer of fashionable novels, or an artist? – No; to each and all of these surmises, there existed some valid objection – 'Then,' said everybody, 'he must be *somebody.*' – 'I should think he must be,' reasoned Mr Malderton, within himself, 'because he perceives our superiority, and pays us so much attention.'

The night succeeding the conversation we have just recorded, was 'assembly night'. The double-fly was ordered to be at the door of Oak Lodge at nine o'clock precisely. The Miss Maldertons were dressed in sky-blue satin trimmed with artificial flowers; and Mrs M. (who was a little fat woman), in ditto ditto, looked like her eldest daughter multiplied by two. Mr Frederick Malderton, the eldest son, in full-dress costume, was the very *beau idéal* of a smart waiter; and Mr Thomas Malderton, the youngest, with his white dress stock, blue coat, bright buttons, and red watch ribbon, strongly resembled the portrait of that interesting but rash young gentleman, George Barnwell. Every member of the party had made up his or her mind to cultivate the acquaintance of Mr Horatio Sparkins. Miss Teresa, of course, was to be as amiable and interesting as ladies of eight-and-twenty on the look-out for a husband, usually are. Mrs Malderton would be all smiles and graces. Miss Marianne would request the favour of some verses for her album. Mr Malderton would patronise the great unknown by asking him to dinner. Tom intended to ascertain the extent of his information on the interesting topics of snuff and cigars. Even Mr Frederick Malderton himself, the family authority on all points of taste, dress, and fashionable arrangement; who had lodgings of his own in town; who had a free admission to Covent Garden theatre; who always dressed according to the fashions of the months; who went up the water twice a week in the season; and who actually had an intimate friend who once knew a gentleman who formerly lived in the Albany, – even he had determined that Mr Horatio Sparkins must be a devilish good fellow, and that he would do him the honour of challenging him to a game at billiards.

The first object that met the anxious eyes of the expectant family on their entrance into the ballroom, was the interesting Horatio, with his hair brushed off his forehead, and his eyes fixed on the ceiling, reclining in a contemplative attitude on one of the seats.

'There he is, my dear,' whispered Mrs Malderton to Mr Malderton.

'How like Lord Byron!' murmured Miss Teresa.

'Or Montgomery!' whispered Miss Marianne.

'Or the portraits of Captain Cook!' suggested Tom.

'Tom – don't be an ass!' said his father, who checked him on all occasions, probably with a view to prevent his becoming 'sharp' – which was very unnecessary.

The elegant Sparkins attitudinised with admirable effect, until the family had crossed the room. He then started up, with the most natural appearance of surprise and delight: accosted Mrs Malderton with the utmost cordiality; saluted the young ladies in the most enchanting manner; bowed to, and shook hands with, Mr Malderton, with a degree of respect amounting almost to veneration; and returned the greetings of the two young men in a half gratified, half patronising manner, which fully convinced them that he must be an important, and, at the same time, condescending personage.

'Miss Malderton,' said Horatio, after the ordinary salutations, and bowing very low, 'may I be permitted to presume to hope that you will allow me to have the pleasure—'

'I don't *think* I am engaged,' said Miss Teresa, with a dreadful affectation of indifference – 'but, really – so many—'

Horatio looked handsomely miserable.

'I shall be most happy,' simpered the interesting Teresa, at last. Horatio's countenance brightened up, like an old hat in a shower of rain.

'A very genteel young man, certainly!' said the gratified Mr Malderton, as the obsequious Sparkins and his partner joined the quadrille which was just forming.

'He has a remarkably good address,' said Mr Frederick.

'Yes, he is a prime fellow,' interposed Tom, who always managed to put his foot in it – 'he talks just like an auctioneer.'

'Tom!' said his father solemnly, 'I think I desired you, before, not to be a fool.' Tom looked as happy as a cock on a drizzly morning.

'How delightful!' said the interesting Horatio to his partner, as they promenaded the room at the conclusion of the set – 'how delightful, how refreshing it is, to retire from the cloudy storms, the vicissitudes, and the troubles of life, even if it be but for a few short fleeting moments: and to spend those moments, fading and evanescent though they be, in the delightful, the blessed society of one individual – whose frowns would be death, whose coldness would be madness, whose falsehood would be ruin, whose constancy would be bliss; the possession of whose affection would be the brightest and best reward that Heaven could bestow on man!'

'What feeling! what sentiment!' thought Miss Teresa, as she leaned more heavily on her companion's arm.

'But enough – enough!' resumed the elegant Sparkins, with a theatrical air. 'What have I said? what have I – I – to do with sentiments like these? Miss Malderton' – here he stopped short – 'may I hope to be permitted to offer the humble tribute of—'

'Really, Mr Sparkins,' returned the enraptured Teresa, blushing in the sweetest confusion, 'I must refer you to papa. I never can, without his consent, venture to—'

'Surely he cannot object—'

'Oh, yes. Indeed, indeed, you know him not!' interrupted Miss Teresa, well knowing there was nothing to fear, but wishing to make the interview resemble a scene in some romantic novel.

'He cannot object to my offering you a glass of negus,' returned the adorable Sparkins, with some surprise.

'Is that all?' thought the disappointed Teresa. 'What a fuss about nothing!'

'It will give me the greatest pleasure, sir, to see you to dinner at Oak Lodge, Camberwell, on Sunday next at five o'clock, if you have no better engagement,' said Mr Malderton, at the conclusion of the evening, as he and his sons were standing in conversation with Mr Horatio Sparkins.

Horatio bowed his acknowledgments, and accepted the flattering invitation.

'I must confess,' continued the father, offering his snuff box to his new acquaintance, 'that I don't enjoy these assemblies half so much as the comfort – I had almost said the luxury – of Oak Lodge. They have no great charms for an elderly man.'

'And after all, sir, what is man?' said the metaphysical Sparkins. 'I say, what is man?'

'Ah! very true,' said Mr Malderton; 'very true.'

'We know that we live and breathe,' continued Horatio; 'that we have wants and wishes, desires and appetites — '

'Certainly,' said Mr Frederick Malderton, looking profound.

'I say, we know that we exist,' repeated Horatio, raising his voice, 'but there we stop; there, is an end to our knowledge; there, is the summit of our attainments; there, is the termination of our ends. What more do we know?'

'Nothing,' replied Mr Frederick – than whom no one was more capable of answering for himself in that particular. Tom was about to hazard something, but, fortunately for his reputation, he caught his father's angry eye, and slunk off like a puppy convicted of petty larceny.

'Upon my word,' said Mr Malderton the elder, as they were returning home in the fly, 'that Mr Sparkins is a wonderful young man. Such surprising knowledge! such extraordinary information! and such a splendid mode of expressing himself'

'I think he must be somebody in disguise,' said Miss Marianne. 'How charmingly romantic!'

'He talks very loud and nicely,' timidly observed Tom, 'but I don't exactly understand what he means.'

'I almost begin to despair of *your* understanding anything, Tom,' said his father, who, of course, had been much enlightened by Mr Horatio Sparkins's conversation.

'It strikes me, Tom,' said Miss Teresa, 'that you have made yourself very ridiculous this evening.'

'No doubt of it,' cried everybody – and the unfortunate Tom reduced himself into the least possible space. That night, Mr and Mrs Malderton had a long conversation respecting their daughter's prospects and future arrangements. Miss Teresa went to bed, considering whether, in the event of her marrying a title, she could conscientiously encourage the visits of her present associates; and dreamed, all night, of disguised noblemen, large routs, ostrich plumes, bridal favours, and Horatio Sparkins.

Various surmises were hazarded on the Sunday morning, as to the mode of conveyance which the anxiously-expected Horatio would adopt. Did he keep a gig? – was it possible he could come on horseback? – or would he patronize the stage? These, and other various conjectures of equal importance, engrossed the attention of Mrs Malderton and her daughters during the whole morning after church.

'Upon my word, my dear, it's a most annoying thing that that vulgar brother of yours should have invited himself to dine here today,' said Mr Malderton to his wife. 'On account of Mr Sparkins's coming down, I purposely abstained from asking any one but Flamwell. And then to think of your brother – a tradesman – it's insufferable! I declare I wouldn't have him mention his shop, before our new guest – no, not for a thousand pounds! I wouldn't care if he had the good sense to conceal the disgrace he is to the family; but he's so fond of his horrible business, that he *will* let people know what he is.'

Mr Jacob Barton, the individual alluded to, was a large grocer; so vulgar, and so lost to all sense of feeling, that he actually never scrupled to avow that he wasn't above his business: 'he'd made his money by it, and he didn't care who know'd it.'

'Ah! Flamwell, my dear fellow, how d'ye do?' said Mr Malderton, as a little spoffish man, with green spectacles, entered the room. 'You got my note?'

'Yes I did; and here I am in consequence.'

'You don't happen to know this Mr Sparkins by name? You know everybody!'

Mr Flamwell was one of those gentlemen of remarkably extensive information whom one occasionally meets in society, who pretend to know everybody but in reality know nobody. At Malderton's, where any stories about great people were received with a greedy air, he was an especial favourite; and, knowing the kind of people he had to deal with, he carried his passion of claiming acquaintance with everybody, to the most immoderate length. He had rather a singular way of telling his greatest lies in a parenthesis, and with an air of self-denial, as if he feared being thought egotistical.

'Why, no, I don't know him by that name,' returned Flamwell, in a low tone, and with an air of immense importance. 'I have no doubt I know him, though. Is he tall?'

'Middle-sized,' said Miss Teresa.

'With black hair?' inquired Flamwell, hazarding a bold guess.

'Yes,' returned Miss Teresa, eagerly.

'Rather a snub nose?'

'No,' said the disappointed Teresa, 'he has a Roman nose.'

'I said a Roman nose, didn't I?' inquired Flamwell. 'He's an elegant young man?'

'Oh, certainly.'

'With remarkably prepossessing manners?'

'Oh, yes!' said all the family together. 'You must know him.'

'Yes, I thought you knew him, if he was anybody,' triumphantly exclaimed Mr Malderton. 'Who d'ye think he is?'

'Why from your description,' said Flamwell, ruminating, and sinking his voice almost to a whisper, 'he bears a strong resemblance to the Honourable Augustus Fitz-Edward Fitz-John Fitz-Osborne. He's a very talented young man, and rather eccentric. It's extremely probable he may have changed his name for some temporary purpose.'

Teresa's heart beat high. Could he be the Honourable Augustus Fitz-Edward Fitz-John Fitz-Osborne! What a name to be elegantly engraved upon two glazed cards, tied together with a piece of white satin ribbon! 'The Honourable Mrs Augustus Fitz-Edward Fitz-John Fitz-Osborne!' The thought was transport.

'It's five minutes to five,' said Mr Malderton, looking at his watch: 'I hope he's not going to disappoint us.'

'There he is!' exclaimed Miss Teresa, as a loud double knock was heard at the door. Everybody endeavoured to look – as people when they particularly expect a visitor always do – as if they were perfectly unsuspicious of the approach of anybody.

The room door opened – 'Mr Barton!' said the servant.

'Confound the man!' murmured Malderton. 'Ah! my dear sir, how d'ye do! Any news?'

'Why no,' returned the grocer, in his usual bluff manner. 'No, none partickler. None that I am much aware of. How d'ye do, gals and boys? Mr Flamwell, sir – glad to see you.'

'Here's Mr Sparkins!' said Tom, who had been looking out at the window, 'on *such* a black horse!' There was Horatio, sure enough, on a large black horse, curvetting and prancing along, like an Astley's supernumerary. After a great deal of reining in, and pulling up, with the accompaniments of snorting, rearing, and kicking, the animal consented to stop at about a hundred yards from the gate, where Mr Sparkins dismounted, and confided him to the care of Mr Malderton's groom. The ceremony of introduction was gone through, in all due form. Mr Flamwell looked from behind his green spectacles at Horatio with an air of mysterious importance; and the gallant Horatio looked unutterable things at Teresa.

'Is he the Honourable Mr Augustus What's-his-name?' whispered Mrs Malderton to Flamwell, as he was escorting her to the dining room.

'Why, no – at least not exactly,' returned that great authority – 'not exactly.'

'Who *is* he then?'

'Hush!' said Flamwell, nodding his head with a grave air, importing that he knew very well; but was prevented, by some grave reasons of state, from disclosing the important secret. It might be one of the ministers making himself acquainted with the views of the people.

'Mr Sparkins,' said the delighted Mrs Malderton, 'pray divide the ladies. John, put a chair for the gentleman between Miss Teresa and Miss Marianne.' This was addressed to a man who, on ordinary occasions, acted as half-groom, half-gardener; but who, as it was important to make an impression on Mr Sparkins, had been forced into a white neckerchief and shoes, and touched up, and brushed, to look like a second footman.

The dinner was excellent; Horatio was most attentive to Miss Teresa, and everyone felt in high spirits, except Mr Malderton, who, knowing the propensity of his brother-in-law, Mr Barton, endured that sort of agony which the newspapers inform us is experienced by the surrounding neighbourhood when a pot boy hangs himself in a hayloft, and which is 'much easier to be imagined than described.'

'Have you seen your friend, Sir Thomas Noland, lately, Flamwell?' inquired Mr Malderton, casting a sidelong look at Horatio, to see what effect the mention of so great a man had upon him.

'Why, no – not very lately. I saw Lord Gubbleton the day before yesterday.'

'Ah! I hope his lordship is very well?' said Malderton, in a tone of the greatest interest. It is scarcely necessary to say that, until that moment, he had been quite innocent of the existence of such a person.

'Why, yes; he was very well – very well indeed. He's a devilish good fellow. I met him in the City, and had a long chat with him. Indeed, I'm rather intimate with him. I couldn't stop to talk to him as long as I could wish, though, because I was on my way to a banker's, a very rich man, and a member of Parliament, with whom I am also rather, indeed I may say very, intimate.'

'I know whom you mean,' returned the host, consequentially – in reality knowing as much about the matter as Flamwell himself. 'He has a capital business.'

This was touching on a dangerous topic.

'Talking of business,' interposed Mr Barton, from the centre of the table. 'A gentleman whom you knew very well, Malderton, before you made that first lucky spec of yours, called at our shop the other day, and—'

'Barton, may I trouble you for a potato?' interrupted the wretched master of the house, hoping to nip the story in the bud.

'Certainly,' returned the grocer, quite insensible of his brother-in-law's object – 'and he said in a very plain manner — '

'*Floury,* if you please,' interrupted Malderton again; dreading the termination of the anecdote, and fearing a repetition of the word 'shop.'

'He said, says he,' continued the culprit, after dispatching the potato; 'says he, how goes on your business? So I said, jokingly – you know my way – says I, I'm never above my business, and I hope my business will never be above me. Ha, ha!'

'Mr Sparkins,' said the host, vainly endeavouring to conceal his dismay, 'a glass of wine?'

'With the utmost pleasure, sir.'

'Happy to see you.'

'Thank you.'

'We were talking the other evening,' resumed the host, addressing Horatio, partly with the view of displaying the conversational powers of his new acquaintance, and partly in the hope of drowning the grocer's stories – 'we were talking the other night about the nature of man. Your argument struck me very forcibly.'

'And me,' said Mr Frederick. Horatio made a graceful inclination of the head.

'Pray, what is your opinion of woman, Mr Sparkins?' inquired Mrs Malderton. The young ladies simpered.

'Man,' replied Horatio, 'man, whether he ranged the bright, gay, flowery plains of a second Eden, or the more sterile, barren, and I may say, commonplace regions, to which we are compelled to accustom ourselves, in times such as these; man, under any circumstances, or in any place – whether he were bending beneath the withering blasts of the frigid zone, or scorching under the rays of a vertical sun – man, without woman, would be – alone.'

'I am very happy to find you entertain such honourable opinions, Mr Sparkins,' said Mrs Malderton.

'And I,' added Miss Teresa. Horatio looked his delight, and the young lady blushed.

'Now, it's my opinion — ' said Mr Barton.

'I know what you're going to say,' interposed Malderton, determined not to give his relation another opportunity, 'and I don't agree with you.'

'What!' inquired the astonished grocer.

'I am sorry to differ from you, Barton,' said the host, in as positive a manner as if he really were contradicting a position which the other had laid down, 'but I cannot give my assent to what I consider a very monstrous proposition.'

'But I meant to say — '

'You never can convince me,' said Malderton, with an air of obstinate determination. 'Never.'

'And I,' said Mr Frederick, following up his father's attack, 'cannot entirely agree in Mr Sparkins's argument.'

'What!' said Horatio, who became more metaphysical, and more argumentative, as he saw the female part of the family listening in wondering delight – 'what! Is effect the consequence of cause? Is cause the precursor of effect?'

'That's the point,' said Flamwell.

'To be sure,' said Mr Malderton.

'Because, if effect is the consequence of cause, and if cause does precede effect, I apprehend you are wrong,' added Horatio.

'Decidedly,' said the toad-eating Flamwell.

'At least,' I apprehend that to be the just and logical deduction?' said Sparkins, in a tone of interrogation.

'No doubt of it.' chimed in Flamwell again. 'It settles the point.'

'Well, perhaps it does,' said Mr Frederick; 'I didn't see it before.'

'I don't exactly see it now,' thought the grocer; 'but I suppose it's all right.'

'How wonderfully clever he is!' whispered Mrs Malderton to her daughters, as they retired to the drawing room.

'Oh, he's quite a love!' said both the young ladies together; 'he talks like an oracle. He must have seen a great deal of life.'

The gentlemen being left to themselves, a pause ensued, during which everybody looked very grave, as if they were quite overcome by the profound nature of the previous discussion. Flamwell, who had made up his mind to find out who and what Mr Horatio Sparkins really was, first broke silence.

'Excuse me, sir,' said that distinguished personage, 'I presume you have studied for the bar? I thought of entering once, myself – indeed, I'm rather intimate with some of the highest ornaments of that distinguished profession.'

'N – no!' said Horatio, with a little hesitation; 'not exactly.'

'But you have been much among the silk gowns, or I mistake?' inquired Flamwell, deferentially.

'Nearly all my life,' returned Sparkins.

The question was thus pretty well settled in the mind of Mr Flamwell. He was a young gentleman 'about to be called'.

'I shouldn't like to be a barrister,' said Tom, speaking for the first time, and looking round the table to find somebody who would notice the remark.

No one made any reply.

'I shouldn't like to wear a wig,' said Tom, hazarding another observation.

'Tom, I beg you will not make yourself ridiculous,' said his father. 'Pray listen, and improve yourself by the conversation you hear, and don't be constantly making these absurd remarks.'

'Very well, father,' replied the unfortunate Tom, who had not spoken a word since he had asked for another slice of beef at a quarter-past five o'clock P.M., and it was then eight.

'Well, Tom,' observed his good-natured uncle, 'never mind! *I* think with you. *I* shouldn't like to wear a wig. I'd rather wear an apron.'

Mr Malderton coughed violently. Mr Barton resumed – 'For if a man's above his business—'

The cough returned with tenfold violence, and did not cease until the unfortunate cause of it, in his alarm, had quite forgotten what he intended to say.

'Mr Sparkins,' said Flamwell, returning to the charge, 'do you happen to know Mr Delafontaine, of Bedford Square?'

'I have exchanged cards with him; since which, indeed, I have had an opportunity of serving him considerably,' replied Horatio, slightly colouring; no doubt, at having been betrayed into making the acknowledgment.

'You are very lucky, if you have had an opportunity of obliging that great man,' observed Flamwell, with an air of profound respect.

'I don't know who he is,' he whispered to Mr Malderton, confidentially, as they followed Horatio up to the drawing room. 'It's quite clear, however, that he belongs to the law, and that he is somebody of great importance, and very highly connected.'

'No doubt, no doubt,' returned his companion.

The remainder of the evening passed away most delightfully. Mr Malderton, relieved from his apprehensions by the circumstance of Mr Barton's falling into a profound sleep, was as affable and gracious as possible. Miss Teresa played the 'Fall of Paris', as Mr Sparkins declared, in a most masterly manner, and both of them, assisted by Mr Frederick, tried over glees and trios without number; they having made the pleasing discovery that their voices harmonised beautifully. To be sure, they all sang the first part; and Horatio, in addition to the slight drawback of having no ear, was perfectly innocent of knowing a note of music; still, they passed the time very agreeably, and it was past twelve o'clock before Mr Sparkins ordered the mourning-coach-looking steed to be brought out – an order which was only complied with on the distinct understanding that he was to repeat his visit on the following Sunday.

'But perhaps Mr Sparkins will form one of our party tomorrow evening?' suggested Mrs M. 'Mr Malderton intends taking the girls to see the pantomime.' Mr Sparkins bowed, and promised to join the party in box 48, in the course of the evening.

'We will not tax you for the morning,' said Miss Teresa, bewitchingly; 'for ma is going to take us to all sorts of places, shopping. I know that gentlemen have a great horror of that employment.' Mr Sparkins bowed again, and declared that he should be delighted, but business of importance occupied him in the morning. Flamwell looked at Malderton significantly. – 'It's term time!' he whispered.

At twelve o'clock on the following morning, the 'fly' was at the door of Oak Lodge, to convey Mrs Malderton and her daughters on their expedition for the day. They were to dine and dress for the play at a friend's house. First, driving thither with their band boxes, they departed on their first errand to make some purchases at Messrs Jones, Spruggins, and Smith's, of Tottenham Court Road; after which, they were to go to Redmayne's in Bond Street; thence, to innumerable places that no one ever heard of. The young ladies beguiled the tediousness of the ride by eulogising Mr Horatio Sparkins, scolding their mamma for taking them so far to save a shilling, and wondering whether they should ever reach their destination. At length, the vehicle stopped before a dirty-looking ticketed linen draper's shop, with goods of all kinds, and labels of all sorts and sizes, in the window. There were dropsical figures of seven with a little three-farthings in the corner, 'perfectly invisible to the naked eye'; three hundred and fifty thousand ladies' boas, *from* one shilling and a penny halfpenny; real French kid shoes, at two and ninepence per pair; green parasols, at an equally cheap rate; and 'every description of goods', as the proprietors said – and they must know best – 'fifty per cent under cost price'.

'Lor! ma, what a place you have brought us to!' said Miss Teresa; 'what *would* Mr Sparkins say if he could see us!'

'Ah! what, indeed!' said Miss Marianne, horrified at the idea.

'Pray be seated, ladies. What is the first article?' inquired the obsequious master of the ceremonies of the establishment, who, in his large white neckcloth and formal tie, looked like a bad 'portrait of a gentleman' in the Somerset House exhibition.

'I want to see some silks,' answered Mrs Malderton.

'Directly, ma'am. – Mr Smith! Where *is* Mr Smith?'

'Here, sir,' cried a voice at the back of the shop.

'Pray make haste, Mr Smith,' said the M.C. 'You never are to be found when you're wanted, sir.'

Mr Smith, thus enjoined to use all possible dispatch, leaped over the counter with great agility, and placed himself before the newly arrived customers. Mrs Malderton uttered a faint scream; Miss Teresa, who had been stooping down to talk to her sister, raised her head, and beheld – Horatio Sparkins!

'We will draw a veil,' as novel writers say, over the scene that ensued. The mysterious, philosophical, romantic, metaphysical Sparkins – he who, to the interesting Teresa, seemed like the embodied idea of the young dukes and poetical exquisites in blue silk dressing gowns, and ditto ditto slippers, of whom she had read and dreamed, but had never expected to behold, was suddenly converted into Mr Samuel Smith, the assistant at a 'cheap shop'; the junior partner in a slippery firm of some three weeks' existence. The dignified evanishment of the hero of Oak Lodge, on this unexpected recognition, could only be equalled by that of a furtive dog with a considerable kettle at his tail. All the hopes of the Maldertons were destined at once to melt away, like the lemon ices at a Company's dinner; Almack's was still to them as distant as the North Pole; and Miss Teresa had as much chance of a husband as Captain Ross had of the northwest passage.

Years have elapsed since the occurrence of this dreadful morning. The daisies have thrice bloomed on Camberwell Green; the sparrows have thrice repeated their vernal chirps in Camberwell Grove; but the Miss Maldertons are still unmated. Miss Teresa's case is more desperate than ever; but Flamwell is yet in the zenith of his reputation; and the family have the same predilection for aristocratic personages, with an increased aversion to anything *low*.

## Chapter Six

### *The Black Veil*

Specially written for the first collected edition of *Sketches* 1836.

One winter's evening, towards the close of the year 1800, or within a year or two of that time, a young medical practitioner, recently established in business, was seated by a cheerful fire in his little parlour, listening to the wind which was beating the rain in pattering drops against the window, or rumbling dismally in the chimney. The night was wet and cold; he had been walking through mud and water the whole day, and was now comfortably reposing in his dressing gown and slippers, more than half asleep and less than half awake, revolving a thousand matters in his wandering imagination. First, he thought how hard the wind was blowing, and how the cold, sharp rain would be at that moment beating in his face, if he were not comfortably housed at home. Then, his mind reverted to his annual Christmas visit to his native place and dearest friends; he thought how glad they would all be to see him, and how happy it would make Rose if he could only tell her that he had found a patient at last, and hoped to have more, and to come down again, in a few months' time, and marry her, and take her home to gladden his lonely fireside, and stimulate him to fresh exertions. Then, he began to wonder when his first patient would appear, or whether he was destined, by a special dispensation of Providence, never to have any patients at all; and then, he thought about Rose again, and dropped to sleep and dreamed about her, till the tones of her sweet merry voice sounded in his ears, and her soft tiny hand rested on his shoulder.

There *was* a hand upon his shoulder, but it was neither soft nor tiny; its owner being a corpulent round-headed boy, who, in consideration of the sum of one shilling per week and his food, was let out by the parish to carry medicine and messages. As there was no demand for the medicine, however, and no necessity for the messages, he usually occupied his unemployed hours – averaging fourteen a day – in abstracting peppermint drops, taking animal nourishment, and going to sleep.

'A lady, sir – a lady!' whispered the boy, rousing his master with a shake.

'What lady?' cried our friend, starting up, not quite certain that his dream was an illusion, and half expecting that it might be Rose herself. – 'What lady? Where?'

'*There,* sir!' replied the boy, pointing to the glass door leading into the surgery, with an expression of alarm which the very unusual apparition of a customer might have tended to excite.

The surgeon looked towards the door, and started himself, for an instant, on beholding the appearance of his unlooked-for visitor.

It was a singularly tall woman, dressed in deep mourning, and standing so close to the door that her face almost touched the glass. The upper part of her figure was carefully muffled in a black shawl, as if for the purpose of concealment; and her face was shrouded by a thick black veil. She stood perfectly erect, her figure was drawn up to its full height, and though the surgeon *felt* that the eyes beneath the veil were fixed on him, she stood perfectly motionless, and evinced, by no gesture whatever, the slightest consciousness of his having turned towards her.

'Do you wish to consult me?' he inquired, with some hesitation, holding open the door. It opened inwards, and therefore the action did not alter the position of the figure, which still remained motionless on the same spot.

She slightly inclined her head, in token of acquiescence.

'Pray walk in,' said the surgeon.

The figure moved a step forward; and then, turning its head in the direction of the boy – to his infinite horror – appeared to hesitate.

'Leave the room, Tom,' said the young man, addressing the boy, whose large round eyes had been extended to their utmost width during this brief interview. 'Draw the curtain, and shut the door.'

The boy drew a green curtain across the glass part of the door, retired into the surgery, closed the door after him, and immediately applied one of his large eyes to the keyhole on the other side.

The surgeon drew a chair to the fire, and motioned the visitor to a seat. The mysterious figure slowly moved towards it. As the blaze shone upon the black dress, the surgeon observed that the bottom of it was saturated with mud and rain.

'You are very wet,' he said.

'I am,' said the stranger, in a low deep voice.

'And you are ill?' added the surgeon, compassionately, for the tone was that of a person in pain.

'I am,' was the reply – 'very ill; not bodily, but mentally. It is not for myself, or on my own behalf,' continued the stranger, 'that I come to you. If I laboured under bodily disease, I should not be out, alone, at such an hour, or on such a night as this; and if I were afflicted with it, twenty-four hours hence, God knows how gladly I would lie down and pray to die. It is for another that I beseech your aid, sir. I may be mad to ask it for him – I think I am; but, night after night, through the long dreary hours of watching and weeping, the thought has been ever present to my mind; and though even *I* see the hopelessness of human assistance availing him, the bare thought of laying him in his grave without it makes my blood run cold!' And a shudder, such as the surgeon well knew art could not produce, trembled through the speaker's frame.

There was a desperate earnestness in this woman's manner, that went to the young man's heart. He was young in his profession, and had not yet witnessed enough of the miseries which are daily presented before the eyes of its members, to have grown comparatively callous to human suffering.

'If,' he said, rising hastily, 'the person of whom you speak, be in so hopeless a condition as you describe, not a moment is to be lost. I will go with you instantly. Why did you not obtain medical advice before?'

'Because it would have been useless before – because it is useless even now,' replied the woman, clasping her hands passionately.

The surgeon gazed, for a moment, on the black veil, as if to ascertain the expression of the features beneath it; its thickness, however, rendered such a result impossible.

'You *are* ill,' he said, gently, 'although you do not know it. The fever which has enabled you to bear, without feeling it, the fatigue you have evidently undergone, is burning within you now. Put that to your lips,' he continued, pouring out a glass of water – 'compose yourself for a few moments, and then tell me, as calmly as you can, what the disease of the patient is, and how long he has been ill. When I know what it is necessary I should know, to render my visit serviceable to him, I am ready to accompany you.'

The stranger lifted the glass of water to her mouth, without raising the veil; put it down again untasted; and burst into tears.

'I know,' she said, sobbing aloud, 'that what I say to you now, seems like the ravings of fever. I have been told so before, less kindly than by you. I am not a young woman; and they do say, that as life steals on towards its final close, the last short remnant, worthless as it may seem to all beside, is dearer to its possessor than all the years that have gone before, connected though they be with the recollection of old friends long since dead, and young ones – children perhaps – who have fallen off from, and forgotten one as completely as if they had died too. My natural term of life cannot be many years longer, and should be dear on that account; but I would lay it down without a sigh – with cheerfulness – with joy – if what I tell you now were only false or imaginary. Tomorrow morning he of whom I speak will be, I *know,* though I would fain think otherwise, beyond the reach of human aid; and yet, tonight, though he is in deadly peril, you must not see, and could not serve, him.'

'I am unwilling to increase your distress,' said the surgeon, after a short pause, 'by making any comment on what you have just said, or appearing desirous to investigate a subject you are so anxious to conceal; but there is an inconsistency in your statement which I cannot reconcile with probability. This person is dying tonight, and I cannot see him when my assistance might possibly avail; you apprehend it will be useless tomorrow, and yet you would have me see him then! If he be, indeed, as dear to you as your words and manner would imply, why not try to save his life before delay and the progress of his disease render it impracticable?'

'God help me!' exclaimed the woman, weeping bitterly, 'how can I hope strangers will believe what appears incredible, even to myself? You will *not* see him then, sir?' she added, rising suddenly.

'I did not say that I declined to see him,' replied the surgeon; 'but I warn you, that if you persist in this extraordinary procrastination, and the individual dies, a fearful responsibility rests with you.'

'The responsibility will rest heavily somewhere,' replied the stranger bitterly. 'Whatever responsibility rests with me, I am content to bear, and ready to answer.'

'As I incur none,' continued the surgeon, 'by acceding to your request, I will see him in the morning, if you leave me the address. At what hour can he be seen?'

'*Nine*,' replied the stranger.

'You must excuse me pressing these inquiries,' said the surgeon. 'But is he in your charge now?'

'He is not,' was the rejoinder.

'Then, if I gave you instructions for his treatment through the night, you could not assist him?'

The woman wept bitterly, as she replied, 'I could not.'

Finding that there was but little prospect of obtaining more information by prolonging the interview; and anxious to spare the woman's feelings, which, subdued at first by a violent effort, were now irrepressible and most painful to witness; the surgeon repeated his promise of calling in the morning at the appointed hour. His visitor, after giving him a direction to an obscure part of Walworth, left the house in the same mysterious manner in which she had entered it.

It will be readily believed that no extraordinary a visit produced a considerable impression on the mind of the young surgeon; and that he speculated a great deal and to very little purpose on the possible circumstances of the case. In common with the generality of people, he had often heard and read of singular instances, in which a presentiment of death, at a particular day, or even minute, had been entertained and realised. At one moment he was inclined to think that the present might be such a case; but then it occurred to him that all the anecdotes of the kind he had ever heard, were of persons who had been troubled with a foreboding of their own death. This woman, however, spoke of another person – a man; and it was impossible to suppose that a mere dream or delusion of fancy would induce her to speak of his approaching dissolution with such terrible certainty as she had spoken. It could not be that the man was to be murdered in the morning, and that the woman, originally a consenting party, and bound to secrecy by an oath, had relented, and, though unable to prevent the commission of some outrage on the victim, had determined to prevent his death if possible, by the timely interposition of medical aid? The idea of such things happening within two miles of the metropolis appeared too wild and preposterous to be entertained beyond the instant. Then, his original impression that the woman's intellects were disordered, recurred; and, as it was the only mode of solving the difficulty with any degree of satisfaction, he obstinately made up his mind to believe that she was mad. Certain misgivings upon this point, however, stole upon his thoughts at the time, and presented themselves again and again through the long dull course of a sleepless night; during which, in spite of all his efforts to the contrary, he was unable to banish the black veil from his disturbed imagination.

The back part of Walworth, at its greatest distance from town, is a straggling miserable place enough, even in these days; but, five-and-thirty years ago, the greater portion of it was little better than a dreary waste, inhabited by a few scattered people of questionable character, whose poverty prevented their living in any better neighbourhood, or whose pursuits and mode of life rendered its solitude desirable. Very many of the houses which have since sprung up on all sides, were not built until some years afterwards; and the great majority even of those which were sprinkled about, at irregular intervals, were of the rudest and most miserable description.

The appearance of the place through which he walked in the morning, was not calculated to raise the spirits of the young surgeon, or to dispel any feeling of anxiety or depression which the singular kind of visit he was about to make, had awakened. Striking off from the high road, his way lay across a marshy common, through irregular lanes, with here and there a ruinous and dismantled cottage fast falling to pieces with decay and neglect. A stunted tree, or pool of stagnant water, roused into a sluggish action by the heavy rain of the preceding night, skirted the path occasionally; and, now and then, a miserable patch of garden-ground, with a few old boards knocked together for a summer house, and old palings imperfectly mended with stakes pilfered from the neighbouring hedges, bore testimony, at once to the poverty of the inhabitants, and the little scruple they entertained in appropriating the property of other people to their own use. Occasionally, a filthy-looking woman would make her appearance from the door of a dirty house, to empty the contents of some cooking utensil into the gutter in front, or to scream after a little slip-shod girl, who had contrived to stagger a few yards from the door under the weight of a sallow infant almost as big as herself; but scarcely anything was stirring around; and so much of the prospect as could be faintly traced through the cold damp mist which hung heavily over it, presented a lonely and dreary appearance perfectly in keeping with the objects we have described.

After plodding wearily through the mud and mire; making many inquiries for the place to which he had been directed; and receiving as many contradictory and unsatisfactory replies in return; the young man at length arrived before the house which had been pointed out to him as the object of his destination. It was a small low building, one story above the ground, with even a more desolate and unpromising exterior than any he had yet passed. An old yellow curtain was closely drawn across the window upstairs, and the parlour shutters were closed, but not fastened. The house was detached from any other, and, as it stood at an angle of a narrow lane, there was no other habitation in sight.

When we say that the surgeon hesitated, and walked a few paces beyond the house, before he could prevail upon himself to lift the knocker, we say nothing that need raise a smile upon the face of the boldest reader. The police of London were a very different body in that day; the isolated position of the suburbs, when the rage for building and the progress of improvement had not yet begun to connect them with the main body of the city and its environs, rendered many of them (and this in particular) a place of resort for the worst and most depraved characters. Even the streets in the gayest parts of London were imperfectly lighted at that time; and such places as these were left entirely to the mercy of the moon and stars. The chances of detecting desperate characters, or of tracing them to their haunts, were thus rendered very few, and their offences naturally increased in boldness, as the consciousness of comparative security became the more impressed upon them by daily experience. Added to these considerations, it must be remembered that the young man had spent some time in the public hospitals of the metropolis, and, although neither Burke nor Bishop had then gained a horrible notoriety, his own observation might have suggested to him how easily the atrocities to which the former has since given his name, might be committed. Be this as it may, whatever reflection made him hesitate, he *did* hesitate: but, being a young man of strong mind and great personal courage, it was only for an instant; – he stepped briskly back and knocked gently at the door.

A low whispering was audible, immediately afterwards, as if some person at the end of the passage were conversing stealthily with another on the landing above. It was succeeded by the noise of a pair of heavy boots upon the bare floor. The door-chain was softly unfastened; the door opened; and a tall, ill-favoured man, with black hair, and a face, as the surgeon often declared afterwards, as pale and haggard as the countenance of any dead man he ever saw, presented himself.

'Walk in, sir,' he said in a low tone.

The surgeon did so, and the man having secured the door again, by the chain, led the way to a small back parlour at the extremity of the passage.

'Am I in time?'

'Too soon!' replied the man. The surgeon turned hastily round, with a gesture of astonishment not unmixed with alarm, which he found it impossible to repress.

'If you'll step in here, sir,' said the man, who had evidently noticed the action – 'if you'll step in here, sir, you won't be detained five minutes, I assure you.'

The surgeon at once walked into the room. The man closed the door, and left him alone.

It was a little cold room, with no other furniture than two deal chairs, and a table of the same material. A handful of fire, unguarded by any fender, was burning in the grate, which brought out the damp if it served no more comfortable purpose, for the unwholesome moisture was stealing down the walls, in long slug-like tracks. The window, which was broken and patched in many places, looked into a small enclosed piece of ground, almost covered with water. Not a sound was to be heard, either within the house or without. The young surgeon sat down by the fireplace, to await the result of his first professional visit.

He had not remained in this position many minutes, when the noise of some approaching vehicle struck his ear. It stopped; the street door was opened; a low talking succeeded, accompanied with a shuffling noise of footsteps, along the passage and on the stairs, as if two or three men were engaged in carrying some heavy body to the room above. The creaking of the stairs, a few seconds afterwards, announced that the newcomers having completed their task, whatever it was, were leaving the house. The door was again closed, and the former silence was restored.

Another five minutes had elapsed, and the surgeon had resolved to explore the house, in search of someone to whom he might make his errand known, when the room door opened, and his last night's visitor, dressed in exactly the same manner, with the veil lowered as before, motioned him to advance. The singular height of her form, coupled with the circumstance of her not speaking, caused the idea to pass across his brain for an instant, that it might be a man disguised in woman's attire. The hysteric sobs which issued from beneath the veil, and the convulsive attitude of grief of the whole figure, however, at once exposed the absurdity of the suspicion; and he hastily followed.

The woman led the way upstairs to the front room, and paused at the door, to let him enter first. It was scantily furnished with an old deal box, a few chairs, and a tent bedstead, without hangings or cross rails, which was covered with a patchwork counterpane. The dim light admitted through the curtain which he had noticed from the outside, rendered the objects in the room so indistinct, and communicated to all of them so uniform a hue, that he did not, at first, perceive the object on which his eye at once rested when the woman rushed frantically past him, and flung herself on her knees by the bedside.

Stretched upon the bed, closely enveloped in a linen wrapper, and covered with blankets, lay a human form, stiff and motionless. The head and face, which were those of a man, were uncovered, save by a bandage which passed over the head and under the chin. The eyes were closed. The left arm lay heavily across the bed, and the woman held the passive hand.

The surgeon gently pushed the woman aside, and took the hand in his.

'My God!' he exclaimed, letting it fall involuntarily – 'the man is dead!'

The woman started to her feet and beat her hands together. 'Oh! don't say so, sir,' she exclaimed, with a burst of passion, amounting almost to frenzy. 'Oh! don't say so, sir! I can't bear it! Men have been brought to life, before, when unskillful people have given them up for lost; and men have died, who might have been restored, if proper means had been resorted to. Don't let him lie here, sir, without one effort to save him! This very moment life may be passing away. Do try, sir, – do, for Heaven's sake!' – And while speaking, she hurriedly chafed, first the forehead, and then the breast, of the senseless form before her; and then, wildly beat the cold hands, which, when she ceased to hold them, fell listlessly and heavily back on the coverlet.

'It is of no use, my good woman,' said the surgeon, soothingly, as he withdrew his hand from the man's breast. 'Stay – undraw that curtain!'

'Why?' said the woman, starting up.

'Undraw that curtain!' repeated the surgeon in an agitated tone.

'*I* darkened the room on purpose,' said the woman, throwing herself before him as he rose to undraw it. – 'Oh! sir, have pity on me! If it can be of no use, and he is really dead, do not expose that form to other eyes than mine!'

'This man died no natural or easy death,' said the surgeon. 'I *must* see the body!' With a motion so sudden, that the woman hardly knew that he had slipped from beside her, he tore open the curtain, admitted the full light of day, and returned to the bedside.

'There has been violence here,' he said, pointing towards the body, and gazing intently on the face, from which the black veil was now, for the first time, removed. In the excitement of a minute before, the female had thrown off the bonnet and veil, and now stood with her eyes fixed upon him. Her features were those of a woman about fifty, who had once been handsome. Sorrow and weeping had left traces upon them which not time itself would ever have produced without their aid; her face was deadly pale; and there was a nervous contortion of the lip, and an unnatural fire in her eye, which showed too plainly that her bodily and mental powers had nearly sunk beneath an accumulation of misery.

'There has been violence here,' said the surgeon, preserving his searching glance.

'There has!' replied the woman.

'This man has been murdered.'

'That I call God to witness he has,' said the woman, passionately; 'pitilessly, inhumanly murdered!'

'By whom?' said the surgeon, seizing the woman by the arm.

'Look at the butchers' marks, and then ask me!' she replied.

The surgeon turned his face towards the bed, and bent over the body which now lay full in the light of the window. The throat was swollen, and a livid mark encircled it. The truth flashed suddenly upon him.

'This is one of the men who were hanged this morning!' he exclaimed, turning away with a shudder.

'It is,' replied the woman, with a cold, unmeaning stare.

'Who was he?' inquired the surgeon.

'*My son*,' rejoined the woman; and fell senseless at his feet.

It was true. A companion, equally guilty with himself, had been acquitted for want of evidence; and this man had been left for death, and executed. To recount the circumstances of the case, at this distant period, must be unnecessary, and might give pain to some persons still alive. The history was an everyday one. The mother was a widow without friends or money, and had denied herself necessaries to bestow them on her orphan boy. That boy, unmindful of her prayers, and forgetful of the sufferings she had endured for him – incessant anxiety of mind, and voluntary starvation of body – had plunged into a career of dissipation and crime. And this was the result; his own death by the hangman's hands, and his mother's shame, and incurable insanity.

For many years after this occurrence, and when profitable and arduous avocations would have led many men to forget that such a miserable being existed, the young surgeon was a daily visitor at the side of the harmless mad woman; not only soothing her by his presence and kindness, but alleviating the rigour of her condition by pecuniary donations for her comfort and support, bestowed with no sparing hand. In the transient gleam of recollection and consciousness which preceded her death, a prayer for his welfare and protection, as fervent as mortal ever breathed, rose from the lips of this poor friendless creature. That prayer flew to Heaven, and was heard. The blessings he was instrumental in conferring, have been repaid to him a thousand fold; but, amid all the honours of rank and station which have since been heaped upon him, and which he has so well earned, he can have no reminiscence more gratifying to his heart than that connected with The Black Veil.

## Chapter Seven

### *The Steam Excursion*

First published in the *Monthly Magazine,* October 1834. For a probable source for many details in this sketch see Kathleen Tillotson, 'Dickens and a Story by John Poole', *The Dickensian,* Vol. 52 (1956) pp. 69–70.

Mr Percy Noakes was a law student, inhabiting a set of chambers on the fourth floor, in one of those houses in Gray's Inn Square which command an extensive view of the gardens, and their usual adjuncts – flaunting nursery maids, and townmade children, with parenthetical legs. Mr Percy Noakes was what is generally termed – 'a devilish good fellow'. He had a large circle of acquaintance, and seldom dined at his own expense. He used to talk politics to papas, flatter the vanity of mammas, do the amiable to their daughters, make pleasure engagements with their sons, and romp with the younger branches. Like those paragons of perfection, advertising footmen out of place, he was always 'willing to make himself generally useful'. If any old lady, whose son was in India, gave a ball, Mr Percy Noakes was master of the ceremonies; if any young lady made a stolen match, Mr Percy Noakes gave her away; if a juvenile wife presented her husband with a blooming cherub, Mr Percy Noakes was either godfather, or deputy godfather; and if any member of a friend's family died, Mr Percy Noakes was invariably to be seen in the second mourning coach, with a white handkerchief to his eyes, sobbing – to use his own appropriate and expressive description – 'like winkin'!'

It may readily be imagined that these numerous avocations were rather calculated to interfere with Mr Percy Noakes's professional studies. Mr Percy Noakes was perfectly aware of the fact, and had, therefore, after mature reflection, made up his mind not to study at all – a laudable determination, to which he adhered in the most praiseworthy manner. His sitting room presented a strange chaos of dress gloves, boxing gloves, caricatures, albums, invitation cards, foils, cricket bats, cardboard drawings, paste, gum, and fifty other miscellaneous articles, heaped together in the strangest confusion. He was always making something for somebody, or planning some party of pleasure, which was his great *forte.* He invariably spoke with astonishing rapidity; was smart, spoffish, and eight-and-twenty.

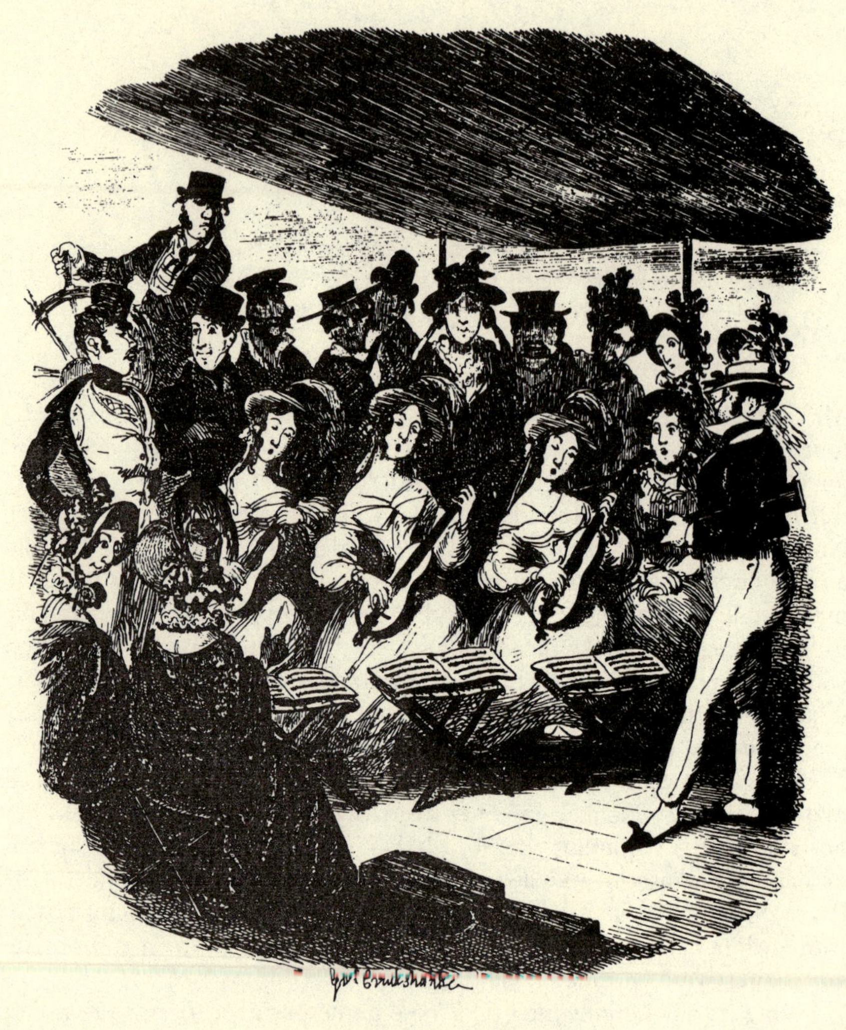

*Steam Excursion (1) (see p. 383)*

'Splendid idea, 'pon my life!' soliloquised Mr Percy Noakes, over his morning's coffee, as his mind reverted to a suggestion which had been thrown out on the previous night, by a lady at whose house he had spent the evening. 'Glorious idea! – Mrs Stubbs.'

'Yes, sir,' replied a dirty old woman with an inflamed countenance, emerging from the bedroom with a barrel of dirt and cinders. – This was the laundress. 'Did you call, sir?'

'Oh! Mrs Stubbs, I'm going out. If that tailor should call again, you'd better say – you'd better say I'm out of town, and shan't be back for a fortnight; and if that bootmaker should come, tell him I've lost his address, or I'd have sent him that little amount. Mind he writes it down; and if Mr Hardy should call – you know Mr Hardy?'

'The funny gentleman, sir?'

'Ah! the funny gentleman. If Mr Hardy should call, say I've gone to Mrs Taunton's about that water party.'

'Yes, sir.'

'And if any fellow calls, and says he's come about a steamer, tell him to be here at five o'clock this afternoon, Mrs Stubbs.'

'Very well, sir.'

Mr Percy Noakes brushed his hat, whisked the crumbs off his inexplicables with a silk handkerchief, gave the ends of his hair a persuasive roll round his forefinger, and sallied forth for Mrs Taunton's domicile in Great Marlborough Street, where she and her daughters occupied the upper part of a house. She was a good-looking widow of fifty, with the form of a giantess and the mind of a child. The pursuit of pleasure, and some means of killing time, were the sole end of her existence. She doted on her daughters, who were as frivolous as herself.

A general exclamation of satisfaction hailed the arrival of Mr Percy Noakes, who went through the ordinary salutations, and threw himself into an easy chair near the ladies' work table, with the ease of a regularly established friend of the family. Mrs Taunton was busily engaged in planting immense bright bows on every part of a smart cap on which it was possible to stick one; Miss Emily Taunton was making a watchguard; Miss Sophia was at the piano, practising a new song – poetry by the young officer, or the police officer, or the custom-house officer, or some other interesting amateur.

'You good creature!' said Mrs Taunton, addressing the gallant Percy. 'You really are a good soul! You've come about the water party, I know.'

'I should rather suspect I had,' replied Mr Noakes, triumphantly. 'Now, come here, girls, and I'll tell you all about it.' Miss Emily and Miss Sophia advanced to the table.

'Now,' continued Mr Percy Noakes, 'it seems to me that the best way will be, to have a committee of ten, to make all the arrangements, and manage the whole set-out. Then, I propose that the expenses shall be paid by these ten fellows jointly.'

'Excellent, indeed!' said Mrs Taunton, who highly approved of this part of the arrangements.

'Then, my plan is, that each of these ten fellows shall have the power of asking five people. There must be a meeting of the committee, at my chambers, to make all the arrangements, and these people shall be then named; every member of the committee shall have the power of black-balling any one who is proposed; and one black ball shall exclude that person. This will ensure our having a pleasant party, you know.'

'What a manager you are!' interrupted Mrs Taunton again.

'Charming!' said the lovely Emily.

'I never did!' ejaculated Sophia.

'Yes, I think it'll do,' replied Mr Percy Noakes, who was now quite in his element. 'I think it'll do. Then you know we shall go down to the Nore, and back, and have a regular capital cold dinner laid out in the cabin before we start, so that everything may be ready without any confusion; and we shall have the lunch laid out, on deck, in those little tea-garden-looking concerns by the paddle boxes – I don't know what you call 'em. Then, we shall hire a steamer expressly for our party, and a band, and have the deck chalked, and we shall be able to dance quadrilles all day; and then, whoever we know that's musical, you know, why they'll make themselves useful and agreeable; and – and – upon the whole, I really hope we shall have a glorious day, you know!'

The announcement of these arrangements was received with the utmost enthusiasm. Mrs Taunton, Emily, and Sophia, were loud in their praises.

'Well, but tell me, Percy,' said Mrs Taunton, 'who are the ten gentlemen to be?'

'Oh! I know plenty of fellows who'll be delighted with the scheme,' replied Mr Percy Noakes, 'of course we shall have—'

'Mr Hardy!' interrupted the servant, announcing a visitor. Miss Sophia and Miss Emily hastily assumed the most interesting attitudes that could be adopted on so short a notice.

'How are you?' said a stout gentleman of about forty, pausing at the door in the attitude of an awkward harlequin. This was Mr Hardy, whom we have before described, on the authority of Mrs Stubbs, as 'the funny gentleman'. He was an Astley-Cooperish Joe Miller – a practical joker, immensely popular with married ladies, and a general favourite with young men. He was always engaged in some pleasure excursion or other, and delighted in getting somebody into a scrape on such occasions. He could sing comic songs, imitate hackney coachmen and fowls, play airs on his chin, and execute concertos on the Jews' harp. He always ate and drank most immoderately, and was the bosom friend of Mr Percy Noakes.

He had a red face, a somewhat husky voice, and a tremendous laugh.

'How *are* you?' said this worthy, laughing, as if it were the finest joke in the world to make a morning call, and shaking hands with the ladies with as much vehemence as if their arms had been so many pump handles.

'You're just the very man I wanted,' said Mr Percy Noakes, who proceeded to explain the cause of his being in requisition.

'Ha! ha! ha!' shouted Hardy, after hearing the statement, and receiving a detailed account of the proposed excursion. 'Oh, capital! glorious! What a day it will be! what fun! – But, I say, when are you going to begin making the arrangements?'

'No time like the present – at once, if you please.'

'Oh, charming!' cried the ladies. 'Pray, do!'

Writing materials were laid before Mr Percy Noakes, and the names of the different members of the committee were agreed on, after as much discussion between him and Mr Hardy as if the fate of nations had depended on their appointment. It was then agreed that a meeting should take place at Mr Percy Noakes's chambers on the ensuing Wednesday evening at eight o'clock, and the visitors departed.

Wednesday evening arrived; eight o'clock came, and eight members of the committee were punctual in their attendance. Mr Loggins, the solicitor, of Boswell Court, sent an excuse, and Mr Samuel Briggs, the ditto of Furnival's Inn, sent his brother: much to his (the brother's) satisfaction, and greatly to the discomfiture of Mr Percy Noakes. Between the Briggses and the Tauntons there existed a degree of implacable hatred, quite unprecedented. The animosity between the Montagues and Capulets, was nothing to that which prevailed between these two illustrious houses. Mrs Briggs was a widow, with three daughters and two sons; Mr Samuel, the eldest, was an attorney, and Mr Alexander, the youngest, was under articles to his brother. They resided in Portland Street, Oxford Street, and moved in the same orbit as the Tauntons – hence their mutual dislike. If the Miss Briggses appeared in smart bonnets, the Miss Tauntons eclipsed them with smarter. If Mrs Taunton appeared in a cap of all the hues of the rainbow, Mrs Briggs forthwith mounted a toque, with all the patterns of the kaleidoscope. If Miss Sophia Taunton learnt a new song, two of the Miss Briggses came out with a new duet. The Tauntons had once gained a temporary triumph with the assistance of a harp, but the Briggses brought three guitars into the field, and effectually routed the enemy. There was no end to the rivalry between them.

Now, as Mr Samuel Briggs was a mere machine, a sort of self-acting legal walking stick; and as the party was known to have originated, however remotely, with Mrs Taunton, the female branches of the Briggs family had arranged that Mr Alexander should attend, instead of his brother; and as the said Mr Alexander was deservedly celebrated for possessing all the pertinacity of a bankruptcy court attorney, combined with the obstinacy of that useful animal which browses on the thistle, he required but little tuition. He was especially enjoined to make himself as disagreeable as possible; and, above all, to black-ball the Tauntons at every hazard.

The proceedings of the evening were opened by Mr Percy Noakes. After successfully urging on the gentlemen present the propriety of their mixing some brandy and water, he briefly stated the object of the meeting, and concluded by observing that the first step must be the selection of a chairman, necessarily possessing some arbitrary – he trusted not unconstitutional – powers, to whom the personal direction of the whole of the arrangements (subject to the approval of the committee) should be confided. A pale young gentleman, in a green stock and spectacles of the same, a member of the honourable society of the Inner Temple, immediately rose for the purpose of proposing Mr Percy Noakes. He had known him long, and this he would say, that a more honourable, a more excellent, or a better-hearted fellow, never existed. – (Hear, hear!) The young gentleman, who was a member of a debating society, took this opportunity of entering into an examination of the state of the English law, from the days of William the Conqueror down to the present period; he briefly adverted to the code established by the ancient Druids; slightly glanced at the principles laid down by the Athenian lawgivers; and concluded with a most glowing eulogium on picnics and constitutional rights.

Mr Alexander Briggs opposed the motion. He had the highest esteem for Mr Percy Noakes as an individual, but he did consider that he ought not to be entrusted with these immense powers – (oh, oh!) – He believed that in the proposed capacity Mr Percy Noakes would not act fairly, impartially, or honourably; but he begged it to be distinctly understood, that he said this without the slightest personal disrespect. Mr Hardy defended his honourable friend, in a voice rendered partially unintelligible by emotion and brandy and water. The proposition was put to the vote, and there appearing to be only one dissentient voice, Mr Percy Noakes was declared duly elected, and took the chair accordingly.

The business of the meeting now proceeded with rapidity. The chairman delivered in his estimate of the probable expense of the excursion, and everyone present subscribed his portion thereof. The question was put that 'The Endeavour' be hired for the occasion; Mr Alexander Briggs moved as an amendment, that the word 'Fly' be substituted for the word 'Endeavour'; but after some debate consented to withdraw his opposition. The important ceremony of balloting then commenced. A tea caddy was placed on a table in a dark corner of the apartment, and everyone was provided with two backgammon men, one black and one white.

The chairman with great solemnity then read the following list of the guests whom he proposed to introduce: – Mrs Taunton and two daughters, Mr Wizzle, Mr Simson. The names were respectively balloted for, and Mrs Taunton and her daughters were declared to be black-balled. Mr Percy Noakes and Mr Hardy exchanged glances.

'Is your list prepared, Mr Briggs?' inquired the chairman.

'It is,' replied Alexander, delivering in the following: – 'Mrs Briggs and three daughters, Mr Samuel Briggs.' The previous ceremony was repeated, and Mrs Briggs and three daughters were declared to be black-balled. Mr Alexander Briggs looked rather foolish, and the remainder of the company appeared somewhat overawed by the mysterious nature of the proceedings.

The balloting proceeded; but one little circumstance which Mr Percy Noakes had not originally foreseen, prevented the system from working quite as well as he had anticipated. Everybody was black-balled. Mr Alexander Briggs, by way of retaliation, exercised his power of exclusion in every instance, and the result was, that after three hours had been consumed in hard balloting, the names of only three gentlemen were found to have been agreed to. In this dilemma what was to be done? either the whole plan must fall to the ground, or a compromise must be effected. The latter alternative was preferable; and Mr Percy Noakes therefore proposed that the form of balloting should be dispensed with, and that every gentleman should merely be required to state whom he intended to bring. The proposal was acceded to; the Tauntons and the Briggses were reinstated; and the party was formed.

The next Wednesday was fixed for the eventful day, and it was unanimously resolved that every member of the committee should wear a piece of blue sarsenet ribbon round his left arm. It appeared from the statement of Mr Percy Noakes, that the boat belonged to the General Steam Navigation Company, and was then lying off the Custom House; and, as he proposed that the dinner and wines should be provided by an eminent city purveyor, it was arranged that Mr Percy Noakes should be on board by seven o'clock to superintend the arrangements, and that the remaining members of the committee, together with the company generally, should be expected to join her by nine o'clock. More brandy and water was dispatched; several speeches were made by the different law students present; thanks were voted to the chairman; and the meeting separated.

The weather had been beautiful up to this period, and beautiful it continued to be. Sunday passed over, and Mr Percy Noakes became unusually fidgety – rushing constantly to and from the Steam Packet Wharf, to the astonishment of the clerks, and the great emolument of the Holborn cabmen. Tuesday arrived, and the anxiety of Mr Percy Noakes knew no bounds. He was every instant running to the window, to look out for clouds; and Mr Hardy astonished the whole square by practising a new comic song for the occasion, in the chairman's chambers.

Uneasy were the slumbers of Mr Percy Noakes that night; he tossed and tumbled about, and had confused dreams of steamers starting off, and gigantic clocks with the hands pointing to a quarter-past nine, and the ugly face of Mr Alexander Briggs looking over the boat's side, and grinning, as if in derision of his fruitless attempts to move. He made a violent effort to get on board, and awoke. The bright sun was shining cheerfully into the bedroom, and Mr Percy Noakes started up for his watch, in the dreadful expectation of finding his worst dreams realised.

It was just five o'clock. He calculated the time – he should be a good half hour dressing himself; and as it was a lovely morning, and the tide would be then running down, he would walk leisurely to Strand Lane, and have a boat to the Custom House.

He dressed himself, took a hasty apology for a breakfast, and sallied forth. The streets looked as lonely and deserted as if they had been crowded, overnight, for the last time. Here and there, an early apprentice, with quenched-looking sleepy eyes, was taking down the shutters of a shop; and a policeman or milkwoman might occasionally be seen pacing slowly along; but the servants had not yet begun to clean the doors, or light the kitchen fires, and London looked the picture of desolation. At the corner of a by-street, near Temple Bar, was stationed a 'street-breakfast'. The coffee was boiling over a charcoal fire, and large slices of bread and butter were piled one upon the other, like deals in a timberyard. The company were seated on a form, which, with a view both to security and comfort, was placed against a neighbouring wall. Two young men, whose uproarious mirth and disordered dress bespoke the conviviality of the preceding evening, were treating three 'ladies' and an Irish labourer. A little sweep was standing at a short distance, casting a longing eye at the tempting delicacies; and a policeman was watching the group from the opposite side of the street. The wan looks and gaudy finery of the thinly-clad women contrasted as strangely with the gay sunlight, as did their forced merriment with the boisterous hilarity of the two young men, who, now and then, varied their amusements by 'bonneting' the proprietor of this itinerant coffee house.

Mr Percy Noakes walked briskly by, and when he turned down Strand Lane, and caught a glimpse of the glistening water, he thought he had never felt so important or so happy in his life.

'Boat, sir?' cried one of the three watermen who were mopping out their boats, and all whistling. 'Boat, sir?'

'No,' replied Mr Percy Noakes, rather sharply; for the inquiry was not made in a manner at all suitable to his dignity.

'Would you prefer a wessel, sir?' inquired another, to the infinite delight of the 'Jack-in-the-water'.

Mr Percy Noakes replied with a look of supreme contempt.

'Did you want to be put on board a steamer, sir?' inquired an old fireman-waterman, very confidentially. He was dressed in a faded red suit, just the colour of the cover of a very old Court guide.

'Yes, make haste – the Endeavour – off the Custom House.'

'Endeavour!' cried the man who had convulsed the 'Jack' before. 'Vy, I see the Endeavour go up half an hour ago.'

'So did I,' said another; 'and I should think she'd gone down by this time, for she's a precious sight too full of ladies and gen'lemen.'

Mr Percy Noakes affected to disregard these representations, and stepped into the boat, which the old man, by dint of scrambling, and shoving, and grating, had brought up to the causeway. 'Shove her off!' cried Mr Percy Noakes, and away the boat glided down the river; Mr Percy Noakes seated on the recently mopped seat, and the watermen at the stairs offering to bet him any reasonable sum that he'd never reach the 'Custum 'us.'

'Here she is, by Jove!' said the delighted Percy, as they ran alongside the Endeavour.

'Hold hard!' cried the steward over the side, and Mr Percy Noakes jumped on board.

'Hope you will find everything as you wished, sir. She looks uncommon well this morning.'

'She does, indeed,' replied the manager, in a state of ecstasy which it is impossible to describe. The deck was scrubbed, and the seats were scrubbed, and there was a bench for the band, and a place for dancing, and a pile of camp stools, and an awning; and then Mr Percy Noakes bustled down below, and there were the pastrycook's men, and the steward's wife, laying out the dinner on two tables the whole length of the cabin; and then Mr Percy Noakes took off his coat and rushed backwards and forwards, doing nothing, but quite convinced he was assisting everybody; and the steward's wife laughed till she cried, and Mr Percy Noakes panted with the violence of his exertions. And then the bell at London Bridge wharf rang; and a Margate boat was just starting; and a Gravesend boat was just starting; and people shouted, and porters ran down the steps with luggage that would crush any men but porters; and sloping boards, with bits of wood nailed on them, were placed between the outside boat and the inside boat; and the passengers ran along them, and looked like so many fowls coming out of an area; and then the bell ceased, and the boards were taken away, and the boats started, and the whole scene was one of the most delightful bustle and confusion.

The time wore on; half-past eight o'clock arrived; the pastrycook's men went ashore; the dinner was completely laid out; and Mr Percy Noakes locked the principal cabin, and put the key in his pocket, in order that it might be suddenly disclosed, in all its magnificence, to the eyes of the astonished company. The band came on board, and so did the wine.

Ten minutes to nine and the committee embarked in a body. There was Mr Hardy, in a blue jacket and waistcoat, white trousers, silk stockings, and pumps – in full aquatic costume, with a straw hat on his head, and an immense telescope under his arm; and there was the young gentleman with the green spectacles, in nankeen inexplicables, with a ditto waistcoat and bright buttons, like the pictures of Paul – not the saint, but he of Virginia notoriety. The remainder of the committee, dressed in white hats, light jackets, waistcoats, and trousers, looked something between waiters and West India planters.

Nine o'clock struck, and the company arrived in shoals. Mr Samuel Briggs, Mrs Briggs, and the Misses Briggs, made their appearance in a smart private wherry. The three guitars, in their respective dark green cases, were carefully stowed away in the bottom of the boat, accompanied by two immense portfolios of music, which it would take at least a week's incessant playing to get through. The Tauntons arrived at the same moment with more music, and a lion – a gentleman with a bass voice and an incipient red moustache. The colours of the Taunton party were pink; those of the Briggses a light blue. The Tauntons had artificial flowers in their bonnets; here the Briggses gained a decided advantage – they wore feathers.

'How d'ye do, dear?' said the Misses Briggs to the Misses Taunton. (The word 'dear' among girls is frequently synonymous with 'wretch'.)

'Quite well, thank you, dear,' replied the Misses Taunton to the Misses Briggs; and then there was such a kissing, and congratulating, and shaking of hands, as might have induced one to suppose that the two families were the best friends in the world, instead of each wishing the other overboard, as they most sincerely did.

Mr Percy Noakes received the visitors, and bowed to the strange gentleman, as if he should like to know who he was. This was just what Mrs Taunton wanted. Here was an opportunity to astonish the Briggses.

'Oh! I beg your pardon,' said the general of the Taunton party, with a careless air. – 'Captain Helves – Mr Percy Noakes – Mrs Briggs – Captain Helves.'

Mr Percy Noakes bowed very low; the gallant captain did the same with all due ferocity, and the Briggses were clearly overcome.

'Our friend, Mr Wizzle, being unfortunately prevented from coming,' resumed Mrs Taunton, 'I did myself the pleasure of bringing the captain, whose musical talents I knew would be a great acquisition.'

'In the name of the committee I have to thank you for doing so, and to offer you welcome, sir,' replied Percy. (Here the scraping was renewed.) 'But pray be seated – won't you walk aft? Captain, will you conduct Miss Taunton? – Miss Briggs, will you allow me?'

'Where could they have picked up that military man?' inquired Mrs Briggs of Miss Kate Briggs, as they followed the little party.

'I can't imagine,' replied Miss Kate, bursting with vexation; for the very fierce air with which the gallant captain regarded the company, had impressed her with a high sense of his importance.

Boat after boat came alongside, and guest after guest arrived. The invites had been excellently arranged: Mr Percy Noakes having considered it as important that the number of young men should exactly tally with that of the young ladies, as that the quantity of knives on board should be in precise proportion to the forks.

'Now, is everyone on board?' inquired Mr Percy Noakes. The committee (who, with their bits of blue ribbon, looked as if they were all going to be bled) bustled about to ascertain the fact, and reported that they might safely start.

'Go on!' cried the master of the boat from the top of one of the paddle boxes.

'Go on!' echoed the boy, who was stationed over the hatchway to pass the directions down to the engineer; and away went the vessel with that agreeable noise which is peculiar to steamers, and which is composed of a mixture of creaking, gushing, clanging, and snorting.

'Hoi – oi – oi – oi – oi – oi – o – i – i – i – i!' shouted half-a-dozen voices from a boat, a quarter of a mile astern.

'Ease her!' cried the captain: 'do these people belong to us, sir?'

'Noakes,' exclaimed Hardy, who had been looking at every object, far and near, through the large telescope, 'it's the Fleetwoods and the Wakefields – and two children with them, by Jove!'

'What a shame to bring children!' said everybody; 'how very inconsiderate!'

'I say, it would be a good joke to pretend not to see 'em, wouldn't it?' suggested Hardy, to the immense delight of the company generally. A council of war was hastily held, and it was resolved that the newcomers should be taken on board, on Mr Hardy solemnly pledging himself to tease the children during the whole of the day.

'Stop her!' cried the captain.

'Stop her!' repeated the boy; whizz went the steam, and all the young ladies, as in duty bound, screamed in concert. They were only appeased by the assurance of the martial Helves, that the escape of steam consequent on stopping a vessel was seldom attended with any great loss of human life.

Two men ran to the side; and after some shouting, and swearing, and angling for the wherry with a boat-hook, Mr Fleetwood, and Mrs Fleetwood, and Master Fleetwood, and Mr Wakefield, and Mrs Wakefield, and Miss Wakefield, were safely deposited on the deck. The girl was about six years old, the boy about four; the former was dressed in a white frock with a pink sash and dog's-eared-looking little spencer: a straw bonnet and green veil, six inches by three and a half; the latter was attired for the occasion in a nankeen frock, between the bottom of which, and the top of his plaid socks, a considerable portion of two small mottled legs was discernible. He had a light blue cap with a gold band and tassel on his head, and a damp piece of gingerbread in his hand, with which he had slightly embossed his countenance.

The boat once more started off; the band played 'Off she goes'; the major part of the company conversed cheerfully in groups; and the old gentlemen walked up and down the deck in pairs, as perseveringly and gravely as if they were doing a match against time for an immense stake. They ran briskly down the Pool; the gentlemen pointed out the Docks, the Thames Police Office, and other elegant public edifices; and the young ladies exhibited a proper display of horror at the appearance of the coal whippers and ballast heavers. Mr Hardy told stories to the married ladies, at which they laughed very much in their pocket handkerchiefs, and hit him on the knuckles with their fans, declaring him to be 'a naughty man – a shocking creature' – and so forth; and Captain Helves gave slight descriptions of battles and duels, with a most bloodthirsty air, which made him the admiration of the women, and the envy of the men. Quadrilling commenced; Captain Helves danced one set with Miss Emily Taunton, and another set with Miss Sophia Taunton. Mrs Taunton was in ecstasies. The victory appeared to be complete; but alas! the inconstancy of man! Having performed this necessary duty, he attached himself solely to Miss Julia Briggs, with whom he danced no less than three sets consecutively, and from whose side he evinced no intention of stirring for the remainder of the day.

Mr Hardy, having played one or two very brilliant fantasias on the Jews' harp, and having frequently repeated the exquisitely amusing joke of slily chalking a large cross on the back of some member of the committee, Mr Percy Noakes expressed his hope that some of their musical friends would oblige the company by a display of their abilities.

'Perhaps,' he said in a very insinuating manner, 'Captain Helves will oblige us?' Mrs Taunton's countenance lighted up, for the captain only sang duets, and couldn't sing them with anybody but one of her daughters.

'Really,' said that warlike individual, 'I should be very happy, but—'

'Oh! pray do,' cried all the young ladies.

'Miss Emily, have you any objection to join in a duet?'

'Oh! not the slightest,' returned the young lady, in a tone which clearly showed she had the greatest possible objection.

'Shall I accompany you, dear?' inquired one of the Miss Briggses, with the bland intention of spoiling the effect.

'Very much obliged to you, Miss Briggs,' sharply retorted Mrs Taunton, who saw through the manœuvre; 'my daughters always sing without accompaniments.'

'And without voices,' tittered Mrs Briggs, in a low tone.

'Perhaps,' said Mrs Taunton, reddening, for she guessed the tenor of the observation, though she had not heard it clearly – 'Perhaps it would be as well for some people, if their voices were not quite so audible as they are to other people.'

'And perhaps, if gentlemen who are kidnapped to pay attention to some persons' daughters, had not sufficient discernment to pay attention to other persons' daughters,' returned Mrs Briggs, 'some persons would not be so ready to display that ill-temper which, thank God, distinguishes them from other persons.'

'Persons!' ejaculated Mrs Taunton.

'Persons,' replied Mrs Briggs.

'Insolence!'

'Creature!'

'Hush! hush!' interrupted Mr Percy Noakes, who was one of the very few by whom this dialogue had been overheard. 'Hush! – pray, silence for the duet.'

After a great deal of preparatory crowing and humming, the captain began the following duet from the opera of 'Paul and Virginia', in that grunting tone in which a man gets down, Heaven knows where, without the remotest chance of ever getting up again. This, in private circles, is frequently designated 'a bass voice'.

> See (sung the captain) from o–ce–an ri–sing
> Bright flames the or–b of d–ay.
> From yon gro–ove, the varied so–ongs–

Here, the singer was interrupted by varied cries of the most dreadful description, proceeding from some grove in the immediate vicinity of the starboard paddle box.

'My child!' screamed Mrs Fleetwood. 'My child! it is his voice – I know it.'

Mr Fleetwood, accompanied by several gentlemen, here rushed to the quarter from whence the noise proceeded, and an exclamation of horror burst from the company; the general impression being, that the little innocent had either got his head in the water, or his legs in the machinery.

'What is the matter?' shouted the agonised father, as he returned with the child in his arms.

'Oh! oh! oh!' screamed the small sufferer again.

'What is the matter, dear?' inquired the father once more – hastily stripping off the nankeen frock, for the purpose of ascertaining whether the child had one bone which was not smashed to pieces.

'Oh! oh! – I'm so frightened!'

'What at, dear? – what at?' said the mother, soothing the sweet infant.

'Oh! he's been making such dreadful faces at me,' cried the boy, relapsing into convulsions at the bare recollection.

'He! – who?' cried everybody, crowding round him.

'Oh! – him!' replied the child, pointing at Hardy, who affected to be the most concerned of the whole group.

The real state of the case at once flashed upon the minds of all present, with the exception of the Fleetwoods and the Wakefields. The facetious Hardy, in fulfilment of his promise, had watched the child to a remote part of the vessel, and, suddenly appearing before him with the most awful contortions of visage, had produced his paroxysm of terror. Of course, he now observed that it was hardly necessary for him to deny the accusation; and the unfortunate little victim was accordingly led below, after receiving sundry thumps on the head from both his parents, for having the wickedness to tell a story.

This little interruption having been adjusted, the captain resumed, and Miss Emily chimed in, in due course. The duet was loudly applauded, and, certainly, the perfect independence of the parties deserved great commendation. Miss Emily sang her part, without the slightest reference to the captain; and the captain sang so loud, that he had not the slightest idea what was being done by his partner. After having gone through the last few eighteen or nineteen bars by himself, therefore, he acknowledged the plaudits of the circle with that air of self-denial which men usually assume when they think they have done something to astonish the company.

'Now,' said Mr Percy Noakes, who had just ascended from the fore-cabin, where he had been busily engaged in decanting the wine, 'if the Misses Briggs will oblige us with something before dinner, I am sure we shall be very much delighted.'

One of those hums of admiration followed the suggestion, which one frequently hears in society, when nobody has the most distant notion what he is expressing his approval of. The three Misses Briggs looked modestly at their mamma, and the mamma looked approvingly at her daughters, and Mrs Taunton looked scornfully at all of them. The Misses Briggs asked for their guitars, and several gentlemen seriously damaged the cases in their anxiety to present them. Then there was a very interesting production of three little keys for the aforesaid cases, and a melodramatic expression of horror at finding a string broken; and a vast deal of screwing and tightening, and winding and turning, during which Mrs Briggs expatiated to those near her on the immense difficulty of playing a guitar, and hinted at the wondrous proficiency of her daughters in that mystic art. Mrs Taunton whispered to a neighbour that it was 'quite sickening!' and the Misses Taunton looked as if they knew how to play, but disdained to do it.

At length, the Misses Briggs began in real earnest. It was a new Spanish composition, for three voices and three guitars. The effect was electrical. All eyes were turned upon the captain, who was reported to have once passed through Spain with his regiment, and who must be well acquainted with the national music. He was in raptures. This was sufficient; the trio was encored; the applause was universal; and never had the Tauntons suffered such a complete defeat.

'Bravo! bravo!' ejaculated the captain; – 'bravo!'

'Pretty? isn't it, sir?' inquired Mr Samuel Briggs, with the air of a self-satisfied showman. By-the-bye, these were the first words he had been heard to utter since he left Boswell Court the evening before.

'De–lightful!' returned the captain, with a flourish and a military cough; – 'de–lightful!'

'Sweet instrument!' said an old gentleman with a bald head, who had been trying all the morning to look through a telescope, inside the glass of which Mr Hardy had fixed a large black wafer.

'Did you ever hear a Portuguese tambourine?' inquired that jocular individual.

'Did *you* ever hear a tom-tom, sir?' sternly inquired the captain, who lost no opportunity of showing off his travels, real or pretended.

'A what?' asked Hardy, rather taken aback.

'A tom-tom.'

'Never!'

'Nor a gum-gum?'

'Never!'

'What *is* a gum-gum?' eagerly inquired several young ladies.

'When I was in the East Indies,' replied the captain – (here was a discovery – he had been in the East Indies!) – 'when I was in the East Indies, I was once stopping a few thousand miles up the country, on a visit at the house of a very particular friend of mine, Ram Chowdar Doss Azuph Al Bowlar – a devilish pleasant fellow. As we were enjoying our hookahs, one evening, in the cool verandah in front of his villa, we were rather surprised by the sudden appearance of thirty-four of his Kit-ma-gars (for he had rather a large establishment there), accompanied by an equal number of Con-su-mars, approaching the house with a threatening aspect, and beating a tom-tom. The Ram started up—'

'Who?' inquired the bald gentleman, intensely interested.

'The Ram – Ram Chowdar—'

'Oh!' said the old gentleman, 'I beg your pardon; pray go on.'

' – Started up and drew a pistol. "Helves," said he, "my boy," – he always called me, my boy – "Helves,' said he, "do you hear that tom-tom?" "I do," said I. His countenance, which before was pale, assumed a most frightful appearance; his whole visage was distorted, and his frame shaken by violent emotions. "Do you see that gum-gum?" said he. "No," said I, staring about me. "You don't?" said he. "No, I'll be damned if I do," said I; "and what's more, I don't know what a gum-gum is," said I. I really thought the Ram would have dropped. He drew me aside, and with an expression of agony I shall never forget, said in a low whisper—'

'Dinner's on the table, ladies,' interrupted the steward's wife.

'Will you allow me?' said the captain, immediately suiting the action to the word, and escorting Miss Julia Briggs to the cabin, with as much ease as if he had finished the story.

'What an extraordinary circumstance!' ejaculated the same old gentleman, preserving his listening attitude.

'What a traveller!' said the young ladies.

'What a singular name!' exclaimed the gentlemen, rather confused by the coolness of the whole affair.

'I wish he had finished the story,' said an old lady. 'I wonder what a gum-gum really is?'

'By Jove!' exclaimed Hardy, who until now had been lost in utter amazement, 'I don't know what it may be in India, but in England I think a gum-gum has very much the same meaning as a hum-bug.'

'How illiberal! how envious!' cried everybody, as they made for the cabin, fully impressed with a belief in the captain's amazing adventures. Helves was the sole lion for the remainder of the day – impudence and the marvellous are pretty sure passports to any society.

The party had by this time reached their destination, and put about on their return home. The wind, which had been with them the whole day, was now directly in their teeth; the weather had become gradually more and more overcast; and the sky, water, and shore, were all of that dull, heavy, uniform lead-colour, which house painters daub in the first instance over a street door which is gradually approaching a state of convalescence. It had been 'spitting' with rain for the last half-hour, and now began to pour in good earnest. The wind was freshening very fast, and the waterman at the wheel had unequivocally expressed his opinion that there would shortly be a squall. A slight emotion on the part of the vessel, now and then, seemed to suggest the possibility of its pitching to a very uncomfortable extent in the event of its blowing harder; and every timber began to creak, as if the boat were an overladen clothes basket. Seasickness, however, is like a belief in ghosts – everyone entertains some misgivings on the subject, but few will acknowledge any. The majority of the company, therefore, endeavoured to look peculiarly happy, feeling all the while especially miserable.

'Don't it rain?' inquired the old gentleman before noticed, when, by dint of squeezing and jamming, they were all seated at table.

'I think it does – a little,' replied Mr Percy Noakes, who could hardly hear himself speak, in consequence of the pattering on the deck.

'Don't it blow?' inquired someone else.

'No, I don't think it does,' responded Hardy, sincerely wishing that he could persuade himself that it did not; for he sat next the door, and was almost blown off his seat.

'It'll soon clear up,' said Mr Percy Noakes, in a cheerful tone.

'Oh, certainly!' ejaculated the committee generally.

'No doubt of it!' said the remainder of the company, whose attention was now pretty well engrossed by the serious business of eating, carving, taking wine, and so forth.

The throbbing motion of the engine was but too perceptible. There was a large, substantial, cold boiled leg of mutton, at the bottom of the table, shaking like blancmange; a previously hearty sirloin of beef looked as if it had been suddenly seized with the palsy; and some tongues, which were placed on dishes rather too large for them, went through the most surprising evolutions; darting from side to side, and from end to end, like a fly in an inverted wine glass. Then, the sweets shook and trembled, till it was quite impossible to help them, and people gave up the attempt in despair; and the pigeon pies looked as if the birds, whose legs were stuck outside, were trying to get them in. The table vibrated and started like a feverish pulse, and the very legs were convulsed – everything was shaking and jarring. The beams in the roof of the cabin seemed as if they were put there for the sole purpose of giving people headaches, and several elderly gentlemen became ill-tempered in consequence. As fast as the steward put the fire-irons up, they *would* fall down again; and the more the ladies and gentlemen tried to sit comfortably on their seats, the more the seats seemed to slide away from the ladies and gentlemen. Several ominous demands were made for small glasses of brandy; the countenances of the company gradually underwent most extraordinary changes; one gentleman was observed suddenly to rush from table without the slightest ostensible reason, and dart up the steps with incredible swiftness: thereby greatly damaging both himself and the steward, who happened to be coming down at the same moment.

The cloth was removed; the dessert was laid on the table; and the glasses were filled. The motion of the boat increased; several members of the party began to feel rather vague and misty, and looked as if they had only just got up. The young gentleman with the spectacles, who had been in a fluctuating state for some time – at one moment bright, and at another dismal, like a revolving light on the sea coast – rashly announced his wish to propose a toast. After several ineffectual attempts to preserve his perpendicular, the young gentleman, having managed to hook himself to the centre leg of the table with his left hand, proceeded as follows:

'Ladies and gentlemen. A gentleman is among us – I may say a stranger – (here some painful thought seemed to strike the orator; he paused, and looked extremely odd) – whose talents, whose travels, whose cheerfulness—'

'I beg your pardon, Edkins,' hastily interrupted Mr Percy Noakes, – 'Hardy, what's the matter?'

'Nothing,' replied the 'funny gentleman', who had just life enough left to utter two consecutive syllables.

'Will you have some brandy?'

'No!' replied Hardy in a tone of great indignation, and looking as comfortable as Temple Bar in a Scotch mist; 'what should I want brandy for?'

'Will you go on deck?'

'No, I will *not.*' This was said with a most determined air, and in a voice which might have been taken for an imitation of anything; it was quite as much like a guinea-pig as a bassoon.

'I beg your pardon, Edkins,' said the courteous Percy; 'I thought our friend was ill. Pray go on.'

A pause.

'Pray go on.'

'Mr Edkins *is* gone,' cried somebody.

'I beg your pardon, sir,' said the steward, running up to Mr Percy Noakes, 'I beg your pardon, sir, but the gentleman as just went on deck – him with the green spectacles – is uncommon bad, to be sure; and the young man as played the wiolin says, that unless he has some brandy he can't answer for the consequences. He says he has a wife and two children, whose werry subsistence depends on his breaking a wessel, and he expects to do so every moment. The flageolet's been werry ill, but he's better, only he's in a dreadful prusperation.'

All disguise was now useless; the company staggered on deck; the gentlemen tried to see nothing but the clouds; and the ladies, muffled up in such shawls and cloaks as they had brought with them, lay about on the seats, and under the seats, in the most wretched condition. Never was such a blowing, and raining, and pitching, and tossing, endured by any pleasure party before. Several remonstrances were sent down below, on the subject of Master Fleetwood, but they were totally unheeded in consequence of the indisposition of his natural protectors. That interesting child screamed at the top of his voice, until he had no voice left to scream with; and then Miss Wakefield began, and screamed for the remainder of the passage.

Mr Hardy was observed, some hours afterwards, in an attitude which induced his friends to suppose that he was busily engaged in contemplating the beauties of the deep; they only regretted that his taste for the picturesque should lead him to remain so long in a position, very injurious at all times, but especially so to an individual labouring under a tendency of blood to the head.

The party arrived off the Custom House at about two o'clock on the Thursday morning, dispirited and worn out. The Tauntons were too ill to quarrel with the Briggses, and the Briggses were too wretched to annoy the Tauntons. One of the guitar cases was lost on its passage to a hackney coach, and Mrs Briggs has not scrupled to state that the Tauntons bribed a porter to throw it down an area. Mr Alexander Briggs opposes vote by ballot – he says from personal experience of its inefficacy; and Mr Samuel Briggs, whenever he is asked to express his sentiments on the point, says he has no opinion on that or any other subject.

Mr Edkins – the young gentleman in the green spectacles – makes a speech on every occasion on which a speech can possibly be made: the eloquence of which can only be equalled by its length. In the event of his not being previously appointed to a judgeship, it is probable that he will practise as a barrister in the New Central Criminal Court.

Captain Helves continued his attention to Miss Julia Briggs, whom he might possibly have espoused, if it had not unfortunately happened that Mr Samuel arrested him, in the way of business, pursuant to instructions received from Messrs. Scroggings and Payne, whose town debts the gallant captain had condescended to collect, but whose accounts, with the indiscretion sometimes peculiar to military minds, he had omitted to keep with that dull accuracy which custom has rendered necessary. Mrs Taunton complains that she has been much deceived in him. He introduced himself to the family on board a Gravesend steam-packet, and certainly, therefore, ought to have proved respectable.

Mr Percy Noakes is as light-hearted and careless as ever.

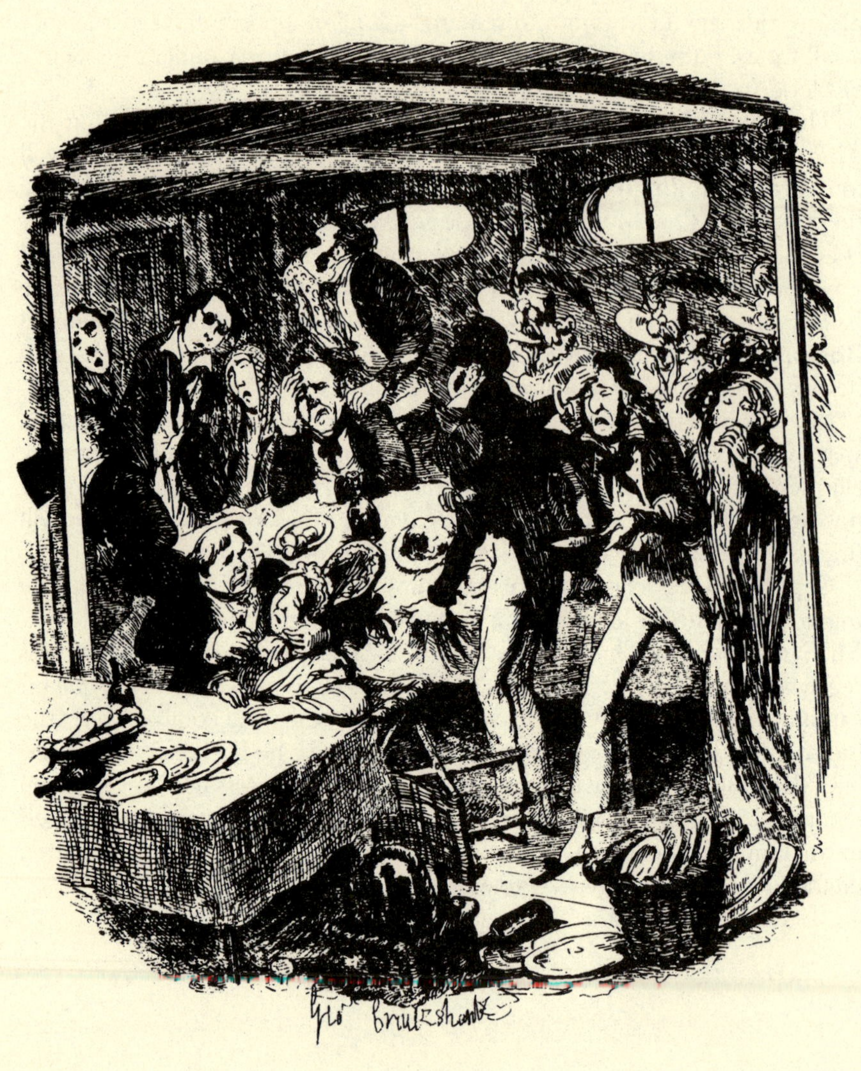

*Steam Excursion (2)*

## Chapter Eight

### *The Great Winglebury Duel*

Originally published in the *First Series,* 1836. In a letter to the publisher Macrone Dickens mentions that 'The Great Winglebury Duel' is due for publication in the *Monthly Magazine* in December 1835, but it did not appear there, perhaps, as the *Pilgrim* editors suggest (*Pilgrim,* Vol. 1, 114) because Dickens had decided to dramatise the story as *The Strange Gentleman.* This was produced at the St James's Theatre with the celebrated comic actor John Pritt Harley in the title role on 29 September 1836 and ran for over fifty performances.

The Boots's knowing comment, 'bit of Sving, eh?', refers to the 'Captain Swing' scare of 1830–2 when farmers who had introduced new agricultural machinery, throwing farm labourers out of work, received anonymous letters signed 'Captain Swing', threatening to burn down their ricks. In several cases these threats were actually put into effect.

The little town of Great Winglebury is exactly forty-two miles and three-quarters from Hyde Park corner. It has a long, straggling, quiet High Street, with a great black and white clock at a small red Town Hall, half-way up – a market place – a cage – an assembly room – a church – a bridge – a chapel – a theatre – a library – an inn – a pump – and a Post Office. Tradition tells of a 'Little Winglebury', down some crossroad about two miles off; and, as a square mass of dirty paper, supposed to have been originally intended for a letter, with certain tremulous characters inscribed thereon, in which a lively imagination might trace a remote resemblance to the word 'Little', was once stuck up to be owned in the sunny window of the Great Winglebury Post Office, from which it only disappeared when it fell to pieces with dust and extreme old age, there would appear to be some foundation for the legend. Common belief is inclined to bestow the name upon a little hole at the end of a muddy lane about a couple of miles long, colonised by one wheelwright, four paupers, and a beer shop; but even this authority, slight as it is, must be regarded with extreme suspicion, inasmuch as the inhabitants of the hole aforesaid concur in opining that it never had any name at all, from the earliest ages down to the present day.

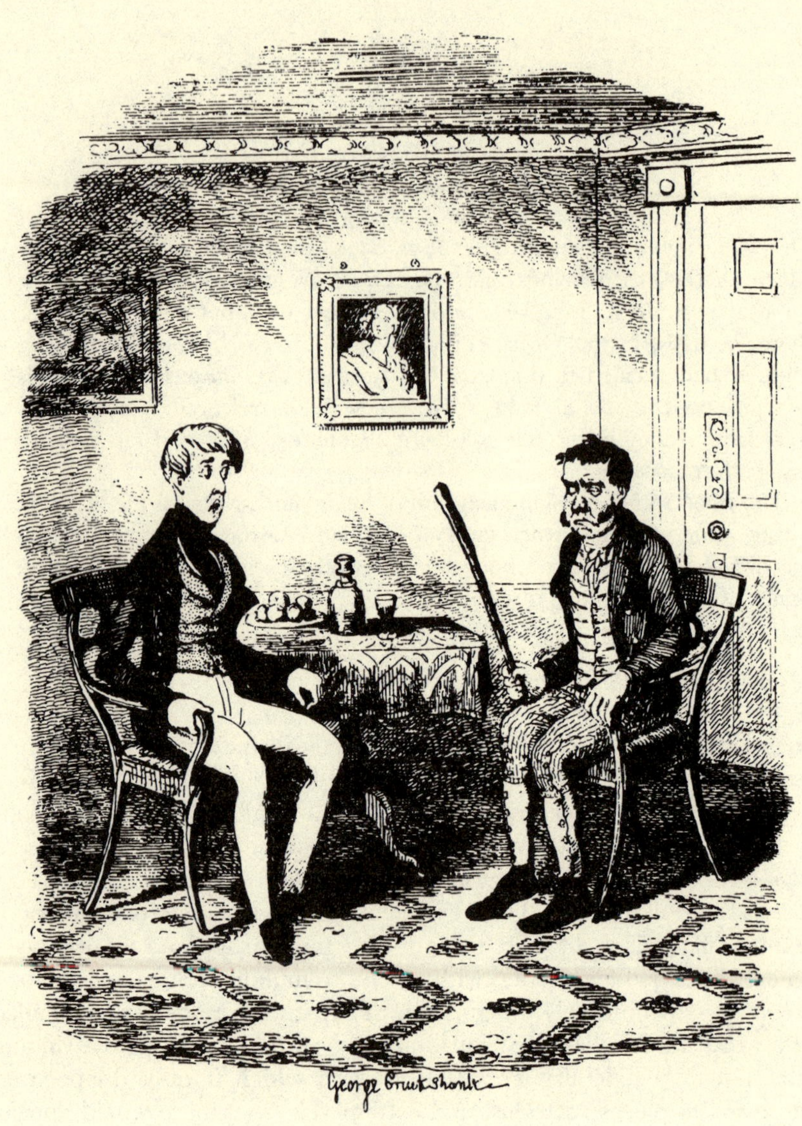

*Under Restraint* *(see p. 401)*

The Winglebury Arms, in the centre of the High Street, opposite the small building with the big clock, is the principal inn of Great Winglebury; – the commercial inn, posting house, and excise office; the 'Blue' house at every election, and the Judges' house at every assizes. It is the headquarters of the Gentlemen's Whist Club of Winglebury Blues (so called in opposition to the Gentlemen's Whist Club of Winglebury Buffs, held at the other house, a little further down): and whenever a juggler, or waxwork man, or concert giver, takes Great Winglebury in his circuit, it is immediately placarded all over the town that Mr So-and-so, 'trusting to that liberal support which the inhabitants of Great Winglebury have long been so liberal in bestowing, has at a great expense engaged the elegant and commodious assembly rooms, attached to the Winglebury Arms.' The house is a large one, with a red brick and stone front; a pretty spacious hall, ornamented with evergreen plants, terminates in a perspective view of the bar, and a glass case, in which are displayed a choice variety of delicacies ready for dressing, to catch the eye of a newcomer the moment he enters, and excite his appetite to the highest possible pitch. Opposite doors lead to the 'coffee' and 'commercial' rooms; and a great wide, rambling staircase, – three stairs and a landing – four stairs and another landing – one step and another landing – half-a-dozen stairs and another landing – and so on – conducts to galleries of bedrooms, and labyrinths of sitting rooms, denominated 'private', where you may enjoy yourself, as privately as you can in any place where some bewildered being walks into your room every five minutes, by mistake, and then walks out again, to open all the doors along the gallery until he finds his own.

Such is the Winglebury Arms, at this day, and such was the Winglebury Arms some time since – no matter when – two or three minutes before the arrival of the London stage. Four horses with cloths on – change for a coach – were standing quietly at the corner of the yard, surrounded by a listless group of post boys in shiny hats and smock frocks, engaged in discussing the merits of the cattle; half-a-dozen ragged boys were standing a little apart, listening with evident interest to the conversation of these worthies; and a few loungers were collected round the horse trough, awaiting the arrival of the coach.

The day was hot and sunny, the town in the zenith of its dullness, and with the exception of these few idlers, not a living creature was to be seen. Suddenly, the loud notes of a key bugle broke the monotonous stillness of the street; in came the coach, rattling over the uneven paving with a noise startling enough to stop even the large faced clock itself. Down got the outsides, up went the windows in all directions, out came the waiters, up started the ostlers, and the loungers, and the post boys, and the ragged boys, as if they were electrified – unstrapping, and unchaining, and unbuckling, and dragging willing horses out, and forcing reluctant horses in, and making a most exhilarating bustle. 'Lady inside, here!' said the guard. 'Please to alight, ma'am,' said the waiter. 'Private sitting room?' interrogated the lady. 'Certainly, ma'am,' responded the chambermaid. 'Nothing but these 'ere trunks, ma'am?' inquired the guard. 'Nothing more,' replied the lady. Up got the outsides again, and the guard, and the coachman; off came the cloths, with a jerk; 'All right,' was the cry; and away they went. The loungers lingered a minute or two in the road, watching the coach until it turned the corner, and then loitered away one by one. The street was clear again, and the town, by contrast, quieter than ever.

'Lady in number twenty-five,' screamed the landlady. – 'Thomas!'

'Yes, ma'am.'

'Letter just been left for the gentleman in number nineteen. Boots at the Lion left it. No answer.'

'Letter for you, sir,' said Thomas, depositing the letter on number nineteen's table.

'For me?' said number nineteen, turning from the window, out of which he had been surveying the scene just described.

'Yes, sir,' – (waiters always speak in hints, and never utter complete sentences) – 'yes, sir, – Boots at the Lion, sir, – Bar, sir, – Missis said number nineteen, sir – Alexander Trott, Esq., sir? – Your card at the bar, sir, I think, sir?'

'My name *is* Trott,' replied number nineteen, breaking the seal. 'You may go, waiter.' The waiter pulled down the window blind, and then pulled it up again – for a regular waiter must do something before he leaves the room – adjusted the glasses on the sideboard, brushed a place that was *not* dusty, rubbed his hands very hard, walked stealthily to the door, and evaporated.

There was, evidently, something in the contents of the letter, of a nature, if not wholly unexpected, certainly extremely disagreeable. Mr Alexander Trott laid it down, and took it up again, and walked about the room on particular squares of the carpet, and even attempted, though unsuccessfully, to whistle an air. It wouldn't do. He threw himself into a chair, and read the following epistle aloud: –

*Blue Lion and Stomach-warmer,*
*Great Winglebury*
*Wednesday Morning.*

'Sir. Immediately on discovering your intentions, I left our counting house, and followed you. I know the purport of your journey; – that journey shall never be completed.

'I have no friend here, just now, on whose secrecy I can rely. This shall be no obstacle to my revenge. Neither shall Emily Brown be exposed to the mercenary solicitations of a scoundrel, odious in her eyes, and contemptible in everybody else's: nor will I tamely submit to the clandestine attacks of a base umbrella-maker.

'Sir. From Great Winglebury church, a footpath leads through four meadows to a retired spot known to the townspeople as Stiffun's Acre.' [Mr Trott shuddered.] 'I shall be waiting there alone, at twenty minutes before six o'clock tomorrow morning. Should I be disappointed in seeing you there, I will do myself the pleasure of calling with a horsewhip.

Horace Hunter.

'PS. There is a gunsmith's in the High Street; and they won't sell gunpowder after dark – you understand me.

'PPS. You had better not order your breakfast in the morning until you have met me. It may be an unnecessary expense.'

'Desperate-minded villain! I knew how it would be!' ejaculated the terrified Trott. 'I always told father, that once start me on this expedition, and Hunter would pursue me like the Wandering Jew. It's bad enough as it is, to marry with the old people's commands, and without the girl's consent; but what will Emily think of me, if I go down there breathless with running away from this infernal salamander? What *shall* I do? What *can* I do? If I go back to the city, I'm disgraced forever – lose the girl – and, what's more, lose the money too. Even if I did go on to the Browns' by the coach, Hunter would be after me in a post-chaise; and if I go to this place, this Stiffun's Acre (another shudder), I'm as good as dead. I've seen him hit the man at the Pall-mall shooting gallery, in the second buttonhole of the waistcoat, five times out of every six, and when he didn't hit him there, he hit him in the head.' With this consolatory reminiscence Mr Alexander Trott again ejaculated, 'What shall I do?'

Long and weary were his reflections, as, burying his face in his hand, he sat, ruminating on the best course to be pursued. His mental direction post pointed to London. He thought of the 'governor's' anger, and the loss of the fortune which the paternal Brown had promised the paternal Trott his daughter should contribute to the coffers of his son. Then the words 'To Brown's' were legibly inscribed on the said direction post, but Horace Hunter's denunciation rung in his ears; – last of all it bore, in red letters, the words, 'To Stiffun's Acre'; and then Mr Alexander Trott decided on adopting a plan which he presently matured.

First and foremost, he dispatched the underboots to the Blue Lion and Stomach-warmer, with a gentlemanly note to Mr Horace Hunter, intimating that he thirsted for his destruction and would do himself the pleasure of slaughtering him next morning, without fail. He then wrote another letter, and requested the attendance of the other boots – for they kept a pair. A modest knock at the room door was heard. 'Come in,' said Mr Trott. A man thrust in a red head with one eye in it, and being again desired to 'come in', brought in the body and the legs to which the head belonged, and a fur cap which belonged to the head.

'You are the upper boots, I think?' inquired Mr Trott.

'Yes, I am the upper boots,' replied a voice from inside a velveteen case, with mother-of-pearl buttons – 'that is, I'm the boots as b'longs to the house; the other man's my man, as goes errands and does odd jobs. Top boots and half boots, I calls us.'

'You're from London?' inquired Mr Trott.

'Driv a cab once,' was the laconic reply.

'Why don't you drive it now?' asked Mr Trott.

'Over-driv the cab, and driv over a 'ooman,' replied the top boots, with brevity.

'Do you know the mayor's house?' inquired Mr Trott.

'Rather,' replied the boots, significantly, as if he had some good reason to remember it.

'Do you think you could manage to leave a letter there?' interrogated Trott.

'Shouldn't wonder,' responded boots.

'But this letter,' said Trott, holding a deformed note with a paralytic direction in one hand, and five shillings in the other – 'this letter is anonymous.'

'A – what?' interrupted the boots.

'Anonymous – he's not to know who it comes from.'

'Oh! I see,' responded the reg'lar, with a knowing wink, but without evincing the slightest disinclination to undertake the charge – 'I see – bit o' Sving, eh?' and his one eye wandered round the room, as if in quest of a dark lantern and phosphorus box. 'But, I say!' he continued, recalling the eye from its search, and bringing it to bear on Mr Trott. 'I say, he's a lawyer, our mayor, and insured in the County. If you've a spite agen him, you'd better not burn his house down – blessed if I don't think it would be the greatest favour you could do him.' And he chuckled inwardly.

If Mr Alexander Trott had been in any other situation, his first act would have been to kick the man downstairs by deputy; or, in other words, to ring the bell, and desire the landlord to take his boots off. He contented himself, however, with doubling the fee and explaining that the letter merely related to a breach of the peace. The top boots retired, solemnly pledged to secrecy; and Mr Alexander Trott sat down to a fried sole, maintenon cutlet, Madeira, and sundries, with greater composure than he had experienced since the receipt of Horace Hunter's letter of defiance.

The lady who alighted from the London coach had no sooner been installed in number twenty-five, and made some alteration in her travelling dress, than she indited a note to Joseph Overton, esquire, solicitor, and mayor of Great Winglebury, requesting his immediate attendance on private business of paramount importance – a summons which that worthy functionary lost no time in obeying; for after sundry openings of his eyes, divers ejaculations of 'Bless me!' and other manifestations of surprise, he took his broad-brimmed hat from its accustomed peg in his little front office, and walked briskly down the High Street to the Winglebury Arms; through the hall and up the staircase of which establishment he was ushered by the landlady, and a crowd of officious waiters, to the door of number twenty-five.

'Show the gentleman in,' said the stranger lady, in reply to the foremost waiter's announcement. The gentleman was shown in accordingly.

The lady rose from the sofa; the mayor advanced a step from the door; and there they both paused, for a minute or two, looking at one another as if by mutual consent. The mayor saw before him a buxom richly dressed female of about forty; the lady looked upon a sleek man, about ten years older, in drab shorts and continuations, black coat, neckcloth, and gloves.

'Miss Julia Manners!' exclaimed the mayor at length, 'you astonish me.'

'That's very unfair of you, Overton,' replied Miss Julia, 'for I have known you long enough not to be surprised at anything you do, and you might extend equal courtesy to me.'

'But to run away – actually run away – with a young man!' remonstrated the mayor.

'You wouldn't have me actually run away with an old one, I presume?' was the cool rejoinder.

'And then to ask me – me – of all people in the world – a man of my age and appearance – mayor of the town – to promote such a scheme!' pettishly ejaculated Joseph Overton; throwing himself into an armchair, and producing Miss Julia's letter from his pocket, as if to corroborate the assertion that he *had* been asked.

'Now, Overton,' replied the lady, 'I want your assistance in this matter, and I must have it. In the lifetime of that poor old dear, Mr Cornberry, who – who —'

'Who was to have married you, and didn't, because he died first; and who left you his property unencumbered with the addition of himself,' suggested the mayor.

'Well,' replied Miss Julia, reddening slightly, 'in the lifetime of the poor old dear, the property had the encumbrance of your management; and all I will say of that, is, that I only wonder *it* didn't die of consumption instead of its master. You helped yourself then: – help me now.'

Mr Joseph Overton was a man of the world, and an attorney; and as certain indistinct recollections of an odd thousand pounds or two, appropriated by mistake, passed across his mind, he hemmed deprecatingly, smiled blandly, remained silent for a few seconds; and finally inquired, 'What do you wish me to do?'

'I'll tell you,' replied Miss Julia – 'I'll tell you in three words. Dear Lord Peter — '

'That's the young man, I suppose — ' interrupted the mayor.

'That's the young Nobleman,' replied the lady, with a great stress on the last word. 'Dear Lord Peter is considerably afraid of the resentment of his family; and we have therefore thought it better to make the match a stolen one. He left town, to avoid suspicion, on a visit to his friend, the Honourable Augustus Flair, whose seat, as you know, is about thirty miles from this, accompanied only by his favourite tiger. We arranged that I should come here alone in the London coach; and that he, leaving his tiger and cab behind him, should come on, and arrive here as soon as possible this afternoon.'

'Very well,' observed Joseph Overton, 'and then he can order the chaise, and you can go on to Gretna Green together, without requiring the presence or interference of a third party, can't you?'

'No,' replied Miss Julia. 'We have every reason to believe – dear Lord Peter not being considered very prudent or sagacious by his friends, and they having discovered his attachment to me – that, immediately on his absence being observed, pursuit will be made in this direction: – to elude which, and to prevent our being traced, I wish it to be understood in this house, that dear Lord Peter is slightly deranged, though perfectly harmless; and that I am, unknown to him, awaiting his arrival to convey him in a post-chaise to a private asylum – at Berwick, say. If I don't show myself much, I dare say I can manage to pass for his mother.'

The thought occurred to the mayor's mind that the lady might show herself a good deal without fear of detection; seeing that she was about double the age of her intended husband. He said nothing, however, and the lady proceeded.

'With the whole of this arrangement dear Lord Peter is acquainted; and all I want you to do is to make the delusion more complete by giving it the sanction of your influence in this place, and assigning this as a reason to the people of the house for my taking the young gentleman away. As it would not be consistent with the story that I should see him until after he has entered the chaise, I also wish you to communicate with him, and inform him that it is all going on well.'

'Has he arrived?' inquired Overton.

'I don't know,' replied the lady.

'Then how am I to know!' inquired the mayor. 'Of course, he will not give his own name at the bar.'

'I begged him, immediately on his arrival, to write you a note,' replied Miss Manners; 'and to prevent the possibility of our project being discovered through its means, I desired him to write anonymously, and in mysterious terms, to acquaint you with the number of his room.'

'Bless me!' exclaimed the mayor, rising from his seat, and searching his pockets – 'most extraordinary circumstance – he *has* arrived – mysterious note left at my house in a most mysterious manner, just before yours – didn't know what to make of it before, and certainly shouldn't have attended to it. – Oh! here it is.' And Joseph Overton pulled out of an inner coat pocket the identical letter penned by Alexander Trott. 'Is this his lordship's hand?'

'Oh yes,' replied Julia; 'good, punctual creature! I have not seen it more than once or twice, but I know he writes very badly and very large. These dear, wild young noblemen, you know, Overton — '

'Aye, aye, I see,' replied the mayor. – 'Horses and dogs, play and wine – grooms, actresses, and cigars – the stable, the green room, the saloon, and the tavern; and the legislative assembly at last.'

'Here's what he says,' pursued the mayor; ' "Sir, – A young gentleman in number nineteen at the Winglebury Arms, is bent on committing a rash act tomorrow morning at an early hour." (That's good – he means marrying.) "If you have any regard for the peace of this town, or the preservation of one – it may be two – human lives" – What the deuce does he mean by that?'

'That he's so anxious for the ceremony, he will expire if it's put off, and that I may possibly do the same,' replied the lady with great complacency.

'Oh! I see – not much fear of that; – well – "two human lives, you will cause him to be removed tonight." (He wants to start at once.) "Fear not to do this on your responsibility: for tomorrow the absolute necessity of the proceeding will be but too apparent. Remember: number nineteen. The name is Trott. No delay; for life and death depend upon your promptitude." Passionate language, certainly. Shall I see him?'

'Do,' replied Miss Julia; 'and entreat him to act his part well. I am half afraid of him. Tell him to be cautious.'

'I will,' said the mayor.

'Settle all the arrangements.'

'I will,' said the mayor again.

'And say I think the chaise had better be ordered for one o'clock.'

'Very well,' said the mayor once more; and, ruminating on the absurdity of the situation in which fate and old acquaintance had placed him, he desired a waiter to herald his approach to the temporary representative of number nineteen.

The announcement, 'Gentleman to speak with you, sir,' induced Mr Trott to pause half way in the glass of port, the contents of which he was in the act of imbibing at the moment; to rise from his chair; and retreat a few paces towards the window, as if to secure a retreat, in the event of the visitor assuming the form and appearance of Horace Hunter. One glance at Joseph Overton, however, quieted his apprehensions. He courteously motioned the stranger to a seat. The waiter, after a little jingling with the decanter and glasses, consented to leave the room; and Joseph Overton, placing the broad-brimmed hat on the chair next him, and bending his body gently forward, opened the business by saying in a very low and cautious tone,

'My lord—'

'Eh?' said Mr Alexander Trott, in a loud key, with the vacant and mystified stare of a chilly somnambulist.

'Hush – hush!' said the cautious attorney: 'to be sure – quite right – no titles here – my name is Overton, sir.'

'Overton?'

'Yes: the mayor of this place – you sent me a letter with anonymous information, this afternoon.'

'I, sir?' exclaimed Trott with ill-dissembled surprise; for, coward as he was, he would willingly have repudiated the authorship of the letter in question. 'I, sir?'

'Yes, you, sir; did you not?' responded Overton, annoyed with what he supposed to be an extreme degree of unnecessary suspicion. 'Either this letter is yours, or it is not. If it be, we can converse securely upon the subject at once. If it be not, of course I have no more to say.'

'Stay, stay,' said Trott, 'it *is* mine; I *did* write it. What could I do, sir? I had no friend here.'

'To be sure, to be sure,' said the mayor, encouragingly, 'you could not have managed it better. Well, sir; it will be necessary for you to leave here tonight in a post-chaise and four. And the harder the boys drive, the better. You are not safe from pursuit.'

'Bless me!' exclaimed Trott, in an agony of apprehension, 'can such things happen in a country like this? Such unrelenting and cold-blooded hostility!' He wiped off the concentrated essence of cowardice that was oozing fast down his forehead, and looked aghast at Joseph Overton.

'It certainly is a very hard case,' replied the mayor with a smile, 'that, in a free country, people can't marry whom they like without being hunted down as if they were criminals. However, in the present instance the lady is willing, you know, and that's the main point, after all.'

'Lady willing,' repeated Trott, mechanically. 'How do you know the lady's willing?'

'Come, that's a good one,' said the mayor, benevolently tapping Mr Trott on the arm with his broad-brimmed hat; 'I have known her, well, for a long time; and if anybody could entertain the remotest doubt on the subject, I assure you I have none, nor need you have.'

'Dear me!' said Mr Trott, ruminating. 'This is *very* extraordinary!'

'Well, Lord Peter,' said the mayor, rising.

'Lord Peter?' repeated Mr Trott.

'Oh – ah, I forgot. Mr Trott, then – Trott – very good, ha! ha! – Well, sir, the chaise shall be ready at half-past twelve.'

'And what is to become of me until then?' inquired Mr Trott, anxiously. 'Wouldn't it save appearances, if I were placed under some restraint?'

'Ah!' replied Overton, 'very good thought – capital idea indeed. I'll send somebody up directly. And if you make a little resistance when we put you in the chaise it wouldn't be amiss – look as if you didn't want to be taken away, you know.'

'To be sure,' said Trott – 'to be sure.'

'Well, my lord,' said Overton, in a low tone, 'until then, I wish your lordship a good evening.'

'Lord – lordship?' ejaculated Trott again, falling back a step or two, and gazing, in unutterable wonder, on the countenance of the mayor.

'Ha-ha! I see, my lord – practising the madman? – very good indeed – very vacant look – capital, my lord, capital – good evening, Mr – Trott – ha! ha! ha!'

'That mayor's decidedly drunk,' soliloquised Mr Trott, throwing himself back in his chair, in an attitude of reflection.

'He is a much cleverer fellow than I thought him, that young nobleman – he carries it off uncommonly well,' thought Overton, as he went his way to the bar, there to complete his arrangements. This was soon done. Every word of the story was implicitly believed, and the one-eyed boots was immediately instructed to repair to number nineteen, to act as custodian of the person of the supposed lunatic until half-past twelve o'clock. In pursuance of this direction, that somewhat eccentric gentleman armed himself with a walking stick of gigantic dimensions, and repaired, with his usual equanimity of manner, to Mr Trott's apartment, which he entered without any ceremony, and mounted guard in, by quietly depositing himself on a chair near the door, where he proceeded to beguile the time by whistling a popular air with great apparent satisfaction.

'What do you want here, you scoundrel?' exclaimed Mr Alexander Trott, with a proper appearance of indignation at his detention.

The boots beat time with his head, as he looked gently round at Mr Trott with a smile of pity, and whistled an *adagio* movement.

'Do you attend in this room by Mr Overton's desire?' inquired Trott, rather astonished at the man's demeanour.

'Keep yourself to yourself, young feller,' calmly responded the boots, 'and don't say nothin' to nobody.' And he whistled again.

'Now, mind!' ejaculated Mr Trott, anxious to keep up the farce of wishing with great earnestness to fight a duel if they'd let him. 'I protest against being kept here. I deny that I have any intention of fighting with anybody. But as it's useless contending with superior numbers, I shall sit quietly down.'

'You'd better,' observed the placid boots, shaking the large stick expressively.

'Under protest, however,' added Alexander Trott, seating himself with indignation in his face, but great content in his heart. 'Under protest.'

'Oh, certainly!' responded the boots; 'anything you please. If you're happy, I'm transported; only don't talk too much – it'll make you worse.'

'Make me worse?' exclaimed Trott, in unfeigned astonishment: 'the man's drunk!'

'You'd better be quiet, young feller,' remarked the boots, going through a threatening piece of pantomime with the stick.

'Or mad!' said Mr Trott, rather alarmed. 'Leave the room, sir, and tell them to send somebody else.'

'Won't do!' replied the boots.

'Leave the room!' shouted Trott, ringing the bell violently: for he began to be alarmed on a new score.

'Leave that 'ere bell alone, you wretched loo-nattic!' said the boots, suddenly forcing the unfortunate Trott back into his chair, and brandishing the stick aloft. 'Be quiet, you miserable object, and don't let everybody know there'a a madman in the house.'

'He *is* a madman! He *is* a madman!' exclaimed the terrified Mr Trott, gazing on the one eye of the red-headed boots with a look of abject horror.

'Madman!' replied the boots, 'dam'me, I think he *is* a madman with a vengeance! Listen to me, you unfort'nate. Ah! would you?' [a slight tap on the head with the large stick, as Mr Trott made another move towards the bell handle] 'I caught you there! did I?'

'Spare my life!' exclaimed Trott, raising his hands imploringly.

'I don't want your life,' replied the boots, disdainfully, 'though I think it 'ud be a charity if somebody took it.'

'No, no, it wouldn't,' interrupted poor Mr Trott, hurriedly; 'no, no, it wouldn't! I – I – 'd rather keep it!'

'O werry well,' said the boots: 'that's a mere matter of taste – ev'ry one to his liking. Hows'ever, all I've got to say is this here: You sit quietly down in that chair, and I'll sit hoppersite you here, and if you keep quiet and don't stir, I won't damage you; but if you move hand or foot till half-past twelve o'clock, I shall alter the expression of your countenance so completely, that the next time you look in the glass you'll ask vether you're gone out of town, and ven you're likely to come back again. So sit down.'

'I will – I will,' responded the victim of mistakes; and down sat Mr Trott and down sat the boots too, exactly opposite him, with the stick ready for immediate action in case of emergency.

Long and dreary were the hours that followed. The bell of Great Winglebury church had just struck ten, and two hours and a half would probably elapse before succour arrived.

For half-an-hour, the noise occasioned by shutting up the shops in the street beneath, betokened something like life in the town, and rendered Mr Trott's situation a little less insupportable; but when even these ceased, and nothing was heard beyond the occasional rattling of a post-chaise as it drove up the yard to change horses, and then drove away again, or the clattering of horses' hoofs in the stables behind, it became almost unbearable. The boots occasionally moved an inch or two, to knock superfluous bits of wax off the candles, which were burning low, but instantaneously resumed his former position; and as he remembered to have heard, somewhere or other, that the human eye had an unfailing effect in controlling mad people, he kept his solitary organ of vision constantly fixed on Mr Alexander Trott. That unfortunate individual stared at his companion in his turn, until his features grew more and more indistinct – his hair gradually less red – and the room more misty and obscure. Mr Alexander Trott fell into a sound sleep, from which he was awakened by a rumbling in the street, and a cry of 'Chaise-and-four for number twenty-five!' A bustle on the stairs succeeded; the room door was hastily thrown open; and Mr Joseph Overton entered, followed by four stout waiters, and Mrs Williamson, the stout landlady of the Winglebury Arms.

'Mr Overton!' exclaimed Mr Alexander Trott, jumping up in a frenzy. 'Look at this man, sir; consider the situation in which I have been placed for three hours past – the person you sent to guard me, sir, was a madman – a madman – a raging, ravaging, furious madman.'

'Bravo!' whispered Overton.

'Poor dear!' said the compassionate Mrs Williamson, 'mad people always thinks other people's mad.'

'Poor dear!' ejaculated Mr Alexander Trott. 'What the devil do you mean by poor dear! Are you the landlady of this house?'

'Yes, yes,' replied the stout old lady, 'don't exert yourself, there's a dear! Consider your health, now; do.'

'Exert myself!' shouted Mr Alexander Trott; 'it's a mercy, ma'am, that I have any breath to exert myself with! I might have been assassinated three hours ago by that one-eyed monster with the oakum head. How dare you have a madman, ma'am – how dare you have a madman, to assault and terrify the visitors to your house?'

'I'll never have another,' said Mrs Williamson, casting a look of reproach at the mayor.

'Capital, capital,' whispered Overton again, as he enveloped Mr Alexander Trott in a thick travelling cloak.

'Capital, sir!' exclaimed Trott, aloud; 'it's horrible. The very recollection makes me shudder. I'd rather fight four duels in three hours, if I survived the first three, than I'd sit for that time face to face with a madman.'

'Keep it up, my lord, as you go downstairs,' whispered Overton, 'your bill is paid, and your portmanteau in the chaise.' And then he added aloud, 'Now, waiters, the gentleman's ready.'

At this signal, the waiters crowded round Mr Alexander Trott. One took one arm; another, the other; a third, walked before with a candle; the fourth, behind with another candle; the boots and Mrs Williamson brought up the rear; and downstairs they went: Mr Alexander Trott expressing alternately at the very top of his voice either his feigned reluctance to go, or his unfeigned indignation at being shut up with a madman.

Mr Overton was waiting at the chaise door, the boys were ready mounted, and a few ostlers and stable nondescripts were standing round to witness the departure of 'the mad gentleman'. Mr Alexander Trott's foot was on the step when he observed (which the dim light had prevented his doing before) a figure seated in the chairs, closely muffled up in a cloak like his own.

'Who's that?' he inquired of Overton, in a whisper.

'Hush, hush,' replied the mayor: 'the other party of course.'

'The other party!' exclaimed Trott, with an effort to retreat.

'Yes, yes; you'll soon find that out, before you go far, I should think – but make a noise, you'll excite suspicion if you whisper to me so much.'

'I won't go in this chaise!' shouted Mr Alexander Trott, all his original fears recurring with tenfold violence. 'I shall be assassinated – I shall be – '

'Bravo, bravo,' whispered Overton. 'I'll push you in.'

'But I won't go,' exclaimed Mr Trott. 'Help here, help! They're carrying me away against my will. This is a plot to murder me.'

'Poor dear!' said Mrs Williamson again.

'Now, boys, put 'em along,' cried the mayor, pushing Trott in and slamming the door. 'Off with you, as quick as you can, and stop for nothing till you come to the next stage – all right!'

'Horses are paid, Tom,' screamed Mrs Williamson; and away went the chaise, at the rate of fourteen miles an hour, with Mr Alexander Trott and Miss Julia Manners carefully shut up in the inside.

Mr Alexander Trott remained coiled up in one corner of the chaise, and his mysterious companion in the other, for the first two or three miles; Mr Trott edging more and more into his corner, as he felt his companion gradually edging more and more from hers; and vainly endeavouring in the darkness to catch a glimpse of the furious face of the supposed Horace Hunter.

'We may speak now,' said his fellow traveller, at length; 'the post boys can neither see nor hear us.'

'That's not Hunter's voice!' – thought Alexander, astonished.

'Dear Lord Peter!' said Miss Julia, most winningly: putting her arm on Mr Trott's shoulder. 'Dear Lord Peter. Not a word?'

'Why, it's a woman!' exclaimed Mr Trott, in a low tone of excessive wonder.

'Ah! Whose voice is that?' said Julia; ''tis not Lord Peter's.'

'No, – it's mine,' replied Mr Trott.

'Yours!' ejaculated Miss Julia Manners; 'a strange man! Gracious heaven! How came you here!'

'Whoever you are, you might have known that I came against my will, ma'am,' replied Alexander, 'for I made noise enough when I got in.'

'Do you come from Lord Peter?' inquired Miss Manners.

'Confound Lord Peter,' replied Trott pettishly. 'I don't know any Lord Peter. I never heard of him before tonight, when I've been Lord Peter'd by one and Lord Peter'd by another, till I verily believe I'm mad, or dreaming—'

'Whither are we going?' inquired the lady tragically.

'How should *I* know, ma'am?' replied Trott with singular coolness; for the events of the evening had completely hardened him.

'Stop! stop!' cried the lady, letting down the front glasses of the chaise.

'Stay, my dear ma'am!' said Mr Trott, pulling the glasses up again with one hand, and gently squeezing Miss Julia's waist with the other. 'There is some mistake here; give me till the end of this stage to explain my share of it. We must go so far; you cannot be set down here alone, at this hour of the night.'

The lady consented; the mistake was mutually explained. Mr Trott was a young man, had highly promising whiskers, an undeniable tailor, and an insinuating address – he wanted nothing but valour, and who wants that with three thousand a year? The lady had this, and more; she wanted a young husband, and the only course open to Mr Trott to retrieve his disgrace was a rich wife. So they came to the conclusion that it would be a pity to have all this trouble and expense for nothing; and that as they were so far on the road already, they had better go to Gretna Green, and marry each other; and they did so. And the very next preceding entry in the Blacksmith's book, was an entry of the marriage of Emily Brown with

Horace Hunter. Mr Hunter took his wife home, and begged pardon, and *was* pardoned; and Mr Trott took *his* wife home, begged pardon too, and was pardoned also. And Lord Peter, who had been detained beyond his time by drinking champagne and riding a steeplechase, went back to the Honourable Augustus Flair's, and drank more champagne, and rode another steeplechase, and was thrown and killed. And Horace Hunter took great credit to himself for practising on the cowardice of Alexander Trott; and all these circumstances were discovered in time, and carefully noted down; and if you ever stop a week at the Winglebury Arms, they will give you just this account of The Great Winglebury Duel.

## Chapter Nine

### *Mrs Joseph Porter*

First published as 'Mrs Joseph Porter "Over the Way"' in the *Monthly Magazine,* January 1834, Dickens's second appearance 'in all the glory of print'. Domestic amateur theatricals had been a prominent activity in the Dickens household during 1833. To honour Shakespeare's birthday on 27 April Dickens organised and starred in an elaborate production of the popular opera *Clari; or, the Maid of Milan* in the family's London lodgings – the evening's entertainment also featured an interlude and a farce. Later in the year he had composed an operatic burlesque *O'Thello* in which his father played the part of 'The Great Unpaid' and other members of the family took parts. For an account of the surviving fragments of this burlesque see *The Dickensian,* Vol. 73 (1977), pp. 67–8.

Most extensive were the preparations at Rose Villa, Clapham Rise, in the occupation of Mr Gattleton (a stockbroker in especially comfortable circumstances), and great was the anxiety of Mr Gattleton's interesting family, as the day fixed for the representation of the Private Play which had been 'many months in preparation', approached. The whole family was infected with the mania for Private Theatricals; the house, usually so clean and tidy, was, to use Mr Gattleton's expressive description, 'regularly turned out o' windows'; the large dining room, dismantled of its furniture and ornaments, presented a strange jumble of flats, flies, wings, lamps, bridges, clouds, thunder and lightning, festoons and flowers, daggers and foil, and various other messes in theatrical slang included under the comprehensive name of 'properties'. The bedrooms were crowded with scenery, the kitchen was occupied by carpenters. Rehearsals took place every other night in the drawing room, and every sofa in the house was more or less damaged by the perseverance and spirit with which Mr Sempronius Gattleton, and Miss Lucina, rehearsed the smothering scene in 'Othello' – it having been determined that that tragedy should form the first portion of the evening's entertainments.

'When we're a *leetle* more perfect, I think it will go admirably,' said Mr Sempronius, addressing his *corps dramatique,* at the conclusion of the hundred and fiftieth rehearsal. In consideration of his sustaining the trifling

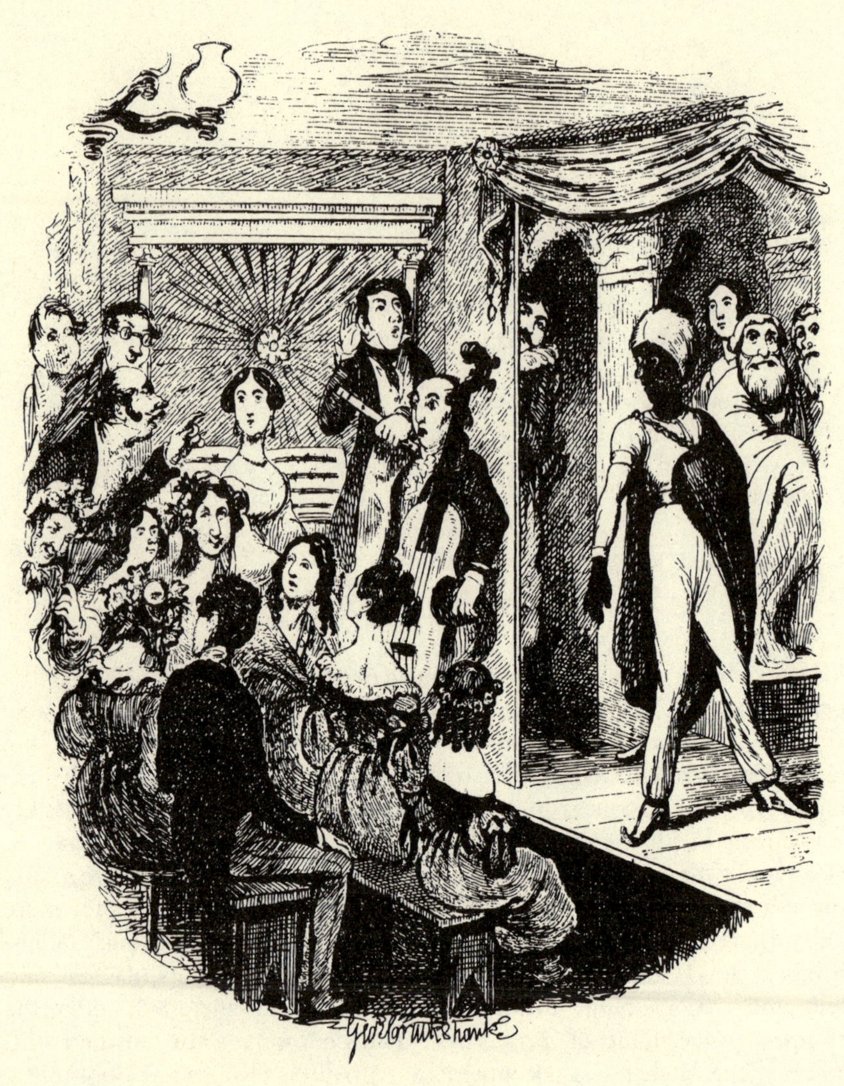

*Mr Sempronius Gattleton as Othello* *(see p. 412)*

inconvenience of bearing all the expenses of the play, Mr Sempronius had been in the most handsome manner, unanimously elected stage manager. 'Evans,' continued Mr Gattleton the younger, addressing a tall, thin, pale young gentleman, with extensive whiskers – 'Evans, you play *Roderigo* beautifully.'

'Beautifully,' echoed the three Miss Gattletons; for Mr Evans was pronounced by all his lady friends to be 'quite a dear'. He looked so interesting, and had such lovely whiskers: to say nothing of his talent for writing verses in albums and playing the flute! *Roderigo* simpered and bowed.

'But I think,' added the manager, 'you are hardly perfect in the – fall – in the fencing scene, where you are – you understand?'

'It's very difficult,' said Mr Evans, thoughtfully; 'I've fallen about a good deal in our counting house lately, for practice, only I find it hurts one so. Being obliged to fall backward you see, it bruises one's head a good deal.'

'But you must take care you don't knock a wing down,' said Mr Gattleton, the elder, who had been appointed prompter, and who took as much interest in the play as the youngest of the company. 'The stage is very narrow, you know.'

'Oh! don't be afraid,' said Mr Evans, with a very self-satisfied air: 'I shall fall with my head "off", and then I can't do any harm.'

'But, egad,' said the manager, rubbing his hands, 'we shall make a decided hit in "Masaniello". Harleigh sings that music admirably.'

Everybody echoed the sentiment. Mr Harleigh smiled, and looked foolish – not an unusual thing with him – hummed 'Behold how brightly breaks the morning', and blushed as red as the fisherman's nightcap he was trying on.

'Let's see,' resumed the manager, telling the number on his fingers, 'we shall have three dancing female peasants, besides *Fenella* and four fishermen. Then, there's our man Tom; he can have a pair of ducks of mine, and a check shirt of Bob's, and a red nightcap, and he'll do for another – that's five. In the choruses, of course, we can sing at the sides; and in the market scene we can walk about in cloaks and things. When the revolt takes place, Tom must keep rushing in on one side and out on the other, with a pickaxe, as fast as he can. The effect will be electrical; it will look exactly as if there were an immense number of 'em. And in the eruption scene we must burn the red fire, and upset the tea trays, and make all sorts of noises – and it's sure to do.'

'Sure! sure!' cried all the performers *unâ voce* – and away hurried, Mr Sempronius Gattleton to wash the burnt cork off his face, and superintend the 'setting up' of some of the amateur painted, but never-sufficiently-to-be-admired, scenery.

Mrs Gattleton, was a kind, good tempered, vulgar soul, exceedingly fond of her husband and children, and entertaining only three dislikes. In the first place, she had a natural antipathy to anybody else's unmarried daughters; in the second, she was in bodily fear of anything in the shape of ridicule; lastly – almost a necessary consequence of this feeling – she regarded, with feelings of the utmost horror, one Mrs Joseph Porter, over the way. However, the good folks of Clapham and its vicinity stood very much in awe of scandal and sarcasm; and thus Mrs Joseph Porter was courted, and flattered, and caressed, and invited, for much the same reason that induces a poor author, without a farthing in his pocket, to behave with extraordinary civility to a twopenny postman.

'Never mind, ma,' said Miss Emma Porter, in colloquy with her respected relative, and trying to look unconcerned; 'if they had invited me, you know that neither you nor pa would have allowed me to take part in such an exhibition.'

'Just what I should have thought from your high sense of propriety,' returned the mother. 'I am glad to see, Emma, you know how to designate the proceeding.' Miss P., by-the-bye, had only the week before made 'an exhibition' of herself for four days, behind a counter at a fancy fair, to all and every of her Majesty's liege subjects who were disposed to pay a shilling each for the privilege of seeing some four dozen girls flirting with strangers, and playing at shop.

'There!' said Mrs Porter, looking out of window; 'there are two rounds of beef and a ham going in – clearly for sandwiches; and Thomas, the pastry cook, says, there have been twelve dozen tarts ordered, besides blancmange and jellies. Upon my word! think of the Miss Gattletons in fancy dresses, too!'

'Oh, it's too ridiculous!' said Miss Porter, hysterically.

'I'll manage to put them a little out of conceit with the business, however,' said Mrs Porter, and out she went on her charitable errand.

'Well, my dear Mrs Gattleton,' said Mrs Joseph Porter, after they had been closeted for some time, and when, by dint of indefatigable pumping, she had managed to extract all the news about the play, 'well, my dear, people may say what they please; indeed we know they will, for some folks are *so* ill-natured. Ah, my dear Miss Lucina, how d'ye do? I was just telling your mamma that I have heard it said that—'

'What?'

'Mrs Porter is alluding to the play, my dear,' said Mrs Gattleton; 'she was, I am sorry to say, just informing me that—'

'Oh, now pray don't mention it,' interrupted Mrs Porter; 'it's most absurd – quite as absurd as young What's-his-name saying he wondered how Miss Caroline, with such a foot and ankle, could have the vanity to play *Fenella*.'

'Highly impertinent, whoever said it,' said Mrs Gattleton, bridling up.

'Certainly, my dear,' chimed in the delighted Mrs Porter; 'most undoubtedly! Because, as I said, if Miss Caroline *does* play *Fenella,* it doesn't follow, as a matter of course, that she should think she has a pretty foot; – and then – such puppies as these young men are – he had the impudence to say, that—'

How far the amiable Mrs Porter might have succeeded in her pleasant purpose, it is impossible to say, had not the entrance of Mr Thomas Balderstone, Mrs Gattleton's brother, familiarly called in the family 'Uncle Tom', changed the course of conversation, and suggested to her mind an excellent plan of operation on the evening of the play.

Uncle Tom was very rich, and exceedingly fond of his nephews and nieces: as a matter of course, therefore, he was an object of great importance in his own family. He was one of the best hearted men in existence: always in a good temper, and always talking. It was his boast that he wore top boots on all occasions, and had never worn a black silk neckerchief; and it was his pride that he remembered all the principal plays of Shakespeare from beginning to end – and so he did. The result of this parrot-like accomplishment was, that he was not only perpetually quoting himself, but that he could never sit by, and hear a misquotation from the 'Swan of Avon' without setting the unfortunate delinquent right. He was also something of a wag; never missed an opportunity of saying what he considered a good thing, and invariably laughed until he cried at anything that appeared to him mirth-moving or ridiculous.

'Well, girls!' said Uncle Tom, after the preparatory ceremony of kissing and how-d'ye-do-ing had been gone through – 'how d'ye get on? Know your parts, eh? – Lucina, my dear, act ii, scene 1 – place, left – cue – "Unknown fate", – What's next, eh? – Go on – "The Heavens—" '

'Oh, yes,' said Miss Lucina, 'I recollect –

The heavens forbid
But that our loves and comforts should increase
Even as our days do grow!" '

'Make a pause here and there,' said the old gentleman, who was a great critic. ' "But that our loves and comforts should increase" – emphasis on the last syllable, "crease", – loud "even", – one, two, three, four; then loud again, "as our days do grow"; emphasis on *days.* That's the way, my dear; trust to your uncle for emphasis. Ah! Sem, my boy, how are you?'

'Very well, thankee, uncle,' returned Mr Sempronius, who had just appeared, looking something like a ringdove with a small circle round each eye: the result of his constant corking. 'Of course we see you on Thursday.'

'Of course, of course, my dear boy.'

'What a pity it is your nephew didn't think of making you prompter, Mr Balderstone!' whispered Mrs Joseph Porter; 'you would have been invaluable.'

'Well, I flatter myself, I *should* have been tolerably up to the thing,' responded Uncle Tom.

'I must bespeak sitting next you on the night,' resumed Mrs Porter; 'and then, if our dear young friends here should be at all wrong, you will be able to enlighten me. I shall be so interested.'

'I am sure I shall be most happy to give you any assistance in my power.'

'Mind, it's a bargain.'

'Certainly.'

'I don't know how it is,' said Mrs Gattleton to her daughters, as they were sitting round the fire in the evening, looking over their parts, 'but I really very much wish Mrs Joseph Porter wasn't coming on Thursday. I am sure she's scheming something.'

'She can't make *us* ridiculous, however,' observed Mr Sempronius Gattleton, haughtily.

The long-looked-for Thursday arrived in due course, and brought with it, as Mr Gattleton, senior, philosophically observed, 'no disappointments to speak of.' True, it was yet a matter of doubt whether *Cassio* would be enabled to get into the dress which had been sent for him from the masquerade warehouse. It was equally uncertain whether the principal female singer would be sufficiently recovered from the influenza to make her appearance; Mr Harleigh, the *Masaniello* of the night, was hoarse, and rather unwell, in consequence of the great quantity of lemon and sugar candy he had eaten to improve his voice; and two flutes and a violoncello had pleaded severe colds. What of that? the audience were all coming. Everybody knew his part; the dresses were covered with tinsel and spangles; the white plumes looked beautiful; Mr Evans had practised falling until he was bruised from head to foot and quite perfect; *Iago* was sure that, in the stabbing scene, he should make 'a decided hit'. A self-taught deaf gentleman, who had kindly offered to bring his flute, would be a most valuable addition to the orchestra; Miss Jenkins's talent for the piano was too well known to be doubted for an instant; Mr Cape had practised the violin accompaniment with her frequently; and Mr Brown, who had kindly undertaken, at a few hours' notice, to bring his violoncello, would, no doubt, manage extremely well.

Seven o'clock came, and so did the audience; all the rank and fashion of Clapham and its vicinity was fast filling the theatre. There were the Smiths, the Gubbinses, the Nixons, the Dixons, the Hicksons, people with all sorts of names, two aldermen, a sheriff in perspective, Sir Thomas

Glumper (who had been knighted in the last reign for carrying up an address on somebody's escaping from nothing); and last, not least, there were Mrs Joseph Porter and Uncle Tom, seated in the centre of the third row from the stage; Mrs P. amusing Uncle Tom with all sorts of stories, and Uncle Tom amusing everyone else by laughing most immoderately.

Ting, ting, ting! went the prompter's bell at eight o'clock precisely, and dash went the orchestra into the overture to 'The Men of Prometheus'. The pianoforte player hammered away with laudable perseverance; and the violoncello, which struck in at intervals, 'sounded very well, considering'. The unfortunate individual, however, who had undertaken to play the flute accompaniment 'at sight', found, from fatal experience, the perfect truth of the old adage, 'out of sight, out of mind'; for being very near-sighted, and being placed at a considerable distance from his music book, all he had an opportunity of doing was to play a bar now and then in the wrong place, and put the other performers out. It is, however, but justice to Mr Brown to say that he did this to admiration. The overture, in fact, was not unlike a race between the different instruments; the piano came in first by several bars, and the violoncello next, quite distancing the poor flute; for the deaf gentleman *too-too'd* away, quite unconscious that he was at all wrong, until apprised, by the applause of the audience, that the overture was concluded. A considerable bustle and shuffling of feet was then heard upon the stage, accompanied by whispers of 'Here's a pretty go! – what's to be done?' &c. The audience applauded again, by way of raising the spirits of the performers; and then Mr Sempronius desired the prompter in a very audible voice, to 'clear the stage, and ring up'.

Ting, ting, ting! went the bell again. Everybody sat down; the curtain shook; rose sufficiently high to display several pair of yellow boots paddling about; and there remained.

Ting! ting, ting! went the bell again. The curtain was violently convulsed, but rose no higher; the audience tittered; Mrs Porter looked at Uncle Tom; Uncle Tom looked at everybody, rubbing his hands, and laughing with perfect rapture. After as much ringing with the little bell as a muffin boy would make in going down a tolerably long street, and a vast deal of whispering, hammering, and calling for nails and cord, the curtain at length rose, and discovered Mr Sempronius Gattleton *solus,* and decked for *Othello.* After three distinct rounds of applause, during which Mr Sempronius applied his right hand to his left breast, and bowed in the most approved manner, the manager advanced and said:

'Ladies and Gentlemen – I assure you it is with sincere regret, that I regret to be compelled to inform you, that *Iago* who was to have played Mr Wilson – I beg your pardon, Ladies and Gentlemen, but I am naturally somewhat agitated (applause) – I mean, Mr Wilson, who was to have played *Iago,* is – that is, has been – or, in other words, Ladies and Gentlemen, the fact is, that I have just received a note, in which I am informed that *Iago* is unavoidably detained at the Post Office this evening. Under these circumstances, I trust – a – a – amateur performance – a – another gentleman undertakes to read the part – request indulgence for a short time – courtesy and kindness of a British audience.' Overwhelming applause. Exit Mr Sempronius Gattleton, and curtain falls.

The audience were, of course, exceedingly good-humoured; the whole business was a joke; and accordingly they waited for an hour with the utmost patience, being enlivened by an interlude of rout cakes and lemonade. It appeared by Mr Sempronius's subsequent explanation, that the delay would not have been so great, had it not so happened that when the substitute *Iago* had finished dressing, and just as the play was on the point of commencing, the original *Iago* unexpectedly arrived. The former was therefore compelled to undress, and the latter to dress for his part; which, as he found some difficulty in getting into his clothes, occupied no inconsiderable time. At last, the tragedy began in real earnest. It went off well enough, until the third scene of the first act, in which *Othello* addresses the Senate: the only remarkable circumstance being, that as *Iago* could not get on any of the stage boots, in consequence of his feet being violently swelled with the heat and excitement, he was under the necessity of playing the part in a pair of Wellingtons, which contrasted rather oddly with his richly embroidered pantaloons. When *Othello* started with his address to the Senate (whose dignity was represented by the *Duke,* a carpenter, two men engaged on the recommendation of the gardener, and a boy), Mrs Porter found the opportunity she so anxiously sought.

Mr Sempronius proceeded:

> 'Most potent, grave, and reverend signiors,
> My very noble and approv'd good masters,
> That I have ta'en away this old man's daughter,
> It is most true; – rude am I in my speech—'

'Is that right?' whispered Mrs Porter to Uncle Tom.

'No.'

'Tell him so, then.'

'I will. Sem!' called out Uncle Tom, 'that's wrong, my boy.'

'What's wrong, uncle?' demanded *Othello,* quite forgetting the dignity of his situation.

'You've left out something. "True I have married—" '

'Oh, ah!' said Mr Sempronius, endeavouring to hide his confusion as much and as ineffectually as the audience attempted to conceal their half-suppressed tittering, by coughing with extraordinary violence –

—"true I have married her; –
The very head and front of my offending
Hath this extent; no more."

(*Aside*) Why don't you prompt, father?'

'Because I've mislaid my spectacles,' said poor Mr Gattleton, almost dead with the heat and bustle.

'There, now it's "rude am I," ' said Uncle Tom.

'Yes, I know it is,' returned the unfortunate manager, proceeding with his part.

It would be useless and tiresome to quote the number of instances in which Uncle Tom, now completely in his element, and instigated by the mischievous Mrs Porter, corrected the mistakes of the performers; suffice it to say that, having mounted his hobby, nothing could induce him to dismount; so, during the whole remainder of the play, he performed a kind of running accompaniment, by muttering everybody's part as it was being delivered, in an undertone. The audience were highly amused, Mrs Porter delighted, the performers embarrassed; Uncle Tom never was better pleased in all his life; and Uncle Tom's nephews and nieces had never, although the declared heirs to his large property, so heartily wished him gathered to his fathers as on that memorable occasion.

Several other minor causes, too, united to damp the ardour of the *dramatis personæ*. None of the performers could walk in their tights, or move their arms in their jackets; the pantaloons were too small, the boots too large, and the swords of all shapes and sizes. Mr Evans, naturally too tall for the scenery, wore a black velvet hat with immense white plumes, the glory of which was lost in 'the flies'; and the only other inconvenience of which was, that when it was off his head he could not put it on, and when it was on he could not take it off. Notwithstanding all his practice, too, he fell with his head and shoulders as neatly through one of the side scenes, as a harlequin would jump through a panel in a Christmas pantomime. The pianoforte player, overpowered by the extreme heat of the room, fainted away at the commencement of the entertainment, leaving the music of 'Masaniello' to the flute and violoncello. The orchestra complained that Mr Harleigh put them out, and Mr Harleigh declared that the orchestra prevented his singing a note. The fishermen, who were hired for the occasion, revolted to the very life, positively refusing to play without an increased allowance of spirits; and, their demand being complied with, getting drunk in the eruption scene as naturally as possible. The red fire, which was burnt at the conclusion of the second act, not only nearly suffocated the audience, but nearly set the house on fire into the bargain; and, as it was, the remainder of the piece was acted in a thick fog.

In short, the whole affair was, as Mrs Joseph Porter triumphantly told everybody, 'a complete failure'. The audience went home at four o'clock in the morning, exhausted with laughter, suffering from severe headaches, and smelling terribly of brimstone and gunpowder. The Messrs Gattleton, senior and junior, retired to rest, with the vague idea of emigrating to Swan River early in the ensuing week.

Rose Villa has once again resumed its wonted appearance; the dining room furniture has been replaced; the tables are as nicely polished as formerly; the horsehair chairs are ranged against the wall, as regularly as ever; Venetian blinds have been fitted to every window in the house to intercept the prying gaze of Mrs Joseph Porter. The subject of theatricals is never mentioned in the Gattleton family, unless, indeed, by Uncle Tom, who cannot refrain from sometimes expressing his surprise and regret at finding that his nephews and nieces appear to have lost the relish they once possessed for the beauties of Shakespeare, and quotations from the works of that immortal bard.

# Chapter Ten

## *A Passage in the Life of Mr Watkins Tottle*

First published in two chapters in the *Monthly Magazine,* January and February 1835. Peter Ackroyd notes in *Dickens,* (1990) p. 160 that the detailed description in the second chapter of Mr Solomon Jacobs's 'lock up' (or 'sponging') house in Cursitor Street was certainly based on unhappy recent experience. Dickens's impecunious father had been arrested for debt in November 1834 and taken to Sloman's sponging house at No. 4 Cursitor Street where Dickens had to go to bail him out (see *Pilgrim,* Vol. 1, 44 f.).

### CHAPTER THE FIRST

Matrimony is proverbially a serious undertaking. Like an overweening predilection for brandy and water, it is a misfortune into which a man easily falls, and from which he finds it remarkably difficult to extricate himself. It is of no use telling a man who is timorous on these points, that it is but one plunge, and all is over. They say the same thing at the Old Bailey, and the unfortunate victims derive as much comfort from the assurance in the one case as in the other.

Mr Watkins Tottle was a rather uncommon compound of strong uxorious inclinations, and an unparalleled degree of anti-connubial timidity. He was about fifty years of age; stood four feet six inches and three-quarters in his socks – for he never stood in stockings at all – plump, clean, and rosy. He looked something like a vignette to one of Richardson's novels, and had a clean-cravatish formality of manner, and kitchen-pokerness of carriage, which Sir Charles Grandison himself might have envied. He lived on an annuity, which was well adapted to the individual who received it, in one respect – it was rather small. He received it in periodical payments on every alternate Monday; but he ran himself out, about a day after the expiration of the first week, as regularly as an eight day clock; and then, to make the comparison complete, his landlady wound him up, and he went on with a regular tick.

Mr Watkins Tottle had long lived in a state of single blessedness, as bachelors say, or single cursedness, as spinsters think; but the idea of matrimony had never ceased to haunt him. Wrapt in profound reveries

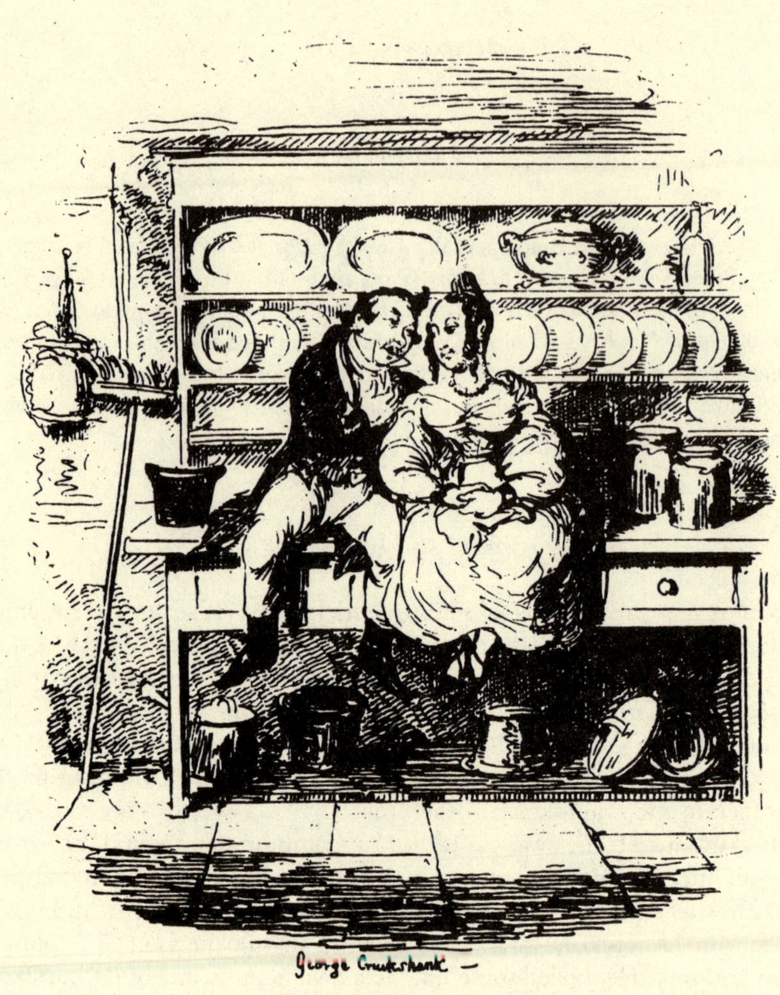


*The Courtship of Mr Parsons* (see p. 425)

on this never failing theme, fancy transformed his small parlour in Cecil Street, Strand, into a neat house in the suburbs; the half-hundredweight of coals under the kitchen stairs suddenly sprang up into three tons of the best Walls-end; his small French bedstead was converted into a regular matrimonial four-poster; and in the empty chair on the opposite side of the fireplace, imagination seated a beautiful young lady, with a very little independence or will of her own, and a very large independence under a will of her father's.

'Who's there?' inquired Mr Watkins Tottle, as a gentle tap at his room door disturbed these meditations one evening.

'Tottle, my dear fellow, how *do* you do?' said a short elderly gentleman with a gruffish voice, bursting into the room, and replying to the question by asking another.

'Told you I should drop in some evening,' said the short gentleman, as he delivered his hat into Tottle's hand, after a little struggling and dodging.

'Delighted to see you, I'm sure,' said Mr Watkins Tottle, wishing internally that his visitor had 'dropped in' to the Thames at the bottom of the street, instead of dropping into his parlour. The fortnight was nearly up, and Watkins was hard up.

'How is Mrs Gabriel Parsons?' inquired Tottle.

'Quite well, thank you,' replied Mr Gabriel Parsons, for that was the name the short gentleman revelled in. Here there was a pause; the short gentleman looked at the left hob of the fireplace; Mr Watkins Tottle stared vacancy out of countenance.

'Quite well,' repeated the short gentleman, when five minutes had expired. 'I may say remarkably well.' And he rubbed the palms of his hands as hard as if he were going to strike a light by friction.

'What will you take?' inquired Tottle, with the desperate suddenness of a man who knew that unless the visitor took his leave, he stood very little chance of taking anything else.

'Oh, I don't know – have you any whiskey?'

'Why,' replied Tottle, very slowly, for all this was gaining time, 'I *had* some capital, and remarkably strong whiskey last week; but it's all gone – and therefore its strength—'

'Is much beyond proof; or, in other words, impossible to be proved,' said the short gentleman; and he laughed very heartily, and seemed quite glad the whiskey had been drunk. Mr Tottle smiled – but it was the smile of despair. When Mr Gabriel Parsons had done laughing, he delicately insinuated that, in the absence of whiskey, he would not be averse to brandy. And Mr Watkins Tottle, lighting a flat candle very ostentatiously; and displaying an immense key, which belonged to the street door, but which, for the sake of appearances, occasionally did duty in an imaginary wine cellar; left the room to entreat his landlady to charge their glasses, and charge them in the bill. The application was successful; the spirits were speedily called – not from the vasty deep, but the adjacent wine vaults. The two short gentlemen mixed their grog; and then sat cosily down before the fire – a pair of shorts airing themselves.

'Tottle,' said Mr Gabriel Parsons, 'you know my way – off-hand, open, say what I mean, mean what I say, hate reserve, and can't bear affectation. One is a bad domino which only hides what good people have about 'em, without making the bad look better; and the other is much about the same thing as pinking a white cotton stocking to make it look like a silk one. Now listen to what I'm going to say.'

Here, the little gentleman paused, and took a long pull at his brandy and water. Mr Watkins Tottle took a sip of his, stirred the fire, and assumed an air of profound attention.

'It's of no use humming and ha'ing about the matter,' resumed the short gentleman – 'You want to get married.'

'Why,' replied Mr Watkins Tottle evasively; for he trembled violently; and felt a sudden tingling throughout his whole frame; 'why – I should certainly – at least, I *think* I should like—'

'Won't do,' said the short gentleman. – 'Plain and free – or there's an end of the matter. Do you want money?'

'You know I do.'

'You admire the sex?'

'I do.'

'And you'd like to be married?'

'Certainly.'

'Then you shall be. There's an end of that.' Thus saying, Mr Gabriel Parsons took a pinch of snuff, and mixed another glass.

'Let me entreat you to be more explanatory,' said Tottle. 'Really, as the party principally interested, I cannot consent to be disposed of in this way.'

'I'll tell you,' replied Mr Gabriel Parsons, warming with the subject, and the brandy and water – 'I know a lady – she's stopping with my wife now – who is just the thing for you. Well educated; talks French; plays the piano; knows a good deal about flowers and shells, and all that sort of thing; and has five hundred a year, with an uncontrolled power of disposing of it, by her last will and testament.'

'I'll pay my addresses to her,' said Mr Watkins Tottle. 'She isn't *very* young – is she?'

'Not very; just the thing for you. I've said that already.'

'What coloured hair has the lady?' inquired Mr Watkins Tottle.

'Egad, I hardly recollect,' replied Gabriel, with coolness. 'Perhaps I ought to have observed at first, she wears a front.'

'A what?' ejaculated Tottle.

'One of those things with curls, along here,' said Parsons, drawing a straight line across his forehead, just over his eyes, in illustration of his meaning. 'I know the front's black; I can't speak quite positively about her own hair; because, unless one walks behind her, and catches a glimpse of it under her bonnet, one seldom sees it; but I should say that it was *rather* lighter than the front – a shade of a greyish tinge, perhaps.'

Mr Watkins Tottle looked as if he had certain misgivings of mind. Mr Gabriel Parsons perceived it, and thought it would be safe to begin the next attack without delay.

'Now, were you ever in love, Tottle?' he inquired.

Mr Watkins Tottle blushed up to the eyes, and down to the chin, and exhibited a most extensive combination of colours as he confessed the soft impeachment.

'I suppose you popped the question more than once when you were a young – I beg your pardon – a younger – man?' said Parsons.

'Never in my life!' replied his friend, apparently indignant at being suspected of such an act. 'Never!' The fact is that I entertain, as you know, peculiar opinions on these subjects. I am not afraid of ladies, young or old – far from it; but I think that, in compliance with the custom of the present day, they allow too much freedom of speech and manner to marriageable men. Now, the fact is that anything like this easy freedom I never could acquire; and as I am always afraid of going too far, I am generally, I dare say, considered formal and cold.'

'I shouldn't wonder if you were,' replied Parsons, gravely; 'I shouldn't wonder. However, you'll be all right in this case; for the strictness and delicacy of this lady's ideas greatly exceed your own. Lord bless you, why when she came to our house, there was an old portrait of some man or other, with two large black staring eyes, hanging up in her bedroom; she positively refused to go to bed there, till it was taken down, considering it decidedly wrong.'

'I think so, too,' said Mr Watkins Tottle; 'certainly.'

'And then, the other night – I never laughed so much in my life' – resumed Mr Gabriel Parsons; 'I had driven home in an easterly wind, and caught a devil of a face ache. Well; as Fanny – that's Mrs Parsons, you know – and this friend of hers, and I, and Frank Ross, were playing a rubber, I said, jokingly, that when I went to bed I should wrap my head in Fanny's flannel petticoat. She instantly threw up her cards, and left the room.'

'Quite right!' said Mr Watkins Tottle; 'she could not possibly have behaved in a more dignified manner. What did you do?'

'Do? – Frank took dummy; and I won sixpence.'

'But didn't you apologise for hurting her feelings?'

'Devil a bit. Next morning at breakfast, we talked it over. She contended that any reference to a flannel petticoat was improper; – men ought not to be supposed to know that such things were. I pleaded my coverture; being a married man.'

'And what did the lady say to that?' inquired Tottle, deeply interested.

'Changed her ground, and said that Frank being a single man, its impropriety was obvious.'

'Noble-minded creature!' exclaimed the enraptured Tottle.

'Oh! both Fanny and I said, at once, that she was regularly cut out for you.'

A gleam of placid satisfaction shone on the circular face of Mr Watkins Tottle, as he heard the prophecy.

'There's one thing I can't understand,' said Mr Gabriel Parsons, as he rose to depart; 'I cannot, for the life and soul of me, imagine how the deuce you'll ever contrive to come together. The lady would certainly go into convulsions if the subject were mentioned.' Mr Gabriel Parsons sat down again, and laughed until he was weak. Tottle owed him money, so he had a perfect right to laugh at Tottle's expense.

Mr Watkins Tottle feared, in his own mind, that this was another characteristic which he had in common with this modern Lucretia. He, however, accepted the invitation to dine with the Parsonses on the next day but one, with great firmness: and looked forward to the introduction, when again left alone, with tolerable composure.

The sun that rose on the next day but one, had never beheld a sprucer personage on the outside of the Norwood stage, than Mr Watkins Tottle; and when the coach drew up before a cardboard-looking house with disguised chimneys, and a lawn like a large sheet of green letter paper, he certainly had never lighted to his place of destination a gentleman who felt more uncomfortable.

The coach stopped, and Mr Watkins Tottle jumped – we beg his pardon – alighted, with great dignity. 'All right!' said he, and away went the coach up the hill with that beautiful equanimity of pace for which 'short' stages are generally remarkable.

Mr Watkins Tottle gave a faltering jerk to the handle of the garden gate bell. He essayed a more energetic tug, and his previous nervousness was not at all diminished by hearing the bell ringing like a fire alarum.

'Is Mr Parsons at home?' inquired Tottle of the man who opened the gate. He could hardly hear himself speak, for the bell had not yet done tolling.

'Here I am,' shouted a voice on the lawn, – and there was Mr Gabriel Parsons in a flannel jacket, running backwards and forwards, from a wicket to two hats piled on each other, and from the two hats to the wicket, in the most violent manner, while another gentleman with his coat off was getting down the area of the house, after a ball. When the gentleman without the coat had found it – which he did in less than ten minutes – he ran back to the hats, and Gabriel Parsons pulled up. Then the gentleman without the coat called out 'play', very loudly, and bowled. Then Mr Gabriel Parsons knocked the ball several yards, and took another run. Then the other gentleman aimed at the wicket, and didn't hit it; and Mr Gabriel Parsons, having finished running on his own account, laid down the bat and ran after the ball, which went into a neighbouring field. They called this cricket.

'Tottle, will you "go in"?' inquired Mr Gabriel Parsons, as he approached him, wiping the perspiration off his face.

Mr Watkins Tottle declined the offer, the bare idea of accepting which made him even warmer than his friend.

"Then we'll go into the house, as it's past four, and I shall have to wash my hands before dinner," said Mr Gabriel Parsons. "Here, I hate ceremony, you know! Timson, that's Tottle – Tottle, that's Timson; bred for the church, which I fear will never be bread for him;" and he chuckled at the old joke. Mr Timson bowed carelessly. Mr Watkins Tottle bowed stiffly. Mr Gabriel Parsons led the way to the house. He was a rich sugar baker, who mistook rudeness for honesty, and abrupt bluntness for an open and candid manner; many besides Gabriel mistake bluntness for sincerity.

Mrs Gabriel Parsons received the visitors most graciously on the steps, and preceded them to the drawing room. On the sofa, was seated a lady of very prim appearance, and remarkably inanimate. She was one of those persons at whose age it is impossible to make any reasonable guess; her features might have been remarkably pretty when she was younger, and they might always have presented the same appearance. Her complexion – with a slight trace of powder here and there – was as clear as that of a well-made wax doll, and her face as expressive. She was handsomely dressed, and was winding up a gold watch.

'Miss Lillerton, my dear, this is our friend Mr Watkins Tottle; a very old acquaintance I assure you,' said Mrs Parsons, presenting the Strephon of Cecil Street, Strand. The Lady rose and made a deep curtsey; Mr Watkins Tottle made a bow.

'Splendid, majestic creature!' thought Tottle.

Mr Timson advanced, and Mr Watkins Tottle began to hate him. Men generally discover a rival, instinctively, and Mr Watkins Tottle felt that his hate was deserved.

'May I beg,' said the reverend gentleman, – 'May I beg to call upon you, Miss Lillerton, for some trifling donation to my soup, coals, and blanket distribution society?'

'Put my name down for two sovereigns, if you please,' responded Miss Lillerton.

'You are truly charitable, madam,' said the Reverend Mr Timson, 'and we know that charity will cover a multitude of sins. Let me beg you to understand that I do not say this from the supposition that you have many sins which require palliation; believe me when I say that I never yet met any one who had fewer to atone for, than Miss Lillerton.'

Something like a bad imitation of animation lighted up the lady's face as she acknowledged the compliment. Watkins Tottle incurred the sin of wishing that the ashes of the Reverend Charles Timson were quietly deposited in the churchyard of his curacy, wherever it might be.

'I'll tell you what,' interrupted Parsons, who had just appeared with clean hands and a black coat, 'it's my private opinion, Timson, that your "distribution society" is rather a humbug.'

'You are so severe,' replied Timson, with a Christian smile: he disliked Parsons, but liked his dinners.

'So positively unjust!' said Miss Lillerton.

'Certainly,' observed Tottle. The lady looked up; her eyes met those of Mr Watkins Tottle. She withdrew them in a sweet confusion, and Mr Watkins Tottle did the same – the confusion was mutual.

'Why,' urged Mr Parsons, pursuing his objections, 'what on earth is the use of giving a man coals who has nothing to cook, or giving him blankets when he hasn't a bed, or giving him soup when he requires substantial food? – 'like sending them ruffles when wanting a shirt.' Why not give 'em a trifle of money, as I do, when I think they deserve it, and let them purchase what they think best? Why? – because your subscribers wouldn't see their names flourishing in print on the church door – that's the reason.'

'Really, Mr Parsons, I hope you don't mean to insinuate that I wish to see *my* name in print, on the church door,' interrupted Miss Lillerton.

'I hope not,' said Mr Watkins Tottle, putting in another word, and getting another glance.

'Certainly not,' replied Parsons. 'I dare say you wouldn't mind seeing it in writing, though, in the church register – eh?'

'Register! What register?' inquired the lady, gravely.

'Why, the register of marriages, to be sure,' replied Parsons, chuckling at the sally, and glancing at Tottle. Mr Watkins Tottle thought he should have fainted for shame, and it is quite impossible to imagine what effect the joke would have had upon the lady, if dinner had not been, at that moment, announced. Mr Watkins Tottle, with an unprecedented effort of gallantry, offered the tip of his little finger; Miss Lillerton accepted it gracefully, with maiden modesty: and they proceeded in due state to the dinner table, where they were soon deposited side by side. The room was very snug, the dinner very good, and the little party in spirits. The conversation became pretty general, and when Mr Watkins Tottle had extracted one or two cold observations from his neighbour, and had taken wine with her, he began to acquire confidence rapidly. The cloth was removed; Mrs Gabriel Parsons drank four glasses of port on the plea of being a nurse just then; and Miss Lillerton took about the same number of sips, on the plea of not wanting any at all. At length, the ladies retired, to the great gratification of Mr Gabriel Parsons, who had been coughing and frowning at his wife, for half-an-hour previously – signals which Mrs Parsons never happened to observe, until she had been pressed to take her ordinary quantum, which, to avoid giving trouble, she generally did at once.

'What do you think of her?' inquired Mr Gabriel Parsons of Mr Watkins Tottle, in an undertone.

'I dote on her with enthusiasm already!' replied Mr Watkins Tottle.

'Gentlemen, pray let us drink "the ladies",' said the Reverend Mr Timson.

'The ladies!' said Mr Watkins Tottle, emptying his glass. In the fullness of his confidence, he felt as if he could make love to a dozen ladies, off-hand.

'Ah!' said Mr Gabriel Parsons, 'I remember when I was a young man – fill your glass, Timson.'

'I have this moment emptied it.'

'Then fill again.'

'I will,' said Timson, suiting the action to the word.

'I remember,' resumed. Mr Gabriel Parsons, 'when I was a younger man, with what a strange compound of feelings I used to drink that toast, and how I used to think every woman was an angel.'

'Was that before you were married?' mildly inquired Mr Watkins Tottle.

'Oh! certainly,' replied Mr Gabriel Parsons. 'I have never thought so since; and a precious milksop I must have been, ever to have thought so at all. But, you know, I married Fanny under the oddest and most ridiculous circumstances possible.'

'What were they, if one may inquire?' asked Timson, who had heard the story, on an average, twice a week for the last six months. Mr Watkins Tottle listened attentively, in the hope of picking up some suggestion that might be useful to him in his new undertaking.

'I spent my wedding night in a back kitchen chimney,' said Parsons, by way of a beginning.

'In a back kitchen chimney!' ejaculated Watkins Tottle. 'How dreadful!'

'Yes, it wasn't very pleasant,' replied the small host. 'The fact is, Fanny's father and mother liked me well enough as an individual, but had a decided objection to my becoming a husband. You see, I hadn't any money in those days, and they had; and so they wanted Fanny to pick up somebody else. However, we managed to discover the state of each other's affections somehow. I used to meet her at some mutual friends' parties; at first we danced together, and talked, and flirted, and all that sort of thing; then I used to like nothing so well as sitting by her side – we didn't talk so much then, but I remember I used to have a great notion of looking at her out of the extreme corner of my left eye – and then I got very miserable and sentimental, and began to write verses, and use Macassar oil. At last, I couldn't bear it any longer, and after I had walked up and down the sunny side of Oxford Street in tight boots for a week – and a devilish hot summer it was too – in the hope of meeting her, I sat down and wrote a letter, and begged her to manage to see me clandestinely, for I wanted to hear her decision from her own mouth. I said I had discovered, to my perfect satisfaction, that I couldn't live without her, and that if she didn't have me, I had made up my mind to take prussic acid, or take to drinking, or emigrate, so as to take myself off in some way or other. Well, I borrowed a pound, and bribed the housemaid to give her a note, which she did.'

'And what was the reply?' inquired Timson, who had found, before, that to encourage the repetition of old stories is to get a general invitation.

'Oh, the usual one! Fanny expressed herself very miserable; hinted at the possibility of an early grave; said that nothing should induce her to swerve from the duty she owed her parents; implored me to forget her, and find out somebody more deserving, and all that sort of thing. She said she could, on no account, think of meeting me unknown to her pa and ma; and entreated me, as she should be in a particular part of Kensington Gardens at eleven o'clock next morning, not to attempt to meet her there.'

'You didn't go, of course?' said Watkins Tottle.

'Didn't I? – Of course I did. There she was, with the identical housemaid in perspective, in order that there might be no interruption. We walked about for a couple of hours; made ourselves delightfully miserable; and were regularly engaged. Then, we began to 'correspond' – that is to say, we used to exchange about four letters a day; what we used to say in 'em I can't imagine. And I used to have an interview, in the kitchen, or the cellar, or some such place, every evening. Well, things went on in this way for some time; and we got fonder of each other every day. At last, as our love was raised to such a pitch, and as my salary had been raised too, shortly before, we determined on a secret marriage. Fanny arranged to sleep at a friend's on the previous night; we were to be married early in the morning; and then we were to return to her home and be pathetic. She was to fall at the old gentleman's feet, and bathe his boots with her tears; and I was to hug the old lady and call her "mother", and use my pocket handkerchief as much as possible. Married we were, the next morning; two girls – friends of Fanny's – acting as bridesmaids; and a man, who was hired for five shillings and a pint of porter, officiating as father. Now, the old lady unfortunately put off her return from Ramsgate, where she had been paying a visit, until the next morning; and as we placed great reliance on her, we agreed to postpone our confession for four-and-twenty hours. My newly made wife returned home, and I spent my wedding day in strolling about Hampstead Heath, and execrating my father-in-law. Of course, I went to comfort my dear little wife at night, as much as I could, with the assurance that our troubles would soon be over. I opened the garden gate, of which I had a key, and was shown by the servant to our old place of meeting – a back kitchen, with a stone floor and a dresser: upon which, in the absence of chairs, we used to sit and make love.'

'Make love upon a kitchen dresser!' interrupted Mr Watkins Tottle, whose ideas of decorum were greatly outraged.

'Ah! On a kitchen dresser!' replied Parsons. 'And let me tell you, old fellow, that, if you were really over head-and-ears in love, and had no other place to make love in, you'd be devilish glad to avail yourself of such an opportunity. However, let me see; – where was I?'

'On the dresser,' suggested Timson.

'Oh – ah! Well, here I found poor Fanny, quite disconsolate and uncomfortable. The old boy had been very cross all day, which made her feel still more lonely; and she was quite out of spirits. So I put a good face on the matter, and laughed it off, and said we should enjoy the pleasures of a matrimonial life more by contrast; and, at length, poor Fanny brightened up a little. I stopped there till about eleven o'clock, and, just as I was taking my leave for the fourteenth time, the girl came running down the stairs, without her shoes, in a great fright, to tell us that the old villain – Heaven forgive me for calling him so, for he is dead and gone now! – prompted I suppose by the prince of darkness, was coming down, to draw his own beer for supper – a thing he had not done before, for six months, to my certain knowledge; for the cask stood in that very back kitchen. If he discovered me there, explanation would have been out of the question; for he was so outrageously violent, when at all excited, that he never would have listened to me. There was only one thing to be done. The chimney was a very wide one; it had been originally built for an oven; went up perpendicularly for a few feet, and then shot backward and formed a sort of small cavern. My hopes and fortune – the means of our joint existence almost – were at stake. I scrambled in like a squirrel; coiled myself up in this recess; and, as Fanny and the girl replaced the deal chimney board, I could see the light of the candle which my unconscious father-in-law carried in his hand. I heard him draw the beer; and I never heard beer run so slowly. He was just leaving the kitchen, and I was preparing to descend, when down came the infernal chimney board with a tremendous crash. He stopped and put down the candle and the jug of beer on the dresser; he was a nervous old fellow, and any unexpected noise annoyed him. He coolly observed that the fireplace was never used, and sending the frightened servant into the next kitchen for a hammer and nails, actually nailed up the board, and locked the door on the outside. So there was I, on my wedding night, in the light kerseymere trousers, fancy waistcoat, and blue coat that I had been married in in the morning, in a back kitchen chimney, the bottom of which was nailed up, and the top of which had been formerly raised some fifteen feet, to prevent the smoke from annoying the neighbours. And there,' added Mr Gabriel Parsons, as he passed the bottle, 'there I remained till half-past seven the next morning, when the housemaid's sweetheart, who was a carpenter, unshelled me. The old dog had nailed me up so securely, that, to this very hour, I firmly believe that no one but a carpenter could ever have got me out.'

'And what did Mrs Parsons's father say, when he found you were married?' inquired Watkins Tottle, who, although he never saw a joke, was not satisfied until he heard a story to the very end.

'Why, the affair of the chimney so tickled his fancy, that he pardoned us off hand, and allowed us something to live on till he went the way of all flesh. I spent the next night in his second floor front, much more comfortably than I had spent the preceding one; for, as you will probably guess—'

'Please, sir, missis has made tea,' said a middle-aged female servant, bobbing into the room.

'That's the very housemaid that figures in my story,' said Mr Gabriel Parsons. 'She went into Fanny's service when we were first married, and has been with us ever since; but I don't think she has felt one atom of respect for me since the morning she saw me released, when she went into violent hysterics, to which she has been subject ever since. Now, shall we join the ladies?'

'If you please,' said Mr Watkins Tottle.

'By all means,' added the obsequious Mr Timson; and the trio made for the drawing room accordingly.

Tea being concluded, and the toast and cups having been duly handed, and occasionally upset, by Mr Watkins Tottle, a rubber was proposed. They cut for partners – Mr and Mrs Parsons; and Mr Watkins Tottle and Miss Lillerton. Mr Timson having conscientious scruples on the subject of card playing, drank brandy and water, and kept up a running spar with Mr Watkins Tottle. The evening went off well; Mr Watkins Tottle was in high spirits, having some reason to be gratified with his reception by Miss Lillerton; and before he left, a small party was made up to visit the Beulah Spa on the following Saturday.

'It's all right, I think,' said Mr Gabriel Parsons to Mr Watkins Tottle as he opened the garden gate for him.

'I hope so,' he replied, squeezing his friend's hand.

'You'll be down by the first coach on Saturday,' said Mr Gabriel Parsons.

'Certainly,' replied Mr Watkins Tottle. 'Undoubtedly.'

But fortune had decreed that Mr Watkins Tottle should not be down by the first coach on Saturday. His adventures on that day, however, and the success of his wooing, are subjects for another chapter.

## CHAPTER THE SECOND

'The first coach has not come in yet, has it, Tom?' inquired Mr Gabriel Parsons, as he very complacently paced up and down the fourteen feet of gravel which bordered the 'lawn', on the Saturday morning which had been fixed upon for the Beulah Spa jaunt.

'No, sir; I haven't seen it,' replied a gardener in a blue apron, who let himself out to do the ornamental for half-a-crown a day and his 'keep'.

'Time Tottle was down,' said Mr Gabriel Parsons, ruminating – 'Oh, here he is, no doubt,' added Gabriel, as a cab drove rapidly up the hill; and he buttoned his dressing gown, and opened the gate to receive the expected visitor. The cab stopped, and out jumped a man in a coarse Petersham great coat, whity-brown neckerchief, faded black suit, gamboge-coloured top boots, and one of those large-crowned hats, formerly seldom met with, but now very generally patronised by gentlemen and costermongers.

'Mr Parsons?' said the man, looking at the superscription of a note he held in his hand, and addressing Gabriel with an inquiring air.

'*My* name is Parsons,' responded the sugar baker.

'I've brought this here note,' replied the individual in the painted tops, in a hoarse whisper: 'I've brought this here note from a gen'lm'n as come to our house this mornin'.'

'I expected the gentleman at my house,' said Parsons, as he broke the seal, which bore the impression of her Majesty's profile as it is seen on a sixpence.

'I've no doubt the gen'lm'n would ha' been here,' replied the stranger, 'if he hadn't happened to call at our house first; but we never trusts no

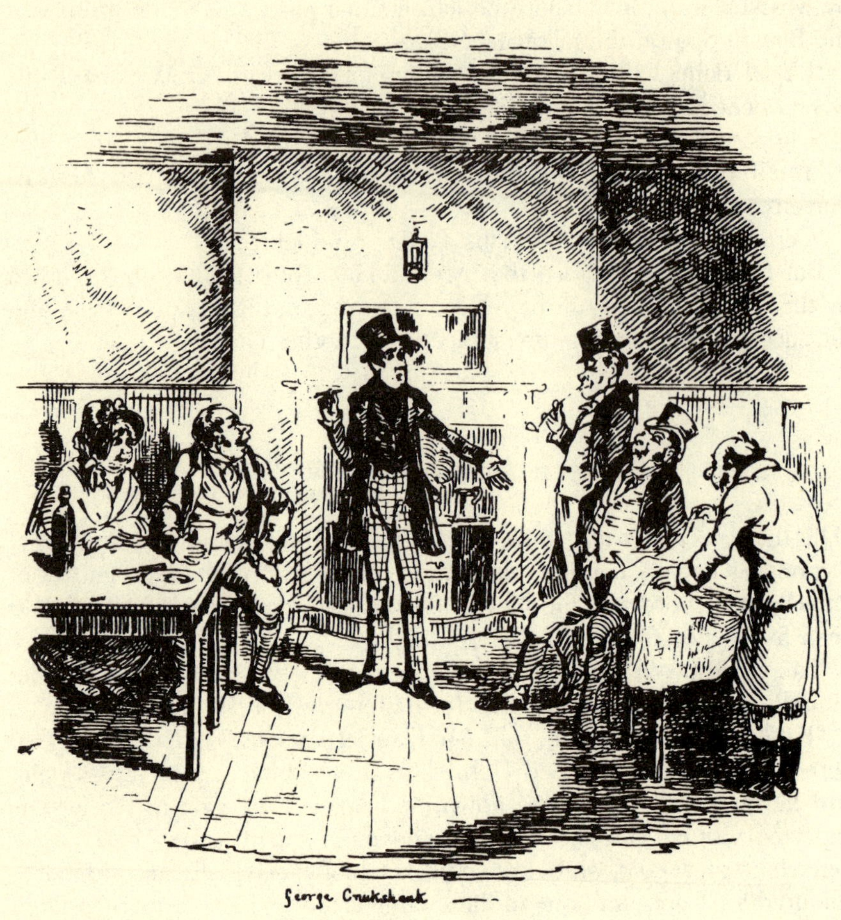

*The Lock-up House*

gen'lm'n furder nor we can see him – no mistake about that there' – added the unknown, with a facetious grin; 'beg your pardon, sir, no offence meant, only – once in, and I wish you may – catch the idea, sir?'

Mr Gabriel Parsons was not remarkable for catching anything suddenly, but a cold. He therefore only bestowed a glance of profound astonishment on his mysterious companion, and proceeded to unfold the note of which he had been the bearer. Once opened and the idea was caught with very little difficulty. Mr Watkins Tottle had been suddenly arrested for 33*l.* 10*s.* 4*d.*, and dated his communication from a lock-up house in the vicinity of Chancery Lane.

'Unfortunate affair this!' said Parsons, refolding the note.

'Oh! nothin' ven you're used to it,' coolly observed the man in the Petersham.

'Tom!' exclaimed Parsons, after a few minutes' consideration, 'just put the horse in, will you? – Tell the gentleman that I shall be there almost as soon as you are,' he continued, addressing the sheriff-officer's Mercury.

'Werry well,' replied that important functionary; adding, in a confidential manner, 'I'd adwise the gen'lm'n's friends to settle. You see it's a mere trifle; and, unless the gen'lm'n means to go up afore the court, it's hardly worth while waiting for detainers, you know. Our governor's wide awake, he is. I'll never say nothin' agin him, nor no man; but he knows what's o'clock, he does, uncommon.' Having delivered this eloquent, and, to Parsons, particularly intelligible harangue, the meaning of which was eked out by divers nods and winks, the gentleman in the boots reseated himself in the cab, which went rapidly off, and was soon out of sight. Mr Gabriel Parsons continued to pace up and down the pathway for some minutes, apparently absorbed in deep meditation. The result of his cogitations seemed to be perfectly satisfactory to himself, for he ran briskly into the house; said that business had suddenly summoned him to town; that he had desired the messenger to inform Mr Watkins Tottle of the fact; and that they would return together to dinner. He then hastily equipped himself for a drive, and mounting his gig, was soon on his way to the establishment of Mr Solomon Jacobs, situate (as Mr Watkins Tottle had informed him), in Cursitor Street, Chancery Lane.

When a man is in a violent hurry to get on, and has a specific object in view, the attainment of which depends on the completion of his journey, the difficulties which interpose themselves in his way appear not only to be innumerable, but to have been called into existence especially for the occasion. The remark is by no means a new one, and Mr Gabriel Parsons had practical and painful experience of its justice in the course of his drive. There are three classes of animated objects which prevent your driving with any degree of comfort or celerity through streets which are but little frequented – they are pigs, children, and old women. On the occasion we are describing, the pigs were luxuriating on cabbage stalks, and the shuttlecocks fluttered from the little deal battledores, and the children played in the road; and women, with a basket in one hand, and the street door key in the other, *would* cross just before the horse's head, until Mr Gabriel Parsons was perfectly savage with vexation, and quite hoarse with hoi-ing and imprecating. Then, when he got into Fleet Street, there was 'a stoppage', in which people in vehicles have the satisfaction of remaining stationary for half an hour, and envying the slowest pedestrians; and where policemen rush about, and seize hold of horses' bridles, and back them into shop windows, by way of clearing the road and preventing confusion. At length Mr Gabriel Parsons turned into Chancery Lane, and having inquired for, and been directed to Cursitor Street (for it was a locality of which he was quite ignorant), he soon found himself opposite the house of Mr Solomon Jacobs. Confiding his horse and gig to the care of one of the fourteen boys who had followed him from the other side of Blackfriars Bridge on the chance of his requiring their services, Mr Gabriel Parsons crossed the road and knocked at an inner door, the upper part of which was of glass, grated like the windows of this inviting mansion with iron bars – painted white to look comfortable.

The knock was answered by a sallow-faced, red-haired, sulky boy, who, after surveying Mr Gabriel Parsons through the glass, applied a large key to an immense wooden excrescence, which was in reality a lock, but which, taken in conjunction with the iron nails with which the panels were studded, gave the door the appearance of being subject to warts.

'I want to see Mr Watkins Tottle,' said Parsons.

'It's the gentleman that come in this morning, Jem,' screamed a voice from the top of the kitchen stairs, which belonged to a dirty woman who had just brought her chin to a level with the passage floor. 'The gentleman's in the coffee room.'

'Upstairs, sir,' said the boy, just opening the door wide enough to let Parsons in without squeezing him, and double locking it the moment he had made his way through the aperture – 'First floor – door on the left.'

Mr Gabriel Parsons thus instructed, ascended the uncarpeted and ill lighted staircase, and after giving several subdued taps at the before mentioned 'door on the left', which were rendered inaudible by the hum of voices within the room, and the hissing noise attendant on some frying operations which were carrying on below stairs, turned the handle, and entered the apartment. Being informed that the unfortunate object of his visit had just gone upstairs to write a letter, he had leisure to sit down and observe the scene before him.

The room – which was a small, confined den – was partitioned off into boxes, like the common room of some inferior eating house. The dirty floor had evidently been as long a stranger to the scrubbing brush as to carpet or floor cloth: and the ceiling was completely blackened by the flare of the oil lamp by which the room was lighted at night. The grey ashes on the edges of the tables, and the cigar ends which were plentifully scattered about the dusty grate, fully accounted for the intolerable smell of tobacco which pervaded the place; and the empty glasses and half saturated slices of lemon on the tables together with the porter pots beneath them, bore testimony to the frequent libations in which the individuals who honoured Mr Solomon Jacobs by a temporary residence in his house indulged. Over the mantelshelf was a paltry looking glass, extending about half the width of the chimneypiece; but by way of counterpoise, the ashes were confined by a rusty fender about twice as long as the hearth.

From this cheerful room itself, the attention of Mr Gabriel Parsons was naturally directed to its inmates. In one of the boxes two men were playing at cribbage with a very dirty pack of cards, some with blue, some with green, and some with red backs – selections from decayed packs. The cribbage board had been long ago formed on the table by some ingenious visitor with the assistance of a pocket knife and a two-pronged fork, with which the necessary number of holes had been made in the table at proper distances for the reception of the wooden pegs. In another box a stout, hearty-looking man, of about forty, was eating some dinner which his wife – an equally comfortable looking personage – had brought him in a basket: and in a third, a genteel-looking young man was talking earnestly, and in a low tone, to a young female, whose face was concealed by a thick veil, but whom Mr Gabriel Parsons immediately set down in his own mind as the debtor's wife. A young fellow of vulgar manners, dressed in the very extreme of the prevailing fashion, was pacing up and down the room, with a lighted cigar in his mouth and his hands in his pockets, ever and anon puffing forth volumes of smoke, and occasionally applying, with much apparent relish, to a pint pot, the contents of which were 'chilling' on the hob.

'Fourpence more, by gum!' exclaimed one of the cribbage players, lighting a pipe, and addressing his adversary at the close of the game; 'one 'ud think you'd got luck in a pepper cruet, and shook it out when you wanted it.'

'Well, that a'n't a bad un,' replied the other, who was a horse dealer from Islington.

'No; I'm blessed if it is,' interposed the jolly-looking fellow, who, having finished his dinner, was drinking out of the same glass as his wife, in truly conjugal harmony, some hot gin and water. The faithful partner of his cares had brought a plentiful supply of the anti-temperance fluid in a large flat stone bottle, which looked like a half gallon jar that had been successfully tapped for the dropsy. 'You're a rum chap, you are, Mr Walker – will you dip your beak into this, sir?'

'Thank'ee, sir,' replied Mr Walker, leaving his box, and advancing to the other to accept the proffered glass. 'Here's your health, sir, and your good 'ooman's here. Gentlemen all – yours, and better luck still. Well, Mr Willis,' continued the facetious prisoner, addressing the young man with the cigar, 'you seem rather down today – floored, as one may say. What's the matter, sir? Never say die, you know.'

'Oh! I'm all right,' replied the smoker. 'I shall be bailed out tomorrow.'

'Shall you, though?' inquired the other. 'Damme, I wish I could say the same. I am as regularly over head and ears as the Royal George, and stand about as much chance of being *bailed out*. Ha! ha! ha!'

'Why,' said the young man, stopping short, and speaking in a very loud key, 'look at me. What d'ye think I've stopped here two days for?'

''Cause you couldn't get out, I suppose,' interrupted Mr Walker, winking to the company. 'Not that you're exactly obliged to stop here, only you can't help it. No compulsion, you know, only you must – eh?'

'A'n't he a rum un?' inquired the delighted individual, who had offered the gin and water, of his wife.

'Oh, he just is!' replied the lady, who was quite overcome by these flashes of imagination.

'Why, my case,' frowned the victim, throwing the end of his cigar into the fire, and illustrating his argument by knocking the bottom of the pot on the table, at intervals, – 'my case is a very singular one. My father's a man of large property, and I am his son.'

'That's a very strange circumstance!' interrupted the jocose Mr Walker, *en passant*.

' – I am his son, and have received a liberal education. I don't owe no man nothing – not the value of a farthing, but I was induced, you see, to put my name to some bills for a friend – bills to a large amount, I may say a very large amount, for which I didn't receive no consideration. What's the consequence?'

'Why, I suppose the bills went out, and you came in. The acceptances weren't taken up, and you were, eh?' inquired Walker.

'To be sure,' replied the liberally-educated young gentleman. 'To be sure; and so here I am, locked up for a matter of twelve hundred pound.'

'Why don't you ask your old governor to stump up?' inquired Walker, with a somewhat sceptical air.

'Oh! bless you, he'd never do it,' replied the other, in a tone of expostulation – 'Never!'

'Well, it is very odd to – be – sure,' interposed the owner of the flat bottle, mixing another glass, 'but I've been in difficulties, as one may say, now for thirty year. I went to pieces when I was in a milk walk, thirty year ago; arterwards, when I was a fruiterer, and kept a spring wan; and arter that again in the coal and 'tatur line – but all that time I never see a youngish chap come into a place of this kind, who wasn't going out again directly, and who hadn't been arrested on bills which he'd given a friend and for which he'd received nothing whatsomever – not a fraction.'

'Oh! it's always the cry,' said Walker. 'I can't see the use on it; that's what makes me so wild. Why, I should have a much better opinion of an individual, if he'd say at once in an honourable and gentlemanly manner as he'd done everybody he possibly could.'

'Aye, to be sure,' interposed the horse dealer, with whose notions of bargain and sale the axiom perfectly coincided, 'so should I.'

The young gentleman, who had given rise to these observations, was on the point of offering a rather angry reply to these sneers, but the rising of the young man before noticed, and of the female who had been sitting by him, to leave the room, interrupted the conversation. She had been weeping bitterly, and the noxious atmosphere of the room acting upon her excited feelings and delicate frame, rendered the support of her companion necessary as they quitted it together.

There was an air of superiority about them both, and something in their appearance so unusual in such a place, that a respectful silence was observed until the *whirr – r – bang* of the spring door announced that they were out of hearing. It was broken by the wife of the ex-fruiterer.

'Poor creetur!' said she, quenching a sigh in a rivulet of gin and water. 'She's very young.'

'She's a nice-looking 'ooman too,' added the horse dealer.

'What's he in for, Ikey?' inquired Walker, of an individual who was spreading a cloth with numerous blotches of mustard upon it, on one of the tables, and whom Mr Gabriel Parsons had no difficulty in recognising as the man who had called upon him in the morning.

'Vy,' responded the factotum, 'it's one of the rummiest rigs you ever heard on. He come in here last Vensday, which by-the-bye he's a-going over the water tonight – hows'ever that's neither here nor there. You see I've been a-going back'ards and for'ards about his business, and ha' managed to pick up some of his story from the servants and them; and so far as I can make it out, it seems to be summat to this here effect—'

'Cut it short, old fellow,' interrupted Walker, who knew from former experience that he of the top boots was neither very concise nor intelligible in his narratives.

'Let me alone,' replied Ikey, 'and I'll ha' vound up, and made my lucky in five seconds. This here young gen'lm'n's father – so I'm told, mind ye – and the father o' the young voman, have always been on very bad, out and out, rig'lar knock me down sort o' terms; but somehow or another, ven he vos a-wisitin' at some gentlefolk's house, as he knowed at college, he came into contract with the young lady. He seed her several times, and then he up and said he'd keep company vith her, if so be as she vos agreeable. Vell, she vos as sweet upon him as he vos upon her, and so I s'pose they made it all right; for they got married 'bout six months arterwards, unbeknown, mind ye, to the two fathers – leastways so I'm told. When they heard on it – my eyes, there vos such a combustion! Starvation vos the very least that vos to be done to 'em. The young gen'lm'n's father cut him off vith a bob, 'cos he'd cut himself off vith a wife; and the young lady's father he behaved even worser and more unnat'ral, for he not only blow'd her up dreadful, and swore he'd never see her again, but he employed a chap as I knows – and as you knows, Mr Valker, a precious sight too well – to go about and buy up the bills and them things on which the young husband, thinking his governor 'ud come round agin, had raised the vind just to blow himself on vith for a time; besides vich, he made all the interest he could to set other people agin him. Consequence vos, that he paid as long as he could; but things he never expected to have to meet till he'd had time to turn himself round, come fast upon him, and he vos nabbed. He vos brought here, as I said afore, last Vensday, and I think there's about – ah, half-a-dozen detainers agin him downstairs now. I have been,' added Ikey 'in the purfession these fifteen year, and I never met vith such windictiveness afore!'

'Poor creeturs!' exclaimed the coal dealer's wife once more: again resorting to the same excellent prescription for nipping a sigh in the bud. 'Ah! when they've seen as much trouble as I and my old man here have, they'll be as comfortable under it as we are.'

'The young lady's a pretty creature,' said Walker, 'only she's a little too delicate for my taste – there ain't enough of her. As to the young cove, he may be very respectable and what not, but he's too down in the mouth for me – he ain't game.'

'Game!' exclaimed Ikey, who had been altering the position of a green handled knife and fork at least a dozen times, in order that he might remain in the room under the pretext of having something to do. 'He's game enough ven there's anything to be fierce about; but who could be game as you call it, Mr Walker, with a pale young creetur like that, hanging about him? – It's enough to drive any man's heart into his boots to see 'em together – and no mistake at all about it. I never shall forget her first comin' here; he wrote to her on the Thursday to come – I know he did, 'cos I took the letter. Uncommon fidgety he vos all day to be sure, and in the evening he goes down into the office, and he says to Jacobs, says he, 'Sir, can I have the loan of a private room for a few minutes this evening, without incurring any additional expense – just to see my wife in?' says he. Jacobs looked as much as to say – 'Strike me bountiful if you ain't one of the modest sort!' but as the gen'lm'n who had been in the back parlour had just gone out, and had paid for it for that day, he says – werry grave – "Sir," says he, "it's agin our rules to let private rooms to our lodgers on gratis terms, but," says he, "for a gentleman, I don't mind breaking through them for once." So then he turns round to me, and says, "Ikey, put two mould candles in the back parlour, and charge 'em to this gen'lm'n's account," vich I did. Vell, by and bye a hackney coach comes up to the door, and there, sure enough, vos the young lady, wrapped up in a hopera cloak, as it might be, and all alone. I opened the gate that night, so I went up ven the coach come, and he vos a-waitin' at the parlour door – and wasn't he a-trembling, neither? The poor creetur see him, and could hardly walk to meet him. "Oh, Harry!" she says "that it should have come to this; and all for my sake," says she, putting her hand upon his shoulder. So he puts his arm round her pretty little waist, and leading her gently a little way into the room, so that he might be able to shut the door, he says, so kind and soft like – "Why, Kate," says he –'

'Here's the gentleman you want,' said Ikey, abruptly breaking off in his story, and introducing Mr Gabriel Parsons to the crestfallen Watkins Tottle, who at that moment entered the room. Watkins advanced with a wooden expression of passive endurance, and accepted the hand which Mr Gabriel Parsons held out.

'I want to speak to you,' said Gabriel, with a look strongly expressive of his dislike of the company.

'This way,' replied the imprisoned one, leading the way to the front drawing room, where rich debtors did the luxurious at the rate of a couple of guineas a day.

'Well, here I am,' said Mr Watkins, as he sat down on the sofa; and placing the palms of his hands on his knees, anxiously glanced at his friend's countenance.

'Yes; and here you're likely to be,' said Gabriel, coolly, as he rattled the money in his unmentionable pockets, and looked out of the window.

'What's the amount with the costs?' inquired Parsons, after an awkward pause.

'37*l.* 3*s.* 10*d.*'

'Have you any money?'

'Nine and sixpence halfpenny.'

Mr Gabriel Parsons walked up and down the room for a few seconds, before he could make up his mind to disclose the plan he had formed; he was accustomed to drive hard bargains, but was always most anxious to conceal his avarice. At length he stopped short, and said, 'Tottle, you owe me fifty pounds.'

'I do.'

'And from all I see, I infer that you are likely to owe it to me.'

'I fear I am.'

'Though you have every disposition to pay me if you could?'

'Certainly.'

'Then,' said Mr Gabriel Parsons, 'listen: here's my proposition. You know my way of old. Accept it – yes or no – I will or I won't. I'll pay the debt and costs, and I'll lend you 10*l.* more (which, added to your annuity, will enable you to carry on the war well) if you'll give me your note of hand to pay me one hundred and fifty pounds within six months after you are married to Miss Lillerton.'

'My dear—'

'Stop a minute – on one condition; and that is, that you propose to Miss Lillerton at once.'

'At once! My dear Parsons, consider.'

'It's for you to consider, not me. She knows you well from reputation, though she did not know you personally until lately. Notwithstanding all her maiden modesty, I think she'd be devilish glad to get married out of hand with as little delay as possible. My wife has sounded her on the subject, and she has confessed.'

'What – what?' eagerly interrupted the enamoured Watkins.

'Why,' replied Parsons, 'to say exactly what she has confessed, would be rather difficult, because they only spoke in hints, and so forth; but my wife, who is no bad judge in these cases, declared to me that what she had confessed was as good as to say that she was not insensible of your merits – in fact, that no other man should have her.'

Mr Watkins Tottle rose hastily from his seat, and rang the bell.

'What's that for?' inquired Parsons.

'I want to send the man for the bill stamp,' replied Mr Watkins Tottle.

'Then you've made up your mind?'

'I have,' – and they shook hands most cordially. The note of hand was given – the debt and costs were paid – Ikey was satisfied for his trouble, and the two friends soon found themselves on that side of Mr Solomon Jacobs's establishment, on which most of his visitors were very happy when they found themselves once again – to wit, the *out*side.

'Now,' said Mr Gabriel Parsons, as they drove to Norwood together – 'you shall have an opportunity to make the disclosure tonight, and mind you speak out, Tottle.'

'I will – I will!' replied Watkins, valorously.

'How I should like to see you together,' ejaculated Mr Gabriel Parsons. – 'What fun!' and he laughed so long and so loudly, that he disconcerted Mr Watkins Tottle, and frightened the horse.

'There's Fanny and your intended walking about on the lawn,' said Gabriel, as they approached the house. 'Mind your eye, Tottle.'

'Never fear,' replied Watkins, resolutely, as he made his way to the spot where the ladies were walking.

'Here's Mr Tottle, my dear,' said Mrs Parsons, addressing Miss Lillerton. The lady turned quickly round, and acknowledged his courteous salute with the same sort of confusion that Watkins had noticed on their first interview, but with something like a slight expression of disappointment or carelessness.

'Did you see how glad she was to see you?' whispered Parsons to his friend.

'Why I really thought she looked as if she would rather have seen somebody else,' replied Tottle.

'Pooh, nonsense!' whispered Parsons again – 'it's always the way with the women, young or old. They never show how delighted they are to see those whose presence makes their hearts beat. It's the way with the whole sex, and no man should have lived to your time of life without knowing it. Fanny confessed it to me, when we were first married, over and over again – see what it is to have a wife.'

'Certainly,' whispered Tottle, whose courage was vanishing fast.

'Well, now, you'd better begin to pave the way,' said Parsons, who, having invested some money in the speculation, assumed the office of director.

'Yes, yes, I will – presently,' replied Tottle, greatly flurried.

'Say something to her, man,' urged Parsons again. 'Confound it! pay her a compliment, can't you?'

'No! not till after dinner,' replied the bashful Tottle, anxious to postpone the evil moment.

'Well, gentlemen,' said Mrs Parsons, 'you are really very polite; you stay away the whole morning, after promising to take us out, and when you do come home, you stand whispering together and take no notice of us.'

'We were talking of the *business*, my dear, which detained us this morning,' replied Parsons, looking significantly at Tottle.

'Dear me! how very quickly the morning has gone,' said Miss Lillerton, referring to the gold watch, which was wound up on state occasions, whether it required it or not.

'*I* think it has passed very slowly,' mildly suggested Tottle.

('That's right – bravo!') whispered Parsons.

'Indeed!' said Miss Lillerton, with an air of majestic surprise.

'I can only impute it to my unavoidable absence from your society, madam,' said Watkins, 'and that of Mrs Parsons.'

During this short dialogue the ladies had been leading the way to the house.

'What the deuce did you stick Fanny into that last compliment for?'

inquired Parsons, as they followed together; 'it quite spoilt the effect.'

'Oh! it really would have been too broad without,' replied Watkins Tottle, 'much too broad!'

'He's mad!' Parsons whispered his wife, as they entered the drawing room, 'mad from modesty.'

'Dear me!' ejaculated the lady, 'I never heard of such a thing.'

'You'll find we have quite a family dinner, Mr Tottle,' said Mrs Parsons, when they sat down to table: 'Miss Lillerton is one of us, and, of course, we make no stranger of you.'

Mr Watkins Tottle expressed a hope that the Parsons family never would make a stranger of him; and wished internally that his bashfulness would allow him to feel a little less like a stranger himself.

'Take off the covers, Martha,' said Mrs Parsons, directing the shifting of the scenery with great anxiety. The order was obeyed, and a pair of boiled fowls, with tongue and et ceteras, were displayed at the top, and a fillet of veal at the bottom. On one side of the table two green sauce-tureens, with ladles of the same, were setting to each other in a green dish; and on the other was a curried rabbit, in a brown suit, turned up with lemon.

'Miss Lillerton, my dear,' said Mrs Parsons, 'shall I assist you?'

'Thank you, no; I think I'll trouble Mr Tottle.'

Watkins started – trembled – helped the rabbit and broke a tumbler. The countenance of the lady of the house, which had been all smiles previously, underwent an awful change.

'Extremely sorry,' stammered Watkins, assisting himself to currie and parsley and butter, in the extremity of his confusion.

'Not the least consequence,' replied Mrs Parsons, in a tone which implied that it was of the greatest consequence possible, – directing aside the researches of the boy, who was groping under the table for the bits of broken glass.

'I presume,' said Miss Lillerton, 'that Mr Tottle is aware of the interest which bachelors usually pay in such cases; a dozen glasses for one is the lowest penalty.'

Mr Gabriel Parsons gave his friend an admonitory tread on the toe. Here was a clear hint that the sooner he ceased to be a bachelor and emancipated himself from such penalties, the better. Mr Watkins Tottle viewed the observation in the same light, and challenged Mrs Parsons to take wine, with a degree of presence of mind which, under all the circumstances, was really extraordinary.

'Miss Lillerton,' said Gabriel, 'may I have the pleasure?'

'I shall be most happy.'

'Tottle, will you assist Miss Lillerton, and pass the decanter. Thank you.' (The usual pantomimic ceremony of nodding and sipping gone through) –

'Tottle, were you ever in Suffolk?' inquired the master of the house, who was burning to tell one of his seven stock stories.

'No,' responded Watkins, adding, by way of a saving clause, 'but I've been in Devonshire.'

'Ah!' replied Gabriel, 'it was in Suffolk that a rather singular circumstance happened to me many years ago. Did you ever happen to hear me mention it?'

Mr Watkins Tottle *had* happened to hear his friend mention it some four hundred times. Of course he expressed great curiosity, and evinced the utmost impatience to hear the story again. Mr Gabriel Parsons forthwith attempted to proceed, in spite of the interruptions to which, as our readers must frequently have observed, the master of the house is often exposed in such cases. We will attempt to give them an idea of our meaning.

'When I was in Suffolk—' said Mr Gabriel Parsons.

'Take off the fowls first, Martha,' said Mrs Parsons. 'I beg your pardon, my dear.'

'When I was in Suffolk,' resumed Mr Parsons, with an impatient glance at his wife, who pretended not to observe it, 'which is now some years ago, business led me to the town of Bury St Edmund's. I had to stop at the principal places in my way, and therefore, for the sake of convenience, I travelled in a gig. I left Sudbury one dark night – it was winter time – about nine o'clock; the rain poured in torrents, the wind howled among the trees that skirted the roadside, and I was obliged to proceed at a foot-pace, for I could hardly see my hand before me, it was so dark—'

'John,' interrupted Mrs Parsons, in a low, hollow voice, 'don't spill the gravy.'

'Fanny,' said Parsons impatiently, 'I wish you'd defer these domestic reproofs to some more suitable time. Really, my dear, these constant interruptions are very annoying.'

'My dear, I didn't interrupt you,' said Mrs Parsons.

'But, my dear, you *did* interrupt me,' remonstrated Mr Parsons.

'How very absurd you are, my love! I must give directions to the servants; I am quite sure that if I sat here and allowed John to spill the gravy over the new carpet, you'd be the first to find fault when you saw the stain tomorrow morning.'

'Well,' continued Gabriel, with a resigned air, as if he knew there was no getting over the point about the carpet, 'I was just saying, it was so dark that I could hardly see my hand before me. The road was very lonely, and I assure you, Tottle (this was a device to arrest the wandering attention of that individual, which was distracted by a confidential communication between Mrs Parsons and Martha, accompanied by the delivery of a large bunch of keys), I assure you, Tottle, I became somehow impressed with a sense of the loneliness of my situation—'

'Pie to your master,' interrupted Mrs Parsons, again directing the servant.

'Now, pray, my dear,' remonstrated Parsons once more, very pettishly. Mrs P. turned up her hands and eyebrows, and appealed in dumb show to Miss Lillerton. 'As I turned a corner of the road,' resumed Gabriel, 'the horse stopped short and reared tremendously. I pulled up, jumped out, ran to his head, and found a man lying on his back in the middle of the road, with his eyes fixed on the sky. I thought he was dead; but no, he was alive, and there appeared to be nothing the matter with him. He jumped up, and putting his hand to his chest, and fixing upon me the most earnest gaze you can imagine, exclaimed—'

'Pudding here,' said Mrs Parsons.

'Oh! it's no use,' exclaimed the host, now rendered desperate. 'Here, Tottle; a glass of wine. It's useless to attempt relating anything when Mrs Parsons is present.'

This attack was received in the usual way. Mrs Parsons talked *to* Miss Lillerton and *at* her better half; expatiated on the impatience of men generally; hinted that her husband was peculiarly vicious in this respect, and wound up by insinuating that she must be one of the best tempers that ever existed, or she never could put up with it. Really what she had to endure sometimes, was more than anyone who saw her in everyday life could by possibility suppose. – The story was now a painful subject, and therefore Mr Parsons declined to enter into any details, and contented himself by stating that the man was a maniac, who had escaped from a neighbouring madhouse.

The cloth was removed; the ladies soon afterwards retired, and Miss Lillerton played the piano in the drawing room overhead, very loudly, for the edification of the visitor. Mr Watkins Tottle and Mr Gabriel Parsons sat chatting comfortably enough, until the conclusion of the second bottle, when the latter, in proposing an adjournment to the drawing room, informed Watkins that he had concerted a plan with his wife for leaving him and Miss Lillerton alone, soon after tea.

'I say,' said Tottle, as they went upstairs, 'don't you think it would be better if we put it off till – till – tomorrow?'

'Don't *you* think it would have been much better if I had left you in that wretched hole I found you in this morning?' retorted Parsons bluntly.

'Well – well – I only made a suggestion,' said poor Watkins Tottle, with a deep sigh.

Tea was soon concluded, and Miss Lillerton, drawing a small work-table on one side of the fire, and placing a little wooden frame upon it, something like a miniature clay mill without the horse, was soon busily engaged in making a watchguard with brown silk.

'God bless me!' exclaimed Parsons, starting up with well-feigned surprise, 'I've forgotten those confounded letters. Tottle, I know you'll excuse me.'

If Tottle had been a free agent, he would have allowed no one to leave the room on any pretence, except himself. As it was, however, he was obliged to look cheerful when Parsons quitted the apartment.

He had scarcely left, when Martha put her head into the room, with – 'Please, ma'am, you're wanted.'

Mrs Parsons left the room, shut the door carefully after her, and Mr Watkins Tottle was left alone with Miss Lillerton.

For the first five minutes there was a dead silence. – Mr Watkins Tottle was thinking how he should begin, and Miss Lillerton appeared to be thinking of nothing. The fire was burning low; Mr Watkins Tottle stirred it, and put some coals on.

'Hem!' coughed Miss Lillerton; Mr Watkins Tottle thought the fair creature had spoken. 'I beg your pardon,' said he.

'Eh?'

'I thought you spoke.'

'No.'

'Oh!'

'There are some books on the sofa, Mr Tottle, if you would like to look at them,' said Miss Lillerton, after the lapse of another five minutes.

'No, thank you,' returned Watkins; and then he added, with a courage which was perfectly astonishing, even to himself, 'Madam, that is Miss Lillerton, I wish to speak to you.'

'To me!' said Miss Lillerton, letting the silk drop from her hands, and sliding her chair back a few paces. – 'Speak – to me!'

'To you, madam – and on the subject of the state of your affections.' The lady hastily rose and would have left the room; but Mr Watkins Tottle gently detained her by the hand, and holding it as far from him as the joint length of their arms would permit, he thus proceeded: 'Pray do not misunderstand me, or suppose that I am led to address you, after so short an acquaintance, by any feeling of my own merits – for merits I have none which could give me a claim to your hand. I hope you will acquit me of any presumption when I explain that I have been acquainted, through Mrs Parsons, with the state – that is, that Mrs Parsons has told me – at least, not Mrs Parsons, but—' here Watkins began to wander, but Miss Lillerton relieved him.

'Am I to understand, Mr Tottle, that Mrs Parsons has acquainted you with my feeling – my affection – I mean my respect, for an individual of the opposite sex?'

'She has.'

'Then, what?' inquired Miss Lillerton, averting her face, with a girlish air, 'what could induce *you* to seek such an interview as this? What can your object be? How can I promote your happiness, Mr Tottle?'

Here was the time for a flourish – 'By allowing me,' replied Watkins, falling bump on his knees, and breaking two brace-buttons and a waistcoat string, in the act – 'By allowing me to be your slave, your servant – in short, by unreservedly making me the confidant of your heart's feelings – may I say for the promotion of your own happiness – may I say, in order that you may become the wife of a kind and affectionate husband?'

'Disinterested creature!' exclaimed Miss Lillerton, hiding her face in a white pocket handkerchief with an eyelet hole border.

Mr Watkins Tottle thought that if the lady knew all, she might possibly alter her opinion on this last point. He raised the tip of her middle finger ceremoniously to his lips, and got off his knees as gracefully as he could. 'My information was correct?' he tremulously inquired, when he was once more on his feet.

'It was.' Watkins elevated his hands, and looked up to the ornament in the centre of the ceiling, which had been made for a lamp, by way of expressing his rapture.

'Our situation, Mr Tottle,' resumed the lady, glancing at him through one of the eyelet holes, 'is a most peculiar and delicate one.'

'It is,' said Mr Tottle.

'Our acquaintance has been of *so* short duration,' said Miss Lillerton.

'Only a week,' assented Watkins Tottle.

'Oh! more than that,' exclaimed the lady, in a tone of surprise.

'Indeed!' said Tottle.

'More than a month – more than two months!' said Miss Lillerton.

'Rather odd, this,' thought Watkins.

'Oh!' he said, recollecting Parson's assurance that she had known him from report, 'I understand. But, my dear madam, pray consider. The longer this acquaintance has existed, the less reason is there for delay now. Why not at once fix a period for gratifying the hopes of your devoted admirer?'

'It has been represented to me again and again that this is the course I ought to pursue,' replied Miss Lillerton, 'but pardon my feelings of delicacy, Mr Tottle – pray excuse this embarrassment – I have peculiar ideas on such subjects, and I am quite sure that I never could summon up fortitude enough to name the day to my future husband.'

'Then allow *me* to name it,' said Tottle eagerly.

'I should like to fix it myself,' replied Miss Lillerton, bashfully, 'but I cannot do so without at once resorting to a third party.'

'A third party!' thought Watkins Tottle; 'who the deuce is that to be, I wonder!'

'Mr Tottle,' continued Miss Lillerton, 'you have made me a most disinterested and kind offer – that offer I accept. Will you at once be the bearer of a note from me to – to Mr Timson?'

'Mr Timson!' said Watkins.

'After what has passed between us,' responded Miss Lillerton, still averting her head, 'you must understand whom I mean; Mr Timson, the – the clergyman.'

'Mr Timson, the clergyman!' ejaculated Watkins Tottle, in a state of inexpressible beatitude, and positive wonder at his own success. 'Angel! Certainly – this moment!'

'I'll prepare it immediately,' said Miss Lillerton, making for the door; 'the events of this day have flurried me so much, Mr Tottle, that I shall not leave my room again this evening; I will send you the note by the servant.'

'Stay, – stay,' cried Watkins Tottle, still keeping a most respectful distance from the lady; 'when shall we meet again?'

'Oh! Mr Tottle,' replied Miss Lillerton, coquettishly, 'when *we* are married, I can never see you too often, nor thank you too much;' and she left the room.

Mr Watkins Tottle flung himself into an armchair, and indulged in the most delicious reveries of future bliss, in which the idea of 'Five hundred pounds per annum, with an uncontrolled power of disposing of it by her last will and testament,' was somehow or other the foremost. He had gone through the interview so well, and it had terminated so admirably, that he almost began to wish he had expressly stipulated for the settlement of the annual five hundred on himself.

'May I come in?' said Mr Gabriel Parsons, peeping in at the door.

'You may,' replied Watkins.

'Well, have you done it?' anxiously inquired Gabriel.

'Have I done it!' said Watkins Tottle. 'Hush – I'm going to the clergyman.'

'No!' said Parsons. 'How well you have managed it!'

'Where does Timson live?' inquired Watkins.

'At his uncle's,' replied Gabriel, 'just round the lane. He's waiting for a living, and has been assisting his uncle here for the last two or three months. But how well you have done it – I didn't think you could have carried it off so!'

Mr Watkins Tottle was proceeding to demonstrate that the Richardsonian principle was the best on which love could possibly be made, when he was interrupted by the entrance of Martha, with a little pink note folded like a fancy cocked hat.

'Miss Lillerton's compliments,' said Martha, as she delivered it into Tottle's hands, and vanished.

'Do you observe the delicacy?' said Tottle, appealing to Mr Gabriel Parsons, '*Compliments*, not *love*, by the servant, eh?'

Mr Gabriel Parsons didn't exactly know what reply to make, so he poked the forefinger of his right hand between the third and fourth ribs of Mr Watkins Tottle.

'Come,' said Watkins, when the explosion of mirth, consequent on this practical jest, had subsided, 'we'll be off at once – let's lose no time.'

'Capital!' echoed Gabriel Parsons; and in five minutes they were at the garden gate of the villa tenanted by the uncle of Mr Timson.

'Is Mr Charles Timson at home?' inquired Mr Watkins Tottle of Mr Charles Timson's uncle's man.

'Mr Charles *is* at home,' replied the man, stammering; 'but he desired me to say he couldn't be interrupted, sir, by any of the parishioners.'

'*I* am not a parishioner,' replied Watkins.

'Is Mr Charles writing a sermon, Tom?' inquired Parsons, thrusting himself forward.

'No, Mr Parsons, sir; he's not exactly writing a sermon, but he is practising the violoncello in his own bedroom, and gave strict orders not to be disturbed.'

'Say I'm here,' replied Gabriel, leading the way across the garden; 'Mr Parsons and Mr Tottle, on private and particular business.'

They were shown into the parlour, and the servant departed to deliver his message. The distant groaning of the violoncello ceased; footsteps were heard on the stairs; and Mr Timson presented himself, and shook hands with Parsons with the utmost cordiality.

'How do you do, sir?' said Watkins Tottle, with great solemnity.

'How do *you* do, sir?' replied Timson, with as much coldness as if it were a matter of perfect indifference to him how he did, as it very likely was.

'I beg to deliver this note to you,' said Watkins Tottle, producing the cocked hat.

'From Miss Lillerton!' said Timson, suddenly changing colour. 'Pray sit down.'

Mr Watkins Tottle sat down; and while Timson perused the note, fixed his eyes on an oyster-sauce-coloured portrait of the Archbishop of Canterbury, which hung over the fireplace.

Mr Timson rose from his seat when he had concluded the note, and looked dubiously at Parsons. 'May I ask,' he inquired, appealing to Watkins Tottle, 'whether our friend here is acquainted with the object of your visit?'

'Our friend is in *my* confidence,' replied Watkins, with considerable importance.

'Then, sir,' said Timson, seizing both Tottle's hands, 'allow me in his presence to thank you most unfeignedly and cordially, for the noble part you have acted in this affair.'

'He thinks I recommended him,' thought Tottle. 'Confound these fellows! they never think of anything but their fees.'

'I deeply regret having misunderstood your intentions, my dear sir,' continued Timson. 'Disinterested and manly, indeed! There are very few men who would have acted as you have done.'

Mr Watkins Tottle could not help thinking that this last remark was anything but complimentary. He therefore inquired, rather hastily, 'When is it to be?'

'On Thursday,' replied Timson, – 'on Thursday morning at half-past eight.'

'Uncommonly early,' observed Watkins Tottle, with an air of triumphant self-denial. 'I shall hardly be able to get down here by that hour.' (This was intended for a joke.)

'Never mind, my dear fellow,' replied Timson, all suavity, shaking hands with Tottle again most heartily, 'so long as we see you to breakfast, you know—'

'Eh!' said Parsons, with one of the most extraordinary expressions of countenance that ever appeared in a human face.

'What!' ejaculated Watkins Tottle, at the same moment.

'I say that so long as we see you to breakfast,' replied Timson, 'we will excuse your being absent from the ceremony, though of course your presence at it would give us the utmost pleasure.'

Mr Watkins Tottle staggered against the wall, and fixed his eyes on Timson with appalling perseverance.

'Timson,' said Parsons, hurriedly, brushing his hat with his left arm, 'when you say "us", whom do you mean?'

Mr Timson looked foolish in his turn, when he replied, 'Why – Mrs Timson that will be this day week: Miss Lillerton that is—'

'Now don't stare at that idiot in the corner,' angrily exclaimed Parsons, as the extraordinary convulsions of Watkins Tottle's countenance excited the wondering gaze of Timson, – 'but have the goodness to tell me in three words the contents of that note.'

'This note,' replied Timson, 'is from Miss Lillerton, to whom I have been for the last five weeks regularly engaged. Her singular scruples and strange feeling on some points have hitherto prevented my bringing the engagement to that termination which I so anxiously desire. She informs me here, that she sounded Mrs Parsons with the view of making her her confidante and go-between, that Mrs Parsons informed this elderly gentleman, Mr Tottle, of the circumstance, and that he, in the most kind and delicate terms, offered to assist us in any way, and even undertook to convey this note, which contains the promise I have long sought in vain – an act of kindness for which I can never be sufficiently grateful.'

'Good night, Timson,' said Parsons, hurrying off, and carrying the bewildered Tottle with him.

'Won't you stay – and have something?' said Timson.

'No, thank ye,' replied Parsons; 'I've had quite enough;' and away he went, followed by Watkins Tottle in a state of stupefaction.

Mr Gabriel Parsons whistled until they had walked some quarter of a mile past his own gate, when he suddenly stopped, and said –

'You are a clever fellow, Tottle, ain't you?'

'I don't know,' said the unfortunate Watkins.

'I suppose you'll say this is Fanny's fault, won't you?' inquired Gabriel.

'I don't know anything about it,' replied the bewildered Tottle.

'Well,' said Parsons, turning on his heel to go home, 'the next time you make an offer, you had better speak plainly, and don't throw a chance away. And the next time you're locked up in a spunging-house, just wait there till I come and take you out, there's a good fellow.'

How, or at what hour, Mr Watkins Tottle returned to Cecil Street is unknown. His boots were seen outside his bedroom door next morning; but we have the authority of his landlady for stating that he neither emerged therefrom nor accepted sustenance for four-and-twenty hours. At the expiration of that period, and when a council of war was being held in the kitchen on the propriety of summoning the parochial beadle to break his door open, he rang his bell, and demanded a cup of milk and water. The next morning he went through the formalities of eating and drinking as usual, but a week afterwards he was seized with a relapse, while perusing the list of marriages in a morning paper, from which he never perfectly recovered.

A few weeks after the last-named occurrence, the body of a gentleman unknown was found in the Regent's canal. In the trousers pockets were four shillings and threepence halfpenny; a matrimonial advertisement from a lady, which appeared to have been cut out of a Sunday paper; a toothpick, and a card case, which it is confidently believed would have led to the identification of the unfortunate gentleman, but for the circumstances of there being none but blank cards in it. Mr Watkins Tottle absented himself from his lodgings shortly before. A bill, which has not been taken up, was presented next morning; and a bill, which has not been taken down, was soon afterwards affixed in his parlour window.

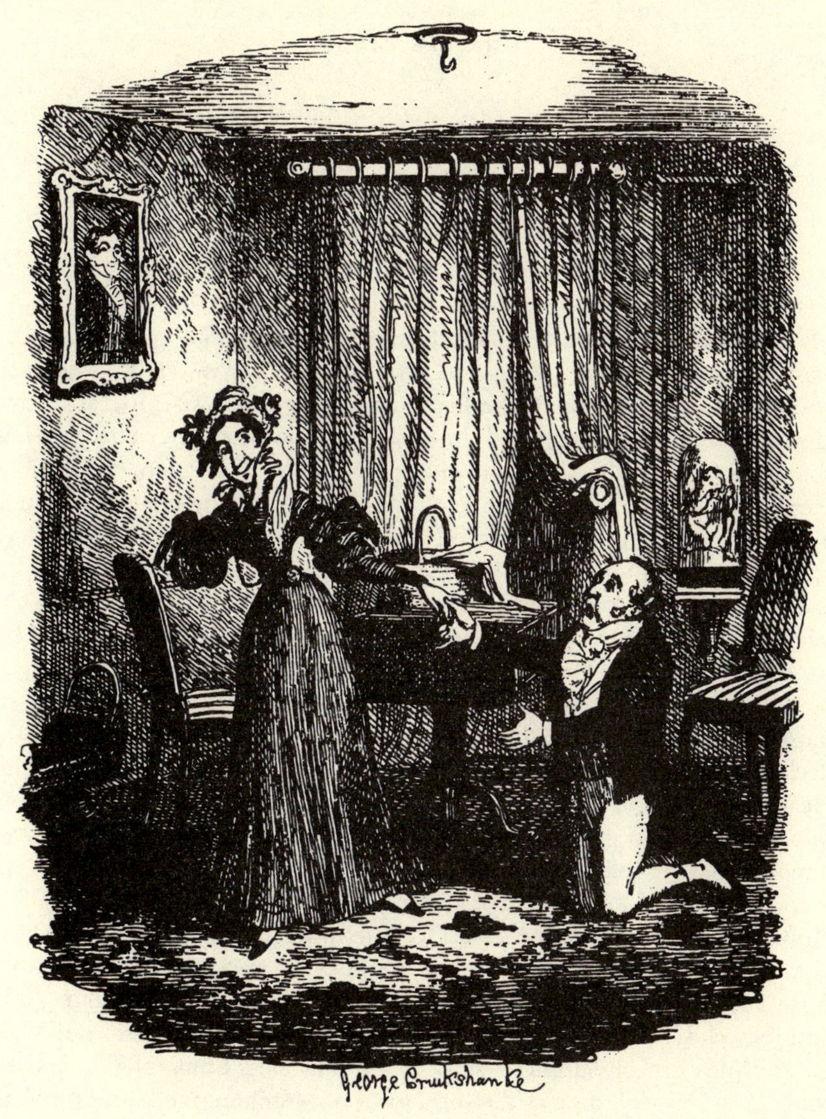


*Mr Watkins Tottle and Miss Lillerton*

## Chapter Eleven

### *The Bloomsbury Christening*

First published in the *Monthly Magazine*, April 1834.

Mr Nicodemus Dumps, or, as his acquaintance called him, 'long Dumps', was a bachelor, six feet high, and fifty years old: cross, cadaverous, odd and ill-natured. He was never happy but when he was miserable; and always miserable when he had the best reason to be happy. The only real comfort of his existence was to make everybody about him wretched – then he might be truly said to enjoy life. He was afflicted with a situation in the Bank worth five hundred a year, and he rented a 'first-floor furnished', at Pentonville, which he originally took because it commanded a dismal prospect of an adjacent churchyard. He was familiar with the face of every tombstone, and the burial service seemed to excite his strongest sympathy. His friends said he was surly – he insisted he was nervous; they thought him a lucky dog, but he protested that he was 'the most unfortunate man in the world'. Cold as he was, and wretched as he declared himself to be, he was not wholly unsusceptible of attachments. He revered the memory of Hoyle, as he was himself an admirable and imperturbable whist player, and he chuckled with delight at a fretful and impatient adversary. He adored King Herod for his massacre of the innocents; and if he hated one thing more than another, it was a child. However, he could hardly be said to hate anything in particular, because he disliked everything in general; but perhaps his greatest antipathies were cabs, old women, doors that would not shut, musical amateurs, and omnibus cads. He subscribed to the 'Society for the Suppression of Vice' for the pleasure of putting a stop to any harmless amusements; and he contributed largely towards the support of two itinerant methodist parsons, in the amiable hope that if circumstances rendered any people happy in this world, they might perchance be rendered miserable by fears for the next.

Mr Dumps had a nephew who had been married about a year, and who was somewhat of a favourite with his uncle, because he was an admirable subject to exercise his misery-creating powers upon. Mr Charles Kitterbell was a small, sharp, spare man, with a very large head, and a

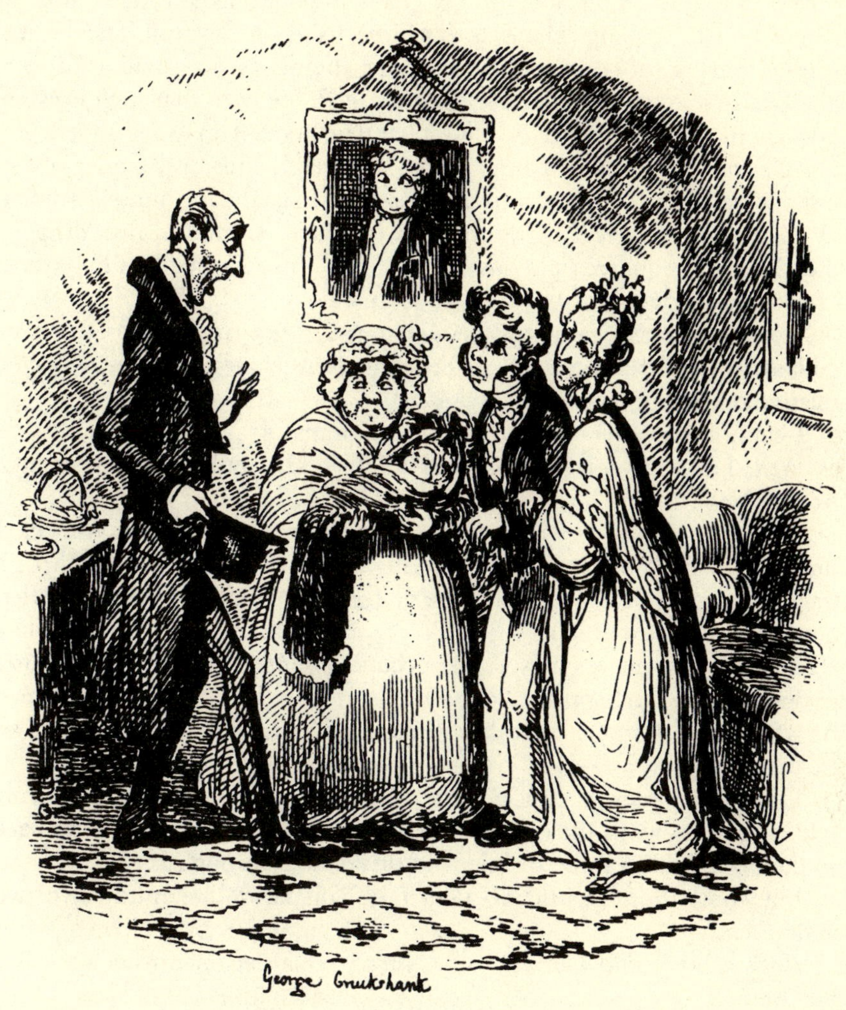


*The Bloomsbury Christening (see p. 456)*

broad, good-humoured countenance. He looked like a faded giant, with the head and face partially restored; and he had a cast in his eye which rendered it quite impossible for anyone with whom he conversed to know where he was looking. His eyes appeared fixed on the wall, and he was staring you out of countenance; in short, there was no catching his eye, and perhaps it is a merciful dispensation of Providence that such eyes are not catching. In addition to these characteristics, it may be added that Mr Charles Kitterbell was one of the most credulous and matter-of-fact little personages that ever took *to* himself a wife, and *for* himself a house in Great Russell Street, Bedford Square. (Uncle Dumps always dropped the 'Bedford Square', and inserted in lieu thereof the dreadful words 'Tottenham Court Road'.)

'No, but, uncle, 'pon my life you must – you must promise to be godfather,' said Mr Kitterbell, as he sat in conversation with his respected relative one morning.

'I cannot, indeed I cannot,' returned Dumps.

'Well, but why not? Jemima will think it very unkind. It's very little trouble.'

'As to the trouble,' rejoined the most unhappy man in existence, 'I don't mind that; but my nerves are in that state – I cannot go through the ceremony. You know I don't like going out. – For God's sake, Charles, don't fidget with that stool so; you'll drive me mad.' Mr Kitterbell, quite regardless of his uncle's nerves, had occupied himself for some ten minutes in describing a circle on the floor with one leg of the office stool on which he was seated, keeping the other three up in the air, and holding fast on by the desk.

'I beg your pardon, uncle,' said Kitterbell, quite abashed, suddenly releasing his hold on the desk, and bringing the three wandering legs back to the floor, with a force sufficient to drive them through it.

'But come, don't refuse. If it's a boy, you know, we must have two godfathers.'

'*If* it's a boy!' said Dumps; 'why can't you say at once whether it *is* a boy or not?'

'I should be very happy to tell you, but it's impossible I can undertake to say whether it's a girl or a boy, if the child isn't born yet.'

'Not born yet!' echoed Dumps, with a gleam of hope lighting up his lugubrious visage. 'Oh, well, it *may* be a girl, and then you won't want me; or if it is a boy, it *may* die before it is christened.'

'I hope not,' said the father that expected to be, looking very grave.

'I hope not,' acquiesced Dumps, evidently pleased with the subject. He was beginning to get happy. '*I* hope not, but distressing cases frequently occur during the first two or three days of a child's life; fits, I am told, are exceedingly common, and alarming convulsions are almost matters of course.'

'Lord, uncle!' ejaculated little Kitterbell, gasping for breath.

'Yes; my landlady was confined – let me see – last Tuesday: an uncommonly fine boy. On the Thursday night the nurse was sitting with him upon her knee before the fire, and he was as well as possible. Suddenly he became black in the face, and alarmingly spasmodic. The medical man was instantly sent for, and every remedy was tried, but—'

'How frightful!' interrupted the horror-stricken Kitterbell.

'The child died, of course. However, your child *may* not die; and if it should be a boy, and should *live* to be christened, why I suppose I must be one of the sponsors.' Dumps was evidently good-natured on the faith of his anticipations.

'Thank you, uncle,' said his agitated nephew, grasping his hand as warmly as if he had done him some essential service. 'Perhaps I had better not tell Mrs K. what you have mentioned.'

'Why, if she's low-spirited, perhaps you had better not mention the melancholy case to her,' returned Dumps, who of course had invented the whole story; 'though perhaps it would be but doing your duty as a husband to prepare her for the *worst*.'

A day or two afterwards, as Dumps was perusing a morning paper at the chop house which he regularly frequented, the following paragraph met his eyes:–

> '*Births*. – On Saturday, the 18th inst., in Great Russell Street, the lady of Charles Kitterbell, Esq., of a son.'

'It *is* a boy!' he exclaimed, dashing down the paper, to the astonishment of the waiters. 'It *is* a boy!' But he speedily regained his composure as his eye rested on a paragraph quoting the number of infant deaths from the bills of mortality.

Six weeks passed away, and as no communication had been received from the Kitterbells, Dumps was beginning to flatter himself that the child was dead, when the following note painfully resolved his doubts:–

*'Great Russell Street,*
*'Monday morning.*

'Dear Uncle, – You will be delighted to hear that my dear Jemima has left her room, and that your future godson is getting on capitally. He was very thin at first, but he is getting much larger, and nurse says he is filling out every day. He cries a good deal, and is a very singular colour, which made Jemima and me rather uncomfortable; but as nurse says it's natural, and as of course we know nothing about these things yet, we are quite satisfied with what nurse says. We think he will be a sharp child; and nurse says she's sure he will, because he never goes to sleep. You will readily believe that we are all very happy, only we're a little worn out for want of rest, as he keeps us awake all night; but this we must expect, nurse says, for the first six or eight months. He has been vaccinated, but in consequence of the operation being rather awkwardly performed, some small particles of glass were introduced into the arm with the matter. Perhaps this may in some degree account for his being rather fractious; at least, so nurse says. We propose to have him christened at twelve o'clock on Friday, at Saint George's church, in Hart Street, by the name of Frederick Charles William. Pray don't be later than a quarter before twelve. We shall have a very few friends in the evening, when of course we shall see you. I am sorry to say that the dear boy appears rather restless and uneasy today: the cause, I fear, is fever.

'Believe me, dear Uncle,
'Yours affectionately,
'CHARLES KITTERBELL.

'P.S. – I open this note to say that we have just discovered the cause of little Frederick's restlessness. It is not fever, as I apprehended, but a small pin, which nurse accidentally stuck in his leg yesterday evening. We have taken it out, and he appears more composed, though he still sobs a good deal.'

It is almost unnecessary to say that the perusal of the above interesting statement was no great relief to the mind of the hypochondriacal Dumps. It was impossible to recede, however, and so he put the best face – that is to say, an uncommonly miserable one – upon the matter; and purchased a handsome silver mug for the infant Kitterbell, upon which he ordered the initials 'F.C.W.K.', with the customary untrained grape-vine-looking flourishes, and a large full stop, to be engraved forthwith.

Monday was a fine day, Tuesday was delightful, Wednesday was equal to either, and Thursday was finer than ever; four successive fine days in London! Hackney coachmen became revolutionary, and crossing-sweepers began to doubt the existence of a First Cause. The *Morning Herald* informed its readers that an old woman in Camden Town had been heard to say that the fineness of the season was 'unprecedented in the memory of the oldest inhabitant'; and Islington clerks, with large families and small salaries, left off their black gaiters, disdained to carry their once green cotton umbrellas, and walked to town in the conscious pride of white stockings and cleanly brushed Bluchers. Dumps beheld all this with an eye of supreme contempt – his triumph was at hand. He knew that if it had been fine for four weeks instead of four days, it would rain when he went out; he was lugubriously happy in the conviction that Friday would be a wretched day – and so it was. 'I knew how it would be,' said Dumps, as he turned round opposite the Mansion House at half-past eleven o'clock on the Friday morning. 'I knew how it would be. *I* am concerned, and that's enough;' – and certainly the appearance of the day was sufficient to depress the spirits of a much more buoyant-hearted individual than himself. It had rained, without a moment's cessation, since eight o'clock; everybody that passed up Cheapside and down Cheapside, looked wet, cold and dirty. All sorts of forgotten and long-concealed umbrellas had been put into requisition. Cabs whisked about, with the 'fare' as carefully boxed up behind two glazed calico curtains as any mysterious picture in any one of Mrs Radcliffe's castles; omnibus horses smoked like steam engines; nobody thought of 'standing up' under doorways or arches; they were painfully convinced it was a hopeless case; and so everybody went hastily along, jumbling and jostling, and swearing and perspiring, and slipping about, like amateur skaters behind wooden chairs on the Serpentine on a frosty Sunday.

Dumps paused; he could not think of walking, being rather smart for the christening. If he took a cab he was sure to be spilt, and a hackney coach was too expensive for his economical ideas. An omnibus was waiting at the opposite corner – it was a desperate case – he had never heard of an omnibus upsetting or running away, and if the cad did knock him down, he could 'pull him up' in return.

'Now, sir!' cried the young gentleman who officiated as 'cad' to the 'Lads of the Village', which was the name of the machine just noticed. Dumps crossed.

'This vay, sir!' shouted the driver of the 'Hark-away', pulling up his vehicle immediately across the door of the opposition – 'This vay, sir – he's full.' Dumps hesitated, whereupon the 'Lads of the Village' commenced pouring out a torrent of abuse against the 'Hark-away'; but the conductor of the 'Admiral Napier' settled the contest in a most satisfactory manner for all parties by seizing Dumps round the waist, and thrusting him into the middle of his vehicle, which had just come up and only wanted the sixteenth inside.

'All right,' said the 'Admiral', and off the thing thundered, like a fire engine at full gallop, with the kidnapped customer inside, standing in the position of a half doubled-up bootjack, and falling about with every jerk of the machine, first on the one side, and then on the other, like a 'Jack-in-the-green', on May day, setting to the lady with a brass ladle.

'For Heaven's sake, where am I to sit?' inquired the miserable man of an old gentleman, into whose stomach he had just fallen for the fourth time.

'Anywhere but on my *chest*, sir,' replied the old gentleman in a surly tone.

'Perhaps the *box* would suit the gentleman better,' suggested a very damp lawyer's clerk, in a pink shirt, and a smirking countenance.

After a great deal of struggling and falling about, Dumps at last managed to squeeze himself into a seat, which, in addition to the slight disadvantage of being between a window that would not shut, and a door that must be open, placed him in close contact with a passenger, who had been walking about all the morning without an umbrella, and who looked as if he had spent the day in a full water butt – only wetter.

'Don't bang the door so,' said Dumps to the conductor, as he shut it after letting out four of the passengers; 'I am very nervous – it destroys me.'

'Did any gen'lm'n say anythink?' replied the cad, thrusting in his head, and trying to look as if he didn't understand the request.

'I told you not to bang the door so!' repeated Dumps, with an expression of countenance like the knave of clubs, in convulsions.

'Oh! vy, it's rather a sing'ler circumstance about this here door, sir, that it von't shut without banging,' replied the conductor; and he opened the door very wide, and shut it again with a terrific bang, in proof of the assertion.

'I beg your pardon, sir,' said a little prim, wheezing old gentleman, sitting opposite Dumps, 'I beg your pardon; but have you ever observed, when you have been in an omnibus on a wet day, that four people out of five always come in with large cotton umbrellas, without a handle at the top, or the brass spike at the bottom?'

'Why, sir,' returned Dumps, as he heard the clock strike twelve, 'it never struck me before; but now you mention it, I—Hollo! hollo!' shouted the persecuted individual, as the omnibus dashed past Drury Lane, where he had directed to be set down – 'Where is the cad?'

'I think he's on the box, sir,' said the young gentleman before noticed in the pink shirt, which looked like a white one ruled with red ink.

'I want to be set down!' said Dumps in a faint voice, overcome by his previous efforts.

'I think these cads want to be *set down*,' returned the attorney's clerk, chuckling at his sally.

'Hollo!' cried Dumps again.

'Hollo!' echoed the passengers. The omnibus passed St Giles's church.

'Hold hard!' said the conductor; 'I'm blowed if we ha'n't forgot the gen'lm'n as vas to be set down at Doory Lane. – Now, sir, make haste, if you please,' he added, opening the door, and assisting Dumps out with as much coolness as if it was 'all right'. Dumps's indignation was for once getting the better of his cynical equanimity. 'Drury Lane!' he gasped, with the voice of a boy in a cold bath for the first time.

'Doory Lane, sir? – yes, sir – third turning on the right-hand side, sir.'

Dumps's passion was paramount: he clutched his umbrella, and was striding off with the firm determination of not paying the fare. The cad, by a remarkable coincidence, happened to entertain a directly contrary opinion, and Heaven knows how far the altercation would have proceeded, if it had not been most ably and satisfactorily brought to a close by the driver.

'Hollo!' said that respectable person, standing up on the box, and leaning with one hand on the roof of the omnibus. 'Hollo, Tom! tell the gentleman if so be as he feels aggrieved, we will take him up to the Edgeer (Edgeware) Road for nothing, and set him down at Doory Lane when we comes back. He can't reject that, anyhow.'

The argument was irresistible: Dumps paid the disputed sixpence, and in a quarter of an hour was on the staircase of No. 14, Great Russell Street.

Everything indicated that preparations were making for the reception of 'a few friends' in the evening. Two dozen extra tumblers, and four ditto wine glasses – looking anything but transparent, with little bits of straw in them – were on the slab in the passage, just arrived. There was a great smell of nutmeg, port wine, and almonds, on the staircase; the covers were taken off the stair carpet, and the figure of Venus on the first landing looked as if she were ashamed of the composition candle in her right hand, which contrasted beautifully with the lamp-blacked drapery of the goddess of love. The female servant (who looked very warm and bustling) ushered Dumps into a front drawing room, very prettily furnished, with a plentiful sprinkling of little baskets, paper table mats, china watchmen, pink and gold albums, and rainbow-bound little books on the different tables.

'Ah, uncle!' said Mr Kitterbell, 'how d'ye do? Allow me – Jemima, my dear – my uncle. I think you've seen Jemima before, sir?'

'Have had the *pleasure*,' returned big Dumps, his tone and look making it doubtful whether in his life he had ever experienced the sensation.

'I'm sure,' said Mrs Kitterbell, with a languid smile, and a slight cough. 'I'm sure – hem – any friend – of Charles's – hem – much less a relation, is—'

'I knew you'd say so, my love,' said little Kitterbell, who, while he appeared to be gazing on the opposite houses, was looking at his wife with a most affectionate air: 'Bless you!' The last two words were accompanied with a simper, and a squeeze of the hand, which stirred up all Uncle Dumps's bile.

'Jane, tell nurse to bring down baby,' said Mrs Kitterbell, addressing the servant. Mrs Kitterbell was a tall, thin young lady, with very light hair, and a particularly white face – one of those young women who almost invariably, though one hardly knows why, recall to one's mind the idea of a cold fillet of veal. Out went the servant, and in came the nurse, with a remarkably small parcel in her arms, packed up in a blue mantle trimmed with white fur. – This was the baby.

'Now, uncle,' said Mr Kitterbell, lifting up that part of the mantle which covered the infant's face, with an air of great triumph, '*who* do you think he's like?'

'He! he! Yes, who?' said Mrs K., putting her arm through her husband's, and looking up into Dumps's face with an expression of as much interest as she was capable of displaying.

'Good God, how small he is!' cried the amiable uncle, starting back with well-feigned surprise; '*remarkably* small indeed.'

'Do you think so?' inquired poor little Kitterbell, rather alarmed. 'He's a monster to what he was – ain't he, nurse?'

'He's a dear,' said the nurse, squeezing the child, and evading the question – not because she scrupled to disguise the fact, but because she couldn't afford to throw away the chance of Dumps's half crown.

'Well, but who is he like?' inquired little Kitterbell.

Dumps looked at the little pink heap before him, and only thought at the moment of the best mode of mortifying the youthful parents.

'I really don't know *who* he's like,' he answered, very well knowing the reply expected of him.

'Don't you think he's like *me*?' inquired his nephew, with a knowing air.

'Oh, *decidedly* not!' returned Dumps, with an emphasis not to be misunderstood. 'Decidedly not like you. – Oh, certainly not.'

'Like Jemima?' asked Kitterbell, faintly.

'Oh, dear no; not in the least. I'm no judge, of course, in such cases; but I really think he's more like one of those little carved representations that one sometimes sees blowing a trumpet on a tombstone!' The nurse stooped down over the child, and with great difficulty prevented an explosion of mirth. Pa and ma looked almost as miserable as their amiable uncle.

'Well!' said the disappointed little father, 'you'll be better able to tell what he's like by-and-bye. You shall see him this evening with his mantle off.'

'Thank you,' said Dumps, feeling particularly grateful.

'Now, my love,' said Kitterbell to his wife, 'it's time we were off. We're to meet the other godfather and the godmother at the church, uncle, – Mr and Mrs Wilson from over the way – uncommonly nice people. My love, are you well wrapped up?'

'Yes, dear.'

'Are you sure you won't have another shawl?' inquired the anxious husband.

'No, sweet,' returned the charming mother, accepting Dumps's proffered arm; and the little party entered the hackney coach that was to take them to the church; Dumps amusing Mrs Kitterbell by expatiating largely on the danger of measles, thrush, teeth-cutting and other interesting diseases to which children are subject.

The ceremony (which occupied about five minutes) passed off without anything particular occurring. The clergyman had to dine some distance from town, and had two churchings, three christenings, and a funeral to perform in something less than an hour. The godfathers and godmother, therefore, promised to renounce the devil and all his works – 'and all that sort of thing' – as little Kitterbell said – 'in less than no time'; and with the exception of Dumps nearly letting the child fall into the font when he handed it to the clergyman, the whole affair went off in the usual business-like and matter-of-course manner, and Dumps re-entered the Bank gates at two o'clock with a heavy heart, and the painful conviction that he was regularly booked for an evening party.

Evening came – and so did Dumps's pumps, black silk stockings, and white cravat which he had ordered to be forwarded, per boy, from Pentonville. The depressed godfather dressed himself at a friend's counting house, from whence, with his spirits fifty degrees below proof, he sallied forth – as the weather had cleared up, and the evening was tolerably fine – to walk to Great Russell Street. Slowly he paced up Cheapside, Newgate Street, down Snow Hill, and up Holborn ditto, looking as grim as the figure head of a man of war, and finding out fresh causes of misery at every step. As he was crossing the corner of Hatton Garden, a man, apparently intoxicated, rushed against him, and would have knocked him down, had he not been providentially caught by a very genteel young man, who happened to be close to him at the time. The shock so disarranged Dumps's nerves, as well as his dress, that he could hardly stand. The gentleman took his arm, and in the kindest manner walked with him as far as Furnival's Inn. Dumps, for about the first time in his life, felt grateful and polite; and he and the gentlemanly-looking young man parted with mutual expressions of goodwill.

'There are at least some well-disposed men in the world,' ruminated the misanthropical Dumps as he proceeded towards his destination.

Rat – tat – ta–ra–ra–ra–ra–rat – knocked a hackney coachman at Kitterbell's door, in imitation of a gentleman's servant, just as Dumps reached it; and out came an old lady in a large toque, and an old gentleman in a blue coat, and three female copies of the old lady in pink dresses, and shoes to match.

'It's a large party,' sighed the unhappy godfather, wiping the perspiration from his forehead, and leaning against the area railings. It was some time before the miserable man could muster up courage to knock at the door, and when he did, the smart appearance of a neighbouring greengrocer (who had been hired to wait for seven and sixpence, and whose calves alone were worth double the money), the lamp in the passage, and the Venus on the landing, added to the hum of many voices, and the sound of a harp and two violins, painfully convinced him that his surmises were but too well founded.

'How are you?' said little Kitterbell, in a greater bustle than ever, bolting out of the little back parlour with a corkscrew in his hand, and various particles of sawdust, looking like so many inverted commas, on his inexpressibles.

'Good God!' said Dumps, turning into the aforesaid parlour to put his shoes on, which he had brought in his coat pocket, and still more appalled by the sight of seven fresh-drawn corks, and a corresponding number of decanters. 'How many people are there upstairs?'

'Oh, not above thirty-five. We've had the carpet taken up in the back drawing room, and the piano and the card tables are in the front. Jemima thought we'd better have a regular sit-down supper in the front parlour, because of the speechifying, and all that. But, Lord! uncle, what's the matter?' continued the excited little man, as Dumps stood with one shoe on, rummaging his pockets with the most frightful distortion of visage. 'What have you lost? Your pocket book?'

'No,' returned Dumps, diving first into one pocket and then into the other, and speaking in a voice like Desdemona with the pillow over her mouth.

'Your card case? snuff box? the key of your lodgings?' continued Kitterbell, pouring question on question with the rapidity of lightning.

'No! no!' ejaculated Dumps, still diving eagerly into his empty pockets.

'Not – not – the *mug* you spoke of this morning?'

'Yes, the *mug*!' replied Dumps, sinking into a chair.

'How *could* you have done it?' inquired Kitterbell. 'Are you sure you brought it out?'

'Yes! yes! I see it all!' said Dumps, starting up as the idea flashed across his mind; 'miserable dog that I am – I was born to suffer. I see it all: it was the gentlemanly-looking young man!'

'Mr Dumps!' shouted the greengrocer in a stentorian voice, as he ushered the somewhat recovered godfather into the drawing room half an hour after the above declaration. 'Mr Dumps!' – everybody looked at the door, and in came Dumps, feeling about as much out of place as a salmon might be supposed to be on a gravel walk.

'Happy to see you again,' said Mrs Kitterbell, quite unconscious of the unfortunate man's confusion and misery; 'you must allow me to introduce you to a few of our friends: – my mamma, Mr Dumps – my papa and sisters.' Dumps seized the hand of the mother as warmly as if she was his own parent, bowed *to* the young ladies, and *against* a gentleman behind him, and took no notice whatever of the father, who had been bowing incessantly for three minutes and a quarter.

'Uncle,' said little Kitterbell, after Dumps had been introduced to a select dozen or two, 'you must let me lead you to the other end of the room, to introduce you to my friend Danton. Such a splendid fellow! – I'm sure you'll like him – this way.' – Dumps followed as tractably as a tame bear.

Mr Danton was a young man of about five-and-twenty, with a considerable stock of impudence, and a very small share of ideas: he was a great favourite, especially with young ladies of from sixteen to twenty-six years of age, both inclusive. He could imitate the French horn to admiration, sang comic songs most inimitably, and had the most insinuating way of saying impertinent nothings to his doting female admirers. He had acquired, somehow or other, the reputation of being a great wit, and accordingly, whenever he opened his mouth, everybody who knew him laughed very heartily.

The introduction took place in due form. Mr Danton bowed, and twirled a lady's handkerchief, which he held in his hand, in a most comic way. Everybody smiled.

'Very warm,' said Dumps, feeling it necessary to say something.

'Yes. It was warmer yesterday,' returned the brilliant Mr Danton. – A general laugh.

'I have great pleasure in congratulating you on your first appearance in the character of a father, sir,' he continued, addressing Dumps – 'godfather, I mean.' – The young ladies were convulsed, and the gentlemen in ecstasies.

A general hum of admiration interrupted the conversation, and announced the entrance of nurse with the baby. A universal rush of the young ladies immediately took place. (Girls are always *so* fond of babies in company.)

'Oh, you dear!' said one.

'How sweet!' cried another, in a low tone of the most enthusiastic admiration.

'Heavenly!' added a third.

'Oh! what dear little arms!' said a fourth, holding up an arm and fist about the size and shape of the leg of a fowl cleanly picked.

'Did you ever!' – said a little coquette with a large bustle, who looked like a French lithograph, appealing to a gentleman in three waistcoats – 'Did you ever!'

'Never, in my life,' returned her admirer, pulling up his collar.

'Oh, *do* let me take it, nurse!' cried another young lady. 'The love!'

'Can it open its eyes, nurse?' inquired another, affecting the utmost innocence. – Suffice it to say, that the single ladies unanimously voted him an angel, and that the married ones, *nem. con.*, agreed that he was decidedly the finest baby they had ever beheld – except their own.

The quadrilles were resumed with great spirit. Mr Danton was universally admitted to be beyond himself; several young ladies enchanted the company and gained admirers by singing 'We met' – 'I saw her at the Fancy Fair' – and other equally sentimental and interesting ballads. 'The young men,' as Mrs Kitterbell said, 'made themselves very agreeable'; the girls did not lose their opportunity; and the evening promised to go off excellently. Dumps didn't mind it: he had devised a plan for himself – a little bit of fun in his own way – and he was almost happy! He played a rubber and lost every point. Mr Danton said he could not have lost every point, because he made a point of losing: everybody laughed tremendously. Dumps retorted with a better joke, and nobody smiled, with the exception of the host, who seemed to consider it his duty to laugh till he was black in the face, at everything. There was only one drawback – the musicians did not play with quite as much spirit as could have been wished. The cause, however, was satisfactorily explained; for it appeared, on the testimony of a gentleman who had come up from Gravesend in the afternoon, that they had been engaged on board a steamer all day, and had played almost without cessation all the way to Gravesend, and all the way back again.

The 'sit-down supper' was excellent; there were four barley-sugar temples on the table, which would have looked beautiful if they had not melted away when the supper began; and a watermill, whose only fault was that instead of going round, it ran over the tablecloth. Then there were fowls, and tongue, and trifle, and sweets, and lobster salad, and potted beef – and everything. And little Kitterbell kept calling out for clean plates, and the clean plates did not come: and then the gentlemen who wanted the plates said they didn't mind, they'd take a lady's; and then Mrs Kitterbell applauded their gallantry, and the greengrocer ran about till he thought his seven and sixpence was very hardly earned; and the young ladies didn't eat much for fear it shouldn't look romantic, and the married ladies ate as much as possible, for fear they shouldn't have enough; and a great deal of wine was drunk, and everybody talked and laughed considerably.

'Hush! hush!' said Mr Kitterbell, rising and looking very important. 'My love (this was addressed to his wife at the other end of the table), take care of Mrs Maxwell, and your mamma, and the rest of the married ladies; the gentlemen will persuade the young ladies to fill their glasses, I am sure.'

'Ladies and gentlemen,' said long Dumps, in a very sepulchral voice and rueful accent, rising from his chair like the ghost in Don Juan, 'will you have the kindness to charge your glasses? I am desirous of proposing a toast.'

A dead silence ensued, and the glasses were filled – everybody looked serious.

'Ladies and gentlemen,' slowly continued the ominous Dumps, 'I' – (here Mr Danton imitated two notes from the French horn, in a very loud key, which electrified the nervous toast proposer, and convulsed his audience.)

'Order! order!' said little Kitterbell, endeavouring to suppress his laughter.

'Order!' said the gentlemen.

'Danton, be quiet,' said a particular friend on the opposite side of the table.

'Ladies and gentlemen,' resumed Dumps, somewhat recovered, and not much disconcerted, for he was always a pretty good hand at a speech – 'In accordance with what is, I believe, the established usage on these occasions, I, as one of the godfathers of Master Frederick Charles William Kitterbell – (here the speaker's voice faltered, for he remembered the mug) – venture to rise to propose a toast. I need hardly say that it is the health and prosperity of that young gentleman, the particular event of whose early life we are here met to celebrate – (applause). Ladies and gentlemen, it is impossible to suppose that our friends here, whose sincere well-wishers we all are, can pass through life without some trials, considerable suffering, severe affliction, and heavy losses!' – Here the arch-traitor paused, and slowly drew forth a long, white pocket handkerchief – his example was followed by several ladies. 'That these trials may be long spared them is my most earnest prayer, my most fervent wish (a distinct sob from the grandmother). I hope and trust, ladies and gentlemen, that the infant whose christening we have this evening met to celebrate, may not be removed from the arms of his parents by premature decay (several cambrics were in requisition): that his young and now *apparently* healthy form may not be wasted by lingering disease. (Here Dumps cast a sardonic glance around, for a great sensation was manifest among the married ladies.) You, I am sure, will concur with me in wishing that he may live to be a comfort and a blessing to his parents. ('Hear, hear!' and an audible sob from Mr Kitterbell.) But should he not be what we could wish – should he forget in after times the duty which he owes to them – should they unhappily experience that distracting truth, "how sharper than a serpent's tooth it is to have a thankless child"' – Here Mrs Kitterbell, with her handkerchief to her eyes, and accompanied by several ladies, rushed from the room, and went into violent hysterics in the passage, leaving her better half in almost as bad a condition, and a general impression in Dumps's favour; for people like sentiment, after all.

It need hardly be added, that this occurrence quite put a stop to the harmony of the evening. Vinegar, hartshorn, and cold water, were now as much in request as negus, rout cakes, and *bonbons* had been a short time before. Mrs Kitterbell was immediately conveyed to her apartment, the musicians were silenced, flirting ceased, and the company slowly departed. Dumps left the house at the commencement of the bustle, and walked home with a light step, and (for him) a cheerful heart. His landlady, who slept in the next room, has offered to make oath that she heard him laugh, in his peculiar manner, after he had locked his door. The assertion, however, is so improbable, and bears on the face of it such strong evidence of untruth, that it has never obtained credence to this hour.

The family of Mr Kitterbell has considerably increased since the period to which we have referred; he has now two sons and a daughter; and as he expects, at no distant period, to have another addition to his blooming progeny, he is anxious to secure an eligible godfather for the occasion. He is determined, however, to impose upon him two conditions. He must bind himself, by a solemn obligation, not to make any speech after supper; and it is indispensable that he should be in no way connected with 'the most miserable man in the world'.

## Chapter Twelve

### *The Drunkard's Death*

Specially written to appear as the last of the tales in *Sketches. Second Series*, 1837.

We will be bold to say, that there is scarcely a man in the constant habit of walking, day after day, through any of the crowded thoroughfares of London, who cannot recollect among the people whom he 'knows by sight', to use a familiar phrase, some being of abject and wretched appearance whom he remembers to have seen in a very different condition, whom he has observed sinking lower and lower, by almost imperceptible degrees, and the shabbiness and utter destitution of whose appearance, at last, strike forcibly and painfully upon him, as he passes by. Is there any man who has mixed much with society, or whose avocations have caused him to mingle, at one time or other, with a great number of people, who cannot call to mind the time when some shabby, miserable wretch, in rags and filth, who shuffles past him now in all the squalor of disease and poverty, was a respectable tradesman, or clerk, or a man following some thriving pursuit, with good prospects, and decent means? – or cannot any of our readers call to mind from among the list of their *quondam* acquaintance, some fallen and degraded man, who lingers about the pavement in hungry misery – from whom everyone turns coldly away, and who preserves himself from sheer starvation, nobody knows how? Alas! such cases are of too frequent occurrence to be rare items in any man's experience; and but too often arise from one cause – drunkenness – that fierce rage for the slow, sure poison, that oversteps every other consideration; that casts aside wife, children, friends, happiness, and station; and hurries its victims madly on to degradation and death.

Some of these men have been impelled, by misfortune and misery, to the vice that has degraded them. The ruin of worldly expectations, the death of those they loved, the sorrow that slowly consumes, but will not break the heart, has driven them wild; and they present the hideous spectacle of madmen, slowly dying by their own hands. But by far the greater part have wilfully, and with open eyes, plunged into the gulf from which the man who once enters it never rises more, but into which he sinks deeper and deeper down, until recovery is hopeless.

Such a man as this once stood by the bedside of his dying wife, while his children knelt around, and mingled low bursts of grief with their innocent prayers. The room was scantily and meanly furnished; and it needed but a glance at the pale form from which the light of life was fast passing away, to know that grief, and want, and anxious care, had been busy at the heart for many a weary year. An elderly woman, with her face bathed in tears, was supporting the head of the dying woman – her daughter – on her arm. But it was not towards her that the wan face turned; it was not her hand that the cold and trembling fingers clasped; they pressed the husband's arm; the eyes so soon to be closed in death rested on his face, and the man shook beneath their gaze. His dress was slovenly and disordered, his face inflamed, his eyes bloodshot and heavy. He had been summoned from some wild debauch to the bed of sorrow and death.

A shaded lamp by the bedside cast a dim light on the figures around, and left the remainder of the room in thick, deep shadow. The silence of night prevailed without the house, and the stillness of death was in the chamber. A watch hung over the mantelshelf; its low ticking was the only sound that broke the profound quiet, but it was a solemn one, for well they knew, who heard it, that before it had recorded the passing of another hour, it would beat the knell of a departed spirit.

It is a dreadful thing to wait and watch for the approach of death; to know that hope is gone, and recovery impossible; and to sit and count the dreary hours through long, long nights – such nights as only watchers by the bed of sickness know. It chills the blood to hear the dearest secrets of the heart – the pent-up, hidden secrets of many years – poured forth by the unconscious helpless being before you; and to think how little the reserve and cunning of a whole life will avail, when fever and delirium tear off the mask at last. Strange tales have been told in the wanderings of dying men; tales so full of guilt and crime, that those who stood by the sick person's couch have fled in horror and affright, lest they should be scared to madness by what they heard and saw; and many a wretch has died alone, raving of deeds the very name of which has driven the boldest man away.

But no such ravings were to be heard at the bedside by which the children knelt. Their half stifled sobs and moanings alone broke the silence of the lonely chamber. And when at last the mother's grasp relaxed, and, turning one look from the children to the father, she vainly strove to speak, and fell backward on the pillow, all was so calm and tranquil that she seemed to sink to sleep. They leant over her; they called upon her name, softly at first, and then in the loud and piercing tones of desperation. But there was no reply. They listened for her breath, but no sound came.

They felt for the palpitation of the heart, but no faint throb responded to the touch. That heart was broken, and she was dead!

The husband sunk into a chair by the bedside, and clasped his hands upon his burning forehead. He gazed from child to child, but when a weeping eye met his, he quailed beneath its look. No word of comfort was whispered in his ear, no look of kindness lighted on his face. All shrunk from and avoided him; and when at last he staggered from the room, no one sought to follow or console the widower.

The time had been when many a friend would have crowded round him in his affliction, and many a heartfelt condolence would have met him in his grief. Where were they now? One by one, friends, relations, the commonest acquaintance even, had fallen off from and deserted the drunkard. His wife alone had clung to him in good and evil, in sickness and poverty, and how had he rewarded her? He had reeled from the tavern to her bedside in time to see her die.

He rushed from the house, and walked swiftly through the streets. Remorse, fear, shame, all crowded on his mind. Stupefied with drink, and bewildered with the scene he had just witnessed, he re-entered the tavern he had quitted shortly before. Glass succeeded glass. His blood mounted, and his brain whirled round. Death! Everyone must die, and why not *she*? She was too good for him; her relations had often told him so. Curses on them! Had they not deserted her, and left her to whine away the time at home? Well – she was dead, and happy perhaps. It was better as it was. Another glass – one more! Hurrah! It was a merry life while it lasted; and he would make the most of it.

Time went on; the three children who were left to him, grew up, and were children no longer. The father remained the same – poorer, shabbier, and more dissolute-looking, but the same confirmed and irreclaimable drunkard. The boys had, long ago, run wild in the streets, and left him; the girl alone remained, but she worked hard, and words or blows could always procure him something for the tavern. So he went on in the old course, and a merry life he led.

One night, as early as ten o'clock – for the girl had been sick for many days, and there was, consequently, little to spend at the public house – he bent his steps homeward, bethinking himself that if he would have her able to earn money, it would be as well to apply to the parish surgeon, or, at all events, to take the trouble of inquiring what ailed her, which he had not yet thought it worthwhile to do. It was a wet December night; the wind blew piercing cold, and the rain poured heavily down. He begged a few halfpence from a passer-by, and having bought a small loaf (for it was his interest to keep the girl alive, if he could), he shuffled onwards as fast as the wind and rain would let him.

At the back of Fleet Street, and lying between it and the waterside, are several mean and narrow courts, which form a portion of Whitefriars: it was to one of these that he directed his steps.

The alley into which he turned might, for filth and misery, have competed with the darkest corner of this ancient sanctuary in its dirtiest and most lawless time. The houses, varying from two stories in height to four, were stained with every indescribable hue that long exposure to the weather, damp, and rottenness can impart to tenements composed originally of the roughest and coarsest materials. The windows were patched with papers, and stuffed with the foulest rags; the doors were falling from their hinges; poles with lines on which to dry clothes, projected from every casement, and sounds of quarrelling or drunkenness issued from every room.

The solitary oil lamp in the centre of the court had been blown out, either by the violence of the wind or the act of some inhabitant who had excellent reasons for objecting to his residence being rendered too conspicuous; and the only light which fell upon the broken and uneven pavement, was derived from the miserable candles that here and there twinkled in the rooms of such of the more fortunate residents as could afford to indulge in so expensive a luxury. A gutter ran down the centre of the alley – all the sluggish odours of which had been called forth by the rain; and as the wind whistled through the old houses, the doors and shutters creaked upon their hinges, and the windows shook in their frames, with a violence which every moment seemed to threaten the destruction of the whole place.

The man whom we have followed into this den, walked on in the darkness, sometimes stumbling into the main gutter, and at others into some branch repositories of garbage which had been formed by the rain, until he reached the last house in the court. The door, or rather what was left of it, stood ajar, for the convenience of the numerous lodgers; and he proceeded to grope his way up the old and broken stair, to the attic story.

He was within a step or two of his room door, when it opened, and a girl, whose miserable and emaciated appearance was only to be equalled by that of the candle which she shaded with her hand, peeped anxiously out.

'Is that you, father?' said the girl.

'Who else should it be?' replied the man gruffly. 'What are you trembling at? It's little enough that I've had to drink today, for there's no drink without money, and no money without work. What the devil's the matter with the girl?'

'I am not well, father – not at all well,' said the girl, bursting into tears.

'Ah!' replied the man, in the tone of a person who is compelled to admit a very unpleasant fact, to which he would rather remain blind, if he could. 'You must get better somehow, for we must have money. You must go to the parish doctor, and make him give you some medicine. They're paid for it, damn 'em. What are you standing before the door for? Let me come in, can't you?'

'Father,' whispered the girl, shutting the door behind her, and placing herself before it, 'William has come back.'

'Who?' said the man, with a start.

'Hush!' replied the girl, 'William; brother William.'

'And what does he want?' said the man, with an effort at composure – 'money? meat? drink? He's come to the wrong shop for that, if he does. Give me the candle – give me the candle, fool – I ain't going to hurt him.' He snatched the candle from her hand, and walked into the room.

Sitting on an old box, with his head resting on his hand, and his eyes fixed on a wretched cinder fire that was smouldering on the hearth, was a young man of about two-and-twenty, miserably clad in an old coarse jacket and trousers. He started up when his father entered.

'Fasten the door, Mary,' said the young man hastily – 'Fasten the door. You look as if you didn't know me, father. It's long enough since you drove me from home; you may well forget me.'

'And what do you want here, now?' said the father, seating himself on a stool, on the other side of the fireplace. 'What do you want here, now?'

'Shelter,' replied the son. 'I'm in trouble: that's enough. If I'm caught I shall swing; that's certain. Caught I shall be, unless I stop here; that's *as* certain. And there's an end of it.'

'You mean to say, you've been robbing, or murdering, then?' said the father.

'Yes, I do,' replied the son. 'Does it surprise you, father?' He looked steadily in the man's face, but he withdrew his eyes, and bent them on the ground.

'Where's your brothers?' he said, after a long pause.

'Where they'll never trouble you,' replied his son: 'John's gone to America, and Henry's dead.'

'Dead!' said the father, with a shudder, which even he could not repress.

'Dead,' replied the young man. 'He died in my arms – shot like a dog, by a gamekeeper. He staggered back, I caught him, and his blood trickled down my hands. It poured out from his side like water. He was weak, and it blinded him, but he threw himself down on his knees, on the grass, and prayed to God, that if his mother was in heaven, He would hear her prayers for pardon for her youngest son. "I was her favourite boy, Will," he said, "and I am glad to think, now, that when she was dying, though I was a very young child then, and my little heart was almost bursting, I knelt down at the foot of the bed, and thanked God for having made me so fond of her as to have never once done anything to bring the tears into her eyes. O Will, why was she taken away, and father left?" There's his dying words, father,' said the young man; 'make the best you can of 'em. You struck him across the face, in a drunken fit, the morning we ran away; and here's the end of it.'

The girl wept aloud; and the father, sinking his head upon his knees, rocked himself to and fro.

'If I am taken,' said the young man, 'I shall be carried back into the country, and hung for that man's murder. They cannot trace me here, without your assistance, father. For aught I know, you may give me up to justice; but unless you do, here I stop, until I can venture to escape abroad.'

For two whole days, all three remained in the wretched room, without stirring out. On the third evening, however, the girl was worse than she had been yet, and the few scraps of food they had were gone. It was indispensably necessary that somebody should go out; and as the girl was too weak and ill, the father went, just at nightfall.

He got some medicine for the girl, and a trifle in the way of pecuniary assistance. On his way back, he earned sixpence by holding a horse; and he turned homewards with enough money to supply their most pressing wants for two or three days to come. He had to pass the public house. He lingered for an instant, walked past it, turned back again, lingered once more, and finally slunk in. Two men whom he had not observed, were on the watch. They were on the point of giving up their search in despair, when his loitering attracted their attention; and when he entered the public house, they followed him.

'You'll drink with me, master,' said one of them, proffering him a glass of liquor.

'And me too,' said the other, replenishing the glass as soon as it was drained of its contents.

The man thought of his hungry children, and his son's danger. But they were nothing to the drunkard. He *did* drink; and his reason left him.

'A wet night, Warden,' whispered one of the men in his ear, as he at length turned to go away, after spending in liquor one half of the money on which, perhaps, his daughter's life depended.

'The right sort of night for our friends in hiding, Master Warden,' whispered the other.

'Sit down here,' said the one who had spoken first, drawing him into a corner. 'We have been looking arter the young un. We came to tell him it's all right now, but we couldn't find him 'cause we hadn't got the precise direction. But that ain't strange, for I don't think he know'd it himself, when he come to London, did he?'

'No, he didn't,' replied the father.

The two men exchanged glances.

'There's a vessel down at the docks, to sail at midnight, when it's high water,' resumed the first speaker, 'and we'll put him on board. His passage is taken in another name, and what's better than that, it's paid for. It's lucky we met you.'

'Very,' said the second.

'Capital luck,' said the first, with a wink to his companion.

'Great,' replied the second, with a slight nod of intelligence.

'Another glass here; quick' – said the first speaker. And in five minutes more, the father had unconsciously yielded up his own son into the hangman's hands.

Slowly and heavily the time dragged along, as the brother and sister, in their miserable hiding place, listened in anxious suspense to the slightest sound. At length, a heavy footstep was heard upon the stair; it approached nearer; it reached the landing; and the father staggered into the room.

The girl saw that he was intoxicated, and advanced with the candle in her hand to meet him; she stopped short, gave a loud scream, and fell senseless on the ground. She had caught sight of the shadow of a man reflected on the floor. They both rushed in, and in another instant the young man was a prisoner, and handcuffed.

'Very quietly done,' said one of the men to his companion, 'thanks to the old man. Lift up the girl, Tom – come, come, it's no use crying, young woman. It's all over now, and can't be helped.'

The young man stooped for an instant over the girl, and then turned fiercely round upon his father, who had reeled against the wall, and was gazing on the group with drunken stupidity.

'Listen to me, father,' he said, in a tone that made the drunkard's flesh creep. 'My brother's blood, and mine, is on your head: I never had kind look or word, or care, from you, and alive or dead, I never will forgive you. Die when you will, or how, I will be with you. I speak as a dead man now, and I warn you, father, that as surely as you must one day stand before your Maker, so surely shall your children be there, hand in hand, to cry for judgment against you.' He raised his manacled hands in a threatening attitude, fixed his eyes on his shrinking parent, and slowly left the room; and neither father nor sister ever beheld him more, on this side of the grave.

When the dim and misty light of a winter's morning penetrated into the narrow court, and struggled through the begrimed window of the wretched room, Warden awoke from his heavy sleep, and found himself alone. He arose, and looked round him; the old flock mattress on the floor was undisturbed; everything was just as he remembered to have seen it last: and there were no signs of anyone, save himself, having occupied the room during the night. He inquired of the other lodgers, and of the neighbours; but his daughter had not been seen or heard of. He rambled through the streets, and scrutinised each wretched face among the crowds that thronged them, with anxious eyes. But his search was fruitless, and he returned to his garret when night came on, desolate and weary.

For many days he occupied himself in the same manner, but no trace of his daughter did he meet with, and no word of her reached his ears. At length he gave up the pursuit as hopeless. He had long thought of the probability of her leaving him, and endeavouring to gain her bread in quiet, elsewhere. She had left him at last to starve alone. He ground his teeth, and cursed her!

He begged his bread from door to door. Every halfpenny he could wring from the pity or credulity of those to whom he addressed himself, was spent in the old way. A year passed over his head; the roof of a jail was the only one that had sheltered him for many months. He slept under archways, and in brickfields – anywhere, where there was some warmth or shelter from the cold and rain. But in the last stage of poverty, disease, and houseless want, he was a drunkard still.

At last, one bitter night, he sunk down on a door step faint and ill. The premature decay of vice and profligacy had worn him to the bone. His cheeks were hollow and livid; his eyes were sunken, and their sight was dim. His legs trembled beneath his weight, and a cold shiver ran through every limb.

And now the long-forgotten scenes of a misspent life crowded thick and fast upon him. He thought of the time when he had a home – a happy, cheerful home – and of those who peopled it, and flocked about him then, until the forms of his elder children seemed to rise from the grave, and stand about him – so plain, so clear, and so distinct they were that he could touch and feel them. Looks that he had long forgotten were fixed upon him once more; voices long since hushed in death sounded in his ears like the music of village bells. But it was only for an instant. The rain beat heavily upon him; and cold and hunger were gnawing at his heart again.

He rose, and dragged his feeble limbs a few paces further. The street was silent and empty; the few passengers who passed by, at that late hour, hurried quickly on, and his tremulous voice was lost in the violence of the storm. Again that heavy chill struck through his frame, and his blood seemed to stagnate beneath it. He coiled himself up in a projecting doorway, and tried to sleep.

But sleep had fled from his dull and glazed eyes. His mind wandered strangely, but he was awake, and conscious. The well-known shout of drunken mirth sounded in his ear, the glass was at his lips, the board was covered with choice rich food – they were before him: he could see them all, he had but to reach out his hand, and take them – and, though the illusion was reality itself, he knew that he was sitting alone in the deserted street, watching the raindrops as they pattered on the stones; that death was coming upon him by inches – and that there were none to care for or help him.

Suddenly he started up, in the extremity of terror. He had heard his own voice shouting in the night air, he knew not what, or why. Hark! A groan! – another! His senses were leaving him: half-formed and incoherent words burst from his lips; and his hands sought to tear and lacerate his flesh. He was going mad, and he shrieked for help till his voice failed him.

He raised his head, and looked up the long dismal street. He recollected that outcasts like himself, condemned to wander day and night in those dreadful streets, had sometimes gone distracted with their own loneliness. He remembered to have heard many years before that a homeless wretch had once been found in a solitary corner, sharpening a rusty knife to plunge into his own heart, preferring death to that endless, weary, wandering to and fro. In an instant his resolve was taken, his limbs received new life; he ran quickly from the spot, and paused not for breath until he reached the riverside.

He crept softly down the steep stone stairs that lead from the commencement of Waterloo Bridge, down to the water's level. He crouched into a corner, and held his breath, as the patrol passed. Never did prisoner's heart throb with the hope of liberty and life half so eagerly as did that of the wretched man at the prospect of death. The watch passed close to him, but he remained unobserved; and after waiting till the sound of footsteps had died away in the distance, he cautiously descended, and stood beneath the gloomy arch that forms the landing place from the river.

The tide was in, and the water flowed at his feet. The rain had ceased, the wind was lulled, and all was, for the moment, still and quiet – so quiet, that the slightest sound on the opposite bank, even the rippling of the water against the barges that were moored there, was distinctly audible to his ear. The stream stole languidly and sluggishly on. Strange and fantastic forms rose to the surface, and beckoned him to approach; dark gleaming eyes peered from the water, and seemed to mock his hesitation, while hollow murmurs from behind urged him onwards. He retreated a few paces, took a short run, desperate leap, and plunged into the river.

Not five seconds had passed when he rose to the water's surface – but what a change had taken place in that short time, in all his thoughts and feelings! Life – life in any form, poverty, misery, starvation – anything but death. He fought and struggled with the water that closed over his head, and screamed in agonies of terror. The curse of his own son rang in his ears. The shore – but one foot of dry ground – he could almost touch the step. One hand's breadth nearer, and he was saved – but the tide bore him onward, under the dark arches of the bridge, and he sank to the bottom.

Again he rose, and struggled for life. For one instant – for one brief instant – the buildings on the river's banks, the lights on the bridge through which the current had borne him, the black water, and the fast-flying clouds, were distinctly visible – once more he sunk, and once again he rose. Bright flames of fire shot up from earth to heaven, and reeled before his eyes, while the water thundered in his ears, and stunned him with its furious roar.

A week afterwards the body was washed ashore, some miles down the river, a swollen and disfigured mass. Unrecognised and unpitied, it was borne to the grave; and there it has long since mouldered away!

# Other Early Papers

# SUNDAY UNDER THREE HEADS

This pamphlet, written by Dickens under the pseudonym Timothy Sparks, was published by Chapman and Hall with three illustrations by Phiz in June 1836, just three months after *Pickwick Papers* had begun to appear in serial form. It was inspired by Dickens's vigorous opposition to the Bill for the Better Observance of Sunday promoted in Parliament by Sir Andrew Agnew (1793–1849), MP for the Scottish county of Wigtonshire 1830–7. Agnew, a baronet, introduced his bill for the third time in May 1836 when it was defeated by only a mere thirty-two votes. Dickens prefaces his pamphlet with a challenging dedication to the Bishop of London, Charles Blomfield (1786–1857), who was a strong proponent of Sunday Observance legislation. Unabashed by Dickens's polemics, Agnew introduced his bill again in 1837 and this time it passed its second reading but was lost when Parliament was dissolved on the death of William IV. Agnew was not re-elected and no one else took up the cause.

# DEDICATION

## TO THE RIGHT REVEREND THE BISHOP OF LONDON

My Lord,

You were among the first, some years ago, to expatiate on the vicious addiction of the lower classes of society, to Sunday excursions; and were thus instrumental in calling forth occasional demonstrations of those extreme opinions on the subject, which are very generally received with derision, if not with contempt.

Your elevated station, my Lord, affords you countless opportunities of increasing the comforts and pleasures of the humbler classes of society – not by the expenditure of the smallest portion of your princely income, but by merely sanctioning with the influence of your example, their harmless pastimes and innocent recreations.

That your Lordship would ever have contemplated Sunday recreations with so much horror, if you had been at all acquainted with the wants and necessities of the people who indulged in them, I cannot imagine possible. That a Prelate of your elevated rank has the faintest conception of the extent of those wants, and the nature of those necessities, I do not believe.

For these reasons, I venture to address this little Pamphlet to your Lordship's consideration. I am quite conscious that the outlines I have drawn, afford but a very imperfect description of the feelings they are intended to illustrate; but I claim for them one merit – their truth and freedom from exaggeration. I may have fallen short of the mark, but I have never overshot it: and while I have pointed out what appears to me to be injustice on the part of others, I hope I have carefully abstained from committing it myself.

I am, My Lord,
Your Lordship's most obedient, humble Servant,
TIMOTHY SPARKS.

*June 1836*

I

## *AS IT IS*

There are few things from which I derive greater pleasure, than walking through some of the principal streets of London on a fine Sunday, in summer, and watching the cheerful faces of the lively groups with which they are thronged. There is something, to my eyes at least, exceedingly pleasing in the general desire evinced by the humbler classes of society to appear neat and clean on this their only holiday. There are many grave old persons, I know, who shake their heads with an air of profound wisdom, and tell you that poor people dress too well nowadays; that when they were children, folks knew their stations in life better; that you may depend upon it, no good will come of this sort of thing in the end, – and so forth: but I fancy I can discern in the fine bonnet of the working man's wife, or the feather-bedizened hat of his child, no inconsiderable evidence of good feeling on the part of the man himself, and an affectionate desire to expend the few shillings he can spare from his week's wages, in improving the appearance and adding to the happiness of those who are nearest and dearest to him. This may be a very heinous and unbecoming degree of vanity, perhaps, and the money might possibly be applied to better uses; it must not be forgotten, however, that it might very easily be devoted to worse: and if two or three faces can be rendered happy and contented, by a trifling improvement of outward appearance, I cannot help thinking that the object is very cheaply purchased, even at the expense of a smart gown, or a gaudy riband. There is a great deal of very unnecessary cant about the over-dressing of the common people. There is not a manufacturer or tradesman in existence, who would not employ a man who takes a reasonable degree of pride in the appearance of himself and those about him, in preference to a sullen slovenly fellow, who works doggedly on, regardless of his own clothing and that of his wife and children, and seeming to take pleasure or pride in nothing.

The pampered aristocrat, whose life is one continued round of licentious pleasures and sensual gratifications; or the gloomy enthusiast, who detests the cheerful amusements he can never enjoy, and envies the healthy feelings he can never know, and who would put down the one and suppress the other, until he made the minds of his fellow beings as besotted and distorted as his own; – neither of these men can by possibility form an adequate notion of what Sunday really is, to those whose lives are spent in sedentary or laborious occupations, and who are accustomed to look forward to it through their whole existence, as their only day of rest from toil, and innocent enjoyment.

The sun that rises over the quiet streets of London on a bright Sunday morning, shines till his setting, on gay and happy faces. Here and there, so early as six o'clock, a young man and woman in their best attire may be seen hurrying along their way to the house of some acquaintance, who is included in their scheme of pleasure for the day; from whence, after stopping to take 'a bit of breakfast', they sally forth, accompanied by several old people, and a whole crowd of young ones, bearing large hand baskets full of provisions, and Belcher handkerchiefs done up in bundles, with the neck of a bottle sticking out at the top, and closely-packed apples bulging out at the sides, – and away they hurry along the streets leading to the steam packet wharfs, which are already plentifully sprinkled with parties bound for the same destination. Their good humour and delight know no bounds – for it is a delightful morning, all blue overhead, and nothing like a cloud in the whole sky; and even the air of the river at London Bridge is something to them, shut up as they have been, all the week, in close streets and heated rooms. There are dozens of steamers to all sorts of places – Gravesend, Greenwich, and Richmond; and such numbers of people, that when you have once sat down on the deck, it is all but a moral impossibility to get up again – to say nothing of walking about, which is entirely out of the question. Away they go, joking and laughing, and eating and drinking, and admiring everything they see, and pleased with everything they hear, to climb Windmill Hill, and catch a glimpse of the rich cornfields and beautiful orchards of Kent; or to stroll among the fine old trees of Greenwich Park, and survey the wonders of Shooter's Hill and Lady James's Folly; or to glide past the beautiful meadows of Twickenham and Richmond, and to gaze with a delight which only people like them can know, on every lovely object in the fair prospect around. Boat follows boat, and coach succeeds coach, for the next three hours; but all are filled, and all with the same kind of people – neat and clean, cheerful and contented.

They reach their places of destination, and the taverns are crowded; but there is no drunkenness or brawling, for the class of men who commit the enormity of making Sunday excursions, take their families with them: and this in itself would be a check upon them, even if they were inclined to dissipation, which they really are not. Boisterous their mirth may be, for they have all the excitement of feeling that fresh air and green fields can impart to the dwellers in crowded cities, but it is innocent and harmless. The glass is circulated, and the joke goes round; but the one is free from excess, and the other from offence; and nothing but good humour and hilarity prevail.

In streets like Holborn and Tottenham Court Road, which form the central market of a large neighbourhood, inhabited by a vast number of mechanics and poor people, a few shops are open at an early hour of the morning; and a very poor man, with a thin and sickly woman by his side, may be seen with their little basket in hand, purchasing the scanty quantity of necessaries they can afford, which the time at which the man receives his wages, or his having a good deal of work to do, or the woman's having been out charing till a late hour, prevented their procuring overnight. The coffee shops too, at which clerks and young men employed in counting houses can procure their breakfasts, are also open. This class comprises, in a place like London, an enormous number of people, whose limited means prevent their engaging for their lodgings any other apartment than a bedroom, and who have consequently no alternative but to take their breakfasts at a coffee shop, or go without it altogether. All these places, however, are quickly closed; and by the time the church bells begin to ring, all appearance of traffic has ceased. And then, what are the signs of immorality that meet the eye? Churches are well filled, and Dissenters' chapels are crowded to suffocation. There is no preaching to empty benches, while the drunken and dissolute populace run riot in the streets.

Here is a fashionable church, where the service commences at a late hour, for the accommodation of such members of the congregation – and they are not a few – as may happen to have lingered at the Opera far into the morning of the Sabbath; an excellent contrivance for poising the balance between God and Mammon, and illustrating the ease with which a man's duties to both may be accommodated and adjusted. How the carriages rattle up, and deposit their richly-dressed burdens beneath the lofty portico! The powdered footmen glide along the aisle, place the richly bound prayer books on the new pew desks, slam the doors, and hurry away, leaving the fashionable members of the congregation to inspect each other through their glasses, and to dazzle and glitter in the eyes of the few shabby people in the free seats. The organ peals forth, the hired singers commence a short hymn, and the congregation condescendingly rise, stare about them, and converse in whispers. The clergyman enters the reading desk, – a young man of noble family and elegant demeanour, notorious at Cambridge for his knowledge of horse-flesh and dancers, and celebrated at Eton for his hopeless stupidity. The service commences. Mark the soft voice in which he reads, and the impressive manner in which he applies his white hand, studded with brilliants, to his perfumed hair. Observe the graceful emphasis with which he offers up the prayers for the King, the Royal Family, and all the Nobility; and the nonchalance with which he hurries over the more uncomfortable portions of the service, the seventh commandment for instance, with a studied regard for the taste and feeling of his auditors, only to be equalled by that displayed by the sleek divine who succeeds him, who murmurs, in a voice kept down by rich feeding, most comfortable doctrines for exactly twelve minutes, and then arrives at the anxiously expected 'Now to God', which is the signal for the dismissal of the congregation. The organ is again heard; those who have been asleep wake up, and those who have kept awake, smile and seem greatly relieved; bows and congratulations are exchanged, the livery servants are all bustle and commotion, bang go the steps, up jump the footmen, and off rattle the carriages: the inmates discoursing on the dresses of the congregation, and congratulating themselves on having set so excellent an example to the community in general, and Sunday pleasurers in particular.

Enter a less orthodox place of religious worship, and observe the contrast. A small close chapel with a white-washed wall, and plain deal pews and pulpit, contains a closely packed congregation, as different in dress as they are opposed in manner, to that we have just quitted. The hymn is sung – not by paid singers, but by the whole assembly at the loudest pitch of their voices, unaccompanied by any musical instrument, the words being given out, two lines at a time, by the clerk. There is something in the sonorous quavering of the harsh voices, in the lank and hollow faces of the men, and the sour solemnity of the women, which bespeaks this a stronghold of intolerant zeal and ignorant enthusiasm: The preacher enters the pulpit. He is a coarse, hard-faced man of forbidding aspect, clad in rusty black, and bearing in his hand a small plain Bible from which he selects some passage for his text, while the hymn is concluding. The congregation fall upon their knees, and are hushed into profound stillness as he delivers an extempore prayer, in which he calls upon the Sacred Founder of the Christian faith to bless his ministry, in terms of disgusting and impious familiarity not to be described. He begins his oration in a drawling tone, and his hearers listen with silent attention. He grows warmer as he proceeds with his subject, and his gesticulation becomes proportionately violent. He clenches his fists, beats the book upon the desk before him, and swings his arms wildly about his head. The congregation murmur their acquiescence in his doctrines: and a short groan occasionally bears testimony to the moving nature of his eloquence. Encouraged by these symptoms of approval, and working himself up to a pitch of enthusiasm amounting almost to frenzy, he denounces sabbath-breakers with the direst vengeance of offended Heaven. He stretches his body half out of the pulpit, thrusts forth his arms with frantic gestures, and blasphemously calls upon the Deity to visit with eternal torments those who turn aside from the word, as interpreted and preached by – himself. A low moaning is heard, the women rock their bodies to and fro, and wring their hands; the preacher's fervour increases, the perspiration starts upon his brow, his face is flushed, and he clenches his hands convulsively, as he draws a hideous and appalling picture of the horrors preparing for the wicked in a future state. A great excitement is visible among his hearers, a scream is heard, and some young girl falls senseless on the floor. There is a momentary rustle, but it is only for a moment – all eyes are turned towards the preacher. He pauses, passes his handkerchief across his face, and looks complacently round. His voice resumes its natural tone, as with mock humility he offers up a thanksgiving for having been successful in his efforts, and having been permitted to rescue one sinner from the path of evil. He sinks back into his seat, exhausted with the violence of his ravings; the girl is removed, a hymn is sung, a petition for some measure for securing the better observance of the Sabbath, which has been prepared by the good man, is read; and his worshipping admirers struggle who shall be the first to sign it.

But the morning service has concluded, and the streets are again crowded with people. Long rows of cleanly dressed charity children, preceded by a portly beadle and a withered schoolmaster, are returning to their welcome dinner; and it is evident, from the number of men with beer trays who are running from house to house, that no inconsiderable portion of the population are about to take theirs at this early hour. The bakers' shops, in the humbler suburbs especially, are filled with men, women, and children, each anxiously waiting for the Sunday dinner. Look at the group of children who surround that working man who has just emerged from the baker's shop at the corner of the street, with the reeking dish, in which a diminutive joint of mutton simmers above a vast heap of half browned potatoes. How the young rogues clap their hands, and dance round their father, for very joy at the prospect of the feast: and how anxiously the youngest and chubbiest of the lot lingers on tiptoe by his side, trying to get a peep into the interior of the dish. They turn up the street, and the chubby faced boy trots on as fast as his little legs will carry him, to herald the approach of the dinner to 'Mother' who is standing with a baby in her arms on the doorstep, and seems almost as pleased with the whole scene as the children themselves; whereupon 'baby' not precisely understanding the importance of the business in hand, but clearly perceiving that it is something unusually lively, kicks and crows most lustily, to the unspeakable delight of all the children and both the parents: and the dinner is borne into the house amidst a shouting of small voices, and jumping of fat legs, which would fill Sir Andrew Agnew with astonishment; as well it might, seeing that Baronets, generally speaking, eat pretty comfortable dinners all the week through, and cannot be expected to understand what people feel, who only have a meat dinner on one day out of every seven.

The bakings being all duly consigned to their respective owners, and the beer man having gone his rounds, the church bells ring for afternoon service, the shops are again closed, and the streets are more than ever thronged with people; some who have not been to church in the morning, going to it now; others who have been to church, going out for a walk; and others – let us admit the full measure of their guilt – going for a walk, who have not been to church at all. I am afraid the smart servant of all work, who has been loitering at the corner of the square for the last ten minutes, is one of the latter class. She is evidently waiting for somebody, and though she may have made up her mind to go to church with him one of these mornings, I don't think they have any such intention on this particular afternoon. Here he is, at last. The white trousers, blue coat, and yellow waistcoat – and more especially that cock of the hat – indicate, as surely as inanimate objects can, that Chalk Farm and not the parish church is their destination. The girl colours up, and puts out her hand with a very awkward affectation of indifference. He gives it a gallant squeeze, and away they walk, arm in arm, the girl just looking back towards her 'place' with an air of conscious self-importance, and nodding to her fellow-servant who has gone up to the two-pair-of-stairs window, to take a full view of 'Mary's young man', which being communicated to William, he takes off his hat to the fellow-servant: a proceeding which affords unmitigated satisfaction to all parties, and impels the fellow-servant to inform Miss Emily confidentially, in the course of the evening, 'that the young man as Mary keeps company with, is one of the most genteelest young men as ever she see.'

The two young people who have just crossed the road, and are following this happy couple down the street, are a fair specimen of another class of Sunday pleasurers. There is a dapper smartness, struggling through very limited means, about the young man, which induces one to set him down at once as a junior clerk to a tradesman or attorney. The girl no one could possibly mistake. You may tell a young woman in the employment of a large dressmaker, at any time, by a certain neatness of cheap finery and humble following of fashion which pervade her whole attire; but unfortunately there are other tokens not to be misunderstood – the pale face with its hectic bloom, the slight distortion of form which no artifice of dress can wholly conceal, the unhealthy stoop, and the short cough – the effects of hard work and close application to a sedentary employment, upon a tender frame. They turn towards the fields. The girl's countenance brightens, and an unwonted glow rises in her face. They are going to Hampstead or Highgate, to spend their holiday afternoon in some place where they can see the sky, the fields, and trees, and breathe for an hour or two the pure air, which so seldom plays upon that poor girl's form, or exhilarates her spirits.

I would to God, that the iron hearted man who would deprive such people as these of their only pleasures, could feel the sinking of heart and soul, the wasting exhaustion of mind and body, the utter prostration of present strength and future hope, attendant upon that incessant toil which lasts from day to day, and from month to month; that toil which is too often protracted until the silence of midnight, and resumed with the first stir of morning. How marvellously would his ardent zeal for other men's souls diminish after a short probation, and how enlightened and comprehensive would his views of the real object and meaning of the institution of the Sabbath become!

The afternoon is far advanced – the parks and public drives are crowded. Carriages, gigs, phaetons, stanhopes, and vehicles of every description, glide smoothly on. The promenades are filled with loungers on foot, and the road is thronged with loungers on horseback. Persons of every class are crowded together, here, in one dense mass. The plebeian, who takes his pleasure on no day but Sunday, jostles the patrician, who takes his from year's end to year's end. You look in vain for any outward signs of profligacy or debauchery. You see nothing before you but a vast number of people, the denizens of a large and crowded city, in the needful and rational enjoyment of air and exercise.

It grows dusk. The roads leading from the different places of suburban resort, are crowded with people on their return home, and the sound of merry voices rings through the gradually darkening fields. The evening is hot and sultry. The rich man throws open the sashes of his spacious dining room, and quaffs his iced wine in splendid luxury. The poor man, who has no room to take his meals in, but the close apartment to which he and his family have been confined throughout the week, sits in the tea garden of some famous tavern, and drinks his beer in content and comfort. The fields and roads are gradually deserted, the crowd once more pour into the streets, and disperse to their several homes; and by midnight all is silent and quiet, save where a few stragglers linger beneath the window of some great man's house, to listen to the strains of music from within, or stop to gaze upon the splendid carriages which are waiting to convey the guests from the dinner party of an Earl.

There is a darker side to this picture, on which, so far from its being any part of my purpose to conceal it, I wish to lay particular stress. In some parts of London, and in many of the manufacturing towns of England, drunkenness and profligacy in their most disgusting forms, exhibit in the open streets on Sunday a sad and a degrading spectacle. We need go no farther than St Giles's, or Drury Lane, for sights and scenes of a most repulsive nature. Women with scarcely the articles of apparel which common decency requires, with forms bloated by disease, and faces rendered hideous by habitual drunkenness – men reeling and staggering along – children in rags and filth – whole streets of squalid and miserable appearance, whose inhabitants are lounging in the public road, fighting, screaming, and swearing – these are the common objects which present themselves in, these are the well known characteristics of, that portion of London to which I have just referred.

And why is it that all well-disposed persons are shocked, and public decency scandalised, by such exhibitions?

These people are poor – that is notorious. It may be said that they spend in liquor, money with which they might purchase necessaries, and there is no denying the fact; but let it be remembered that even if they applied every farthing of their earnings in the best possible way, they would still be very, very poor. Their dwellings are necessarily uncomfortable, and to a certain degree unhealthy. Cleanliness might do much, but they are too crowded together, the streets are too narrow, and the rooms too small, to admit of their ever being rendered desirable habitations. They work very hard all the week. We know that the effect of prolonged and arduous labour is to produce, when a period of rest does arrive, a sensation of lassitude which it requires the application of some stimulus to overcome. What stimulus have they? Sunday comes, and with it a cessation of labour. How are they to employ the day, or what inducement have they to employ it in recruiting their stock of health? They see little parties, on pleasure excursions, passing through the streets; but they cannot imitate their example, for they have not the means. They may walk, to be sure, but it is exactly the inducement to walk that they require. If every one of these men knew that by taking the trouble to walk two or three miles he would be enabled to share in a good game of cricket, or some athletic sport, I very much question whether any of them would remain at home.

But you hold out no inducement, you offer no relief from listlessness, you provide nothing to amuse his mind, you afford him no means of exercising his body. Unwashed and unshaven, he saunters moodily about, weary and dejected. In lieu of the wholesome stimulus he might derive from nature, you drive him to the pernicious excitement to be gained from art. He flies to the gin shop as his only resource; and when, reduced to a worse level than the lowest brute in the scale of creation, he lies wallowing in the kennel, your saintly lawgivers lift up their hands to heaven, and exclaim for a law which shall convert the day intended for rest and cheerfulness, into one of universal gloom, bigotry, and persecution.

## II

### *As Sabbath Bills Would Make It*

The provisions of the bill introduced into the House of Commons by Sir Andrew Agnew, and thrown out by that House on the motion for the second reading, on the 18th of May in the present year, by a majority of 32, may very fairly be taken as a test of the length to which the fanatics, of which the honourable Baronet is the distinguished leader, are prepared to go. No test can be fairer; because while on the one hand this measure may be supposed to exhibit all that improvement which mature reflection and long deliberation may have suggested, so on the other it may very reasonably be inferred, that if it be quite as severe in its provisions, and to the full as partial in its operation, as those which have preceded it, and experienced a similar fate, the disease under which the honourable Baronet and his friends labour, is perfectly hopeless, and beyond the reach of cure.

The proposed enactments of the bill are briefly these:— All work is prohibited on the Lord's day, under heavy penalties, increasing with every repetition of the offence. There are penalties for keeping shops open – penalties for drunkenness – penalties for keeping open houses of entertainment – penalties for being present at any public meeting or assembly – penalties for letting carriages, and penalties for hiring them – penalties for travelling in steam-boats, and penalties for taking passengers – penalties on vessels commencing their voyage on Sunday – penalties on the owners of cattle who suffer them to be driven on the Lord's day – penalties on constables who refuse to act, and penalties for resisting them when they do. In addition to these trifles, the constables are invested with arbitrary, vexatious, and most extensive powers; and all this in a bill which sets out with a hypocritical and canting declaration that 'nothing is more acceptable to God than the *true and sincere* worship of Him according to His holy will, and that it is the bounden duty of Parliament to promote the observance of the Lord's day, by protecting every class of society against being required to sacrifice their comfort, health, religious privileges, and conscience, for the convenience, enjoyment, or supposed advantage of any other class on the Lord's day'! The idea of making a man truly moral through the ministry of constables, and sincerely religious under the influence of penalties, is worthy of the mind which could form such a mass of monstrous absurdity as this bill is composed of.

The House of Commons threw the measure out certainly, and by so doing retrieved the disgrace – so far as it could be retrieved – of placing among the printed papers of Parliament, such an egregious specimen of legislative folly; but there was a degree of delicacy and forbearance about the debate that took place, which I cannot help thinking as unnecessary and uncalled for, as it is unusual in Parliamentary discussions. If it had been the first time of Sir Andrew Agnew's attempting to palm such a measure upon the country, we might well understand, and duly appreciate, the delicate and compassionate feeling due to the supposed weakness and imbecility of the man, which prevented his proposition being exposed in its true colours, and induced this Hon. Member to bear testimony to his excellent motives, and that Noble Lord to regret that he could not – although he had tried to do so – adopt any portion of the bill. But when these attempts have been repeated again and again; when Sir Andrew has renewed them session after session, and when it has become palpably evident to the whole House that

> His impudence of proof in every trial,
> Kens no polite, and heeds no plain denial–

it really becomes high time to speak of him and his legislation, as they appear to deserve, without that gloss of politeness, which is all very well in an ordinary case, but rather out of place when the liberties and comforts of a whole people are at stake.

In the first place, it is by no means the worst characteristic of this bill, that it is a bill of blunders: it is, from beginning to end, a piece of deliberate cruelty, and crafty injustice. If the rich composed the whole population of this country, not a single comfort of one single man would be affected by it. It is directed exclusively, and without the exception of a solitary instance, against the amusements and recreations of the poor. This was the bait held out by the Hon. Baronet to a body of men, who cannot be supposed to have any very strong sympathies in common with the poor, because they cannot understand their sufferings or their struggles. This is the bait, which will in time prevail, unless public attention is awakened, and the public feeling exerted, to prevent it.

Take the very first clause, the provision that no man shall be allowed to work on Sunday – 'That no person, upon the Lord's day, shall do, or hire, or employ any person to do any manner of labour, or any work of his or her ordinary calling.' What class of persons does this affect? The rich man? No. Menial servants, both male and female, are specially exempted from the operation of the bill. 'Menial servants' are among the poor people. The bill has no regard for them. The Baronet's dinner must be cooked on Sunday, the Bishop's horses must be groomed, and the Peer's carriage must be driven. So the menial servants are put utterly beyond the pale of grace; – unless indeed, they are to go to heaven through the sanctity of their masters, and possibly they might think even that rather an uncertain passport.

There is a penalty for keeping open houses of entertainment. Now, suppose the bill had passed, and that half-a-dozen adventurous licensed victuallers, relying upon the excitement of public feeling on the subject, and the consequent difficulty of conviction (this is by no means an improbable supposition), had determined to keep their houses and gardens open, through the whole Sunday afternoon, in defiance of the law. Every act of hiring or working, every act of buying or selling, or delivering, or causing anything to be bought or sold, is specifically made a separate offence – mark the effect. A party, a man and his wife and children, enter a tea garden, and the informer stations himself in the next box, from whence he can see and hear everything that passes. 'Waiter!' says the father. 'Yes, Sir.' 'Pint of the best ale!' 'Yes, Sir.' Away runs the waiter to the bar, and gets the ale from the landlord. Out comes the informer's notebook – penalty on the father for hiring, on the waiter for delivering, and on the landlord for selling, on the Lord's day. But it does not stop here. The waiter delivers the ale, and darts off, little suspecting the penalties in store for him. 'Hollo,' cries the father, 'waiter!' 'Yes, Sir.' 'Just get this little boy a biscuit will you?' 'Yes, Sir.' Off runs the waiter again, and down goes another case of hiring, another case of delivering, and another case of selling; and so it would go on *ad infinitum*, the sum and substance of the matter being, that every time a man or woman cried 'Waiter!' on Sunday, he or she would be fined not less than forty shillings, nor more than a hundred; and every time a waiter replied, 'Yes, Sir,' he and his master would be fined in the same amount: with addition of a new sort of window duty on the landlord, to wit, a tax of twenty shillings an hour for every hour beyond the first one, during which he should have his shutters down on the Sabbath.

With one exception, there are perhaps no clauses in the whole bill, so strongly illustrative of its partial operation, and the intention of its framer, as those which relate to travelling on Sunday. Penalties of ten, twenty, and thirty pounds, are mercilessly imposed upon coach proprietors who shall run their coaches on the Sabbath; one, two, and ten pounds upon those who hire, or let to hire, horses and carriages upon the Lord's day, but not one syllable about those who have no necessity to hire, because they have carriages and horses of their own; not one word of a penalty on liveried coachmen and footmen. The whole of the saintly venom is directed against the hired cabriolet, the humble fly, or the rumbling hackney coach, which enables a man of the poorer class to escape for a few hours from the smoke and dirt, in the midst of which he has been confined throughout the week: while the escutcheoned carriage and the dashing cab may whirl their wealthy owners to Sunday feasts and private oratorios, setting constables, informers, and penalties, at defiance. Again, in the description of the places of public resort which it is rendered criminal to attend on Sunday, there are no words comprising a very fashionable promenade. Public discussions, public debates, public lectures and speeches, are cautiously guarded against; for it is by their means that the people become enlightened enough to deride the last efforts of bigotry and superstition. There is a stringent provision for punishing the poor man who spends an hour in a news room, but there is nothing to prevent the rich one from lounging away the day in the Zoological Gardens.

There is, in four words, a mock proviso, which affects to forbid travelling 'with any animal' on the Lord's day. This, however, is revoked, as relates to the rich man, by a subsequent provision. We have then a penalty of not less than fifty, nor more than one hundred pounds, upon any person participating in the control, or having the command of any vessel which shall commence her voyage on the Lord's day, should the wind prove favourable. The next time this bill is brought forward (which will no doubt be at an early period of the next session of Parliament) perhaps it will be better to amend this clause by declaring, that from and after the passing of the act, it shall be deemed unlawful for the wind to blow at all upon the Sabbath. It would remove a great deal of temptation from the owners and captains of vessels.

The reader is now in possession of the principal enacting clauses of Sir Andrew Agnew's bill, with the exception of one, for preventing the killing or taking of '*fish, or other wild animals*', and the ordinary provisions which are inserted for form's sake in all acts of Parliament. I now beg his attention to the clauses of exemption.

They are two in number. The first exempts menial servants from any rest, and all poor men from any recreation: outlaws a milkman after nine o' clock in the morning, and makes eating-houses lawful for only two hours in the afternoon; permits a medical man to use his carriage on Sunday, and declares that a clergyman may either use his own, or hire one.

The second is artful, cunning, and designing; shielding the rich man from the possibility of being entrapped, and affecting at the same time, to have a tender and scrupulous regard for the interests of the whole community. It declares, 'that nothing in this act contained, shall extend to works of piety, charity, or necessity'.

What is meant by the word 'necessity' in this clause? Simply this – that the rich man shall be at liberty to make use of all the splendid luxuries he has collected around him, on any day in the week, because habit and custom have rendered them 'necessary' to his easy existence; but that the poor man who saves his money to provide some little pleasure for himself and family at lengthened intervals, shall not be permitted to enjoy it. It is not 'necessary' to him: – Heaven knows, he very often goes long enough without it. This is the plain English of the clause. The carriage and pair of horses, the coachman, the footman, the helper, and the groom, are 'necessary' on Sundays, as on other days, to the bishop and the nobleman; but the hackney coach, the hired gig, or the taxed cart, cannot possibly be 'necessary' to the working man on Sunday, for he has it not at other times. The sumptuous dinner and the rich wines are 'necessaries' to a great man in his own mansion: but the pint of beer and the plate of meat degrade the national character in an eating house.

Such is the bill for promoting the true and sincere worship of God according to his Holy Will, and for protecting every class of society against being required to sacrifice their health and comfort on the Sabbath. Instances in which its operation would be as unjust as it would be absurd, might be multiplied to an endless amount; but it is sufficient to place its leading provisions before the reader. In doing so, I have purposely abstained from drawing upon the imagination for possible cases; the provisions to which I have referred, stand in so many words upon the bill as printed by order of the House of Commons; and they can neither be disowned nor explained away.

Let us suppose such a bill as this to have actually passed both branches of the legislature; to have received the royal assent; and to have come into operation. Imagine its effect in a great city like London.

Sunday comes, and brings with it a day of general gloom and austerity. The man who has been toiling hard all the week, has been looking towards the Sabbath, not as to a day of rest from labour, and healthy recreation, but as one of grievous tyranny and grinding oppression. The day which his Maker intended as a blessing, man has converted into a curse. Instead of being hailed by him as his period of relaxation, he finds it remarkable only as depriving him of every comfort and enjoyment. He has many children about him, all sent into the world at an early age to struggle for a livelihood; one is kept in a warehouse all day, with an interval of rest too short to enable him to reach home, another walks four or five miles to his employment at the docks, a third earns a few shillings weekly as an errand boy, or office messenger; and the employment of the man himself, detains him at some distance from his home from morning till night. Sunday is the only day on which they could all meet together, and enjoy a homely meal in social comfort; and now they sit down to a cold and cheerless dinner: the pious guardians of the man's salvation having, in their regard for the welfare of his precious soul, shut up the bakers' shops. The fire blazes high in the kitchen chimney of these well fed hypocrites, and the rich steams of the savoury dinner scent the air. What care they to be told that this class of men have neither a place to cook in – nor means to bear the expense, if they had?

Look into your churches – diminished congregations, and scanty attendance. People have grown sullen and obstinate, and are becoming disgusted with the faith which condemns them to such a day as this, once in every seven. And as you cannot make people religious by Act of Parliament, or force them to church by constables, they display their feeling by staying away.

Turn into the streets, and mark the rigid gloom that reigns over everything around. The roads are empty, the fields are deserted, the houses of entertainment are closed. Groups of filthy and discontented-looking men are idling about at the street corners, or sleeping in the sun; but there are no decently-dressed people of the poorer class passing to and fro. Where should they walk to? It would take them an hour, at least, to get into the fields, and when they reached them they could procure neither bite nor sup without the informer and the penalty. Now and then a carriage rolls smoothly on, or a well mounted horseman, followed by a liveried attendant, canters by; but with these exceptions, all is as melancholy and quiet as if a pestilence had fallen on the city.

Bend your steps through the narrow and thickly-inhabited streets, and observe the sallow faces of the men and women who are lounging at the doors, or lolling from the windows. Regard well the closeness of these crowded rooms, and the noisome exhalations that rise from the drains and kennels; and then laud the triumph of religion and morality, which condemns people to drag their lives out in such stews as these and makes it criminal for them to eat or drink in the fresh air, or under the clear sky. Here and there, from some half-opened window, the loud shout of drunken revelry strikes upon the ear, and the noise of oaths and quarrelling – the effect of the close and heated atmosphere – is heard on all sides. See how the men all rush to join the crowd that are making their way down the street, and how loud the execrations of the mob become as they draw nearer. They have assembled round a little knot of constables, who have seized the stock-in-trade, heinously exposed on Sunday, of some miserable walking stick seller, who follows clamouring for his property. The dispute grows warmer and fiercer, until at last some of the more furious among the crowd rush forward to restore the goods to their owner. A general conflict takes place; the sticks of the constables are exercised in all directions; fresh assistance is procured; and half a dozen of the assailants are conveyed to the station house struggling, bleeding, and cursing. The case is taken to the police office on the following morning; and after a frightful amount of perjury on both sides, the men are sent to prison for resisting the officers, their families to the workhouse to keep them from starving: and there they both remain for a month afterwards, glorious trophies of the sanctified enforcement of the Christian Sabbath. Add to such scenes as these the profligacy, idleness, drunkenness, and vice, that will be committed to an extent which no man can foresee, on Monday, as an atonement for the restraint of the preceding day; and you have a very faint and imperfect picture of the religious effects of this Sunday legislation, supposing it could ever be forced upon the people.

But let those who advocate the cause of fanaticism reflect well upon the probable issue of their endeavours. They may by perseverance, succeed with Parliament. Let them ponder on the probability of succeeding with the people. You may deny the concession of a political question for a time, and a nation will bear it patiently. Strike home to the comforts of every man's fireside – tamper with every man's freedom and liberty – and one month, one week, may rouse a feeling abroad which a king would gladly yield his crown to quell, and a peer would resign his coronet to allay.

It is the custom to affect a deference for the motives of those who advocate these measures, and a respect for the feelings by which they are actuated. They do not deserve it. If they legislate in ignorance, they are criminal and dishonest; if they do so with their eyes open, they commit wilful injustice; in either case, they bring religion into contempt. But they do NOT legislate in ignorance. Public prints, and public men, have pointed out to them again and again the consequences of their proceedings. If they persist in thrusting themselves forward, let those consequences rest upon their own heads, and let them be content to stand upon their own merits.

It may be asked, what motives can actuate a man who has so little regard for the comfort of his fellow-beings, so little respect for their wants and necessities, and so distorted a notion of the beneficence of his Creator. I reply, an envious, heartless, ill-conditioned dislike to seeing those whom fortune has placed below him, cheerful and happy – an intolerant confidence in his own high worthiness before God, and a lofty impression of the demerits of others – pride, selfish pride, as inconsistent with the spirit of Christianity itself, as opposed to the example of its Founder upon earth.

To these may be added another class of men – the stern and gloomy enthusiasts, who would make earth a hell, and religion a torment: men who, having wasted the earlier part of their lives in dissipation and depravity, find themselves when scarcely past its meridian, steeped to the neck in vice, and shunned like a loathsome disease. Abandoned by the world, having nothing to fall back upon, nothing to remember but time mis-spent, and energies misdirected, they turn their eyes and not their thoughts to Heaven, and delude themselves into the impious belief, that in denouncing the lightness of heart of which they cannot partake, and the rational pleasures from which they never derived enjoyment, they are more than remedying the sins of their old career, and – like the founders of monasteries and builders of churches, in ruder days – establishing a good set claim upon their Maker.

## III

### *As It Might Be Made*

The supporters of Sabbath Bills, and more especially the extreme class of Dissenters, lay great stress upon the declarations occasionally made by criminals from the condemned cell or the scaffold, that to Sabbath breaking they attribute their first deviation from the path of rectitude; and they point to these statements, as an incontestable proof of the evil consequences which await a departure from that strict and rigid observance of the Sabbath, which they uphold. I cannot help thinking that in this, as in almost every other respect connected with the subject, there is a considerable degree of cant, and a very great deal of wilful blindness. If a man be viciously disposed – and with very few exceptions, not a man dies by the executioner's hands, who has not been in one way or other a most abandoned and profligate character for many years – if a man be viciously disposed, there is no doubt that he will turn his Sunday to bad account, that he will take advantage of it to dissipate with other bad characters as vile as himself; and that in this way he may trace his first yielding to temptation, possibly his first commission of crime, to an infringement of the Sabbath. But this would be an argument against any holiday at all. If his holiday had been Wednesday instead of Sunday, and he had devoted it to the same improper uses, it would have been productive of the same results. It is too much to judge of the character of a whole people by the confessions of the very worst members of society. It is not fair to cry down things which are harmless in themselves, because evil disposed men may turn them to bad account. Who ever thought of deprecating the teaching poor people to write because some porter in a warehouse had committed forgery? Or into what man's head did it ever enter, to prevent the crowding of churches because it afforded a temptation for the picking of pockets?

When the Book of Sports, for allowing the peasantry of England to divert themselves with certain games in the open air, on Sundays, after evening service, was published by Charles the First, it is needless to say the English people were comparatively rude and uncivilised. And yet it is extraordinary to how few excesses it gave rise, even in that day, when men's minds were not enlightened, or their passions moderated, by the influence of education and refinement. That some excesses were committed through its means, in the remoter parts of the country, and that it was discontinued in those places in consequence, cannot be denied: but generally speaking, there is no proof whatever on record, of its having had any tendency to increase crime, or to lower the character of the people.

The Puritans of that time were as much opposed to harmless recreations and healthful amusements as those of the present day, and it is amusing to observe that each in their generation advance precisely the same description of arguments. In the British Museum there is a curious pamphlet got up by the Agnews of Charles's time, entitled 'A Divine Tragedie lately acted, or a Collection of sundry memorable examples of God's Judgements upon Sabbath Breakers, and other like Libertines in their unlawful Sports, happening within the realme of England, in the compass only of two yeares last past, since the Booke (of Sports) was published, worthy to be knowne and considered of all men, especially such who are guilty of the sinne, or archpatrons thereof.' This amusing document contains some fifty or sixty veritable accounts of balls of fire that fell into churchyards and upset the sporters, and sporters that quarrelled and upset one another, and so forth: and among them is one anecdote containing an example of a rather different kind, which I cannot resist the temptation of quoting, as strongly illustrative of the fact, that this blinking of the question has not even the recommendation of novelty.

'A woman about Northampton, the same day that she heard the booke for sports read, went immediately, and having 3. pence in her purse, hired a fellow to goe to the next towne to fetch a Minstrell, who coming, she with others fell a dauncing, which continued within night; at which time shee was got with child, which at the birth shee murthering, was detected and apprehended, and being convented before the justice, shee confessed it, and withal told the occasion of it, saying it was her falling to sport on the Sabbath, upon the reading of the Booke, so as for this treble sinfull act, her presumptuous profaning of the Sabbath, w$^{h.}$ brought her adultory and that murther. Shee was according to the Law both of God and man, put to death. Much sinne and misery followeth upon Sabbath breaking.'

It is needless to say that if the young lady near Northampton had 'fallen to sport' of such a dangerous description, on any other day but Sunday, the first result would probably have been the same: it never having been distinctly shown that Sunday is more favourable to the propagation of the human race than any other day in the week. The second result – the murder of the child – does not speak very highly for the amiability of her natural disposition; and the whole story, supposing it to have had any foundation at all, is about as much chargeable upon the Book of Sports, as upon the Book of Kings. Such 'sports' have taken place in Dissenting Chapels before now; but religion has never been blamed in consequence;

not has it been proposed to shut up the chapels on that account.

The question, then, very fairly arises, whether we have any reason to suppose that allowing games in the open air on Sundays, or even providing the means of amusement for the humbler classes of society on that day, would be hurtful and injurious to the character and morals of the people.

I was travelling in the west of England a summer or two back, and was induced by the beauty of the scenery, and the seclusion of the spot, to remain for the night in a small village, distant about seventy miles from London. The next morning was Sunday; and I walked out towards the church. Groups of people – the whole population of the little hamlet apparently – were hastening in the same direction. Cheerful and good-humoured congratulations were heard on all sides, as neighbours overtook each other, and walked on in company. Occasionally I passed an aged couple, whose married daughter and her husband were loitering by the side of the old people, accommodating their rate of walking to their feeble pace, while a little knot of children hurried on before; stout young labourers in clean round frocks; and buxom girls with healthy, laughing faces, were plentifully sprinkled about in couples, and the whole scene was one of quiet and tranquil contentment, irresistibly captivating. The morning was bright and pleasant, the hedges were green and blooming, and a thousand delicious scents were wafted on the air, from the wild flowers which blossomed on either side of the footpath. The little church was one of those venerable simple buildings which abound in the English counties; half overgrown with moss and ivy, and standing in the centre of a little plot of ground, which, but for the green mounds with which it was studded, might have passed for a lovely meadow. I fancied that the old clanking bell which was now summoning the congregation together, would seem less terrible when it rung out the knell of a departed soul, than I had ever deemed possible before – that the sound would tell only of a welcome to calmness and rest, amidst the most peaceful and tranquil scene in nature.

I followed into the church – a low-roofed building with small arched windows, through which the sun's rays streamed upon a plain tablet on the opposite wall, which had once recorded names, now as undistinguishable on its worn surface, as were the bones beneath, from the dust into which they had resolved. The impressive service of the Church of England was spoken – not merely *read* – by a grey-headed minister, and the responses delivered by his auditors, with an air of sincere devotion as far removed from affectation or display, as from coldness or indifference. The psalms were accompanied by a few instrumental performers, who were stationed in a small gallery extending across the church at the lower end, over the door: and the voices were led by the clerk, who it was evident derived no slight pride and gratification from this portion of the service. The discourse was plain, unpretending, and well adapted to the comprehension of the hearers. At the conclusion of the service, the villagers waited in the churchyard to salute the clergyman as he passed; and two or three, I observed, stepped aside, as if communicating some little difficulty, and asking his advice. This, to guess from the homely bows, and other rustic expressions of gratitude, the old gentleman readily conceded. He seemed intimately acquainted with the circumstances of all his parishioners; for I heard him inquire after one man's youngest child, another man's wife, and so forth; and that he was fond of his joke, I discovered from overhearing him ask a stout, fresh-coloured young fellow, with a very pretty bashful-looking girl on his arm, 'when those banns were to be put up?' – an inquiry which made the young fellow more fresh-coloured, and the girl more bashful, and which, strange to say, caused a great many other girls who were standing round, to colour up also, and look anywhere but in the faces of their male companions.

As I approached this spot in the evening about half an hour before sunset, I was surprised to hear the hum of voices, and occasionally a shout of merriment from the meadow beyond the churchyard; which I found, when I reached the stile, to be occasioned by a very animated game of cricket, in which the boys and young men of the place were engaged, while the females and old people were scattered about: some seated on the grass watching the progress of the game, and others sauntering about in groups of two or three, gathering little nosegays of wild roses and hedge flowers. I could not but take notice of one old man in particular, with a bright-eyed granddaughter by his side, who was giving a sunburnt young fellow some instructions in the game, which he received with an air of profound deference, but with an occasional glance at the girl, which induced me to think that his attention was rather distracted from the old gentleman's narration of the fruits of his experience. When it was his turn at the wicket, too, there was a glance towards the pair every now and then, which the old grandfather very complacently considered as an appeal to his judgment of a particular hit, but which a certain blush in the girl's face, and a downcast look of the bright eye, led me to believe was intended for somebody else than the old man, – and understood by somebody else, too, or I am much mistaken.

I was in the very height of the pleasure which the contemplation of this scene afforded me, when I saw the old clergyman making his way towards us. I trembled for an angry interruption to the sport, and was almost on the point of crying out, to warn the cricketers of his approach; he was so close upon me, however, that I could do nothing but remain still, and anticipate the reproof that was preparing. What was my agreeable surprise to see the old gentleman standing at the stile, with his hands in his pockets, surveying the whole scene with evident satisfaction! And how dull I must have been, not to have known till my friend the grandfather (who, by-the-bye, said he had been a wonderful cricketer in his time) told me, that it was the clergyman himself who had established the whole thing: that it was his field they played in; and that it was he who had purchased stumps, bats, ball, and all!

It is such scenes as this I would see near London on a Sunday evening. It is such men as this who would do more in one year to make people properly religious, cheerful, and contented, than all the legislation of a century could ever accomplish.

It will be said – it has been very often – that it would be matter of perfect impossibility to make amusements and exercises succeed in large towns, which may be very well adapted to a country population. Here, again, we are called upon to yield to bare assertions on matters of belief and opinion, as if they were established and undoubted facts. That there is a wide difference between the two cases, no one will be prepared to dispute; that the difference is such as to prevent the application of the same principle to both, no reasonable man, I think, will be disposed to maintain. The great majority of the people who make holiday on Sunday now, are industrious, orderly, and well behaved persons. It is not unreasonable to suppose that they would be no more inclined to an abuse of pleasures provided for them, than they are to an abuse of the pleasures they provide for themselves; and if any people, for want of something better to do, resort to criminal practices on the Sabbath as at present observed, no better remedy for the evil can be imagined, than giving them the opportunity of doing something which will amuse them, and hurt nobody else.

The propriety of opening the British Museum to respectable people on Sunday, has lately been the subject of some discussion. I think it would puzzle the most austere of the Sunday legislators to assign any valid reason for opposing so sensible a proposition. The Museum contains rich specimens from all the vast museums and repositories of Nature, and rare and curious fragments of the mighty works of art, in bygone ages: all calculated to awaken contemplation and inquiry, and to tend to the enlightenment and improvement of the people. But attendants would be necessary, and a few men would be employed upon the Sabbath. They certainly would; but how many? Why, if the British Museum, and the National Gallery, and the Gallery of Practical Science, and every other exhibition in London, from which knowledge is to be derived and information gained, were to be thrown open on a Sunday afternoon, not fifty people would be required to preside over the whole: and it would take treble the number to enforce a Sabbath bill in any three populous parishes.

I should like to see some large field, or open piece of ground, in every outskirt of London, exhibiting each Sunday evening on a larger scale, the scene of the little country meadow. I should like to see the time arrive, when a man's attendance to his religious duties might be left to that religious feeling which most men possess in a greater or less degree, but which was never forced into the breast of any man by menace or restraint. I should like to see the time when Sunday might be looked forward to, as a recognised day of relaxation and enjoyment, and when every man might feel, what few men do now, that religion is not incompatible with rational pleasure and needful recreation.

How different a picture would the streets and public places then present! The museums, and repositories of scientific and useful inventions, would be crowded with ingenious mechanics and industrious artisans, all anxious for information, and all unable to procure it at any other time. The spacious saloons would be swarming with practical men: humble in appearance, but destined, perhaps, to become the greatest inventors and philosophers of their age. The labourers who now lounge away the day in idleness and intoxication, would be seen hurrying along, with cheerful faces and clean attire, not to the close and smoky atmosphere of the public house, but to the fresh and airy fields. Fancy the pleasant scene. Throngs of people, pouring out from the lanes and alleys of the metropolis, to various places of common resort at some short distance from the town, to join in the refreshing sports and exercises of the day – the children gambolling in crowds upon the grass, the mothers looking on, and enjoying themselves the little game they seem only to direct; other parties strolling along some pleasant walks, or reposing in the shade of the stately trees; others again intent upon their different amusements. Nothing should be heard on all sides, but the sharp stroke of the bat as it sent the ball skimming along the ground, the clear ring of the quoit, as it struck upon the iron peg: the noisy murmur of many voices, and the loud shout of mirth and delight, which would awaken the echoes far and wide, till the fields rung with it. The day would pass away in a series of enjoyments which would awaken no painful reflections when night arrived; for they would be calculated to bring with them only health and contentment. The young would lose that dread of religion, which the sour austerity of its professors too often inculcates in youthful bosoms; and the old would find less difficulty in persuading them to respect its observances. The drunken and dissipated, deprived of any excuse for their misconduct, would no longer excite pity but disgust. Above all, the more ignorant and humble class of men, who now partake of many of the bitters of life, and taste but few of its sweets, would naturally feel attachment and respect for that code of morality, which, regarding the many hardships of their station, strove to alleviate its rigours, and endeavoured to soften its asperity.

This is what Sunday might be made, and what it might be made without impiety or profanation. The wise and beneficent Creator who places men upon earth, requires that they shall perform the duties of that station of life to which they are called, and He can never intend that the more a man strives to discharge those duties, the more he shall be debarred from happiness and enjoyment. Let those who have six days in the week for all the world's pleasures, appropriate the seventh to fasting and gloom, either for their own sins or those of other people, if they like to bewail them; but let those who employ their six days in a worthier manner, devote their seventh to a different purpose. Let divines set the example of true morality: preach it to their flocks in the morning, and dismiss them to enjoy true rest in the afternoon; and let them select for their text. and let Sunday legislators take for their motto, the words which fell from the lips of that Master, whose precepts they misconstrue, and whose lessons they pervert – 'The Sabbath was made for man, and not man to serve the Sabbath.'

# PAPERS FROM *BENTLEY'S MISCELLANY*

## *The Pantomime Of Life*

First published in *Bentley's Miscellany* in March 1837 under the general title 'Stray Chapters by Boz'. Dickens had been editing *Bentley's* since January and was committed to supplying sixteen pages of his own writing to each number. The instalments of *Oliver Twist* (begun in the February number) were running short of this total, hence the makeweight 'Stray Chapters'. English pantomime had taken over the personages of the old *commedia dell'arte* – Harlequin, Columbine, Pantaloon and Clown – and Dickens refers to them all in this piece. Harlequin was always armed with a magic wand, at the touch of which characters, props and whole stage sets could be transformed. He was the most prominent character in the piece until the genius of Joseph Grimaldi (1778–1837), resulted in the Clown's replacing him in this respect. Grimaldi retired in 1823 and it was not long before people began saying, as Leigh Hunt wrote in December 1831, 'Pantomimes are not what they were'. Dickens vigorously disagreed: 'our relish for the entertainment still remains unimpaired', he declared in the introductory chapter he wrote for the 1838 edition of Grimaldi's *Memoirs* that he undertook for Bentley. He talks also there of the 'strong veneration for Clowns' that he conceived in his earliest years.

The satire on Parliamentary politicians at the end of this piece reflects the contempt he had come to feel for them during his time as a reporter in the Commons (see headnote to 'A Parliamentary Sketch', above, p. 151).

Before we plunge headlong into this paper, let us at once confess to a fondness for pantomimes – to a gentle sympathy with clowns and pantaloons – to an unqualified admiration of harlequins and columbines – to a chaste delight in every action of their brief existence, varied and many-coloured as those actions are, and inconsistent though they occasionally be with those rigid and formal rules of propriety which regulate the proceedings of meaner and less comprehensive minds. We revel in pantomimes – not because they dazzle one's eyes with tinsel and gold leaf;

not because they present to us, once again, the well-beloved chalked faces and goggle eyes of our childhood; not even because, like Christmas-day and Twelfth-night, and Shrove-Tuesday, and one's own birthday, they come to us but once a year; – our attachment is founded on a graver and a very different reason. A pantomime is to us a mirror of life; nay more, we maintain that it is so to audiences generally, although they are not aware of it, and that this very circumstance is the secret cause of their amusement and delight.

Let us take a slight example. The scene is a street: an elderly gentleman, with a large face and strongly marked features, appears. His countenance beams with a sunny smile, and a perpetual dimple is on his broad, red cheek. He is evidently an opulent elderly gentleman, comfortable in circumstances, and well-to-do in the world. He is not unmindful of the adornment of his person, for he is richly, not to say gaudily, dressed; and that he indulges to a reasonable extent in the pleasures of the table may be inferred from the joyous and oily manner in which he rubs his stomach, by way of informing the audience that he is going home to dinner. In the fulness of his heart, in the fancied security of wealth, in the possession and enjoyment of all the good things of life, the elderly gentleman suddenly loses his footing and stumbles. How the audience roar! He is set upon by a noisy and officious crowd, who buffet and cuff him unmercifully. They scream with delight! Every time the elderly gentleman struggles to get up, his relentless persecutors knock him down again. The spectators are convulsed with merriment! And when at last the elderly gentleman does get up, and staggers away, despoiled of hat, wig, and clothing, himself battered to pieces, and his watch and money gone, they are exhausted with laughter, and express their merriment and admiration in rounds of applause.

Is this like life? Change the scene to any real street; – to the Stock Exchange, or the City banker's; the merchant's counting house, or even the tradesman's shop. See any one of these men fall, – the more suddenly, and nearer the zenith of his pride and riches, the better. What a wild hallo is raised over his prostrate carcase by the shouting mob; how they whoop and yell as he lies humbled beneath them! Mark how eagerly they set upon him when he is down; and how they mock and deride him as he slinks away. Why, it is the pantomime to the very letter.

Of all the pantomimic *dramatis personae*, we consider the pantaloon the most worthless and debauched. Independent of the dislike one naturally feels at seeing a gentleman of his years engaged in pursuits highly unbecoming his gravity and time of life, we cannot conceal from ourselves the fact that he is a treacherous, worldly-minded old villain, constantly enticing his younger companion, the clown, into acts of fraud or petty larcency, and generally standing aside to watch the result of the enterprise.

If it be successful, he never forgets to return for his share of the spoil; but if it turn out a failure, he generally retires with remarkable caution and expedition, and keeps carefully aloof until the affair has blown over. His amorous propensities, too, are eminently disagreeable; and his mode of addressing ladies in the open street at noon-day is downright improper, being usually neither more nor less than a perceptible tickling of the aforesaid ladies in the waist, after committing which, he starts back, manifestly ashamed (as well he may be) of his own indecorum and temerity; continuing, nevertheless, to ogle and beckon to them from a distance in a very unpleasant and immoral manner.

Is there any man who cannot count a dozen pantaloons in his own social circle? Is there any man who has not seen them swarming at the west end of the town on a sunshiny day or a summer's evening, going through the last-named pantomimic feats with as much liquorish energy, and as total an absence of reserve, as if they were on the very stage itself? We can tell upon our fingers a dozen pantaloons of our acquaintance at this moment – capital pantaloons, who have been performing all kinds of strange freaks, to the great amusement of their friends and acquaintance, for years past; and who to this day are making such comical and ineffectual attempts to be young and dissolute, that all beholders are like to die with laughter.

Take that old gentleman who has just emerged from the *Café de l'Europe* in the Haymarket, where he has been dining at the expense of the young man upon town with whom he shakes hands as they part at the door of the tavern. The affected warmth of that shake of the hand, the courteous nod, the obvious recollection of the dinner, the savoury flavour of which still hangs upon his lips, are all characteristics of his great prototype. He hobbles away humming an opera tune, and twirling his cane to and fro, with affected carelessness. Suddenly he stops – 'tis at the milliner's window. He peeps through one of the large panes of glass; and, his view of the ladies within being obstructed by the India shawls, directs his attentions to the young girl with the band box in her hand, who is gazing in at the window also. See! he draws beside her. He coughs; she turns away from him. He draws near her again; she disregards him. He gleefully chucks her under the chin, and, retreating a few steps, nods and beckons with fantastic grimaces, while the girl bestows a contemptuous and supercilious look upon his wrinkled visage. She turns away with a flounce, and the old gentleman trots after her with a toothless chuckle. The pantaloon to the life!

But the close resemblance which the clowns of the stage bear to those of everyday life is perfectly extraordinary. Some people talk with a sigh of the decline of pantomime, and murmur in low and dismal tones the name of Grimaldi. We mean no disparagement to the worthy and excellent old man when we say that this is downright nonsense. Clowns that beat Grimaldi all to nothing turn up every day, and nobody patronizes them – more's the pity!

'I know who you mean,' says some dirty-faced patron of Mr. Osbaldistone's, laying down the Miscellany when he has got thus far, and bestowing upon vacancy a most knowing glance; 'you mean C.J. Smith as did Guy Fawkes, and George Barnwell at the Garden.' The dirty-faced gentleman has hardly uttered the words, when he is interrupted by a young gentleman in no shirt-collar and a Petersham coat. 'No, no,' says the young gentleman; 'he means Brown, King, and Gibson, at the 'Delphi.' Now, with great deference both to the first-named gentleman with the dirty face, and the last-named gentleman in the non-existing shirt-collar, we do *not* mean either the performer who so grotesquely burlesqued the Popish conspirator, or the three unchangeables who have been dancing the same dance under different imposing titles, and doing the same thing under various high-sounding names for some five or six years last past. We have no sooner made this avowal, than the public, who have hitherto been silent witnesses of the dispute, inquire what on earth it is we *do* mean; and, with becoming respect, we proceed to tell them.

It is very well known to all playgoers and pantomime-seers, that the scenes in which a theatrical clown is at the very height of his glory are those which are described in the play-bills as 'Cheesemonger's shop and Crockery warehouse,' or 'Tailor's shop, and Mrs Queertable's boarding-house,' or places bearing some such title, where the great fun of the thing consists in the hero's taking lodgings which he has not the slightest intention of paying for, or obtaining goods under false pretences, or abstracting the stock-in-trade of the respectable shopkeeper next door, or robbing warehouse porters as they pass under his window, or to shorten the catalogue, in his swindling everybody he possibly can, it only remaining to be observed that, the more extensive the swindling is, and the more barefaced the impudence of the swindler, the greater the rapture and ecstasy of the audience. Now it is a most remarkable fact that precisely this sort of thing occurs in real life day after day, and nobody sees the humour of it. Let us illustrate our position by detailing the plot of this portion of the pantomime – not of the theatre, but of life.

The Honourable Captain Fitz-Whisker Fiercy, attended by his livery servant Do'em – a most respectable servant to look at, who has grown grey in the service of the captain's family – views, treats for, and ultimately obtains possession of, the unfurnished house, such a number, such a street. All the tradesmen in the neighbourhood are in agonies of competition for the captain's custom; the captain is a good-natured, kind-hearted, easy man, and, to avoid being the cause of disappointment to any, he most handsomely gives orders to all. Hampers of wine, baskets of provisions, cart loads of furniture, boxes of jewellery, supplies of luxuries of the costliest description, flock to the house of the Honourable Captain Fitz-Whisker Fiercy, where they are received with the utmost readiness by the highly respectable Do'em; while the captain himself struts and swaggers about with that compound air of conscious superiority and general bloodthirstiness which a military captain should always, and does most times, wear, to the admiration and terror of plebeian men. But the tradesmen's backs are no sooner turned, than the captain, with all the eccentricity of a mighty mind, and assisted by the faithful Do'em whose devoted fidelity is not the least touching part of his character, disposes of everything to great advantage; for, although the articles fetch small sums, still they are sold considerably above cost price, the cost to the captain having been nothing at all. After various manoeuvres, the imposture is discovered, Fitz-Fiercy and Do'em are recognized as confederates, and the police office to which they are both taken is thronged with their dupes.

Who can fail to recognize in this, the exact counterpart of the best portion of a theatrical pantomime – Fitz-Whisker Fiercy by the clown; Do'em by the pantaloon; and supernumeraries by the tradesmen? The best of the joke, too, is that the very coal-merchant who is loudest in his complaints against the person who defrauded him, is the identical man who sat in the centre of the very front row of the pit last night and laughed the most boisterously at this very same thing, – and not so well done either. Talk of Grimaldi, we say again! Did Grimaldi, in his best days, ever do anything in this way equal to Da Costa?

The mention of this latter justly celebrated clown reminds us of his last piece of humour, the fraudulently obtaining certain stamped acceptances from a young gentleman in the army. We had scarcely laid down our pen to contemplate for a few moments this admirable actor's performance of that exquisite practical joke, than a new branch of our subject flashed suddenly upon us. So we take it up again at once.

All people who have been behind the scenes, and most people who have been before them, know that in the representation of a pantomime, a good many men are sent upon the stage for the express purpose of being cheated, or knocked down, or both. Now, down to a moment ago, we had never been able to understand for what possible purpose a great number of odd, lazy, large-headed men, whom one is in the habit of meeting here, and there, and everywhere, could ever have been created. We see it all, now. They are the supernumeraries in the pantomime of life; the men who have been thrust into it, with no other view than to be constantly tumbling over each other, and running their heads against all sorts of strange things. We sat opposite to one of these men at the supper-table, only last week. Now we think of it, he was exactly like the gentlemen with the pasteboard heads and faces, who do the corresponding business in the theatrical pantomimes; there was the same broad stolid simper – the same dull leaden eye – the same unmeaning, vacant stare; and whatever was said, or whatever was done, he always came in at precisely the wrong place, or jostled against something that he had not the slightest business with. We looked at the man across the table again and again; and could not satisfy ourselves what race of beings to class him with. How very odd that this never occurred to us before!

We will frankly own that we have been much troubled with the harlequin. We see harlequins of so many kinds in the real living pantomime, that we hardly know which to select as the proper fellow of him of the theatres. At one time we were disposed to think that the harlequin was neither more nor less than a young man of family and independent property, who had run away with an opera-dancer, and was fooling his life and his means away in light and trivial amusements. On reflection, however, we remembered that harlequins are occasionally guilty of witty and even clever acts, and we are rather disposed to acquit our young men of family and independent property, generally speaking, of any such misdemeanours. On a more mature consideration of the subject, we have arrived at the conclusion that the harlequins of life are just ordinary men, to be found in no particular walk or degree, on whom a certain station, or particular conjunction of circumstances, confers the magic wand. And this brings us to a few words on the pantomime of public and political life, which we shall say at once, and then conclude – merely premising in this place that we decline any reference whatever to the columbine, being in no wise satisfied of the nature of her connection with her parti-coloured lover, and not feeling by any means clear that we should be justified in introducing her to the virtuous and respectable ladies who peruse our lucubrations.

We take it that the commencement of a Session of Parliament is neither more nor less than the drawing up of the curtain for a grand comic pantomime, and that his Majesty's most gracious speech on the opening thereof may be not inaptly compared to the clown's opening speech of 'Here we are!' 'My lords and gentlemen, here we are!' appears, to our mind at least, to be a very good abstract of the point and meaning of the propitiatory address of the ministry. When we remember how frequently this speech is made, immediately after *the change* too, the parallel is quite perfect, and still more singular.

Perhaps the cast of our political pantomime never was richer than at this day. We are particularly strong in clowns. At no former time, we should say, have we had such astonishing tumblers, or performers so ready to go through the whole of their feats for the amusement of an admiring throng. Their extreme readiness to exhibit, indeed, has given rise to some ill-natured reflections; it having been objected that by exhibiting gratuitously through the country when the theatre is closed, they reduce themselves to the level of mountebanks, and thereby tend to degrade the respectability of the profession. Certainly Grimaldi never did this sort of thing; and though Brown, King, and Gibson have gone to the Surrey in vacation time, and Mr C.J. Smith has ruralised at Sadler's Wells, we find no theatrical precedent for a general tumbling through the country, except in the gentleman, name unknown, who threw summersets on behalf of the late Mr Richardson, and who is no authority either, because he had never been on the regular boards.

But laying aside this question, which after all is a mere matter of taste, we may reflect with pride and gratification of heart on the proficiency of our clowns as exhibited in the season. Night after night will they twist and tumble about, till two, three, and four o'clock in the morning; playing the strangest antics, and giving each other the funniest slaps on the face that can possibly be imagined, without evincing the smallest tokens of fatigue. The strange noises, the confusion, the shouting and roaring, amid which all this is done, too, would put to shame the most turbulent sixpenny gallery that ever yelled through a boxing night.

It is especially curious to behold one of these clowns compelled to go through the most surprising contortions by the irresistible influence of the wand of office, which his leader or harlequin holds above his head. Acted upon by this wonderful charm he will become perfectly motionless, moving neither hand, foot, nor finger, and will even lose the faculty of speech at an instant's notice; or on the other hand, he will become all life and animation if required, pouring forth a torrent of words without sense or meaning, throwing himself into the wildest and most fantastic contortions, and even grovelling on the earth and licking up the dust. These exhibitions are more curious than pleasing; indeed, they are rather disgusting than otherwise, except to the admirers of such things, with whom we confess we have no fellow feeling.

Strange tricks – very strange tricks – are also performed by the harlequin who holds for the time being the magic wand which we have just mentioned. The mere waving it before a man's eyes will dispossess his brains of all the notions previously stored there, and fill it with an entirely new set of ideas; one gentle tap on the back will alter the colour of a man's coat completely; and there are some expert performers who, having this wand held first on one side and then on the other, will change from side to side, turning their coats at every evolution, with so much rapidity and dexterity, that the quickest eye can scarcely detect their motions. Occasionally, the genius who confers the wand, rests it from the hand of the temporary possessor, and consigns it to some new performer; on which occasions all the characters change sides, and then the race and the hard knocks begin anew.

We might have extended this chapter to a much greater length – we might have carried the comparison into the liberal professions – we might have shown, as was in fact our original purpose, that each is in itself a little pantomime with scenes and characters of its own, complete; but as we fear we have been quite lengthy enough already, we shall leave this chapter just where it is. A gentleman, not altogether unknown as a dramatic poet, wrote thus a year or two ago –

> 'All the world's a stage,
> And all the men and women merely players:'

and we, tracking out his footsteps at the scarcely-worth-mentioning little distance of a few millions of leagues behind, venture to add, by way of new reading, that he meant a Pantomime, and that we are all actors in The Pantomime of Life.

## *Some Particulars Concerning a Lion*

The second and last of the 'Stray Chapters by Boz' (see headnote to 'The Pantomime of Life', above, p. 500). 'Some Particulars ...' appeared in May 1837 (Vol. 1, pp. 515–18). The lionising of writers and other artists in the public eye was very prevalent in the 1830s and was denounced by Harriet Martineau (who had suffered from it) in an article. 'Literary Lionism', written in 1837 and reprinted in Vol. 1 of her *Autobiography* (1877). She noted that 'lionisers' were a new phenomenon, 'not because an inhuman disregard of the feelings of the sensitive, the foibles of the vain, the privileges of the endowed, is new: but because it is somewhat new to see the place of cards, music, masks, my lord's fool, and my lady's monkey, supplied by authors in virtue of their authorship'. Dickens had already made hilarious literary capital out of the fashion in his portrait of Mrs Leo Hunter and her *fête champêtre* in *Pickwick Papers*, ch. 15 (1836).

We have a great respect for lions in the abstract. In common with most other people, we have heard and read of many instances of their bravery and generosity. We have duly admired that heroic self-denial and charming philanthropy which prompts them never to eat people except when they are hungry, and we have been deeply impressed with a becoming sense of the politeness they are said to display towards unmarried ladies of a certain state. All natural histories teem with anecdotes illustrative of their excellent qualities; and one old spelling book in particular recounts a touching instance of an old lion, of high moral dignity and stern principle, who felt it his imperative duty to devour a young man who had contracted a habit of swearing, as a striking example to the rising generation.

All this is extremely pleasant to reflect upon, and, indeed, says a very great deal in favour of lions as a mass. We are bound to state, however, that such individual lions as we have happened to fall in with have not put forth any very striking characteristics, and have not acted up to the chivalrous character assigned them by their chroniclers. We never saw a lion in what is called his natural state, certainly; that is to say, we have never met a lion out walking in a forest, or crouching in his lair under a tropical sun, waiting till his dinner should happen to come by, hot from the baker's. But we have seen some under the influence of captivity, and the pressure of misfortune; and we must say that they appeared to us very apathetic, heavy-headed fellows.

The lion at the Zoological Gardens, for instance. He is all very well; he has an undeniable mane, and looks very fierce; but, Lord bless! what of that? The lions of the fashionable world look just as ferocious, and are the most harmless creatures breathing. A box-lobby lion or a Regent Street animal will put on a most terrible aspect, and roar fearfully if you affront him; but he will never bite, and, if you offer to attack him manfully, will fairly turn tail and sneak off. Doubtless these creatures roam about sometimes in herds, and if they meet any especially meek-looking and peaceably-disposed fellow, will endeavour to frighten him; but the faintest show of a vigorous resistance is sufficient to scare them even then. These are pleasant characteristics, whereas we make it matter of distinct charge against the Zoological lion and his brethren at the fairs, that they are sleepy, dreamy, sluggish quadrupeds.

We do not remember to have ever seen one of them perfectly awake, except at feeding time. In every respect we uphold the biped lions against their four-footed namesakes, and we boldly challenge controversy upon the subject.

With these opinions it may be easily imagined that our curiosity and interest were very much excited the other day, when a lady of our acquaintance called on us and resolutely declined to accept our refusal of her invitation to an evening party; 'for,' said she, 'I have got a lion coming.' We at once retracted our plea of a prior engagement, and became as anxious to go, as we had previously been to stay away.

We went early, and posted ourselves in an eligible part of the drawing room, from whence we could hope to obtain a full view of the interesting animal. Two or three hours passed, the quadrilles began, the room filled; but no lion appeared. The lady of the house became inconsolable, – for it is one of the peculiar privileges of these lions to make solemn appointments and never keep them, – when all of a sudden there came a tremendous double rap at the street door, and the master of the house, after gliding out (unobserved as he flattered himself) to peep over the banisters, came into the room, rubbing his hands together with great glee, and cried out in a very important voice, 'My dear, Mr— (naming the lion) has this moment arrived.'

Upon this, all eyes were turned towards the door, and we observed several young ladies, who had been laughing and conversing previously with great gaiety and good humour, grow extremely quiet and sentimental; while some young gentlemen, who had been cutting great figures in the facetious and small-talk way, suddenly sank very obviously in the estimation of the company, and were looked upon with great coldness and indifference. Even the young man who had been ordered from the music shop to play the pianoforte was visibly affected, and struck several false notes in the excess of his excitement.

All this time there was a great talking outside, more than once accompanied by a loud laugh, and a cry of 'Oh! capital! excellent!' from which we inferred that the lion was jocose, and that these exclamations were occasioned by the transports of his keeper and our host. Nor were we deceived; for when the lion at last appeared, we overheard his keeper, who was a little prim man, whisper to several gentlemen of his acquaintance, with uplifted hands, and every expression of half-suppressed admiration, that — (naming the lion again) was in *such* cue tonight!

The lion was a literary one. Of course there were a vast number of people present who had admired his roarings, and were anxious to be introduced to him; and very pleasant it was to see them brought up for the purpose, and to observe the patient dignity with which he received all their patting and caressing. This brought forcibly to our mind what we had so often witnessed at country fairs, where the other lions are compelled to go through as many forms of courtesy as they chance to be acquainted with, just as often as admiring parties happen to drop in upon them.

While the lion was exhibiting in this way, his keeper was not idle, for he mingled among the crowd, and spread his praises most industriously. To one gentleman he whispered some very choice thing that the noble animal had said in the very act of coming upstairs, which, of course, rendered the mental effort still more astonishing; to another he murmured a hasty account of a grand dinner that had taken place the day before, where twenty-seven gentlemen had got up all at once to demand an extra cheer for the lion; and to the ladies he made sundry promises of interceding to procure the majestic brute's sign-manual for their albums. Then there were little private consultations in different corners, relative to the personal appearance and stature of the lion; whether he was shorter than they had expected to see him, or taller, or thinner, or fatter, or younger, or older; whether he was like his portrait, or unlike it; and whether the particular shade of his eyes was black, or blue, or hazel, or green, or yellow, or mixture. At all these consultations the keeper assisted; and, in short, the lion was the sole and single subject of discussion till they sat him down to whist, and then people relapsed into their old topics of conversation – themselves and each other.

We must confess that we looked forward with no slight impatience to the announcement of supper; for if you wish to see a tame lion under particularly favourable circumstances, feeding time is the period of all others to pitch upon. We were therefore very much delighted to observe a sensation among the guests, which we well knew how to interpret, and immediately afterwards to behold the lion escorting the lady of the house downstairs. We offered our arm to an elderly female of our acquaintance, who – dear old soul! – is the very best person that ever lived, to lead down to any meal; for, be the room ever so small, or the party ever so large, she is sure, by some intuitive perception of the eligible, to push and pull herself and conductor close to the best dishes on the table; – we say we offered our arm to this elderly female, and, descending the stairs shortly after the lion, were fortunate enough to obtain a seat nearly opposite him.

Of course the keeper was there already. He had planted himself at precisely that distance from his charge which afforded him a decent pretext for raising his voice, when he addressed him, to so loud a key as could not fail to attract the attention of the whole company, and immediately began to apply himself seriously to the task of bringing the lion out, and putting him through the whole of his manoeuvres. Such flashes of wit as he elicited from the lion! First of all, they began to make puns upon a salt cellar, and then upon the breast of a fowl, and then upon the trifle; but the best jokes of all were decidedly on the lobster salad, upon which latter subject the lion came out most vigorously, and, in the opinion of the most competent authorities, quite out-shone himself. This is a very excellent mode of shining in society, and is founded, we humbly conceive, upon the classic model of the dialogues between Mr Punch and his friend the proprietor, wherein the latter takes all the uphill work, and is content to pioneer to the jokes and repartees of Mr P. himself, who never fails to gain great credit and excite much laughter thereby. Whatever it be founded on, however, we recommend it to all lions, present and to come; for in this instance it succeeded to admiration, and perfectly dazzled the whole body of hearers.

When the salt cellar, and the fowl's breast, and the trifle, and the lobster salad were all exhausted, and could not afford standing room for another solitary witticism, the keeper performed that very dangerous feat which is still done with some of the caravan lions, although in one instance it terminated fatally, of putting his head in the animal's mouth, and placing himself entirely at its mercy. Boswell frequently presents a melancholy instance of the lamentable results of this achievement, and other keepers and jackals have been terribly lacerated for their daring. It is due to our lion to state that he condescended to be trifled with in the most gentle manner, and finally went home with the showman in a hack cab: perfectly peaceable, but slightly fuddled.

Being in a contemplative mood, we were led to make some reflections upon the character and conduct of this genus of lions as we walked homewards, and we were not long in arriving at the conclusion that our former impression in their favour was very much strengthened and confirmed by what we had recently seen. While the other lions receive company and compliments in a sullen, moody, not to say snarling manner, these appear flattered by the attentions that are paid them; while those conceal themselves to the utmost of their power from the vulgar gaze, these court the popular eye, and unlike their brethren, whom nothing short of compulsion will move to exertion, are ever ready to display their acquirements to the wondering throng. We have known bears of undoubted ability who, when the expectations of a large audience have been wound up to the utmost pitch, have peremptorily refused to dance; well-taught monkeys, who have unaccountably objected to exhibit on the slack wire; and elephants of unquestioned genius, who have suddenly declined to turn the barrel organ; but we never once knew or heard of a biped lion, literary or otherwise, – and we state it as a fact which is highly creditable to the whole species, – who, occasion offering, did not seize with avidity on any opportunity which was afforded him, of performing to his heart's content on the first violin.

## *Full Report Of The First Meeting Of The Mudfog Association For the Advancement of Everything*

First published in *Bentley's Miscellany* in October 1837 (Vol. 2, pp. 397–413). Dickens had invented the name 'Mudfog' for the town in which Oliver Twist was born (*Bentley's*, February 1837). The Mudfog Association satirises the British Association for the Advancement of Science which had held its inaugural meeting in York in 1831. Founded to 'obtain a greater degree of national attention to the objects of science', its increasingly florid publicity, the self-importance of many of the speakers, and the emphasis on banqueting as well as lecturing had already attracted considerable mockery – for example, from Cruikshank in his *Comic Almanack* for 1835 (from which Dickens borrowed the comic pub name of the Pig and Tinder-box). Dickens himself had already guyed it in the opening chapter of *Pickwick Papers* (April 1836) when the Pickwick Club congratulates Mr Pickwick on his paper on the Hampstead Ponds 'with Some Observations on the Theory of Tittlebats') and again at the end of ch. 39 (May 1837) with the over-excitable 'scentific gentleman' and his fatuous 'treatise' on electricity. For a full discussion of Dickens's satire see G. A. Chaudhry's 'The Mudfog Papers' in *The Dickensian*, Vol. 70 (1974), pp. 104–112. Dr Chaudhry notes that, while the British Association undoubtedly 'did much to popularise science', it was 'indiscriminate in its confusion between science, technology, social statistics and sheer crankiness'; he also shows that Dickens's parody of elaborate newspaper reporting of the assemblage of participants is very little exaggerated.

Dickens's paper has many very topical references, as Chaudhry shows. Among them is the parachute joke (below, p. 522); a man had just been killed jumping from a balloon over Vauxhall Gardens, using a parachute 'in the form of an umbrella reversed' (the *Examiner*, 30 July 1837). Dickens's satire on statistics and on those who would restrict children's reading to factual and 'improving' material (below, pp. 526) clearly looks forward to his full-scale onslaught on such educationalists in *Hard Times* (1854).

We have made the most unparalleled and extraordinary exertions to place before our readers a complete and accurate account of the proceedings at the late grand meeting of the Mudfog Association, holden in the town of Mudfog; it affords us great happiness to lay the result before them, in the shape of various communications received from our able, talented and graphic correspondent, expressly sent down for the purpose, who has immortalized us, himself, Mudfog, and the association, all at one and the same time. We have been, indeed, for some days unable to determine who will transmit the greatest name to posterity; ourselves, who sent our correspondent down; our correspondent, who wrote an account of the matter; or the association, who gave our correspondent something to write about. We rather incline to the opinion that we are the greatest man of the party, inasmuch as the notion of an exclusive and authentic report originated with us; this may be prejudice: it may arise from a prepossession on our part in our own favour. Be it so. We have no doubt that every gentleman concerned in this mighty assemblage is troubled with the same complaint in a greater or less degree; and it is a consolation to us to know that we have at least this feeling in common with the great scientific stars, the brilliant and extraordinary luminaries, whose speculations we record.

We give our correspondent's letters in the order in which they reached us. Any attempt at amalgamating them into one beautiful whole, would only destroy that glowing tone, that dash of wildness, and rich vein of picturesque interest, which pervade them throughout.

*'Mudfog, Monday night, seven o'clock.*

'We are in a state of great excitement here. Nothing is spoken of, but the approaching meeting of the association. The inn doors are thronged with waiters anxiously looking for the expected arrivals; and the numerous bills which are wafered up in the windows of private houses, intimating that there are beds to let within, give the streets a very animated and cheerful appearance, the wafers being of a great variety of colours, and the monotony of printed inscriptions being relieved by every possible size and style of handwriting. It is confidently rumoured that Professors Snore, Doze, and Wheezy have engaged three beds and a sitting room at the Pig and Tinder-box. I give you the rumour as it has reached me; but I cannot, as yet, vouch for its accuracy. The moment I have been enabled to obtain any certain information upon this interesting point, you may depend upon receiving it.'

*'Half-past seven.*

'I have just returned from a personal interview with the landlord of the Pig and Tinder-box. He speaks confidently of the probability of Professors Snore, Doze, and Wheezy taking up their residence at his house during the sitting of the association, but denies that the beds have been yet engaged; in which representation he is confirmed by the chambermaid – a girl of artless manners, and interesting appearance. The boots denies that it is at all likely that Professors Snore, Doze, and Wheezy will put up here; but I have reason to believe that this man has been suborned by the proprietor of the Original Pig, which is the opposition hotel. Amidst such conflicting testimony it is difficult to arrive at the real truth; but you may depend upon receiving authentic information upon this point the moment the fact is ascertained. The excitement still continues. A boy fell through the window of the pastrycook's shop at the corner of the High Street about half an hour ago, which has occasioned much confusion. The general impression is that it was an accident. Pray heaven it may prove so!'

*'Tuesday, noon.*

'At an early hour this morning the bells of all the churches struck seven o'clock; the effect of which, in the present lively state of the town, was extremely singular. While I was at breakfast, a yellow gig, drawn by a dark grey horse, with a patch of white over his right eyelid, proceeded at a rapid pace in the direction of the Original Pig stables; it is currently reported that this gentleman has arrived here for the purpose of attending the association, and, from what I have heard, I consider it extremely probable, although nothing decisive is yet known regarding him. You may conceive the anxiety with which we are all looking forward to the arrival of the four o'clock coach this afternoon.

'Notwithstanding the excited state of the populace, no outrage has yet been committed, owing to the admirable discipline and discretion of the police, who are nowhere to be seen. A barrel-organ is playing opposite my window, and groups of people, offering fish and vegetables for sale, parade the streets. With these exceptions everything is quiet, and I trust will continue so.'

*'Five o'clock.*

'It is now ascertained, beyond all doubt, that Professors Snore, Doze, and Wheezy will *not* repair to the Pig and Tinder-box, but have actually engaged apartments at the Original Pig. This intelligence is *exclusive*; and I leave you and your readers to draw their own inferences from it. Why Professor Wheezy, of all people in the world, should repair to the Original Pig in preference to the Pig and Tinder-box, it is not easy to conceive. The professor is a man who should be above all such petty feelings. Some people here openly impute treachery, and a distinct breach of faith to Professors Snore and Doze; while others, again, are disposed to acquit them of any culpability in the transaction, and to insinuate that the blame rests solely with Professor Wheezy. I own that I incline to the latter opinion; and although it gives me great pain to speak in terms of censure or disapprobation of a man of such transcendent genius and acquirements, still I am bound to say that, if my suspicions be well founded, and if all the reports which have reached my ears be true, I really do not well know what to make of the matter.

'Mr. Slug, so celebrated for his statistical researches, arrived this afternoon by the four o'clock stage. His complexion is a dark purple, and he has a habit of sighing constantly. He looked extremely well, and appeared in high health and spirits. Mr Woodensconce also came down in the same conveyance. The distinguished gentleman was fast asleep on his arrival, and I am informed by the guard that he had been so the whole way. He was, no doubt, preparing for his approaching fatigues; but what gigantic visions must those be that flit through the brain of such a man when his body is in a state of torpidity!

'The influx of visitors increases every moment. I am told (I know not how truly) that two post-chaises have arrived at the Original Pig within the last half-hour, and I myself observed a wheelbarrow, containing three carpet bags and a bundle, entering the yard of the Pig and Tinder-box no longer ago than five minutes since. The people are still quietly pursuing their ordinary occupations; but there is a wildness in their eyes, and an unwonted rigidity in the muscles of their countenances, which shows to the observant spectator that their expectations are strained to the very utmost pitch. I fear, unless some very extraordinary arrivals take place to-night, that consequences may arise from this popular ferment, which every man of sense and feeling would deplore.'

*'Twenty minutes past six.*

'I have just heard that the boy who fell through the pastrycook's window last night has died of the fright. He was suddenly called upon to pay three and sixpence for the damage done, and his constitution, it seems, was not strong enough to bear up against the shock. The inquest, it is said, will be held tomorrow.'

*'Three-quarters past seven.*

'Professors Muff and Nogo have just driven up to the hotel door; they at once ordered dinner with great condescension. We are all very much delighted with the urbanity of their manners, and the ease with which they adapt themselves to the forms and ceremonies of ordinary life. Immediately on their arrival they sent for the head waiter, and privately requested him to purchase a live dog, – as cheap a one as he could meet with, – and to send him up after dinner, with a pie board, a knife and fork, and a clean plate. It is conjectured that some experiments will be tried upon the dog tonight; if any particulars should transpire, I will forward them by express.'

*'Half-past eight.*

'The animal has been procured. He is a pug dog, of rather intelligent appearance, in good condition, and with very short legs. He has been tied to a curtain peg in a dark room, and is howling dreadfully.'

*'Ten minutes to nine.*

'The dog has just been rung for. With an instinct which would appear almost the result of reason, the sagacious animal seized the waiter by the calf of the leg when he approached to take him, and made a desperate, though ineffectual resistance. I have not been able to procure admission to the apartment occupied by the scientific gentlemen; but, judging from the sounds which reached my ears when I stood upon the landing-place outside the door, just now, I should be disposed to say that the dog had retreated growling beneath some article of furniture, and was keeping the professors at bay. This conjecture is confirmed by the testimony of the ostler, who, after peeping through the key-hole, assures me that he distinctly saw Professor Nogo on his knees, holding forth a small bottle of prussic acid, to which the animal, who was crouched beneath an arm-chair, obstinately declined to smell. You cannot imagine the feverish state of irritation we are in, lest the interests of science should be sacrificed to the prejudices of a brute creature, who is not endowed with sufficient sense to foresee the incalculable benefits which the whole human race may derive from so very slight a concession on his part.'

*'Nine o'clock.*

'The dog's tail and ears have been sent downstairs to be washed: from which circumstances we infer that the animal is no more. His forelegs have been delivered to the boots to be brushed, which strengthens the supposition.'

*'Half after ten.*

'My feelings are so overpowered by what has taken place in the course of the last hour and a half, that I have scarcely strength to detail the rapid succession of events which have quite bewildered all those who are cognizant of their occurrence. It appears that the pug dog mentioned in my last was surreptitiously obtained, – stolen, in fact, – by some person attached to the stable department, from an unmarried lady resident in this town. Frantic on discovering the loss of her favourite, the lady rushed distractedly into the street, calling in the most heart-rending and pathetic manner upon the passengers to restore her, her Augustus, – for so the deceased was named, in affectionate remembrance of a former lover of his mistress, to whom he bore a striking personal resemblance, which renders the circumstances additionally affecting. I am not yet in a condition to inform you what circumstance induced the bereaved lady to direct her steps to the hotel which had witnessed the last struggles of her *protégé*. I can only state that she arrived there, at the very instant when his detached members were passing through the passage on a small tray. Her shrieks still reverberate in my ears! I grieve to say that the expressive features of Professor Muff were much scratched and lacerated by the injured lady; and that Professor Nogo, besides sustaining several severe bites, has lost some handfuls of hair from the same cause. It must be some consolation to these gentlemen to know that their ardent attachment to scientific pursuits has alone occasioned these unpleasant consequences; for which the sympathy of a grateful country will sufficiently reward them. The unfortunate lady remains at the Pig and Tinder-box and up to this time is reported in a very precarious state.

'I need scarcely tell you that this unlooked-for catastrophe has cast a damp and gloom upon us in the midst of our exhilaration; natural in any case, but greatly enhanced in this, by the amiable qualities of the deceased animal, who appears to have been much and deservedly respected by the whole of his acquaintance.'

*'Twelve o'clock.*

'I take the last opportunity before sealing my parcel to inform you that the boy who fell through the pastrycook's window is not dead, as was universally believed, but alive and well. The report appears to have had its origin in his mysterious disappearance. He was found half an hour since on the premises of a sweet-stuff maker, where a raffle had been announced for a second-hand sealskin cap and a tambourine; and where – a sufficient number of members not having been obtained at first – he had patiently waited until the list was completed. This fortunate discovery has in some degree restored our gaiety and cheerfulness. It is proposed to get up a subscription for him without delay.

'Everybody is nervously anxious to see what tomorrow will bring forth. If anyone should arrive in the course of the night, I have left strict directions to be called immediately. I should have sat up, indeed, but the agitating events of this day have been too much for me.

'No news yet of either of the Professors Snore, Doze, or Wheezy. It is very strange!'

*'Wednesday afternoon.*

'All is now over; and, upon one point at least, I am at length enabled to set the minds of your readers at rest. The three professors arrived at ten minutes after two o'clock, and, instead of taking up their quarters at the Original Pig, as it was universally understood in the course of yesterday that they would assuredly have done, drove straight to the Pig and Tinder-box, where they threw off the mask at once, and openly announced their intention of remaining. Professor Wheezy *may* reconcile this very extraordinary conduct with *his* notions of fair and equitable dealing, but I would recommend Professor Wheezy to be cautious how he presumes too far upon his well-earned reputation. How such a man as Professor Snore, or, which is still more extraordinary, such an individual as Professor Doze, can quietly allow himself to be mixed up with such proceedings as these, you will naturally inquire. Upon this head, rumour is silent; I have my speculations, but forbear to give utterance to them just now.'

*'Four o'clock.*

'The town is filling fast; eighteenpence has been offered for a bed and refused. Several gentlemen were under the necessity last night of sleeping in the brick fields, and on the steps of doors, for which they were taken before the magistrates in a body this morning, and committed to prison as vagrants for various terms. One of these persons I understand to be a highly-respectable tinker, of great practical skill, who had forwarded a paper to the President of Section D. Mechanical Science, on the construction of pipkins with copper bottoms and safety valves, of which report speaks highly. The incarceration of this gentleman is greatly to be regretted, as his absence will preclude any discussion on the subject.

'The bills are being taken down in all directions, and lodgings are being secured on almost any terms. I have heard of fifteen shillings a week for two rooms, exclusive of coals and attendance, but I can scarcely believe it. The excitement is dreadful. I was informed this morning that the civil authorities, apprehensive of some outbreak of popular feeling, had commanded a recruiting sergeant and two corporals to be under arms; and that, with the view of not irritating the people unnecessarily by their presence, they had been requested to take up their position before daybreak in a turnpike, distant about a quarter of a mile from the town. The vigour and promptness of these measures cannot be too highly extolled.

'Intelligence has just been brought me, that an elderly female, in a state of inebriety, has declared in the open street her intention to "do" for Mr Slug. Some statistical returns compiled by that gentleman, relative to the consumption of raw spirituous liquors in this place, are supposed to be the cause of the wretch's animosity. It is added that this declaration was loudly cheered by a crowd of persons who had assembled on the spot; and that one man had the boldness to designate Mr Slug aloud by the opprobrious epithet of 'Stick-in-the-mud!' It is earnestly to be hoped that now, when the moment has arrived for their interference, the magistrates will not shrink from the exercise of that power which is vested in them by the constitution of our common country.'

*'Half-past ten.*

'The disturbance, I am happy to inform you, has been completely quelled, and the ringleader taken into custody. She had a pail of cold water thrown over her, previous to being locked up, and expresses great contrition and uneasiness. We are all in a fever of anticipation about tomorrow; but now that we are within a few hours of the meeting of the association, and at last enjoy the proud consciousness of having its illustrious members amongst us, I trust and hope everything may go off peaceably. I shall send you a full report of tomorrow's proceedings by the night coach.'

*'Eleven o'clock.*

'I open my letter to say that nothing whatever has occurred since I folded it up.'

*'Thursday*

'The sun rose this morning at the usual hour. I did not observe anything particular in the aspect of the glorious planet, except that he appeared to me (it might have been a delusion of my heightened fancy) to shine with more than common brilliancy, and to shed a refulgent lustre upon the town, such as I had never observed before. This is the more extraordinary, as the sky was perfectly cloudless, and the atmosphere peculiarly fine. At half-past nine o'clock the general committee assembled, with the last year's president in the chair. The report of the council was read; and one passage, which stated that the council had corresponded with no less than three thousand five hundred and seventy-one persons, (all of whom paid their own postage,) on no fewer than seven thousand two hundred and forty-three topics, was received with a degree of enthusiasm which no efforts could suppress. The various committees and sections having been appointed, and the more formal business transacted, the great proceedings of the meeting commenced at eleven o'clock precisely. I had the happiness of occupying a most eligible position at that time, in

'SECTION A. – ZOOLOGY AND BOTANY.

GREAT ROOM, PIG AND TINDER-BOX.

*President* – Professor Snore. *Vice-Presidents* – Professors Doze and Wheezy.

'The scene at this moment was particularly striking. The sun streamed through the windows of the apartments, and tinted the whole scene with its brilliant rays, bringing out in strong relief the noble visages of the professors and scientific gentlemen, who, some with bald heads, some with red heads, some with brown heads, some with grey heads, some with black heads, some with block heads, presented a *coup d'œil* which no eye-witness will readily forget. In front of these gentlemen were papers and inkstands; and round the room, on elevated benches extending as far as the forms could reach, were assembled a brilliant concourse of those lovely and elegant women for which Mudfog is justly acknowledged to be without a rival in the whole world. The contrast between their fair faces and the dark coats and trousers of the scientific gentlemen I shall never cease to remember while Memory holds her seat.

'Time having been allowed for a slight confusion, occasioned by the falling down of the greater part of the platforms, to subside, the president called on one of the secretaries to read a communication entitled, "Some remarks on the industrious fleas, with considerations on the importance of establishing infant schools among that numerous class of society; of directing their industry to useful and practical ends; and of applying the surplus fruits thereof, towards providing for them a comfortable and respectable maintenance in their old age."

'The Author stated that, having long turned his attention to the moral and social condition of these interesting animals, he had been induced to visit an exhibition in Regent Street, London, commonly known by the designation of 'The Industrious Fleas.' He had there seen many fleas, occupied certainly in various pursuits and avocations, but occupied, he was bound to add, in a manner which no man of well-regulated mind could fail to regard with sorrow and regret. One flea, reduced to the level of a beast of burden, was drawing about a miniature gig, containing a particularly small effigy of His Grace the Duke of Wellington; while another was staggering beneath the weight of a golden model of his great adversary Napoleon Buonaparte. Some, brought up as mountebanks and ballet dancers, were performing a figure dance (he regretted to observe that, of the fleas so employed, several were females); others were in training, in a small cardboard box, for pedestrians, – mere sporting characters – and two were actually engaged in the cold-blooded and barbarous occupation of duelling; a pursuit from which humanity recoiled with horror and disgust. He suggested that measures should be immediately taken to employ the labour of these fleas as part and parcel of the productive power of the country, which might easily be done by the establishment among them of infant schools and houses of industry, in which a system of virtuous education, based upon sound principles, should be observed, and moral precepts strictly inculcated. He proposed that every flea who presumed to exhibit, for hire, music, or dancing, or any species of theatrical entertainment, without a licence, should be considered a vagabond, and treated accordingly; in which respect he only placed him upon a level with the rest of mankind. He would further suggest that their labour should be placed under the control and regulation of the state, who should set apart from the profits, a fund for the support of superannuated or disabled fleas, their widows and orphans. With this view, he proposed that liberal premiums should be offered for the three best designs for a general almshouse; from which – as insect architecture was well known to be in a very advanced and perfect state – we might possibly derive many valuable hints for the improvement of our metropolitan universities, national galleries, and other public edifices.

'The President wished to be informed how the ingenious gentleman proposed to open a communication with fleas generally, in the first instance, so that they might be thoroughly imbued with a sense of the advantages they must necessarily derive from changing their mode of life, and applying themselves to honest labour. This appeared to him the only difficulty.

'The Author submitted that this difficulty was easily overcome, or rather that there was no difficulty at all in the case. Obviously the course to be pursued, if her Majesty's government could be prevailed upon to take up the plan, would be, to secure at a remunerative salary the individual to whom he had alluded as presiding over the exhibition in Regent Street at the period of his visit. That gentleman would at once be able to put himself in communication with the mass of the fleas, and to instruct them in pursuance of some general plan of education, to be sanctioned by Parliament, until such time as the more intelligent among them were advanced enough to officiate as teachers to the rest.

'The President and several members of the section highly complimented the author of the paper last read, on his most ingenious and important treatise. It was determined that the subject should be recommended to the immediate consideration of the council.

'Mr Wigsby produced a cauliflower somewhat larger than a chaise-umbrella, which had been raised by no other artificial means than the simple application of highly-carbonated soda water as manure. He explained that by scooping out the head, which would afford a new and delicious species of nourishment for the poor, a parachute, in principle something similar to that constructed by M. Garnerin, was at once obtained; the stalk of course being kept downwards. He added that he was perfectly willing to make a descent from a height of not less than three miles and a quarter; and had in fact already proposed the same to the proprietors of Vauxhall Gardens, who in the handsomest manner at once consented to his wishes, and appointed an early day next summer for the undertaking; merely stipulating that the rim of the cauliflower should be previously broken in three or four places to ensure the safety of the descent.

'The President congratulated the public on the *grand gala* in store for them, and warmly eulogised the proprietors of the establishment alluded to, for their love of science, and regard for the safety of human life, both of which did them the highest honour.

'A member wished to know how many thousand additional lamps the royal property would be illuminated with, on the night after the descent.

'Mr Wigsby replied that the point was not yet finally decided; but he believed it was proposed, over and above the ordinary illuminations, to exhibit in various devices eight millions and a half of additional lamps.

'The Member expressed himself much gratified with this announcement.

'Mr Blunderum delighted the section with a most interesting and valuable paper "on the last moments of the learned pig", which produced a very strong impression on the assembly, the account being compiled from the personal recollections of his favourite attendant. The account stated in the most emphatic terms that the animal's name was not Toby, but Solomon; and distinctly proved that he could have no near relatives in the profession, as many designing persons had falsely stated, inasmuch as his father, mother, brothers and sisters, had all fallen victims to the butcher at different times. An uncle of his indeed, had with very great labour been traced to a sty in Somers Town; but as he was in a very infirm state at the time, being afflicted with measles, and shortly afterwards disappeared, there appeared too much reason to conjecture that he had been converted into sausages. The disorder of the learned pig was originally a severe cold, which, being aggravated by excessive trough indulgence, finally settled upon the lungs, and terminated in a general decay of the constitution. A melancholy instance of a presentiment entertained by the animal of his approaching dissolution was recorded. After gratifying a numerous and fashionable company with his performances, in which no falling off whatever was visible, he fixed his eyes on the biographer, and, turning to the watch which lay on the floor, and on which he was accustomed to point out the hour, deliberately passed his snout twice round the dial. In precisely four-and-twenty hours from that time he had ceased to exist!

'Professor Wheezy inquired whether, previous to his demise, the animal had expressed, by signs or otherwise, any wishes regarding the disposal of his little property.

'Mr Blunderum replied that, when the biographer took up the pack of cards at the conclusion of the performance, the animal grunted several times in a significant manner, and nodding his head as he was accustomed to do when gratified. From these gestures it was understood that he wished the attendant to keep the cards, which he had ever since done. He had not expressed any wish relative to his watch, which had accordingly been pawned by the same individual.

'The President wished to know whether any Member of the section had ever seen or conversed with the pig-faced lady, who was reported to have worn a black velvet mask, and to have taken her meals from a golden trough.

'After some hesitation a Member replied that the pig-faced lady was his mother-in-law, and that he trusted the President would not violate the sanctity of private life.

'The President begged pardon. He had considered the pig-faced lady a public character. Would the honourable member object to state, with a view to the advancement of science, whether she was in any way connected with the learned pig?

'The Member replied in the same low tone that, as the question appeared to involve a suspicion that the learned pig might be his half-brother, he must decline answering it.

## 'Section B. – Anatomy and Medicine.

### COACH HOUSE, PIG AND TINDER-BOX.

*President* – Dr Toorell. *Vice-Presidents* – Professors Muff and Nogo.

'Dr Kutankumagen (of Moscow) read to the section a report of a case which had occurred within his own practice, strikingly illustrative of the power of medicine, as exemplified in his successful treatment of a virulent disorder. He had been called in to visit the patient on the 1 April 1837. He was then labouring under symptoms peculiarly alarming to any medical man. His frame was stout and muscular, his step firm and elastic, his cheeks plump and red, his voice loud, his appetite good, his pulse full and round. He was in the constant habit of eating three meals *per diem*, and of drinking at least one bottle of wine, and one glass of spirituous liquors diluted with water, in the course of the four-and-twenty hours. He laughed constantly, and in so hearty a manner that it was terrible to hear him. By dint of powerful medicine, low diet, and bleeding, the symptoms in the course of three days perceptibly decreased. A rigid perseverance in the same course of treatment for only one week, accompanied with small doses of water-gruel, weak broth, and barley-water, led to their entire disappearance. In the course of a month he was sufficiently recovered to be carried downstairs by two nurses, and to enjoy an airing in a close carriage, supported by soft pillows. At the present moment he was restored so far as to walk about, with the slight assistance of a crutch and a boy. It would perhaps be gratifying to the section to learn that he ate little, drank little, slept little, and was never heard to laugh by any accident whatever.

'Dr W. R. Fee, in complimenting the honourable member upon the triumphant cure he had effected, begged to ask whether the patient still bled freely?

'Dr Kutankumagen replied in the affirmative.

'Dr W. R. Fee – And you found that he bled freely during the whole course of the disorder?

'Dr Kutankumagen. – Oh dear, yes; most freely.

'Dr Neeshawts supposed that if the patient had not submitted to be bled with great readiness and perseverance, so extraordinary a cure could never, in fact, have been accomplished. Dr Kutankumagen rejoined, certainly not.

'Mr Knight Bell (MRCS) exhibited a wax preparation of the interior of a gentleman who in early life had inadvertently swallowed a door key. It was a curious fact that a medical student of dissipated habits, being present at the *post mortem* examination, found means to escape unobserved from the room, with that portion of the coats of the stomach upon which an exact model of the instrument was distinctly impressed, with which he hastened to a locksmith of doubtful character, who made a new key from the pattern so shown to him. With this key the medical student entered the house of the deceased gentleman, and committed a burglary to a large amount, for which he was subsequently tried and executed.

'The President wished to know what became of the original key after the lapse of years. Mr Knight Bell replied that the gentleman was always much accustomed to punch, and it was supposed the acid had gradually devoured it.

'Dr Neeshawts and several of the members were of opinion that the key must have lain cold and heavy upon the gentleman's stomach.

'Mr Knight Bell believed it did at first. It was worthy of remark, perhaps, that for some years the gentleman was troubled with a nightmare, under the influence of which he always imagined himself a wine-cellar door.

'Professor Muff related a very extraordinary and convincing proof of the wonderful efficacy of the system of infinitesimal doses, which the section were doubtless aware was based upon the theory that the very minutest amount of any given drug, properly dispersed through the human frame, would be productive of precisely the same result as a very large dose administered in the usual manner. Thus, the fortieth part of a grain of calomel was supposed to be equal to a five-grain calomel pill, and so on in proportion throughout the whole range of medicine. He had tried the experiment in a curious manner upon a publican who had been brought into the hospital with a broken head, and was cured upon the infinitesimal system in the incredibly short space of three months. This man was a hard drinker. He (Professor Muff) had dispersed three drops of rum through a bucket of water, and requested the man to drink the whole. What was the result? Before he had drunk a quart, he was in a state of beastly intoxication; and five other men were made dead drunk with the remainder.

'The President wished to know whether an infinitesimal dose of soda water would have recovered them? Professor Muff replied that the twenty-fifth part of a teaspoonful, properly administered to each patient, would have sobered him immediately. The President remarked that this was a most important discovery, and he hoped the Lord Mayor and Court of Aldermen would patronize it immediately.

'A Member begged to be informed whether it would be possible to administer – say, the twentieth part of a grain of bread and cheese to all grown-up paupers, and the fortieth part to children, with the same satisfying effect as their present allowance.

'Professor Muff was willing to stake his professional reputation on the perfect adequacy of such a quantity of food to the support of human life – in workhouses; the addition of the fifteenth part of a grain of pudding twice a week would render it a high diet.

'Professor Nogo called the attention of the section to a very extraordinary case of animal magnetism. A private watchman, being merely looked at by the operator from the opposite side of a wide street, was at once observed to be in a very drowsy and languid state. He was followed to his box, and being once slightly rubbed on the palms of the hands, fell into a sound sleep, in which he continued without intermission for ten hours.

## 'Section C. – Statistics.

### HAY LOFT, ORIGINAL PIG.

*President* – Mr Woodensconce. *Vice-Presidents* – Mr Ledbrain and Mr Timbered.

'Mr Slug stated to the section the result of some calculations he had made with great difficulty and labour, regarding the state of infant education among the middle classes of London. He found that, within a circle of three miles from the Elephant and Castle, the following were the names and numbers of children's books principally in circulation: –

| | |
|---|---|
| 'Jack the Giant-killer | 7,943 |
| Ditto and Beanstalk | 8,621 |
| Ditto and Eleven Brothers | 2,845 |
| Ditto and Jill | 1,998 |
| Total | 21,407 |

'He found that the proportion of Robinson Crusoes to Philip Quarlls was as four and a half to one; and that the preponderance of Valentine and Orsons over Goody Two Shoeses was as three and an eighth of the former to half a one of the latter; a comparison of Seven Champions with Simple Simons gave the same result. The ignorance that prevailed was lamentable. One child, on being asked whether he would rather be Saint George of England or a respectable tallow-chandler, instantly replied, 'Taint George of Ingling'. Another, a little boy of eight years old, was found to be firmly impressed with a belief in the existence of dragons, and openly stated that it was his intention when he grew up, to rush forth sword in hand for the deliverance of captive princesses, and the promiscuous slaughter of giants. Not one child among the number interrogated had ever heard of Mungo Park, – some inquiring whether he was at all connected with the black man that swept the crossing; and others whether he was in any way related to the Regent's Park. They had not the slightest conception of the commonest principles of mathematics, and considered Sindbad the Sailor the most enterprising voyager that the world had ever produced.

'A Member strongly deprecating the use of all the other books mentioned, suggested that Jack and Gill might perhaps be exempted from the general censure, inasmuch as the hero and heroine, in the very outset of the tale, were depicted as going *up* a hill to fetch a pail of water, which was a laborious and useful occupation, – supposing the family linen was being washed, for instance.

'Mr Slug feared that the moral effect of this passage was more than counterbalanced by another in a subsequent part of the poem, in which very gross allusion was made to the mode in which the heroine was personally chastised by her mother

'"For laughing at Jack's disaster;"

besides, the whole work had this one great fault, *it was not true.*

'The President complimented the honourable member on the excellent distinction he had drawn. Several other members, too, dwelt upon the immense and urgent necessity of storing the minds of children with nothing but facts and figures; which process the President very forcibly remarked, had made them (the section) the men they were.

'Mr Slug then stated some curious calculations respecting the dogs'-meat barrows of London. He found that the total number of small carts and barrows engaged in dispensing provision to the cats and dogs of the metropolis was one thousand seven hundred and forty-three. The average number of skewers delivered daily with the provender, by each dogs'-meat cart or barrow, was thirty-six. Now, multiplying the number of skewers so delivered by the number of barrows, a total of sixty-two thousand seven hundred and forty-eight skewers daily would be obtained. Allowing that, of these sixty-two thousand seven hundred and forty-eight skewers, the odd two thousand seven hundred and forty-eight were accidentally devoured with the meat, by the most voracious of the animals supplied, it followed that sixty thousand skewers per day, or the enormous number of twenty-one millions nine hundred thousand skewers annually, were wasted in kennels and dustholes of London; which, if collected and warehoused, would in ten years' time afford a mass of timber more than sufficient for the construction of a first-rate vessel of war for the use of her Majesty's navy, to be called "The Royal Skewer", and to become under that name the terror of all the enemies of this island.

'Mr X. Ledbrain read a very ingenious communication, from which it appeared that the total number of legs belonging to the manufacturing population of one great town in Yorkshire was, in round numbers, forty thousand, while the total number of chair and stool legs in their houses was only thirty thousand, which, upon the very favourable average of three legs to a seat, yielded only ten thousand seats in all. From this calculation it would appear, – not taking wooden or cork legs into the account, but allowing two legs to every person, – that ten thousand individuals (one-half of the whole population) were either destitute of any rest for their legs at all, or passed the whole of their leisure time in sitting upon boxes.

'SECTION D. – MECHANICAL SCIENCE.

COACH-HOUSE, ORIGINAL PIG.

*President* – Mr Carter. *Vice-Presidents* – Mr Truck and Mr Waghorn.

'Professor Queerspeck exhibited an elegant model of a portable railway, neatly mounted in a green case, for the waistcoat pocket. By attaching this beautiful instrument to his boots, any Bank or public-office clerk could transport himself from his place of residence to his place of business, at the easy rate of sixty-five miles an hour, which, to gentlemen of sedentary pursuits, would be an incalculable advantage.

'The President was desirous of knowing whether it was necessary to have a level surface on which the gentleman was to run.

'Professor Queerspeck explained that City gentlemen would run in trains, being handcuffed together to prevent confusion or unpleasantness. For instance, trains would start every morning at eight, nine, and ten o'clock, from Camden Town, Islington, Camberwell, Hackney, and various other places in which City gentlemen are accustomed to reside. It would be necessary to have a level, but he had provided for this difficulty by proposing that the best line that the circumstances would admit of, should be taken through the sewers which undermine the streets of the metropolis, and which, well lighted by jets from the gas pipes which run immediately above them, would form a pleasant and commodious arcade, especially in winter-time, when the inconvenient custom of carrying umbrellas, now so general, could be wholly dispensed with. In reply to another question, Professor Queerspeck stated that no substitute for the purposes to which these arcades were at present devoted had yet occurred to him, but that he hoped no fanciful objection on this head would be allowed to interfere with so great an undertaking.

'Mr Jobba produced a forcing machine on a novel plan, for bringing joint-stock railway shares prematurely to a premium. The instrument was in the form of an elegant gilt weather-glass, of most dazzling appearance, and was worked behind, by strings, after the manner of a pantomime trick, the strings being always pulled by the directors of the company to which the machine belonged. The quicksilver was so ingeniously placed, that when the acting directors held shares in their pockets, figures denoting very small expenses and very large returns appeared upon the glass; but the moment the directors parted with these pieces of paper, the estimate of needful expenditure suddenly increased itself to an immense extent, while the statements of certain profits became reduced in the same proportion. Mr Jobba stated that the machine had been in constant requisition for some months past, and he had never once known it to fail.

'A Member expressed his opinion that it was extremely neat and pretty. He wished to know whether it was not liable to accidental derangement? Mr Jobba said that the whole machine was undoubtedly liable to be blown up, but that was the only objection to it.

'Professor Nogo arrived from the anatomical section to exhibit a model of a safety fire-escape, which could be fixed at any time, in less than half an hour, and by means of which, the youngest or most infirm persons (successfully resisting the progress of the flames until it was quite ready) could be preserved if they merely balanced themselves for a few minutes on the sill of their bedroom window, and got into the escape without falling into the street. The Professor stated that the number of boys who had been rescued in the daytime by this machine from houses which were not on fire, was almost incredible. Not a conflagration had occurred in the whole of London for many months past to which the escape had not been carried on the very next day, and put in action before a concourse of persons.

'The President inquired whether there was not some difficulty in ascertaining which was the top of the machine, and which the bottom, in cases of pressing emergency.

'Professor Nogo explained that of course it could not be expected to act quite as well when there was a fire, as when there was not a fire; but in the former case he thought it would be of equal service whether the top were up or down.'

With the last section our correspondent concludes his most able and faithful Report, which will never cease to reflect credit upon him for his scientific attainments, and upon us for our enterprising spirit. It is needless to take a review of the subjects which have been discussed; of the mode in which they have been examined; of the great truths which they have elicited. They are now before the world, and we leave them to read, to consider, and to profit.

The place of meeting for next year has undergone discussion, and has at length been decided, regard being had to, and evidence being taken upon, the goodness of its wines, the supply of its markets, the hospitality of its inhabitants, and the quality of its hotels. We hope at this next meeting our correspondent may again be present, and that we may be once more the means of placing his communications before the world. Until that period we have been prevailed upon to allow this number of our Miscellany to be retailed to the public, or wholesaled to the trade, without any advance upon our usual price.

We have only to add, that the committees are now broken up, and that Mudfog is once again restored to its accustomed tranquillity, – that Professors and Members have had balls, and *soirées*, and suppers, and great mutual complimentations, and have at length dispersed to their several homes, – whither all good wishes and joys attend them, until next year!

Signed Boz.

## *Full Report of the Second Meeting of the Mudfog Association For the Advancement of Everything*

First published in *Bentley's Miscellany* September 1838 (Vol. 4, pp. 209–27) where it substituted for an instalment of *Oliver Twist* – see Kathleen Tillotson's introduction to the Clarendon Edition of *Oliver*, 1966, p. xxii. The British Association for the Advancement of Science held its 1838 meeting in Newcastle 20 August–15 September. Cruikshank suggested the automaton police office idea to Dickens, who was delighted by it (see *Pilgrim*, Vol. 1, p. 418). Many members of the Association travelled to Newcastle by boat, which was all grist to Dickens's satiric mill. The exhibition of the skull of the murderer James Greenacre, executed for killing Hannah Brown in 1837, by 'Professor John Ketch' ('Jack Ketch' being the nickname for the public hangman), below, p. 549, refers to a lecture at the Association reported in the *Examiner* on 26 August: a Dr Inglis had lectured on the skull of the famous scholar-murderer Eugene Aram (executed 1759), seeking to prove by 'phrenological observations' that he had been innocent. Some members of the audience expressed considerable doubt as to whether the skull was, in fact, Aram's.

In October last, we did ourselves the immortal credit of recording, at an enormous expense, and by dint of exertions unparalleled in the history of periodical publication, the proceedings of the Mudfog Association for the Advancement of Everything, which in that month held its first great half yearly meeting, to the wonder and delight of the whole empire. We announced at the conclusion of that extraordinary and most remarkable Report, that when the Second Meeting of the Society should take place, we should be found again at our post, renewing our gigantic and spirited endeavours, and once more making the world ring with the accuracy, authenticity, immeasurable superiority, and intense remarkability of our account of its proceedings. In redemption of this pledge, we caused to be dispatched per steam to Oldcastle (at which place this second meeting of the Society was held on the 20th instant), the same superhumanly-endowed gentleman who furnished the former report, and who, – gifted by nature with transcendent abilities, and furnished by us with a body of assistants scarcely inferior to himself, – has forwarded a series of letters which, for faithfulness of description, power of language, fervour of thought, happiness of expression, and importance of subject-matter, have no equal in the epistolary literature of any age or country. We give this gentleman's correspondence entire, and in the order in which it reached our office.

*'Saloon of Steamer, Thursday night, half-past eight.*

'When I left New Burlington Street this evening in the hackney cabriolet, number four thousand two hundred and eighty-five, I experienced sensations as novel as they were oppressive. A sense of the importance of the task I had undertaken, a consciousness that I was leaving London, and, stranger still, going somewhere else, a feeling of loneliness and a sensation of jolting, quite bewildered my thoughts, and for a time rendered me even insensible to the presence of my carpet bag and hat box. I shall ever feel grateful to the driver of a Blackwall omnibus who, by thrusting the pole of his vehicle through the small door of the cabriolet, awakened me from a tumult of imaginings that are wholly indescribable. But of such materials is our imperfect nature composed!

'I am happy to say that I am the first passenger on board, and shall thus be enabled to give you an account of all that happens in the order

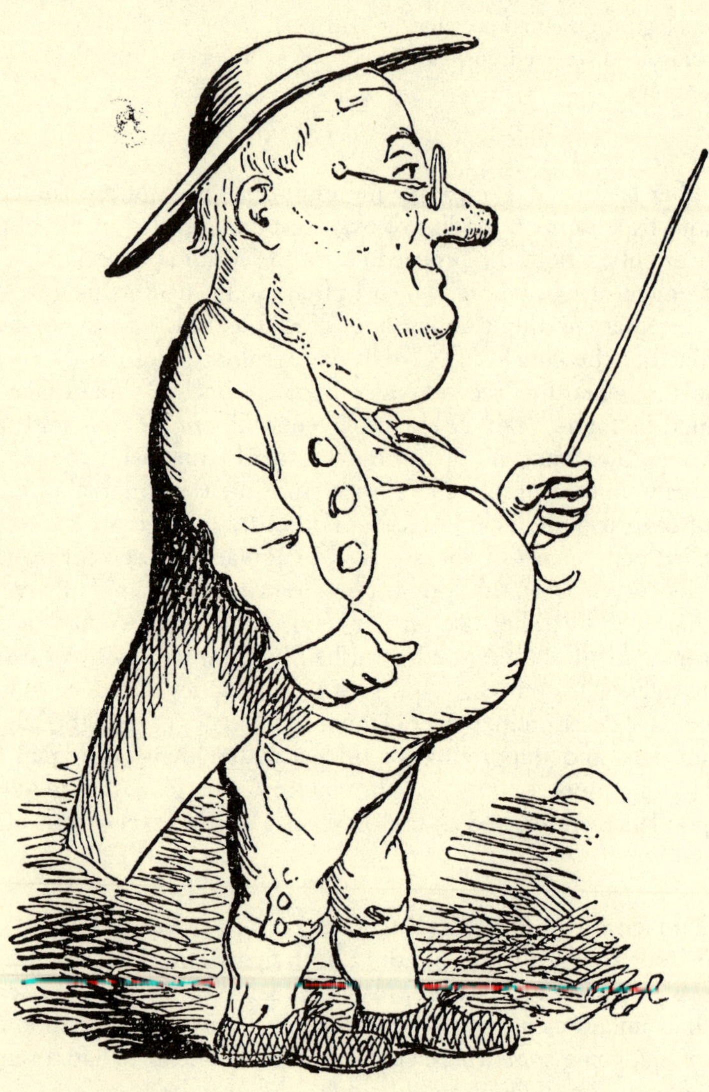

*The Tyrant Sowster* *(see p. 540)*

of its occurrence. The chimney is smoking a good deal, and so are the crew; and the captain, I am informed, is very drunk in a little house upon deck, something like a black turnpike. I should infer from all I hear that he has got the steam up.

'You will readily guess with what feelings I have just made the discovery that my berth is in the same closet with those engaged by Professor Woodensconce, Mr Slug and Professor Grime. Professor Woodensconce has taken the shelf above me, and Mr Slug and Professor Grime the two shelves opposite. Their luggage has already arrived. On Mr Slug's bed is a long tin tube of about three inches in diameter, carefully closed at both ends. What can this contain? Some powerful instrument of a new construction, doubtless.'

*'Ten minutes past nine.*

'Nobody has yet arrived, nor has anything fresh come in my way except several joints of beef and mutton, from which I conclude that a good plain dinner has been provided for tomorrow. There is a singular smell below, which gave me some uneasiness at first; but as the steward says it is always there, and never goes away, I am quite comfortable again. I learn from this man that the different sections will be distributed at the Black Boy and Stomach-ache, and the Boot-jack and Countenance. If this intelligence be true (and I have no reason to doubt it), your readers will draw such conclusions as their different opinions may suggest.

'I write down these remarks as they occur to me, or as the facts come to my knowledge, in order that my first impressions may lose nothing of their original vividness. I shall dispatch them in small packets as opportunities arise.'

*'Half-past nine.*

'Some dark object has just appeared upon the wharf. I think it is a travelling carriage.'

*'A quarter to ten.*

'No, it isn't.'

*'Half-past ten.*

'The passengers are pouring in every instant. Four omnibuses full have just arrived upon the wharf, and all is bustle and activity. The noise and confusion are very great. Cloths are laid in the cabins, and the steward is placing blue platesful of knobs of cheese at equal distances down the centre of the tables. He drops a great many knobs; but, being used to it, picks them up again with great dexterity, and, after wiping them on his sleeve, throws them back into the plates. He is a young man of exceedingly prepossessing appearance – either dirty or a mulatto, but I think the former.

'An interesting old gentleman, who came to the wharf in an omnibus, has just quarrelled violently with the porters, and is staggering towards the vessel with a large trunk in his arms. I trust and hope that he may reach it in safety; but the board he has to cross is narrow and slippery. Was that a splash? Gracious powers!

'I have just returned from the deck. The trunk is standing upon the extreme brink of the wharf, but the old gentleman is nowhere to be seen. The watchman is not sure whether he went down or not, but promises to drag for him the first thing tomorrow morning. May his humane efforts prove successful!

'Professor Nogo has this moment arrived with his night-cap on under his hat. He has ordered a glass of cold brandy and water, with a hard biscuit and a bason, and has gone straight to bed. What can this mean?

'The three other scientific gentlemen to whom I have already alluded have come on board, and have all tried their beds, with the exception of Professor Woodensconce, who sleeps in one of the top ones, and can't get into it. Mr Slug, who sleeps in the other top one, is unable to get out of his, and is to have his supper handed up by a boy. I have had the honour to introduce myself to these gentlemen, and we have amicably arranged the order in which we shall retire to rest; which it is necessary to agree upon, because, although the cabin is very comfortable, there is not room for more than one gentleman to be out of bed at a time, and even he must take his boots off in the passage.

'As I anticipated, the knobs of cheese were provided for the passengers' supper, and are now in course of consumption. Your readers will be surprised to hear that Professor Woodensconce has abstained from cheese for eight years, although he takes butter in considerable quantities. Professor Grime having lost several teeth, is unable, I observe, to eat his crusts without previously soaking them in his bottled porter. How interesting are these peculiarities!'

*'Half-past eleven.*

'Professors Woodensconce and Grime, with a degree of good humour that delights us all, have just arranged to toss for a bottle of mulled port. There has been some discussion whether the payment should be decided by the first toss or the best out of three. Eventually the latter course has been determined on. Deeply do I wish that both gentlemen could win; but that being impossible, I own that my personal aspirations (I speak as an individual, and do not compromise either you or your readers by this expression of feeling) are with Professor Woodensconce. I have backed that gentleman to the amount of eighteenpence.'

*'Twenty minutes to twelve.*

'Professor Grime has inadvertently tossed his half-crown out of one of the cabin windows, and it has been arranged that the steward shall toss for him. Bets are offered on any side to any amount, but there are no takers.

'Professor Woodensconce has just called "woman"; but the coin having lodged in a beam, is a long time coming down again. The interest and suspense of this one moment are beyond anything that can be imagined.'

*'Twelve o'clock.*

'The mulled port is smoking on the table before me, and Professor Grime has won. Tossing is a game of chance; but on every ground, whether of public or private character, intellectual endowments, or scientific attainments, I cannot help expressing my opinion that Professor Woodensconce *ought* to have come off victorious. There is an exultation about Professor Grime incompatible, I fear, with true greatness.'

*'A quarter past twelve.*

'Professor Grime continues to exult, and to boast of his victory in no very measured terms, observing that he always does win, and that he knew it would be a "head" beforehand, with many other remarks of a similar nature. Surely this gentleman is not so lost to every feeling of decency and propriety as not to feel and know the superiority of Professor Woodensconce? Is Professor Grime insane? or does he wish to be reminded in plain language of his true position in society, and the precise level of his acquirements and abilities? Professor Grime will do well to look to this.'

*'One o'clock.*

'I am writing in bed. The small cabin is illuminated by the feeble light of a flickering lamp suspended from the ceiling; Professor Grime is lying on the opposite shelf on the broad of his back, with his mouth wide open. The scene is indescribably solemn. The rippling of the tide, the noise of the sailors' feet overhead, the gruff voices on the river, the dogs on the shore, the snoring of the passengers, and a constant creaking of every plank in the vessel, are the only sounds that meet the ear. With these exceptions, all is profound silence.

'My curiosity has been within the last moment very much excited. Mr Slug, who lies above Professor Grime, has cautiously withdrawn the curtains of his berth, and, after looking anxiously out, as if to satisfy himself that his companions are asleep, has taken up the tin tube of which I have before spoken, and is regarding it with great interest. What rare mechanical combination can be obtained in that mysterious case? It is evidently a profound secret to all.'

*'A quarter past one.*

'The behaviour of Mr Slug grows more and more mysterious. He has unscrewed the top of the tube, and now renews his observations upon his companions, evidently to make sure that he is wholly unobserved. He is clearly on the eve of some great experiment. Pray heaven that it be not a dangerous one; but the interests of science must be promoted, and I am prepared for the worst.'

*'Five minutes later.*

'He has produced a large pair of scissors, and drawn a roll of some substance, not unlike parchment in appearance, from the tin case. The experiment is about to begin. I must strain my eyes to the utmost, in the attempt to follow its minutest operation.'

*'Twenty minutes before two.*

'I have at length been enabled to ascertain that the tin tube contains a few yards of some celebrated plaster, recommended – as I discover on regarding the label attentively through my eye-glass – as a preservative against sea sickness. Mr Slug has cut it up into small portions, and is now sticking it over himself in every direction.'

*'Three o'clock.*

'Precisely a quarter of an hour ago we weighed anchor, and the machinery was suddenly put in motion with a noise so appalling, that Professor Woodensconce (who had ascended to his berth by means of a platform of carpet bags arranged by himself on geometrical principles) darted from his shelf head foremost, and, gaining his feet with all the rapidity of extreme terror, ran wildly into the ladies' cabin, under the impression that we were sinking, and uttering loud cries for aid. I am assured that the scene which ensued baffles all description. There were one hundred and forty-seven ladies in their respective berths at the time.

'Mr Slug has remarked, as an additional instance of the extreme ingenuity of the steam engine as applied to purposes of navigation, that in whatever part of the vessel a passenger's berth may be situated, the machinery always appears to be exactly under his pillow. He intends stating this very beautiful, though simple discovery, to the association.'

*'Half-past three.*

'We are still in smooth water; that is to say, in as smooth water as a steam vessel ever can be, for, as Professor Woodensconce (who has just woke up) learnedly remarks, another great point of ingenuity about a steamer is, that it always carries a little storm with it. You can scarcely conceive how exciting the jerking pulsation of the ship becomes. It is a matter of positive difficulty to get to sleep.'

*'Friday afternoon, six o'clock.*

'I regret to inform you that Mr Slug's plaster has proved of no avail. He is in great agony, but has applied several large additional pieces notwithstanding. How affecting is this extreme devotion to science and pursuit of knowledge under the most trying circumstances!

'We were extremely happy this morning, and the breakfast was one of the most animated description. Nothing unpleasant occurred until noon, with the exception of Doctor Foxey's brown silk umbrella and white hat becoming entangled in the machinery while he was explaining to a knot of ladies the construction of the steam engine. I fear the gravy soup for lunch was injudicious. We lost a great many passengers almost immediately afterwards.'

*'Half-past six.*

'I am again in bed. Anything so heart rending as Mr Slug's sufferings it has never yet been my lot to witness.'

*'Seven o'clock.*

'A messenger has just come down for a clean pocket handkerchief from Professor Woodensconce's bag, that unfortunate gentleman being quite unable to leave the deck, and imploring constantly to be thrown overboard. From this man I understand that Professor Nogo, though in a state of utter exhaustion, clings feebly to the hard biscuit and cold brandy and water, under the impression that they will yet restore him. Such is the triumph of mind over matter.

'Professor Grime is in bed, to all appearance quite well; but he *will* eat, and it is disagreeable to see him. Has this gentleman no sympathy with the sufferings of his fellow creatures? If he has, on what principle can he call for mutton chops – and smile?'

*'Black Boy and Stomach-ache,*
*Oldcastle, Saturday noon.*

'You will be happy to learn that I have at length arrived here in safety. The town is excessively crowded, and all the private lodgings and hotels are filled with *savans* of both sexes. The tremendous assemblage of intellect that one encounters in every street is in the last degree overwhelming.

'Notwithstanding the throng of people here, I have been fortunate enough to meet with very comfortable accommodation on very reasonable terms, having secured a sofa in the first floor passage at one guinea per night, which includes permission to take my meals in the bar, on condition that I walk about the streets at all other times, to make room for other gentlemen similarly situated. I have been over the outhouses intended to be devoted to the reception of the various sections, both here and at the Boot-jack and Countenance, and am much delighted with the arrangements. Nothing can exceed the fresh appearance of the sawdust with which the floors are sprinkled. The forms are of unplaned deal, and the general effect, as you can well imagine, is extremely beautiful.'

*'Half-past nine*

'The number and rapidity of the arrivals are quite bewildering. Within the last ten minutes a stagecoach has driven up to the door, filled inside and out with distinguished characters, comprising Mr Muddlebranes, Mr Drawley, Professor Muff, Mr X. Misty, Mr X. X. Misty, Mr Purblind, Professor Rummun, The Honourable and Reverend Mr Long Eers, Professor John Ketch, Sir William Joltered, Doctor Buffer, Mr Smith (of London), Mr Brown (of Edinburgh), Sir Hookham Snivey, and Professor Pumpkinskull. The ten last-named gentlemen were wet through, and looked extremely intelligent.'

*'Sunday, two o'clock, pm.*

'The Honourable and Reverend Mr Long Eers, accompanied by Sir William Joltered, walked and drove this morning. They accomplished the former feat in boots, and the latter in a hired fly. This has naturally given rise to much discussion.

'I have just learnt that an interview has taken place at the Boot-jack and Countenance between Sowster, the active and intelligent beadle of this place, and Professor Pumpkinskull, who, as your readers are doubtless aware, is an influential member of the council. I forbear to communicate any of the rumours to which this very extraordinary proceeding has given rise until I have seen Sowster, and endeavoured to ascertain the truth from him.'

*'Half-past six.*

'I engaged a donkey chaise shortly after writing the above, and proceeded at a brisk trot in the direction of Sowster's residence, passing through a beautiful expanse of country, with red brick buildings on either side, and stopping in the market place to observe the spot where Mr Kwakley's hat was blown off yesterday. It is an uneven piece of paving, but has certainly no appearance which would lead one to suppose that any such event had recently occurred there. From this point I proceeded – passing the gas works and tallow melter's – to a lane which had been pointed out to me as the beadle's place of residence; and before I had driven a dozen yards further, I had the good fortune to meet Sowster himself advancing towards me.

'Sowster is a fat man, with a more enlarged development of that peculiar conformation of countenance which is vulgarly termed a double chin than I remember to have ever seen before. He has also a very red nose, which he attributes to a habit of early rising – so red, indeed, that but for this explanation I should have supposed it to proceed from occasional inebriety. He informed me that he did not feel himself at liberty to relate what had passed between himself and Professor Pumpkinskull, but had no objection to state that it was connected with a matter of police regulation, and added with peculiar significance "Never wos sitch times!"

'You will easily believe that this intelligence gave me considerable surprise, not wholly unmixed with anxiety, and that I lost no time in waiting on Professor Pumpkinskull, and stating the object of my visit. After a few moments' reflection, the Professor, who, I am bound to say, behaved with the utmost politeness, openly avowed (I mark the passage in italics) *that he had requested Sowster to attend on the Monday morning at the Boot-jack and Countenance, to keep off the boys; and that he had further desired that the under-beadle might be stationed, with the same object, at the Black Boy and Stomach-ache!*

'Now I leave this unconstitutional proceeding to your comments and the consideration of your readers. I have yet to learn that a beadle, without the precincts of a church, churchyard, or workhouse, and acting otherwise than under the express orders of churchwardens and overseers in council assembled, to enforce the law against people who come upon the parish, and other offenders, has any lawful authority whatever over the rising youth of this country I have yet to learn that a beadle can be called out by any civilian to exercise a domination and despotism over the boys of Britain. I have yet to learn that a beadle will be permitted by the commissioners of poor law regulation to wear out the soles and heels of his boots in illegal interference with the liberties of people not proved poor or otherwise criminal. I have yet to learn that a beadle has power to stop up the Queen's highway at his will and pleasure, or that the whole width of the street is not free and open to any man, boy, or woman in existence, up to the very walls of the houses – aye, be they Black Boys and Stomach-aches, or Boot-jacks and Countenances, I care not.'

*'Nine o'clock.*

'I have procured a local artist to make a faithful sketch of the tyrant Sowster, which, as he has acquired this infamous celebrity, you will no doubt wish to have engraved for the purpose of presenting a copy with every copy of your next number. I enclose it. The under-beadle has consented to write his life, but it is to be strictly anonymous.

'The accompanying likeness is of course from the life, and complete in every respect. Even if I had been totally ignorant of the man's real character, and it had been placed before me without remark, I should have shuddered involuntarily. There is an intense malignity of expression in the features, and a baleful ferocity of purpose in the ruffian's eye, which appals and sickens. His whole air is rampant with cruelty, nor is the stomach less characteristic of his demoniac propensities.'

*'Monday.*

'The great day has at length arrived. I have neither eyes, nor ears, nor pens, nor ink, nor paper, for anything but the wonderful proceedings that have astounded my senses. Let me collect my energies and proceed to the account.

### 'Section A. – Zoology and Botany.

#### FRONT PARLOUR, BLACK BOY AND STOMACH-ACHE.

*President* – Sir William Joltered. *Vice Presidents* – Mr Muddlebranes and Mr Drawley.

'Mr X. X. Misty communicated some remarks on the disappearance of dancing bears from the streets of London, with observations on the exhibition of monkeys as connected with barrel organs. The writer had observed, with feelings of the utmost pain and regret, that some years ago a sudden and unaccountable change in the public taste took place with reference to itinerant bears, who, being discountenanced by the populace, gradually fell off one by one from the streets of the metropolis, until not one remained to create a taste for natural history in the breasts of the poor and uninstructed. One bear, indeed – a brown and ragged animal, – had lingered about the haunts of his former triumphs, with a worn and dejected visage and feeble limbs, and had essayed to wield his quarter staff for the amusement of the multitude; but hunger, and an utter want of any due recompense for his abilities, had at length driven him from the field, and it was only too probable that he had fallen a sacrifice to the rising taste for grease. He regretted to add that a similar, and no less lamentable, change had taken place with reference to monkeys. These delightful animals had formerly been almost as plentiful as the organs on the tops of which they were accustomed to sit; the proportion in the year

1829 (it appeared by the parliamentary return) being as one monkey to three organs. Owing, however, to an altered taste in musical instruments, and the substitution, in a great measure, of narrow boxes of music for organs, which left the monkeys nothing to sit upon, this source of public amusement was wholly dried up. Considering it a matter of the deepest importance, in connection with national education, that the people should not lose such opportunities of making themselves acquainted with the manners and customs of two most interesting species of animals, the author submitted that some measures should be immediately taken for the restoration of these pleasing and truly intellectual amusements.

'The President inquired by what means the honourable member proposed to attain this most desirable end?

'The Author submitted that it could be most fully and satisfactorily accomplished, if her Majesty's Government would cause to be brought over to England, and maintained at the public expense, and for the public amusement, such a number of bears as would enable every quarter of the town to be visited – say at least by three bears a week. No difficulty whatever need be experienced in providing a fitting place for the reception of these animals, as a commodious bear-garden could be erected in the immediate neighbourhood of both Houses of Parliament; obviously the most proper and eligible spot for such an establishment.

'Professor Mull doubted very much whether any correct ideas of natural history were propagated by the means of which the honourable member had so ably adverted. On the contrary, he believed that they had been the means of diffusing very incorrect and imperfect notions on the subject. He spoke from personal observation and personal experience, when he said that many children of great abilities had been induced to believe, from what they had observed in the streets, at and before the period to which the honourable gentleman had referred, that all monkeys were born in red coats and spangles, and that their hats and feathers also came by nature. He wished to know distinctly whether the honourable gentleman attributed the want of encouragement the bears had met with to the decline of public taste in that respect, or to a want of ability on the part of the bears themselves?

'Mr X. X. Misty replied that he could not bring himself to believe but that there must be a great deal of floating talent among the bears and monkeys generally; which, in the absence of any proper encouragement, was dispersed in other directions.

'Professor Pumpkinskull wished to take that opportunity of calling the attention of the section to a most important and serious point. The author of the treatise just read had alluded to the prevalent taste for bears' grease as a means of promoting the growth of hair, which undoubtedly was diffused to a very great and (as it appeared to him) very alarming extent.

No gentleman attending that section could fail to be aware of the fact that the youth of the present age evinced, by their behaviour in the streets, and at all places of public resort, a considerable lack of that gallantry and gentlemanly feeling which, in more ignorant times, had been thought becoming. He wished to know whether it were possible that a constant outward application of bears' grease by the young gentlemen about town had imperceptibly infused into those unhappy persons something of the nature and quality of the bear. He shuddered as he threw out the remark; but if this theory, on inquiry, should prove to be well founded, it would at once explain a great deal of unpleasant eccentricity of behaviour, which, without some such discovery, was wholly unaccountable.

'The President highly complimented the learned gentleman on his most valuable suggestion, which produced the greatest effect upon the assembly; and remarked that only a week previous he had seen some young gentlemen at a theatre eyeing a box of ladies with a fierce intensity, which nothing but the influence of some brutish appetite could possibly explain. It was dreadful to reflect that our youth were so rapidly verging into a generation of bears.

'After a scene of scientific enthusiasm it was resolved that this important question should be immediately submitted to the consideration of the council.

'The President wished to know whether any gentleman could inform the section what had become of the dancing dogs?

'A Member replied, after some hesitation, that on the day after three glee-singers had been committed to prison as criminals by a late most zealous police magistrate of the metropolis, the dogs had abandoned their professional duties, and dispersed themselves in different quarters of the town to gain a livelihood by less dangerous means. He was given to understand that since that period they had supported themselves by lying in wait for and robbing blind men's poodles.

'Mr Flummery exhibited a twig, claiming to be a veritable branch of that noble tree known to naturalists as the SHAKSPEARE, which has taken root in every land and climate, and gathered under the shade of its broad green boughs the great family of mankind. The learned gentleman remarked that the twig had been undoubtedly called by other names in its time; but that it had been pointed out to him by an old lady in Warwickshire, where the great tree had grown, as a shoot of the genuine SHAKSPEARE, by which name he begged to introduce it to his countrymen.

'The President wished to know what botanical definition the honourable gentleman could afford of the curiosity.

'Mr Flummery expressed his opinion that it was A DECIDED PLANT.

'SECTION B. – DISPLAY OF MODELS AND MECHANICAL SCIENCE

LARGE ROOM, BOOT-JACK AND COUNTENANCE.

*President* – Mr Mallett. *Vice Presidents* – Messrs Leaver and Scroo.

'Mr Crinkles exhibited a most beautiful and delicate machine, of little larger size than an ordinary snuff box, manufactured entirely by himself, and composed exclusively of steel, by the aid of which more pockets could be picked in one hour than by the present slow and tedious process in four-and-twenty. The inventor remarked that it had been put into active operation in Fleet Street, the Strand, and other thoroughfares, and had never been once known to fail.

'After some slight delay, occasioned by the various members of the section buttoning their pockets,

'The President narrowly inspected the invention, and declared that he had never seen a machine of more beautiful or exquisite construction. Would the inventor be good enough to inform the section whether he had taken any and what means for bringing it into general operation?

'Mr Crinkles stated that, after encountering some preliminary difficulties, he had succeeded in putting himself in communication with Mr Fogle Hunter, and other gentlemen connected with the swell mob, who had awarded the invention the very highest and most unqualified approbation. He regretted to say, however, that these distinguished practitioners, in common with a gentleman of the name of Gimlet-eyed Tommy, and other members of a secondary grade of the profession whom he was understood to represent, entertained an insuperable objection to its being brought into general use, on the ground that it would have the inevitable effect of almost entirely superseding manual labour, and throwing a great number of highly deserving persons out of employment.

'The President hoped that no such fanciful objections would be allowed to stand in the way of such a great public improvement.

'Mr Crinkles hoped so too; but he feared that if the gentlemen of the swell mob persevered in their objection, nothing could be done.

'Professor Grime suggested that surely, in that case, her Majesty's Government might be prevailed upon to take it up.

'Mr Crinkles said that if the objection were found to be insuperable he should apply to parliament, which he thought could not fail to recognise the utility of the invention.

'The President observed that, up to this time parliament had certainly got on very well without it; but, as they did their business on a very large scale, he had no doubt they would gladly adopt the improvement. His only fear was that the machine might be worn out by constant working.

'Mr Coppernose called the attention of the section to a proposition of great magnitude and interest, illustrated by a vast number of models, and stated with much clearness and perspicuity in a treatise entitled "Practical Suggestions on the necessity of providing some harmless and wholesome relaxation for the young noblemen of England." His proposition was, that a space of ground of not less than ten miles in length and four in breadth should be purchased by a new company, to be incorporated by Act of Parliament, and inclosed by a brick wall of not less than twelve feet in height. He proposed that it should be laid out with highway roads, turnpikes, bridges, miniature villages, and every object that could conduce to the comfort and glory of Four-in-hand Clubs, so that they might be fairly presumed to require no drive beyond it. This delightful retreat would be fitted up with most commodious and extensive stables, for the convenience of such of the nobility and gentry as had a taste for ostlering, and with houses of entertainment furnished in the most expensive and handsome style. It would be further provided with whole streets of door knockers and bell handles of extra size, so constructed that they could be easily wrenched off at night, and regularly screwed on again, by attendants provided for the purpose, every day. There would also be gas lamps of real glass, which could be broken at a comparatively small expense per dozen, and a broad and handsome foot pavement for gentlemen to drive their cabriolets upon when they were humorously disposed – for the full enjoyment of which feat live pedestrians would be procured from the workhouse at a very small charge per head. The place being inclosed, and carefully screened from the intrusion of the public, there would be no objection to gentlemen laying aside any article of their costume that was considered to interfere with a pleasant frolic, or, indeed, to their walking about without any costume at all, if they liked that better. In short, every facility of enjoyment would be afforded that the most gentlemanly person could possibly desire. But as even these advantages would be incomplete unless there were some means provided of enabling the nobility and gentry to display their prowess when they sallied forth after dinner, and as some inconvenience might be experienced in the event of their being reduced to the necessity of pummelling each other, the inventor had turned his attention to the construction of an entirely new police force, composed exclusively of automaton figures, which, with the assistance of the ingenious Signor Gagliardi, of Windmill Street, in the Haymarket, he had succeeded in making with such nicety, that a policeman, cab driver, or old woman, made upon the principle of the models exhibited, would walk about until knocked down like any real man; nay, more, if set upon and beaten by six or eight noblemen or gentlemen, after it was down, the figure would utter divers groans, mingled with entreaties for mercy, thus rendering the illusion complete, and the enjoyment perfect. But the invention did not stop even here; for station houses would be built, containing good beds for noblemen and gentlemen during the night, and in the morning they would repair to a commodious police office, where a pantomimic investigation would take place before the automaton magistrates, – quite equal to life, – who would fine them in so many counters, with which they would be previously provided for the purpose. This office would be furnished with an inclined plane, for the convenience of any nobleman or gentleman who might wish to bring in his horse as a witness; and the prisoners would be at perfect liberty, as they were now, to interrupt the complainants as much as they pleased, and to make any remarks that they thought proper. The charge for these amusements would amount to very little more than they already cost, and the inventor submitted that the public would be much benefited and comforted by the proposed arrangement.

'Professor Nogo wished to be informed what amount of automaton police force it was proposed to raise in the first instance.

'Mr Coppernose replied, that it was proposed to begin with seven divisions of police of a score each, lettered from A to G inclusive. It was proposed that not more than half this should be placed on active duty, and that the remainder should be kept on shelves in the police office ready to be called out at a moment's notice.

'The President, awarding the utmost merit to the ingenious gentleman who had originated the idea, doubted whether the automaton police would quite answer the purpose. He feared that noblemen and gentlemen would perhaps require the excitement of thrashing living subjects.

'Mr Coppernose submitted that as the usual odds in such cases were ten noblemen or gentlemen to one policeman or cab driver, it could make very little difference in point of excitement whether the policeman or cab driver were a man or a block. The great advantage would be, that a policeman's limbs might be all knocked off, and yet he would be in a condition to do duty next day. He might even give his evidence next morning with his head in his hand, and give it equally well.

'Professor Muff. – Will you allow me to ask you, sir, of what materials it is intended that the magistrates' heads shall be composed?

'Mr Coppernose. – The magistrates will have wooden heads, of course, and they will be made of the toughest and thickest materials that can possibly be obtained.

'Professor Muff. – I am quite satisfied. This is a great invention.

'Professor Nogo. – I see but one objection to it. It appears to me that the magistrates ought to talk.

'Mr Coppernose no sooner heard this suggestion than he touched a small spring in each of the two models of magistrates which were placed upon the table; one of the figures immediately began to exclaim with great volubility that he was sorry to see gentlemen in such a situation, and the other to express a fear that the policeman was intoxicated.

'The section, as with one accord, declared with a shout of applause that the invention was complete; and the President, much excited, retired with Mr Coppernose to lay it before the council. On his return,

'Mr Tickle displayed his newly invented spectacles, which enabled the wearer to discern, in very bright colours, objects at a great distance, and rendered him wholly blind to those immediately before him. It was, he said, a most valuable and useful invention, based strictly upon the principle of the human eye.

'The President required some information upon this point. He had yet to learn that the human eye was remarkable for the peculiarities of which the honourable gentleman had spoken.

'Mr Tickle was rather astonished to hear this, when the President could not fail to be aware that a large number of most excellent persons and great statesmen could see, with the naked eye, most marvellous horrors on West India plantations, while they could discern nothing whatever in the interior of Manchester cotton mills. He must know, too, with what quickness of perception most people could discover their neighbour's faults, and how very blind they were to their own. If the President differed from the great majority of men in this respect, his eye was a defective one, and it was to assist his vision that these glasses were made.

'Mr Blank exhibited a model of a fashionable annual, composed of copper plates, gold leaf, and silk boards, and worked entirely by milk and water.

'Mr Prosee, after examining the machine, declared it to be so ingeniously composed, that he was wholly unable to discover how it went on at all.

'Mr Blank. – Nobody can, and that is the beauty of it.

### 'Section C. – Anatomy and Medicine.

BAR ROOM, BLACK BOY AND STOMACH-ACHE.

*President* – Dr Soemup. *Vice Presidents* – Messrs Pessell and Mortair.

'Dr Grummidge stated to the section a most interesting case of monomania, and described the course of treatment he had pursued with perfect success. The patient was a married lady in the middle rank of life, who, having seen another lady at an evening party in a full suit of pearls, was suddenly seized with a desire to possess a similar equipment, although her husband's finances were by no means equal to the necessary outlay. Finding her wish ungratified, she fell sick, and the symptoms soon became so alarming, that he (Dr Grummidge) was called in. At this period the prominent tokens of the disorder were sullenness, a total indisposition to perform domestic duties, great peevishness, and extreme languor, except when pearls were mentioned, at which times the pulse quickened, the eyes grew brighter, the pupils dilated, and the patient, after various incoherent exclamations, burst into a passion of tears, and exclaimed that nobody cared for her, and that she wished herself dead. Finding that the patient's appetite was affected in the presence of company, he began by ordering a total abstinence from all stimulants, and forbidding any sustenance but weak gruel; he then took twenty ounces of blood, applied a blister under each ear, one upon the chest, and another on the back; having done which, and administered five grains of calomel, he left the patient to her repose. The next day she was somewhat low, but decidedly better, and all appearances of irritation were removed. The next day she improved still further, and on the next again. On the fourth there was some appearance of a return of the old symptoms, which no sooner developed themselves, than he administered another dose of calomel, and left strict orders that, unless a decidedly favourable change occurred within two hours, the patient's head should be immediately shaved to the very last curl. From that moment she began to mend, and, in less than four-and-twenty hours was perfectly restored. She did not now betray the least emotion at the sight or mention of pearls or any other ornaments. She was cheerful and good humoured, and a most beneficial change had been effected in her whole temperament and condition.

'Mr Pipkin (MRCS) read a short but most interesting communication in which he sought to prove the complete belief of Sir William Courtenay, otherwise Thom, recently shot at Canterbury, in the Homœopathic system. The section would bear in mind that one of the Homœopathic doctrines was, that infinitesimal doses of any medicine which would occasion the disease under which the patient laboured, supposing him to be in a healthy state, would cure it. Now, it was a remarkable circumstance – proved in the evidence – that the deceased Thom employed a woman to follow him about all day with a pail of water, assuring her that one drop (a purely homœopathic remedy, the section would observe), placed upon his tongue, after death, would restore him. What was the obvious inference? That Thom, who was marching and countermarching in osier beds, and other swampy places, was impressed with a presentiment that he should be drowned; in which case, had his instructions been complied with, he could not fail to have been brought to life again instantly by his own prescription. As it was, if this woman, or any other person, had administered an infinitesimal dose of lead and gunpowder immediately after he fell, he would have recovered forthwith. But unhappily the woman concerned did not possess the power of reasoning by analogy, or carrying out a principle, and thus the unfortunate gentleman had been sacrificed to the ignorance of the peasantry.

## 'Section D. – Statistics.

### OUT-HOUSE, BLACK BOY AND STOMACH-ACHE.

*President* – Mr Slug. *Vice Presidents* – Messrs Noakes and Styles.

'Mr Kwakley stated the result of some most ingenious statistical inquiries relative to the difference between the value of the qualification of several members of Parliament as published to the world, and its real nature and amount. After reminding the section that every member of Parliament for a town or borough was supposed to possess a clear freehold estate of three hundred pounds per annum, the honourable gentleman excited great amusement and laughter by stating the exact amount of freehold property possessed by a column of legislators, in which he had included himself. It appeared from the table, that the amount of such income possessed by each was 0 pounds, 0 shillings, and 0 pence, yielding an average of the same. (Great laughter.) It was pretty well known that there were accommodating gentlemen in the habit of furnishing new members with temporary qualifications, to the ownership of which they swore solemnly – of course as a mere matter of form. He argued from these *data* that it was wholly unnecessary for members of Parliament to possess any property at all, especially as when they had none the public could get them so much cheaper.

## 'Supplementary Section, E – Umbugology and Ditchwaterisics.

*President* – Mr Grub *Vice Presidents* – Messrs Dull and Dummy.

'A paper was read by the secretary descriptive of a bay pony with one eye, which had been seen by the author standing in a butcher's cart at the corner of Newgate Market. The communication described the author of the paper as having, in the prosecution of a mercantile pursuit, betaken himself one Saturday morning last summer from Somers Town to Cheapside; in the course of which expedition he had beheld the extraordinary appearance above described. The pony had one distinct eye, and it had been pointed out to him by his friend Captain Blunderbore, of the Horse Marines, who assisted the author in his search, that whenever he winked this eye he whisked his tail (possibly to drive the flies off), but that he always winked and whisked at the same time. The animal was lean, spavined, and tottering; and the author proposed to constitute it of the family of *Fitfordogsmeataurious*. It certainly did occur to him that there was no case on record of a pony with one clearly defined and distinct organ of vision, winking and whisking at the same moment.

'Mr Q. J. Snuffletoffle had heard of a pony winking his eye, and likewise of a pony whisking his tail, but whether they were two ponies or the same pony he could not undertake positively to say. At all events, he was acquainted with no authentic instance of a simultaneous winking and whisking, and he really could not but doubt the existence of such a marvellous pony in opposition to all those natural laws by which ponies were governed. Referring, however, to the mere question of his one organ of vision, might he suggest the possibility of this pony having been literally half asleep at the time he was seen, and having closed only one eye.

'The President observed that, whether the pony was half asleep or fast asleep, there could be no doubt that the association was wide awake, and therefore that they had better get the business over, and go to dinner. He had certainly never seen anything analogous to this pony, but he was not prepared to doubt its existence; for he had seen many queerer ponies in his time, though he did not pretend to have seen any more remarkable donkeys than the other gentleman around him.

'Professor John Ketch was then called upon to exhibit the skull of the late Mr Greenacre, which he produced from a blue bag, remarking, on being invited to make any observations that occurred to him, "that he'd pound it as that 'ere 'spectable section had never seed a more gamerer cove nor he vos."

'A most animated discussion upon this interesting relic ensued; and, some difference of opinion arising respecting the real character of the deceased gentleman, Mr Blubb delivered a lecture upon the cranium before him, clearly showing that Mr Greenacre possessed the organ of destructiveness to a most unusual extent, with a most remarkable development of the organ of carveativeness. Sir Hookham Snivey was proceeding to combat this opinion, when Professor Ketch suddenly interrupted the proceedings by exclaiming, with great excitement of manner, "Walker!"

'The President begged to call the learned gentleman to order.

'Professor Ketch. – "Order be blowed! you've got the wrong un, I tell you. It ain't no 'ed at all; it's a coker-nut as my brother-in-law has been a-carvin', to hornament his new baked tatur-stall wots a-comin' down 'ere vile the 'sociation's in the town. Hand over, vill you?"

'With these words, Professor Ketch hastily repossessed himself of the cocoa-nut, and drew forth the skull, in mistake for which he had exhibited it. A most interesting conversation ensued; but as there appeared some doubt ultimately whether the skull was Mr Greenacre's, or a hospital patient's, or a pauper's, or a man's, or a woman's, or a monkey's, no particular result was obtained.'

'I cannot,' says our talented correspondent in conclusion, 'I cannot close my account of these gigantic researches and sublime and noble triumphs without repeating a *bon mot* of Professor Woodensconce's, which shows how the greatest minds may occasionally unbend when truth can be presented to listening ears, clothed in an attractive and playful form. I was standing by, when, after a week of feasting and feeding, that learned gentleman, accompanied by the whole body of wonderful men, entered the hall yesterday, where a sumptuous dinner was prepared; where the richest wines sparkled on the board, and fat bucks – propitiatory sacrifices to learning – sent forth their savoury odours. "Ah!" said Professor Woodensconce, rubbing his hands, "this is what we meet for; this is what inspires us; this is what keeps us together, and beckons us onward; this is the *spread* of science, and a glorious spread it is." '

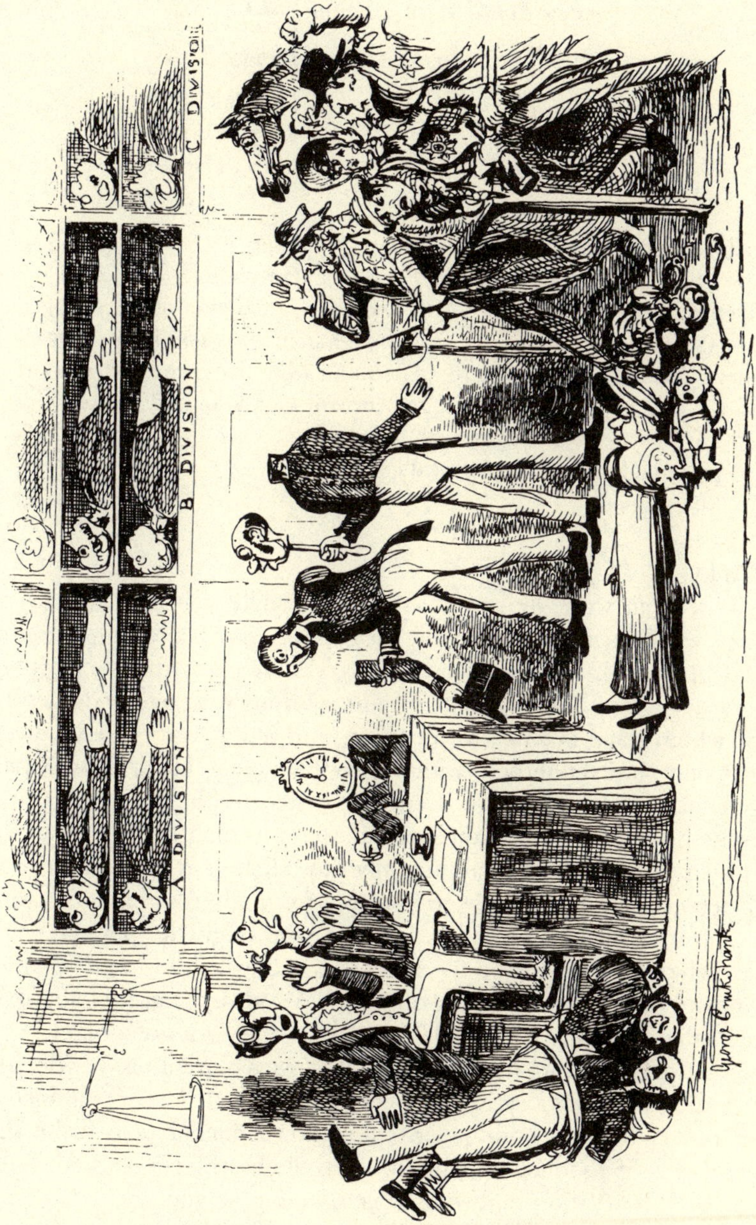

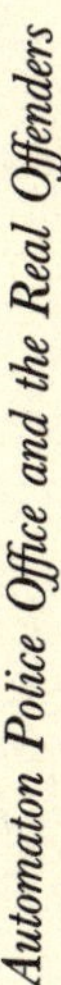

*Automaton Police Office and the Real Offenders*

## *Familiar Epistle From a Parent to a Child Aged Two Years and Two Months*

Dickens's editorial farewell to his readers published in *Bentley's Miscellany* February 1839 (Vol. 5, pp. 219–20). For the background to this piece see introduction above, pp. xix–xxii. With Dickens's description of the changed status of the mail guard compare the comments in *London on Wheels* (British Transport Commission, 1962), p. 6: 'The mails were the cream of transport . . . and the mail guards – at first equipped with blunderbusses, but later, as the highwaymen were put down, with long copper coach-horns – were men of great pride and prestige in their calling.'

My Child,

To recount with what trouble I have brought you up – with what an anxious eye I have regarded your progress, – how late and how often I have sat up at night working for you, – and how many thousand letters I have received from, and written to your various relations and friends, many of whom have been of a querulous and irritable turn, – to dwell on the anxiety and tenderness with which I have (as far as I possessed the power) inspected and chosen your food; rejecting the indigestible and heavy matter which some injudicious but well-meaning old ladies would have had you swallow, and retaining only those light and pleasant articles which I deemed calculated to keep you free from all gross humours, and to render you an agreeable child, and one who might be popular with society in general, – to dilate on the steadiness with which I have prevented your annoying any company by talking politics – always assuring you that you would thank me for it yourself some day when you grew older, – to expatiate, in short, upon my own assiduity as a parent, is beside my present purpose, though I cannot but contemplate your fair appearance – your robust health, and unimpeded circulation (which I take to be the great secret of your good looks) without the liveliest satisfaction and delight.

It is a trite observation, and one which, young as you are, I have no doubt you have often heard repeated, that we have fallen upon strange times, and live in days of constant shiftings and changes. I had a melancholy instance of this only a week or two since. I was returning from Manchester to London by the Mail Train, when I suddenly fell into another train – a mixed train – of reflection, occasioned by the dejected and disconsolate demeanour of the Post Office Guard. We were stopping at some station where they take in water, when he dismounted slowly from the little box in which he sits in ghastly mockery of his old condition with pistol and blunderbuss beside him, ready to shoot the first highwayman (or railwayman) who shall attempt to stop the horses, which now travel (when they travel at all) *inside* and in a portable stable invented for the purpose, – he dismounted, I say, slowly and sadly, from his post, and looking mournfully about him as if in dismal recollection of the old roadside public-house – the blazing fire – the glass of foaming ale – the buxom handmaid and admiring hangers-on of tap-room and stable, all honoured by his notice; and, retiring a little apart, stood leaning against a signal-post, surveying the engine with a look of combined affliction and disgust which no words can describe. His scarlet coat and golden lace were tarnished with ignoble smoke; flakes of soot had fallen on his bright green shawl – his pride in days of yore – the steam condensed in the tunnel from which we had just emerged, shone upon his hat like rain. His eye betokened that he was thinking of the coachman; and as it wandered to his own seat and his own fast-fading garb, it was plain to see that he felt his office and himself had alike no business there, and were nothing but an elaborate practical joke.

As we whirled away, I was led insensibly into an anticipation of those days to come, when mail-coach guards shall no longer be judges of horse flesh – when a mail-coach guard shall never even have seen a horse – when stations shall have superseded stables, and corn shall have given place to coke. 'In those dawning times,' thought I, 'exhibition rooms shall teem with portraits of her Majesty's favourite engine, with boilers after Nature by future Landseers. Some Amburgh, yet unborn, shall break wild horses by his magic power; and in the dress of a mail-coach guard exhibit his TRAINED ANIMALS in a mock mail-coach. Then shall wondering crowds observe how that, with the exception of his whip, it is all his eye; and crowned heads shall see them fed on oats, and stand alone unmoved and undismayed, while courtiers flee affrighted when the coursers neigh!'

Such, my child, were the reflections from which I was only awakened then, as I am now, by the necessity of attending to matters of present through minor importance. I offer no apology to you for the digression, for it brings me very naturally to the subject of change, which is the very subject of which I desire to treat.

In fact, my child, you have changed hands. Henceforth I resign you to the guardianship and protection of one of my most intimate and valued friends, Mr Ainsworth, with whom, and with you, my best wishes and warmest feelings will ever remain. I reap no gain or profit by parting from you, nor will any conveyance of your property be required, for, in this respect, you have always been literally 'Bentley's' Miscellany, and never mine.

Unlike the driver of the old Manchester mail, I regard this altered state of things with feelings of unmingled pleasure and satisfaction. Unlike the guard of the new Manchester mail, *your* guard is at home in his new place, and has roystering highwaymen and gallant desperadoes ever within call. And if I might compare you, my child, to an engine; (not a Tory engine, nor a Whig engine, but a brisk and rapid locomotive;) your friends and patrons to passengers; and he who now stands towards you *in loco parentis* as the skilful engineer and supervisor of the whole, I would humbly crave leave to postpone the departure of the train on its new and auspicious course for one brief instant, while, with hat in hand, I approach side by side with the friend who travelled with me on the old road, and presume to solicit favour and kindness in behalf of him and his new charge, both for their sakes and that of the old coachman,

Boz.

# INDEX AND GLOSSARY

*NOTE:* this Index and Glossary covers only Dickens's text; it does not index editorial matter such as headnotes. The following abbreviations have been used: coll. = colloquial; dem. = demolished; obs. = obsolete; sl. = slang.

on the Sabbath could indulge in lawful recreations afterwards; reissued by Charles I (1633) 493f.

BOORS CAROUSING allusion to the kind of genre painting of peasants drinking associated with such Dutch and Flemish artists as Adriaen Brouwer (1605/6–38) and Adriaen van Ostade (1610–84) 188

BOOTS inn servant employed to clean guests' shoes and generally make himself useful 394

BOSOM FRIEND (sl.) warm clothing to protect the chest, a comforter 12

BOSWELL James Boswell (1740–95) friend and biographer of Dr Johnson who would sometimes provoke the great man into verbally crushing him 511

BOSWELL COURT street in Bloomsbury, London 373

BOULOGNE port and resort town on the northern coast of France, very popular with the English in the nineteenth century, especially when they were in financial difficulties 287

BOUQUET bunch of sweet-smelling herbs placed in front of judges in court to protect them from being infected by 'gaol fever' (i.e., typhus) carried by prisoners at the bar 196

BOW STREET in Covent Garden, London, famous for its magistrates' court (established 1740) 148, 270

BRAMAH, PATENT type of lock invented by Joseph Bramah (1748–1814), patented in 1784 268

'BRAVE OLD HOAK, THE' popular song, words by Henry Chorley (1808–72), music by E.J. Loder (1813–65) 59

BREACH OF PROMISE OF MARRIAGE 286f.

BRIGHTON fashionable seaside resort town in Sussex 330

BRILLIANT OF THE FIRST WATER a diamond of the finest cut and quality 11

BRITISH ASSOCIATION FOR THE ADVANCEMENT OF SCIENCE caricatured as Mudfog Association for the Advancement of Everything 513ff.

BRITISH MUSEUM Great Russell Street, London, opened 1759 and rebuilt 1823–47 (the Round Reading Room dates from 1852–7) 188, 262, 275, 494, 497

BRIXTON newly-developed south-western suburb of London, much favoured by City businessmen 345

BROKER dealer in second-hand furniture 26ff.; BROKER'S SHOPS 177ff.

BROOKES'S gentlemen's club in the West End of London (founded 1674) 215

BROWN, KING AND GIBSON performers at the Adelphi Theatre 503, 506

BUCELLAS Portuguese white wine resembling hock 280

BUCKLERSBURY City of London street, just south of the Royal Exchange 213

BURKE William Burke (1792–1829) Irish criminal executed in Edinburgh for conspiring with William Hare to murder people whose bodies they then sold to an anatomist 364

BURTON ALE pale ale brewed at Burton on Trent, Staffordshire 219

BURY ST EDMUNDS town in Suffolk 439

BUTCHERS' COMPANY one of the City Livery Companies (craft guilds) 162

BYRON Lord Byron (1788–1824), poet 276ff., 348: *see also* *CHILDE HAROLD, DON JUAN*

CAB-HORSES 144

CABMEN 214, 278, 394

CABS 87 and *passim*

CAD conductor of an omnibus 139ff., and *passim*

'CAMBERVEL' i.e., Camberwell Fair 118

CAMBERWELL middle-class south-eastern suburb of London 345, 358, 528

CAMBRIDGE UNIVERSITY 479

CAMDEN TOWN working-class north-western suburb of London (home of

great danger, returned to his farm 148

CITY ROAD east London thoroughfare 231

CITY THEATRE converted chapel in Milton Street, Finsbury (north London) 267

CIVIL SERVICE qualities requisite in a senior civil servant 224: *see also* CLERKS, GOVERNMENT

CLAPHAM prosperous south London suburb 405ff. (CLAPHAM RISE is a fictitious street-name)

CLAPTON eastern suburb of London, now part of the borough of Hackney; in the nineteenth century a very respectable residential district 94

CLARE MARKET (dem.) London slum area west of Lincoln's Inn Fields (*q.v.*) 182

CLERGYMEN 11ff., 479f. 496

CLERKS, CITY 53f. and *passim*

CLERKS, GOVERNMENT 222, 294, 306

CLOWNS 175, 500ff.

COACHES *see* STAGE-COACH TRAVEL

COAL WHIPPERS dockers who hoisted coal on and off ships and barges by means of pulleys 380

COBURG THEATRE the Royal Coburg Theatre in the Waterloo Road, opened 1818, which changed its name to the Royal Victoria 1833: *see* VICTORIA THEATRE

COLD BATH FIELDS (dem.) prison in Clerkenwell, London, built 1794 and officially known as the Middlesex House of Correction; the SILENT SYSTEM (*q.v.*) was strictly enforced here 272

COLEMAN STREET in the City of London 231

COLLEGE OF PHYSICIANS 201

COLOSSEUM place of entertainment in Regent's Park, London, opened 1829, the brainchild of Thomas Horner (*q.v.*); its principal attraction was a huge panorama of London, Paris, etc. 115

COLOSSUS, THE BRAZEN the Colossus of Rhodes, one of the Seven Wonders of the ancient world, a huge bronze statue that straddled the entrance to Rhodes Harbour 90

COLUMBINE pantomime heroine, deriving from the *Commedia dell'Arte* 256, 292, 500, 505

'COME THE DOUBLE MONKEY' unidentified theatrical accomplishment 58

COMMONS, HOUSE OF *see* PARLIAMENT

COOK, CAPTAIN James Cook (1728–79), circumnavigator 348

COPENHAGEN HOUSE (dem.) famous tea-garden in Islington, north London, opened in the mid-eighteenth century 174

CORNWALL, THAT PLACE IN by the early nineteenth century Cornwall had become a byword for electoral corruption; of its 28 Parliamentary seats in 1830, 18 were 'pocket boroughs', i.e., owned by individuals; the particular 'place' Dickens alludes to here is probably Grampound which returned 2 members to Parliament until it was disfranchised for flagrant corruption in 1821 233

CORPORATION BILL the Municipal Corporations Act of 1835 103

COSMORAMAS an elaborate form of peep-show where one looked through a series of windows (each one being, in fact, a convex lens) at pictures of great monuments or natural phenomena like volcanic eruptions or great waterfalls, the subjects seeming to be full-scale as a result of the lens; in 1821 the first Cosmorama Room opened in London 129

COURTENAY, SIR WILLIAM name assumed by a lunatic called Thom or Tom (1799–1838) who also proclaimed himself the Messiah and attracted a large following among the Kentish peasantry; he was shot by the military in May 1838 during a bloody affray at Blaen Wood, near Canterbury 547

arrived in London once a week 58, 329

DOUBLE-MILLED extra strong, closely woven 18

DRAB whitey-brown in colour; DRABS trousers of this colour *passim*

DRAMATISTS, HACK 87

DRAWING ROOM formal reception held by the sovereign 296

DRUIDS ancient British priests 374

DRUMMOND STREET in north-west London, between Regent's Park and Euston Station 247, 250

DRURY LANE ancient London thoroughfare leading from Holborn south to the Strand (*q.v.*) *passim*

DRURY LANE THEATRE one of the two London theatres established by royal patent in Charles II's reign, rebuilt 1812 13, 107, 243

DUBLIN 295

DUCROW Andrew Ducrow (1793–1842), famous equestrian performer 108, 111, 135

DUKE, A Frederick, Duke of York (1763–1827) 68

DUKE OF YORK'S COLUMN commemorative column erected by public subscription 1830–1 to honour Frederick, Duke of York, for many years Commander-in-Chief of the British Army 170

DUTCH CLOCK wooden German wall-clock, 'Dutch' being a corruption of 'deutsch' 29, 154, 279

DWARFS 118f.

EAGLE TAVERN tea-garden off the City Road, east London, which became a prototype music hall in 1825, later a theatre and finally a Salvation Army centre; dem. 1901 when a public house was built on the site 228f.

EAST INDIES 383

EASTERN DESCENT, OF i.e., Muslim and thus able to have more than one wife 17

EATON SQUARE part of Belgravia in south-west London, begun 1827 43

EDGWARE ROAD runs north from Oxford Street (*q.v.*) to St John's Wood 455

EDUCATION female 97, 316ff.; Dame's school 106: *see also* NATIONAL SCHOOL

ELEPHANT AND CASTLE London district south of the Thames, the junction of several major roads leading to Kent and Surrey; named after a tavern which stood there in the 1760s 526

ELEPHANTS, PERFORMING 512

ENVY AND HATRED ... AND ALL UNCHARITABLENESS quotation from the Litany in the Book of Common Prayer 24

EPISTLE, THE a reading from one of the Apostolic letters in the New Testament forming part of the Anglican Communion Service 12

*L'ÉTÉ* unidentified piano piece 321

ETON Public School founded 1440 479

EUSTON SQUARE Bloomsbury 247

EXCHANGE, THE the Royal Exchange 347, 501: *see also* 'CHANGE

EXECUTION, AN in legal terminology forcible possession by officials of a debtor's house and goods which are then sold off to pay the debt; 'to be taken in execution' to find oneself in this situation 33

EXETER 'CHANGE building on the north side of the Strand (*q.v.*) dating from the late seventeenth century with shops on the ground floor and an exhibition hall above which a menagerie was housed 215

EXETER HALL built in the Strand (*q.v.*) 1830–1 (site now occupied by the Strand Palace Hotel); used for religious and scientific meetings, especially the great May meetings of the Evangelicals for the promotion of charitable and missionary work 40

EYE, MIND YOUR (coll.) be careful 436

'FALL OF PARIS, THE' 'The Surrender

of Paris, a descriptive fantasia for the pianoforte' by L. Jensen (1816) 356

FALSTAFF the jovial glutton in Shakespeare's *Henry IV* plays 160

FANCY FAIRS charitable events 63, 94, 279, 408

FARRINGDON STREET east London street on the fringe of the City 141

FATES, THE THREE in Greek mythology the three goddesses who control the destinies of men and women 17

FATIMA Bluebeard's bride, a type of feminine curiosity 147

FERGUSON'S FIRST in his autobiography, the astronomer James Ferguson (1710–76) gives an account of his early attempts at watch-making: 'a watch with wooden wheels and a whale-bone spring ... I enclosed the whole in a wooden case very little bigger than a breakfast cup' 188

FETTER LANE street in the City of London running between Fleet Street and Holborn Circus 253

FINSBURY SQUARE rectangular square with the City Road running through the east side, built 1777–92 231

FIRE-FIGHTING 8

'FIRE-WORSHIPPERS, THE' one of the four verse romances included in Thomas Moore's *Lallah Rookh* (1817); another is 'Paradise and the Peri' 281

FITZROY SQUARE imposing square west of north Tottenham Court Road (*q.v.*) built 1790–1829 86

FLEAS, PERFORMING exhibitions of performing fleas were a favourite entertainment at fairs; drawing a little carriage was a favourite trick 520f.

FLEET PRISON known to have been a debtors' prison as early as 1290, it was burnt down in the Gordon Riots of 1780, and rebuilt on the original site off Farringdon Lane in east London 287

FLEET STREET connects the Strand (*q.v.*) with Ludgate Hill in the City of London 145 and *passim*

'FLOW ON, THOU SHINING RIVER' from Thomas Moore's *National Airs* (1815), where it appears as 'Portuguese Air'; set to music as a duet by Sir J.A. Stevenson (1760–1833) 296

FLOWER-POT INN, THE public house in Bishopsgate, in the City of London, the starting-point of the Norwich coach 310

FLY, A light, double-seated one-horse carriage; the term came to be used of any vehicle let out for hire 333; DOUBLE FLY 348

'FLY, FLY FROM THE WORLD' one of Thomas Moore's songs: 'Fly from the world, O Bessy, to me,/Thou wilt never find any sincerer' 59

FOGLE (sl.) handkerchief 543

FOUNDLING, THE the Foundling Hospital established in 1739 by Captain Coram (?1668–1751) 289

FOX Charles James Fox (1749–1806), brilliant Whig opponent of the Tory Pitt 155

FRANK until the introduction of the Penny Post MPs enjoyed the privilege of 'franking' letters, i.e., signing the envelope or outer fold, thereby enabling it to go post-free 155, 294

FREE SEATS seats in the parish church reserved for those too poor to be able to rent their own pew 11, 37, 480

FREEMASON'S, THE i.e., Freemasons' Hall, Great Queen Street, Holborn, west London, a frequent venue for public dinners 162

FRENCH LAMPS i.e., argand lamps, a greatly improved kind of oil lamp with a tubular wick, invented by the Swiss Aimé Argand (1755–1803) 222

FROCK, ROUND a smock 65

FROGS ornamental fastenings or tasselled buttons on a coat or cloak 45, 109

FRY, MRS Elizabeth Fry (1780–1845), a Quaker who visited Newgate Prison in 1813 and was so horrified by the conditions there that she devoted the rest of her life to prison reform 195

until 1940 runaway couples could get married here (subject to 21 days' Scottish residence by one or other of the parties) simply by declaring to a blacksmith, toll-keeper, etc., their willingness to marry 396, 403

GRIMALDI Joseph Grimaldi (1778–1837), celebrated clown and star of early nineteenth-century pantomime 502ff.

GROSVENOR SQUARE fashionable square in the West End of London, east of Park Lane 171

GUERNSEY SHIRTS closely-knitted blue woollen tunics worn by sailors 101

GUILDHALL situated in Gresham Street in the City of London and meeting place of the Common Council 162

GUINNESS'S STOUT the Dublin brewing firm of Guinness was founded in 1759; its stout soon became celebrated 292

HACKNEY north-eastern suburb of London 94, 528

HACKNEY COACHES 83ff. and *passim*; HACKNEY-COACHMEN 194

HALF-BAPTISE truncated form of the baptism service carried out when the full service could not be performed, e.g., in an emergency when a baby's imminent death was expected 12

*HAMLET* 283

HAMMERSMITH west London; HAMMERSMITH SUSPENSION BRIDGE, a bridge linking Hammersmith on the north side of the Thames with Barnes on the south – the bridge referred to by Dickens, completed in 1827, was replaced by the present one in 1883 81

HAMPSTEAD now part of north London but in Dickens's time still a village 482; HAMPSTEAD HEATH, an open area of heath and woodland in north London 425; HAMPSTEAD ROAD 96

HAMPTON COURT a Royal Palace in Middlesex built by Cardinal Wolsey, and presented to Henry VIII in 1526; the famous maze was constructed in the reign of William III (1689–1702) 70

'HARF-A-CROWN' two shillings and six pence, an eighth of a pound in old money 114

HARLEQUIN pantomime character whose magic bat or wand had the power to change people and things into something completely different 505f. and *passim*

'HARMONIC MEETINGS' sing-songs held in the upper room of a public house with professional singers and the audience joining in the choruses – forerunner of the music-hall 59f., 255, 262

HART STREET former street in Bloomsbury, now Bloomsbury Way 452

HATTON GARDEN situated in north London, being the whole area between Leather Lane, Saffron Hill, Holborn and Hatton Wall, originally the gardens of the Elizabethan Hatton House 457

HAVANNAH CIGARS 266ff.

HAYMARKET, THE street in the West End of London connecting Pall Mall East with the east end of Piccadilly Circus; formerly it was a centre for the sale of farm produce 148, 502, 544

HEBE in Greek mythology the goddess of youth, cup-bearer to the gods 159

*HERALD see MORNING HERALD*

HEROD King of the Jews (37–4 BC) notorious for his massacre of the innocents (*Matt.* 2: 16) 448

HESSIAN BOOTS high boots with short tassels in front at the top; made of hessian, and first worn by troops in Hesse, Germany, they became fashionable in England in the nineteenth century 214

HIGHFLIER, ALFRED one of the leading characters in Thomas Morton's comedy *A Roland for an Oliver* (1819) 124

HIGHGATE north London suburb, adjacent to Hampstead, and still a village in Dickens's day 482

HIGH-LOWS laced ankle-boots 24, 312

'HIS FIRST APPEARANCE IN THAT CHARACTER' playbill terminology 286

'HIS IMPUDENCE OF PROOF . . .' unidentified quotation 486

HOBLER, MR Francis Hobler, for many years the Lord Mayor's Clerk at the Mansion House, evidently an incorrigibly facetious individual 7, 145

HOGARTH, WILLIAM (1697–1764), English painter and graphic artist 286

HOLBORN London thoroughfare running west from the City 145 and *passim*; HOLBORN HILL, name given to the stretch of Holborn between Farringdon Street and Fetter Lane

HOLLAND, BROWN coarse linen cloth, first manufactured in the Netherlands, much used in furnishing 13

HOLLOWAY north London suburb 142

HOLYHEAD Anglesey, north Wales; port of embarkation for Ireland 134

HOLYWELL STREET formerly a narrow London street of squalid houses in the vicinity of the Strand, well known for its vendors of old clothes 76

HOMOEOPATHY 547

HORACE (65–8 BC), Roman poet 298

HORNER, LITTLE JACK hero of the well-known nursery rhyme 115

HORNER, MR in 1821–2 Thomas Hornor (*sic*; d. 1844), made a series of detailed sketches of the panoramic view of London, which made up a huge continuous painting on a strip of canvas, 64 feet high, and was displayed on the walls of the great rotunda of the Colosseum in Regent's Park 115

HORSE GUARDS (coll.) the War Office, which in the nineteenth century was located in the mid-eighteenth-century Horse Guards building in Whitehall 215

HOSPITALS 236ff.

HOUSE, THE (coll.) the Workhouse (*q.v.*)

HOUSE OF CORRECTION FOR MIDDLESEX also known as Cold Bath Fields (*q.v.*) a prison in Clerkenwell, London (dem. 1889), built in 1794 and regarded as one of the strictest, where the SILENT SYSTEM (*q.v.*) was enforced 146

'HOW SHARPER THAN A SERPENT'S TOOTH . . .' Shakespeare, *King Lear*, I.iv. 461

HOYLE Edmund Hoyle (1672–1769), leading authority on whist, the rules of which he standardised in his *Short Treatise on Whist* (1742) 448

HULKS, THE prison-ships 204

HUMMUMS (dem.) a one-time famous London inn situated in Covent Garden 52

HUNGERFORD MARKET formerly a large two-storeyed building in the Charing Cross area of west London erected in 1833 as a replacement for the earlier market of 1680 68

'I AM A FRIAR' song by J. O'Keeffe (1747–1833) 251

'I SAW HER AT THE FANCY FAIR' perhaps an inaccurate recollection of Thomas Haynes Bayly's humorous poem, 'I saw her as, I fancied, fair' about the unreliability of ladies' cosmetics 460

'I WISH YOU MAY GET IT' slang phrase current in the early nineteenth century roughly equivalent to our modern 'You'll be lucky!' 24, 429

IMPERENCE Cockney pronunciation of 'impertinence' 82, 229

'INCREASE AND MULTIPLY' a paraphrase of *Gen.* 1: 28, 'Be fruitful and multiply and replenish the earth' 74

INDIA 369, 383; (EAST INDIES) INDIA HOUSE East India House in Leadenhall Street (dem. 1862), the headquarters of the East India Company

INDIANS, STAGE 144

INEXPLICABLES euphemism for 'trousers' 306, 371, 378; 'INEXPRESSIBLES' 285, 294

INNS OF COURT four legal societies possessing the exclusive right of calling persons to the bar (i.e., enabling them

a strap or bow 80, 172; KNEE-SHORTS 90; KNEE-SMALLS 142

KNIGHTSBRIDGE street leading from Hyde Park Corner to Kensington 51

KYE-BOSK (sl.) kyebosh or kibosh: to 'put the kibosh' on someone means to crush them 73

LADY JAMES'S FOLLY a Gothic tower on Shooters Hill (*q.v.*) built for Lady James in 1784 to celebrate her husband's capture of the island of Saxerndroog off Malabar 478

LAMPS, THE (sl.) footlights 110

LANDSEER, EDWIN HENRY (1802–73), famous animal painter 553

LEOPOLD, PRINCE (1790–1865) Prince of Saxe-Coburg who married Charlotte, heiress-apparent to the British throne (*q.v.*), and later became first King of the Belgians 13, 345

LETHE-WATER in Greek mythology, the souls of the dead were obliged to drink from Lethe, one of the rivers of Hades, so that they should forget their earthly lives 185

LIBRARIES circulating libraries were centres of social life in resort towns often having concert and gaming rooms attached 94, 279, 340f.

LICENSED VICTUALLERS one of the City of London livery companies 162

'LIGHT GUITAR, THE' song by H.S. Van Dyke set to music by John Barnett (1802–90) 293

'LIKE SENDING THEM RUFFLES . . .' quotation from Goldsmith's *Haunch of Venison* (1776) 422

LILLIPUTIAN tiny (from Lilliput in Swift's *Gulliver's Travels*) 65

LINCOLN'S INN FIELDS residential square in west London adjacent to Lincoln's Inn, laid out by Inigo Jones in the early seventeenth century 141

LIONS 508f.

LISSON GROVE north-west London 149

LIST (SHOES) coarse woollen cloth 81

LITANY, THE prayers of intercession that on certain days form part of part of the Morning Service in the Church of England 12

LITTLE RUSSELL STREET west London 266

LLOYD'S London company of shipowners, underwriters and merchants which originated in Edward Lloyd's coffee-house in Lombard Street in the eighteenth century 94, 347

LONDON BRIDGE leads across the Thames from the City to Southwark; a new bridge was built in the 1820s (opened 1831) and therefore some of Dickens's references are to Old London Bridge and some to the newer one 67, 327; LONDON BRIDGE WHARF 103, 377

LONDON UNIVERSITY its original site was at the northern end of Gower Street, Bloomsbury, where the building which is now University College was begun in 1827 281

LONG ACRE west London, street running east-west just to the north of Covent Garden (*q.v.*) 176, 261

LORD MAYOR OF LONDON 67, 145, 162, 196, 526

LUCINIAN MYSTERIES those connected with childbirth; from Lucina, the name of the Roman goddess of light and the patroness of childbirth 147

LUCKY, MADE MY (thieves' sl.) escaped, got away 433

LUCRETIA, THIS MODERN legendary wife of a Roman consul; she committed suicide after having been raped by Sextus Tarquinius 420; LUCRETIAN 115

'LUNGS OF LONDON, THE' the parks of London were first so-called by Lord Chatham (1708–78) 112

MACASSAR OIL *see* ROWLAND'S MACASSAR OIL

'MACAULAY, THAT YOUNG' Thomas Babington Macaulay (1800–59) entered Parliament as a Liberal MP in 1830, and in 1834 accepted the position of

legal adviser to the supreme council of India 155

*MACBETH* produced at a private theatre 125

MAGISTRATES class prejudice of 545f.

MAIDEN LANE not the famous Maiden Lane in Covent Garden but the street now known as York Way in Holloway, which was then in the northern outskirts of London 174

MANCHESTER cotton mills in 546

MANCHESTER BUILDINGS a double row of private houses in south-west London, between Cannon Row and the river, near Westminster Bridge 158

MANSION HOUSE official residence of the Lord Mayor of London 145, 453

MANTUA-MAKING making of ladies' gowns and dresses (expression probably originated from a confusion of French *manteau*, cloak, with Mantua, the city in Italy) 19, 287

MARGATE coastal resort in Kent 330; MARGATE PACKET 103, 337

MARRIAGE 415

MARSH GATE district on the Surrey side of the Thames near where Waterloo Station now stands 57, 62

MARTIN, RICHARD Richard Martin (1754–1834), MP, co-founder of the Society for Prevention of Cruelty of Animals, popularly known as 'Humanity Martin'; introduced the Act for Protecting the Rights of Animals 1822 which bore heavily on costermongers (street-traders selling fruit, fish, etc., from a barrow) who ill-treated their horses 85

*MASANIELLO* James Kenny's 1829 adaptation of Auber's opera *Masaniello* was enormously popular and often revived 407

MELODRAMA 117f., 319

*MEN OF PROMETHEUS* ballet (1801) by Salvatore Vigano (1769–1821) for which Beethoven (1770–1827) wrote the music 411

MERCURY in Classical mythology the messenger of the gods 429

METHODISTS 448

MILLBANK *see* PENITENTIARY

MILLBANK STREET in Westminster, just south of the Houses of Parliament 158

MILTON John Milton (1608–74), poet 277

MILTON STREET *see* CITY THEATRE

MINOR THEATRES theatres other than the 'legitimate' theatres of Covent Garden, Drury Lane and the Haymarket which were the only ones legally allowed to present regular dramas; the 'Minors' became the home of melodrama, 'burlettas', farce etc. 110, 111, 122; MINOR PLAY-BILL PHRASEOLOGY 73

MISSIONARIES 38

MONKEYS, PERFORMING 512, 540f.

MONMOUTH STREET former thoroughfare in west-central London famed for its old clothes shops; became part of Shaftesbury Avenue (the present Monmouth Street, formerly Little and Great St Andrews Streets, was re-named in the 1930s) 76ff.

MONTAGUES AND CAPULETS the rival families in Shakespeare's *Romeo and Juliet* 373

MONTGOMERY probably an allusion to the Revd Robert Montgomery (1807–55), poet 348

MOORE, THOMAS (1780–1852) Irish poet whose popularity rivalled Byron's (*q.v.*) and Scott's (*q.v.*) in the early nineteenth century 281

*MORNING HERALD* London newspaper first published in 1780; very much a staid 'family' paper 136, 452

MOSCHELES Ignaz Moscheles (1794–1870), Czech pianist and composer, a pupil of Beethoven; taught Dickens's sister Fanny at the Royal Academy of Music 322

MOSCOW 524

MPs 68, 151ff., 318ff; property qualifications of 548

PARACHUTES 522

*PARADISE AND THE PERI* *see* 'FIRE-WORSHIPPERS, THE'

PARK, MUNGO (1771–1806) African explorer whose *Travels* appeared in 1799 527

PARKS, THE usually meaning Hyde Park, Green Park, and St James's Park, three of the Royal Parks in London 112

PARLIAMENT 152ff., 505f., 541: *see also* MPs

PARLIAMENT STREET continuation of Whitehall 68

PATENT SHOT MANUFACTORY (dem. 1950), the tower of Messrs Watts's factory, 140 feet high, was a London landmark; built in 1789, it stood to the south-east of Waterloo Bridge and was preserved as a feature of the 1951 Festival of Britain site 67

PATENT THEATRES Covent Garden and Drury Lane Theatres were independent of the Lord Chamberlain's authority, to which other theatres were subject; their licence derived from letters of patent granted directly by the sovereign 249

PATTENS raised wooden overshoe worn in wet or muddy weather 19, 53

*PAUL ET VIRGINIE* a sentimental prose idyll, first published in 1789, by Bernardin de Saint-Pierre, friend and disciple of Rousseau 378; a ballad-opera based on the book (words by J. Cobb, music by W. Reeve and J. Mazzinghi) was produced in 1800, *Paul and Virginia* 381

PAUL PRY TO CALEB WILLIAMS Pry is a central figure in a comedy of that name by John Poole (1825), and Caleb Williams is the eponymous hero of a novel by William Godwin (1794); Pry was an inquisitive busybody, but Williams was a faithful servant who kept his master's guilty secret as long as possible 172

PAUL'S CHAIN street in central London; name derived from a chain that used to be thrown across the roadway to prevent its use during divine service in St Paul's Cathedral 89

PAUPERS *see* POVERTY

PAWNBROKERS 186ff.

PEDLARS' ACRE formerly an area on the north bank of the Thames between Waterloo and Westminster bridges, belonging from ancient times to the borough of Lambeth; according to legend, bequeathed to the borough by a pedlar on condition that his portrait, and that of his dog, should be preserved for ever in one of the parish church's stained glass windows 68

PEGWELL BAY pleasure-beach adjacent to the resort town of Ramsgate, Kent 337ff.

PELISSE woman's outer garment, with armholes or sleeves, reaching to the ankles 98, 130, 289

PEMBROKE TABLE one with hinged leaves or flaps which can be folded; said to have been named after an eighteenth-century Earl of Pembroke 44, 177

PENITENTIARY, THE early name of Millbank Prison (completed 1821, dem. 1903) for convicted criminals awaiting transportation; the prison stood on the site now occupied by the Tate Gallery 100, 148

PENSIONERS [GREENWICH] naval veterans 115

PENTONVILLE north London suburb, lying just to the north of Clerkenwell; prosperous and fashionable in Dickens's day but went down in the world in the late nineteenth century 53, 228, 231, 448

PERCEVAL Spencer Perceval, British prime minister assassinated in 1812 158

PERCY STREET off Tottenham Court Road (*q.v.*) 253

PERKING (obs.) inquisitive 20

PETERSHAM GREAT-COAT type of heavy overcoat named after Viscount Petersham (d. 1851), a leader of fashion in early nineteenth-century sporting circles 135, 427, 429, 593

house forming part of Newgate Prison 201

SEVEN CHAMPIONS a romance called *The Famous History of the Seven Champions of Christendom* written about 1597 by Richard Johnson (1573–1659?) 527

SEVEN DIALS part of the slum area of St Giles's, west London, between Bloomsbury and Covent Garden, so named because it is the point of convergence of seven streets 70ff.

SHAKESPEARE 542: *see also HAMLET, RICHARD III, MACBETH*, MONTAGUES, *OTHELLO*, SHYLOCK, YORICK; quoted 461, 507, 521

'SHAY' CART (coll.) a chaise, a light, open, two-wheeled carriage for two 114

SHED, ... WHICH ... LOVE TENANTED allusion to song in Thomas Moore's comic opera *MP or the Blue Stocking*: 'Young Love once lived in a humble shed' 174

SHEPPARD, JACK (1702–24) housebreaker and highway robber, famous as the only prisoner who ever escaped twice from Newgate gaol; died on the scaffold 201

SHERIDAN, RICHARD BRINSLEY (1751–1816) dramatist and politician 154, 158, 160, 313, 315

SHERIFF'S POUNDAGE (obs.) fee based on the value (calculated at 1s. in the pound up to £100 and 6d. thereafter) on goods distrained by a broker, payable to a sheriff's officer for his services in court 31

SHOE LANE street in east London partially demolished 1869 when Holborn Viaduct was constructed 141

SHOOTER'S HILL south London district between Greenwich Park and Blackheath 478

SHORTS knee-breeches 418

SHROVE TUESDAY the last day before Lent begins on Ash Wednesday, Pancake Day 501

SHRUB drink made from the juice of lemons, currants, and raspberries mixed with spirits, e.g., rum 184, 228

SHYLOCK the villain of Shakespeare's *Merchant of Venice*, one of Kean's great parts 123

SIAMESE TWINS two Chinese boys born in Siam (Thailand) in 1811, joined together at the breast bone; exhibited all over the world, appearing in London in 1829; died in 1871 17

SIDDONS, MRS Sarah Siddons (1755–1831), the great tragedienne whose career lasted from 1774 to 1812 125

SILENT SYSTEM prison system under which prisoners worked together and used the same dormitories, but were forbidden to speak to one another or communicate in any other way; they were, therefore, under constant surveillance day and night 146

SIMPSON, THE LATE MR C. H. Simpson, for 37 years the popular Master of Ceremonies at Vauxhall Gardens, celebrated for his extraordinarily obsequious manner 129

SINDBAD THE SAILOR Sindbad was the sailor-hero of a sequence of marvellous stories in *The Arabian Nights* 527

SLAP-BANG (sl.) cheap eating-houses were sometimes called 'Slap-bangs' from the off-hand way in which food was served up to their customers 265

SLAVES, EMANCIPATION OF THE 233

SLIPS the ends or rear-stage extremities of gallery seats in a theatre 267

SMITH, C. J. Covent Garden actor who played Guido Fawkes in *Harlequin Guy Fawkes* during the 1835–6 season and Georgy Barnwell (later Clown) in *Harlequin and Georgy Barnwell* during the 1836–7 one 503, 506

SMITHFIELD area on the north-eastern boundary of the City of London; the capital's principal meat market 156

SMOKE-JACK apparatus for turning a spit, which is rotated by the air current in the chimney 301

SNOW-HILL a street off Holborn Viaduct, east London 457

SOCIABLE open four-wheeled carriage in which the two pairs of occupants face each other 114

SOCIETY FOR SUPPRESSION OF VICE founded 1801 448

SOLOMON King of Israel 115

SOMERS TOWN lower-middle-class residential area of north-west London, north of the Euston Road stretching towards Hampstead, and including Euston, St Pancras, and King's Cross within its limits 53 and *passim*

SOMERSET HOUSE a palace in the Strand (*q.v.*), west London, built in the mid-sixteenth century, demolished and rebuilt in the late eighteenth century as government offices 222, 306; the Royal Academy was located there 1771–1836 – allusion to its exhibitions 357

SPELLING BOOK, AN OLD probable allusion to Daniel Fenning's *Universal Spelling Book* (1756) which features a bad boy called Harry who ultimately becomes 'a Prey to Wild Beasts' 508

SPENCER close-fitting bodice or jacket 131, 380

SPOFFISH (sl.) bustling, officious 351, 369

SPONTANEOUS COMBUSTION a medical myth widely received in the early nineteenth century, the idea being that the chemical elements of the human body could become so corrupted that the victim could suddenly perish in a self-generated conflagration cf. *Bleak House* chs. 32–3, 52

SPOUT, UP THE 'Spout' was the slang term for the chute by which articles left at a pawnbroker's were removed from the shop to a basement store-room; to say that something had gone 'up the spout' therefore meant it had been lost to its owner, probably for ever 189

SPRING GARDENS west of Trafalgar Square 253

STAGE-COACH TRAVEL 52, 133ff., 310f. 391f., 553

STAMFORD HILL prosperous north London suburb 94, 306

STAMP DUTY tax levied on newspapers and other periodicals (called 'a tax on knowledge') 20

STANHOPES light, open-seated carriage, with two or four wheels; called after Fitzroy Stanhope (1787–1864) for whom the first was made 483

STANLEY, LORD Edward, Lord Stanley, later Earl of Derby (1799–1869), who entered Parliament in 1820, and quickly established a reputation for himself as a speaker 155

STATISTICS 526ff.

STEAMBOATS 103ff.

STERNE, LAURENCE (1713–68), novelist 61

STOCK neckband, often made of glazed leather, and uncomfortable to wear 263

'STONE JUG' (sl.) Newgate Prison 271

STRAND, THE the street, just over ¾ mile long, which extends from Charing Cross to the Law Courts and thus links Westminster to the City 65, 215; STRAND LANE 376

STREPHON archetypal pastoral lover, from the character of that name in *Arcadia* by Sir Philip Sidney (1554–86) 421

STUMPY (sl.) money 149

SUDBURY town in Suffolk 439

SUFFOLK 439

SUN FIRE OFFICE insurance company whose plaque (plate), like those of similar firms, was shown on the wall of the insured person's house to enable the company's fire brigade to identify the premises 178

SURFACE, CHARLES hero of Sheridan's *School for Scandal* (1777) 123

SURREY THEATRE (dem. 1934) theatre in the Blackfriars Road on the south bank of the Thames; built for equestrian entertainments in 1782, burned down and rebuilt 1803, converted into a

TURPIN Dick Turpin (1706–39) famous highwayman, hanged in York 201

TWELFTH NIGHT 6 January, the official last day of the Christmas festivities 501

TWICKENHAM Thames-side village in Middlesex 100, 478

TWO PAIR BACK/FRONT a back or front room on the second (American, third) floor up two flights or 'pairs' of stairs 74, 110, 246

TWOPENNY POSTMAN before the introduction of the Penny Post in 1840 the charge for local delivery of letters in London was twopence 287, 408

UNITARIAN Mrs Bloss's malapropism for 'valetudinarian' 290

UNMENTIONABLES euphemism for trousers 134, 263, 435 f.; *cf.* INEXPLICABLES

VACCINATION 452

VALENTINE & ORSON an old French romance which became a favourite children's story in England after its translation into English in the sixteenth century; twin princes are born in a forest near Orleans and one, Orson, is carried off by a bear and becomes a wild man, whilst the other, Valentine, is taken by the king and brought up at court 294, 527

VAUXHALL BRIDGE links Pimlico north of the Thames with Vauxhall (completed 1816) 102

VAUXHALL GARDENS London pleasure-gardens 126ff., 299, 522

VENUS 445

VICTORIA THEATRE the Old Vic theatre in the Waterloo Road (south bank of the Thames); opened as the Royal Coburg in 1818, it became the Royal Victoria in 1833; famous for its melodramas 57, 171 (Royal Coburg)

VIVISECTION 516ff.

VURKIS i.e., workhouse (*q.v.*) 171

WAFER thin adhesive disc, made of a baked flour-and-water paste, used for sealing letters before the introduction of gummed envelopes 289

WAITERS 392

WAITHMAN'S MONUMENT obelisk formerly standing at Ludgate Circus, east London, erected in 1833 to the memory of Robert Waithman (1764–1833), a linen-draper who was Lord Mayor of London in 1823 and also MP for the City 170

WALKER! (sl.) an interjection expressing derisive incredulity 549

WALKING GENTLEMEN theatrical supernumeraries of genteel appearance 110, 276

WALLSEND coal from Wallsend, Northumberland 417

WALWORTH a village south of London, now part of the borough of Southwark 305, 363f.

WANDERING JEW legendary figure condemned to wander the earth until Christ's second coming 275, 393

WANDSWORTH suburb of London south of the River Thames between Putney and Battersea 345

'WARM WITH-' i.e., hot and with sugar 229

WARREN, MR Robert Warren, manufacturer of blacking with premises at 30 Strand (*q.v.*), who advertised his wares with rhyming jingles 74

WATCH-BOX (HOUSE) a kind of sentry-box used by night-watchman 12

WATCHING-RATES tax levied on parishioners for the upkeep of local watchman 20

WATER, OF THE FIRST *see* BRILLIANT

WATERLOO BRIDGE crosses the Thames between the Blackfriars and Westminster bridges; completed in 1817 (dem. 1936 and reconstructed 1937–42) 67, 122, 471

WATERLOO PLACE begun in 1816 as a termination of Nash's Regent Street